Handbook of Pharmaceutical Controlled Release Technology

Handbook of Pharmaceutical Controlled Release Technology

executive editor
Donald L. Wise
*Cambridge Scientific, Inc.
Cambridge, Massachusetts*

associate editors

Lisa Brannon-Peppas
*Biogel Technology, Inc.
Indianapolis, Indiana*

**Alexander M. Klibanov
Robert S. Langer**
*Massachusetts Institute of Technology
Cambridge, Massachusetts*

Antonios G. Mikos
*Rice University
Houston, Texas*

Nicholas A. Peppas
*Purdue University
West Lafayette, Indiana*

Debra J. Trantolo
*Cambridge Scientific, Inc.
Cambridge, Massachusetts*

Gary E. Wnek
*Virginia Commonwealth University
Richmond, Virginia*

Michael J. Yaszemski
*Mayo Clinic
Rochester, Minnesota*

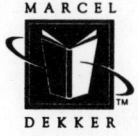

Marcel Dekker, Inc.   New York • Basel

Second Indian Reprint 2008

ISBN-10: 0-8247-0369-3
ISBN-13: 978-0-8247-0369-1

Headquarters
Marcel Dekker, Inc.
270 Madison Avenue, New York, NY 10016
tel: 212-696-9000; fax: 212-685-4540

World Wide Web
http://www.dekker.com

Copyright © 2000 by Marcel Dekker, Inc. All Rights Reserved.

Neither this book nor any part may be reproduced or transmitted in any form or by any means, electronic or mechanical, including photocopying, microfilming, and recording, or by any information storage and retrieval system, without permission in writing from the publisher.

Printed and bound by Replika Press Pvt. Ltd., India.

FOR SALE IN INDIAN SUBCONTINENT ONLY.

Preface

The ways in which medicinal chemicals or the newer biologicals are administered have gained increasing attention in the past three decades. Normally, a medicinal chemical or biological (i.e., "drug") is administered in high dose at a given time—and then that dose has to be repeated several hours or days later. This often results in damaging side effects and leads to poor control of drug therapy. As a consequence, increasing attention has been focused on methods for giving these biologically active agents continuously for prolonged time periods and in a controlled fashion. The primary method of accomplishing this controlled release has been through incorporating the biologically active agents within polymers (i.e., biopolymers).

The purpose of this book is to review controlled release technology primarily as it relates to medicinal applications, but chapters on agricultural broadcast applications and animal care are included for completeness. We should perhaps begin with a definition of a controlled release system, and contrast it to a sustained release system. Ideally, in a controlled release system the rate of release is determined largely by the design of the device itself (which could be a polymer system or pump), and is not dependent on environmental conditions (e.g., pH of the gastrointestinal tract). In contrast, a sustained release system provides prolonged action but the release rate is significantly affected by environmental conditions. Since there is no perfectly clear-cut distinction between controlled and sustained release, our intention in this book has been to focus principally on controlled release formulations but to include sustained release systems when it is appropriate for complete coverage of a particular topic.

The goal of this book is threefold. It is intended to be a handbook on the design, fabrication, methods of controlling release, and theoretical considerations of various classes of drug delivery systems (matrixes, membrane controlled reservoir systems, bioerodible systems, and pendant chain systems). In addition, chapters cover the application of these systems for oral and transdermal delivery, providing information that will enable those new to the field to understand a particular kind of delivery system and how to modify it to achieve desired release kinetics. The methods of determining parameters critical to performance evaluations are discussed in detail.

This volume also covers medical usage of controlled release polymers. Several chapters present a particular area of interest (ophthalmology, bone repair, etc.) and give a critical analysis of both the advantages and disadvantages of controlled release systems from such standpoints as expense, comfort, control of disease, possibility of side effects, and patient compliance. These chapters review the successes and failures of controlled release technology in conducted studies and clinical evaluations, discuss ongoing studies, and assess future projects. The types of drug delivery systems used in these applications are discussed, and the types of constraints one would want to impose on the design of systems for practical clinical applications are evaluated. Such topics as mathematical modeling and pharmacokinetic and bioavailability considerations are discussed.

Each chapter presents a complete view of a particular topic. There is therefore a minor amount of repetition; for example, diffusion equations are discussed in several chapters. This was done to provide continuity within each chapter and to facilitate the understanding of when a controlled release system would be useful for a particular application, what system to choose, and how to formulate and evaluate that system.

This text has evolved from decades of background in developing biopolymeric systems for the controlled release of biologically active agents. A bit of personal reminiscing and even nostalgia may be appropriate here. The work of the several associate editors has been largely focused on developing biopolymers for implantable/injectable controlled release systems for special situations in which patient compliance has been the major driving force (i.e., situations in which conventional administration of biologically active agents was not practical, not acceptable, or simply not carried out for a patient's personal reasons). The funding for this development work was provided almost totally by private foundations, agencies of the U.S. government, and international organizations. Because of the pointed problems of patient compliance and funding sources, the very first development programs were for controlled release systems for fertility control, treatment of narcotic addiction, and malaria prophylaxis. All this work was initiated at about the same time—in the early 1970s. Although treatment of alcoholism, for example, was cited early as having potential for a controlled release application, funding (and therefore development) was not initiated until fairly recently.

Work on several biopolymeric systems other than implantable/injectable systems was also initiated in the early 1970s in which the controlled release of biologically active agents was integral to the overall objectives. For example, work was initiated to develop a synthetic biopolymeric burn wound covering as a replacement for cadaver skin that incorporated suitable biologically active agents, for example, bactericides. Also, development work on new biopolymeric composite materials for such applications as fixation of orthopedic surgical implants and repair of avulsive combat-type maxillofacial injuries always implied the ultimate incorporation of selected biologically active agents into the biopolymeric matrix, even if initial development work focused on the synthesis and evaluation of the biopolymeric material. Biopolymeric systems for controlled release of biologically active agents have also been used in broadcast applications such as herbicides, larvicides, and molluscicides. In broadcast applications the cost of the biopolymeric materials is of significance; for human implants the biopolymer cost is almost not a consideration at all.

The selection of the biopolymer has been of special interest. Early development work focused on the synthesis of copolymers of lactic and glycolic acids (i.e., PLGA), because they were known at the time to be biodegradable (i.e., to hydrolyze and be metabolized). Therefore, these products of glycolysis were used early in the development of controlled release systems simply because they presented a practical starting point for investigating the concept of controlled release. Later, other monomers of human metabolism were investigated as ones to be synthesized into polymers for use as biodegradable implants. For example, work was initiated on using monomers of the Krebs cycle and on using selected amino acids to synthesize biopolymers that would break down to the parent monomer (e.g., the polymer polypropylene fumarate). The reasoning in using all these monomers (i.e., using products of glycolysis such as lactic and glycolic acid, using Krebs cycle monomers, using amino acids, etc.) was that, upon synthesis, these biopolymers would maintain what was termed biocompatibility (i.e., tissue reaction would be minimum). Clearly, for broadcast applications the question of tissue compatibility is not a problem, but environmental acceptance is a question to be addressed.

Mechanism of release is a further consideration in the design of biopolymeric systems for the controlled release of biologically active agents. The development work has primarily been focused on matrix-type systems as well as microencapsulation. In the matrix system the biopolymer and the biologically active agent are intimately mixed in a physical matrix much as gravel or sand is mixed in cement. Further, diffusion of the active agent and hydrolysis of the polymer occur simultaneously to achieve the controlled release. As a result, a mathematical

Preface

description of the mechanism has been difficult, and essentially empirical relationships have evolved for predicting release. With the microencapsulation system, the biopolymer is made to envelope the active agent, much like an eggshell.

It is anticipated that this text will be most useful as a guide to industrial and academic research directors and program managers who are exploring the potential of biopolymeric controlled release for application to their own problems. For this reason as much detail as possible has been preserved. This has been done so that people actually involved in system development and in problem-solving may be able to follow well the topical material presented.

Donald L. Wise

Contents

Preface   iii

Part I: Polymers as Drug Delivery Carriers

1. Hydrophilic Cellulose Derivatives as Drug Delivery Carriers: 1
   Influence of Substitution Type on the Properties of Compressed Matrix Tablets
   Carmen Ferrero Rodriguez, Nathalie Bruneau, Jérôme Barra, Dorothée Alfonso, and Eric Doelker

2. Poly(Vinyl Alcohol) as a Drug Delivery Carrier   31
   Surya K. Mallapragada and Shannon McCarthy-Schroeder

3. Development of Acrylate and Methacrylate Polymer Networks for   47
   Controlled Release by Photopolymerization Technology
   Robert Scott, Jennifer H. Ward, and Nicholas A. Peppas

4. Smart Polymers for Controlled Drug Delivery   65
   Joseph Kost and Smadar A. Lapidot

5. Complexing Polymers in Drug Delivery   89
   Anthony M. Lowman

6. Polylactic and Polyglycolic Acids as Drug Delivery Carriers   99
   Lisa Brannon-Peppas and Michel Vert

7. Use of Infrared and Raman Spectroscopy for Characterization of   131
   Controlled Release Systems
   A. B. Scranton, B. Drescher, E. W. Nelson, and J. L. Jacobs

8. Accurate Models in Controlled Drug Delivery Systems   155
   Balaji Narasimhan

Part II: Mechanism-Based Classification of Controlled Release Devices

9. Drug Release from Swelling-Controlled Systems   183
   Paolo Colombo, Patrizia Santi, Ruggero Bettini, Christopher S. Brazel, and Nicholas A. Peppas

10. Superporous Hydrogels as a Platform for Oral Controlled Drug Delivery 211
    Jun Chen, Haesun Park, and Kinam Park

11. Osmotic Implantable Delivery Systems 225
    Cynthia L. Stevenson, Felix Theeuwes, and Jeremy C. Wright

12. Bioadhesive Controlled Release Systems 255
    Nicholas A. Peppas, Monica D. Little, and Yanbin Huang

Part III: Micro- and Nanoparticulate Release Systems

13. Microencapsulation Technology: Interfacial Polymerization Method 271
    A. Atïlla Hıncal and H. Süheyla Kaş

14. Nanoparticulate Controlled Release Systems for Cancer Therapy 287
    C. Dubernet, E. Fattal, and P. Couvreur

15. Microencapsulation Using Coacervation/Phase Separation: An Overview of the Technique and Applications 301
    H. Süheyla Kaş and Levent Öner

16. Microsphere Preparation by Solvent Evaporation Method 329
    A. Atïlla Hıncal and Sema Çalış

17. Nanosuspensions: A Formulation Approach for Poorly Soluble and Poorly Bioavailable Drugs 345
    R. H. Müller, B. H. L. Böhm, and M. J. Grau

18. Large-Scale Production of Solid Lipid Nanoparticles (SLN) and Nanosuspensions (DissoCubes) 359
    R. H. Müller, A. Dingler, T. Schneppe, and S. Gohla

19. Solid Lipid Nanoparticles (SLN) as a Carrier System for the Controlled Release of Drugs 377
    R. H. Müller, A. Lippacher, and S. Gohla

20. Stability of Encapsulated Substances in Poly(Lactide-co-Glycolide) Delivery Systems 393
    Steven P. Schwendeman, Anna Shenderova, Gaozhong Zhu, and Wenlei Jiang

21. Development of Polysaccharide Nanoparticles as Novel Drug Carrier Systems 413
    C. Vauthier and P. Couvreur

Part IV: Classification of Controlled Release Devices According to Administration Site

22. An Overview of Controlled Release Systems 431
    S. Venkatraman, N. Davar, A. Chester, and L. Kleiner

Contents

23. Research and Development Aspects of Oral Controlled-Release Dosage Forms 465
    Yihong Qiu and Guohua Zhang

24. A Gastrointestinal Retentive Microparticulate System to Improve Oral Drug Delivery 505
    Y. Kawashima, H. Takeuchi, and H. Yamamoto

25. In Vitro–In Vivo Correlations in the Development of Solid Oral Controlled Release Dosage Forms 527
    Yihong Qiu, Emil E. Samara, and Guoliang Cao

26. Gamma Scintigraphy in the Analysis of the Behavior of Controlled Release Systems 551
    C. G. Wilson and N. Washington

27. Electrically Assisted Transdermal Delivery of Drugs 567
    Ajay K. Banga

28. A Novel Method Based on Artificial Neural Networks for Optimizing Transdermal Drug Delivery Systems 583
    Kozo Takayama and Tsuneji Nagai

29. Transdermal Drug Delivery by Skin Electroporation 597
    Tani Chen, Robert Langer, and James C. Weaver

30. Enhancement of Transdermal Transport Using Ultrasound in Combination with Other Enhancers 607
    Samir Mitragotri, Robert Langer, and Joseph Kost

31. Electrotransport Systems for Transdermal Delivery: A Practical Implementation of Iontophoresis 617
    Erik R. Scott, J. Bradley Phipps, J. Richard Gyory, and Rama V. Padmanabhan

Part V: Peptide and Protein Release Systems

32. Controlled Release Protein Therapeutics: Effects of Process and Formulation on Stability 661
    Paul A. Burke

33. Solid-State Chemical Stability of Peptides and Proteins: Application to Controlled Release Formulations 693
    Elizabeth M. Topp, Yuan Song, Ashley Wilson, Rong Li, Michael J. Hageman, and Richard L. Schowen

34. Growth Factor Release from Biodegradable Hydrogels to Induce Neovascularization 725
    Yoshito Ikada and Yasuhiko Tabata

35. Biopolymers for Release of Interleukin-2 for Treatment of Cancer 743
   *Debra J. Trantolo, Joseph D. Gresser, A. Ganiyu Jimoh, Donald L. Wise,
   and James C. Yang*

Part VI: Medical Applications of Drug Delivery

36. Osmotic Drug Delivery from Asymmetric Membrane Film-Coated 751
   Dosage Forms
   *Mary Tanya am Ende, Scott M. Herbig, Richard W. Korsmeyer,
   and Mark B. Chidlaw*

37. Controlled Release Pain Management Systems 787
   *Vasif Hasirci, Dilek Sendil, Leonidas C. Goudas, Daniel B. Carr,
   and Donald L. Wise*

38. Biodegradable Systems for Long-Acting Nestorone 807
   *Debra J. Trantolo, Donald L. Wise, A. J. Moo-Young, Yung-Yueh Hsu,
   and Joseph D. Gresser*

39. Preparation and Evaluation of Buprenorphine Microspheres 821
   for Parenteral Administration
   William R. Ravis, Yuh-Jing Lin, and Ram Murty

40. Prolonged Release of Hydromorphone from a Novel Poly(Lactic-co-Glycolic) 837
   Acid Depot System: Initial In Vitro and In Vivo Observations
   *Leonidas C. Goudas, Daniel B. Carr, Richard M. Kream, Louis Shuster,
   William M. Vaughan, Joseph D. Gresser, Donald L. Wise,
   and Debra J. Trantolo*

41. Incorporation of an Active Agent into a Biodegradable Cement: 849
   Encapsulation of the Agent as Protection from Chemical Degradation
   During Cure and Effect on Release Profile
   *Joseph D. Gresser, Debra J. Trantolo, Pattisapu R. J. Gangadharam,
   Hisanori X. Nagaoka, Yung-Yueh Hsu, and Donald L. Wise*

42. The Pharmacoeconomic Value of Controlled Release Dosage Forms 865
   Laura B. Gardner

Index 873

1
Hydrophilic Cellulose Derivatives as Drug Delivery Carriers:
Influence of Substitution Type on the Properties of Compressed Matrix Tablets

Carmen Ferrero Rodriguez,* Nathalie Bruneau, Jérôme Barra, Dorothée Alfonso, and Eric Doelker
University of Geneva, Geneva, Switzerland

I. INTRODUCTION

Today, compressed hydrophilic matrices have become most popular as modified release dosage forms for oral administration. Among the swellable polymers used to prolong drug release, cellulose ethers, in particular hydroxypropylmethylcellulose (HPMC), provoked considerable interest because most display good compression characteristics, including when directly compressed, and have adequate swelling properties that allow rapid formation of an external gel layer controlling drug release. They are available in several substitution and viscosity (molecular mass) grades and are well characterized in compendia. Furthermore, most of them have U.S. GRAS status (Generally Recognized As Safe) (1–6).

Since the first disclosure of the principle of compressed hydrophilic matrices in the open literature, much attention has been paid to the drug (solute) release mechanism. Thus, Huber et al. (7) suggested that drug release was controlled both by diffusion of the drug and attrition of the gel layer formed gradually around the tablets. However, the first basic work on release kinetics was that of Lapidus and Lordi (8,9) who demonstrated the applicability of diffusion equations for a semi-infinite medium. Since then, various theoretical models have been proposed for drug release from swellable systems and some have been experimentally checked with compressed cellulose ether systems. Peppas et al. (10) published a model that accounts for both volume change of the swellable matrix and countercurrent diffusion of the solvent. Lee (11) provided analytical solutions for erodible swellable systems, where zero-order release is achieved when the movements of the diffusing front (solid drug–drug solution interface) and the eroding front (rubbery polymer–solvent interface) are synchronized. Later, Peppas and Franson (12) proposed the concept of swelling-controlled release systems where solute release is governed by the penetration velocity of the solvent (swelling front). In those systems, constant release is observed when the solvent penetration is much slower than drug diffusion in the

---

Current affiliation: University of Seville, Seville, Spain

swollen gel (case 2, transport). Lee and Peppas (13) were able to predict the thickness of the gel layer as a function of time, rate of swelling, and velocity of the eroding front. Harland et al. (14) established that the gel thickness is proportional to the square root of time as long as the swelling front moves more rapidly than the eroding front, but synchronization of both fronts may occur leading to constant drug release. More recently, Colombo et al. (15) stressed the importance of a third front, the diffusion front, identifying the interface between the still undissolved (solid) drug and the dissolved drug in the gel layer. The existence of this front was first reported by Lee (11) and Lee and Kim (16). Drug release is a function of the dissolved drug gel layer that separates the diffusion front from the erosion front. Figure 1 depicts the relative position of the three moving fronts in a swellable matrix. The diffusion front is present as long as the concentration of the undissolved drug exceeds its solubility in the swollen polymer matrix.

In other attempts to analyze release data from hydrophilic matrix systems, Möckel and Lippold (17) and Kätzhendler et al. (18) assumed purely erosion-controlled release. Using model-independent moment analysis, Tahara et al. (19,20) postulated that the rate-limiting factor for release of a poorly water-soluble drug is the erosion of the matrix tablet, whereas the infiltration (penetration) rate of water in the matrix is the key for highly soluble drugs. Both water penetration rate and matrix erosion rate are the controlling factors for drugs with intermediate solubilities. Finally, Ju et al. (21–23) developed scaling laws for predicting polymer and drug release from hydrophilic matrices. Interestingly, these laws allow calculation of the release profiles for new formulations from the release profile of a known formulation.

Basic studies dealing with release mechanisms from compressed cellulose ethers have essentially reported only on HPMC. However, it is well known that other derivatives, e.g., methylcellulose (MC), hydroxyethylcellulose (HEC), and hydroxypropylcellulose (HPC), behave quite differently with regard to drug release. Thus, it was the aim of this study to elucidate which physicochemical properties of these closely related cellulose derivatives could explain the observed differences and to ascertain which mechanisms(s), among the several proposed, may be considered as governing release of water-soluble drugs. For that purpose, six nonionic ethers were selected, varying by their substitution type (HPMC, MC, HEC, and HPC) or degree of

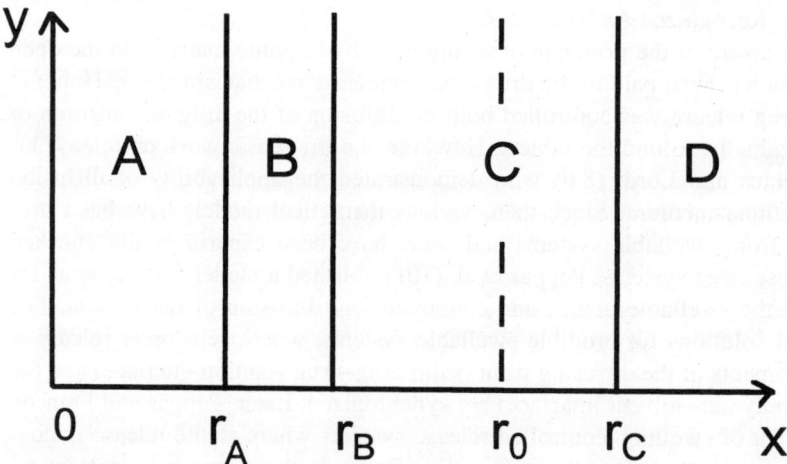

Figure 1 Schematic representation of the swelling front at r_A, the diffusion front at r_B, the original position of the matrix surface at r_0, and the erosion front at r_C. The abcissa x is the distance along the tablet radius r. (A) Glassy polymer with undissolved drug; (B) gel layer with undissolved drug; (C) gel layer with dissolved drug; and (D) dissolution medium.

substitution (USP HPMC 2208, 2906, and 2910). All were of similar viscosity grades (4000–5000 mPas)—although not of identical molecular masses—and were characterized for their hydrophilicity by various parameters. Phenylpropanolamine hydrochloride was selected as water-soluble model drug, and was used at various loadings. In addition, two other drugs were also used to investigate the effect of solute solubility on the release mechanism. Compressed matrices made of pure polymers and drugs were assessed for their swelling, erosion, and release properties.

II. EXPERIMENTAL

A. Materials

The cellulose ethers used were USP/NF grades and were kindly donated by Dow Stade (Stade, Germany) and Colorcon (Orpington, UK) for Methocel A4M Prem. (MC), Methocel K4M Prem. CR.GR (HPMC 2208), Methocel F4M Prem. EP (2906) and Methocel E4MCR Prem. EP (HPMC 2910), and from Aqualon (Wilmington, DE) for Natrosol 250 M Pharm (HEC) and Klucel 99MF (HPC). All materials had a moisture content of less than 5%. Size fractions of less than 63 μm were used to minimize the lag time observed during drug release with coarse fractions (24). The degree of substitution, molar substitution (for HEC and HPC), nominal viscosity (2% aqueous solution), and molecular weight values of the derivatives are reported in Table 1.

Phenylpropanolamine hydrochloride (PPA), theophylline (THP), pseudoephedrine hydrochloride (PED), and anthrone were purchased from Fluka (Buchs, Switzerland).

B. Polymer Molecular Weight

Gel permeation chromatography was used to determine the molecular weight of the six derivatives tested, as necessary to estimate the polymer disentanglement concentration. The chromatographic equipment consisted of a Waters 600E system controller (Milford, MA), a Waters 717 Plus autosampler, a Waters 410 differential refractometer, and a polymethacrylate-based Ultrahydrogel linear column (7.5 mm × 30 cm, Waters). The mobile phase was a mixture of 0.05 M sodium nitrate and acetonitrile (80:20). The flow rate was set at 0.5 mL/min and temperature at 25°C. Approximately 150 μL of 0.1% polymer solution in the mobile phase was injected. Pullulans and sodium polystyrenesulfonates were used as standards.

Table 1 Average Degree of Substitution, DS, and Molar Substitution, MS, and Nominal Viscosity Grade Weight-Average Molecular Weight, M_w, Molecular Weight of the Repeating Unit M_0, Weight-Average Degree of Polymerization DP_w of the Cellulose Ethers Used (Manufacturer's Data)

Material	Methoxyl DS	Hydroxyethoxyl DS	Hydroxyethoxyl MS	Hydroxypropyl[a] DS	Hydroxypropyl[a] MS	Viscosity grade[a] (mPa·s)	M_w^b	M_n^c	M_w/M_n^c	M_0^d	DP_w
MC	1.8	—	—	—	—	4000	676900[d]	305080	2.22	158.5	4270
HPMC 2208	1.4	—	—	0.21	—	4000	636360[d]	241770	2.63	181.1	3510
2906	1.8	—	—	0.13	—	4000	684770[d]	196230	3.49	180.4	3800
2910	1.9	—	—	0.23	—	4000	696720[d]	246990	2.82	185.5	3760
HEC	—	1.3	2.5	—	—	5000	926880	293570	3.16	200.5	4620
HPC	—	—	—	2.5	4.0	5000	1061780	330050	3.22	394.2	2690

[a]Viscosity of a 2% aqueous solution.
[b]Gel permeation chromatography data.
[c]Calculated from the substitution.
[d]Calculated from the number-average molecular weight M_n, assuming a polydispersity index M_w/M_n of 3.

C. Polymer Hydrophilicity

Hydrophilicity of the materials was principally assessed by evaluating the solubility parameters, first by means of the group contribution method. Solubility parameters and molar volumes were calculated according to Hoy (25) and Fedors (26), respectively. The calculations were run assuming the substituent distributions obtained from nuclear magnetic resonance (NMR) data by Rossel (27) for MC, by Tezuka et al. (28) for HPMC, by Lindberg et al. (29) for HEC, and by Lee and Perlin (30) for HPC. Solubility parameters were also evaluated experimentally, as described elsewhere (31). Hydrophilicity can also be estimated through hygroscopicity. In this respect, values of moisture content of the materials exposed for 30 days at 74% relative humidity were determined [results published elsewhere (32)].

D. Compact Preparation

Polymer and drug (in a 80:20 weight ratio) were mixed for 15 min (Turbula TA2 blender, W. Bachofen, Basel, Switzerland) and 500 mg of mixture was directly compressed at 10 kN in a 15-mm die using a hydraulic press (Graseby Specac, Orpington, UK) equipped with flat-faced punches.

E. Swelling and Front Movements

The position of the fronts upon water penetration inside the tablets, the drug release behavior, and the polymer dissolution were studied at 37°C using the circular device described by Bettini et al. (33), allowing the water to enter only from the lateral side. The cylindrical matrix was locked between two transparent poly(methyl methacrylate) disks and the assembly placed in a USP 23 dissolution apparatus 2. Tests were carried out at 37°C with the paddle rotating at 75 rpm and using 400 mL dissolution medium. Methylene blue (0.004%) was added to water to improve the visualization of the three concentric circles corresponding to the swelling, diffusion, and erosion fronts, respectively.

F. Drug Release and Polymer Dissolution

Polymer dissolution and drug release were studied under the same conditions as previously, except that pure water was used. Samples (5 mL) were withdrawn at defined time intervals and replaced by fresh medium. The amount of polymer entering into solution was quantified colorimetrically by means of the anthrone method (34). No interaction occurred with PPA. In addition, the swollen tablets were removed from the medium after 4 h, dried to a constant weight, and the mass balance established by taking into account the initial weight of the tablet, the released drug, and the dissolved polymer.

The drug concentration was determined spectrophotometrically at 256 nm for PPA, 272 nm for THP, and 257 nm for PED. All of the experiments were performed in triplicate.

G. Polymer Disentanglement Concentration

Matrix erosion is described as the dissolution of the disentangled macromolecules from the rubbery polymer. Polymer disentanglement occurs beyond a critical concentration C_d, depending on the molecular weight of the chains, and on their conformation in a given solvent and at a given temperature. Actually, the disentanglement concentration C_d is hard to estimate with accuracy, in contrast to another closely related critical concentration describing chain entanglement, the coil overlap concentration C_p^*, beyond which polymer chain disentanglement commences. Overlap concentrations were obtained by low shear viscometry.

The low-shear Newtonian viscosities of aqueous solutions ranging from 0.1% to 2.0% were measured at 37°C using an Ubbelhode capillary viscosimeter (Schott, Mainz, Germany). Measurements were made at 37°C on pure aqueous solutions and, in the case of MC and HPC, also in the presence of 2% PPA. It is expected that electrolytes may change the conformation of macromolecules, especially at temperatures close to the θ temperature. The coil overlap concentration C_p^* is equivalent to the transition concentration on a double logarithmic plot of the viscosity η against polymer concentration C. This is attributed to the transition from dilute solution conditions, where individual polymer macromolecules are present as isolated coils, to concentrated solution conditions, where the total hydrodynamic volume of chains exceeds the volume of solution. Thus, C_p^* marks the onset of coil overlap and interpenetration (35–38).

III. POLYMER HYDROPHILICITY

Parameters describing the hydrophilicity of the cellulose ethers tested are listed in Table 2. The total solubility parameter δ_t was divided into the dispersion component δ_d, the polar component δ_p, and the hydrogen-bonding component δ_h. Values of fractional polarity x_p were calculated from the relation $x_p = 1 - (\delta_d/\delta_t)^2$ (39) or $x_p = (\delta_a/\delta_t)^2$, where δ_a is the solubility parameter usually used to describe the association interactions ($\delta_a^2 = \delta_p^2 + \delta_h^2$).

As expected, the solubility parameters of the cellulose ethers only varied significantly in their polar and hydrogen-bonding components and, thus, in their association interaction components and fractional polarities. When considering the calculated parameters, the differences between the three HPMCs were negligible. HEC exhibited the highest δ_t and δ_a values and thus the highest polarity x_p. As for MC and HPC they lay on the opposite side. Experimental determination of the solubility parameters only allowed the identification of two groups of materials: MC, HPMC 2208, and HEC were more polar than HPMC 2906, HPMC 2910, and HPC. This is due to the difficulty of finding discriminating solvents for the determination. Several experimental values have been reported in the literature for cellulose ethers (see Ref. 32), but they deal only with total solubility parameters. The only partial solubility parameters published, to our knowledge, are those by Archer (40,41) concerning MC and HPMCs and those by Choi et al. (42) concerning HPC. Incidentally, the latter authors have stressed that the group contribution methods are particularly weak in predicting the polar component δ_p. As in the present study, differences in the values obtained by Archer et al. (40,41) were quite small with the notable exception of HPC.

The hydrophilicity of the materials was also assessed by their ability to absorb water vapor. The same sequence of moisture content after 30 days at 74% relative humidity was observed as for x_p.

Taking into consideration all data presented in Table 2, hydrophilicity can be estimated as increasing in the order HPC ≅ MC < HPMC 2910 ≅ HPMC 2906 < HPMC 2208 < HEC.

IV. EFFECT OF SUBSTITUTION TYPE ON MATRIX CHARACTERISTICS

A. Swelling Characteristics

When the tablets containing PPA and the cellulose derivatives were in contact with water (containing methylene blue), the swelling, the diffusion, and the erosion fronts could be seen and their position evaluated. Figure 2 shows the positions of the three fronts. Position 0 at the beginning of the experiment corresponds to the interface between the matrix and water.

Table 2 Solubility Parameters and Hygroscopicities of the Cellulose Derivatives Tested

Material		Calculated solubility parameters (MPa$^{1/2}$)					Experimental solubility parameters (MPa$^{1/2}$)					Moisture content (%)[a]
		δ_d	δ_p	δ_h	δ_t	δ_a	x_p	δ_d	δ_p	δ_h	δ_t	δ_a	x_p	
MC		16.3	12.7	12.1	23.9	17.5	0.54	16.0	17.0	15.7	28.1	23.1	0.67	12.6
HPMC	2208	15.3	16.5	18.0	28.8	24.4	0.72	15.8	17.0	16.2	28.4	23.5	0.69	14.0
	2906	15.4	16.1	17.3	28.2	23.6	0.70	18.1	14.0	13.3	26.4	19.2	0.53	11.0
	2910	15.4	15.9	16.8	27.8	23.1	0.69	18.1	14.0	13.2	26.4	19.2	0.53	11.8
HEC		15.3	17.4	19.6	30.3	26.2	0.75	17.3	19.9	15.1	30.4	25.0	0.68	21.7
HPC		16.4	13.4	13.3	25.1	18.9	0.57	18.1	14.0	13.2	26.4	19.2	0.53	10.9

[a] At 74% relative humidity.

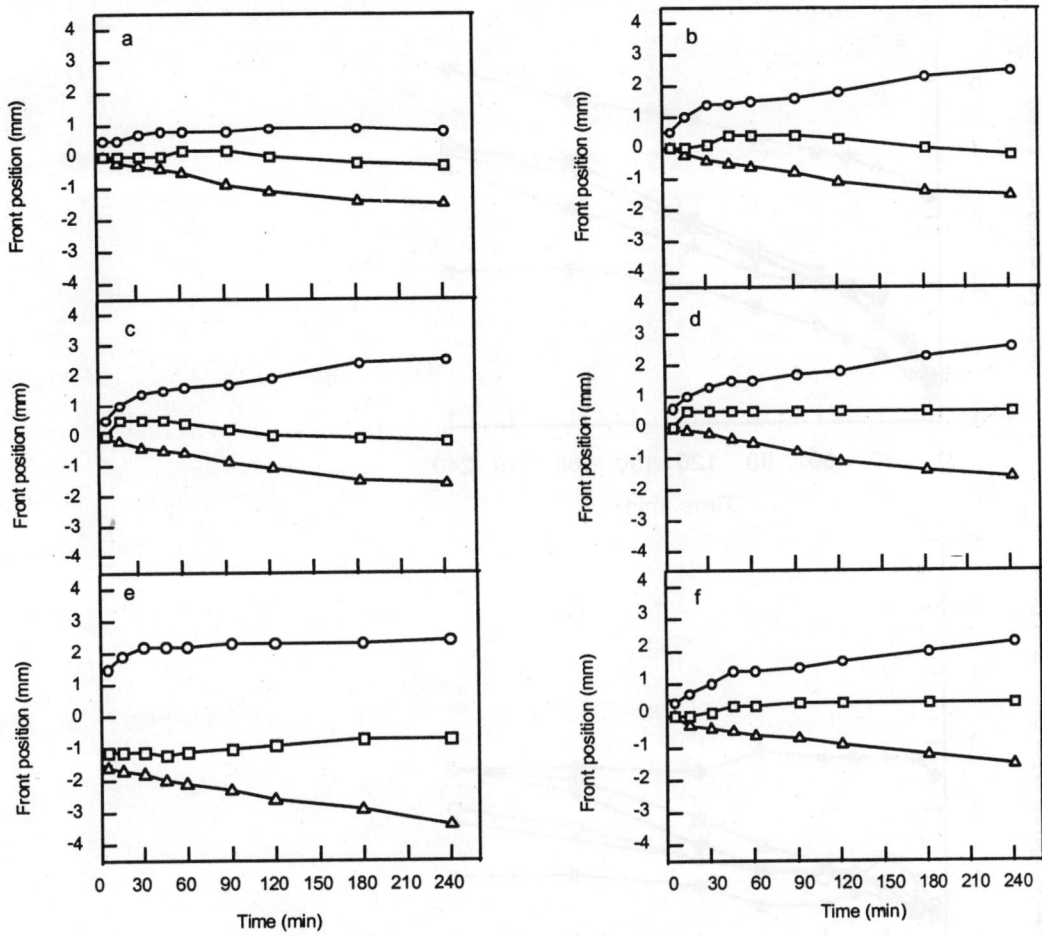

Figure 2 Swelling (△), diffusion (□), and erosion (○) front positions vs. time in matrices prepared with MC (a), HPMC 2208 (b), HPMC 2906 (c), HPMC 2910 (d), HEC (e), and HPC (f).

A rapid initial inward movement of the swelling front was sometimes noted (especially for the very hydrophilic HEC), but the general tendency was a constant rate, as reported, for instance, by Colombo et al. (15) for HPMCs 2208 of varying molecular mass. The diffusion front was rather steady relative to the initial position. A slight outward movement was even observed, resulting from an inwardly moving front compensated by the expansion of the matrix upon swelling. The erosion front exhibited a rapid initial movement for all derivatives (this movement was spectacular for HEC), followed by an almost linear change. No recession of the erosion front was observed over the duration of the experiment, which would have indicated predominant erosion.

Better appreciation of the movement of either the swelling or the diffusion front is possible by calculating the thickness of the gel layer ($r_C - r_A$) and that of the dissolved drug, or diffusion layer ($r_B - r_C$). As shown in Fig. 3a, a rapid increase in gel layer thickness was observed early on for all derivatives; then the gel layers grew at approximately the same rate. The initial increase was drastic for HEC and less pronounced for MC. The HPMCs and HPC displayed similar intermediate patterns of change. Incidentally, Mitchell et al. (43) using thermomechanical

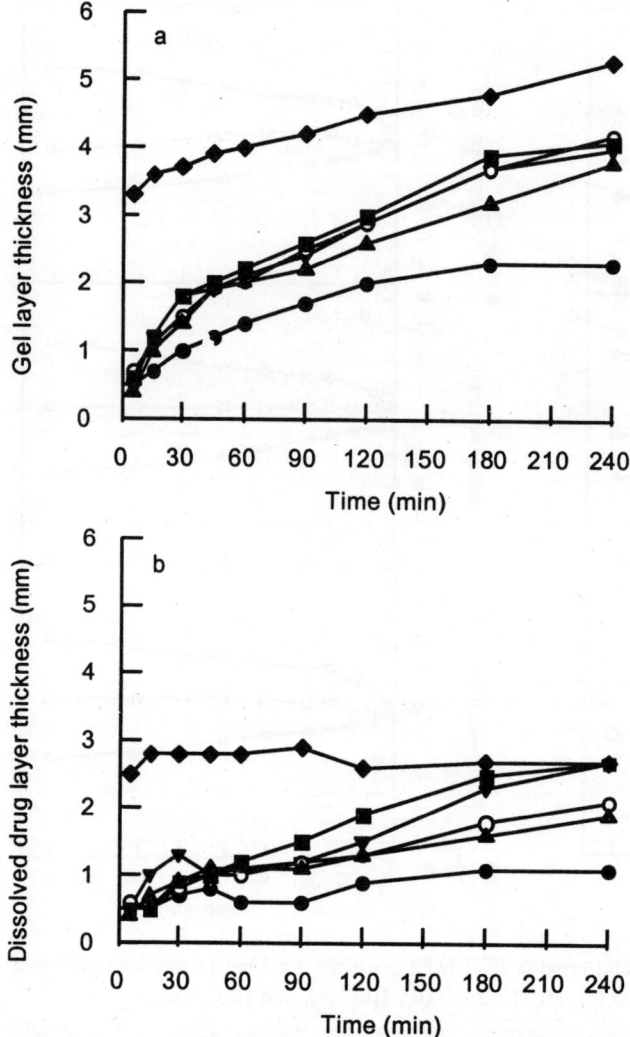

Figure 3 Gel layer thickness (a) and dissolved drug layer thickness (b) vs. time in matrices prepared with MC (●), HPMC 2208 (▼), HPMC 2906 (■), HPMC 2910 (○), HEC (◆), and HPC (▲).

analysis and Rajabi-Siahboomi et al. (44) using NMR imaging also noticed an equal development of the gel layer for the same three HPMC grades. The absence of synchronization between the movements of the two front movements, which would result in a constant gel layer thickness, should preclude constant release, in accordance with Harland's model (14).

The profiles of change of the dissolved drug layer thickness with time had different aspects (Fig. 3b). The thickness reaches constant values very rapidly for MC and HEC. According to Lee (11), this synchronization of the diffusion and erosion fronts could be indicative of constant solute release. In contrast, the thickness of the dissolved drug layer increased steadily for HPMCs and HPC.

Further insight may be gained in the mechanism of water penetration in the systems by plotting the normalized thickness as a function of the square root of time (Fig. 4). The normalized gel layer is defined as $(r_C - r_A)/r_0$, whereas the normalized dissolved drug layer is given

Hydrophilic Cellulose Derivatives

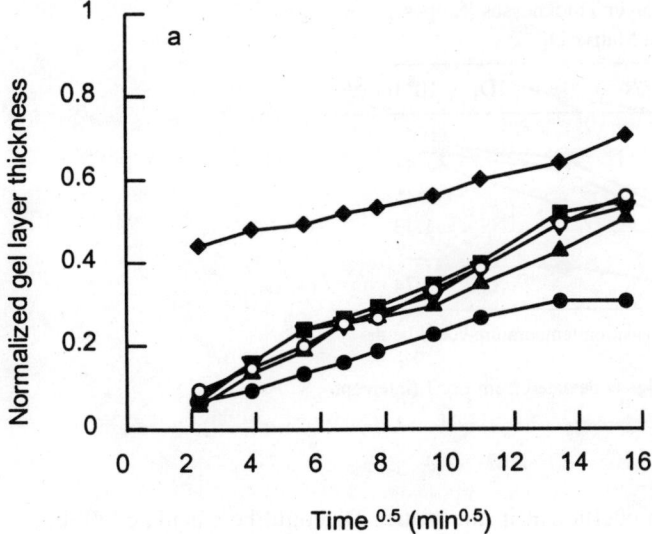

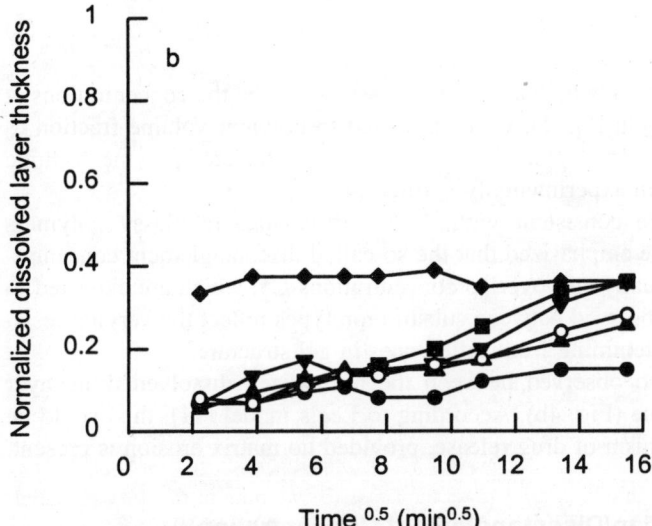

Figure 4 Normalized gel layer thickness (a) and normalized diffusion layer thickness (b) vs. square root of time in matrices prepared with MC (●), HPMC 2208 (▼), HPMC 2906 (■), HPMC 2910 (○), HEC (♦), and HPC (▲).

by $(r_C - r_B)/r_0$, where r_0 is the initial tablet radius. In case of the normalized gel layer thickness (Fig. 4a), a linear relationship was observed, at least at first glance, for five of the six derivatives, as predicted by the model of Lee and Peppas (13) for Fickian diffusion. The glassy to rubbery state transition occurs faster than polymer dissolution. The model is not respected for HEC because of acceleration in change of the swelling front (Fig. 2). From the slope of the lines in Fig. 4a, the disentanglement polymer volume fraction c_d as determined under Sec. B, and the polymer volume fraction at the rubbery/glassy interface c^* [at r_A in Fig. 1) as calculated

Table 3 Rates of Growth of the Gel Layer Thicknesses (Slopes of Fig. 4a) and Water Diffusivities in the Matrix D_1

Material		Slope × 10^4 (cm/s$^{0.5}$)	D_1 × 10^8 (cm^2/s)
MC		2.58	0.60
HPMC	2208	4.38	1.51
	2906	4.53	—[a]
	2910	4.57	1.43
HEC		—[b]	—[b]
HPC		4.13	0.74

[a] Could not be calculated because no glass transition temperature could be detected for this derivative.
[b] Was not calculated because the profile in Fig. 4a deviated from Eq. 1 (intercept different from zero).

previously (45), the water diffusion coefficient in the matrix D_1 could be calculated (Table 3) by use of Eq. 1 (13):

$$D_1 = \frac{\text{slope}^2 (1 - c^*) r_0^2}{2 (2 - c^*)(c^* - c_d)} \tag{1}$$

The disentanglement concentrations C_d, which are actually assumed to be the concentrations at the polymer–solvent interface (at r_C in Fig. 1), were converted to polymer volume fraction c_d taking a polymer true density of 1.3 g/cm^3. Note that the previously calculated polymer volume fraction c^* for HPMC 2910 has been experimentally verified (46).

The calculated D_1 values are consistent with water diffusivities in glassy polymers [10^{-8}–10^{-9} cm^2/s (47)]. It should be emphasized that the so-called disentanglement concentrations C_d as determined here are actually coil overlap concentrations C_p^*, which are expected to be lower than C_d. The differences observed between substitution types reflect the varying resistance to water diffusion, probably stemming from differences in gel structure.

A linear relationship was also observed between the normalized dissolved drug layer thickness and the square root of time (Fig. 4b). According to Lee's model (11), this would be in agreement with a Fickian mechanism of drug release, provided no matrix erosion is present.

B. Polymer Erosion and Overlap/Disentanglement Concentration

It has long been reported that hydrophilic matrices prepared with cellulose ethers undergo erosion upon contact with dissolution media (7). Erosion profiles have been published, to the authors' knowledge, only for HPMC (18–21, 48–51) and HPC (52) grades. Figure 5 presents such results for the six derivatives tested, when mixed with 20% PPA.

Polymer dissolution was the highest for HEC and MC, and then for the other derivatives. Concerning the three HPMC grades, erosion was slowest for type 2906 as observed by Bonferoni et al. (48). The two other types dissolved at the same rate, in contrast to the findings of the previous authors with matrices of pure polymers.

The observed differences in polymer dissolution rates can be explained in terms of the differences between the polymer disentanglement concentration C_d values (the concentration at which polymer chains detach from the matrix and traverse the boundary diffusion layer toward the bulk dissolution medium). Based on the Levich theory, the polymer dissolution flux, J_p, is assumed to take the form (21–23):

Hydrophilic Cellulose Derivatives

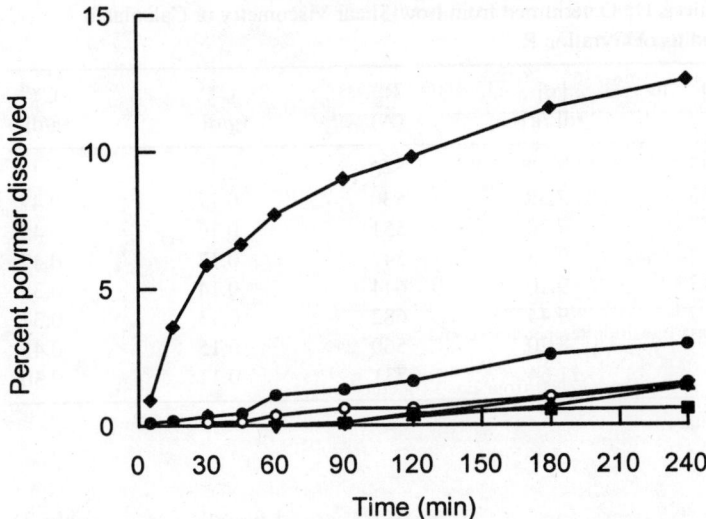

Figure 5 Polymer dissolution profiles from matrices containing 20% PPA prepared with MC (●), HPMC 2208 (▼), HPMC 2906 (■), HPMC 2910 (○), HEC (♦), and HPC (▲).

$$J_p = f_p <D_p>^{2/3} \nu^{-1/6} \omega_{app}^{1/2} C_d \qquad (2)$$

where f_p is a constant depending on the experimental setting, $<D_p>$ is an averaged diffusivity of the polymer in the dissolution medium, ν is the solvent kinematic viscosity, and ω is the apparent stirring rate. Thus, assuming constant hydrodynamic conditions and diffusion coefficient (all derivatives had rather similar molecular weights), only C_d, specific for a given polymer/system and temperature, could account for the differences in polymer flux.

Beside its determination through low shear viscometry (see G.), the overlap concentration is also obtainable through knowledge of the conformation and the molecular weight of the polymer chains (21,53):

$$C_p^* = \frac{3M_w}{4\pi N_A R_g^3} \qquad (3)$$

where M_w is the weight-average molecular weight, N_A Avogadro's number, and R_g the radius of gyration of the polymer in the given conditions. The radius of gyration can be calculated from the intrinsic viscosity $[\eta]$, with the aid of the Flory-Fox equation (54):

$$R_g^3 = \frac{[\eta]M_w}{6^{3/2}\Phi} \qquad (4)$$

where Φ is a universal constant. The theoretical value of Φ is 3.62×10^{21}, but the empirical value originally recommended by Flory and Fox (2.1–2.2×10^{21}) was used here. The viscosity data were thus also used to determine the intrinsic viscosity. The linear extrapolation to obtain (μ) was made by the Kraemer equation:

$$\frac{\ln \eta_{rel}}{C} = [\eta] + k[\eta]^2 C \qquad (5)$$

where η_{rel} is the relative viscosity, k a constant, and C the polymer concentration.

Table 4 Coil Overlap Concentrations C_p^* Determined from Low-Shear Viscometry or Calculated from Intrinsic Viscosity $[\eta]$ and Radius of Gyration R_g

Material	C_p^{*a} (g/dL)	$[\eta]$ (dL/g)	R_g^b (Å)	C_p^{*c} (g/dL)	C_p^{*d} (g/dL)
MC	0.50	7.37	540	0.17	0.47
HPMC 2208	0.43	7.39	530	0.17	0.47
2906	0.49	7.70	551	0.16	0.45
2910	0.54	7.43	547	0.17	0.47
HEC	1.15	9.10	644	0.14	0.38
HPC	0.49	9.44	682	0.13	0.37
MC + 2% PPA	0.51	8.20	560	0.15	0.43
HPC + 2% PPA	0.80	11.64	731	0.11	0.30

^aDirectly from low-shear viscometry data.
^bCalculated using Eq. 4.
^cCalculated using Eq. 3.
^dCalculated using Eq. 7.

Table 4 lists the coil overlap concentrations C_p^* as determined by direct extrapolation of the viscosity data. As expected, HEC and, to a lesser extent, MC detach from the matrix at a higher concentration, leading to a higher mass transfer flux.

Table 4 also reports values of the gyration radius R_g and the coil overlap concentration C_p^*, as calculated from the intrinsic viscosity $[\eta]$ and the molecular weight M_w. Note that knowledge of the molecular weight of the polymer is not necessary for the calculation of C_p^* from the intrinsic viscosity as substitution of Eq. 4 into Eq. 3 leads to:

$$C_p^* = \frac{3 \cdot 6^{3/2} \Phi}{4\pi N_A [\eta]} \quad (6)$$

Such coil overlap concentrations are systematically lower than those directly determined by extrapolation. This may arise from taking a universal value for Φ. Better correlation with directly determined values is obtained from (37):

$$C_p^* = 3.5/[\eta] \quad (7)$$

except for the cases of HEC and HPC in the presence of 2% PPA.

No C_p^*, $[\eta]$, and R_g values seem to have been published in the literature for the same derivatives (same degree of substitution and molecular weight as those used here at 37°C). Only Kato et al. (55) reported radii of gyration of 840Å for a 4600 mPas viscosity grade HPMC 2906 and of 980Å for a 4900 mPas viscosity grade HPMC 2910, using light scattering at room temperature for M_w determination. The corresponding C_p^* values (calculated using Eq. 3) were 3.2 and 2.8 g/dL. The gyration radii are in reasonable agreement with the values reported here, taking into account that the coil dimensions decrease with increasing temperature. Data have been published on the effect of temperature on the radius of gyration of HEC in aqueous solution (56) and on the intrinsic viscosity of MC (57). It should also be noted that lower R_g values are obtained when calculated from the intrinsic viscosities reported by Kato et al. (55), as compared to the experimentally determined radii of gyration.

As for adding 2% PPA to the aqueous solutions of the derivatives, it had no appreciable influence on either the coil overlap concentration C_p^* or on the intrinsic viscosity $[\eta]$ in the case of MC, whose θ temperature is approximately 47°C (58). In contrast, a significant increase in

C_p^* was noted for HPC, with a θ temperature of 41°C (59), i.e., very close to the experimental temperature.

Results on the effect of electrolytes on the intrinsic viscosity and radius of gyration of MC (of low molecular weight) at room temperature have been reported. Neely (60) did not observe any change in [η] and R_g on addition of 0.5 M NaCl. In contrast, a decrease in [η] and R_g was found by Marriott and John (61) when adding NaCl or other electrolytes. Mitchell et al. (62) observed a slight increase at 20°C of the intrinsic viscosity of HPMC 2208 (4000 mPas) in the presence of propranolol hydrochloride or tetracycline hydrochloride.

In parallel, electrolytes have been shown to affect the gelation temperature or the cloud point of cellulose ethers. Touitou and Donbrow (63) noticed that large cationic and anionic drugs raised the gelation temperature of HPMC 2208 gels. According to Mitchell et al. (62,64), salts were found to lower the cloud point of the same polymer, whereas large drug molecules increased the cloud point or had little effect.

From the present findings it can be anticipated that the drug eventually present at the gel layer–dissolution medium interface will not affect the overlap concentration C_p^*, and thus the disentanglement concentration C_d, of polymers with θ temperatures far from the experimental temperature, in particular polymers such as HEC with a θ temperature of approximately 300°C (65). This assertion is backed up by the fact that at this interface the solute concentration is probably close to zero.

Above all, the main feature is that HEC and MC are more prone to chain disentanglement, and thus to erosion, than the other cellulose ethers, with the probable result of more rapid drug release. It is also worth recalling that not all derivatives possess similar molecular weights due to varying degrees of substitution.

C. Drug Release

Release profiles of PPA are shown in Fig. 6. Although differences in drug release were not pronounced because of reduced tablet release surface area exposed to the dissolution medium,

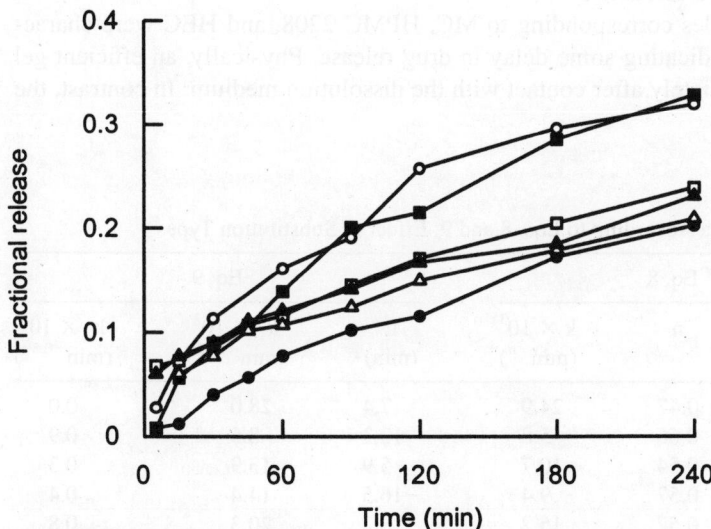

Figure 6 PPA fractional release from 20% drug-loaded matrices prepared with MC (●), HPMC 2208 (▼), HPMC 2906 (■), HPMC 2910 (○), HEC (♦), and HPC (▲).

fractional release could be observed to increase significantly in the order HPMC 2208 < HPMC 2906 ≅ HPMC 2910 ≅ HPC < HEC ≅ MC. Release differed markedly during the early time points. This can be ascribed to whether or not the polymer can rapidly form a continuous gel layer at the matrix surface and so prevent initial dissolution of the surface. The ability to form quickly a continuous gelified barrier is related to the hydrophilicity of the polymer (see Table 2), as exemplified by HEC and HPMC 2208.

Insight into the release mechanism could be gained by fitting the release data to the following expression (66):

$$M_t/M_\infty = k(t - L)^n \tag{8}$$

Here M_t/M_∞ is the fractional drug released at time t (the drug loading was considered as M_∞) and L is a so-called lag time. Equation 8 is a modified form of the semiempirical equation proposed by Peppas (67), intended to account for a delay before drug release or, as observed here with some derivatives, for a burst release, with the consequence of L being either positive or negative. The constant k is a kinetic constant measuring the velocity of drug release and n is a diffusional exponent that depends on the release mechanism and the shape of the matrix tested. Here, as drug release occurred only from the lateral surface of the matrix, one-dimensional radial release (cylindrical geometry) was considered. Fickian diffusion is thus defined by n = 0.45, anomalous (non-Fickian) transport by 0.45 < n < 0.89, and case II transport (relaxation- or swelling-controlled systems) by n = 0.89 (68,69). In the latter case, one has to realize that an erosion-controlled system would also lead to a kinetics similar to that of case II transport.

The relative Fickian (F) and relaxational (R) (or erosional) contributions to drug release were evaluated using the heuristic model developed by Peppas and Sahlin (70), as extended by Ford et al. (66) by introducing a lag time:

$$M_t/M_\infty = k_1 (t - L)^{0.45} + k_2 (t - L)^{0.89} \tag{9}$$

where k_1 and k_2 are the rate constants of the Fickian and the relaxational (erosional) contributions, respectively.

Values of the various corresponding parameters, determined using a nonlinear least squares fitting method, are listed in Table 5.

Using both models, profiles corresponding to MC, HPMC 2208, and HEC were characterized by positive L values, indicating some delay in drug release. Physically, an efficient gel barrier has been formed immediately after contact with the dissolution medium. In contrast, the

Table 5 Analysis of Release Data According to Eqs. 8 and 9: Effect of Substitution Type

Polymer and drug		Eq. 8			Eq. 9		
		L (min)	n	$k \times 10^3$ (min^{-n})	L (min)	$k_1 \times 10^3$ $(min^{-0.45})$	$k_2 \times 10^3$ $(min^{-0.89})$
MC		6.1	0.47	24.9	7.4	28.0	0.0
HPMC	2208	11.6	0.66	5.8	13.3	8.5	0.9
	2906	−9.4	0.54	10.7	−5.9	13.9	0.3
	2910	−24.7	0.57	9.4	−16.5	14.4	0.4
HEC		6.1	0.57	15.2	8.2	20.3	0.8
HPC		−16.3	0.57	9.9	11.1	14.4	0.5

negative L values observed for HPMC 2906, HPMC 2910, and HPC indicate burst release due to delayed formation of the gel barrier and thus immediate release of the surface drug.

Considering Eq. 8, pure Fickian diffusion appears to be the controlling release mechanism only for MC (with n close to 0.45), whereas non-Fickian transport prevails for all other cellulose derivatives (0.45 < n < 0.89).

Based on the pioneering work of Lapidus and Lordi (8,9), drug release from compressed hydrophilic matrices has been traditionally analyzed using Higuchi's equations, assuming planar diffusion. More recently, frequent use has been made of the semiempirical equation $M_t/M_\infty = kt^n$ and non-Fickian release has been reported for matrix systems prepared with various viscosity grades of HPMC 2208 (76,71–78) and HPC (79). Note that some release experiments were carried out using the same cell as described here (6,77) or with matrix tablets partially coated with impermeable membranes, making them similar to the setting used here (75–78). Generally, partially swelling- or erosion-controlled release has been invoked. Here the exponent n values observed for HPMC 2208 and HPC are in line with those reported in previous studies.

The time dependence of the ratio of relaxational (R) (or erosional) and Fickian (F) contributions was calculated as:

$$R/F = k_2(t - L)^{0.45}/k_1 \tag{9}$$

Figure 7 clearly shows that the relaxational or erosional contribution increased with time. When examining more deeply the nature of the non-Fickian contribution, it came out that significant erosion-controlled release (Fig. 5) could operate only for HEC. Macromolecular relaxation is thus most probably the mechanism complementary to Fickian diffusion for the other five derivatives.

One could add that Ford et al. (66) also deduced from the observed decrease in activation energy with increasing HPMC 2208 (1500 mPa/s) content in promethazine hydrochloride tablets that diffusion was not the only factor controlling the release rate.

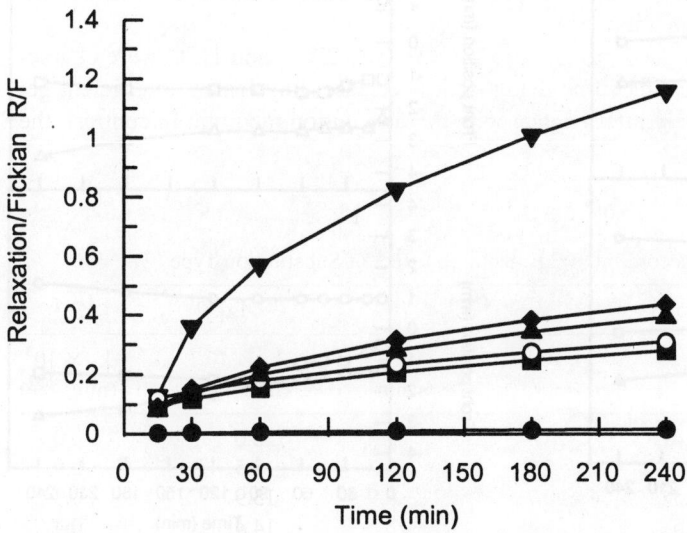

Figure 7 R/F ratio values vs. time for PPA release from matrices prepared with MC (●), HPMC 2208 (▼), HPMC 2906 (■), HPMC 2910 (○), HEC (♦), and HPC (▲).

IV. EFFECT OF DRUG LOADING ON MATRIX CHARACTERISTICS

Data presented so far have dealt with matrices loaded with 20% PPA, but it is common knowledge that drug loading may alter the release mechanism. This effect was examined by selecting the two polymers with extreme release characteristics, namely HPMC 2208 and HEC, and by incorporating 40% and 60% of PPA. Figure 8 shows the front movements upon water penetration. Data corresponding to 20% drug-loaded matrices have also been included to facilitate comparison.

Drug loading had very little influence on front movements in HPMC 2208 matrices. At most the swelling front moved more quickly, probably due to an osmotic effect (80). The effect was much more pronounced for HEC matrices, especially with regard to the diffusion and erosion fronts. The diffusion front moved faster as the proportion of drug increased, whereas the observed erosion front movements were small as the proportion of PPA increased, due to more marked polymer dissolution (see later).

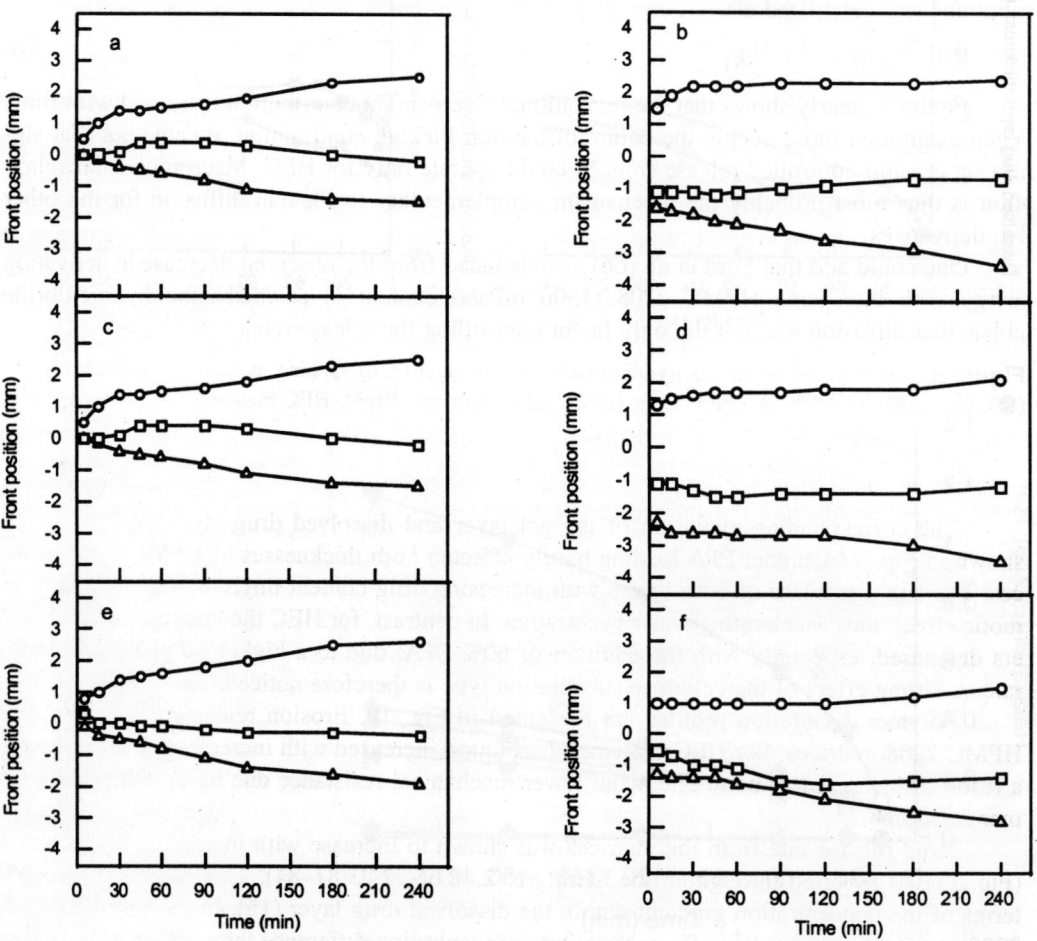

Figure 8 Swelling (Δ), diffusion (□), and erosion (○) front positions vs. time in matrices loaded with 20% (a, b) or 40% (c, d) or 60% (e, f) PPA. Left: HPMC 2208 matrices. Right: HEC matrices.

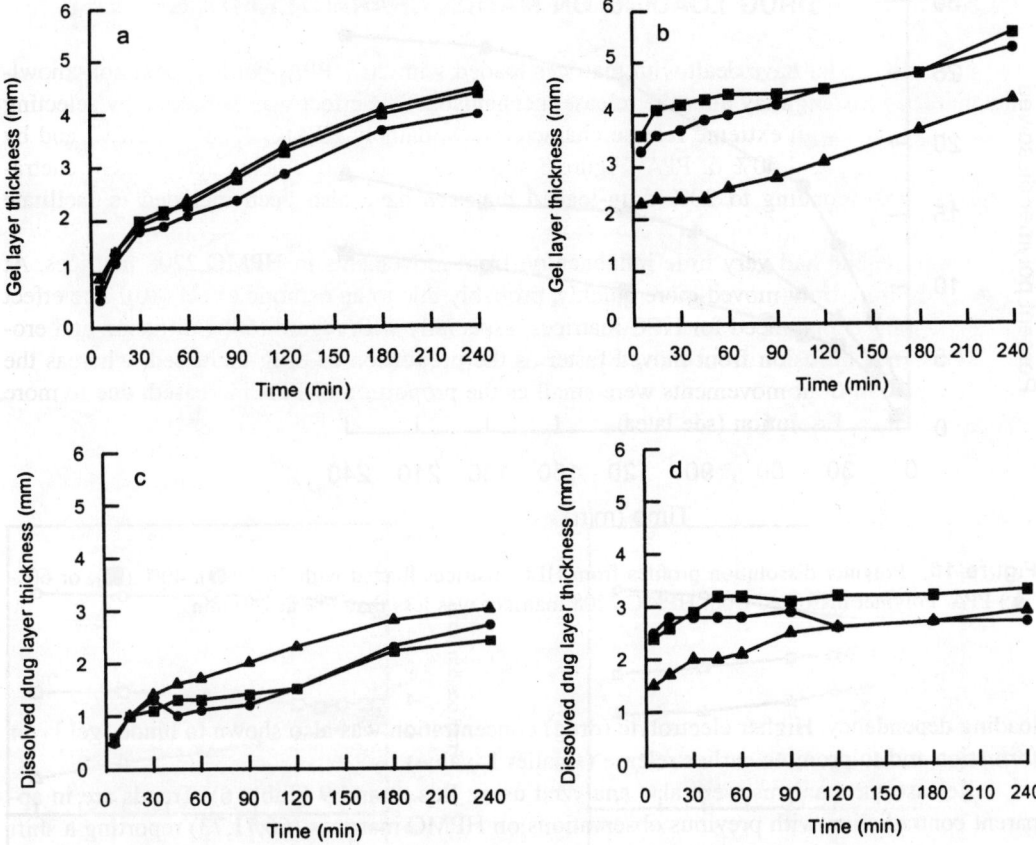

Figure 9 Gel layer thickness (a, b) and dissolved drug layer (c, d) vs. time in matrices loaded with 20% (●), (40% (■), or 60% (▲) PPA. Left: HPMC 2208 matrices. Right: HEC matrices.

The corresponding evolution of the gel layer and dissolved drug layer thicknesses are shown in Fig. 9. A higher PPA loading hardly affected both thicknesses of HPMC 2208 matrices. The slight increase of both layers with increasing drug content might be due to higher osmotic effect, thus accelerating water penetration. In contrast, for HEC the thickness of both layers decreased, especially with the addition of 60% PPA, due to a higher polymer dissolution rate. A strong effect of the cellulose substitution type is therefore noticed.

Polymer dissolution profiles are presented in Fig. 10. Erosion remained very low with HPMC 2208 matrices. For HEC, polymer dissolution increased with increasing drug content as a result of increased osmotic effect and lower mechanical resistance due to a diminished polymer fraction.

Drug release rate from the matrices was shown to increase with increasing drug content (Fig. 11), as reported throughout the literature (2,46,66,71,73,81–84). This can be analyzed in terms of the concentration gradient within the dissolved drug layer (15). In the case of HPMC 2208 matrices, drug loading affects the solute concentration difference through the layer but not the gel thickness. For HEC, drug loading both increases the solute concentration difference (for a highly soluble drug) and diminishes the layer thickness by erosion, leading to the strongest

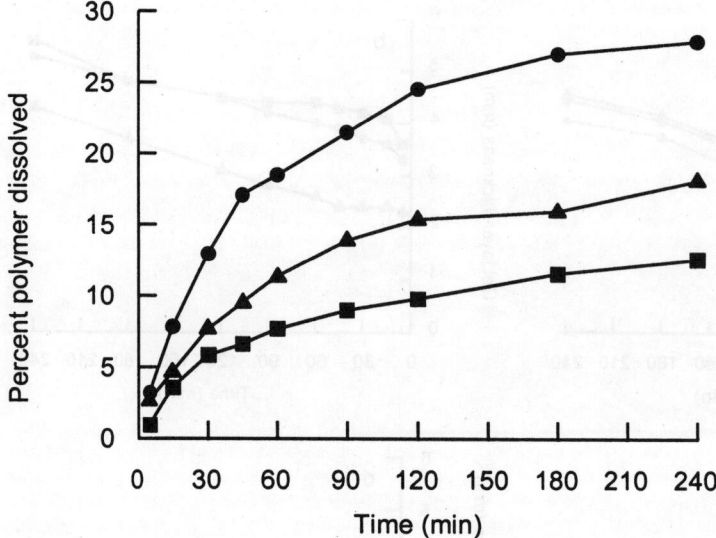

Figure 10 Polymer dissolution profiles from HEC matrices loaded with 20% (●), 40% (■), or 60% (▲) PPA. Polymer dissolved from HPMC 2208 matrices was less than 6% at 240 min.

loading dependency. Higher electrolyte (drug) concentration was also shown to hinder gel layer formation and to promote earlier release (smaller L value).

Release mechanisms were also analyzed using Eqs. 8 and 9 (Table 6). Trends are in apparent contradiction with previous observations on HPMC matrices (66,71,73) reporting a shift to more anomalous transport with increasing drug loading. It must be stressed that these authors did not introduce an L term in their fitting equation, even though L is affected by drug loading. For HEC matrices, purely Fickian diffusion was observed even at 60% PPA loading. Additionally, the profiles shown in Fig. 12, drawn from Eq. 9, show that the relaxation (HPMC 2208) and erosional (HEC) contributions again increased with time but that they are not dependent on drug loading.

Table 6 Analysis of Release Data According to Eqs. 8 and 9: Effect of Drug Loading

Polymer and PPA loading	Eq. 8			Eq. 9		
	L (min)	n	$k \times 10^3$ ($\min^{-n}$)	L (min)	$k_1 \times 10^3$ ($\min^{-0.45}$)	$k_2 \times 10^3$ ($\min^{-0.89}$)
HPMC 2208						
20%	11.6	0.66	5.8	13.3	8.5	0.9
40%	2.8	0.68	5.2	6.9	8.6	0.9
60%	6.7	0.66	7.1	9.5	10.8	1.0
HEC						
20%	6.1	0.57	15.2	8.2	20.3	0.8
40%	−4.3	0.58	16.4	−0.4	23.6	1.0
60%	−8.8	0.42	48.2	−9.8	44.8	0.0

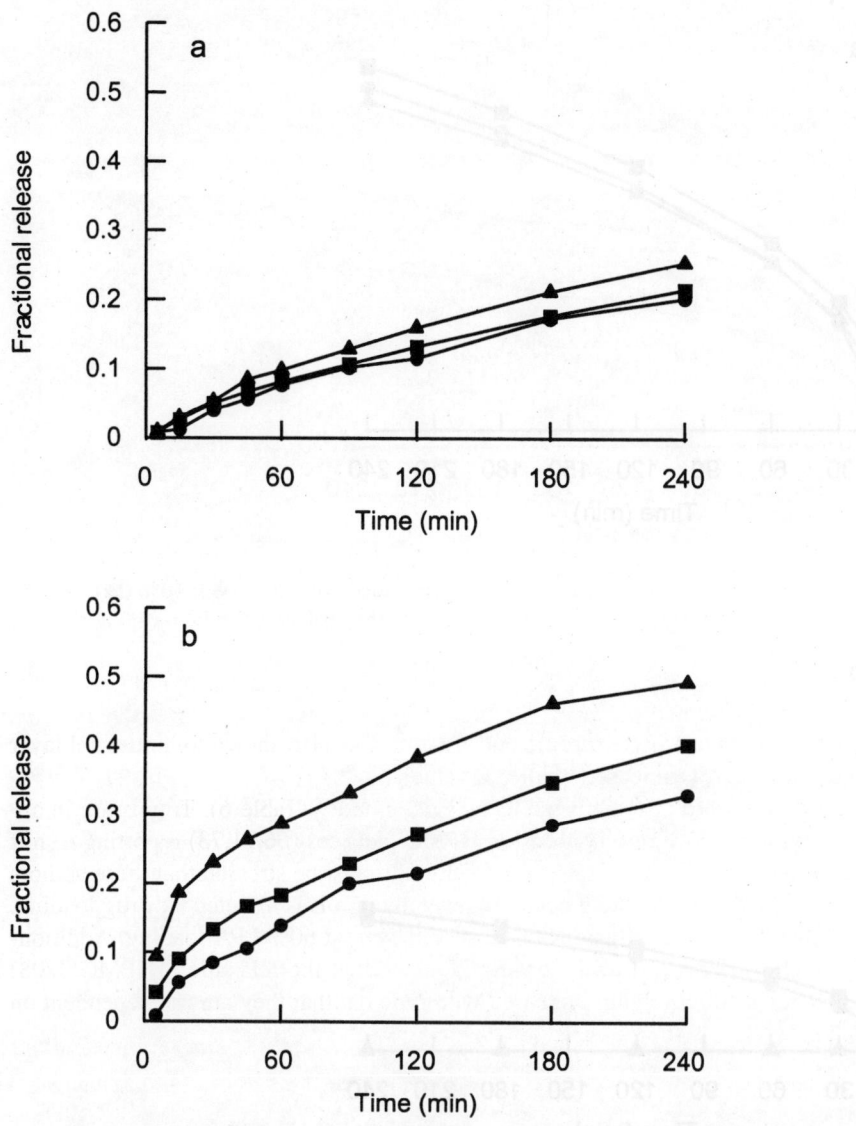

Figure 11 PPA fractional release from HPMC 2208 (a) and HEC (b) matrices loaded with 20% (●), 40% (■), or 60% (▲) PPA.

V. EFFECT OF DRUG SOLUBILITY ON MATRIX CHARACTERISTICS

In addition to drug loading, drug solubility is certainly capable of altering water penetration, erosion, and hence drug release. So far the available data have been limited to PPA with a solubility in water at 37°C of 410 mg/mL. Two other drugs with similar diffusivities (molecular weights) but different solubilities were thus selected to investigate the effect of this factor. Theophylline (THP) was less soluble (11 mg/mL) than PPA, whereas pseudoephedrine hydrochloride (PED) had twice the solubility (860 mg/mL). Both drugs were incorporated at 20% loading again in HPMC 2208 and HEC. Front movements are shown in Fig. 13.

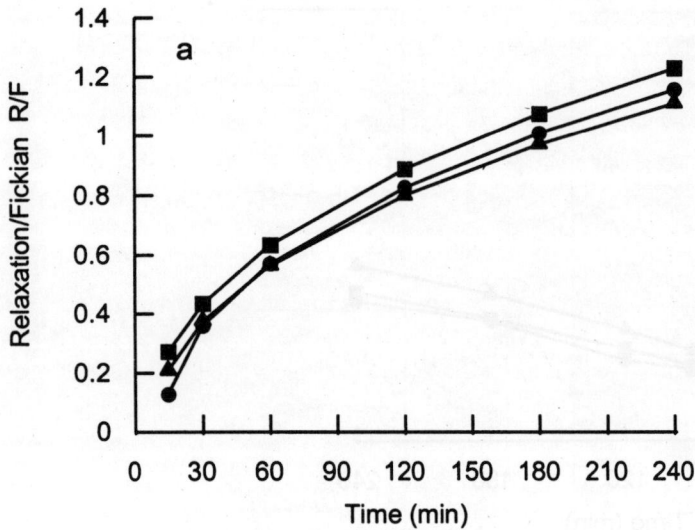

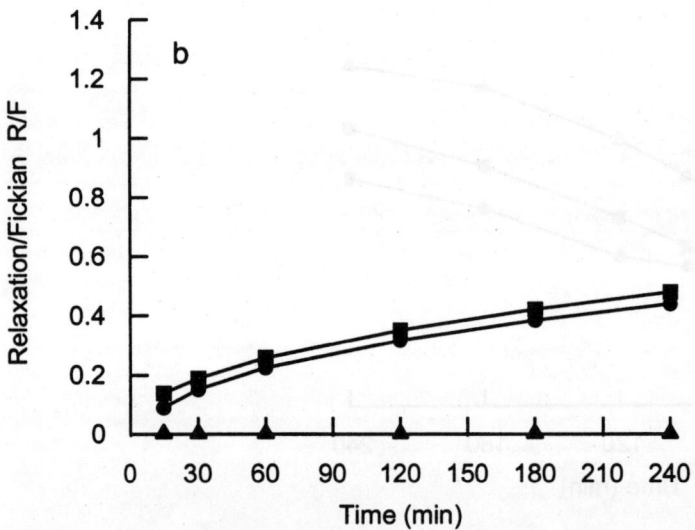

Figure 12 R/F ratio values vs. time for PPA release from HPMC 2208 (a) and HEC (b) matrices loaded with 20% (●), 40% (■), or 60% (▲) PPA.

Drug solubility appears to have some influence on front movements in HPMC 2208 matrices (Fig. 13a, c, e). The swelling front exhibited more rapid movements with increasing drug solubility due to osmotic effect. When the solubility increased, the diffusion front also moved faster. In the case of HEC matrices, more peculiar front movements were observed with increasing drug solubility (Fig. 13b, d, f). The advancement of the swelling front was not very much affected. Note that a diffusion front was always present, even when the highly soluble PED was incorporated in the matrices. The peculiar evolution of the diffusion front in the matrix containing THP was explained as follows: At early times, as a result of rapid swelling, the

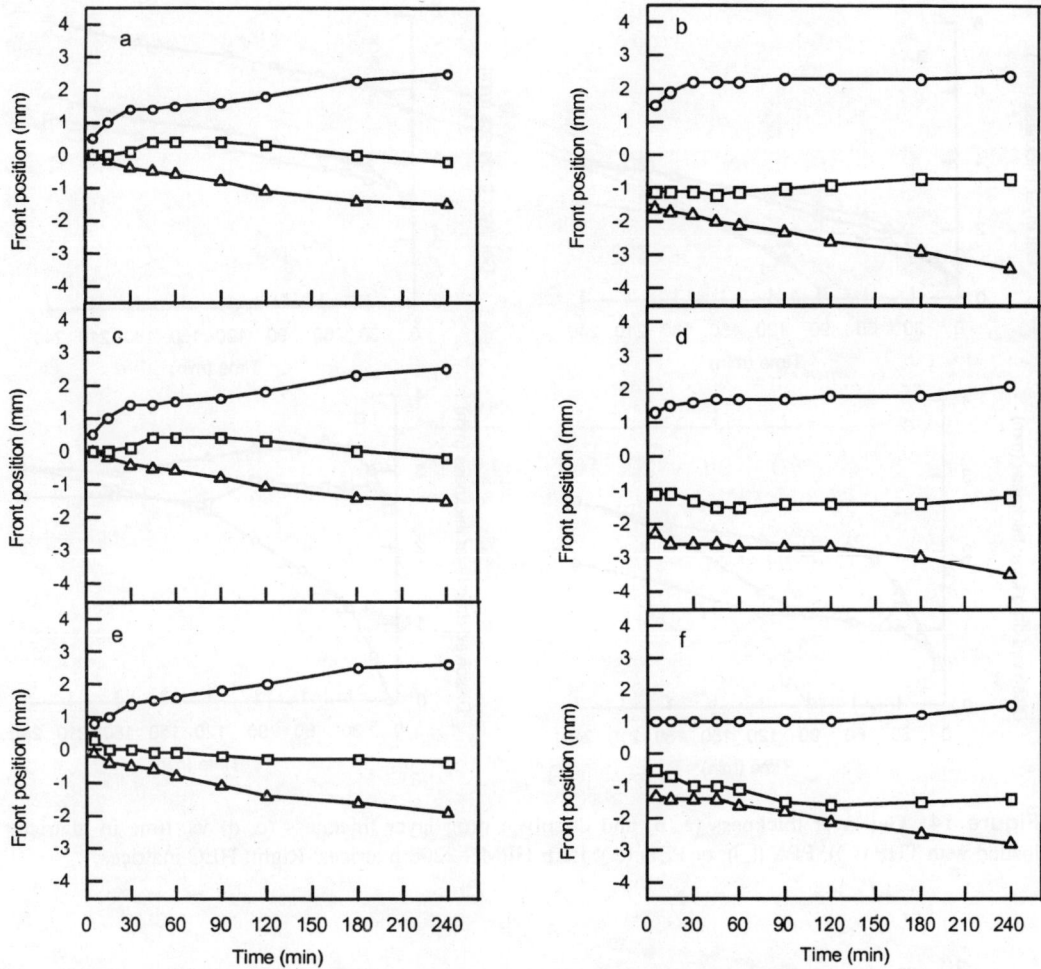

Figure 13 Swelling (△), diffusion (□), and erosion (○) front positions vs. time in matrices loaded with THP (a, b), PPA (c, d), and PED (e, f). Left: HPMC 2208 matrices. Right: HEC matrices.

tablet expanded outwardly pulling the diffusion front. Then, upon dissolution of the drug, the diffusion front moved inward, while the erosion front remained stable due to erosion.

The evolution of the resulting gel layer and dissolved drug layer thicknesses are presented in Fig. 14. In HPMC 2208 matrices, the thicknesses are least for the poorly soluble THP. In the case of HEC matrices, the thicknesses are oppositely affected due to differences in polymer dissolution. The gel layer is the thickest when THP is incorporated, with the thickness of the dissolved drug layer being the thinnest.

With HPMC 2208 polymer dissolution remained negligible within 8 h, whatever the drug incorporated (Fig. 15), but erosion of the HEC matrices was enhanced when loaded with the highly soluble PED due to an osmotic effect.

Corresponding release profiles are illustrated in Fig. 16. As reported by several authors (2,9,15,17,19,71,73,74,79,83), increased solubility resulted in higher release rate. The larger concentration gradient through the gel layer (although the thickness increased slightly with increasing solubility) accounts for this (15).

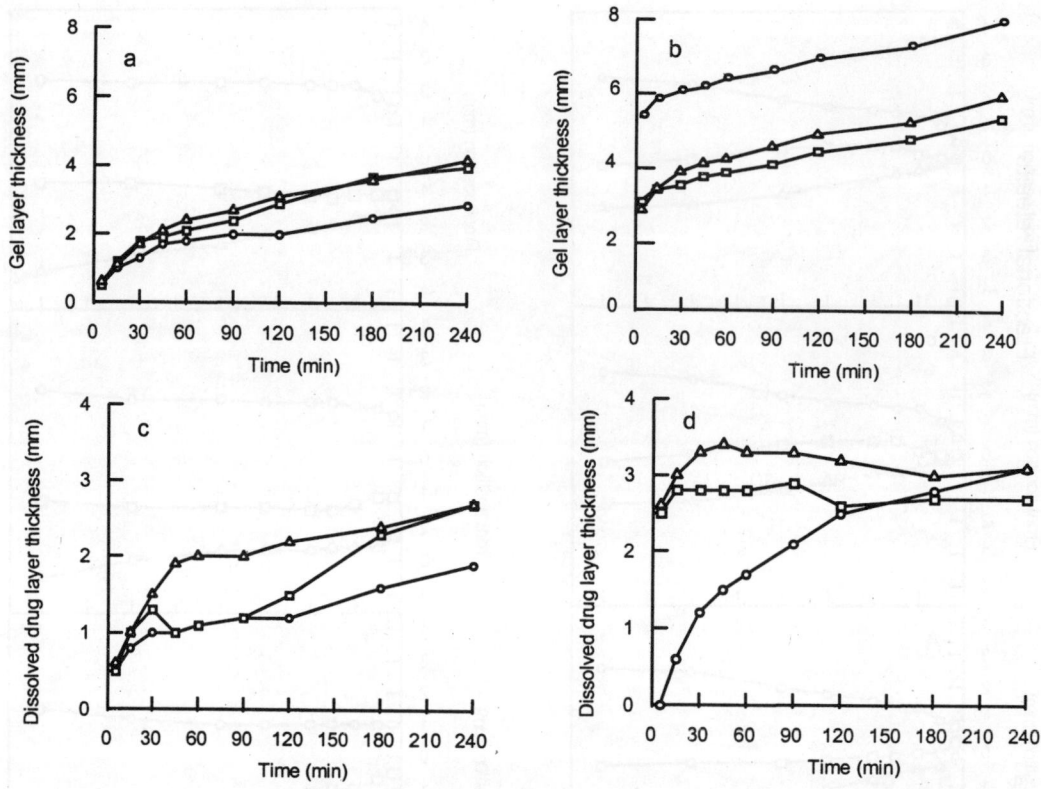

Figure 14 Gel layer thickness (a, b) and dissolved drug layer thickness (c, d) vs. time in matrices loaded with THP (○), PPA (□), or PED (△). Left: HPMC 2208 matrices. Right: HEC matrices.

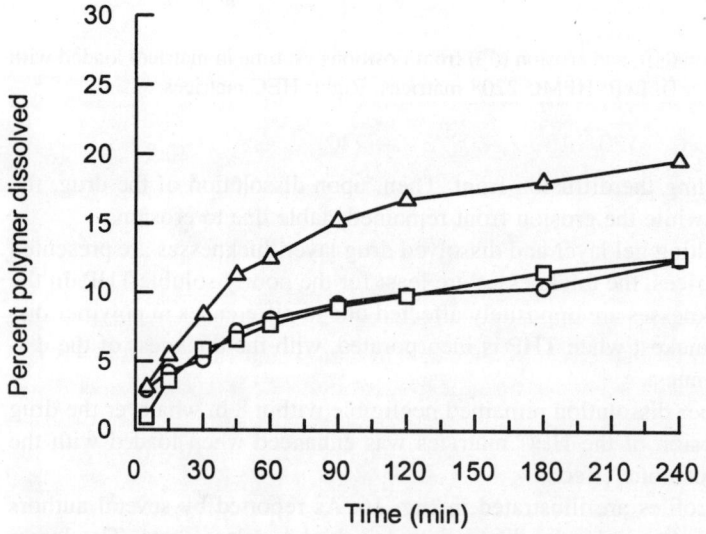

Figure 15 Polymer dissolution profiles from HEC matrices loaded with 20% THP (○), PPA (□), and PED (△). Polymer dissolved from HPMC 2208 matrices was less than 2% at 240 min.

Hydrophilic Cellulose Derivatives

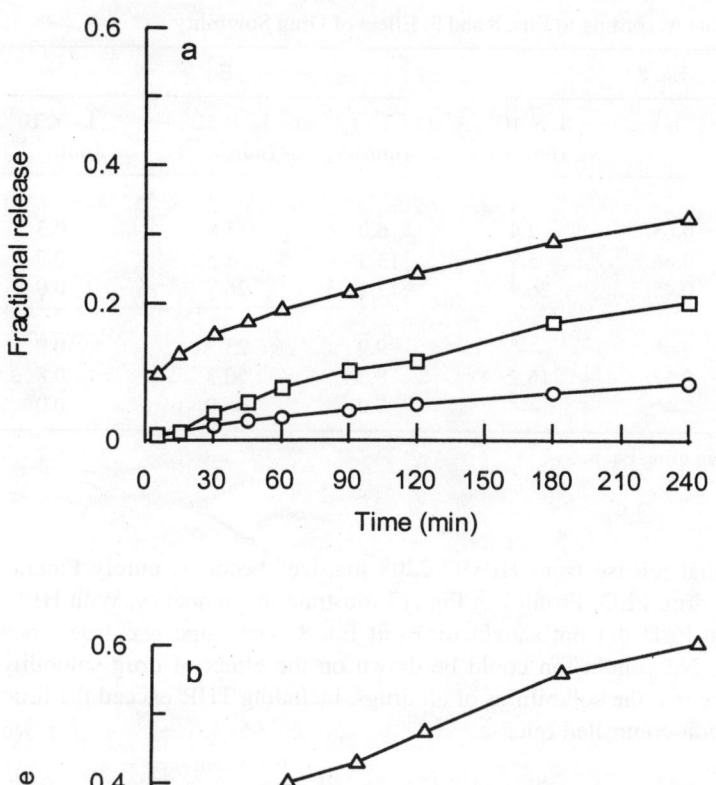

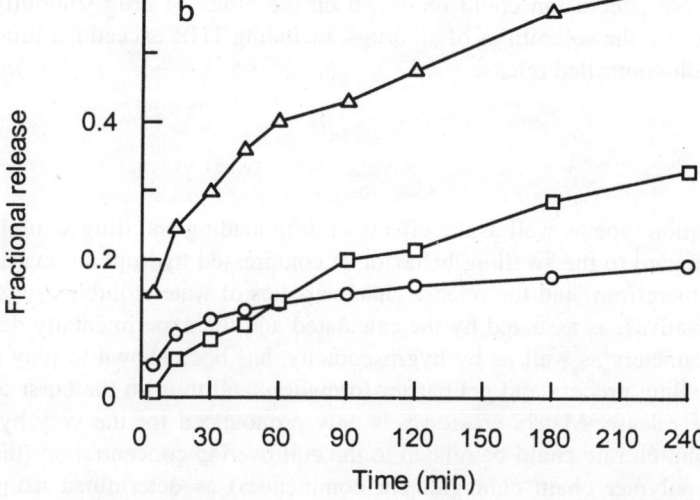

Figure 16 Fractional release of THP (◯), PPA (□), and PED (△) from HPMC 2208 (a) and HEC (b) matrices.

The effect of drug solubility on the release mechanism was examined through Eqs 8 and 9 (Table 7, Fig. 17). As far as the dependence of the exponent n of Eq. 8 on drug solubility is concerned, authors (19,71,73,74) have generally observed that n departs from Fickian diffusion for very poorly soluble drugs. It is argued that matrix erosion becomes the rate-limiting factor. Thus, a deviation was seen by Tahara et al. (19) only for a drug of 0.07 mg/mL. A solubility limit of 330 mg/mL (diazepam) can be estimated from the data of Ford (71). In contrast, Colombo et al. (15) did not notice any change in n values (with HPMC 2208 matrices) when the solubility of buflomedil pyridoxal phosphate was decreased to 1 mg/mL by lowering the pH of the dissolution medium.

Table 7 Analysis of Release Data According to Eqs. 8 and 9: Effect of Drug Solubility

Polymer and drug	Eq. 8			Eq. 9		
	L (min)	n	$k \times 10^3$ ($\min^{-n}$)	L (min)	$k_1 \times 10^3$ ($\min^{-0.45}$)	$k_2 \times 10^3$ ($\min^{-0.89}$)
HPMC 2208						
THP	2.4	0.65	2.4	6.0	3.8	0.3
PPA	11.6	0.66	5.8	13.3	8.5	0.9
PED	−16.9	0.45	26.7	−17.2	26.7	0.0
HEC						
THP	—[a]	—[a]	—[a]	−9.9	25.3	0.0
PPA	6.1	0.57	15.2	8.2	20.3	0.8
PED	—[a]	—[a]	—[a]	−7.0	66.9	0.0

[a]No satisfactory fit was observed when using Eq. 8.

Here it was observed that release from HPMC 2208 matrices becomes purely Fickian with the highly water-soluble drug PED. Profiles in Fig. 17 illustrate this tendency. With HEC, release data of both THP and PED did not satisfactorily fit Eq. 8. The same was true when deleting the L term in Eq. 8. No conclusion could be drawn on the effect of drug solubility when using Eq. 9. Finally, note that the solubilities of all drugs, including THP, exceed the limit generally recognized for erosion-controlled release.

VI. CONCLUSION

The effect of cellulose substitution type as well as the effects of drug loading and drug solubility have been addressed with regard to the swelling behavior of compressed hydrophilic matrices, the polymer erosion rate therefrom, and the release characteristics of water-soluble drugs. The hydrophilicity of the derivatives, as assessed by the calculated and the experimentally determined partial solubility parameters as well as by hygroscopicity, has been shown to play a role only in the very early swelling process and gel barrier formation, and thus on the burst or lag eventually observed in the release. Matrix erosion was only pronounced for the very hydrophilic HEC. Polymer dissolution rate could be related to the coil overlap concentration (the concentration beyond which polymer chain entanglement commences) as determined using low-shear viscosimetry.

Drug release from the matrices was examined using a device allowing perfect radial swelling. Release mechanism of phenylpropanolamine hydrochloride was shown to be dependent on the polymer substitution type, using known release equations modified to account for a burst or lag in release. Fickian diffusion was the govering factor only for MC. Non-Fickian (anomalous) transport was observed for all other cellulose ethers. However, if some macromolecular relaxation-controlled release may be invoked for the HPMCs and HPC, leading to a time-dependent increase in diffusion coefficient due to continuous polymer swelling (84), erosion is probably the contributing factor in the case of HEC compensating the continuous decline in release rate due to diffusion. The influence of drug loading and that of drug solubility (theophylline, pseudoephedrine hydrochloride) on the matrix performances were also examined. Changes in the release rate were observed but the release kinetics were generally only slightly affected.

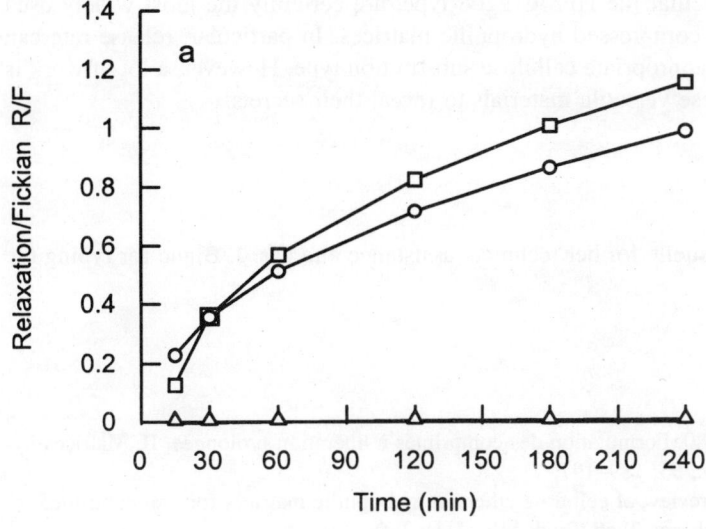

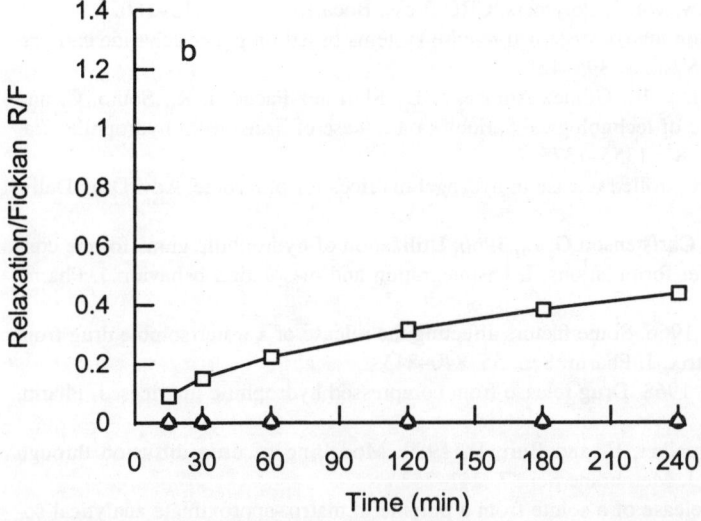

Figure 17 R/F ratio values vs. time for release of THP (○), PPA (□), and PED (△) from HPMC 2208 (a) and HEC (b) matrices.

Countless experimental results and theories have been published in the literature, but still a lot of independent studies remain to be conducted to ascertain the release mechanisms prevailing in these swellable systems. In this respect, it is possible that compensatory effects are responsible for the apparent kinetics. Thus, it would be of interest to carry out more extensive studies on water and drug diffusivity in gels using independent techniques (85,86). Measurements of the distribution and interaction of water with the material (87–89), as related to the substitution type, would also be beneficial for the elucidation of the solute release mechanism. It is also known that cellulose derivatives, at least HPC (90), form mesophases that can complicate solute transport. Finally, chain relaxation–controlled release would certainly be substantiated when performing independent mechanical relaxation studies.

Cellulose ethers, in particular the HPMC 2208 type, are certainly the most widely used polymers in the production of compressed hydrophilic matrices. In particular, release rate can be modulated by selecting the appropriate cellulose substitution type. However, a lot of work is still to be done in order for these versatile materials to reveal their secrets.

ACKNOWLEDGMENTS

The authors thank Ms. D. Massuelle for her technical assistance and Ms. J. Blanc for typing the manuscript.

REFERENCES

1. Buri, P. and Doelker, E., 1980. Formulation des comprimés à libération prolongée. II. Matrices hydrophiles. Pharm. Acta Helv., 55: 189–197.
2. Aldermann, D. A., 1984. A review of cellulose ethers in hydrophilic matrices for oral controlled release dosage forms. Int. J. Pharm. Tech. Prod. Mfr., 5(3): 1–9.
3. Doelker, E., 1987. Water-swollen cellulose derivatives in pharmacy. In: N. A. Peppas (Ed.), Hydrogels in Medicine and Pharmacy, Vol. 2, Polymers, CRC Press, Boca Raton, pp. 115–160.
4. Melia, C. D., 1991. Hydrophilic matrix sustained release systems based on polysaccharide carriers. Crit. Rev. Ther. Drug Carrier Syst., 8: 395–421.
5. Vasquez, M. J., Pérez-Marcol, J. B., Gómez-Amoza, J. L., Martinez-Pacheco, R., Souto, C. and Concheiro, A., 1992. Influence of technological variables on release of drugs from hydrophilic matrices. Drug Dev. Ind. Pharm., 81: 1355–1375.
6. Colombo P., 1993. Swelling-controlled release in hydrogel matrices for oral route. Adv. Drug Deliv. Rev., 11: 37–57.
7. Huber, H. E., Dale, L. B. and Christenson G. L., 1966. Utilization of hydrophilic gums for the control of drug release from tablet formulations, I. Disintegration and dissolution behavior. J. Pharm. Sci., 55: 974–976.
8. Lapidus, H. and Lordi, N. G., 1966. Some factors affecting the release of a water-soluble drug from a compressed hydrophilic matrix. J. Pharm. Sci., 55: 840–843.
9. Lapidus, H. and Lordi, N. G., 1968. Drug release from compressed hydrophilic matrices. J. Pharm. Sci., 57: 1292–1301.
10. Peppas, N. A., Gurny, R., Doelker, E. and Buri, P., 1980. Modelling of drug diffusion through swellable polymeric systems. J. Membrane Sci., 7: 241–253.
11. Lee, P. I., 1980. Diffusional release of a solute from a polymeric matrix-approximate analytical solutions. J. Membrane Sci., 7: 255–275.
12. Peppas, N. A. and Franson, N. M., 1983. The swelling interface number as a criterion for prediction of diffusional solute release mechanisms in swellable polymers. J. Polym. Sci. Polym Phys., 121: 983–997.
13. Lee, P. I. and Peppas, N. A., Prediction of polymer dissolution in swellable controlled-release systems, J. Controlled Rel., 6 (1987) 207–215.
14. Harland, R. S., Gazzaniga, A., Sangalli, M. E., Colombo, P. and Peppas, N. A., 1988. Drug/polymer matrix swelling and dissolution. Pharm. Res., 5: 488–494.
15. Colombo, P., Bettini, R., Massimo, G., Catellani, P. L. Santi, P. and Peppas, N. A., 1995. Drug diffusion front movement is important in drug release control from swellable matrix tablets. J. Pharm. Sci., 84: 991–997.
16. Lee, P. I. and Kim, C. -J., 1991. Probing the mechanisms of drug release from hydrogels, J. Controlled Rel., 16: 229–236.
17. Möckel, J. E. and Lippold, B. C., 1993. Zero-order drug release from hydrocolloid matrices, Pharm. Res., 10: 1066–1070.

18. Katzhendler, I., Hoffman, A., Goldenberger, A. and Friedman, M., 1997. Modeling of drug release from erodible tablets, J. Pharm. Sci., 86: 110–115.
19. Tahara K., Yamamoto K. and Nishihata T., 1996. Application of model-independent and model analysis for the investigation of effect of drug solubility on its release rate from hydroxypropyl methylcellulose sustained release tablets. Int. J. Pharm., 133: 17–27.
20. Tahara, K., Yamamoto, K. and Nishihata, T., 1995. Overall mechanism behind matrix sustained release (SR) tablets prepared with hydroxypropyl methylcellulose 2910. J. Controlled Rel., 35: 59–66.
21. Ju, R. T. C., Nixon, P. R., M. V. and Patel M. V., 1995. Drug release from hydrophilic matrices. 1. New scaling laws for predicting polymer and drug release based on the polymer disentanglement concentration and the diffusion layer. J. Pharm. Sci., 84: 1455–1463.
22. Ju R. T. C., Nixon P. R. and Patel M. V., 1995. Drug release from hydrophilic matrices. 2. A mathematical model based on the polymer desentanglement concentration and the diffusion layer. J. Pharm. Sci., 83: 1464–1477.
23. Ju, R. T. C., Nixon, P. R. and Patel, M. V., 1997. Diffusion coefficients of polymer chains in the diffusion layer adjacent to a swollen hydrophilic matrix. J. Pharm. Sci., 86: 1293–1297.
24. Salomon, J. -L., Doelker, E. and Buri, P., 1979. Sustained release of a water-soluble drug from hydrophilic compressed dosage forms. Pharm. Ind., 41: 799–802.
25. Hoy, K. L., 1989. Solubility parameter as a design parameter for water borne polymers and coatings. J. Coated Fabr., 19: 53–67.
26. Fedors, R. F., 1974. A method for estimating both the solubility parameters and molar volumes of liquids. Polym. Eng. Sci., 14: 147–154.
27. Rosell, K. G., 1988, Distribution of substituents in methylcellulose. J. Carbohyd. Chem., 7: 525–536.
28. Tezuka, Y., Imai, K., Oshima T. M. and Chiba, T., 1990. Determination of substituent distribution in cellulose ethers by means of a ^{13}C NMR study on their acetylated derivatives, 4. O-methyl-O-hydroxyalkylcelluloses. Makromol. Chem., 191: 681–690.
29. Lindberg, B. and Lindquist, U., 1987, Distribution of substituents in O-(2-hydroxyethyl)-cellulose. Carbohydr. Res., 170: 207–214.
30. Lee, D. -S. and Perlin, A. S., 1982. ^{13}C-N.M.R.-spectral and related studies on the distribution of substituents in O-(2-hydroxypropyl)cellulose. Carbohydr. Res., 106: 1–19.
31. Bruneau N., Barra J., Buri P. and Doelker E., 2000. Solubility parameters and surface free energies of water-soluble cellulose derivatives as a function of substitution type. Eur. J. Pharm. Biopharm. (submitted).
32. Doelker, E., 1994. Cellulose derivatives. Adv. Polym. Sci., 107: 199–265.
33. Bettini, R., Colombo, P., Massimo, G., Catellani, P. L. and Vitali, T., 1994. Swelling and drug release in hydrogel matrices: polymer viscosity and matrix porosity effects. Eur. J. Pharm. Sci., 2: 218–219.
34. Morris, D. L., 1948. Quantitative determination of carbohydrates with Dreywood's anthrone reagent. Science, 107: 254–255.
35. Porter, R. S. and Johnson, J. F., 1966. The entanglement concept in polymer systems. Chem. Rev., 66: 1–27.
36. Morris, E. R., Cutler, A. N., Boss-Murphy, S. B., Rees, D. A. and Price, J., 1981. Concentration and shear rate dependence of viscosity in random coil polysaccharide solutions. Carbohyd. Polym., 1: 5–21.
37. Tomioka, M. and Matsumura, G., 1987. Effects of concentration and degree of polymerization on the rheological properties of methylcellulose aqueous solution. Chem. Pharm. Bull., 35: 2510–2518.
38. Schmidt, J., Weigel, R., Burchard, W. and Richtering, W., 1997. Methylhydroxypropyl cellulose: shear induced birefringence measurements in the semi-dilute regime. Macromol. Symp., 120: 247–257.
39. Rowe, R. C., 1988. Binder–substrate interactions in tablets: a theoretical approach based on solubility parameters. Acta Pharm. Technol., 34: 144–146.
40. Archer, W. L., 1991. Determination of Hansen solubility parameters for selected cellulose ether derivatives. Ind. Eng. Chem. Res., 30: 2292–2298.

41. Archer, W. L., 1992. Hansen solubility parameters for selected cellulose ether derivatives and their use in the pharmaceutical industry. Drug Dev. Ind. Pharm., 18: 599–616.
42. Choi, P., Kavassalis, T. A. and Rudin, A., 1994. Estimation of Hansen solubility parameters for (hydroxyethyl)- and (hydroxypropyl)cellulose through molecular simulation. Ind. Eng. Chem. Res., 33: 3154–3159.
43. Mitchell, K., Ford, J. L., Armstrong, D. J., Elliott, P. N. C. Hogan, J. E. and Rostron, C., 1993. The influence of substitution type on the performance of methylcellulose and hydroxypropylmethylcellulose in gels and matrices. Int. J. Pharm., 100: 143–154.
44. Rajabi-Siahboomi, A. R., Bowtell, R. W., Mansfield, P., Henderson, A., Davies, M. C. and C. D. Melia, 1994. Structure and behaviour in hydrophilic matrix sustained release dosage forms: 2. NMR-imaging studies of dimensional changes in the gel layer and core of HPMC tablets undergoing hydration. J. Controlled Rel., 31: 121–128.
45. Doelker, E., 1990. Swelling behavior of water-soluble cellulose derivatives. In: L. Brannon-Peppas and R. S. Harland (Eds.), Absorbent Polymer Technology, Elsevier, Amsterdam, pp. 125–145.
46. Hancock, B. and Zografi, G., 1994. The relationship between the glass transition temperature and the water content of amorphous pharmaceutical solids. Pharm. Res., 11: 471–477.
47. Barrie, J. A., 1968, Water in polymer. In: J. Crank and G. S. Park (Eds.), Diffusion in Polymers, Academic Press, London, pp. 259–313.
48. Bonferoni, M. C., Rossi, S., Ferrari, F., Bertoni, M., Sinistus, R. and Caramella, C., 1995. Characterization of three hydroxypropylmethylcellulose substitution types: rheological properties and dissolution behaviour. Eur. J. Pharm. Biopharm., 41: 242–246.
49. Skoug, J. W., Mikelsons, M. V., Vigneron, C. N. and Stemm, N. L., 1993. Qualitative evaluation of the mechanism of release of matrix sustained release dosage forms by measurement of polymer release. J. Controlled Rel., 27: 227–245.
50. Kim, H. and Fassihi, R., 1997. A new ternary polymeric matrix system for controlled drug delivery of highly soluble drugs: I. Diltiazem hydrochloride. Pharm. Res., 14: 1415–1421.
51. Abrahamsson, B., Alpsten, M., Bake, B., Larsson, A. and Sjögren, J., 1998. In vitro and in vivo erosion of two different hydrophilic gel matrix tablets. Eur. J. Pharm. Biopharm., 46: 69–75.
52. Grabowski, L. A., Bondi, J. V. and Harwood, R. J., 1985. Dissolution rate studies of compression-molded units made from hydroxypropyl cellulose films. J. Pharm. Sci., 74: 540–544.
53. Munch, J. P., Lemaréchal, P., Candau, S. and Herz, J., 1977. Light scattering spectroscopy of polydimethylsiloxane-toluene gels. J. Phys., 38: 1499–1509.
54. Flory, P. J., 1986. Principle of Polymer Chemistry, Cornell University Press, Ithaca, p. 1953.
55. Kato, T., Asami, H. and Takashi, A., 1986. Adsorption of hydroxypropyl methylcellulose onto aluminia surfaces. Kobunshi Robunshu, 43: 399–404.
56. Brown, W., Henley, D. and Öhman, J., 1963. Studies on cellulose derivatives. Part II. The influence of solvent and temperature on the configuration and hydrodynamic behaviour of hydroxyethylcellulose in dilute solution. Makromol. Chem., 64: 49–67.
57. Amari, T. and Nakamura, M., 1974. Viscoelastic properties of dilute aqueous solution of methylcellulose at ultrasonic frequencies. J. Appl. Polym. Sci., 18: 3329–3344.
58. Kato, T., Yokoyama, M. and Takahashi, A., 1978. Melting temperatures of thermally reversible gels. Colloid Polym. Sci., 256: 15–21.
59. Bergman, R. and Sundlöf, L. -O., 1977. Diffusion transport and thermodynamic properties in concentrated water solutions of hydroxypropyl cellulose at temperature up to phase separation. Eur. Polym. J., 13: 881–889.
60. Neely, W. B., 1963. Solution properties of polysaccharides. IV. Molecular weight and aggregate formation in methylcellulose solutions, J. Polym. Sci, A 1: 311–320.
61. Marriott, P. H. and John, E. G., 1973. Influence of electrolytes on the hydration of methylcellulose in solution. J. Pharm. Pharmacol., 25: 633–639.
62. Mitchell, K., Ford, J. L., Armstrong, D. J., Elliott, P. N. C., Hogan, E. and Rostron, C., 1993. The influence of drugs on the properties of gels and swelling characteristics of matrices containing methylcellulose or hydroxypropylmethylcellulose. Int. J. Pharm., 100: 165–173.
63. Touitou, E. and Donbrow, M., 1982. Drug release from non-disintegrating hydrophilic matrices: sodium salicylate as a model drug. Int. J. Pharm., 11: 355–364.

64. Mitchell, K., Ford, J. L., Armstrong, D. J., Elliott, P. N. C., Rostron, C. and Hogan J. E., 1990. The influence of additives on the cloud point, disintegration and dissolution of hydroxypropylmethylcellulose gels and matrix tablets. Int. J. Pharm., 66: 233–242.
65. Brown, W. and Henley, D., 1964. Studies on cellulose derivatives. Part III. Unperturbed dimensions of hydroxyethylcellulose and other derivatives in aqueous solvents. Macromol. Chem., 75: 179–188.
66. Ford, J. L., Mitchell, K., Rowe, P., Armstrong, D. J., Elliott, P. N. C., Rostron, C. and Hogan, J. E., 1991. Mathematical modelling of drug release from hydroxypropylmethylcellulose matrices: effect of temperature. Int. J. Pharm., 71: 95–104.
67. Peppas, N. A., 1985. Analysis of Fickian and non-Fickian drug release from polymer. Pharm. Acta Helv., 60: 110–111.
68. Ritger, P. L. and Peppas, N. A., A simple equation for description of solute release. I. Fickian and non-Fickian release from non-swellable devices in the form of slabs, spheres, cylinders or discs. J. Controlled Rel., 5: 23–36.
69. Ritger, P. L. and Peppas, N. A., 1987. A simple equation for description of solute release. II. Fickian and anomalous release from swellable devices. 5: 37–42.
70. Peppas, N. A. and Sahlin, J. J., 1989. A simple equation for the description of solute release. III. Coupling of diffusion and relaxation. Int. J. Pharm., 57: 169–172.
71. Ford, J. L., Rubinstein, M. H., McCaul, F., Hogan, J. E. and Edgar, J. E., 1987. Importances of drug type, tablet shape and added diluents on drug release kinetics from hydroxypropylmethylcellulose matrix tablets. Int. J. Pharm., 40: 223–234.
72. Catellani, P., Vaona, G., Plazzi, P. and Colombo, P., 1988. Compressed matrices: formulation and drug release kinetics. Acta Pharm. Technol., 34: 38–41.
73. Hogan, J. E., 1989. Hydroxypropylmethylcellulose sustained release technology. Drug Dev. Ind. Pharm., 15: 975–999.
74. Ranga Rao, K. V., Padmalatha Devi, K. and Buri, P., 1990. Influence of molecular size and water solubility of the solute on its release from swelling and erosion controlled polymeric matrices. J. Controlled Rel., 12: 133–141.
75. Colombo, P., Conte, U., Gazzaniga, A., Maggi, L., Sangalli, M. E., Peppas, N. A. and La Manna, A., 1990. Drug release modulation by physical restrictions of matrix swelling. Int. J. Pharm., 63: 43–48.
76. Colombo, P., Catellani, P. L., Peppas, N. A., Maggi, L. and Conte, U., 1992. Swelling characteristics of hydrophilic matrices for controlled release. New dimensionless number to describe the swelling and release behavior. Int. J. Pharm., 88: 99–109.
77. Bettini, R., Colombo, P., Massimo, G., Catellani, P. L. and Vitali, T., 1994. Swelling and drug release in hydrogel matrices: polymer viscosity and matrix porosity effects. Eur. J. Pharm. Sci., 2: 213–219.
78. Peppas, N. A. and Colombo, P., 1997. Analysis of drug release behavior from swellable polymer carriers using the dimensionality index. J. Controlled Rel., 45: 35–40.
79. Ranga Rao, K. V., Padmalatha Devi, K. and Buri, P., 1988. Cellulose matrices for zero-order release of soluble drugs. Drug Dev. Ind. Pharm., 14: 2299–2320.
80. Pham, A. T. and Lee P. I., 1994. Probing the mechanisms of drug release from hydroxypropylmethyl cellulose matrices. Pharm. Res., 11: 1379–1384.
81. Salomon, J. -L., Doelker, E. and Buri, P., 1979. Importance de la technologie et de la formulation pour le mécanisme de libération du chlorure de potassium contenu dans des matrices hydrophiles. 1. Influence de la viscosité et du pourcentage de gélifiant. Pharm. Acta Helv., 54: 82–89.
82. Ford, J. L., Rubinstein, M. H. and Hogan, J. E., 1985. Formulation of sustained release promethazine hydrochloride tablets using hydroxypropylmethylcellulose matrices. Int. J. Pharm., 24: 327–338.
83. Ford, J. L., Rubinstein, M. H. and Hogan J. E., 1985. Propranolol hydrochloride and aminophylline release from matrix tablets containing hydroxypropylmethylcellulose. Int. J. Pharm., 24: 339–350.
84. Lee P. I. L., 1987. Interpretation of drug-release kinetics from hydrogel matrices in terms of time-dependent diffusion coefficients. In: P. I. L. Lee and W. R. Good (Eds.), Controlled-Release Technology: Pharmaceutical Applications, ACS Symposium Series, Vol. 348, American Chemical Society, Washington, DC, pp. 71–83.

85. Rajabi-Siahboomi, A. R., Bowtell, R. W., Mansfield, P., Davies, M. C. and Melia, C. D., 1996. Structure and behavior in hydrophilic matrix sustained release dosage forms: 4. Studies of water mobility and diffusion coefficients in the gel layer of HPMC tablets using NMR imaging. Pharm. Res., 13: 376–380.
86. Gao, P. and Fagerness, P. E., 1995. Diffusion in HPMC gels. I. Determination of drug and water diffusivity by pulsed-field-gradient spin-echo NMR. Pharm. Res., 12: 955–964.
87. Joshi, H. N. and Wilson, T. D., 1993. Calorimetric studies of dissolution of hydroxypropyl methylcellulose E5 (HPMC E5) in water. J. Pharm. Sci, 82: 1033–1038
88. McCrystal, C. B., Ford, J. L. and Rajabi-Siahboomi, A. R., 1997. A study on the interaction of water and cellulose ethers using differential scanning calorimetry. Thermochim. Acta, 294: 91–98.
89. Nokhodchi, A., Ford, J. L. and Rubinstein, M. H., 1997. Studies on the interaction between water and (hydroxypropyl)methylcellulose. J. Pharm. Sci., 86: 608–615.
90. Guido, S., 1995. Phase behavior of aqueous solutions of hydroxypropylcellulose. Macromolecules, 28: 4530–4539.

2
Poly(Vinyl Alcohol) as a Drug Delivery Carrier

Surya K. Mallapragada and Shannon McCarthy-Schroeder
Iowa State University, Ames, Iowa

I. INTRODUCTION

Hermann and Haehnel first synthesized poly(vinyl alcohol) (PVA) in 1924 (1). Today it has become one of the most important polymers in industry and is used in a variety of applications, including textile fibers, paper-coating agents, emulsion stabilizers, and biomedical applications (2). PVA is synthesized by polymerizing not a vinyl alcohol monomer but a vinyl acetate monomer. This monomer is polymerized into poly(vinyl acetate) and then hydrolyzed (3) to produce PVA:

$$\sim[CH_2\text{-}CH(OH)]_n\sim$$

PVA is therefore a copolymer of vinyl acetate and vinyl alcohol, and the degree of hydrolysis indicates the percentage of vinyl alcohol in the copolymer. The first method used to produce PVA was a base-promoted hydrolysis called alkaline saponification (1). This method of producing PVA could not be used for large-scale production. So today many continuous polymerizations are carried out in ester interchange systems (1). PVA is commercially available with a variety of degrees of hydrolysis and crystallinity. This chapter will focus on the characteristics of PVA systems that have been used as drug delivery devices. Both experimental and mathematical modeling approaches will be presented to describe drug release kinetics from PVA systems.

II. BIOCOMPATIBILITY ISSUES IN PVA-BASED SYSTEMS

Poly(vinyl alcohol) is a hydrophilic, semicrystalline polymer. The polymer's biocompatibility makes it an excellent material for use in medical applications. PVA systems have been explored for use in biomedical applications such as drug delivery devices (4,5), contact lenses (6), and artificial organs (7). Formalin-treated PVA (Ivalon®) has been used in prosthetics and as hemodialyzer membranes (5). Numerous studies have been conducted to evaluate polymer biocompatibility. PVA hydrogels were implanted into vitreous bodies of rabbits (8). No abnormalities were found in the cornea or lens, which indicates good biocompatibility for clinical usage of the PVA hydrogel. PVA hydrogels prepared by using a freeze-thaw technique were implanted intramuscularly and subcutaneously in the backs of rabbits for 1 month (5). The gel blocks were covered with several layers of connective tissue. No adhesion to the surrounding tissue was observed.

Artificial articular cartilage implants made of crystalline PVA showed very slight inflammatory reactions of all tissues in response to the implant (7). Platelet adhesion measurement studies were conducted with heat-treated PVA surfaces and the platelets were found to be largely nonadherent to the hydrogels. However, the platelets became more adherent to the hydrogels as their water content was lowered by annealing. PVA hydrogels annealed in the presence of glycerol showed reduced protein adsorption in vitro and reduced platelet adhesion both in vitro and ex vivo compared with that obtained without the addition of glycerol (9).

A number of studies have been conducted to improve the blood compatibility of PVA. The blood compatibility of PVA has been shown to improve by attachment of the natural anticoagulant heparin to the PVA biomaterial surface (10–12). These heparinized surfaces have been shown to exhibit nonthrombogenicity. Platelet adhesion on PVA has also been partially inhibited by incorporating a layer of acetylsalicylic acid on the PVA surface (13). PVA has also been grafted with methyl methacrylate and acrylamide and in vitro blood coagulation tests have shown enhanced antithrombogenicity compared to pure PVA surfaces (14).

III. POLY(VINYL ALCOHOL)-BASED CONTROLLED DRUG DELIVERY DEVICES

Controlled release systems offer a number of advantages over conventional methods (15,16) of drug delivery. A controlled release device maintains the drug concentration within the targeted range for a specific amount of time. The device can be implanted or applied to a specific area of the body to provide localized delivery of the drug and can deliver medication for long time periods. Another advantage of this type of drug delivery system is that it is usually a one-time application or implantation, which reduces the follow-up care required and improves patient compliance.

Poly(vinyl alcohol) has been used in various forms to fabricate controlled drug delivery devices. By changing the degree of hydrolysis, it is possible to control the polymer's dissolution characteristics in water, enabling water-soluble as well as insoluble PVA devices. PVA can also be easily crosslinked to produce insoluble networks or hydrogels that swell in water. The degree of crystallinity also has a significant effect on the diffusion coefficient of drugs through the polymer. The degree of crystallinity of PVA can be easily altered by heat treatment as well as by mechanical techniques. Various delivery routes, such as oral, transdermal, rectal, and nasal, have been explored. The copolymeric nature of PVA provides the polymer with unique gelling characteristics, which in turn are responsible for its adhesive properties. This makes PVA suitable for transdermal or transmucosal delivery applications. The polymer solubility and gelling characteristics can be manipulated to control the rate of diffusion of drugs from PVA devices. Blends of PVA with other polymers can also be used to alter release mechanisms (17).

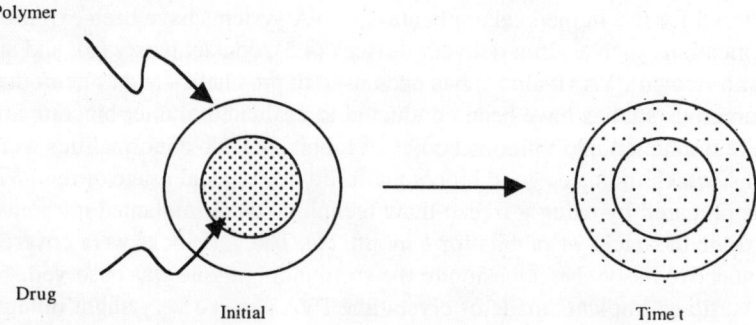

Figure 1 Drug release from a reservoir system. (From Ref. 15.)

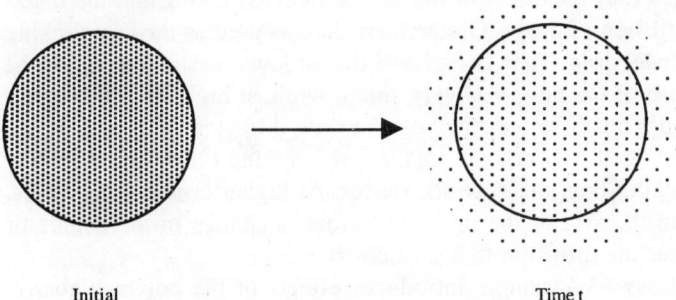

Figure 2 Drug release from a matrix system. (From Ref. 15.)

Poly(vinyl alcohol)-based drug delivery systems can be either reservoir or matrix systems (15). In reservoir systems, a polymer film surrounds a drug core, and the drug diffuses across the film over time as shown in Fig. 1. In matrix systems, the drug is uniformly dissolved or dispersed through the polymer. Figure 2 shows the release of the drug from the matrix. Langer discusses in detail a number of different types of controlled release devices (16) based on the drug release mechanism. The various mechanisms of drug release from the PVA-based systems can be classified as swelling-controlled, polymer dissolution–controlled, crystal dissolution–controlled, and modulated.

A. Swelling-Controlled Release Systems

When PVA is exposed to water, it begins to swell (Fig. 3) and the extent of swelling controls the release of drug from such systems. Swelling-controlled systems can be either matrix or reservoir devices. These systems can be classified according to the fabrication technique.

1. Chemically Crosslinked Devices

This technique produces PVA networks that swell in water but do not dissolve. Various crosslinking agents used include formaldehyde, glutaraldehyde, dicarboxylic acids, and ketones (18). Chemical crosslinking allows good control of the molecular weight between crosslinks by the amount of crosslinking agent added to the solution (19). This makes it possible to control the crosslinked structure and reduce the number of entanglements. Crosslinked PVA membranes have been synthesized and diffusion experiments carried out to measure drug diffusivities and permeabilities to help characterize these systems (13,20).

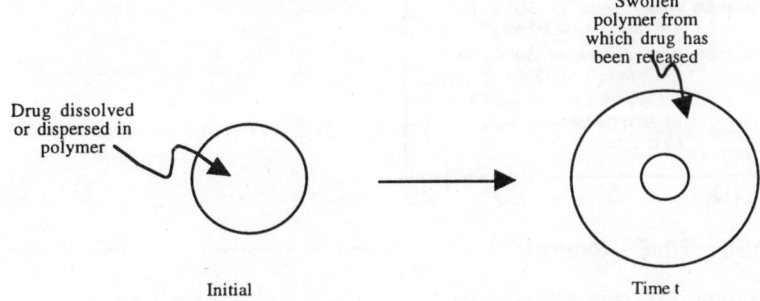

Figure 3 Swelling–controlled drug release mechanism. (From Ref. 15.)

Researchers have investigated (21) the effect of the degree of crosslinking and the relaxation properties of PVA on the diffusion of drugs. Glutaraldehyde was used as the crosslinking agent and theophylline was the model drug. They discovered that at low crosslinking ratios the effect of crosslinking on the release of the drug was very small, while at high crosslinking ratios the degree of crosslinking had a much larger effect on the drug diffusion. This was attributed to the mesh size of the crosslinked network. At smaller crosslinking ratios, the diffusing drug particles are significantly smaller than the network spaces. At higher crosslinking ratios, the network mesh size is closer to the size of the drug. Therefore, a change in the degree of crosslinking in this range influences the diffusion to a greater extent.

Release of drugs from a glassy PVA sample introduces effects of the polymer glassy-rubbery transition into the release kinetics considerations. Korsmeyer and Peppas (21) studied theophylline release from polymeric matrices that were predried at various temperatures and times. The glass-to-rubber relaxations were found to shift the mechanism of release from Fickian to anomalous diffusion (Fig. 4). The effect of drying became larger as the degree of crosslinking increased, and the fraction of the drug released decreased substantially. Gander and co-workers (22) obtained similar results. Both the crosslink density and the particle size greatly influenced the delivery rate of proxyphylline. They studied micromatrices, which released the drug in less than 20 min, and monolithic slabs which released only 40–60% of proxyphylline after 8 h. In the monoliths, release of the drug was found to be controlled by the transition of the polymer from the glassy to the rubbery state.

Crosslinked PVA devices fabricated in the form of microspheres have been extensively investigated. Glutaraldehyde was used as the crosslinking agent for PVA microspheres and the ef-

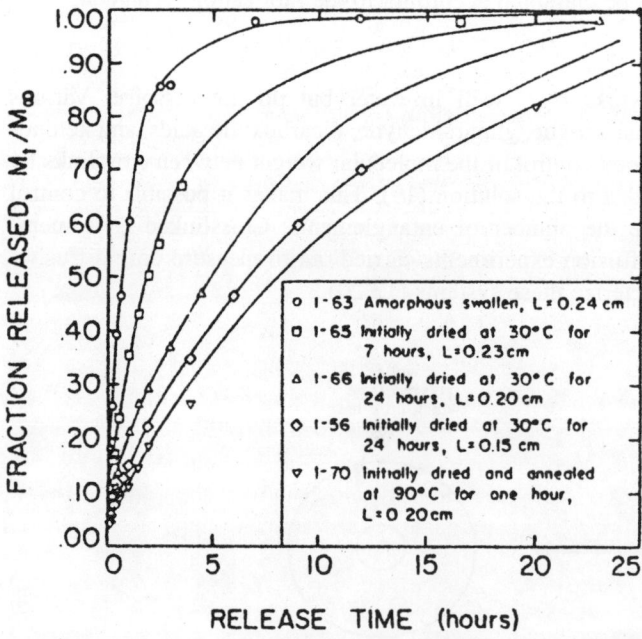

Figure 4 Fractional release of theophylline from amorphous swollen and originally dried gels with crosslinking ratio X = 0.10 at 37°C. (From Ref. 17.)

fect of a number of different variables on the release rate of protease enzymes from these devices was studied (19,23,24). The crosslink density was found to predominantly control the release rate, but other characteristics, such as ionic strength, pH, and particle size, were also found to affect the release rate to some degree. As the ionic strength was increased, the rate of release decreased due to the decrease in swelling of the hydrogel particle. Also, the release rate increased as the size of the particle decreased and increased with increasing pH and degree of hydrolysis of PVA.

Swellable micromatrices were formed by compression followed by external crosslinking by soaking in formaldehyde (25). The release of diprophylline from these crosslinked minimatrix tablets was investigated. Crosslinked PVA microspheres have also been fabricated to release gentamicin (26). Composite PVA beads were fabricated for drug delivery by stepwise saponification of poly(vinyl acetate) suspension polymerization beads and subsequent stepwise crosslinking of PVA core and shell with glutaraldehyde (27). This yielded PVA microspheres with highly crosslinked outer shells and lightly crosslinked inner shells. The outer membrane was found to be the rate-controlling layer for acetaminophen and proxyphylline release from these devices.

Blending PVA with other materials can significantly affect the release characteristics of the device. Glutaraldehyde was used as the chemical crosslinking agent for a PVA film for comparison with a combination of PVA and β-cyclodextrin (β-CD) (28). In the PVA hydrogel, the degree of crosslinking seemed to be the primary controlling factor. When β-CD was added, the crosslink density increased slightly while the drug release from the gel substantially decreased. This is believed to be mostly due to the well-known ability of β-CD to form inclusion complexes. Analysis of the release data showed that the release of theophylline predominantly followed a Fickian mechanism and that the diffusion coefficient decreased as the crosslinking ratio increased.

2. Crosslinking by Irradiation

Most of the chemical crosslinking agents are toxic, and the unreacted crosslinking agent has to be completely removed from the device before the polymer can be implanted. Various methods of physically crosslinking PVA without the use of chemicals have been studied, including the use of irradiation to produce PVA networks.

Poly(vinyl alcohol) can be physically crosslinked by exposure to UV radiation or thermal energy. Colombo and co-workers (25) showed that these methods of preparation produced swellable minimatrices demonstrating non-Fickian anomalous release. This suggests that effective diffusivity of the drug is affected by the swelling of the polymer. They also discovered that the polymer crosslinked by UV radiation showed higher drug release rates than those exposed to thermal energy.

The major problem associated with these polymers crosslinked by irradiation is their weak mechanical properties. Peppas and Merrill (29,30) investigated aqueous solutions of PVA crosslinked via electron beam and γ irradiation, and found that annealing the irradiated hydrogels produces crystallites, which strengthens the material. The annealing time and temperature along with the initial concentration of PVA were found to directly affect the degree of crystallinity. These studies showed that improved mechanical properties such as tensile strength and tear resistance could be obtained.

3. Crosslinking Using a Freeze-Thaw Technique

When PVA is exposed to a number of freeze–thaw cycles, it takes on the physical characteristics of crosslinked PVA (31). The freezing and thawing procedure produces crystals that act as physical crosslinks. This is a totally benign method of fabricating these gels, which is a significant advantage over chemically crosslinked systems. PVA prepared in this manner does not, however, possess the long-term stability that chemically crosslinked gels have.

The properties of PVA hydrogels are largely dependent on the molecular weight, concentration of the solution, time and temperature of freezing, and number of freeze–thaw cycles (32). As the molecular weight and the number of freeze–thaw cycles increases, the gel structure becomes denser (33). In his early work, Peppas (32) found that the number of crystallites increased with an increase of the concentration of PVA in the solution. It was also discovered that an increase in the freezing time caused an increase in the crystallinity of the system.

Syndiotactic and atactic samples were compared. For every cycle the syndiotactic-rich PVA gels were found to exhibit better gelation and lower flow points than atactic-rich PVA gels due to differences in stereoregularity (34). Lower PVA concentrations were required to form these gels compared to atactic-rich PVA (35). These syndiotactic-rich PVA gels were formed even at room temperature, even without undergoing any freeze–thaw procedure. Syndiotactic-rich PVA gels were used to release indomethacin. A number of studies have been conducted to investigate the effect of adding various substances to solutions of PVA (prepared by the freeze–thaw method) on the drug release and the properties of the polymer. Drug release rates from these freeze–thaw gels was decreased by adding sodium alginate or Pluronic® L-62 (36). The strength of the gels was also increased using this technique. The in vitro release of bovine serum albumin from PVA microparticles produced by dispersing PVA in an oil phase and physically crosslinking it using a freeze–thaw procedure was investigated (37). The concentration of the PVA and the particle sizes were found to be important factors in controlling the release rate.

Poly(vinyl alcohol) gel spheres containing drugs (cephalexin and insulin) were prepared by emulsion polymerization and crosslinked by a freeze–thaw technique. These spheres were evaluated as oral drug delivery systems and found to prolong the contact time of drugs with the gastrointestinal wall and improve the absorption characteristics by increasing the effective absorption time (38). PVA freeze–thaw microspheres were investigated for oral administration of insulin. Absorption enhancers were used to overcome poor membrane permeabilities. Prolonged residence times in the ileum were observed (39). PVA gels were loaded with indomethacin and used as rectal suppositories in dogs and rats (40,41). Drug levels in plasma remained at steady plateau levels for up to 9 h.

Some drugs are difficult to take orally because of enzymatic degradation as the drug passes through the liver (36). Since the skin is a fairly impenetrable barrier, only a few drugs inherently possess the properties that allow transdermal drug delivery. In order for a drug to penetrate the skin at significant rates, it must be a low molecular weight material and be soluble in water and oil (42). PVA freeze–thaw gels were used to deliver ketanserin transdermally for wound healing (43). These gels were also tested for buccal mucoadhesive delivery of ergotamine tartrate (44). The mucoadhesive strength of these gels was tested.

4. Heat-Treated Devices

Heat-treated or annealed PVA films are crystalline and cold water–insoluble (45). These have much better mechanical properties compared to the irradiated or the freeze–thaw gels. In fact, some freeze–thaw gels have been subjected to annealing to improve their mechanical properties (30). PVA films loaded with sulfathiazole were cast and heat-treated (46). Heat treatment temperatures above the glass transition temperatures caused significant changes in the drug release rates while temperatures below the glass transition temperature did not alter drug release rates significantly. These films also showed good tear resistance and have potential as transdermal delivery systems. However, the blood compatibility of these devices is found to decrease due to increase in platelet adhesion as the water content of the polymer decreases (47) as a result of annealing. However, this problem can be overcome by annealing the hydrogels in the presence of glycerol, which was found to lower both protein adsorption and platelet adhesion on these surfaces (9).

B. Polymer Dissolution–Controlled Release Systems

In these systems, unlike the crosslinked PVA systems, the polymer dissolves and is excreted by the body. The polymer dissolution rate controls the drug release rate (Fig. 5). This eliminates the need to remove a polymer implant after the drug is released. PVA distribution in the body was measured after intravenous administration in mice. The half-life of dissolved PVA in the body was found to be much longer than for other water-soluble polymers of similar molecular weights such as poly(ethylene glycol) or dextran (48). PVA was found to be located in most organs but with very small accumulation. Minor insignificant interactions of PVA with cell components such as macrophages and blood cells were observed. The excretion rate of PVA reduced rapidly around 30,000 Da.

The swelling and dissolution rates of PVA-poly(sodium acrylate) composite hydrogels were examined. These systems do not involve use of crosslinking agents; the mechanical strength and structural integrity are maintained by a localized saturated solution of poly(sodium acrylate) (49). Compressed tablets of PVA with another water-soluble polymer such as poly(N-vinylpyrrolidone) or poly(ethylene glycol) were investigated as potential soluble drug delivery devices for release of different agents. The incorporation of different polymers was found to cause changes in the mechanisms of solute release from these polymer systems (17).

The effects of blending PVA and polyglycolic acid-co-lactic acid were investigated and the release of myoglobin and cytochrome from spheres coated with this blend (50) also investigated. Compressed PVA-polycaprolactone mixtures were used as models to evaluate erodible implants for sustained drug delivery (51). They showed that this blend provided a way of controlling water content, thus permeability, of hydrophilic and high molecular weight solutes. The release of theophylline from compressed tablets of PVA and methyl acrylate polymer was investigated (52). An oral dosage form using this was found to provide sustained release in dogs for a period of over 16 h and the release was compared with commercially available Theo-Dur systems for theophylline delivery (Fig. 6). PVA microparticles were produced by spray drying and spray desolvation for drug delivery (53). The particles produced by spray drying yielded hollow spheres with sizes greater than 200 μm which were found unsuitable for nasal delivery. However, the spray desolvation technique produces particles with an average diameter of about 50 μm, which are expected to deposit in the nasal cavity and are ideal for nasal delivery.

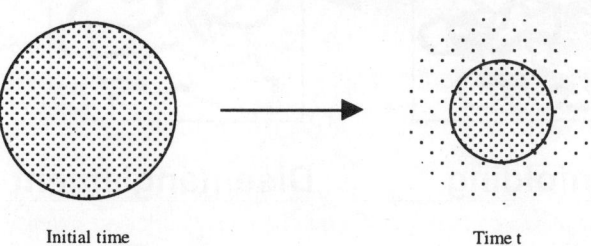

Figure 5 Polymer dissolution–controlled release mechanism.

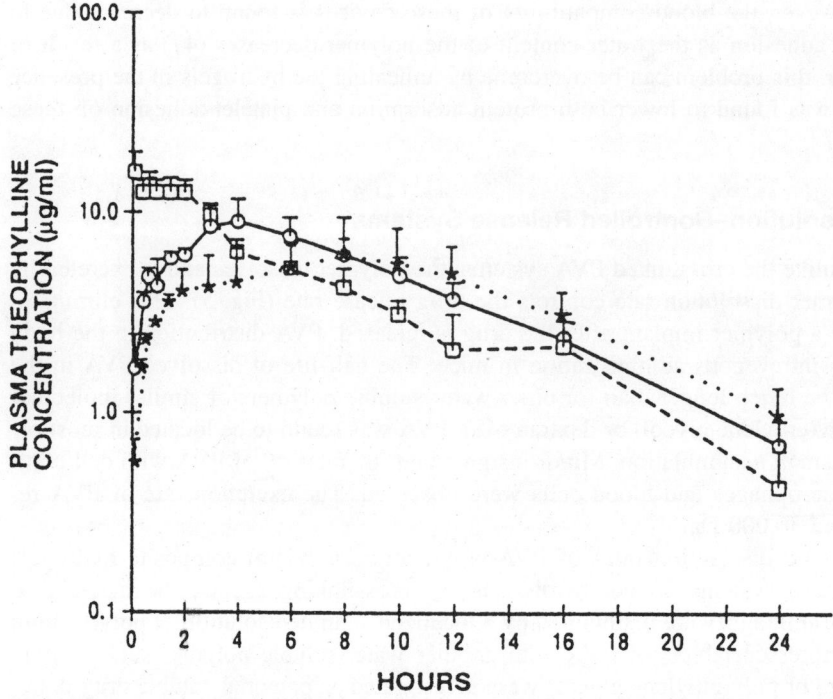

Figure 6 Average plasma theophylline concentrations in three dogs administered 85 mg of theophylline (□) and 100 mg orally as a commercial Theo-Dur tablet (○) and as the PVA blend tablet formulation (*). (From Ref. 52.)

C. Crystal Dissolution–Controlled Release Systems

In crystal dissolution–controlled release systems, the phase erosion process is the rate-controlling step (54,55). Here the release rate is controlled by the change in phase of the polymer from the crystalline to the amorphous phase (Fig. 7). The advantage of these systems is the ease of

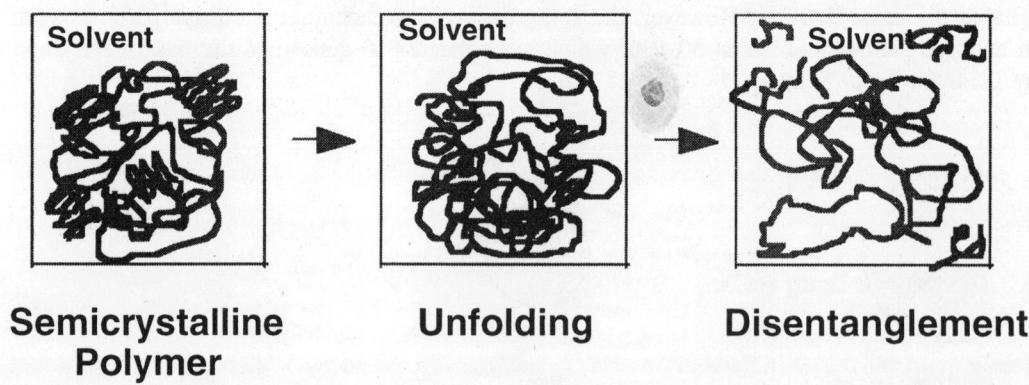

Figure 7 Crystal dissolution–controlled release mechanism. (From Ref. 64.)

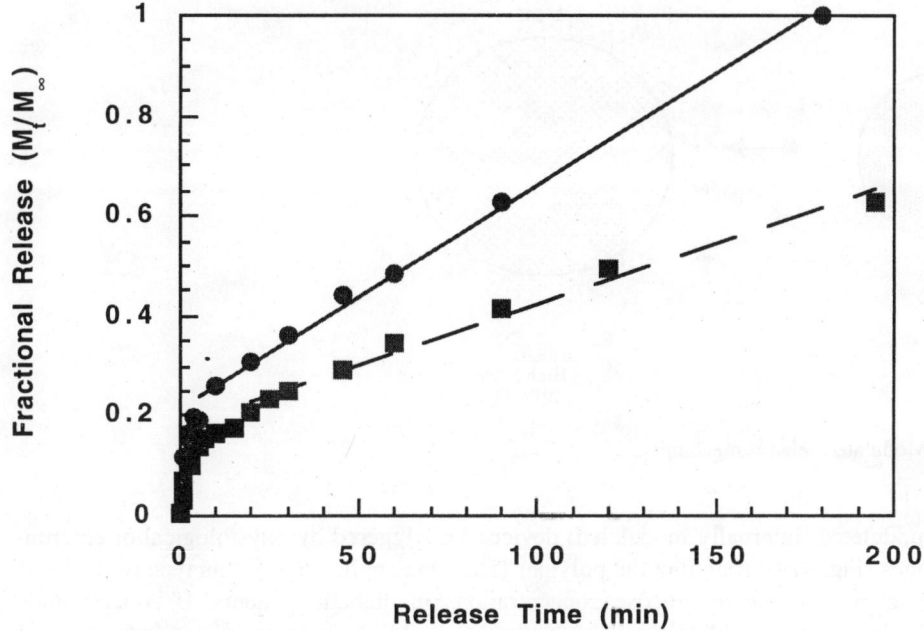

Figure 8 Influence of annealing conditions on metronidazole release at 37°C from PVA controlled release systems (PVA $\overline{M}_n$ = 17,600; metronidazole loading 2 wt %); (●) annealed at 110°C for 20 min (M_t/M_∞ = 0.18 + 0.002 t, r^2 = 0.99124) (■) annealed at 120°C for 1 h (M_t/M_∞ = 0.22 + 0.004 t, r^2 = 0.99663). (From Ref. 54.)

controlling the release rate by annealing temperature and the elimination of toxic crosslinking agents in the device.

As the initial degree of crystallinity increases, the rate of drug released decreases since the crystals are a barrier to diffusion. As the drug is released from these devices, the amount of drug in the device decreases, thereby decreasing the driving force for drug diffusion. However, simultaneously the degree of crystallinity of the polymer decreases due to conversion from crystalline to amorphous phase, leading to an increase in diffusion coefficient of the drug. These two competing effects can be synchronized to obtain a zero-order drug release rate using these systems. Zero-order release of metronidazole (Fig. 8) was achieved from crystal dissolution–controlled PVA systems (54).

Multilayered devices of this type have also been studied for the delivery of multiple drugs or for higher release rates of a single drug. Systems such as these can simplify and facilitate treatment, as well as maintain more consistent levels of medication. Mallapragada and Chin (55) found that annealing the various layers at different times and temperatures can control the release rates of multiple drugs. They also demonstrated that the multilayering technique could increase the amount of drug delivered without significantly affecting the degree of crystallinity of the polymer.

D. Modulated Drug Release Systems

Externally modulated devices are activated by an external stimulus such as application of an electric field (56). PVA-poly(sodium acrylate) composite freeze–thaw gels in electrolyte solutions have been shown to bend and deform in an sinusoidal electric field due to changes in osmotic pressure based on differences in ion concentrations (57).

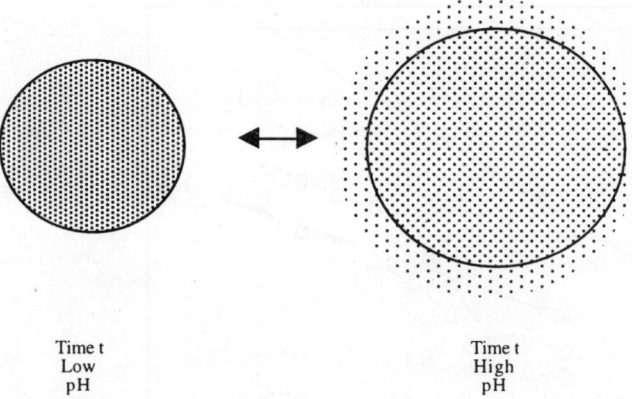

Figure 9 Modulated release mechanism.

Self-modulated (internally modulated) devices are triggered by physiological or environmental changes (Fig. 9) surrounding the polymer (56). One application of this type of device is insulin release in response to glucose concentrations in diabetic patients. PVA-acrylamide blends containing glucose oxidase were synthesized to yield glucose-sensitive membranes that increase their permeability when glucose levels increase (18). The controlled release of riboflavin and insulin through a blend of crosslinked PVA and chitosan has been studied (58). Glucose oxidase was used to impart glucose sensitivity to the membrane for insulin delivery. The amount of riboflavin released over 12 h showed a linear release while the pH changes significantly affected the permeability of the insulin through the polymer blend. An intelligent PVA/poly(N-vinyl pyrrolidone-co-phenylboronic acid) systems was developed for delivering insulin in response to glucose changes in the body (59). PVA was chosen because it can form reversible complexes with borate compounds and the system acts as a sensor molecule for glucose. The viscosity of the gel was found to change steeply in the presence of glucose, thereby enabling a stimuli-responsive polymer.

Studies have shown that hydrogels composed of PVA and poly(acrylic acid) crosslinked by UV radiation (60) followed by a number of freeze–thaw cycles can produce pH/temperature-sensitive drug delivery systems. Indomethacin release from these devices was found to be controlled by changes in pH and temperature. At higher temperatures, the rate of release increased due to the hydrogen bonding between the PVA and poly(acrylic acid). Increases in the pH level also led to higher release rates (Fig. 10).

IV. MATHEMATICAL MODELING

A number of theoretical and empirical relations have been proposed to try to explain the release behavior from PVA drug delivery devices. The following empirical equation was proposed by Ritger and Peppas (61) to describe the fractional drug released from a PVA device that exhibits moderate degrees of swelling:

$$M_t/M_\infty = kt^n \tag{1}$$

where M_t/M_∞ is the drug fraction released, t is time, and k and n are constants for the specific system. Different exponent values indicate whether the diffusion is Fickian, non-Fickian, or, more specifically, zero-order release. They extended this approach to systems that swell to a

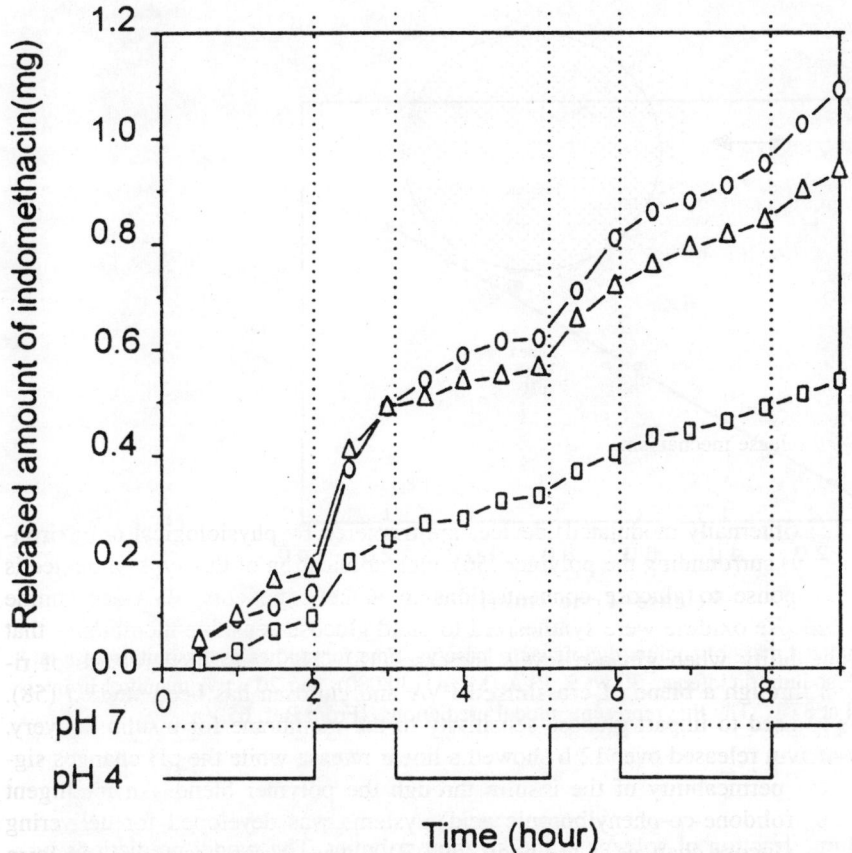

Figure 10 Release change of indomethacin from IPN hydrogels in response to stepwise pH change between pH 4 and 7: (○) IPN46; (△) IPN55; (□) IPN 64. (From Ref. 60.)

large extent in water by using a moving boundary approach for various geometries including plane sheets, cylinders, and spheres. They showed that the diffusional exponent of Eq. 1 is an indication of the mechanism of drug release and takes on various values depending on the geometry of the release device.

A more detailed theoretical model was developed for describing spherical solute diffusion through highly swollen crosslinked polymeric networks. This model predicts that the solute diffusion coefficient is a function of solute size and the network structure. Experimental results with polymeric networks were shown to support this theoretical model (62). This theory was modified to account accurately for the dependence of the diffusion coefficient on the molecular weight between crosslinks. It was shown that the mesh size is an indicator for separations using nonporous membranes where a high degree of swelling is not sufficient for the transport of large macromolecules (63).

Crystal dissolution–controlled release systems were modeled by combining diffusion and crystallization/decrystallization theories (64). The diffusion coefficient of the drug through such systems was assumed to be dependent on the degree of crystallinity of the polymer, the tortu-

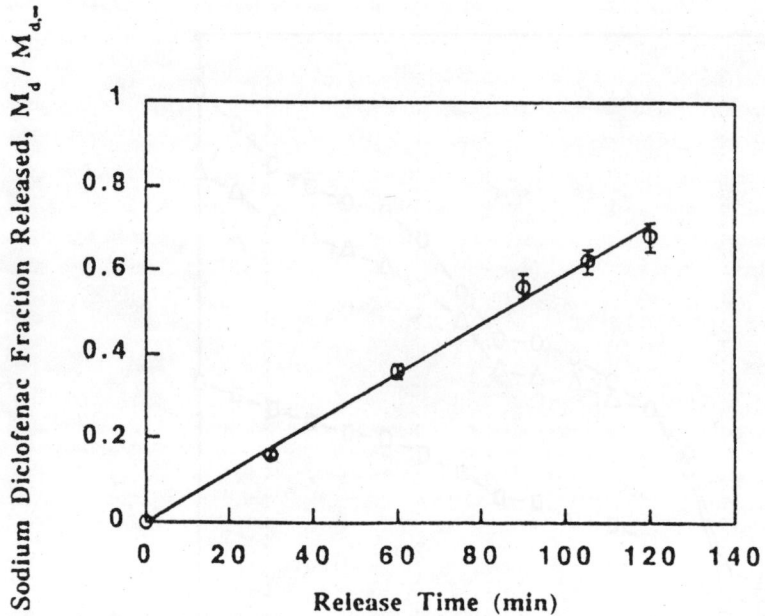

Figure 11 Normalized mass of sodium diclofenac release vs. time for studies of dissolution of a tablet containing 50 wt % sodium diclofenac, 30 wt % PVA (M_n = 130,000), and 20 wt % mannitol in intestinal simulating fluid at 37°C. The line represents model predictions. (From Ref. 65.)

osity, and the volume fraction of solvent in the swollen polymer. The model predictions were found to agree reasonably well with experimental results for release of metronidazole from crystal dissolution–controlled PVA systems.

Dissolution-controlled PVA systems were modeled using a combination of diffusion and reptation theories that account for disentanglement of the polymer chains (65). The results from the model indicate that polymer molecular weight, diffusion coefficients of the drug and water, as well as the water–polymer interaction parameter control the rate of drug release. Based on these, conditions for obtaining zero-order release were established and were found to agree well with experimental results (Fig. 11).

V. CONCLUSIONS

Poly(vinyl alcohol) is a useful material for medical applications due to its biocompatibility and hydrophilic nature. PVA biocompatibility can also be enhanced by immobilizing heparin and other compounds onto PVA surfaces. PVA drug delivery devices can be classified as swelling-controlled, polymer dissolution–controlled, crystal dissolution–controlled, or modulated based on the mechanism of release.

Swelling-controlled devices do not dissolve and can be further classified according to the fabrication process into chemically crosslinked, physically crosslinked, and heat-treated devices. One advantage of the chemically crosslinked form of PVA is that there are a number of ways to control the degree of crosslinking which in turn controls the release rate of the drug. This type of preparation may, however, leave toxic residues that can be harmful and must be removed. Physically crosslinked PVA has the characteristics of chemically crosslinked PVA but does not contain any harmful crosslinking agents. The disadvantage of this form of PVA is that it does not have the long-term stability that chemically crosslinked PVA possesses.

Polymer dissolution–controlled systems cannot use very high PVA molecular weights since the polymer needs to be readily excreted by the body. However, these systems eliminate the need to remove implants from the body after the drug is released. Crystal dissolution–controlled devices do not require the use of any toxic crosslinking agents and the release rate can be controlled by the annealing conditions. The additional advantage of these systems is the ability to obtain zero-order drug release. These devices might not be suitable in cases where the drugs are sensitive to heat treatment. Blending other polymers with PVA can provide some interesting delivery properties and lead to environmentally sensitive drug delivery systems. Mathematical models have been developed to predict drug release from various kinds of PVA systems exhibiting different release mechanisms. These studies demonstrate that PVA has enormous potential for drug delivery applications.

REFERENCES

1. Winkler, H., 1973. Historical development of polyvinyl alcohol. In: Finch, C. A. (Ed.), Polyvinyl Alcohol, Wiley, London, pp. 1–13.
2. Finch, C. A., 1973. Polyvinyl Alcohol, Wiley, London, pp. 622.
3. Noro, K., 1973. Manufacture of polyvinyl acetate for polyvinyl alcohol. In: Finch, C. A. (Ed.), Polyvinyl Alcohol, Wiley, London, pp. 67–71.
4. Aleyamma, A. J. and Sharma, C. P., 1991. Poly(vinyl alcohol) as a biomaterial. In: Sharma, C. P, and Szycher (Ed.), Blood Compatible Materials and Devices. Technomic, Lancaster, PA, pp. 123–130.
5. Tamura, K., Ike, O., Hitomi, S., Isobe, J., Shimizu, Y. and Nambu, M., 1986. A new hydrogel and its medical application. Trans. Am. Soc. Artif. Organs, 32: 605–608.
6. Hyon, S.-H., Cha, W.-I., Ikada, Y., Kita, M., Ogura, Y. and Honda, Y., 1994. Poly(vinyl alcohol) as a soft contact lens material. J. Biomater. Sci. Polym. Ed., 5: 397–406.
7. Noguchi, T., Yamamuro, T., Oka, M., Kumar, P., Kotoura, Y., Hyon, S.-H. and Ikada, Y., 1991. Poly(vinyl alcohol) hydrogel as an artificial articular cartilage: evaluation of biocompatibility. J. Appl. Biomater., 2: 101–107.
8. Kodama, M., Wang, B., Mu, G., Yamaguchi, A., Matsura, T., Hara, Y. and Saishin, M., 1996. PVA hydrogel as an artificial vitreous body. In: Ogata, N., Kim, S. W., Feijen, J. and Okano, T. (Eds.), Advanced Biomaterials in Biomedical Engineering and Drug Delivery Systems, Springer-Verlag, Tokyo, pp. 255–256.
9. Fujimoto, K., Minato, M. and Ikada, Y., 1984. Poly(vinyl alcohol) hydrogels prepared under different annealing conditions and their interactions with blood components. In: Shalaby, S. W., Ikada, Y., Langer, R., and Williams, J. (Eds.), Polymers of Biological and Biomedical Significance. ACS Symposium Series, Vol. 540. American Chemical Society. Washington, D.C., pp. 229–241.
10. Peppas, N. A. and Gehr, T. W. B., 1978. New hydrophilic copolymers for biomedical applications. Trans. Am. Soc. Artif. Intern. Organs., 24: 404–410.
11. Peppas, N. A. and Merrill, E. W., 1977. Development of semicrystalline PVA hydrogels for biomedical applications. J. Biomed. Mater. Res., 11: 423–430.
12. Sefton, M. V., 1988. Blood, guts and chemical engineering. Can. J. Chem. Eng., 67: 706–712.
13. Paul, W. and Sharma, C. P., 1997. Acetylsalicylic acid loaded poly(vinyl alcohol) hemodialysis membranes: effect of drug release on blood compatibility and permeability. J. Biomater. Sci. Polym. Ed., 8: 755–764.
14. Mathew, J. and Kodama, M., 1992. Study of blood compatible polymers I. modification of poly(vinyl alcohol). Polym. J., 24: 31–41.

15. Langer, R., 1990. New methods of drug delivery. Science, 249: 1527–1533.
16. Langer, R., 1993. Polymer-controlled drug delivery systems. Acc. Chem. Res., 26: 537–542.
17. Korsmeyer, R. W., Gurny, R., Doelker, E., Buri, P. and Peppas, N. A., 1983. Mechanisms of solute release from porous hydrophilic polymers. Int. J. Pharm., 15: 25–35.
18. Chandy, T. and Sharma, C. P., 1992. Glucose-responsive insulin release from poly(vinyl alcohol)-blended polyacrylamide membranes containing glucose oxidase. J. Appl. Polym. Sci., 46: 1159–1167.
19. Bachtsi, A. R. and Kiparissides, C., 1995. An experimental investigation of enzyme release from poly(vinyl alcohol) crosslinked microspheres. J. Microencap., 12: 23–25.
20. Uragami, T., Furukawa, T. and Sugihara, M., 1984. Studies on syntheses and permeabilities of special polymer membranes: 57. Permeability of solute through polymer membranes and state of water in their membranes. Polym. Comm., 25: 30–33.
21. Korsmeyer, R. W. and Peppas, N. A., 1981. Effect of the morphology of hydrophilic polymeric matrices on the diffusion and release of water soluble drugs, J. Membr. Sci., 9: 211–227.
22. Gander, B., Beltrami, V., Gurny, R. and Doelker, E., 1990. Effects of the method of drug incorporation and the size of the monolith on drug release from cross-linked polymers. Int. J. Pharm., 58: 63–71.
23. Bachtsi, A. R., Boutris, C. J. and Kiparissides, C., 1996. Production of oil containing cross-linked poly(vinyl alcohol) microcapsules by phase separation—effect of process parameters on the capsule size distribution. J. Appl. Polym. Sci., 60: 9–20.
24. Bachtsi, A. R. and Kiparissides, C., 1996. Synthesis and release studies of oil-containing poly(vinyl alcohol) microcapsules prepared by coacervation. J. Controlled Rel., 38: 49–58.
25. Colombo, P., Conte, U., Caramella, C., Gazzaniga, A. and La Manna, A., 1985. Compressed polymeric mini-matrices for drug release control. J. Controlled Rel., 1: 283–289.
26. Suzuki, S., Charlton, J. F., and Lim, J. K., 1992. Gentamicin microcapsules in polyvinyl alcohol hydrogel for controlled release. Invest. Ophthalmol. Vis. Sci., 33: 1013.
27. Kim, C. J. and Lee, P. I., 1992. Composite poly(vinyl alcohol) beads for controlled drug delivery. Pharm. Res., 9: 10–16.
28. Sreenivasan, K., 1997. On the restriction of the release of water-soluble component from polyvinyl alcohol by blending β-cyclodextrin. J. Appl. Polym. Sci., 65: 1829–1832.
29. Peppas, N. A. and Merrill, E. W., 1977. Crosslinked poly(vinyl alcohol) membranes as swollen elastic networks. J. Appl. Polym. Sci., 21: 1763–1772.
30. Peppas, N. A. and Merrill, E. W., 1976. Poly(vinyl alcohol) hydrogels: reinforcement of radiation-crosslinked networks by crystallization, J. Polym. Sci., 14: 441–457.
31. Nambu, M. 1987. Process for preparing a hydrogel. U.S. Patent 4,664,857.
32. Peppas, N. A., 1975. Turbidimetric studies of aqueous poly(vinyl alcohol) solutions. Makromol. Chem., 176: 3433–3440.
33. Peppas, N. A. and Scott, J. E., 1992. Controlled release from poly(vinyl alcohol) gels prepared by freezing-thawing processes, J. Controlled Rel., 18: 95–100.
34. Yamaura, K., Karasawa, K.-I., Tanigami, T. and Matsuzawa, S., 1994. Gelation of PVA solutions at low temperatures (20 to −78°C) and properties of gels. J. Appl. Polym. Sci., 51: 2041–2046.
35. Horiike, S. and Matsuzawa, S. 1995. Application of syndiotacticity-rich PVA hydrogels to drug delivery systems. J. Appl. Polym. Sci., 58: 1335–1340.
36. Takamura, A., Ishii, F. and Hidaka, H., 1992. Drug release from poly(vinyl alcohol) gel prepared by freeze-thaw procedure. J. Controlled Rel., 20: 21–28.
37. Ficek, B. J. and Peppas, N. A., 1993. Novel preparation of poly(vinyl alcohol) microparticles without crosslinking agent for controlled drug delivery of proteins. J. Controlled Rel., 27: 259–264.
38. Kurosaki, Y., Murakami, T., Nakayama, T. and Kimura, T., 1992. Evaluation of PVA-gel spheres as GI transit time controlling oral drug delivery systems. Proc. Int. Symp. Control. Rel. Bioact. Mater., 19: 273–274.
39. Kimura, T., Sato, K., Sugimoto, K., Tao, R., Murakami, T., Kurosaki, Y. and Nakayama, T., 1996. Oral administration of insulin as poly(vinyl alcohol) gel spheres in diabetic rats. Biol. Pharm. Bull., 19: 897–900.

40. Morimoto, K., Fukanoki, S., Morisaka, K., Hyon, S. H. and Ikada, Y., 1989. Design of polyvinyl alcohol hydrogel as a controlled release vehicle for rectal administration of DL-propranolol-HC1 and atenolol. Chem. Pharm. Bull., 37: 2491–2495.
41. Morimoto, K., Nagayasu, A., Fukanoki, S., Morisaka, K., Hyon, S. H. and Ikada, Y., 1989. Evaluation of polyvinyl alcohol hydrogel as a sustained release vehicle for rectal administration of indomethacin. Pharm. Res., 6: 338–341.
42. Yang, X. and Robinson, J. R., 1988. Bioadhesion in mucosal drug delivery. In: Okano, T. (Ed.), Biorelated Polymers and Gels, Academic Press, Boston, p. 164.
43. Mongia, N. K., Anseth, K. S. and Peppas, N. A., 1996. Mucoadhesive poly(vinyl alcohol) hydrogels produced by freezing/thawing processes—applications in the development of wound healing systems. J. Biomater. Sci., Polym. Ed., 7: 1055–1064.
44. Tsutsumi, K., Takayama, K., Machida, Y., Ebert, C. D., Nakatomi, I. and Nagai, T., 1994. Formulation of buccal mucoadhesive dosage form of ergomine tartrate. S. T. P. Pharm. Sci., 4: 230–234.
45. Lee, P. I., 1993. Poly(vinyl alcohol) membrane systems for the controlled release of chlorinated isocyanurates. J. Appl. Polym. Sci., 50: 941–947.
46. Wan, L. S. C. and Lim, L. Y., 1992. Drug release from heat-treated polyvinyl alcohol films. Drug Dev. Ind. Pharm., 18: 1895–1906.
47. Ko, J. H., Ericson, D., Tucker, J. and Walker, R., 1994. Effect of annealing on the physical properties and blood compatibility of poly(vinyl alcohol) hydrogels. ANTEC, 2651–2655.
48. Yamaoka, T., Tabata, Y. and Ikada, Y., 1995. Comparison of body distribution of poly(vinyl alcohol) with other water soluble polymers after intravenous administration. J. Pharm. Pharmacol., 47: 479–486.
49. Graiver, D., Hyon, S.-H. and Ikada, Y. 1995. Poly(vinyl alcohol)–poly(sodium acrylate) composite hydrogels. 1. Kinetics of swelling and dehydration. J. Appl. Polym. Sci., 57: 1299–1310.
50. Pitt, C. G., Cha, Y., Shah, S. S. and Zhu, K. J., 1992. Blends of PVA and PGLA: control of the permeability of degradability of hydrogels by blending. J. Controlled Rel., 19: 189–200.
51. Wang, P. Y., 1989. Compressed poly(vinyl alcohol)–polycaprolactone admixture as a model to evaluate erodible implants for sustained drug delivery. J. Biomed. Mater. Res., 23: 91–104.
52. DiLuccio, R. C., Hussain, M. A., Coffin-Beach, D., Torosian, G., Shefter, E. and Hurwitz, A. R., 1994. Sustained release oral delivery of theophylline by use of polyvinyl alcohol–methyl acrylate polymers. J. Pharm. Sci., 83: 104–106.
53. Ting, T. Y., Gonda, I., and Gipps, E. M., 1992. Microparticles of polyvinyl alcohol for nasal delivery. 1. Generation by spray drying and spray-desolvation. Pharm. Res., 9: 1330–1335.
54. Mallapragada, S. K., Peppas, N. A. and Colombo, P., 1997. Crystal dissolution–controlled release systems: II. Metronidazole release from semicrystalline poly(vinyl alcohol) systems. J. Biomed. Mater. Res., 36: 125–130.
55. Mallapragada, S. K. and Chin, S., 1998. Multilayered semicrystalline polymeric controlled release systems. ACS Symposium Series (709: 176–184).
56. Heller, J., 1993. Modulated release from drug delivery devices. Crit. Rev. Ther. Drug Deliv. Syst., 10: 253–305.
57. Shiga, T., Hirose, Y., Okada, A. and Kurauchi, T., 1993. Bending of ionic polymer gel caused by swelling under sinusoidally varying electric fields. J. Appl. Polym. Sci., 47: 113–119.
58. Kim, J. H., Kim, J. Y., Lee, Y. M. and Kim K. Y., 1992. Controlled release of riboflavin and insulin through crosslinked poly(vinyl alcohol)/chitosan blend membrane. J. Appl. Polym. Sci., 44: 1823–1828.
59. Kitano, S., Koyama, Y., Kataoka, K., Okano, T. and Sakurai, Y., 1992. A novel drug delivery system utilizing a glucose responsive complex between poly(vinyl alcohol) and poly(n-vinyl-2-pyrrolidone) with a phenylboronic acid moiety. J. Controlled Rel., 19: 162–170.
60. Shin, H. S., Kim, S. Y. and Lee, Y. M., 1997. Indomethacin release behaviors from pH and thermoresponsive poly(vinyl alcohol) and poly(acrylic acid) IPN hydrogels for site-specific drug delivery. J. Appl. Polym. Sci., 65: 685–693.
61. Ritger, P. L. and Peppas, N. A., 1987. A simple equation for description of solute release II. Fickian and anomalous release from swellable devices. J. Controlled Rel., 5: 37–42.

62. Peppas, N. A. and Reinhart, C. T., 1983. Solute diffusion in swollen membranes. Part I. A new theory. J. Membr. Sci., 15: 275–287.
63. Reinhart, C. T. and Peppas, N. A., 1984. Solute diffusion in swollen membranes. Part II. Influence of crosslinking on diffusive properties. J. Membr. Sci., 18: 227–239.
64. Mallapragada, S. K. and Peppas, N. A., 1997. Crystal dissolution-controlled release systems: I. Physical characteristics and modeling analysis, J. Controlled Rel., 45: 87–94.
65. Narasimhan, B. and Peppas, N. A., 1997. Molecular analysis of drug delivery systems controlled by dissolution of the polymer carrier. J. Pharm. Sci., 86: 297–304.

3
Development of Acrylate and Methacrylate Polymer Networks for Controlled Release by Photopolymerization Technology

Robert Scott, Jennifer H. Ward, and Nicholas A. Peppas
Purdue University, West Lafayette, Indiana

I. STRUCTURE AND APPLICATIONS OF HIGHLY CROSSLINKED POLYMULTI(METH)ACRYLATES

Polymulti(meth)acrylates belong to a class of materials known as highly crosslinked polymer networks. These insoluble polymers are formed by free radical polymerization of multi(meth)acrylate monomers. Multi(meth)acrylate monomers have a variety of structures, as indicated in Fig. 1. Di(meth)acrylate monomers are tetrafunctional in that their two double bonds may participate in a total of four radical propagation steps. Similarly, tri(meth)acrylate monomers are hexafunctional.

Poly(meth)acrylates can also be rendered hydrophilic by copolymerization with acrylic acid (AA) or methacrylic acid (MAA). For example, Fig. 2 shows the network structure of a highly crosslinked poly(diacrylate-co-acrylic acid) network. The figure shows that polymultiacrylates are characterized by a polyacrylate backbone (A), built up over the course of the polymerization by radical propagation through monomer double bonds. If all double bonds are assumed to have reacted, each repeating unit along the poly(meth)acrylate backbone is linked by a molecular bridge to at least one other backbone site, depending on the monomer functionality. These molecular bridges represent crosslinks (B). When the conversion of double bonds is incomplete or when cyclization reactions occur, the crosslinking efficiency is less than unity, and a number of repeating units are substituted with pendant double bonds as shown in Fig. 2 or with cycles.

Due to their highly crosslinked nature, polymulti(meth)acrylates are characterized by a high degree of dimensional stability. These polymers are therefore frequently used in applications that demand high-strength materials with time-independent structure and properties. For example, Kloosterboer et al. (1–3) have reported on the use of polymultiacrylates in laser video disks, optical fiber coatings, and aspherical lenses. However, more recently, such materials have been used in optical waveguides, wire coatings, and adhesives (3), and dental materials (4).

Their mechanical stability, versatility of functional groups, wide range of hydrophilicity/hydrophobicity, and ability to crosslink at a wide range of conditions make these materials prime candidates for biomedical (4–6) and pharmaceutical applications (7–11).

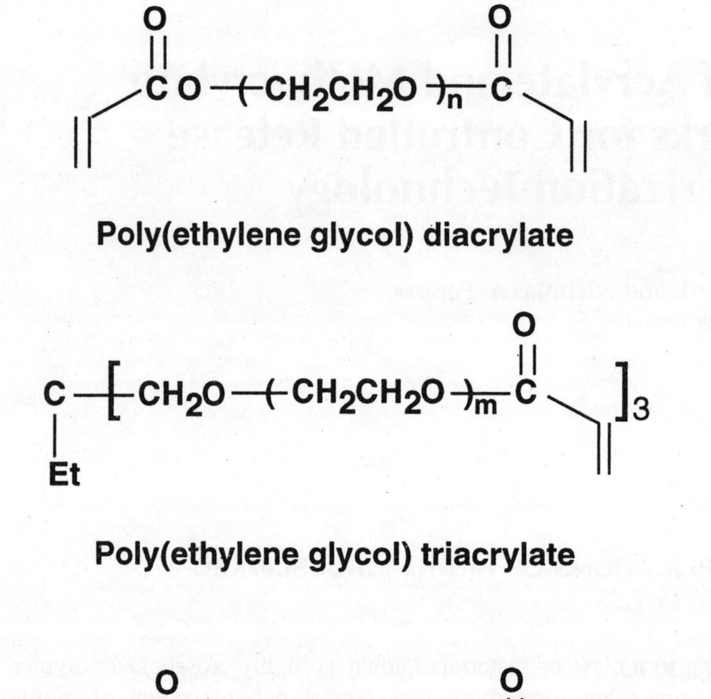

Figure 1 Structures of various multi(meth)acrylate monomers.

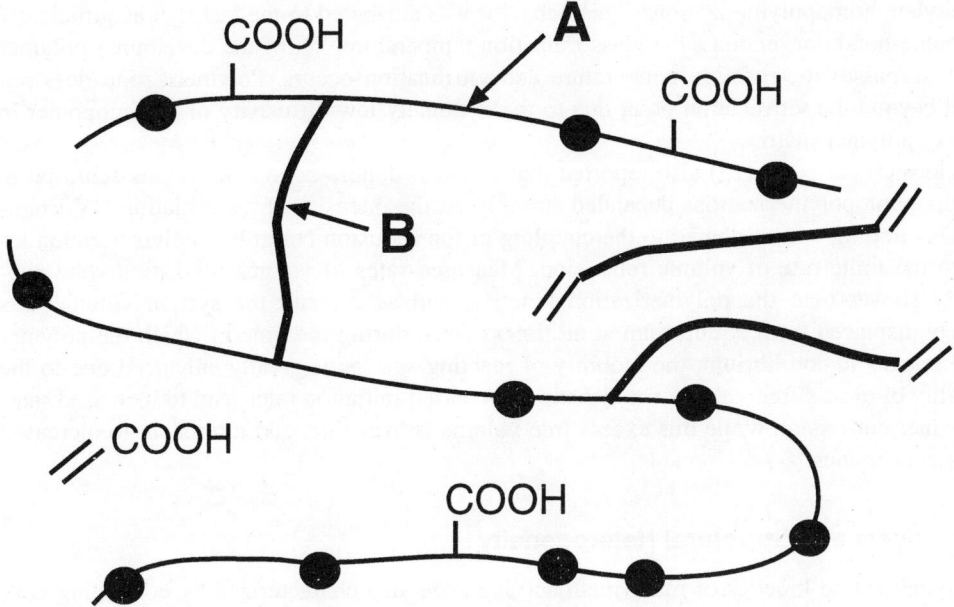

Figure 2 Schematic representation of the network structure in polymulti(meth)acrylates. For clarity, additional sites along the backbone where the diacrylate is incorporated are indicated by ●.

II. PREPARATION OF POLYMULTI(METH)ACRYLATES

Polymulti(meth)acrylates are most often prepared by bulk photopolymerization techniques (2). In such reactions, monomers are mixed in the absence of solvent, a photoinitiator is added, and polymerization is initiated by exposure to UV light. The rapidly changing nature of the reaction medium over the course of the polymerization, as the densely crosslinked network is formed, leads to anomalous polymerization behavior. Among the very important issues that arise during bulk crosslinking polymerizations of multi(meth)acrylates are volume relaxation, incomplete conversion of monomer and/or double bonds, and structural heterogeneity (12–18).

A. Diffusional Effects During Polymerization

The most prominent feature of bulk polymerization reactions involving multifunctional monomers is the strong influence of diffusional effects arising due to the formation of an infinite network. In bulk crosslinking polymerizations, the viscosity of the reaction medium increases greatly over the course of polymerization (and from the beginning of the reaction), creating a significant diffusional resistance to the bimolecular macroradical termination reaction. As a result, the rate coefficient, k_t, which describes the kinetics of the termination reaction, decreases over time. The polymerization rate, which scales as $k_t^{-1/2}$, increases even as reactive double bonds are consumed. This autoacceleration of the polymerization rate due to diffusional effects is known as the Trommsdorff or gel effect (19).

Much of the pioneering work in characterizing diffusional effects on the polymerization kinetics of multi(meth)acrylates was carried out by Kloosterboer and collaborators (13–18). For example, Kloosterboer et al. (13,14) reported final double-bond conversions lower than 100%

for diacrylate homopolymerizations. This behavior was attributed to the fact that at sufficiently high double-bond conversions, the glass transition temperature, T_g, of the developing polymer network surpasses the reaction temperature and vitrification occurs. Polymerization does not proceed beyond the vitrification point due to the extremely low diffusivity of free monomer in the glassy polymer matrix.

Kloosterboer et al. (13) also reported that the final double-bond conversions achieved in diacrylate photopolymerizations depended strongly on the intensity of the initiating UV irradiation. This finding was attributed to the coupling of the diffusion-controlled polymerization kinetics to the finite rate of volume relaxation. Measured rates of volume relaxation were substantially slower than the polymerization kinetics, and as a result the system volume was positively displaced from equilibrium at all times. Thus, during the time in which the polymer volume relaxes to equilibrium, the mobility of reacting species is greatly enhanced due to the availability of excess free volume for diffusion. Increased initiation rates lead to increased rates of monomer conversion while this excess free volume is available, and ultimately to increased limiting conversions.

B. Microgels and Structural Heterogeneity

The polymerization kinetics of multi(meth)acrylates are also characterized by competing contributions to the overall reactivity from free and pendant double bonds. Free double bonds are those attached to unreacted monomer. Pendant double bonds are those attached to the polymer network, formed when a free double bond reacts. For example, during polymerization of a triacrylate, reaction of a free double bond leads to the formation of two pendant double bonds.

The unequal reactivities of free and pendant double bonds may have significant effects on the polymerization kinetics and the polymer network structure. Horie et al. (12) observed rate behavior suggestive of the formation of densely crosslinked microgels during the copolymerization of methyl methacrylate with ethylene dimethacrylate. Subsequently, Kloosterboer et al. (14–16) cited the presence of trapped radicals during di(meth)acrylate homopolymerizations as evidence of microgel formation and structural heterogeneity. The researchers used percolation models to demonstrate that microgel formation is promoted early in the polymerization by the enhanced reactivity of pendant double bonds. Thus, at low conversions the polymerization process is characterized by a preponderance of primary and secondary cyclization reactions that lead to a heterogeneous network structure. Later in the polymerization, the relative reactivities of free and pendant double bonds are reversed.

Kloosterboer et al. (15,16) also showed that the glass transition temperature, T_g, increased greatly with the application of a thermal postcuring process. This behavior indicated the presence of trapped radicals. Calorimetric studies of the aftercure process showed that additional polymerization was due to free monomer and to pendant double bonds. The researchers also observed that T_g depended on the total dose of initiating radiation, regardless of the light intensity. This behavior indicated that polymerization proceeded efficiently even under conditions of low light intensity, although the rate was undetectable by calorimetry measurements and despite the fact that the effects of excess free volume were minimal.

C. Polymerization Kinetics

A systematic examination of the relationship between multi(meth)acrylate monomer structure and the polymerization kinetics was carried out by Moore (20). Photocalorimetry was used to study the polymerization kinetics of a number of multi(meth)acrylate monomers. Steric effects were shown to greatly affect the limiting double-bond conversions.

Subsequently, Hubca and collaborators (21–23) examined the polymerization kinetics of various oligo(ethylene glycol) dimethacrylates as a function of the oligo(ethylene glycol) chain length. Over the range of one to four ethylene glycol units, the polymerization rate was shown to increase with increasing oligo(ethylene glycol) chain length. Hubca et al. (23) also studied the conversion dependence of the copolymer composition in copolymerizations of dimethacrylates with styrene.

Miyazaki and Horibe (24) conducted a more exhaustive series of experiments, in which the length and composition of the chain between functional groups was varied for a series of dimethacrylates and diacrylates. Again, an increasing dependence of the polymerization rate on the length of the spacer between double bonds was observed. Also, monomers with flexible spacers were shown to have faster polymerization rates than those with rigid spacers, and diacrylates were shown to have faster polymerization rates than dimethacrylates of similar structure.

Bowman and Peppas (25) studied the polymerization behavior of oligo(ethylene glycol) dimethacrylates. Specifically, structural effects on the volume shrinkage accompanying polymerization and on the polymerization rate were examined. The volume shrinkage was shown to decrease with increasing monomer size, while the polymerization rate was shown to increase as the oligo(ethylene glycol) chain length was increased.

Scranton et al. (26) studied dimethacrylate homo- and copolymerizations as functions of the dimethacrylate monomer concentration, the solvent concentration, and the dimethacrylate monomer structure. The polymerization kinetics were shown to depend strongly on the double-bond mobility. Increasing the length of the oligo(ethylene glycol) spacer between double bonds on the dimethacrylate monomer, increasing the solvent concentration, or decreasing the dimethacrylate concentration in copolymerizations led to a decrease in the maximum rate of polymerization and a shift in the onset of the gel effect to longer times. These results reflected the dependence of the diffusional characteristics of the system on the network structure and degree of ovation.

The photopolymerization kinetics of oligo(ethylene glycol) diacrylates were studied by Kurdikar and Peppas (27,28). Their rate data indicated that increasing the oligo(ethylene glycol) chain length led to an increase in the reactivity of pendant double bonds and a decease in the reactivity of free double bonds. Strong oxygen inhibition effects and a distribution of radical lifetimes were also demonstrated.

Anseth et al. (4,29–32) studied the polymerization kinetics of multi(meth)acrylate monomers, including trimethylol propane triacrylate, trimethylol propane trimethacrylate, pentaerythritol tetraacrylate, and dipentaerythritol monohydroxypentaacrylate. The volume shrinkage and limiting conversions for these materials were shown to decrease with increasing monomer functionality.

D. Rate Coefficients

The rate coefficients are necessary in order to independently predict the three-dimensional behavior of the produced network. Anseth et al. (29,30) measured the kinetic rate coefficients, k_p and k_t, as a function of double-bond conversion for the various multi(meth)acrylate monomers. This analysis was based on steady-state and non-steady-state measurements of the polymerization rate. The steady-state measurements were performed isothermally with constant light intensity to facilitate calculation of the quantity $k_p/k_t^{1/2}$, where k_p is the rate coefficient for propagation and k_t is the rate coefficient for termination.

Non-steady-state measurements were performed by closing the shutter to the UV light and monitoring the polymerization rate in the absence of initiation (29,30,33). Anseth et al. (29,30) calculated conversion-dependent values of k_p and k_t for the various polymulti(meth)acrylates.

Rate coefficients were substantially higher for multiacrylates than for multimethacrylates and decreased with increasing monomer functionality. Diffusional effects on the polymerization kinetics were reflected in a three-stage dependence on double-bond conversion for k_p and k_t. During the first stage, early in the polymerization, k_t, the rate coefficient for termination, decreased rapidly by one to two orders of magnitude, due to diffusional limitations on bulky macroradicals. During this first stage, the kinetic constant k_p, which describes the propagation reaction, remained relatively constant, since diffusional effects on unreacted monomer were substantially smaller. This decrease in k_t with constant k_p led to the observed gel effect.

When the translational diffusion of macroradicals became sufficiently hindered, the dependence of k_p and k_t on conversion changed, reflecting a change in the termination mechanism. The second stage was then characterized by a proportional dependence of k_t on k_p, arising due to termination by reaction diffusion (29–32). When termination is dominated by reaction diffusion, macroradicals approach one another for termination not by translational diffusion through the intervening space in the reaction medium but by "stepwise" reaction through double bonds in the intervening space.

At high double-bond conversions, diffusion of unreacted monomer through the reaction medium was hindered, leading to autodeceleration. The rate coefficients k_p and k_t decreased rapidly to negligibly small values, and the polymerization stopped prior to incorporation of all available double bonds. This kinetic study (29–32) represented a quantitative examination of the effects leading to limiting conversions in bulk crosslinking polymerizations.

Anseth et al. (34) also measured the conversion-dependent rate coefficients for various oligo(ethylene glycol) dimethacrylates. The rate data supported a reaction diffusion mechanism of termination. Additionally, volume relaxation effects on the polymerization kinetics were measured as a function of oligo(ethylene glycol) chain length. The coupling of the kinetics to the volume relaxation rate was shown to be strongest for short oligo(ethylene glycol) chain lengths.

Efforts to model multi(meth)acrylate polymerizations have relied heavily on free volume approaches. Bowman and Peppas (35) coupled free volume–derived expressions for diffusion-controlled k_p and k_t values (36–38) to expressions describing the time-dependent evolution of the system free volume (39–42) in order to predict multimethacrylate homopolymerization behavior using three adjustable parameters. This model was later expanded by Anseth et al. (31) to accommodate termination based on reaction diffusion.

Kurdikar and Peppas (43) used the Vrentas-Duda (44–51) free volume theory of diffusion and the Smoluchowski (52) expression for diffusion-controlled reaction rate coefficients to develop a first-principles approach for describing multiacrylate polymerization behavior. This model also accounted for the finite rate of volume relaxation and additionally allowed for diffusional effects on the initiator efficiency (53). Both the Bowman-Peppas and the Kurdikar-Peppas approaches relied on the assumption that pendant and free double bonds react with equal probability over the entire course of the polymerization.

Thakur et al. (54) studied the dependence of the nonisothermal polymerization kinetics of oligo(ethylene glycol) diacrylates on various parameters. Average activation energies and heats of polymerization were calculated. Strong diffusional effects on the polymerization rate were observed, and the effects of oxygen inhibition were quantified.

Chiu and Lee (55) examined the microgel formation process during the polymerization of ethylene glycol dimethacrylate using a combination of calorimetric studies, dynamic light scattering, and Fourier transform infrared spectroscopy. Their results indicated a bimodal distribution of structure sizes from the beginning of the polymerization, corresponding to microgel regions and groups of microgel regions. The sizes of these structures were shown to depend strongly on the reaction temperature and on the initiator concentration.

Venhoven et al. (56) examined the effects of varying the initiator concentration in multimethacrylate formulations used in dental resins. They showed that manipulation of the initiator concentration provided a means of controlling the cure rates and the performance properties of the crosslinked polymers without affecting the final double-bond conversion.

III. NETWORK STRUCTURE AND MECHANICAL PROPERTIES

The mechanical stability and the three-dimensional structure of such networks are of utmost importance in pharmaceutical and biomedical applications. For example, knowledge of the three-dimensional network structure helps in controlling not only the elastic modulus and other mechanical properties, but also the effective crosslinking density and mesh size, ξ, of the network. The last parameter in turn affects the drug diffusion coefficient when such systems are used in drug delivery carriers.

A. Rubber Elasticity Analysis

Tobolsky and collaborators (57–60) studied the dynamic mechanical behavior of highly crosslinked copolymers of alkyl acrylates and poly(ethylene glycol) dimethacrylate. The systems examined exhibited well-defined glassy, transition, and rubbery plateau regions, even at high dimethacrylate concentrations. The researchers analyzed the compositional dependence of the rubbery shear modulus, using rubber elasticity theory (57–60):

$$G = \Phi n RT \quad (1)$$

Here G is the rubbery plateau value of the shear modulus, Φ is the front factor, R is the gas constant, and T is the temperature. An expression for the concentration, n, of network chains was developed (58), which accounted for elastic contributions due to the oligo(ethylene glycol) chain of the dimethacrylate monomer:

$$n = c[2x + 3(1 - x)] \quad (2)$$

Here c is the molar concentration of the dimethacrylate crosslinking monomer, while $(1 - x)$ is the mole fraction of the crosslinking monomer in the comonomer mixture. Using Eqs. 1 and 2, Tobolsky and collaborators (57–60) found that the front factor was nearly equal to unity for all compositions.

B. Dynamic Mechanical Behavior

Turner and collaborators (61–64) studied the dynamic mechanical behavior of polydimethacrylate networks typically used in dental restorations. Polymer samples prepared by γ irradiation at various doses exhibited multiple transitions suggestive of a heterogeneous network structure. The researchers postulated the existence of regions of varying mobilities. Additionally, Wilson and Turner (61) demonstrated that photopolymerized dimethacrylate dental materials may exhibit time-dependent mechanical properties in the oral cavity.

Kloosterboer and Lijten (65) demonstrated that photopolymerized 1,6-hexanediol diacrylate exhibited a T_g value 70 K higher than the temperature at which the polymerization was performed. This finding indicated a significant increase in double-bond conversion subsequent to vitrification and therefore suggested that a substantial quantity of free monomer remained at the vitrification point. The authors also suggested the importance of a tertiary hydrogen abstraction mechanism for radical motion in the heterogeneous polymer network.

Simon et al. (66) studied the polymerization kinetics and network structure of copolymers of various oligo(ethylene glycol) dimethacrylates. Thermal scanning calorimetry experiments indicated a heterogeneous polymerization process for all copolymer systems. Copolymers prepared from monomers with widely varying oligo(ethylene glycol) chain lengths exhibited dual glass transition temperatures, suggesting phase separation of the two types of repeating units. Copolymers prepared from monomers with similar oligo(ethylene glycol) chain lengths exhibited a smooth compositional dependence of the dynamic mechanical properties.

Anseth et al. (67) studied the dynamic mechanical T_g of photopolymerized trimethylolpropane triacrylate, pentaerythritol tetraacrylate, and dipentaerythritol monohydroxy pentaacrylate. Measured T_g values decreased with increasing monomer functionality, most likely reflecting the lower limiting double-bond conversions obtained for more highly functional monomers. Extremely broad damping peaks were observed, indicative of a heterogeneous network structure. An increase in T_g was observed for all systems subsequent to a thermal aftertreatment. This behavior demonstrated the presence of trapped radicals in the highly crosslinked polymer matrix.

C. Volume Shrinkage and Aging

Kurdikar and Peppas (68) examined the composition-dependent volume shrinkage behavior for a series of oligo(ethylene glycol) diacrylates. The measured volume shrinkage decreased as the oligo(ethylene glycol) chain length was increased. Also, systems with the shortest oligo(ethylene glycol) chain length exhibited enhanced thermal stability due to their more highly crosslinked nature. All samples exhibited multiple thermal transitions, indicating a heterogeneous network structure.

Bland and Peppas (5) exhaustively studied the dependence of the volume shrinkage behavior of multi(meth)acrylates on the monomer structure. Their findings indicated that bulkier monomers exhibited the least volume shrinkage. Also, volume shrinkage was shown to decrease with increasing monomer functionality. Dietz and Peppas (69) demonstrated substantial aging effects on the mechanical properties of the polymulti(meth)acrylates due to radical trapping.

D. Glass Transition Temperatures

Priola and collaborators (70) systematically examined the dependence of T_g on the oligo(ethylene glycol) chain length in a series of polydiacrylates. The monomer molecular weight was varied over the range of 200–2000 g/mol. The measured T_g values showed a linear dependence on $1/M_c$, where the molecular weight between crosslinks, M_c, was equated with the oligo(ethylene glycol) molecular weight. A similar dependence of T_g on the length of the oligomer chain between reactive double bonds was observed for oligo(tetramethylene ether) (71) and oligo(propylene glycol) (72) diacrylates.

Priola and collaborators (73) also examined the T_g behavior of diacrylate systems with rigid aromatic spacers between acrylate double bonds. In this work, 4,4′-hexafluoroisopropylidenediphenoldihydroxyethylether diacrylate was copolymerized with the corresponding hydrogenated monomer. Measured T_g values showed a linear dependence on the fluorinated monomer content, indicating a random incorporation of the two copolymers into the polymer network.

Lesser and Crawford (74) examined the crosslinking density dependence of T_g in a series of condensation polymers with well-defined values of M_c. Measured T_g values were shown to depend linearly on $1/M_c$, with a slope that depended on the crosslink functionality.

E. Control of the Structure of Highly Crosslinked Polymers

In order to minimize effects due to the thermally induced polymerization of trapped radicals during the study of highly crosslinked networks, Bowman and collaborators (75,76) developed synthesis techniques based on the use of iniferters. Iniferter molecules dissociate to give two low molecular weight radicals: a carbon radical and a sulfur radical. The carbon radicals initiate polymerization; the sulfur radicals terminate living polymer chains in a bimolecular reaction. Because of the availability of this additional termination mechanism in iniferter-initiated polymerizations, radical trapping is avoided. Bowman and collaborators (76) examined the compositional dependence of the relaxation time distribution in dimethacrylate copolymers formed using iniferters.

Presently, work is being conducted to examine the effect of this iniferter on the molecular structure of a crosslinked network. Upon further exposure to UV light, the living polymer chains terminated by the sulfur radical dissociate to form a living polymer chain and a sulfur radical. Experiments conducted on poly(ethylene glycol) dimethacrylates indicate that the polymerization rates of the iniferter-initiated systems are drastically smaller, and an autoacceleration is not observed when compared to the same materials initiated with the conventional initiator, 2,2-dimethoxy-2-phenylacetophenone (DMPA). It is therefore expected that the structures will depend on the type of initiator.

IV. EQUILIBRIUM SWELLING BEHAVIOR OF POLYMULTI(METH)ACRYLATES

Measurements of the equilibrium swelling in thermodynamically compatible penetrants are often used to probe the network structure of crosslinked polymers. By balancing the thermodynamic forces associated with polymer swelling with the elastic forces exerted by the network of polymer chains, Flory and Rehner (77) derived an expression for the average molecular weight between crosslinks, $\overline{M}_c$:

$$\frac{1}{\overline{M}_c} = \frac{2}{\overline{M}_n} - \frac{(\overline{v}/V_1)[\ln(1 - v_{2,s}) + v_{2,s} + \chi v_{2,s}^2]}{\left[v_{2,s}^{1/3} - \frac{v_{2,s}}{2}\right]} \tag{3}$$

Here $\overline{M}_n$ is the number-average molecular weight in the absence of crosslinking, $\overline{v}$ is the polymer specific volume, V_1 is the molar volume of the penetrant, $v_{2,s}$ is the equilibrium polymer volume fraction in the swollen state, and χ is the polymer–solvent interaction parameter. Mikos and Peppas (78) generated experimental data for a series of hydrophilic copolymers to facilitate prediction of χ values in cases where specific polymer–solvent interactions, such as hydrogen bonding, predominate

The equilibrium swelling equation was modified by Peppas and Lucht (79) to account for the effects of a non-Gaussian chain length distribution:

$$\frac{1}{\overline{M}_c} = \frac{2}{\overline{M}_n} - \frac{(\overline{v}/V_1)[\ln(1 - v_{2,s}) + v_{2,s} + \chi v_{2,s}^2]\left[1 - \frac{1}{N} v_{2,s}^{2/3}\right]^3}{\left[v_{2,s}^{1/3} - \frac{v_{2,s}}{2}\right]\left[1 + \frac{1}{N} v_{2,s}^{1/3}\right]^2} \tag{4}$$

Here N is the number of rotatable bonds between crosslinks.

Modifications of Eq. 3 by Barr-Howell and Peppas (80) and by Barar et al. (81) incorporated the effects of variable crosslink functionality and ionization along the polymer network backbone, respectively:

$$\frac{1}{\overline{M}_c} = \frac{2}{\overline{M}_n} - \frac{(\overline{v}/V_1)[\ln(1 - v_{2,s}) + v_{2,s} + \chi v_{2,s}^2]\left[1 - \frac{1}{N} v_{2,s}^{2/3}\right]^3}{A_\phi [v_{2,s}^{1/3} - \omega v_{2,s}]\left[1 + \frac{1}{N} v_{2,s}^{1/3}\right]^2} \quad (5)$$

Here the terms A_ϕ and ω are functionality-dependent structure factors (80).

$$\frac{V_1}{4I}\left[\frac{v_{2,s}}{\overline{v}}\right]^2 \left[\frac{K_a}{10^{-pH} + K_a}\right]^2 = [\ln(1 - v_{2,s}) + v_{2,s} + \chi v_{2,s}^2] + \left[\frac{V_1}{\overline{v} \overline{M}_c}\right]\left[1 - 2\frac{\overline{M}_c}{\overline{M}_n}\right]\left[v_{2,s}^{1/3} - \frac{v_{2,s}}{2}\right] \quad (6)$$

This equation is for anionic networks (81). The parameter I is the ionic strength of the swelling medium, while K_a is the dissociation constant of the ionizable moiety.

Previous efforts (68,69–72,82) to probe the crosslinked structure of polymulti(meth)acrylates using techniques based on penetrant diffusion have been limited to calculations of the crosslinking density from measured equilibrium swelling values. Extremely low equilibrium swelling ratios were observed in all cases due to the highly crosslinked nature of these materials.

For oligo(ethylene glycol) di(meth)acrylates, Bowman et al. (82) reported an increasing dependence of the equilibrium penetrant content on the length of the poly(ethylene glycol) chain in the di(meth)acrylate monomer. An analysis based on Eq. 4 indicated an extremely highly crosslinked network structure.

Kurdikar and Peppas (68) studied the equilibrium swelling behavior of various oligo(ethylene glycol) diacrylates. Mesh sizes ranging from 10.8 Å to 22.7 Å were reported as the oligo(ethylene glycol) chain length was varied over the range of one to nine ethylene glycol units. Also, the equilibrium degree of swelling was shown to increase as the oligo(ethylene glycol) chain length was increased. A similar monomer size dependence of the equilibrium swelling behavior was reported by Priola and collaborators (70–72) for various polydiacrylate systems and by Dietz and Peppas (69) for various polymultiacrylates

V. KINETIC GELATION SIMULATIONS OF NETWORK STRUCTURE

In order to provide predictive information regarding the interdependence of the multi(meth)acrylate polymerization kinetics and the heterogeneous network structure, lattice-based simulation techniques have been developed (83–86). These kinetic gelation simulations provide structural information that is inaccessible by purely kinetic models (87).

For example, Bowman and Peppas (85,86) developed simulation techniques for dimethacrylate monomers that incorporated realistic models of the radical initiation and termination mechanism. The simulations provided information regarding the trapping of radicals, the relative reactivities of free and pendant double bonds, and structural heterogeneity. Kurdikar and Peppas (88) developed off-lattice techniques for prediction of the diffusion-controlled kinetics, including nonconstant initiator efficiency, and structural evolution during diethylene glycol diacrylate photopolymerization.

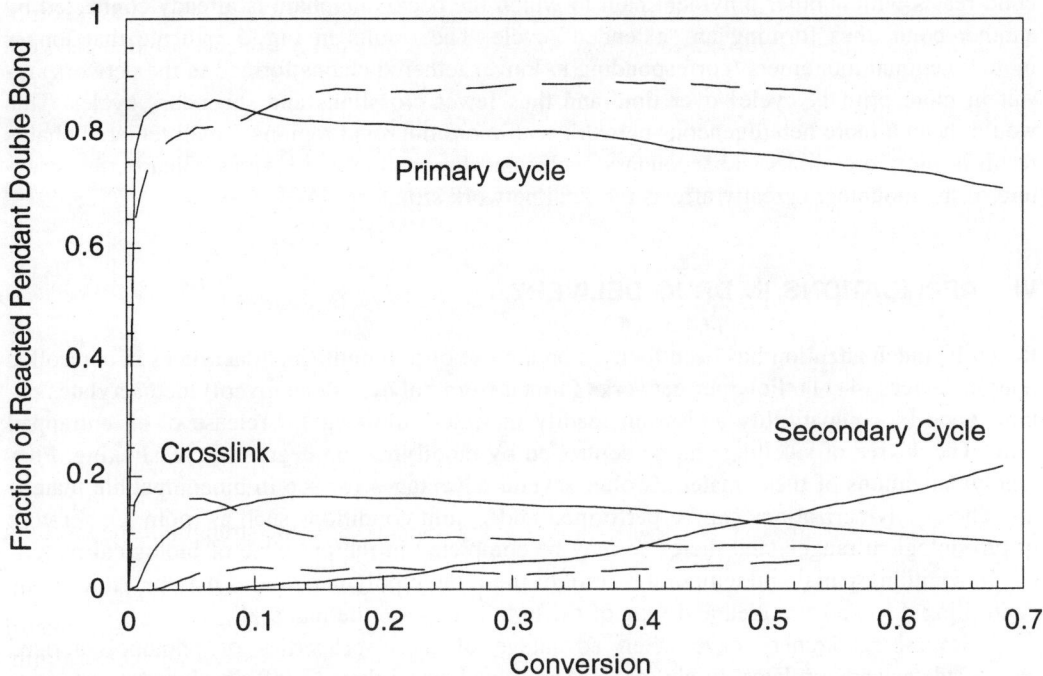

Figure 3 The fraction of the pendant double bonds that react and form primary cycles, secondary cycles, and crosslinks as a function of conversion for a copolymerization with a three-site monofunctional monomer (solid line) and a five-site monofunctional monomer (dashed line).

Anseth et al. (89) developed complementary experimental techniques to quantify the distribution of free volume in polymerizing multi(meth)acrylate systems using mobility-sensitive photochromic probes. This work demonstrated the heterogeneous manner in which the polymer network is assembled, as predicted by the kinetic gelation simulations (83–88).

Presently, the kinetic gelation simulations have been used to determine the effect of the monomer structure on the polymer network. In particular, in gels developed for drug delivery, tethered chains are often used to stabilize proteins and enhance the network (8,9). These tethered chains are a concern in the network formation because they may effect the limiting conversion and the structural heterogeneity. A simulation was thus conducted to examine the evolving structure of a network formed with a crosslinker and a monofunctional monomer of varying length.

Figure 3 displays the results of the network formation for two simulations with different lengths of tethered chains. In these simulations, the initial solution contains 1% initiator, 33% crosslinker which is represented by two sites on the lattice and each site is reactive, and 65% of a monofunctional monomer. In this particular figure, the solid line represents a monofunctional monomer occupying three sites with only one end being reactive; the dashed line represents a monofunctional monomer occupying five sites with only one end being reactive. To gain insight into the network structure, the reactivity of the pendant double bonds is examined. The pendant double bonds formed in the network react to form either a primary cycle, a crosslink, or a secondary cycle. A primary cycle is defined as a pendant double bond that reacts back on its backbone chain forming a small cycle. A crosslink is defined as a pendant double bond that reacts with a separate polymer chain. Finally, a secondary cycle is formed when a pendant double bond reacts with another polymer chain to which the backbone chain is already connected by another bond, thus forming an "extended" cycle. The results in Fig. 3 indicate that longer monofunctional monomers (corresponding to longer tethered chains formed in the network) result in more primary cycles over time and thus fewer crosslinks and secondary cycles. This would mean a more heterogeneous network with more microgel regions. Small tethered chains result in more crosslinks and secondary cycles and fewer microgel regions. Clearly, the structure of the monomers greatly affects the final network structure.

VI. APPLICATIONS IN DRUG DELIVERY

Recently, much attention has been focused on the use of polymulti(meth)acrylates in controlled release devices (4–11). Polymer networks formed from poly(ethylene glycol) methacrylates exhibit good biocompatibility and swell readily in water, allowing for release of an entrapped drug. The degree of swelling can be controlled by modifying the degree of crosslinking. Photopolymerizations of these materials offer several advantages for use in biocompatible materials. These polymerizations can be performed under mild conditions such as room temperature or physiological ranges, and therefore may be completed in the presence of biological materials. In addition, spatial and temporal control of these rapid polymerizations may be achieved by controlling the exposure area and time of the light source on the material.

Several researchers have taken advantage of these properties of photopolymerized methacrylates and acrylates. In particular, Anseth and co-workers (7,90) developed a technique for making drug delivery devices with laminated layers. Each layer incorporated a different drug concentration, which allowed for a more uniform rate of diffusion of the drug or encapsulated substance and decreased the burst effect. The materials used in this unique device were 2-hydroxyethyl methacrylate (HEMA) and diethylene glycol dimethacrylate (DEGDMA) (crosslinker).

Lowman and Peppas (8,9,91–93) developed drug delivery materials composed of poly(methacrylic acid) grafted with poly(ethylene glycol) [P(MAA-g-EG)]. Typically, these materials were photopolymerized in thin films from the monomers of methacrylic acid, poly(ethylene glycol) methacrylate, and the crosslinker tetraethylene glycol dimethacrylate. The P(MAA-g-EG) material is pH-sensitive because it is a complexing system. Additional crosslinks form in this material due to the hydrogen bonding occurring between the ether groups of the poly(ethylene glycol) grafts and the protonated pendant group of the PMAA backbone. In an acidic environment, the material is in the complexed state and has a small pore size because of the additional crosslinks. Thus, there will be no drug diffusion out of the polymer. As the pH of the environment decreases, the complexes dissociate therefore increasing the pore size and releasing the drug by diffusion. Figure 4 displays the effect of the complexation on the mesh size, ξ.

Lowman and Peppas (94,95) applied these materials to the delivery of insulin. These materials were prepared as microparticles by thermal polymerization instead of a photopolymerization in order to increase the response of the materials for in vivo experiments. In this particular application, the complexation nature of this methacrylate material is an advantage because of the pH-sensitive swelling behavior. In the acidic environment of the stomach, the complexation prevents the diffusion of the insulin. Instead, the insulin diffuses out in the less acidic environments encountered after passing through the stomach. In addition, the poly(ethylene glycol) grafts stabilize the insulin and prevent it from binding to the ionizable backbone chain.

Networks made of acrylated poly(ethylene glycol) star polymers have also been developed for drug release devices (96). In their work, Keys et al. prepared hydrogels of acrylated poly(ethylene glycol) stars and poly(ethylene glycol) dimethacrylate by UV polymerization.

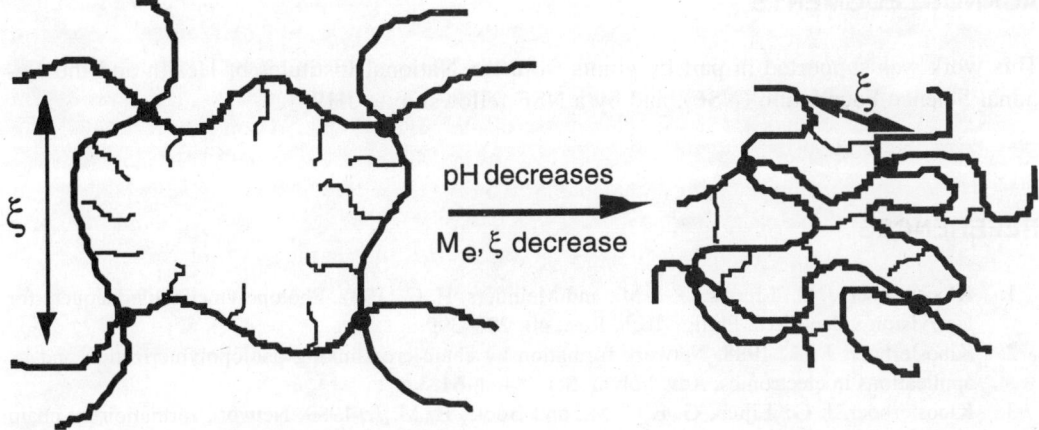

Figure 4 Effect of complexation on the mesh size, ξ, and the effective molecular weight between crosslinks, M_e, in graft copolymer networks with permanent chemical crosslinks (●).

The advantage of the star polymers is the existence of numerous functional groups in a small volume. Therefore, more biologically active molecules can be incorporated into the network. Another application of these materials would be in molecular imprinting where the structure of a biological molecule is replicated inside the network and it "remembers" the original molecule. The large number of functional groups in the star hydrogels is advantageous in molecular imprinting because they can be modified to give the gel-specific properties.

Schwarte and Peppas (11,97) also developed materials composed of methacrylates for drug delivery. Diethylaminoethyl methacrylate (DEAEM) and poly(ethylene glycol) monomethacrylate (PEGMA) were used to form pH-sensitive cationic gels. Normally, under the acidic conditions of performance, cationic gels cannot be used for protein delivery. However, in this system, poly(ethylene glycol) improves the conditions of protein stability. Release studies were conducted on these gels with proxyphylline, vitamin B_{12}, and various dextrans to determine solute diffusion coefficients and the effect of the gel mesh size.

Podual and Peppas (11,98–100) further modified these ionic hydrogels for the glucose-sensitive release of insulin. The enzyme glucose oxidase (GOD) is immobilized into the polymer matrix to incorporate glucose-responsive properties. The glucose oxidase converts surrounding glucose to gluconic acid, thus decreasing the pH in the microenvironment of the hydrogel. In a cationic hydrogel, the decrease in pH causes the gel to swell and the imbibed insulin to diffuse out. In an anionic hydrogel, the opposite occurs in that the gel mesh size decreases in response to a lower pH and squeezes out the insulin.

Polymethacrylates also have also been used in biomaterials. Specifically, Leobandung et al. (101) developed a tract of a transjugular intrahepatic portsystemic shunt (TIPS) made of the polymer P(PEGMA-co-PEGDMA). In their technique, the photopolymerization occurs within the parenchymal tract of a TIPS, thus eliminating the need for an additional stent. This is accomplished by delivering the liquid monomer through a catheter and shining the light source directly on the area to be polymerized. The polymer gel must be strong enough to withstand the force of balloon angioplasty. In addition, the copolymerization with a dimethacrylate reduces the mesh size so that it is small enough to prevent bile leakage and migration of metaplastic biliary epithelial cells.

Clearly, photopolymerizations are an emerging method for preparation of well-characterized, uniform, controlled drug delivery carriers.

ACKNOWLEDGMENTS

This work was supported in part by grants from the National Institutes of Health and the National Science Foundation (NSF), and by a NSF fellowship to JHW.

REFERENCES

1. Kloosterboer, J. G., Lippits, G. J. M., and Meinders, H. C., 1982. Photopolymerizable lacquers for laservision video discs. Philips Tech. Rev., 40: 298–309.
2. Kloosterboer, J. G., 1988. Network formation by chain crosslinking photopolymerization and its applications in electronics. Adv. Polym. Sci., 84: 1–61.
3. Kloosterboer, J. G., Lijten, G. F. C. M., and Boots, H. M. J., 1989. Network formation by chain crosslinking photopolymerization and some applications in electronics. Makromol. Chem., Macromol. Symp., 24: 223–230.
4. Anseth, K. S., Newman, S. M. and Bowman, C. N., 1995. Polymeric dental composites: properties and reaction behavior of multimethacrylate dental restorations. Adv. Polym. Sci., 122: 177–217.
5. Bland, M. H. and Peppas, N. A., 1996. Photopolymerized multifunctional (meth)acrylates as model polymers for dental applications. Biomaterials, 17: 1109–1114.
6. Yang, J.-M., 1998. Study of polymerization of acrylic bone cement: effect of HEMA and EGDMA. J. Biomed. Mater. Res., 43: 54–61.
7. Lu, S. X. and Anseth, K. S., 1999. Photopolymerization of multilaminated poly(HEMA) hydrogels for controlled release. J. Controlled Release, 57: 291–300.
8. Lowman, A. M. and Peppas, N. A., 1997. Design of oral delivery systems for peptides and proteins using complexation graft copolymer networks. In: N. A. Peppas, D. J. Mooney, A. G. Mikos, and L. Brannon-Peppas (Eds.), Biomaterials, Carriers for Drug Delivery and Scaffolds for Tissue Engineering, AIChE, New York, pp. 21–23.
9. Peppas, N. A., Keys, K. B., Torres-Lugo, M. and Lowman, A. M. Poly(ethylene glycol)-containing hydrogels in drug delivery. J. Controlled Release 62: 81–87.
10. Podual, K., Doyle, F. J. and Peppas, N. A., 1997. Glucose-sensitive cationic hydrogels: preparation, characterization, and modeling of swelling properties. In: N. A. Peppas, D. J. Mooney, A. G. Mikos, and L. Brannon-Peppas (Eds.), Biomaterials, Carriers for Drug Delivery and Scaffolds for Tissue Engineering, AIChE, New York, pp 190–192.
11. Schwarte, L. M., Podual, K. and Peppas, N. A., 1998. Cationic hydrogels for controlled release of proteins and other macromolecules. In: I. McCullough and S. Shalaby (Eds.), Materials for Controlled Release Applications, ACS Symposium Series, ACS, Washington, DC.
12. Horie, K., Otagawa, A., Muraoka, M., and Mita, I., 1975. Calorimetric investigation of polymerization reactions. V. Crosslinked copolymerization of methyl methacrylate with ethylene dimethacrylate. J. Polym. Sci., Polym. Chem. Ed., 13: 445–454.
13. Kloosterboer, J. G., van de Hei, G. M. M., Gossink, R. G., and Dortant, G. C. M., 1984. The effects of volume relaxation and thermal mobilization of trapped radicals on the final conversion of photopolymerized diacrylates. Polym. Commun., 25: 322–325.
14. Kloosterboer, J. G., van de Hei, G. M. M., and Boots, H. M. J., 1984. Inhomogeneity during the photopolymerization of diacrylates: DSC experiments and percolation theory. Polym. Commun., 25: 354–357.
15. Kloosterboer, J. G., and Lijten, G. F. C. M., 1987. Thermal and mechanical analysis of a photopolymerization process. Polymer, 28: 1149–1155.
16. Kloosterboer, J. G., and Lijten, G. F. C. M., 1987. Thermal and mechanical analysis of the chain crosslinking polymerization of tetra-ethyleneglycol diacrylate. Polym. Mater. Sci. Eng. Proc. 56: 759–763.
17. Kloosterboer, J. G., Lijten, G. F. C. M., and Zegers, C. P. G., 1989. Formation of densely crosslinked polymer glasses by photopolymerization. Polym. Mater. Sci. Eng. Proc. 60: 122–126.

18. Kloosterboer, J. G., and Lijten, G. F. C. M., 1987. Chain crosslinking photopolymerization of tetra-ethyleneglycol diacrylate. In R. A. Dickie, S. S. Labana, and R. S. Bauer (Eds.), Crosslinked Polymers: Chemistry, Properties, and Applications. American Chemical Society, Washington, D.C., pp. 759–763.
19. Odian, G., 1991. Principles of Polymerization, 3rd Ed. Wiley, New York, p. 286.
20. Moore, J. E., 1977. Photopolymerization of multifunctional acrylates and methacrylates. In: S. S. Labana (Ed.), Chemistry and Properties of Crosslinked Polymers. Academic Press, New York, pp. 535–546.
21. Hubca, G. H., Oprescu, C. R., Dråagan, G. H., and Dimonie, M., 1982. Synthesis and polymerization of polyethylene glycol dimethacrylates. IV. Rev. Roumaine Chim., 27: 433–442.
22. Drågan, G. H., Hubca, G. H., Oprescu, C. R., and Dimonie, M., 1982. Synthesis and polymerization of polyethylene glycol dimethacrylates. V. Rev. Roumaine Chim., 27: 585–590.
23. Hubca, G. H., Oprescu, C. R., Cragheorgheopol, A., Caldararu, H., Racoti, D., and Dimonie, M., 1988. Synthesis and polymerization of polyethylene glycol dimethacrylates. VI. Rev. Roumaine Chim., 27: 659–666.
24. Miyazaki, K. and Takashi, H., 1988. Polymerization of multifunctional methacrylates and acrylates. J. Biomed. Mater. Res., 22: 1011–1022.
25. Bowman, C. N. and Peppas, N. A., 1991. Polymers for information storage systems. 2. polymerization kinetics for preparation of highly crosslinked polydimethacrylates. J. Appl. Polym. Sci., 42: 2013–2018.
26. Scranton, A. B., Bowman, C. N., Klier, J., and Peppas, N. A., 1992. Polymerization reaction dynamics of ethylene glycol methacrylates and dimethacrylates by calorimetry. Polymer, 33: 1683–1689.
27. Kurdikar, D. L. and Peppas, N. A., 1993. Highly crosslinked polymers in information technology applications. Polym. Mater. Sci. Eng. Proceed., 68: 91–92.
28. Kurdikar, D. L. and Peppas, N. A., 1994. A kinetic study of diacrylate photopolymerizations. Polymer, 35: 1004–1011.
29. Anseth, K. S., Wang, C. M., and Bowman, C. N., 1994. Reaction behaviour and kinetic constants for photopolymerizations of multi(meth)acrylate monomers. Polymer, 35: 3243–3250.
30. Anseth, K. S., Bowman, C. N., and Peppas, N. A., 1994. Polymerization kinetics and volume relaxation behavior of photopolymerized multifunctional monomers producing highly crosslinked networks. J. Polym. Sci., Polym. Chem., 32: 139–147.
31. Anseth, K. S. and Bowman, C. N., 1992–93. Reaction diffusion enhanced termination in polymerizations of multifunctional monomers. Polym. React. Eng., 1: 499–520.
32. Anseth, K. S., Wang, C. M., and Bowman, C. N., 1994. Kinetic evidence of reaction diffusion during the polymerization of multi(meth)acrylate monomers. Macromolecules, 27: 650–655.
33. Tryson, G. R. and Shultz, A. R., 1979. A calorimetric study of acrylate photopolymerization. J. Polym. Sci., Polym. Phys. Ed., 17: 2059–2075.
34. Anseth, K. S., Kline, L. M., Walker, T. A., Anderson, K. J., and Bowman, C. N., 1995. Reaction kinetics and volume relaxation during polymerizations of multiethylene glycol dimethacrylates. Macromolecules, 28: 2491–2499.
35. Bowman, C. N. and Peppas, N. A., 1991. Coupling of kinetics and volume relaxation during polymerizations of multiacrylates and multimethacrylates. Macromolecules, 24: 1914–1920.
36. Marten, F. and Hamielec, A., 1978. High-conversion diffusion-controlled polymerization," in polymerization reactors and processes. In: J. Henderson and J. Bouton (Eds.), American Chemical Socirty, Washington, D.C., pp. 43–70.
37. Marten, F. and Hamielec, A., 1982. High-conversion diffusion-controlled polymerization of styrene. J. Appl. Polym. Sci., 27: 489–495.
38. Bueche, F., 1962. Physical Properties of Polymers, Interscience, London.
39. Kovacs, A., 1958. La contraction isotherme du volume des polymères amorphes. J. Polym. Sci., 30: 131–147.
40. Kovacs, A., 1963. Transition vitreuse dans les polymères amorphes. Etude phénoménologique. Fortschr. Hochpolym.-Forsch., 3: 394–507.
41. Hutchinson, J. and Kovacs, A., 1976. A simple phenomenlolgical approach to the thermal behavior of glasses during uniform heating or cooling. J. Polym. Sci., Polym. Phys. Ed., 14: 1575–1599.

42. Kovacs, A., Aklonis, J., Hutchinson, J., and Ramos, A., 1979. Isobaric volume and enthelpy recovery of glasses. 2. Transparent multi-parameter theory J. Polym. Sci., Polym. Phys. Ed., 17: 1097–1162.
43. Kurdikar, D. L. and Peppas, N. A., 1994. Method of determination of initiator efficiency: application to uv polymerizations using 2,2-dimethoxy-2-phenylacetophenone. Macromolecules, 27: 733–738.
44. Vrentas, J. S., and Duda, J. L., 1977. Diffusion in polymer-solvent systems. 1. Reexamination of the free-volume theory. J. Polym. Sci., Polym. Phys. Ed., 15: 403–416.
45. Vrentas, J. S. and Duda, J. L., 1977. Diffusion in polymer-solvent systems. 2. A predictive theory for the dependence of diffusion coefficients on temperature, concentration, and molecular weight. J. Polym. Sci., Polym. Phys. Ed., 15: 417–439.
46. Vrentas, J. S. and Vrentas, C. M., 1991. Solvent self-diffusion in crosslinked polymers. J. Appl. Polym. Sci., 42: 1931–1937.
47. Vrentas, J. S., Liu, H. T., and Duda, J. L., 1980. Estimation of diffusion coefficients for trace amounts of solvents in glassy and molten polymers. J. Appl. Polym. Sci., 25: 1297–1310.
48. Vrentas, J. S., Liu, H. T., and Duda, J. L., 1980. Effect of solvent size on diffusion in polymer–solvent systems. J. Appl. Polym. Sci., 25: 1793–1797.
49. Duda, J. L., Vrentas, J. S., Ju, S. T., and Liu, H. T., 1982. Prediction of diffusion coefficients for polymer solvent systems. AIChE J., 28: 279–285.
50. Vrentas, J. S. and Chu, C.-H., 1989. Predictive capabilities of a free-volume theory for solvent self-diffusion coefficients. J. Poly. Sci., Poly. Phys. Ed., 27: 1179–1184.
51. Zielinski, J. M. and Duda, J. L., 1992. Predicting polymer/solvent diffusion coefficients using free-volume theory. AIChE J., 38: 405–415.
52. Rice, S., 1985. Diffusion-limited reactions. In: C. H. Bamford, C. F. H. Tipper, and R. G. Compton (Eds.), Diffusion Reactions, Elsevier, New York, p. 3.
53. Kurdikar, D. L. and Peppas, N. A., 1994. A kinetic model for diffusion-controlled bulk crosslinking photopolymerizations. Macromolecules, 27: 4084–4092.
54. Thakur, A., Banthia, A. K., and Maiti, B. R., 1995. Studies on the kinetics of free-radical bulk polymerization of multifunctional acrylates by dynamic differential scanning calorimetry. J. Appl. Polym. Sci., 58: 959–966.
55. Chiu, Y. Y., and Lee, J., 1995. Microgel formation in the free radical crosslinking polymerization of ethylene glycol dimethacrylate (EGDMA). I. Experimental. J. Polym. Sci., Polym. Chem., 33: 257–267.
56. Venhoven, B. A. M., de Gee, A. J., and Davidson, C. L., 1996. Light initiation of dental resins. Biomaterials, 24: 2313–2318.
57. Tobolsky, A. V., Katz, D., Thach, R., and Schaffhauser R., 1962. Rubber elasticity in a highly crosslinked system. J. Polym. Sci., 62: S176–S177.
58. Katz, D. and Tobolsky, A. V., 1964. Rubber elasticity in highly crosslinked polyesters. J. Polym. Sci.: Part A, 2: 1587–1594.
59. Katz, D., and Tobolsky, A. V., 1964. Rubber elasticity in highly crosslinked polyethyl acrylate. J. Polym. Sci.: Part A, 2: 1595–1605.
60. Tobolsky, A. V., Katz, D., Takahashi, M., and Schaffhauser, R., 1964. Rubber Elasticity in highly crosslinked systems: crosslinked styrene, methyl methacrylate, ethyl acrylate, and octyl acrylate. J. Polym. Sci.: Part A, 2: 2749–2758.
61. Wilson, T. W. and Turner, D. T., 1987. Characterization of polydimethacrylates and their composites by dynamic mechanical analysis. J. Dent. Res., 66: 1032–1035.
62. Turner, D. T., Haque, Z. U., Kalachandra, S., and Wilson, T. W., 1987. Structure and properties of polydimethacrylates: dental applications. Polym. Mater. Sci. Eng. Proc., 56: 769–773.
63. Turner, D. T., Haque, Z. U., Kalachandra, S., and Wilson, T. W., 1987. Structure and properties of dimethacrylates. In: R. A. Dickie, S. S. Labana, and R. S. Bauer (Eds.), Crosslinked Polymers: Chemistry, Properties, and Applications, American Chemical Society, Washington, D.C., pp. 427–438.
64. Wilson, T. W. and Turner, D. T., 1988. Characterization of highly crosslinked networks by dynamic mechanical analysis: poly(triethylene glycol dimethacrylate). Polym. Mater. Sci. Eng. Proc., 59: 413–417.

65. Kloosterboer, J. G. and Lijten, G. F. C. M., 1990. Photopolymers exhibiting a large difference between glass transition and curing temperatures. Polymer, 31: 95–101.
66. Simon, G. P., Allen, P. E. M., and Williams, D. R. G., 1991. Properties of dimethacrylate copolymers of varying crosslink density. Polymer, 32: 2577–2587.
67. Anseth, K. S., Bowman, C. N., and Peppas, N. A., 1993. Dynamic mechanical studies of the glass transition temperature of photopolymerized multifunctional acrylates. Polym. Bull., 31: 229–233.
68. Kurdikar, D. L. and Peppas, N. A., 1995. The volume shrinkage, thermal and sorption behaviour of polydiacrylates. Polymer, 36: 2249–2255.
69. Dietz, J. E. and Peppas, N. A., 1997. Reaction kinetics and chemical changes during polymerization of multifunctional (meth)acrylates for the production of highly crosslinked polymers used in information storage systems. Polymer, 38: 3767–3781.
70. Priola, A., Gozzelino, G., Ferrero, F., and Malucelli, G., 1993. Properties of polymeric films obtained from u.v. cured poly(ethylene glycol) diacrylates. Polymer, 34: 3653–3657.
71. Malucelli, G., Gozzelino, G., Bongiovanni, R., and Priola, A., 1996. Photopolymerization of poly(tetramethylene ether) glycol diacrylates and properties of the obtained networks. Polymer, 37: 2565–2571.
72. Malucelli, G., Gozzelino, G., Ferrero, F., Bongiovanni, R., and Priola, A., 1997. Synthesis of poly (propylene glycol diacrylates) and properties of the photocured networks. J. Appl. Polym. Sci., 65: 491–497.
73. Bongiovanni, R., Malucelli, G., Pollicino, A., and Priola, A., 1997. Properties of films obtained by uv curing 4,4'-hexafluoroisopropylidenephenoldihydroxyethylether diacrylate and its mixture with the hydrogenated homologue. J. Appl. Polym. Sci., 63: 979–983.
74. Lesser, A. J., and Crawford, E., 1997. Role of network architecture on the glass transition temperature of epoxy resins. J. Appl. Polym. Sci., 66: 387–395.
75. Kannurpatti, A. R., Anderson, K. J., Anseth, J. W., and Bowman, C. N., 1996. Use of inifiters to study the structural evolution and properties of highly crosslinked polymer networks. Polym. Mater. Sci. Eng. Proc., 74: 100–101.
76. Kannurpatti, A. R., Lu, S., and Bowman, C. N., 1996. Reaction behavior and kinetic modeling studies of inifiter photopolymerizations. Polym. Mater. Sci. Eng. Proc., 74: 358–359.
77. Flory, P. J. and Rehner, R., 1943. Statistical mechanics of cross-linked polymer networks II. Swelling. J. Chem. Phys., 11: 521.
78. Mikos, A. G. and Peppas, N. A., 1988. The Flory interaction parameter χ for hydrophilic copolymers with water. Biomaterials, 9: 419–423.
79. Peppas, N. A. and L. M. Lucht, L. M., 1984. Macromolecular structure of coals. I. The organic phase of bituminous coals as a macromolecular network. Chem. Eng. Commun., 30: 291–310.
80. Barr-Howell. B. D. and Peppas, N. A., 1985. Importance of junction functionality in highly crosslinked polymers. Polym. Bull., 13: 91–96.
81. Barar, D. G., Staller, K. P., and Peppas, N. A., 1983. Friedel-Crafts crosslinking methods for polystyrene modification. IV. Macromolecular structure of crosslinked particles. J. Polym. Sci., Polym. Chem., 21: 1013–1024.
82. Bowman, C. N., Carver, A. L., Kennett, S. N., Williams, M. M., and Peppas, N. A., 1990. Polymers for information storage systems III. Crosslinked structure of polydimethacrylates. Polymer, 31: 135–139.
83. Kloosterboer, J. G., van de Hei, G. M. M., and Boots, H. M. J., 1984. Inhomogeneity during the photopolymerization of diacrylates: DSC experiments and percolation theory. Polym. Commun., 25: 354–357.
84. Boots, H. M. J., Kloosterboer, J. G., van de Hei, G. M. M., and Pandey, R. B., 1985. Inhomogeneity during the bulk polymerization of divinyl compounds: differential scanning calorimetry experiments and percolation theory. Br. Polym. J., 17: 219–223.
85. Bowman, C. N. and Peppas, N. A., 1991. Initiation and termination mechanisms in kinetic gelation simulations. J. Polym. Sci., Polym. Chem., 29: 1575–1583.
86. Bowman, C. N. and Peppas, N. A. 1992. A kinetic gelation method for the simulation of free-radical polymerizations. Chem. Eng. Sci., 47: 1411–1419.

87. Kinney, A. B. and A. B. Scranton, A. B., 1994. Formation and structure of crosslinked polyacrylates: methods for modeling network Formation. In: N. A. Peppas and F. L. Buchholz (Eds.), Advances in Superabsorbent Polymers, American Chemical Society, Washington, D.C., pp. 2–26.
88. Kurdikar, D. L., Somvarsky, J., Dusek, K., and Peppas, N. A. 1995. Development and evaluation of a Monte Carlo technique for the simulation of multifunctional polymerizations. Macromolecules, 28: 5910–5920.
89. Anseth, K. S., Rothenberg, M. D., and Bowman, C. N., 1994. A photochromic technique to study polymer network volume distributions and microstructure evolution. Macromolecules, 27: 2890.
90. Lu, S. X., Rameriez, W. F. and Anseth, K. S., 1998. Modeling and optimization of drug release from laminated polymer matrix devices. AICHE J., 44: 1689–1696.
91. Peppas, N. A. and Lowman, A. M., 1998. Protein delivery from novel bioadhesive complexation hydrogels. In: S. Frøkjaer, L. Christrup, and P. Krogsgaard-Larsen (Eds.). Peptide and Protein Drug Delivery, Munksgaard, Copenhagen, pp. 206–216.
92. Lowman, A. M. and Peppas, N. A. Pulsatile drug delivery based on a complexation/decomplexation mechanism. In: S. Dinh and J. DeNuzzio (Eds.), Intelligent Materials and Novel Concepts for Controlled Release Technologies, ACS Symposium Series, ACS, Washington, D.C. Vol. 728, pp. 30–42.
93. Lowman, A. M., Peppas, N. A., Morishita, M. and Nagai, T., 1998. Novel bioadhesive complexation networks for oral protein drug delivery. In: I. McCullough and S. Shalaby (Eds.), Materials for Controlled Release Applications, ACS Symposium Series, ACS, Washington, D.C.
94. Morishita, M., Takayama, K., Nagai, T., Lowman, A. M. and Peppas, N. A., 1997. Application of a pH-responsive polymer to an insulin oral dosage form. Yakuzaigaku, 57 Suppl., 96–97, in Japanese.
95. Lowman, A. M., Morishita, M., Nagai, T. and Peppas, N. A., Oral delivery of insulin using pH-responsive complexation gels. J. Pharm. Sci. 88: 933–937.
96. Keys, K. B., Andreopoulos, F. M. and Peppas, N. A., 1998. Poly(ethylene glycol) star polymer hydrogels. Macromolecules, 31: 8149–8156.
97. Schwarte, L. M. and Peppas, N. A., 1998. Novel poly(ethylene glycol)-grafted, cationic hydrogels: preparation, characterization and diffusive properties. Polymer, 39: 6057–6066.
98. Podual, K., Doyle, F. J., III, and Peppas, N. A., in press. Preparation and characterization of the dynamic response of cationic copolymer hydrogels containing glucose oxidase. Polymer.
99. Podual, K., Doyle, F. J., III, and Peppas, N. A., in press. Dynamic behavior of glucose-oxidase-containing microparticles of poly(ethylene glycol)-grafted cationic hydrogels in an environment of changing pH. Biomaterials.
100. Podual, K., Doyle, F. J., III, and Peppas, N. A., in press. Glucose-sensitivity of glucose oxidase–containing cationic copolymer hydrogels having poly(ethylene glycol) grafts. J. Controlled Release.
101. Leobandung, W., McLennan, G., Patel, N., Moresco, K. P. and Peppas, N. A., 1999. The characterization of P(PEGMA-co-PEGDMA) gels for use in coating the tract of a transjugular intrahepatic porto-systemic shunt. Polym. Pepr., 40: 337–338.

4
Smart Polymers for Controlled Drug Delivery

Joseph Kost and Smadar A. Lapidot
Ben-Gurion University of the Negev, Beer Sheva, Israel

I. INTRODUCTION

Since the beginning of recorded history, natural polymers have been utilized by humans to promote health and healing. For example, early Egyptians used linen for suturing wounds. In the twentieth century, not long after the development of synthetic polymers, use of polymers in a broad range of biomedical applications has been the focus of many researchers and clinicians (1). The rapid advancement of biomedical research led to many creative applications for biocompatible polymers. As modern medicine discerns more mechanisms both of physiology and of pathophysiology, the approach to healing is to mimic or, if possible, recreate the physiology of healthy functioning.

While development of newer and more powerful drugs continues, increasing attention is being given to methods for administering these active substances. In conventional drug delivery, the drug concentration in the blood rises when the drug is taken, then peaks and declines. Maintaining drug in the desired therapeutic range with just a single dose, and targeting the drug to a specific area (lowering the systemic drug level), are goals that have been successfully attained with commercially available controlled release devices (2). However, there are many clinical situations where the approach of a constant drug delivery rate is insufficient, such as the delivery of insulin for patients with diabetes mellitus, antiarrhythmics for patients with heart rhythm disorders, gastric acid inhibitors for ulcer control, nitrates for patients with angina pectoris, as well as selective β-blockade, birth control, general hormone replacement, immunization, and cancer chemotherapy. Furthermore, studies in the field of chronopharmacology indicate that at onset certain diseases exhibit strong circadian temporal dependence. Thus treatment of these diseases could be optimized through the use of responsive delivery systems (3).

In fact, when healthy, it is "smart" biopolymers that maintain proper function. A cell membrane, a phospholipid bilayer, embedded with receptors, pumps, channels, etc., responds to voltage changes, to changes in concentrations of ions and other molecules, by secreting proteins and hormones, by regulating the synthesis of proteins, by activating an action potential, etc. The body's functioning is based on biological feedback control systems, whether it is the autonomic nervous system with parasympathetic and sympathetic nerves, or β-pancreatic cells secreting insulin in response to elevated blood glucose levels. Responsive drug delivery in essence is a man-made imitation of healthy functioning.

"Smart," or "Intelligent," controlled release devices can be classified as open or closed loop systems, as is seen in Figure 1. Open loop systems are those where information about the controlled variable is not automatically used to adjust the system inputs to compensate for the

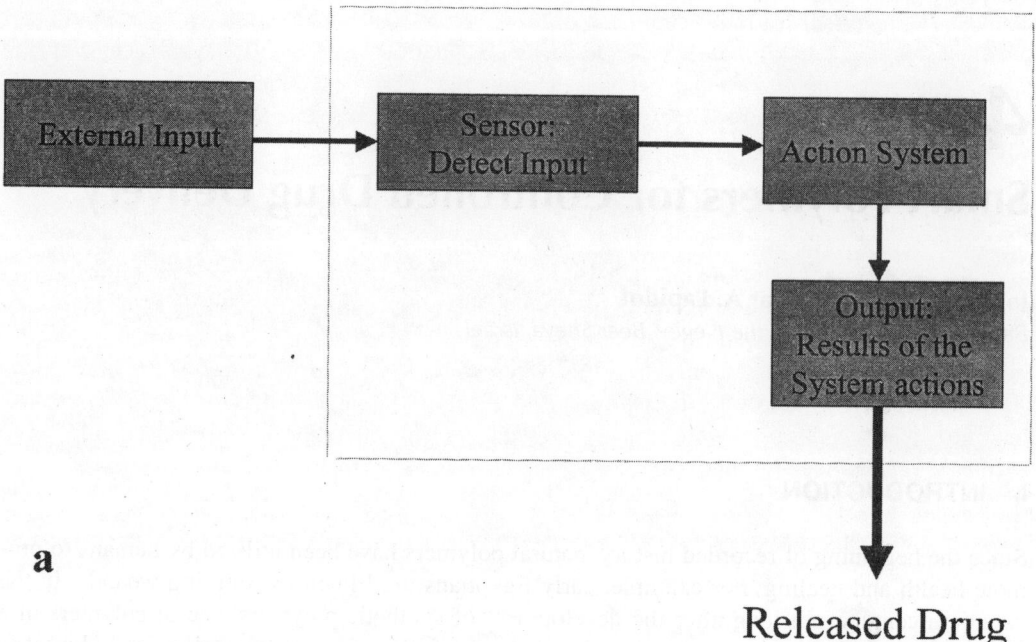

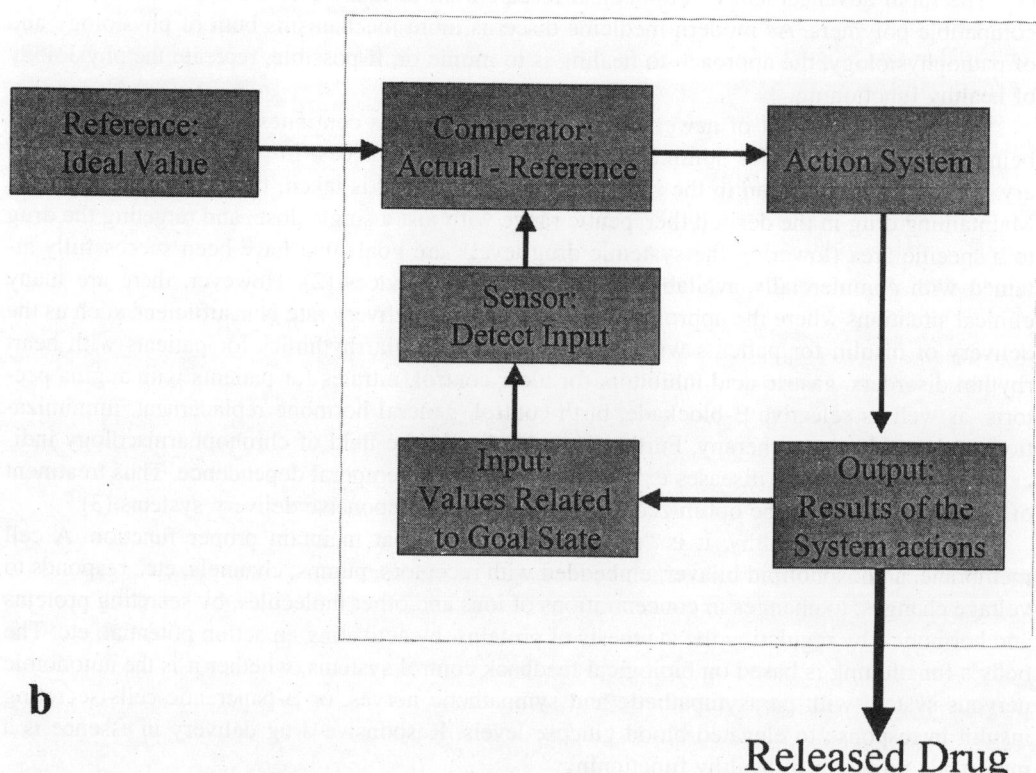

Figure 1 Schematic representation of drug delivery systems and their control mechanisms. (a) Open loop system, (b) closed loop system.

change in the process variables. In the controlled drug delivery field, open loop systems are known as pulsatile or externally regulated. The externally controlled devices apply external triggers for pulsatile delivery such as magnetic, ultrasonic, thermal, or electric irradiation.

Closed loop control systems, on the other hand, are defined as systems where the controlled variable is detected and as a result the system output is adjusted accordingly. Closed loop systems are known as self-regulated in the controlled drug delivery field. In the self-regulated devices the release rate is controlled by feedback information, without any external intervention, as is demonstrated in Fig. 1b. The self-regulated systems utilize several approaches for the rate control mechanisms, such as pH-sensitive polymers, enzyme–substrate reactions, pH-sensitive drug solubility, competitive binding, antibody interactions, and metal concentration–dependent hydrolysis.

Many approaches for mimicking the physiological healthy state are undergoing research. The focus of this review is on smart polymers; therefore, other important work such as using pumps for controlled drug delivery or the microencapsulation of living cells is not covered. This chapter outlines the fundamental principles of both pulsatile and self-regulated systems for drug delivery.

II. PULSATILE SYSTEMS

A. Magnetically Stimulated Systems

1. Feasibility

Drug molecules and magnetic beads are uniformly distributed within a solid polymeric matrix in magnetically triggered systems. Although drug is released by diffusion when the device is exposed to fluids, a much higher release rate is obtained in the presence of an external oscillating magnetic field. The magnetic system was characterized in vitro (4–6). Subsequent in vivo (7) studies showed that when polymeric matrices, made of ethylene–vinyl acetate copolymer (EVAc) containing insulin and magnetic beads, were placed subcutaneously in diabetic rats for 2 months, glucose levels can be repeatedly and reproducibly decreased on demand by application of an oscillating magnetic field.

2. Mechanisms

The two principle parameters controlling the release rates in these systems are the magnetic field characteristics and the mechanical properties of the polymer matrix. It was found that when the frequency of the applied field was increased from 5 to 11 Hz, the release rate of bovine serum albumin (BSA) from EVAc copolymer matrices rose in a linear fashion (4). Saslawski et al. (8) investigated the effect of magnetic field frequency and repeated field application on insulin release from alginate matrices and found that with repeated applications inverse effects can occur: high frequencies gave a significant release enhancement for the second magnetic field application. Subsequent stimulation resulted in decreased enhancement due to the faster depletion at the high frequencies.

The mechanical properties of the polymeric matrix also affect the extent of magnetic enhancement (4). For example, the modulus of elasticity of the EVAc copolymer can be easily altered by changing the vinyl acetate content of the copolymer. The release rate enhancement induced by the magnetic field increases as the modulus of elasticity of EVAc decreases. A similar phenomenon was observed for the crosslinked alginate matrices: higher release rate enhancement for less rigid matrices (8). Edelman et al. (9) also showed that enhanced release rates observed in response to an electromagnetic field (50 G, 60 Hz) applied for 4 min were independent of the duration of the interval between repeated pulses.

B. Ultrasonically Stimulated Systems

1. Feasibility

Release rates of substances can be repeatedly modulated at will from a position external to the delivery system by ultrasonic irradiation (10). Both bioerodible and nonerodible polymers were used as drug carrier matrices.

The bioerodible polymers evaluated were polyglycolide, polylactide, poly[bis(p-carboxyphenoxy)]alkane anhydrides and their copolymers with sebacic acid. Both the polymer erosion and drug release rates were enhanced when the bioerodible samples were exposed to ultrasound. The system's response to the ultrasonic triggering was rapid (within 2 min) and reversible. The releasing agents p-nitroaniline, p-aminohippurate, BSA, and insulin were tested for integrity following exposure to ultrasonic energy and were found to be intact.

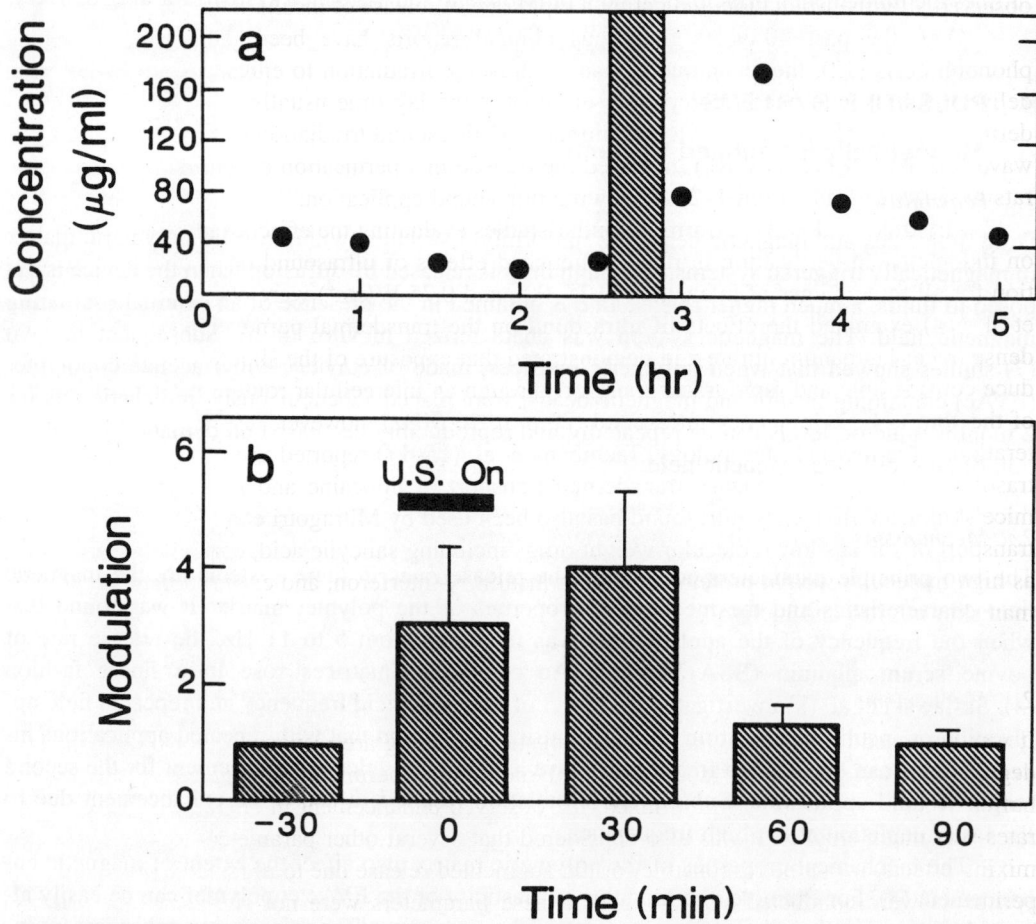

Figure 2 (a) Paraaminohippuric acid (PAH) concentration in the urine of Sprague-Dawley rats as a function of time before, during, and after 20 min exposure to ultrasound (hatched area). (b) Modulation vs. time expressed as a mean and standard deviation of four experimental rats. (Modulation was defined as the ratio of PAH concentration during and after ultrasound exposure to the mean of the PAH concentration prior to exposure) (10).

The enhanced release was also observed in nonerodible systems exposed to ultrasound where the release is diffusion-dependent. Release rates of zinc bovine insulin from EVAc copolymer matrices were 15 times higher when exposed to ultrasound compared to the unexposed periods.

In vivo studies (10) have suggested the feasibility of ultrasound-mediated drug release enhancement. Implants composed of polyanhydride polymers loaded with 10% para-aminohippuric acid (PAH) were implanted subcutaneously in the back of catheterized rats. When exposed to ultrasound, a significant increase in the PAH concentration in urine was detected (400%) (Figure 2). Rat's skin histopathology of the ultrasound treated area after an exposure of 1 h at 5 W/cm^2 did not reveal any differences between treated and untreated skin.

Similar phenomena were observed by Miyazaki et al. (11) who evaluated the effect of ultrasound (1 MHz) on the release rates of insulin from ethylene–vinyl alcohol copolymer matrices and reservoir-type drug delivery systems. When diabetic rats, receiving implants containing insulin, were exposed to ultrasound (1 W/cm^2 for 30 min) a sharp drop in blood glucose levels was observed after the irradiation, indicating a rapid rate of release of insulin in the implanted site.

Over the past 40 years numerous clinical reports have been published concerning phonophoresis (12), the technique of using ultrasonic irradiation to enhance transdermal drug delivery. Ultrasound nearly completely eliminated the lag time usually associated with transdermal delivery of drugs. Three to five minutes of ultrasound irradiation (1.5 W/cm^2 continuous wave or 3 W/cm^2 pulsed wave) increased the transdermal permeation of inulin and mannitol in rats by 5- to 20-fold within 1–2 h following ultrasound application.

Miyazaki et al. (13) performed similar studies evaluating the effect of ultrasound (1 MHz) on indomethacin permeation in rats. Pronounced effects of ultrasound on transdermal absorption for all three ranges of intensities (0.25, 0.5, and 0.75 W/cm^2) were observed. Bommannan et al. (14) examined the effects of ultrasound on the transdermal permeation of the electron-dense tracer lanthanum nitrate and demonstrated that exposure of the skin to ultrasound can induce considerable and rapid tracer transport through an intercellular route. Prolonged exposure of the skin to high-frequency ultrasound (20 min, 16 MHz), however, resulted in structural alterations of epidermal morphology. Tachibana et al. (15–17) reported use of low-frequency ultrasound (48 KHz) to enhance transdermal transport of lidocaine and insulin across hairless mice skin. Low-frequency ultrasound has also been used by Mitragotri et al. (18,19) to enhance transport of various low molecular weight drugs including salicylic acid, corticosterone, as well as high molecular weight proteins including insulin, γ-interferon, and erythropoietin across human skin in vitro and in vivo.

2. Mechanisms

It was proposed (10) that cavitation and acoustic streaming are responsible for the augmented degradation and release of bioerodible polymers. In experiments conducted in a degassed buffer, where cavitation was minimized, the observed enhancement in degradation and release rates was much smaller. It was also considered that several other parameters (temperature and mixing effects) might be responsible for the augmented release due to ultrasound. However, experiments were conducted suggesting that these parameters were not significant. It has also been demonstrated that the extent of release rate enhancement can be regulated by the intensity, frequency, or duty cycle of the ultrasound.

Miyakazi et al. (11) speculate that the ultrasound caused increased temperatures in their delivery system, which may facilitate diffusion.

Mitragotri et al. (20) evaluated the role played by various ultrasound-related phenomena, including cavitation, thermal effects, generation of convective velocities, and mechanical effects during phonophoresis. The authors' experimental findings suggest that among all the ultrasound-related phenomena evaluated, cavitation plays the dominant role in sonophoresis using therapeutic ultrasound (frequency, 1–3 MHz, intensity 0–2 W/cm^2). Confocal microscopy results indicate that cavitation occurs in the keratinocytes of the stratum corneum upon ultrasound exposure. The authors hypothesized that oscillations of the cavitation bubbles induce disorder in the stratum corneum lipid bilayers, thereby enhancing transdermal transport. The theoretical model developed to describe the effect of ultrasound on transdermal transport predicts that sonophoretic enhancement depends most directly on the passive permeant diffusion coefficient in water and not on the permeant diffusion coefficient through the skin.

C. Electrically Stimulated Systems

1. Feasibility

Electrically controlled systems provide drug release by the action of an applied electric field on a rate-limiting membrane and/or directly on the solute, thus controlling its transport across the membrane. The electrophoretic migration of a charged macrosolute within a hydrated membrane results from the combined response to the electrical forces on the solute and its associated counterions in the adjacent electrolyte solution (21).

Electrically controlled membrane permeability has also been of interest in the field of electrically controlled or enhanced transdermal drug delivery (e.g., iontophoresis, electroporation) (22,23).

Anionic gels as vehicles for electrically modulated drug delivery were studied by Hsu and Block (24). Agarose and a combination of agarose with anionic polymers (polyacrylic acid; xanthan gum) were evaluated. The authors conclude that the use of carbomer (polyacrylic acid) in conjunction with agarose enables the formulator to achieve zero-order release with electrical application. Increased anisotropicity of a gel system due to the application of electrical current could alter the effectiveness of the drug delivery system.

D'Emanuele and Staniforth (25) proposed a drug delivery device consisting of a polymer reservoir with a pair of electrodes placed across the rate-limiting membrane. By altering the magnitude of the electric field between the electrodes the authors proposed to modulate the drug release rates in a controlled and predictable manner. A linear relationship was found between current and propanolol HCl permeability through poly(2-hydroxyethyl methacrylate) (PHEMA) membranes crosslinked with ethylene glycol dimethacrylate (1% v/v). Buffer ionic strength, drug reservoir concentration, as well as electrode polarity were found to have significant effects on drug permeability (26).

Labhasetwar et al. (27) propose a similar approach for cardiac drug delivery modulation. The authors studied a cardiac drug implant in dogs that is capable of electric current modulation. Cation exchange membrane was used as an electrically sensitive rate-limiting barrier on the cardiac-contacting surface of the implant. The cardiac implant demonstrated in vitro drug release rates that were responsive to current modulation. In vivo results in dogs have confirmed that electrical modulation resulted in regional coronary enhancement of the drug levels with current responsive increase in drug concentration.

A different approach for electrochemical controlled release is based on polymers that bind and release bioactive compounds in response to an electric signal (28). The polymer has two redox states, only one of which is suitable for ion binding. Drug ions are bound in one redox state and released from the other. The attached electrodes serve to switch the redox states and the amount of current passed can control the amount of ions released.

Hepel and Fijalek (29) propose to use this method of electrochemical pulse stimulation on a novel composite polpyrrole film for delivery of cationic drugs directly to the central nervous system (CNS).

2. Mechanisms

Grimshaw (30) reported four different mechanisms for the transport of proteins and neutral solutes across hydrogel membranes: (a) electrically and chemically induced swelling of a membrane to alter the effective pore size and permeability; (b) electrophoretic augmentation of solute flux within a membrane; (c) electrosmotic augmentation of solute flux within a membrane; and (d) electrostatic partitioning of charged solutes into charged membranes.

Kwon et al. (31) studied the effect of electric current on solute release from crosslinked poly(2-acrylamido-2-methylpropanesulfonic acid-co-n-butylmethacrylate). Edrophonium chloride, a positively charged solute, was released in an on–off pattern from a matrix (monolithic) device by an electric field. The mechanism was explained as an ion exchange between positive solute and hydroxonium ion, followed by fast release of the charged solute from the hydrogel. The fast release was attributed to the electrostatic force, the squeezing effect, and the electroosmosis of the gel. However, the release of neutral solute was controlled by diffusion effected by swelling and deswelling of the gel.

D. Photostimulated Systems

1. Feasibility

Photoinduced phase transition of gels was reported by Mamada et al. (32). Copolymer gels of N-isopropylacrylamide and the photosensitive molecule bis(4-dimethylaminophenyl) (4-vinylphenyl)methyl leucocyanide showed a discontinuous volume phase transition upon UV irradiation, caused by osmotic pressure of cyanide ions created by the UV irradiation.

Yui et al. (33) proposed photoresponsive degradation of heterogeneous hydrogels composed of crosslinked hyaluronic acid and lipid microspheres for temporal drug delivery. Visible light induced degradation of crosslinked hyaluronic acid gels by photochemical oxidation using methylene blue as the photosensitizer. [The hyaluronic acid gels were also proposed by the authors to be inflammation-responsive (34).]

2. Mechanisms

Photoresponsive gels reversibly change their physical or chemical properties upon photoradiation. A photoresponsive polymer consists of a photoreceptor, usually a photochromic chromophore, and a functional part. The optical signal is captured by the photochromic molecules and then the isomerization of the chromophores in the photoreceptor converts it to a chemical signal.

Suzuki and Tanaka (35) reported a phase transition in polymer gels induced by visible light, where the transition mechanism is due only to the direct heating of the network polymer by light.

III. SELF-REGULATED SYSTEMS

A. Environmentally Responsive Systems

Polymers that alter their characteristics in response to changes in their environment have been of great recent interest. Several research groups have been developing drug delivery systems based on these responsive polymers that more closely resemble the normal physiological process. In these devices drug delivery is regulated by means of an interaction with the surrounding environment (feedback information) without any external intervention. The most commonly studied polymers having environmental sensitivity are either pH- or temperature-sensitive; there are also inflammation-sensitive systems.

1. Temperature-Sensitive Systems

Temperature-sensitive polymers can be classified into two groups based on the origin of the thermosensitivity in aqueous media. The first is based on polymer–water interactions, especially specific hydrophobic/hydrophilic balancing effects and the configuration of side groups. The other is based on polymer–polymer interactions in addition to polymer–water interactions. When polymer networks swell in a solvent, there is usually a negligible or small positive enthalpy of mixing or dilution. Although a positive enthalpy change opposes the process, the large gain in the entropy drives it. In aqueous polymer solutions the opposite is often observed. This unusual behavior is associated with a phenomenon of polymer phase separation as the temperature is raised to a critical value, known as the lower critical solution temperature (LCST). N-Alkyl acrylamide homopolymers and their copolymers, including acidic or basic comonomers, show this LCST (36,37). Polymers characterized by LCST usually shrink, as the temperature is increased through the LCST. Lowering the temperature below LCST results in the swelling of the polymer. Bioactive agents such as drugs, enzymes, and antibodies may be immobilized on or in the temperature-sensitive polymers. Examples of such utilizations will be discussed below. Responsive drug release patterns regulated by temperature changes have been recently demonstrated by several groups (36,40–49).

2. pH-Sensitive Systems

The pH range of fluids in various segments of the gastrointestinal tract may provide environmental stimuli for responsive drug release. Studies by several research groups (50–62) have been performed on polymers containing weakly acidic or basic groups in the polymeric backbone. The charge density of the polymers depends on pH and ionic composition of the outer solution (the solution into which the polymer is exposed). Altering the pH of the solution will cause swelling or deswelling of the polymer. Thus drug release from devices made from these polymers will display release rates that are pH-dependent. Polyacidic polymers will be unswollen at low pH, since the acidic groups will be protonated and hence un-ionized. With increasing pH, polyacid polymers will swell. The opposite holds for polybasic polymers, since the ionization of the basic groups will increase with decreasing pH. Siegel et al. (63) found that the swelling properties of the polybasic gels are also influenced by buffer composition (concentration and pK_a). A practical consequence proposed is that these gels may not reliably mediate pH-sensitive swelling–controlled release in oral applications, since the levels of buffer acids in the stomach (where swelling and release are expected to occur) generally cannot be controlled. However, the gels may be useful as mediators of pH-triggered release when precise rate control is of secondary importance.

Annaka and Tanaka (51) reported that more than two phases (swollen and collapsed) can be found in gels consisting of copolymers of randomly distributed positively and negatively charged groups. In these gels, polymer segments interact with each other through attractive or repulsive electrostatic interactions and through hydrogen bonding. The combination of these forces seems to result in the existence of several phases, each characterized by a distinct degree of swelling, with abrupt jumps between them. The existence of these phases presumably reflects the ability of macromolecular systems to adopt different stable conformations in response to changes in environmental conditions. For copolymer gels prepared from acrylic acid (the anionic constituent) and methacrylamidopropyltrimethylammonium chloride (460 mmol/240 mmol) the largest number of phases was seven. A similar approach was proposed by Bell and Peppas (61); membranes made from grafted poly(methacrylic acid-g-ethylene glycol) copolymer showed pH sensitivity due to complex formation and dissociation. Uncomplexed equilibrium swelling ratios were 40–90 times higher than those of complexed states and varied according to copolymer composition and polyethylene glycol graft length.

Giannos et al. (64) proposed temporally controlled drug delivery systems, coupling pH oscillators with membrane diffusion properties. By changing the pH of a solution relative to the pK_a, a drug may be rendered charged or uncharged. Since only the uncharged form of a drug can permeate lipophilic membranes, a temporally modulated delivery profile may be obtained with a pH oscillator in the donor solution.

Heller and Trescony (65) were the first to propose the use of pH-sensitive bioerodible polymers. In their approach, described in the section on systems utilizing enzymes, an enzyme–substrate reaction produces a pH change that is used to modulate the erosion of pH-sensitive polymer containing a dispersed therapeutic agent.

Bioerodible hydrogels containing azoaromatic moieties were synthesized by Ghandehari et al. (66). Hydrogels with lower crosslinking density underwent a surface erosion process and degraded at a faster rate. Hydrogels with higher crosslinking densities degraded at a slower rate by a process whereby the degradation front moved inward to the center of the polymer.

Recently, recombinant DNA methods were used to create artificial proteins that undergo reversible gelation in response to changes in pH or temperature (67). The proteins consist of terminal leucine zipper domains flanking a central, flexible, water-soluble polyelectrolyte segment. Formation of coiled-coil aggregates of the terminal domains in near-neutral aqueous solutions triggers formation of a three-dimensional polymer network, with the polyelectrolyte segment retaining solvent and preventing precipitation of the chain. Dissociation of the coiled-coil aggregates through elevation of pH or temperature causes dissolution of the gel and a return to the viscous behavior that is characteristic of polymer solutions. The authors suggest that these hydrogels have potential in bioengineering applications requiring encapsulation or controlled release of molecules and cellular species.

3. Inflammation-Responsive Systems

Yui et al. (34) proposed an inflammation-responsive drug delivery system based on biodegradable hydrogels of crosslinked hyaluronic acid. Hyaluronic acid is specifically degraded by hydroxyl radicals, which are produced by phagocytic cells such as leukocytes and macrophages, locally at inflammatory sites. In their approach drug-loaded lipid microspheres were dispersed in degradable matrices of crosslinked hyaluronic acid.

B. Systems Utilizing Specific Binding Interactions

All of the following drug delivery systems utilize a specific binding interaction to manipulate the microenvironment of the device and thus modulate the rate of drug release from the polymer. Basic principles of binding and competitive binding are the underlying mechanism of function of these systems. Note that due to the vast amount of literature on the subject, glucose-responsive insulin delivery systems will be discussed in a separate section.

1. Systems Utilizing Antibody Interactions

Pitt et al. (68) proposed utilizing hapten–antibody interactions to suppress enzymatic degradation and permeability of polymeric reservoirs or matrix drug delivery systems. The delivery device consists of naltrexone contained in a polymeric reservoir or dispersed in a polymeric matrix configuration. The device is coated by covalently grafting morphine to the surface. Exposure of the grafted surface to antibodies to morphine results in coating of the surface by the antibodies, a process that can be reversed by exposure to exogenous morphine. The presence of the antibodies on the surface or in the pores of the delivery device will block or impede the permeability of naltrexone in a reservoir configuration or enzyme-catalyzed surface degradation and concomitant release of the drug from a matrix device. A similar approach was proposed for responsive release of a contraceptive agent. The β subunit of human chorionic gonadotropin (HCG) is grafted to the surface of the polymer, which is then exposed to antibodies to β-HCG. The appearance of HCG in the circulatory system (indication of pregnancy) will cause release of a contraceptive drug. (HCG competes for the polymer-bound antibodies to HCG and initiates release of the contraceptive drug.)

Pitt et al. (68,69) also proposed a hypothetical reversible antibody system for controlled release of ethinyl estradiol (EE). EE stimulates biosynthesis of sex hormone–binding globulin (SHBG). High serum levels of EE stimulate the production of SHBG, which increases the concentration of SHBG bound to the polymer surface and reduces the EE release rate. When the EE serum level falls, the SHBG level falls, as does binding of the SHBG to the polymer surface, producing an automatic increase in the EE release rate.

2. Systems Utilizing Chelation

Self-regulated delivery of drugs that function by chelation was also suggested (70). These include certain antibiotics and drugs for the treatment of arthritis, as well as chelators used for the treatment of metal poisoning. The concept is based on the ability of metals to accelerate the hydrolysis of carboxylate or phosphate esters and amides by several orders of magnitude. Attachment of the chelator to a polymer chain by a covalent ester or amide link serves to prevent its premature loss by excretion and reduces its toxicity. In the presence of the specific ion, a complex with the bound chelating agent will form, followed by metal-accelerated hydrolysis and subsequent elimination of the chelated metal. Measurement of the rates of hydrolysis of polyvinyl alcohol coupled with quinaldic acid chelator (PVA-QA) in the presence of Co (II), Zn(II), Cu(II), and Ni(II) confirmed that it is possible to retain the susceptibility of the esters to metal-promoted hydrolysis in a polymer environment.

3. Systems Utilizing Enzymes

In this approach, the mechanism is based on an enzymatic reaction. One possible approach studied is an enzyme reaction that results in a pH change and a polymer system that can respond to that change.

a. Urea-Responsive Delivery. Heller et al. (65) were the first to attempt using immobilized enzymes to alter local pH and thus cause changes in polymer erosion rates. The proposed system is based on the conversion of urea to NH_4HCO_3 and NH_4OH by the action of urease. As this reaction causes a pH increase, a polymer that is subjected to increased erosion at high pH is required.

The authors suggested a partially esterified copolymer of methyl vinyl ether and maleic anhydride. This polymer displays release rates that are pH-dependent. The polymer dissolves by ionization of the carboxylic acid group. The pH-sensitive polymer containing dispersed hydrocortisone is surrounded by urease immobilized in a hydrogel prepared by crosslinking a mixture of urease and BSA with glutaraldehyde. When urea diffuses into the hydrogel, its interaction with the enzyme leads to a pH increase, resulting in enhanced erosion of the pH-sensitive polymer with concomitant changes in the release rate of hydrocortisone.

Figure 3 shows release of hydrocortisone from the described device. Although the device has no therapeutic relevance, it established the feasibility of creating a self-responsive delivery system.

Ishihara et al. (71,72) suggested a nonerodible system based on a similar idea. The system comprises a pH-sensitive membrane, by copolymerizing 4-carboxyacrylanilide with methacrylate, sandwiched within a membrane containing urease immobilized in free radically crosslinked N,N-methylenebisacrylamide. The permeation of a model substance [1,4-bis(2-hydroxyethoxy)benzene] varied with the urea concentration in the external solution.

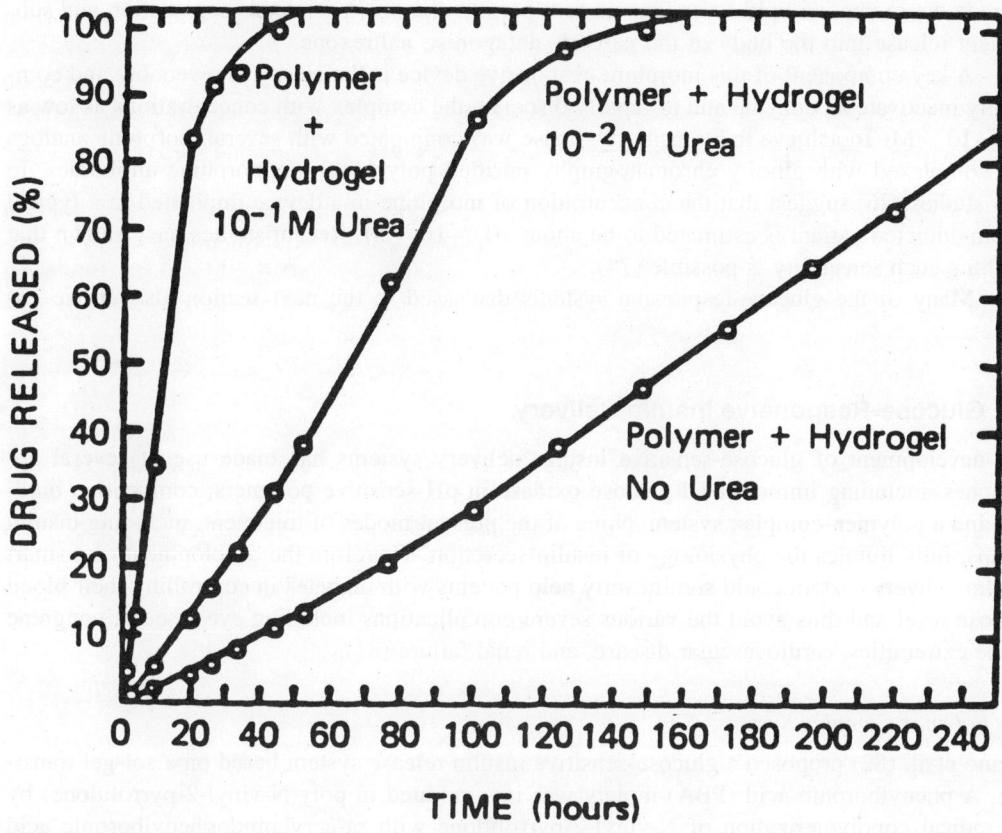

Figure 3 Hydrocortisone release from the N-hexyl ester of methyl vinyl ether and maleic anhydride disks coated with immobilized urease, in the presence and absence of external urea, 35°C, pH 6.25, hydrocortisone loading 10 wt % (65).

b. Morphine-Triggered Naltrexone Delivery System. Heller and co-workers [73–80] have been developing a naltrexone drug delivery system that would be passive until drug release is initiated by the appearance of morphine external to the device. Naltrexone is a long-acting opiate antagonist that blocks opiate-induced euphoria, and thus the intended use of this device is in the treatment of heroin addiction. Activation is based on the reversible inactivation of enzymes achieved by the covalent attachment of hapten close to the active site of the enzyme-hapten conjugate with the hapten antibody. Because the antibodies are large molecules, access of the substrate to the enzyme's active site is sterically inhibited, thus effectively rendering the enzyme inactive. Triggering of drug release is initiated by the appearance of morphine (hapten) in the tissue and dissociation of the enzyme–heptan–antibody complex rendering the enzyme active. This approach is being developed by incorporating the naltrexone in a bioerodible polymer. The polymer matrix is then covered by a lipid layer that prevents water entry, thus preventing its degradation and therefore the release of naltroxane. The system is placed in a dialysis bag. The bag contains lipase (enzyme) that is covalently attached to morphine and reversibly inactivated by antimorphine complexation. Thus, when morphine is present in the tissues surrounding the device, morphine diffuses into the dialysis bag and displaces the lipase-morphine conjugate from the antibody, allowing the now activated enzyme to degrade the protective lipid layer. This in turn permits the polymeric core degradation and subsequent release into the body of the narcotic antagonist, naltrexone.

A key component of this morphine-responsive device is the ability to reversibly and completely inactivate an enzyme and to rapidly disociate the complex with concentrations as low as 10^{-8}–10^{-9} M. To achieve this sensitivity, lipase was conjugated with several morphine analogs and complexed with affinity chromatography purified polyclonal antimorphine antibodies. In vivo studies (76) suggest that the concentration of morphine in a device implanted in a typical heroin-addicted patient is estimated to be about 10^{-7}–10^{-8} M. Recent studies have shown that reaching such sensitivity is possible (74).

Many of the glucose-responsive systems discussed in the next section also utilize enzymes.

C. Glucose-Responsive Insulin Delivery

The development of glucose-sensitive insulin delivery systems has made use of several approaches, including immobilized glucose oxidase in pH-sensitive polymers, competitive binding, and a polymer–complex system. None of the present modes of treatment, including insulin pumps, fully mimics the physiology of insulin secretion. Therefore the development of a smart insulin delivery system could significantly help patients with diabetes in controlling their blood glucose level and thus avoid the various severe complications including eye disease, gangrene of the extremities, cardiovascular disease, and renal failure (81).

1. Polymer Complex System

Kitano et al. (82) proposed a glucose-sensitive insulin release system based on a sol-gel transition. A phenylboronic acid (PBA) moiety was incorporated in poly(N-vinyl-2-pyrrolidone) by the radical copolymerization of N-vinyl-2-pyrrolidone with m-acrylamidophenylboronic acid (poly(NVP-co-PBA)). Insulin was incorporated into a polymer gel formed by a complex of poly(vinyl alcohol) with poly(NVP-co-PBA). PBA can form reversible covalent complexes with molecules having diol units, such as glucose or PVA. With the addition of glucose PVA in the PVA–boronate complex is replaced by glucose. This leads to a transformation of the system from gel to sol state facilitating the release of insulin from the polymeric complex. The same group (83) modified the approach suggesting glucose-responsive gels based on the complexation between polymers having phenylboronic acid groups and PVA. The introduction of an amino group into phenylborate polymers was effective for increasing the complexation ability and the glucose responsivity at physiological pH.

Shiino et al. (84) attached gluconic acids to insulin. The modified insulin, containing two gluconic acid units per insulin (G-Ins), was bound to a PBA gel column and the G-Ins release profile in response to varying concentrations of glucose was studied. Concentration of released G-Ins from PBA gel responded to concentration changes of the eluting glucose. These polymeric complexes have been applied as interpenetrating polymer networks to achieve pulsatile insulin release in response to glucose concentration changes.

2. Competitive Binding

The basic principle of competitive binding and its application to controlled drug delivery was first presented by Brownlee and Cerami (85) who suggested the preparation of glycosylated insulins, which are complementary to the major combining site of carbohydrate-binding proteins such as concanavalin A (Con A). Con A is immobilized on Sepharose beads. The glycosylated insulin, which is biologically active, is displaced from the Con A by glucose in response to, and proportional to, the amount of glucose present which competes for the same binding sites. Kim et al. (86–93) found that the release rate of insulin also depends on the binding affinity of an insulin derivative to the Con A and can be influenced by the choice of saccharide group in glycosylated insulin. By encapsulating the glycosylated insulin-bound Con A with a suitable polymer that is permeable to both glucose and insulin, the glucose influx and insulin efflux would be controlled by the encapsulation membrane.

It was found (87) that the glycosylated insulins are more stable against aggregation than commercial insulin and are also biologically active. The functionality of the intraperitoneally implanted device was tested in pancreatectomized dogs by an intravenous glucose tolerance test (IVGTT). The effect of an administered 500 mg/kg dextrose bolus on blood glucose level was compared with normal and pancreatectomized dogs without an implant. Figure 4 shows the results of this study (92). In addition, the blood glucose profile for a period of 2 days demonstrated that a diabetic dog, implanted with the self-regulating insulin delivery system, was capable of maintaining acceptable glucose levels (50–180 mg/dL) for the majority of the experiment (40 h) (89–91). Makino et al. (86) proposed a modification based on hydrophilic nylon microcapsules containing Con A and succinylamidophenylglucopyranoside insulin. The thin wall of these microcapsules and large surface area resulted in rapid diffusion of glucose and glycosylated insulin, and therefore a much shorter lag time.

In order to limit the leakage of Con A (which is toxic) and allow preparation of porous microspheres, Pai et al. (99) crosslinked the Con A by first blocking the sugar binding sites and then reacting with glutaraldehyde. The porous microspheres demonstrated a rapid exchange between succinylamidophenylglucopyranoside insulin and glucose, with a short response time.

Kokufata et al. (94) reported a gel system that swells and shrinks in response to specific saccharides. The gel consists of a covalently crosslinked polymer network of N-isopropylacrylamide

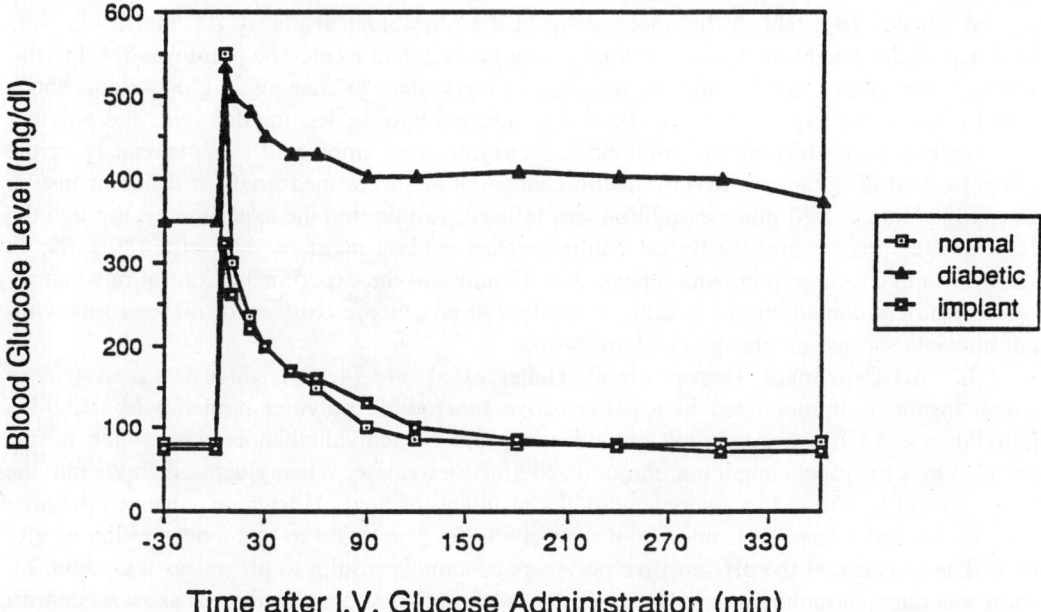

Figure 4 Peripheral blood glucose profiles of dogs administered bolus dextrose (500 mg/kg) during an intravenous glucose tolerance test. Blood glucose levels at t = −30 min show the overnight fasting level 30 min prior to bolus injection of dextrose (93).

in which the lecitin, Con A, is immobilized. Con A displays selective binding affinities for certain saccharides. For example, when the saccharide dextran sulfate is added to the gel, it swells to a volume up to fivefold the original volume. Replacing dextran sulfate with nonionic saccharide α-methyl-D-mannopyranoside brings about collapse of the gel, back almost to its native volume. The process is reversible and repeatable.

Taylor et al. (95) proposed a similar approach for the delivery of insulin. The self-regulating delivery device, responsive to glucose, has been shown to operate in vitro. The device comprises a reservoir of insulin and a gel membrane that determines the delivery rates of insulin. The gel consists of a synthetic polysucrose and lectin, Con A. The mechanism is one of displacement of the branched polysaccharide from the lectin receptors by incoming glucose. The gel loses its high viscosity as a result, but reforms upon removal of glucose, thus providing the rate-controlling barrier for the diffusion of insulin or any other antihyperglycemic drugs.

A very similar approach was also presented by Park et al. (96–98) who synthesized glucose-sensitive membranes based on the interaction between polymer-bound glucose and Con A.

3. Immobilized Glucose Oxidase in pH-Sensitive Polymers

Responsive drug delivery systems based on pH-sensitive polymers have been developed along three different approaches: pH-dependent swelling, degradation, and solubility.

a. pH-Dependent Solubility. Glucose-dependent insulin release was proposed by Langer and co-workers (100–102) based on the fact that insulin solubility is pH-dependent. Insulin was incorporated into EVAc copolymer matrices in solid form. Thus, the release was governed by its dissolution and diffusion rates. Glucose oxidase was immobilized to Sepharose beads which were incorporated along with insulin into EVAc matrices. When glucose entered the matrix, the produced gluconic acid caused a rise in insulin solubility and consequently enhanced release. To establish this mechanism in the physiological pH of 7.4, the insulin was modified by three additional lysine groups so that the resultant isoelectric point was 7.4. In vitro and in vivo studies demonstrated the response of the system to changes in glucose concentration. In the in vivo experiments a catheter was inserted into the left jugular vein, and polymer matrices containing insulin and immobilized enzyme were implanted subcutaneously in the lower back of diabetic rats. Serum insulin concentrations were measured for different insulin matrix implants. A 2 M glucose solution was infused, 15 min into the experiments, through the catheter. Rats that received trilysine insulin/glucose oxidase matrices showed a 180% rise in serum insulin concentration, which peaked at 45 min into the experiment. Control rats that received matrices containing no insulin, or insulin but no glucose oxidase, or diabetic rats without implants showed no change in serum insulin.

b. pH-Dependent Degradation. Heller et al. (73,74,103) suggested a system in which insulin is immobilized in a pH-sensitive bioerodible polymer prepared from 3,9-bis [ethylidene-2,4,8,10-tetraoxaspirol(5,5)undecane] and N-methyldiethanolamine, which is surrounded by a hydrogel containing immobilized glucose oxidase. When glucose diffuses into the hydrogel and is oxidized to gluconic acid, the resultant lowered pH triggers enhanced polymer degradation and release of insulin from the polymer in proportion to the concentration of glucose. The response of the pH-sensitive polymers containing insulin to pH pulses was rapid. Insulin was released rapidly when the pH decreased from 7.4 to 5.0. Insulin release was shut off when the pH increased. The amount of insulin released showed dependence on the pH change. However, when the in vitro studies were repeated in physiological buffer, response of the device was only minimal, even at very low pH pulses. The authors found that the synthesized amine containing polymer undergoes general acid catalysis where the catalyzing species is not hydronium ion but rather the specific buffer molecules used. Therefore, further development of this system will require the development of a bioerodible polymer that not only has adequate pH sensitivity but also undergoes specific ion catalysis.

c. **pH-Dependent Swelling.** Systems based on pH-sensitive polymers consist of immobilized glucose oxidase in a pH-responsive hydrogel, enclosing a saturated insulin solution or incorporated with insulin (104–112). As glucose diffuses into the hydrogel, glucose oxidase catalyzes its conversion to gluconic acid, thereby lowering the pH in the microenvironment of the hydrogel and causing swelling (Fig. 5). Since insulin should permeate the swelled hydrogel more rapidly, faster delivery of insulin in the presence of glucose is anticipated. As the glucose concentration decreases in response to the released insulin, the hydrogel should contract and decrease the rate of insulin delivery.

Horbett and co-workers (104–111) immobilized glucose oxidase in a crosslinked hydrogel made from N,N-dimethylaminoethyl methacrylate (DMA), hydroxyethyl methacrylate (HEMA), and tetraethylene glycol dimethacrylate (TEGDMA). Membranes were prepared at −70°C by radiation polymerization, previously shown to retain the enzymatic activity (113). To obtain sufficient insulin permeability through the gels, porous HEMA/DMA gels were prepared by polymerization under conditions that induce a separation into two phases during polymerization: one phase rich in polymer and the other rich in solvent plus unreacted monomer. When gelation occurs after the phase separation, the areas where the solvent/monomer phase existed become fixed in place as pores in the polymer matrix. The authors used a dilute monomer solution in order to obtain a porous gel, typically 1–10 μm in diameter (105).

The rate of insulin permeation through the membranes was measured in the absence of glucose in a standard transport cell; then glucose was added to one side of the cell to a concentration of 400 mg/dL while the permeation measurement was continued. The results indicated that the insulin transport rate is enhanced significantly by the addition of glucose. The average

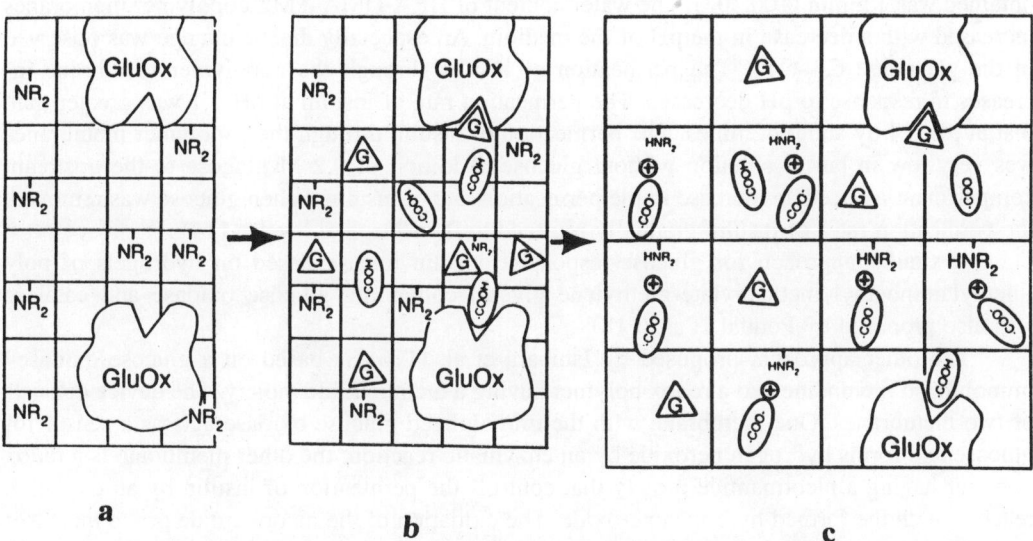

Figure 5 Mechanism of action of glucose-sensitive polymeric hydrogel. (a) In the absence of glucose, at physiologic pH, few of the amine groups are protonated. (b) In the presence of glucose, the glucose oxidase produces gluconic acid that can (c) protonate the amine groups. The fixed positive charge on the polymeric network led to electrostatic repulsion and membrane swelling, and therefore enhanced insulin release (111).

permeability after addition of 400 mg/dL glucose was 2.4–5.5 times higher than before glucose was added. When insulin permeabilities through the porous gels were measured in a flowing system, where permeabilities were measured with fluid flowing continuously past one side of the membrane, no effect of glucose concentration on insulin permeabilities could be detected. The authors propose that inappropriate design of the membranes used in the experiments is the explanation for their lack of response to glucose concentration (104).

A mathematical model describing these glucose-responsive hydrogels demonstrates two important points (104,105): (a) Progressive response to glucose concentration over a range of glucose concentrations can be achieved only with a sufficiently low glucose oxidase loading; otherwise, depletion of oxygen causes the system to become insensitive to glucose. (b) A significant pH decrease in the membrane, with resultant swelling, can be achieved only if the amine concentration is sufficiently low that pH changes are not prevented by the buffering of the amines.

While the great advantage of reservoir systems is the ease with which they can be designed to produce constant release rate kinetics, their main disadvantage are leaks, which are dangerous as all of the incorporated drug could be rapidly released. In attempt to overcome this problem, Goldraich and Kost (112) proposed incorporating the drug (insulin) and the enzyme (glucose oxidase) into the pH-responsive polymeric matrices.

Ishihara et al. (71,72,114–117) investigated two approaches for glucose responsive insulin delivery systems; one approach is similar to that investigated by Horbett et al. (110). The polymers were prepared from 2-hydroxyethyl acrylate (HEA)–N,N-dimethylaminoethyl methacrylate (DMA), 4-trimethylsilylstyrene (TMS), by radical polymerization of the corresponding monomers in dimethylformamide (DMF). The mole fractions of HEA, DMA, and TMS in the copolymer were 0.6, 0.2, and 0.2, respectively. Membranes were prepared by solvent casting. Capsules containing insulin and glucose oxidase were prepared by an interfacial precipitation method using gelatin as an emulsion stabilizer. The average diameter of the polymer capsules obtained was 1.5 mm (100,103). The water content of HEA-DMA-TMS copolymer membranes increased with a decrease in the pH of the medium. An especially drastic change was observed in the pH range 6.3–6.15. The permeation of insulin through the copolymer membrane increases in response to pH decreases. The permeation rate of insulin at pH 6.1 was greater than that at pH 6.4 by about 42 times. The permeation of insulin through the copolymer membranes was very low in buffer solution without glucose. Addition of 0.2 M glucose to the upstream compartment induced an increase in the permeation rate of insulin. When glucose was removed, the permeation rates of insulin gradually returned to their original levels (114).

A similar approach for glucose-responsive insulin release based on hydrogels of poly (diethylaminoethyl methacrylate-g-ethylene glycol) containing glucose oxidase and catalase was also proposed by Podual et al. (118).

The other approach, proposed by Ishihara et al. (116), is based on a glucose oxidase–immobilized membrane and a redox polymer having a nicotinamide moiety. The device consists of two membranes. One membrane with the immobilized glucose oxidase acts as a sensor for glucose and forms hydrogen peroxide by an enzymatic reaction; the other membrane is a redox polymer having a nicotinamide moiety that controls the permeation of insulin by an oxidation reaction with the formed hydrogen peroxide. The oxidation of the nicotinamide group increases hydrophilicity and therefore should enhance the permeability to water-soluble molecules such as insulin. The results showed relatively small increases in insulin permeability.

Iwata et al. (119,120) pretreated porous poly(vinylidene fluoride) membranes (average pore size 0.22 μm) by air plasma and subsequently acrylamide was graft-polymerized on the treated surface. The polyacrylamide was then hydrolyzed to poly(acrylic acid). In the pH range 5–7, grafted poly(acrylic acid) chains are solvated and dissolved, but cannot diffuse into the solution phase because they are grafted to the porous membrane. Thus they effectively close the membrane pores. In the pH range 1–5, the chains collapse and the permeability increases. To achieve the sensitivity of the system to glucose, glucose oxidase was immobilized onto a poly(2-hydroxyethyl methacrylate) gel.

Ito et al. (121) adopted the approach proposed by Iwata et al. (120) using a porous cellulose membrane with surface-grafted poly(acrylic acid) as a pH-sensitive membrane. By immobilization of glucose oxidase onto the poly(acrylic acid)–grafted cellulose membrane, it became responsive to glucose concentrations. The permeation coefficient after glucose addition was about 1.7 times that before the addition of glucose. The authors suggest improving the proposed system (sensitivity of insulin permeability to glucose concentrations) by modification of the graft chain: density, length, and size or density of pores.

Siegel and co-workers (122,123) proposed an implantable "mechanochemical" pump that functions by converting changes in blood glucose activity to a mechanical force, generated by the swelling polymer that pumps insulin out of the device.

More recently, Siegel (124) proposed self-regulating oscillatory drug delivery based on a polymeric membrane whose permeability to the substrate of an enzyme-catalyzed reaction is inhibited by the product of that reaction. This negative feedback system can, under certain conditions, lead to oscillations in membrane permeability and in the levels of substrate and product in the device. Any one of these oscillating variables can then be used to drive a cyclic delivery process. The product concentration in the chamber inhibitorily affects the permeability of the membrane to the substrate. That is, increasing product concentration causes decreasing flux of substrate into the device. Siegel proposed several means of controlled drug delivery based on this idea. Drug solubility could be affected by substrate or product concentration, which oscillates. Alternatively, the drug permeability of the membrane can oscillate with time along with the substrate permeability.

IV. CONCLUDING REMARKS

During the last three decades, polymeric controlled drug delivery has become an important area of research and development. In this short time, a number of systems displaying constant or decreasing release rates have progressed from the laboratory to the clinic and clinical products. Although these polymeric controlled delivery systems are advantageous compared to the conventional methods of drug administration, they are insensitive to the changing metabolic state. In order to more closely control the physiological requirements of the specific drugs, responsive mechanisms must be provided. The approaches discussed represent attempts conducted over the past two decades to achieve pulsatile release. It should be pointed out that these drug delivery systems are still in the developmental stage and much research will have to be conducted for such systems to become practical clinical alternatives. Critical considerations are the biocompatibility and toxicology of these multicomponent polymer-based systems, the response times of these systems to stimuli, the ability to provide practical levels of the desired drug, and addressing necessary formulation issues in dosage or design (e.g., shelf life, sterilization, reproducibility). A key issue in the practical utilization of the pulsatile, externally triggered systems (i.e., magnetic, ultrasound, electrically regulated, and photoresponsive) will be the design of small portable trigger units that the patient can use easily. Ideally, such systems could be worn by the patient, such as a wristwatch-like system, and either it could be preprogrammed to go on and off at specific times, or the patient could turn it on when needed. Critical issues in the development of responsive, self-regulated systems such as those containing enzymes or antibodies are the stability and/or potential leakage and possible immunogenicity of these bioactive agents. The successful development of responsive polymer delivery systems will be a significant challenge. Nevertheless, the considerable pharmacological benefit these systems could potentially provide, particularly given ongoing research in biotechnology, pharmacology, and medicine, which may provide new insights on the desirability and requirements for pulsatile release, should make this an important and fruitful area for future research.

REFERENCES

1. Shalaby, S. W., Hoffman, A. S., Ratner, B. D., and Horbett, T. A. (Eds), Polymers as Biomaterials. Plenum Press, New York (1984).
2. Langer, R., Drug delivery and targeting, Nature, 392, 5–10 (1998).
3. Kost, J., and Langer, R., Responsive polymeric delivery systems, Adv. Drug Deliv. Rev., 6, 19–50 (1991).
4. Kost, J., Noecker, R., Kunica, E., and Langer, R., Magnetically controlled-release systems: effect of polymer composition, J. Biomed. Mater. Res., 19, 935 (1986).
5. Edelman, E., Kost, J., Bobeck, H., and Langer, R., Regulation of drug release from polymer matrices by oscillating magnetic fields., J. Biomed. Mater. Res., 67 (1985).
6. Hsieh, D., Langer, R., and Folkman, J., Magnetic modulation of release of macromolecules from polymers., Proc. Natl. Acad. Sci. USA, 78, 1863 (1981).
7. Kost, J., Wolfrum, J., and Langer, R., Magnetically enhanced insulin release in diabetic rats., J. Biomed. Mater. Res., 21, 1367 (1987).
8. Saslawski, O., Couvrer, P., and Peppas, N., Alginate magnetic release systems: crosslinked structure, swelling and release studies. In: Controlled Release of Bioactive Materials, Heller. J, Harris, F., Lohmann, H., Merkle, H., and Robinson, J. (Eds.), Controlled Release Society, Basel, p. 26 (1988).
9. Edelman, E., Brown, L., Taylor, J., and Langer, R., In vitro and in vivo kinetics of regulated drug release from polymer matrices by oscillating magnetic fields, J. Biomed. Mater. Res., 21, 229 (1987).
10. Kost, J., Leong, K., and Langer, R., Ultrasound-enhanced polymer degradation and release of incorporated substances., Proc. Natl. Acad. Sci. USA, 86, 7663–7666 (1989).
11. Miyazaki, S., Yokouchi, C., and Takada, M., External control of drug release: controlled release of insulin from a hydrophilic polymer implants by ultrasound irradiation in diabetic rats, J. Pharm. Pharmacol., 40, 716–717 (1988).
12. Kost, J., Phonophoresis. In: Electronically Controlled Drug Delivery, Berner, B., and Dinh, S. (Eds.), CRC Press, Boca Raton (1998).
13. Miyazaki, S., Mizuoka, O., and Takada, M., External control of drug release and penetration: enhancement of the transdermal absorption of indomethacin by ultrasound irradiation, J. Pharm. Phrmacol., 43, 115–116 (1990).
14. Bommannan, D., Menon, G., Okuyama, H., Elias, P., and Guy, R., Sonophoresis II: Examination of the mechanism(s) of ultrasound-enhanced transdermal drug delivery., Pharm. Res., 9, 1043–1047 (1992).
15. Tachibana, K., Transdermal delivery of insulin to alloxan-diabetic rabits by ultrasound exposure, Pharm. Res., 9, 952–954 (1992).
16. Tachibana, K., and Tachibana, S., Use of ultrasound to enhance the local anesthetic effect of topically applied aqueous lidocaine, Anesthesiology, 78, 1091–1096 (1993).
17. Tachibana, K., and Tachibana, S., Transdermal delivery of insulin by ultrasonic vibration, J. Pharm. Pharmacol., 43, 270–271 (1991).
18. Mitragotri, S., Blankschtein, D., and Langer, R., Transdermal drug delivery using low-frequency sonophoresis, Pharm. Res., 13, 411–420 (1996).
19. Mitragotri, S., Blankschtein, D., and Langer, R., Ultrasound-mediated transdermal protein delivery, Science, 269, 850–853 (1995).

20. Mitragotri, S., Edwards, D., Blankschtein, D., and Langer, R., A mechanistic study of ultrasonically enhanced transdermal drug delivery, J. Pharm. Sci., 84, 697–706 (1995).
21. Grodzinsky, A. J., and Grimshaw, P. E., Electrically and chemically controlled hydrogels for drug delivery. In: Pulsed and Self-Regulated Drug Delivery, Kost, J. (Ed.), CRC Press, Boca Raton, pp. 47–64 (1990).
22. Prausnitz, M., Bose, R., Langer, R., and Weaver, J., Electroporation of mammalian skin: a new mechanism to enhance transdermal drug delivery, Proc. Natl. Acad. Sci. USA, 90, 10504–10508 (1993).
23. Rolf, D., Chemical and physical methods of enhancing transdermal drug delivery, Pharm. Technol., 12, 130–140 (1988).
24. Hsu, C., and Block, L., Anionic gels as vehicles for electrically-modulated drug delivery. I. Solvent and drug transport phenomena, Pharm. Res., 13, 1865–1870 (1996).
25. D'Emanuele, A., and Staniforth, J. N., An electrically modulated drug delivery device, Pharm. Res., 8, 913–918 (1991).
26. D'Emanuele, A., and Staniforth, J. N., An electrically modulated drug delivery device. II. Effect of ionic strength, drug concentration and temperature, Pharm. Res., 9, 215–219 (1992).
27. Labhasetwar, V., Underwood, T., Schwendemann, S., and Levy, R., Iontophoresis for modulation of cardiac drug delivery in dogs, Proc. Natl. Acad. Sci. USA, 92, 2612–2616 (1995).
28. Miller, L. L., Smith, G. A., Chang, A., and Zhou, Q., Electrochemically controlled release, J. Controlled Release, 6, 293–296 (1987).
29. Hepel, M. and Fijalek, Z, Electrorelease of drugs from composite polymer films. In: Polymeric Drugs and Drug Administration, (Raphael M. Offenbrite, Ed.), American Chemical Society, Washington, DC, pp. 79–97. (1994).
30. Grimshaw, P. E., Grodzinsky, A. J., Yarmush, M. L., and Yarmush, D. M., Dynamic membranes for protein transport: chemical and electrical control, Chem. Eng. Sci., 104, 827–840 (1989).
31. Kwon, I. C., Bae, Y. H., T., O., and Kim, S. W., Drug release from electric current sensitive polymers, J. Controlled Release, 17, 149–156 (1991).
32. Mamada, A., Tanaka, T., Kugwatchkakun, D., and Irie, M., Photoinduced phase transition of gels, Macromolecules, 23, 1517–1519 (1990).
33. Yui, N., Okano, T., and Sakurai, Y., Photo-responsive degradation of heterogeneous hydrogels comprising crosslinked hyaluronic acid and lipid microspheres for temporal drug delivery, J. Controlled Release, 26, 141–145 (1993).
34. Yui, N., Okano, T., and Sakurai, Y., Inflamation responsive degradation of crosslinked hyaluronic acid gel, J. Controlled Release, 22, 105–116 (1992).
35. Suzuki, A., and Tanaka, T., Phase transition in polymer geks induced by visible light, Nature, 346, 345–347 (1990).
36. Hoffman, A. S., Applications of thermally reversible polymers and hydrogels in therapeutics and diagnostics, J. Controlled Release, 6, 297–305 (1987).
37. Tanaka, T., Gels. In: Encyclopedia of Polymer Science and Technology, Vol. 7, Mark, H. F., and Kroschwotz, J. I. (Eds.), Wiley, New York, pp. 514–531 (1985).
38. Ueda, T., Ishihara, K., and Nakabayashi, N., Thermally responsive release of 5-fluorouracil from a biocompatible hydrogel membrane with phospholipid structure, Macromol. Chem. Rapid Commun., 11, 345 (1990).
39. Urry, D. W., Haynes, B., Zhang, H., Harris, R. D., and Prasad, K. U., Mechanochemical coupling in synthetic polypeptides by modulation of inverse temperature transition, Proc. Natl. Acad. Sci. USA, 85, 3407–3411 (1988).
40. Yoshida, M., Asano, M., Kumakura, M., Kataki, R., Mashimo, T., Yuasa, H., and Yamanaka, H., Thermo-responsive hydrogels based on acrylo-l-proline methyl ester and their use in long-acting testosterone delivery systems, Drug Design Deliv., 7, 159–174 (1991).
41. Palasis, M., and Gehrke, H., Permeability of responsive poly(N-isopropylacrylamide) gel to solutes, J. Controlled Release, 18, 1–12 (1992).
42. Okano, T., Bae, Y. H., and Kim, S. W., Temperature responsive controlled drug delivery. In: Pulsed and Self-Regulated Drug Delivery, Kost, J. (Ed.), CRC Press, Boca Raton, pp. 17–46 (1990).
43. Okahata, Y., Noguchi, H., and Seki, T., Thermo-selective permeation from a polymer-grafted capsule membrane, Macromolecules, 19, 493–494 (1986).

44. Katano, H., Maruyama, A., Sanui, K., Ogata, N., Okano, T., and Sakurai, Y., Thermoresponsive swelling and drug release switching of interpenetrating polymer networks composed of poly(acrylamide-co-butyl methacrylate) and poly(acrylic acid), J. Controlled Release, 16, 215–228 (1991).
45. Vakalanka, S., Brazel, C., and Peppas, N., Temperature and pH-sensitive terpolymers for modulated delivery of streptokinase, J. Biomater. Sci. Polym. Ed., 8, 119–129 (1996).
46. Serres, A., Baudys, M., and Kim, S., Temperature and pH-sensitive polymers for human calcitonin delivery, Pharm. Res., 13, 196–201 (1996).
47. Ogata, N., A marriage between natural and synthetic polymers: novel temperature-sensitive bioconjucgates, Journal of Controlled Release, 48, 149–155 (1997).
48. Chung, J. E., Yokoyama, T., Aoyagi, T. S., Y., and Okano, T., Effect of molecular architecture of hydrophobically modified poly(N-isopropylamide) on the formation of thermoresponsive core-shell micellar drug carriers, J. Controlled Release, 53, 119–130 (1998).
49. Baundys, M., Serres, A., Ramkisoon, C., and Kim, S. W., Temperature and pH-sensitive polymers for polypeptide drug delivery, J. Controlled Release, 48, 304–305 (1997).
50. Brannon-Peppas, L., and Peppas, N. A., Solute and penetrant diffusion in swellable polymers. IX. The mechanism of drug release from pH sensitive swelling-controlled systems, J. Controlled Release, 8, 267–274 (1989).
51. Annaka, M., and Tanaka, T., Multiple phases of polymer gels, Nature, 355, 430–432 (1992).
52. Firestone, B. A., and Siegel, R. A., Dynamic pH-dependent swelling properties of hydrophobic polyelectrolyte gel, Polym. Commun., 29, 204–208 (1988).
53. Dong, L.-C., and Hoffman, A. S., Controlled enteric release of macromolecules from pH sensitive, macroporous heterogels, Proc. Int. Symp. Control. Bioact. Mater., 17, 325–326 (1990).
54. Kou, J. H., Fleisher, D., and Amidon, G., Modeling drug release from dynamically swelling poly(hydroxyethyl methacrylate-co-methacrylic acid) hydrogels, J. Controlled Release, 12, 241–250 (1990).
55. Pradny, M., and Kopecek, J., Hydrogels for site-specific oral delivery. Poly(acrylic acid)-co-(butyl acrylate) crosslinked with 4,4'-bis(methacryloamino)azobenzene, Makromol. Chem., 191, 1887–1897 (1990).
56. Siegel, R. A., Falmarzian, M., Firestone, B. A., and Moxley, B. C., pH-Controlled release from hydrophobic/polyelectrolyte hydrogels, J. Controlled Release, 8, 179–182 (1988).
57. Kono, K., Tabata, F., and Takagishi, T., pH-responsive permeability of poly(acrylic acid)–poly(ethylenimine) complex capsule membrane, J. Membr. Sci., 76, 233–243 (1993).
58. Hariharan, D., and Peppas, N. A., Modelling of water transport and solute release in physiologically sensitive gels, J. Controlled Release, 23, 123–136 (1993).
59. Siegel, R. A., and Firestone, B. A., pH-dependent equilibrium swelling of hydrophobic polyelectrolyte copolymer gels, Macromolecules, 21, 3254–3259 (1988).
60. Allcock, H., and Ambrosio, A., Synthesis and characterization of pH-sensitive poly(organophosphazene) hydrogels, Biomaterials, 17, 2295–2302 (1996).
61. Bell, C., and Peppas, N., Water, solute and protein diffusion in physiologically responsive hydrogels of poly(methacrylic acid-g-ethylene glycol), Biomaterials, 17, 1201–1218 (1996).
62. Jarvinen, K., Akerman, S., Svarfvar, B., Tarvainen, T., Viinikka, P., and Paronen, P., Drug release from pH and ionic strength responsive poly(acrylic acid) grafted poly(vinylidenefluoride) membrane bags in vitro, Pharm. Res., 15, 802–805 (1998).
63. Siegel, R. A., Johannes, I., Hunt, A., and Firestone, B. A., Buffer effects on swelling kinetics in polybasic gels, Pharm. Res., 9, 76–81 (1992).
64. Giannos, S., Dinh, S., and Berner, B., Temporally controlled drug delivery systems: coupling of pH oscillators with membrane diffusion, J. Pharm. Sci., 84, 539–543 (1995).
65. Heller, J., and Trescony, P. V., Controlled drug release by polymer dissolution. II. An enzyme mediated delivery system, J. Pharm. Sci., 68, 919–921 (1979).
66. Ghandehari, H., Kopeckova, P., and Kopecek, J., In vitro degradation of pH-sensitive hydrogels containing aromatic azo bonds, Biomaterials, 18, 861–872 (1997).
67. Petka, W., Harden, J., McGrath, K., Wirtz, D., and Tirrell, D., Reversible hydrogels from self-assembling artificial proteins, Science, 281, 389–392 (1998).

68. Pitt, C. G., Gu, Z.-W., Hendren, R. W., Thompson, J., and Wani, M. C., Triggered drug delivery systems, J. Controlled Release, 2, 363–374 (1985).
69. Pitt, C. G., Self-regulated and triggered drug delivery systems, Pharm. Int., 88–91 (1986).
70. Pitt, C. G., Bao, T. T., Gu, Z. W., Wani, M. C., and Zhu, Z. H., The self-regulated delivery of chelating agents. In: Pulsed and Self-Regulated Drug Delivery, Kost, J. (Ed.), CRC Press, Boca Raton, pp. 117–127 (1985).
71. Ishihara, K., Muramoto, N., Fuji, H., and Shinohara, I., pH-induced reversible permeability control of the 4-carboxy acryanilide-methyl methacrylate copolymer membrane, J. Polym. Sci., Polym. Chem. Ed., 23, 2841–2850 (1985).
72. Ishihara, K., Muramoto, N., Fuji, H., and Shinohara, I., Preparation and permeability of urea-responsive membrane consisting of immobilized urease and poly(aromatic carboxylic acid), J. Polym. Sci., Polym. Lett. Ed., 23, 531–535 (1985).
73. Heller, J., Sparer, R. V., and Zenter, G. M., Poly(ortho esters). In: Biodegradable Polymers as Drug Delivery Systems, Chasin, M., and Langer, R., (Eds.), Dekker, New York, pp. 121–161 (1990).
74. Heller, J., Feedback-controlled drug delivery. In: Controlled Drug Delivery: Challenges and Strategies, Park, K. (Ed.), American Chemical Society, pp. 127–146 (1997).
75. Roskos, K., Tefft, V., and Heller, J., J. Clin. Mater., 13, 109–119 (1993).
76. Roskos, K. V., Fritzinger, B. K., Tefft, J. A., and Heller, Biocompatibility and in vivo morphine diffusion into a placebo morphine-triggered naltrexone delivery device in rabbits, J., Biomater., 16, 1235–1239 (1995).
77. Roskos, K. V., Tefft, J. A., Fritzinger, B. K., and Heller, J., Development of a morphine-triggered naltrexone delivery system, J. Controlled Release, 19, 145–160 (1992).
78. Tefft, J. A., Roskos, K. V., and Heller, J., The effect of lipase on the release of naltrexone from triglyceride-coated cellulose acetate phthalate microspheres, J. Biomed. Mater. Res., 26, 713–724 (1992).
79. Nakayama, G. R., Roskos, K. V., Fritzinger, B. K., and Heller, J., A study of reversibily inactivated lipases for use in morphine-triggered naltrexone delivery system, J. Biomed. Mater. Res., 29, 1389–1396 (1995).
80. Heller, J., Chang, A. C., Rodd, G., and Grodsky, G. M., Release of insulin from a pH-sensitive poly(ortho ester), J. Controlled Release, 13, 295–304 (1990).
81. Kost, J., Glucose responsive polymers (medical applications). In: Polymeric Materials Encyclopedia, Salamone, J. C. (Ed.), Vol. 4, CRC Press, Boca Raton, pp. 2825–2829 (1996).
82. Kitano, S., Koyama, Y., Kataoka, K., Okano, T., and Sakurai, Y., A novel drug delivery system utilizing a glucose responsive polymer complex between poly(vinyl alcohol) and poly(N-vinyl-2-pyrrolidone) with phenylboronic acid moiety, J. Controlled Release, 19, 161–170 (1992).
83. Hisamitsu, I., Kataoka, K., T., O., and Sakurai, Y., Glucose-responsive gel from phenylborate polymer and poly(vinyl alcohol): prompt response at physiological pH through the interaction of borate with amino group in the gel, Pharm. Res., 14, 289–293 (1997).
84. Shiino, D. et al., Amine containing phenylboronic acid gel for glucose-responsive insulin release under physiological pH., J. Controlled Release, 37, 269–276, (1995).
85. Brownlee, M., and Cerami, A., A glucose-controlled insulin-delivery system: semisynthetic insulin bound to lectin, Science, 26, 1190–1191 (1979).
86. Makino, K., Mack, E. J., Okano, T., and Kim, S. W., A microcapsule self-regulating delivery system for insulin, J. Controlled Release, 12, 235–239 (1990).
87. Sato, S., Jeong, S. Y., McRea, J. C., and Kim, S. W., Self-regulating insulin delivery systems. II. In vitro studies, J. Controlled Release, 67–77 (1984).
88. Sato, S., Jeong, S. Y., McRea, J. C., and Kim, S. W., Glucose stimulated insulin delivery system, Pure Appl. Chem., 56, 1323–1328 (1984).
89. Seminoff, L., Olsen, G., Zheng, J., Wilson, D., and Kim, S. W., Self-regulated insulin release. Proc. 15th Int. Symp. on Controlled Release of Bioactive Mat., Controlled Release Society, Basel, Switzerland, Vol. 15, p. 161 (1988).
90. Seminoff, L., and Kim, S. W., A self-regulating insulin delivery system based on competitive binding of glucose and glycosylated insulin. In: Pulsed and Self-Regulated Drug Delivery, Kost, J. (Ed.), CRC Press, Boca Raton (1990).

91. Kim, S. W., Pai, C. M., Makino, L. A., Seminoff, L. A., Holmberg, D. L., Gleeson, J. M., Wilson, D. E., and Mack, E. J., Self regulated glycosalated insulin delivery, J. Controlled Release, 11, 193–201 (1990).
92. Jeong, S. Y., Kim, S. W., Holemberg, D., and McRea, J. C., Self-regulating insulin delivery systems. III. In vivo studies, J. Controlled Release, 2, 143–152 (1985).
93. Jeong, S. Y., Kim, S. W., Eenink, M. J. D., and Feijen, J., Self-regulating insulin delivery systems. I. Synthesis and characterization of glycosylated insulin, J. Controlled Release, 1, 57–66 (1984).
94. Kokufata, E., Zhang, Y.-Q., and Tanaka, T., Saccharide-sensitive phase transition of a lectin-loaded gel, Nature, 351, 302–304 (1991).
95. Taylor, M., Tanna, S., Taylor, P., and Adams, G., The delivery of insulin from aqueous and non-aqueous reservoir governed by glucose sensitive gel membrane, J. Drug. Target., 3, 209–216 (1995).
96. Obaidat, A., and K., P., Characterization of protein release through glucose-sensitive hydrogel membranes, Biomaterials, 11, 801–806 (1997).
97. Obaidat, A., and Park, K., Characterization of glucose dependent gel-sol phase transition of the polymeric glucose-concanavalin A hydrogel system, Pharm Res., 13, 998–995 (1996).
98. Lee, S., and Park, K., Synthesis and characterization of sol-gel phase-reversible hydrogels sensitive to glucose, J. Mol. Recog., 9, 549–557 (1996).
99. Pai, C. M., et al., J. Pharm. Sci. 81, 532, (1992).
100. Brown, L., Ghodsian, F., and Langer, R., A glucose mediated insulin delivery system, Proc. Int. Symp. Controlled Rel. Bioact. Mater., 116–167 (1988).
101. Brown, L., Edelman, E., Fishel-Ghodsian, F., and Langer, R., Characterization of glucose-mediated insulin release from implantable polymers, J. Pharm. Sci., 85, 1341–1345 (1996).
102. Fischel-Ghodsian, F., Brown, L., Mathiowitz, E., Brandenburg, D., and Langer, R., Enzymatically controlled drug delivery, Proc. Natl. Acad. Sci. USA, 2403–2466 (1995).
103. Heller, J., Polymers for controlled parenteral delivery of peptides and proteins, Adv. Drug Deliv. Rev., 10, 163–204 (1993).
104. Albin, G., Horbett, T., and Ratner, B., Glucose-sensitive membranes for controlled release of insulin. In: Pulsed and Self-Regulated Drug Delivery, Kost, J. (Ed.), CRC Press, Boca Raton, pp. 159–185 (1990).
105. Albin, G., Horbett, T. A., Miller, S. R., and Ricker, N. L., Theoretical and experimental studies of glucose sensitive membranes, J. Controlled Release, 6, 267–291 (1987).
106. Albin, G., Horbett, T. A., and Ratner, B. D., Glucose sensitive membranes for controlled delivery of insulin: insulin transport studies, J. Controlled Release, 3, 153–164 (1985).
107. Klumb, L. A., and Horbett, T. A., Design of insulin delivery devices based on glucose sensitive membranes, J. Control. Release, 18, 59–80 (1992).
108. Klumb, L. A., and Horbett, T. A., The effect of hydronium ion on the transient behavior of glucose sensitive membranes, J. Controlled Release, 27, 95–114 (1993).
109. Kost, J., Horbett, T. A., Ratner, B. D., and Singh, M., Glucose sensitive membranes containing glucose oxidase: activity, swelling, and permeability studies, J. Biomed. Mater. Res., 19, 1117–1133 (1985).
110. Horbett, T., Kost, J., and Ratner, B., Swelling behavior of glucose sensitive membranes, Am. Chem. Soc., Div. Polym. Chem., 24, 34–35 (1983).
111. Horbett, T., Kost, J., and Ratner, B., Swelling behavior of glucose sensitive membranes. In: Polymers as Biomaterials, Shakaby, S., Hoffman, A., Horbett, T., and Ratner, B. (Eds.), Plenum Press, New York, pp. 193–207 (1984).
112. Goldraich, M., and Kost, J., Glucose-sensitive polymeric matrices for controlled delivery of therapeutics, Clin. Mater., 13, 135–142 (1993).
113. Kaetsu, I., Kumakura, M., and Yoshida, M., Enzyme immobilization by radiation-induced polymerization of 2-hydroxyethyl methacrylate at low temperatures, Biotechnol. Bioeng., 21, 847–861 (1979).
114. Ishihara, K., Glucose responsive polymers for controlled insulin release. Proc. 15th Int. Symp. Controlled Release Society, Basel, Switzerland, Controlled Release of Bioactive Mat., Vol. 15, pp. 168–169 (1988).

115. Ishihara, K., Kobayashi, M., and Shonohara, I., Control of insulin permeation through a polymer membrane with responsive function for glucose, Macromol. Chem., Rapid Commun., 4, 327–331 (1983).
116. Ishihara, K., Kobayashi, M., Ishimaru, N., and Shinohara, I., Glucose induced permeation control of insulin through a complex membrane consisting of immobilized glucose oxidase and a polyamine, Polym. J., 16, 625–631 (1984).
117. Ishihara, K., and Matsui, K., Glucose responsive insulin release from polymer capsule, J. Polym. Sci., Polym. Lett. Ed., 24, 413–417 (1986).
118. Podual, K., Peppas, N., and Doyle, F., Insulin release from pH-sensitive cationic hydrogels. Proc. The 25th International Symposium on Controlled Release of Bioactive Materials, Controlled Release Society, Volume 25, Las Vegas, pp. 135–136 (1998).
119. Iwata, H., and Matsuda, T., Preparation and properties of novel environment-sensitive membranes prepared by graft polymerization onto a porous membrane, J. Membr. Sci., 38, 185–199 (1988).
120. Iwata, H., Amemiya, H., Hata, T., Matsuda, T., Takano, H., and Akutsu, T., Development of novel semipermeable membranes for self-regulated insulin delivery systems, Proc. Int. Symp. Controlled Rel. Bioact. Mater., 15, 170–171 (1988).
121. Ito, Y., Casolaro, M., Kono, K., and Imanishi, Y., An insulin-releasing system that is responsive to glucose, J. Controlled Release, 10, 195–203 (1989).
122. Siegel, R., pH-sensitive gels: swelling equilibria, kinetics and applications for drug delivery. In: Pulsed and Self-Regulated Drug Delivery, Kost, J. (Ed.), CRC Press, Boca Raton, pp. 129–157 (1990).
123. Siegel, R. A., and Firestone, B. A., Mechanochemical approaches to self-regulating insulin pump design, J. Controlled Release, 11, 181–192 (1990).
124. Siegel, R., Modeling of self-regulating oscillatory drug delivery. In: Controlled Release: Challenges and Strategies, Park, K. (Ed.), American Chemical Society (1997).

5
Complexing Polymers in Drug Delivery

Anthony M. Lowman
Drexel University, Philadelphia, Pennsylvania

I. INTRODUCTION

Polymer complexes are insoluble, macromolecular structures formed by the non-covalent association of polymers with an affinity for one another. The complexes form due to association of repeating units on different chains (interpolymer complexes) or on separate regions of the same chain (intrapolymer complexes). Polymer complexes are classified by the nature of the association. The major classes of polymer complexes are stereocomplexes, polyelectrolyte complexes, and hydrogen-bonded complexes (1–4).

Stereocomplexes are formed by the nonionic association of stereoisomers by van der Waals interactions. One example of this type of complex is the interaction of iso- and syndiotactic poly(methyl methacrylate) (PMMA) (1). van der Waals complexes can also form between PMMA and poly(methacrylic acid) (PMAA) (2).

Polyelectrolyte complexes form readily between most polyanions and polycations (3,5). These complexes are formed by ionic association of repeating units on the polymer chains. Some of polymers that exhibit polyelectrolyte complexation include poly(acrylic acid) (PAA) and PMAA with poly(ethyleneimine) (6–10) and PAA with chitosan (11). Polyelectrolytes have been identified for use as desalination and ultrafiltration membranes, dialysis membranes, and peptide stabilizers (12,13).

Interpolymer complexes stabilized by hydrogen bonds form between polymers containing electron-donating protons, typically poly(carboxylic acids), and polymers containing electron-donating groups such as poly(ethylene glycol), polypyrollidones, or alcohols. Some examples of polymer systems that form complexes due to hydrogen bonding include PAA and polyacrylamide (14), PAA and poly(vinyl alcohol) (15–19), PAA and poly(ethylene glycol) (20–23), PMAA and poly(vinyl pyrrolidone) (24–26), and PMAA and poly(ethylene glycol) (PEG) (20,27–50). Previous work has established that complexes of PMAA and poly(vinyl pyrrolidone) are the most stable of the hydrogen-bonded complexes (2,23,24).

Hydrogen-bonded complexes generally form in aqueous media within a narrow range of solvent composition, pH, and ionic strength. Additionally, the complexes are stabilized by the composition and structure of the copolymer, as well as hydrophobic interactions. The stability of hydrogen-bonded complexes is also dependent on many environmental factors such as temperature, nature of the solvent, pH, or ionic strength. Hydrogen-bonded complexes involving polyacids only form when the pH of the solution is sufficiently low for substantial protonation of the acidic. Additionally, this type of interpolymer complex is reversible in nature.

Because of their nature, hydrogen-bonded complexation polymer systems have the ability to function in a wide variety of applications. These materials have been identified for use in sensing applications and chemomechanical systems (30,31,34). However, one application for which these systems have received significant interest is in drug delivery. In particular, complexation copolymers of PMAA/PEG have been studied in great detail for use as drug delivery systems (37,41–43,45,48–50). In this chapter, the use of hydrogen-bonded complexation copolymers of PMAA/PEG as drug delivery systems will be reviewed.

II. COMPLEXATION BETWEEN POLY(METHACRYLIC ACID)/POLY(ETHYLENE GLYCOL)

In copolymers of PMAA/PEG, interpolymer complexes form in acidic media due to hydrogen bonding between protonated carboxylic acid groups and the PEG ether groups (Fig. 1). These complexes dissociate in neutral or basic media due to ionization of the acid groups. In these copolymers, this complexation/decomplexation behavior is reversible in nature.

Copolymers of PMAA/PEG have been one of the most widely studied complexing systems. Beginning with the work of the group of Kabanov in the late 1960s (27,28), pH-responsive complexation in these copolymers have been extensively studied using linear polymers and polymer networks.

A. Complexation in Linear Polymers

In solutions of linear PMAA and PEG, interpolymer complexes form in acidic media due to hydrogen bonding between the PMAA carboxyl protons and the PEG ether group. Antipina et al. (27) studied PMAA and PEG in solution using viscometry and potentiometry. They determined that complex formation was strongly dependent on the length of interacting chains. Papisov et al. (28) studied the thermodynamics of complexation using calorimetry. They observed stabilization of the complexes due to hydrophobic interactions and increased chain length. Osada and Sato (29) used viscometry to study complexation in different solvents. They found that complexation did not occur in methanol or ethanol due to disruption of the hydrophobic interactions. Osada (30) determined that complexation did not occur in polymer solutions containing PEG of molecular weight less than 2000.

Hemker et al. (32) studied complexation in labeled PEG and PMAA. Complexation in this system was verified using pH and fluorescence measurements. Hemker and Frank (33) also studied complexation using light scattering techniques. In systems where complexation occurred, the particle size of the complexes was strongly dependent on the pH of the solution. The largest particles were observed in solutions of pH less than 3.2. As the pH was increased above this point, the size of the particles decreased rapidly. The next major contribution in complexing polymer solutions was made by Klier et al. (36). They observed the molecular level complexation in PMAA/PEG solutions using nuclear Overhauser enhancement NMR spectroscopy.

Eagland et al. (38) also studied the importance of PEG molecular weight on the stability of polymer complexes. They reported results similar to what was previously seen. The group of Baranovsky (40,46) studied complexation in PMAA and hydrophobically modified PEG. They found that complexation was enhanced significantly by the presence of the hydrophobic groups along the PEG.

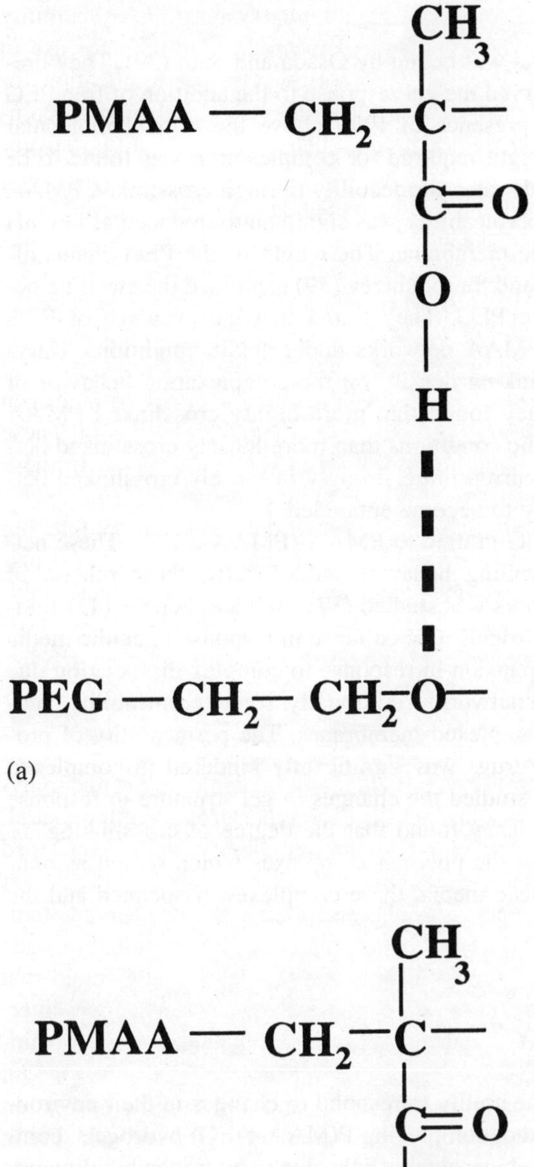

Complexing Polymers in Drug Delivery

(a)

PMAA—CH$_2$—C(CH$_3$)—C(=O)—O—H ⋮ PEG—CH$_2$—CH$_2$—O—

(b)

PMAA—CH$_2$—C(CH$_3$)—C(=O)—O$^-$ PEG—CH$_2$—CH$_2$—O—

Figure 1 Schematic of the complexation/decomplexation behavior of PMAA/PEG (a) in acidic media when the acid group is protonated and (b) in neutral or basic media when the acid group is ionized.

B. Complexation in Polymer Networks

The study of complexation in polymer networks was begun by Osada and Sato (29). They prepared crosslinked PMAA membranes and observed the gel response to the addition of free PEG chains. PMAA membranes collapsed in the presence of PEG above the critical molecular weight. Additionally, the critical molecular weight required for complexation was found to be lower in network structures. Osada (31) studied water permeability through crosslinked PMAA membranes in the presence of free PEG. The permeability was significantly reduced at low pH where complexation resulted in collapse of the membrane. The length of the PEG chains affected the rate of network collapse. Phillapova and Starodubtzev (39) examined the swelling behavior of PMAA gels in the presence of free PEG. They found that the presence of PEG strongly decreased the swelling behavior of PMAA networks under acidic conditions. Karybiants et al. (44) studied the effects of crosslinking density on the complexation behavior of PMAA networks in the presence of PEG. They found that more highly crosslinked PMAA networks swelled to a higher degree under acidic conditions than more loosely crosslinked networks. They determined that complexation occurred more strongly in loosely crosslinked networks as the hydrophilic PEG was not as likely to become entangled.

Klier et al. (35) prepared networks of PEG grafted to PMAA (PMAA-g-EG). These networks exhibited reversible, pH-dependent swelling behavior. Additionally, these release of small molecular weight drugs from these networks was studied (37). Bell and Peppas (41) studied the oscillatory nature of P(MAA-g-EG) hydrogels. Gel collapse in response to acidic media was found to be 5–8.5 times faster than gel expansion in response to complex dissociation due to the decreased permeability of the complexed network. Additionally, solute permeability studies were performed using complexed and uncomplexed membranes. The permeability of proteins (lysozyme) and small molecular weight drugs was significantly hindered in complexed membranes (42,45). Lowman and Peppas (47) studied the changes in gel structure in response to pH changes using rubber elasticity studies. They found that the degree of crosslinking increased in acidic media due to the formation of the polymer complexes which served as nonpermanent physical crosslinks. In neutral or basic media, these complexes dissociated and the crosslink density was decreased.

III. APPLICATIONS IN DRUG DELIVERY

Copolymer networks of P(MAA-g-EG) have the ability to respond to changes in their environmental conditions. In these covalently crosslinked, complexing P(MAA-g-EG) hydrogels, complexation results in the formation of temporary physical crosslinks due to hydrogen bonding between the PEG grafts and the PMAA pendant groups. The physical crosslinks are reversible in nature and dependent on the pH and ionic strength of the environment. Thus, the number of crosslinks, both chemical and physical, the effective molecular weight of the polymer chains between these crosslinks, M_e, and the end-to-end distance of the polymer chains between these crosslinks or mesh size, ξ, are strongly dependent on the pH and ionic strength of the surrounding environment. In acidic media, such systems are relatively unswollen due to the formation of the intermacromolecular complexes. In basic solutions, the pendant groups ionize and the complexes dissociate.

As a result of this behavior, P(MAA-g-EG) hydrogels exhibit drastic changes in their mesh size over small changes of pH (Fig. 2). The ratio of the effective hydrodynamic diameter of the drug, d_h, to the network mesh size is critical in determining the ability of the drug to diffuse through the network (51–53). In complexed gels, this ratio decreases significantly from the

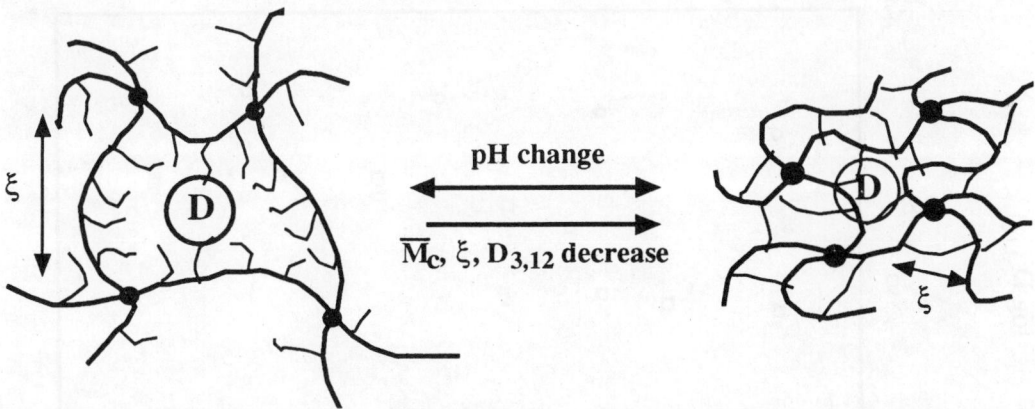

Figure 2 The effect of interpolymer complexation on the correlation length, ξ, and the effective molecular weight between crosslinks, $\overline{M}_c$, in P(MAA-g-EG) graft copolymer networks with permanent chemical crosslinks (●)(48).

uncomplexed case. Because the network mesh size varies widely over small pH changes, P(MAA-g-EG) hydrogels can be used to alter the diffusional characteristics of various sized solutes, including protein- and peptide-drug, based on the pH of the swelling medium. Using this type of carrier, drugs could be delivered in a pulsatile manner or one in which the drug is released at desired rates for specified intervals to maintain the drug concentration in the body at therapeutic levels for longer time periods. The group of Peppas (48–50) has investigated the pH-dependent, diffusional behavior of various sized drugs through P(MAA-g-EG) complexation gels.

The ability of the P(MAA-g-EG) gels to control the rates of diffusion is strongly dependent on the size of the solute and the pH of the environmental fluids. The diffusion coefficients for proxyphylline, vitamin B_{12}, and FITC-dextran in P(MAA-g-EG) hydrogels are plotted as a function of the swelling solution pH in Fig. 3. For gels in the complexed state, the diffusion coefficients were greatest for the smallest molecular weight solute, proxyphylline. For this relatively small molecular weight drug (MW = 238, r_h = 2.2 Å), the diffusion coefficient was on the order of 10^{-8}. As the size of the solute was increased, the diffusion coefficient was severely reduced as the ratio of the solute radius to the network mesh size was increased. For the largest drug studied, FITC-dextran (MW = 4400, r_h = 22.1 Å), the diffusion coefficients for the drug in complexed gels were on the order of 10^{-10}.

For gels swollen in higher pH solutions in which no complexation occurs, the diffusion coefficients for proxyphylline were on the order of 10^{-8}. However, for the case of the larger drugs, the diffusion coefficient was similar for the two solutes and an order of magnitude lower than the diffusion coefficient of proxyphylline. In this case, the diffusion coefficient was reduced because the ratio of the solute radius to network mesh size was sufficiently large to substantially hinder the diffusion of the drug in the highly swollen network.

Because the diffusion coefficient of many solutes in P(MAA-g-EG) vary strongly based on the pH of the environmental fluid, such systems may be able to deliver drugs in a pulsatile or on–off type of manner. This type of behavior is shown in Fig. 4 for vitamin B_{12} in P(MAA-g-EG) gel (49). For the first 24 h of the release of vitamin B_{12} from P(MAA-g-EG) gels swollen in pH = 3.2 buffer solutions was examined. During this period, the gels were in the highly complexed state and only 15% of the drug was released due to the presence of the physical crosslinks.

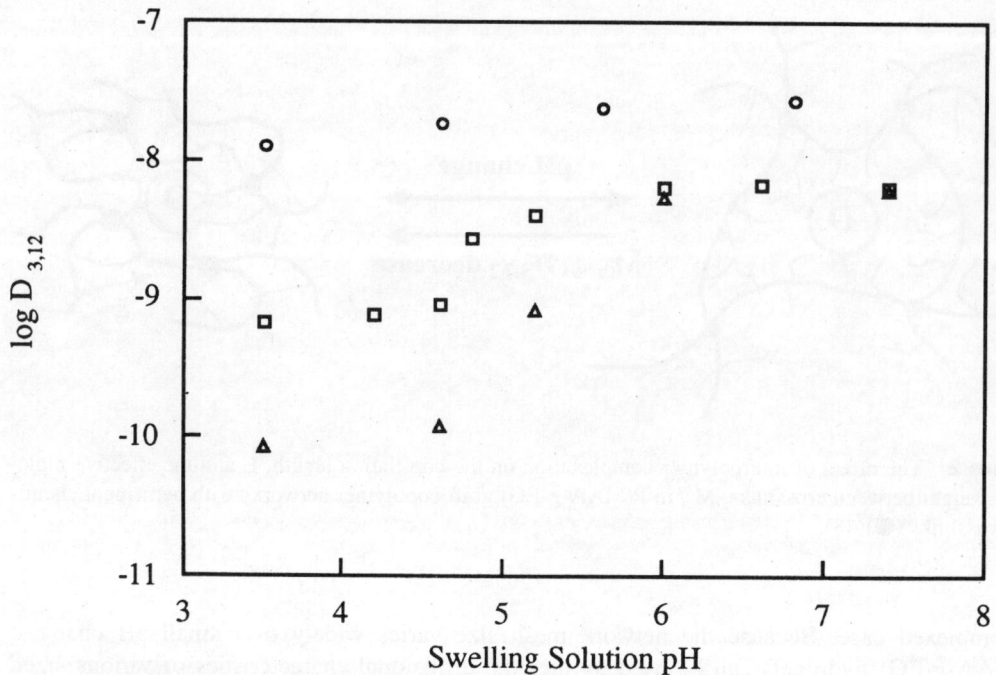

Figure 3 Diffusion coefficients for (○) proxyphylline, (□) vitamin B_{12}, and (△) FITC-dextran in P(MAA-g-EG) hydrogels plotted as a function of the swelling solution pH at 37° C (48).

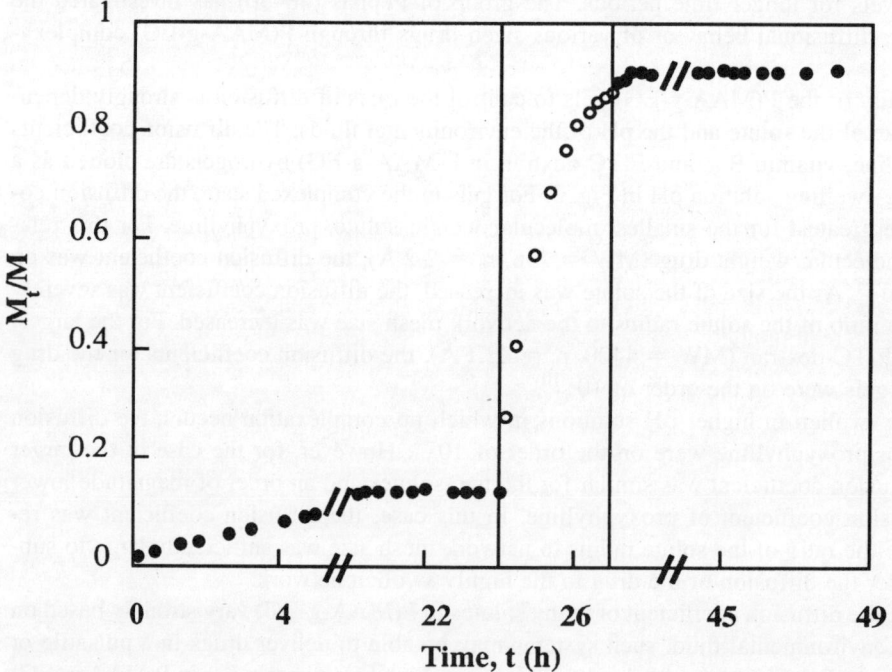

Figure 4 Pulsatile release of vitamin B_{12} from gels containing PEG grafts of MW 1000 and an EG/MAA molar ratio of 1/1 in DMGA-buffered saline solutions (I = 0.1) of pH of (○) 7.1 and (●) 3.2 at 37°C (49).

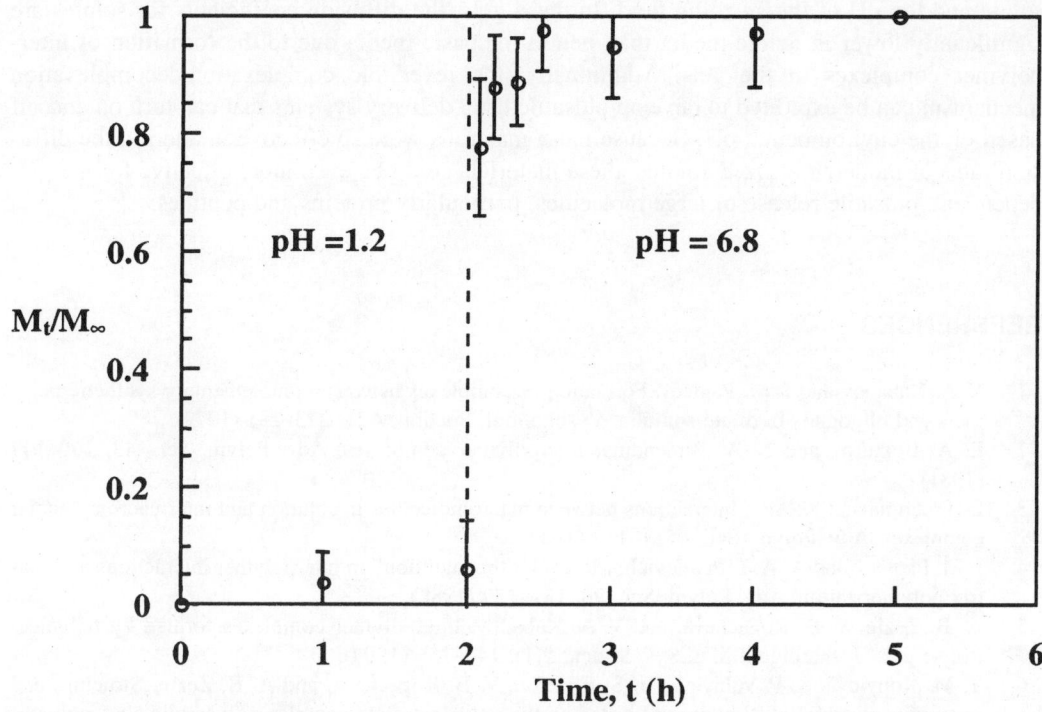

Figure 5 Controlled release of insulin in vitro from P(MAA-g-EG) microparticles simulated gastric fluid (pH = 1.2) for the first 2 h and phosphate-buffered saline solutions (pH = 6.8) for the remaining 3 h at 37°C (49).

However, after 24 h, the hydrogels were placed in environments with pH above the network pK_a (pH = 7.4 buffer solution), resulting in complex dissociation and a more rapid drug release. Under these conditions, 60% of the remaining drug released was in only 2 h. The release was shut off immediately by returning the materials to an acidic solution. In this case, the release was halted due to rapid gel collapse in response to complexation.

Another interesting characteristic of this system is that the hydrogels have the ability to serve as carriers for protein- and peptide-drugs such as insulin (48). One particularly promising application would be for oral delivery of insulin and other protein-based drugs. The release behavior of insulin from P(MAA-g-EG) microgels is shown in Fig. 5. When the particles were swollen in acid media similar to stomach pH, less than 10% of the drug was released. However, when the particles were transferred to a slightly basic solution like that found in the small intestine, all of the drug was released rapidly. This type of release behavior would be ideal for targeted delivery of the macromolecules to the small intestine.

IV. CONCLUSIONS

The formation of complexes due to macromolecular associations in polymer networks has a significant effect on the structure and properties of the material. The ability of complexation hydrogels gels to control the diffusional rates of solutes is strongly dependent on the size of the solute and the pH of the swelling fluid. In these gels, the diffusion coefficients for solutes are significantly lower in acidic media than neutral or basic media due to the formation of interpolymer complexes in the gels. Additionally, the reversible complexation/decomplexation mechanism can be exploited to develop pulsatile drug delivery systems that can turn on and off based on the environmental pH. Because these materials were so effective in altering the diffusion rates of moderately sized solutes, these materials could be even more effective for the pH-dependent, pulsatile release of large molecules, particularly proteins and peptides.

REFERENCES

1. V. A. Kabanov and I. M. Papisov, Formation of complexes between complementary synthetic polymers and oligomers in dilute solution. Vysokolmol. Soedin., A21, 243–281 (1979).
2. E. A. Bekturov and L. A. Bimendina, Interpolymer complexes. Adv. Polym. Sci., 43, 100–147 (1981).
3. E. Tsuchida and K. Abe, Interactions between macromolecules in solution and intermacromolecular complexes. Adv. Polym. Sci., 45, 1–119 (1982).
4. I. M. Papisov and A. A. Litmanovich, Molecular "recognition" in interpolymer interactions and matrix polymerization. Adv. Polym. Sci., 90, 139–179 (1988).
5. A. B. Zezin, V. B. Rogacheva, and V. A. Kabanov, Interpolymer complexes formed by polyelectrolyte gels. J. Intelligent Mat. Sys. Struct., 5(1), 144–156 (1994).
6. Y. M. Kopylova, S. P. Valuyeva, B. S. Eltsefon, V. B. Rogacheva, and A. B. Zezin, Structure and properties of crosslinked hydrogels based on the polyelectrolyte complex polyacrylic acid–polyethyleneimine. Vysokomol. Soedin., A29, 517–524 (1987).
7. K. Kono, F. Tabata, and T. Takagashi, pH-responsive permeability of poly(acrylic acid)–poly(ethylenimine) complex capsule membranes. J. Membr. Sci., 76, 233–243 (1993).
8. S. K. Chatterjee, V. Dureja, and S. Nigam, Interpolymer association between phenolic copolymers and poyelectrolytes: effects of copolymer structure and hydrophobic interactions on the stability of polycomplexes. Polym. Bull., 37, 265–272 (1996).
9. S. K. Chatterjee and N. Misra, Interpolymer complexes of a graft copolymer with polyelectrolytes and equivalent blends of binary homopolymer complexes: a comparative study of their stability and thermodynamic parameters. Macromol. Chem. Phys., 197, 4193–4206 (1996).
10. S. K. Chatterjee and N. Misra, Interpolymer association between random and graft acrylic copolymers with poly(ethylene imine): effects of copolymer structure. Polymer, 38(6), (1997).
11. H. Wang, W. Li, Y. Lu, Z. Wang, and W. Zhong, Studies of chitosan and poly(acrylic acid) interpolymer complex. II. Solution behaviors of the mixture of water-soluble chitosan and poly(acrylic acid). J. Appl. Polym. Sci., 61, 2221–2224 (1996).
12. G. V. Samsonov, Polymeric complexes on synthetic polyelectrolytes and physiologically active components. Vysokomol. Soedin., A21, 723–733 (1979).
13. C. L. Bell and N. A. Peppas, Biomedical membranes from hydrogels and interpolymer complexes. Adv. Polym. Sci., 122, 125–175 (1995).
14. M. A. Moharram, L. S. Balloomal, and H. M. El-gendy, Infrared study of the complexation of polyl(acrylic acid) with poly(acrylamide). J. Appl. Polym. Sci., 59, 987–990 (1996).
15. N. G. Bel'nikevich, T. V. Budtova, N. P. Ivanova, Ye.F. Panarin, Yu.N. Panov, and S. Ya. Frenkel, Complex-formation in aqueous solutions of mixtures of polyacrylic acid and polyvinylalcohol and its copolymers. Vysokomol. Soedin., A31, 1691–1696 (1989).
16. Y. M. Lee, S. H. Kim, and C. S. Cho, Synthesis and swelling characteristics of pH and thermoresponsive interpenetrating polymer network hydrogel composed of poly(vinyl alcohol) and poly(acrylic acid). J. Appl. Polym. Sci., 62, 301–311 (1996).
17. J. Byun, Y. M. Lee, and C. S. Cho, Swelling of thermosensitive interpenetrating polymer networks composed of poly(vinyl alcohol) and poly(acrylic acid). J. Appl. Polym. Sci., 61, 697–702 (1996).

18. H. S. Shin, S. Y. Kim, and Y. M. Lee, Indomethacin release behaviors from pH and Thermoresponsive poly(vinyl alcohol) and poly(acrylic acid) ipn hydrogels for site-specific drug delivery. J. Appl. Polym. Sci., 65, 685–693 (1997).
19. Q. Wang, L. He, and J. Huang, Supermolecular structure and mechanical properties of p(an-am-a)/pva intermacromolecular complex formed through hydrogen bonding. J. Appl. Polym. Sci., 64, 2089–2096 (1997).
20. Y. Osada, Equilibrium study of polymer–polymer complexation of poly(methacrylic acid) and poly(acrylic acid) with complementary polymers through cooperative hydrogen bonding. J. Polym. Sci., Polym. Chem. Ed., 17, 3485–3498 (1979).
21. S. Nishi and T. Kotaka, Complex-forming poly(oxyethylene):poly(acrylic acid) interpenetrating polymer networks. 1. Preparation, structure, and viscoelastic properties. Macromolecules, 18(8), 1519–1525 (1985).
22. S. Nishi and T. Kotaka, Complex-forming poly(oxyethylene):poly(acrylic acid) interpenetrating polymer networks. 2. Function as a chemical valve. Macromolecules, 19(4), 978–984 (1986).
23. M. J. Krupers, F. J. Van der Gaag, and J. Feijen, Complexation of poly(ethylene oxide) with poly(acrylic acid-co-hydroxyethyl methacrylate)s. Eur. Polym. J., 32(6), 785–790 (1996).
24. L. A. Bimendina, V. V. Roganov, and E. A. Bekturov, Hydrodynamic properties of polymethacrylic acid–polyvinylpyrrolidone complexes in solution. Vysokomol. Soedin., A16, 2810–2814 (1974).
25. H. Ohno, K. Abe, and E. Tsuchida, Solvent effect on the formation of poly(methacrylic acid)–poly(n-vinyl pyrrolidone) complex through hydrogen bonding. Makromol. Chem., 179, 755–763 (1978).
26. A. Usaitis, S. L. Maunu, and H. Tenhu, Aggregation of the interpolymer complex of poly(methacrylic acid) and poly(vinyl pyrrolidone) in aqueous solutions. Eur. Polym. J., 33(2), 219–223 (1997).
27. A. D. Antipina, V. Yu Baranovsky, I. M. Papisov, and V. A. Kabanov, Equilibrium peculiarities in the complexing of polymeric acids with poly(ethylene glycol). Vysokomol. Soyed., A14, 941–949 (1972).
28. I. M. Papisov, V. Yu Baranovsky, Y. I. Sergieva, A. D. Antipina, and V. A. Kabanov, Thermodynamics of complex formation between poly(methacrylic acid) and polyethylene glycols. Calculation of temperatures of breakdown of complexes of oligomers and matrices. Vysokomol. Soedin., A16, 1133–1141 (1974).
29. Y. Osada and M. Sato, Thermal equilbrium of the intermacromolecular complexes of polycarboxylic acids realized by cooperative hydrogen bonding. J. Polym. Sci., Polym. Letters Ed., 14, 129–134 (1976).
30. Y. Osada, Effects of polymers and their chain lengths on the contraction of poly(methacrylic acid) network. J. Polym. Sci., Polym. Letters Ed., 18, 281–286 (1980).
31. Y. Osada, K. Honda, and M. Ohta, Control of water permeability by mechanochemical contraction of poly(methacrylic acid)–grafted membranes. J. Membr. Sci., 27, 339–347 (1986).
32. D. J. Hemker, V. Garza, and C. W. Frank, Complexation of poly(methacrylic acid) and pyrene end-labelled poly(ethylene glycol). pH and fluorescence measurements. Macromolecules, 23, 4411–4418 (1987).
33. D. J. Hemker and C. W. Frank, Dynamic light scattering studies of the fractal aggregation of poly(methacrylic acid) and poly(ethylene glycol). Macromolecules, 23, 4404–4410 (1987).
34. Y. Osada, Conversion of chemical energy into mechanical energy by synthetic polymers (chemomechanical systems). Adv. Polym. Sci., 82, 1–46 (1987).
35. J. Klier and N. A. Peppas, Structure and swelling behavior of poly(ethylene glycol)/poly(methacrylic acid) complexes. In: L. Brannon-Peppas and R. S. Harland (Eds.), Absorbent Polymer Technology, Elsevier, Amsterdam, 1990, pp. 147–169.
36. J. Klier, A. B. Scranton, and N. A. Peppas, Self-associating networks of poly(methacrylic acid-g-ethylene glycol). Macromolecules, 23, 4944–4949 (1990).
37. N. A. Peppas and J. Klier, Controlled release by using poly(methacrylic acid-g-ethylene glycol) hydrogels. J. Controlled Release, 16, 203–214 (1991).

38. D. Eagland, N. J. Crowther, and C. J. Butler. Complexation between polyoxyethylene and polymethacrylic acid-The importance of the molar mass of polyoxyethylene. Eur. Polym. J., 30(7), 767–773 (1994).
39. O. E. Philippova and S. G. Starodubtzev, Intermacromolecular complexation between poly(methacrylic acid) hydrogels and poly(ethylene glycol). J. Membr. Sci., Pure Appl. Chem., A32, 1893–1902 (1995).
40. V. Yu Baranovsky and S. Shenkov, Competitive complex forming reactions between monosubstituted and nonsubstituted poly(ethylene glycol)s with poly(methacrylic) acid. J. Polym. Sci., Polym. Chem. Ed., 34, 163–167 (1996).
41. C. L. Bell and N. A. Peppas, Water, solute and protein diffusion in physiologically responsive hydrogels of poly(methacrylic acid-g-ethylene glycol. Biomaterials, 17, 1203–1218 (1996).
42. C. L. Bell and N. A. Peppas, Swelling/syneresis phenomena in gel-forming interpolymer complexes. J. Biomater. Sci., Polym. Ed., 7(8), 671–683 (1996).
43. B. O. Haglund, R. Joshi, and K. J. Himmelstein, An in situ gelling system for parenteral delivery. J. Controlled Rel., 41, 229–235 (1996).
44. N. S. Karybiants, O. E. Phillippova, S. G. Starodubtzev, and A. R. Khoklov, Conformational transitions in poly(methacrylic acid) gel/poly(ethylene glycol) complexes. Effect of the gel cross-linking density. Macromol. Chem. Phys., 197, 2373–2378 (1996).
45. C. L. Bell and N. A. Peppas, Modulation of drug permeation through interpolymer complexed hydrogels for drug delivery applications. J. Controlled Release, 39, 201–207 (1997).
46. V. Doseva, S. Shenkov, and V. Yu Baranovsky, Complex formation between polymethacrylic acid and copolymers of adipic acid with poly(ethylene glycol) in aqueous solution. Polymer, 38(6), 1339–1344 (1997).
47. A. M. Lowman and N. A. Peppas, Analysis of the complexation/decomplexation phenomena in graft copolymer networks. Macromolecules, 30, 4959–4965 (1997).
48. A. M. Lowman, and N. A. Peppas, Solute transport analysis in pH-responsive, complexing hydrogels of poly(methacrylic acid-g-ethylene glycol. J. Biomater. Sci. Polymer Edn., 10, 999–1009 (1999).
49. A. M. Lowman, N. A. Peppas, M. Morishita, and T. Nagai, Novel bioadhesive complexation networks for oral protein drug delivery. In: I. McCulloch and S. W. Shalaby (Eds.), Tailored Polymeric Materials for Controlled Delivery Systems. American Chemical Society Symposium Series #709, ACS, Washington, D.C., 1998 pp. 156–164.
50. A. M. Lowman and N. A. Peppas, Pulsatile drug delivery based on a complexation/decomplexation mechanism. In: S. M. Dinh, J. D. DeNuzzio, and A. R. Comfort (Eds.), Intelligent Materials for Controlled Release. American Chemical Society Symposium Series #728, ACS, Washington, D.C., 1998, pp. 30–42.
51. N. A. Peppas and C. T. Rheinhart, Solute diffusion in swollen membranes. Part I. A new theory. J. Membr. Sci., 15, 275–287 (1983).
52. W. M. Deen, Hindered transport of large macromolecules in liquid filled pores. AIChE J., 33, 1409–1425 (1987).
53. A. P. Sassi, H. W. Blanch, and J. M. Prausnitz, Characterization and size-exclusion effects in highly swollen hydrogels: correlation and prediction. J. Appl. Polym. Sci., 59, 1337–1346 (1996).

6
Polylactic and Polyglycolic Acids as Drug Delivery Carriers

Lisa Brannon-Peppas
Biogel Technology, Inc. Indianapolis, Indiana

Michel Vert
ESA CNRS, University Montpellier 1, Montpellier, France

I. INTRODUCTION: A BRIEF HISTORY OF THE USE OF POLYLACTIC AND POLYGLYCOLIC ACIDS IN MEDICAL APPLICATIONS

The first synthetic polymers designed specifically for use in the body as resorbable materials were the polyglycolides, also known as poly(glycolic acid)s (1), which were used to make the Dexon sutures in 1970. In parallel, research on aliphatic polyesters derived from lactic acid was initiated and led to the first lactic/glycolic copolymer (PLAGA) exploited as the Vicryl suture (2). The PLAGA-based sutures, which did not require surgical removal after healing, paved the way for many other applications known as temporary therapeutic applications, i.e., applications requiring the help of a prosthetic device for a limited period of time, namely, the healing time.

Research on PLAGA polymers, copolymers, and stereocopolymers has been extensive, resulting in many preparation, formulation, and characterization techniques for both implantable and injectable controlled delivery systems. It did not take researchers long to realize the utility of these biodegradable sutures as materials for drug delivery. A 1974 patent, filed in 1971, by American Cyanamid describes resins containing polyglycolic acid units for water-degradable packaging and slow release materials (3). By the late 1980s, the number of patents for lactide- and glycolide-based implants and other devices had escalated significantly (4–6). Currently, both implantable and injectable controlled delivery systems are largely dependent on degradation and removal of the delivery device with few to no adverse biological reactions.

Both academic and industrial researchers have focused on understanding the biodegradation mechanisms of these polymers and the effect on their performance of preparation, processing, and sterilization procedures (7–13). Lactide/glycolide copolymers have had such strong success in drug delivery formulations because their degradation can range from 3 weeks to over a year, depending on the composition of the copolymer as well as the method of preparation and formulation (7,14). The fastest degradation is seen for copolymers with a 50:50 ratio of lactide to glycolide and with low molecular weights. Decreasing the degree of crystallinity will also increase the degradation rate of the resulting polymer.

The ability of PLAGA polymers to dissolve in a variety of organic solvents as well as to be extruded into a number of shapes has been instrumental in exploring their use from biodegradable sutures into implants, microparticles, nanoparticles, and fibers for an ever-increasing number of controlled release formulations and devices. In the new field of tissue engineering, PLAGA is unquestionably the polymer of choice for building the scaffolds on which and in which new organs are grown.

Here we will present an overview of these techniques as well as delve into the newest research areas and possibilities using these biodegradable materials. Attention will be paid to the main characteristics and properties that make PLAGA polymers difficult to handle and to master.

II. PREPARATION OF PLAGA POLYMERS

In the minds of most users, PLAGA are simple polymers that you can buy and use as any polymeric compounds. The situation is actually much more complicated as indicated as early as 1981 (14). Basically, the PLAGA aliphatic polyester family includes an almost infinite number of compounds depending on the gross composition, on the distribution of chiral and achiral repeating units, and on molecular weights (Table 1).

Amid all of the corresponding compounds, one can find amorphous or semicrystalline and rigid or waxy polymers with variable lifetime (6). Although many of these forms have been tested, only a few of the PLAGA polymers have reached the stage of commercialization as bioresorbable devices in drug delivery. For the sake of better reflecting the composition in chiral and achiral units, PLA stereocopolymers and PLAGA copolymers will be identified in this

Table 1 Structure of the Main Members of the Aliphatic Polyester Family

Polymer	Structure
Poly(glycolic acid) PGA	$+[O-CH_2-CO]_n$
Poly(L-lactic acid) PLA100	$+[O-CH(CH_3)-CO]_n$ (H up, CH$_3$ down)
Poly(DL-lactic acid) (stereocopolymers) PLAX [X=m/(m+p)]	$+[O-CH(CH_3)-CO]_m[O-CH(H)-CO]_p$ with CH$_3$ below first, H below second
Poly(L-lactic-co-glycolic acids) PLA100-YGAY [Y=p/(m+p)]	$+[O-CH(CH_3)-CO]_m[O-CH_2-CO]_p$
Poly(L-lactic-co-D-lactic-co-glycolic acids) PLAXGAY [X=m/(m+p+q); Y=q/(m+p+q)]	$+[O-CH(CH_3)-CO]_m[O-CH(H)-CO]_p[O-CH_2-CO]_q$

paper by acronyms PLA_X or PLA_XGA_Y where X is the percentage of L-lactic acid (L-LA) units present in the monomer feed, Y is that of glycolic acid (GA) units, and (100-X-Y) is the percentage of D-lactic acid (D-LA) units (14), except when authors of the cited reference did not use these acronyms. Unfortunately, many papers present in literature are completely void of this kind of information. The absence of precise information on the polymers can be dramatic when one wants to compare data and systems or simply reproduce experiments with a new batch or an aged batch of polymer. On the other hand, giving information on the main influencing factors is no longer enough because it is now known that degradation characteristics of PLAGA polymers depend also on many other factors as we will see later on (15). The synthesis route is one of the latest factors to be identified.

There are various routes to synthesize aliphatic polyesters of the PLAGA-type, namely, step growth polymerization of lactic acid enantiomers and/or glycolic acid, postcondensation of macromonomers, and ring opening polymerization of 1,4-dioxane-2,5-diones (Fig. 1). The literature contains examples where the condensation of lactic acids is carried out without

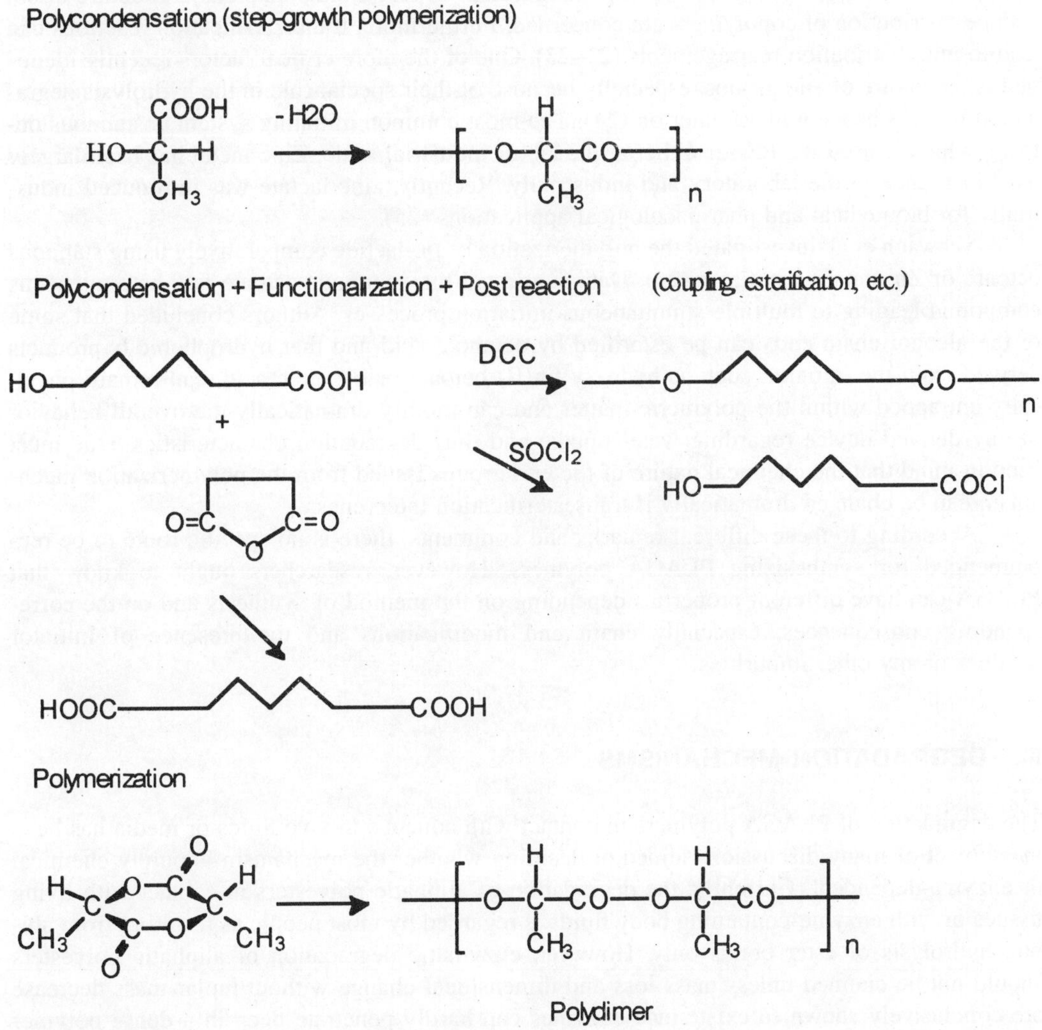

Figure 1 Routes to synthesize poly(lactic-co-glycolic) acid polymers.

(16) and with catalyst (ZnO or p-toluenesulfonic acid, for instance). This route leads to rather low molecular weight compounds (MW < 5000), which can be more or less deformable or rigid depending on the stereoregularity (17). The lower oligomers, namely those with a degree of polymerization (DPn) less than 9, can be soluble in water, the critical DPn being dependent on the pH of the medium (18). High molecular weight PLAGA polymers issued from step growth polycondensation of α-hydroxy acids are also mentioned in the literature. The process consists of condensing oligomers taken as macromonomers by postcondensation using a coupling reagent such as dicyclohexylcarbodiimide (DCC) (19). Postcondensation of oligomers can also be achieved in the presence of bifunctional reagents such as diisocyanates.

However, the main route to high molecular weight PLAGA polymers is ring opening polymerization of heterocyclic monomers composed of two lactic or two glycolic acid units, namely, lactide and glycolide, respectively (20). This kind of polymerization requires the use of an initiating system. Polymerization of 1,4-dioxane 2,5-diones can be achieved according to different initiation mechanisms, namely, anionic, cationic, and insertion-coordination. In some cases, coinitiators are used such as alcohols (14). Each route has specific consequences insofar as molar mass, molar mass distribution, configuration of lactyl units, and chain structure or sequence distribution of copolymers are concerned. Furthermore, transesterification reactions can lead to unit distribution rearrangements (21–23). One of the more critical factors recently identified is the nature of end groups, especially because of their special role in the hydrolysis degradation process as we will see later on (24). The most common initiating system is stannous octoate, which is used worldwide either at the lab or industrial scale. Zinc metal has been largely used in France in the laboratory and industrially. Recently, zinc lactate was introduced industrially for biomedical and pharmacological applications (25).

Schwach et al. investigated the polymerization of DL-lactide comparatively using stannous octoate or Zn metal as initiator (26). Data suggested that stannous octoate is a heterogeneous compound leading to multiple simultaneous initiation processes. Authors concluded that some of the alcohol chain ends can be esterified by octanoic acid and that hydrophobic byproducts derived from the initiator, such as hydroxy tin(II) octoate or octanoic acid, can remain physically entrapped within the polymeric matter and can modify dramatically the overall behavior of any derived device regarding water uptake and thus degradation characteristics. One must keep in mind that the chemical nature of the end groups issued from the polymerization mechanism can be changed dramatically if transesterification intervenes.

According to these different remarks and comments, there is no specific route to be recommended for synthesizing PLAGA polymers. However, researchers ought to know that PLAGA can have different properties depending on the method of synthesis and on the corresponding consequences, especially chain end modifications and the presence of initiator residues or any other impurities.

III. DEGRADATION MECHANISMS

The degradation of PLAGA polymers in contact with aqueous in vivo fluids or media has been the subject of many discussions aimed at deciding whether the mechanism is purely chemical or enzyme-dependent. Currently, the degradation of aliphatic polyesters in contact with living tissues or with enzyme-containing body fluids is regarded by most people as resulting from abiotic hydrolysis of ester bonds only. However, enzymatic degradation of aliphatic polyesters should not be claimed unless mass loss and dimensional change without molar mass decrease are conclusively shown to exist since enzymes can hardly penetrate deep in a dense polymer matrix. One must keep in mind that if, for any reason, surface degradation occurs because the rate of degradation is greater than the rate of diffusion of water into the polymeric mass, surface erosion is observed and thus confusion is possible between enzymatic surface degradation and abiotic, hydrolytic surface degradation. This is unlikely in the case of PLAGA for which water uptake is always rather fast as compared with the degradation rate.

The absence of attack of devices by enzymes does not mean that the hydrolytic process is simple. From the macroscopic viewpoint, degradation of aliphatic polyesters was regarded as homogeneous (bulk erosion) (27), although surface erosion was claimed in a few cases (8). This was primarily due to the fact that molecular weight changes were monitored by viscometry. During the last 10 years, the understanding of the hydrolytic degradation of PLAGA polymers advanced significantly due to the use of size exclusion chromatography (SEC), which revealed the presence of two populations of partially degraded PLAGA devices of rather large sizes. This discovery led to the introduction of the concept of heterogeneous degradation related to diffusion-reaction-dissolution correlated phenomena (28,29).

To summarize, once a PLAGA device is placed in contact with an aqueous medium, water penetrates into the specimen and the hydrolytic cleavage of ester bonds starts. Each ester bond cleavage generates a new carboxyl end group that, in principle, can catalyze the hydrolytic reaction of other ester bonds as proposed in the case of the homogeneous degradation mechanism (27). For a time the partially degraded macromolecules remain insoluble in the surrounding aqueous medium, regardless of its nature, and the degradation proceeds homogeneously. However, as soon as the molecular weight of some of the partially degraded macromolecules becomes low enough to allow dissolution in the aqueous medium, diffusion starts within the whole bulk, with the soluble compounds moving slowly to and off the surface while they continue to degrade. This process combining diffusion, chemical reaction, and dissolution phenomena results in a differentiation between the rates of the degradations at surface and the interior of the matrix. Indeed, oligomers can escape from the surface before total degradation, in contrast to those oligomers that are far inside. The result is a smaller autocatalytic effect at the COOH-depressed surface with respect to the bulk. In buffered media, neutralization of terminal carboxyl might also contribute to discriminate the surface degradation rate. This mechanism accounted well for the formation of two populations of partially degraded macromolecules with different molecular weight and thus the observation of bimodal SEC traces. At the end, hollow structures were observed occasionally, especially in the case of amorphous polymers (28,30). In contrast, in the case of crystallizable polyesters, no hollow structures can be formed due to the crystallization of degradation products (31).

The discovery of this phenomenon helped in understanding the effect of many factors, namely, matrix morphology, chemical composition and configurational structure, molar mass, size and shape, distribution of chemically reactive compounds within the matrix, and nature of the degradation media (32). It also contributed significantly in explaining the effect of entrapped drug on the degradation and release characteristics, depending on the hydrophile–hydrophobe balance. Considering the interdependence of degradation and drug release in controlled drug delivery systems, all these factors also influence the characteristics of drug release, as will be shown.

Table 2 presents the various factors that have been identified as influential on the behavior of PLAGA polymers in aqueous media and on drug release characteristics as discussed in detail in recent reviews (6,13).

According to the general degradation mechanism of PLAGA polymers, there are four main factors that condition the diffusion-reaction-dissolution phenomena: (a) the hydrolysis rate constant of the ester bond; (b) the diffusion coefficient of water within the matrix; (c) the diffusion coefficient of chain fragments within the polymeric matrix; and (d) the solubility of degradation products, generally oligomers, within the surrounding liquid medium from which

Table 2 Factors Affecting the Hydrolytic Degradation of Aliphatic Polyesters

Chemical composition
Molecular weight
Molecular weight distribution
Distribution of counits
Distribution of chiral units
Chain defects
Presence of low molecular weight compounds (monomer, oligomers, solvents, initiators, drugs)
Processing history
Morphology (annealing, quenching, microstructures, residual stresses, porosity)
Storage history
Shape and sizes
Aging conditions (temperature, ionic strength, ion exchange, pH)
Absorption and adsorption of compounds (water, lipids, ions)
Physical property changes (shape, size, diffusion coefficients, stresses, cracks)
Presence of enzymes

penetrating water is issued. Any additional factors, such as temperature, additives in the polymeric matrix, additives in the surrounding medium, pH, buffering capacity, size and processing history, quenching or annealing, steric hindrance, porosity, and other variables, affect the general balance through their effects on the main factors listed above (29).

The effects of chemical composition, molecular weight, molecular weight and repeating units distributions, and crystallinity are now well documented in the literature. Herein we wish to focus the comments on some more recent findings dealing with secondary factors like size and shape, or the ionic character of the entrapped drug, or the initiator used to make PLAGA polymers.

A. Size, Shape, and Porosity

The size of polymer samples has been mentioned occasionally in the literature (33). It is only recently that, on the basis of the heterogeneous degradation mechanism, Grizzi et al. accounted for the differences in degradation rates observed when comparing the degradation characteristics of films, powder, and microspheres issued from the same batch of PLA_{50} polymer (34) showing conclusively that the smaller the polymer size, the slower the degradation rate. From the same logic, one can conclude that porous systems degrade at a slower rate than plain ones, especially if dimensions of the considered device are millimetric.

B. Effect of the Presence of Ionic Drugs

According to the heterogeneous degradation mechanism, any electrostatic interaction between a PLAGA matrix and acidic, basic, or amphoteric drug molecules can drastically affect the degradation characteristics by changing the natural acid–base equilibrium of the matrix due to the presence of chain end carboxylic groups. For acidic drugs, one can expect faster hydrolysis of ester bonds. In contrast, in the case of basic drugs, two effects were observed: base catalysis of ester bond cleavage when the drug is in excess with respect to acid chain ends, and decrease of degradation rate in the contrary (35).

C. Polymerization Initiator

Recently, attention was paid to the effects of the initiator on the degradation characteristics of some PLAGA polymers. It has been shown that dramatic differences in repeating unit distribution can be observed in the case of stereocopolymers such as PLA_{50} (36). On the other hand, it was suggested that stannous octoate causes more or less chain end modification by esterification of alcoholic end groups by octanoic acid and generates hydrophobic residues that resist purification of PLAGA by precipitation from an organic solution with ethanol or water (37). Such modifications do not occur in the case of zinc metal or zinc lactate initiations. Whether similar effects can be observed and contribute to degradation in the case of tiny particles such as micro- and nanospheres or in the case of initiation in the presence of alcohols is still unknown.

In the literature, papers usually do not provide accurate information on the structure and the history of PLAGA-based formulations. Therefore, it is rather difficult to imagine how much the various factors mentioned above contribute to the degradation and the release characteristics. It is strongly suggested that researchers keep in mind that degradation and release characteristics of PLAGA depend on the experimental conditions and on the device's history much more than any other type of polymeric matrix.

As for modeling in vivo conditions, it is recommended to take into account physiological pH, ionic strength and osmolarity, and temperature as much as possible. Using 0.13 M pH 7.4 isosmolar phosphate buffer at 37°C is a convenient choice. However, it is suggested to compare PBS with another pH 7.4 buffer anytime there is a risk of interaction between the drug and phosphate ions. If phosphate ions can perturb the system, the use of any other pH 7.4 isoosmolar buffered medium, including cell culture media, is possible. However, one must keep in mind that in such media, species can be present that can diffuse and modify the matrix physical characteristics and the chain end chemistry, thus affecting the general behavior through the various interrelated factors mentioned above.

IV. CONTROLLED DRUG DELIVERY USING IMPLANTS OF PLAGA

The implants discussed here are those that have been investigated for controlled drug delivery as opposed to devices whose function is primarily structural. Structural implants can include those used for orthopedic applications (38–42) as well as nerve guides (43), in neuronal transplantation (44), as intravascular stents (45), and for repair of articular cartilage (46). Implants prepared from PLAGA are usually in the form of fibers, pressed tablets, extruded forms, or films.

A. Fibers

Biodegradable fibers are usually prepared from poly(L-lactide) (PLA_{100}) using spinning techniques and can be made as solid fibers (47,48) or as hollow fibers (49,50). These fibers can be administered subcutaneously using smaller needles than are necessary for other types of implants. Hollow fiber systems may be made with a wide range of porosities using phase inversion techniques coupled with spinning processes. Parameters such as the bore medium flow rate, spinning dope extrusion rate, fiber take-up rate, spinning height, solvent/nonsolvent pair, and processing temperature will all affect the dimensions and porosity of the final fibers.

Drug delivery studies from these fibers can be accomplished by filling the center of the hollow fibers with a drug solution and sealing the ends of the fibers. The drug delivery rates are strongly dependent on the membrane structure of the hollow fiber wall. Zero-order release of levonorgestrel at rates between 0.1 and 10 µg/cm/day have been achieved in vitro for over 180 days (49). Studies in vivo in rabbits showed that constant levonorgestrel blood levels could be achieved for up to 210 days. Other in vitro release studies of 3-ketodesogestrel also showed relatively constant release for up to 200 days (50). However, similar studies of the release of cisplatin and adriamycin showed release rates that decrease over time. While these hollow fiber systems are interesting because of their ease of administration and their ability to release, in a controlled manner, nearly any drug which may be made in an aqueous solution, such reservoir systems always carry the risk that the membrane may fail and the contents of the reservoir will be released all at once.

B. Tablets

A fairly common method of preparing tablets or pellets of PLAGA for implantation is by direct compression, at either ambient or elevated temperatures, and with or without added solvent. Most of these compression methods are based on classical pharmaceutical tableting techniques. Unless a solvent is used, these techniques are limited to use with low molecular weight polymers whose low glass transition temperatures (~30°C) allow fusion of individual particles and integration of polymer and drug upon compression (51–53). Pressed tablet formulations from low molecular weight poly(DL-lactic acid) (PLA) with number-average molecular weights of 2000 and less have shown time-dependent drug delivery both in vitro and in vivo for a wide range of drugs, including quinidine sulfate, propanolol hydrochloride (51), a luteinizing hormone–releasing agonist (52,53), and calcitonin (54). For tablets prepared from higher molecular weight PLA_{100}, a lag in the degradation and drug release was seen. As formulations were varied from 100% low molecular weight PLA to 100% high molecular weight PLA, in vivo degradation times increased from 5 weeks to 20 weeks with an initial lag time increasing from zero to 10 weeks.

A variation on this technique is a double-layered implant formulation for insulin delivery (55). The two layers in these formulations consisted of a thin layer of PLA_{50} alone and a 1-mm-thick layer of PLA and insulin. The implants were tested in vivo and up to 15 days of activity was seen. The performance of the implants was dependent on the insulin loading rate and the presence of the second PLA layer as well as the thickness of that PLA layer.

C. Extruded Implants

Extruded matrix delivery systems are usually prepared from a concentrated polymer solution in a solvent such as acetone, in which the drug is either dispersed or dissolved (56–58), or using elevated temperatures and solid materials (59–61). These devices are often in the form of cylinders, and can be used as monolithic matrix release systems (59,61) or coated with PLA to further restrict the degradation and subsequent drug release (56,57,60,61). Uncoated cylinders, especially those with higher drug loadings of 30% and 40%, showed primarily diffusion-controlled release. Coated cylinders with drug loadings of 15% or less showed primarily osmotically controlled release, with the actual release being proportional to the square root of time. However, uncoated cylinders with very low drug loadings, 2–10%, showed an initial lag time followed by a rather fast release (61). The duration of this lag time was dependent on the molecular weight of the PLAGA used, with lower molecular weight polymers showing shorter lag times before release began. Drugs that have been studied in these extruded systems include albumin (56), vacomycin hydrochloride, gentamicin sulfate, cefazolin sodium (57,58), isoniazid (59), testosterone, estradiol (60), and melanotan (61).

D. Films

Films of PLA containing a variety of drugs may also be prepared by simply dissolving the polymer in an appropriate solvent, adding drug to prepare a mutual solution or suspension, casting the polymer/drug solution into a desired shape, and allowing the solvent to dry. The solvents used to prepare such films include acetone (62,63), chloroform (64), dichloromethane, ethyl acetate, and others. For films containing gentamicin sulfate at loading rates of 0–30 wt % prepared using acetone (62), 3 days of drying the films under vacuum gave films with less than 1% residual acetone. In addition to varying the drug loading, these films were also prepared with different ratios of low (M_n = 2000) and high (M_n = 170,000) molecular weight PLA. While all samples showed an initial burst of release of 10–20%, the most constant in vitro release was seen for formulations of 70% high molecular weight PLA, 20% low molecular weight PLA, and 10 wt % gentamicin sulfate. Further studies of films prepared by blending high molecular weight PLA (M_n = 133,000) with PLA oligomers at 0, 10, and 30 wt % have shown that the presence of the PLA oligomers accelerates the PLA film degradation (63). In addition, the mechanism of that degradation was strongly dependent on the amount of oligomer present in the polymer films.

Other films of PLA_{100} containing antisense oligonucleotides for treatment of cancer and viral diseases have been prepared using chloroform (64). For these systems, with 2 wt % drug loading and a polymer number average molecular weight of 690,000, residual chloroform levels were approximately 0.026% after drying for 48 h. The release behavior of these films showed an initial release burst of up to 75% of the incorporated drug with slower but measurable release in vitro for at least 28 days. The nature of the oligonucleotide chemistry and sequence length had a more significant effect on the release behavior, including decreasing the initial burst of release, than did the drug loading.

E. Other Implantable Systems

Other less typical forms of PLAGA implants include capsules that will burst and release their drug contents at predetermined times (65) and in situ–forming implants (66,67). A pulsed-releasing capsule consisting of a hollow cylinder of PLA_{50} closed at one end and having a permeable $PLA_{37.5}GA_{25}$ membrane covering the other end of the cylinder has been studied by Jimoh and collaborators (65). Drug and an effervescent agent are contained in the core of the cylinder. As water passes through the membrane, pressure is built up within the cylinder until the membrane ruptures, thereby releasing the follicle-stimulating hormone that had been contained in the core of the PLAGA cylinder.

A number of research groups have studied the possibility of an injectable PLAGA delivery system that will solidify into an implant after injection. The basic principle here is the use of a solvent for the PLAGA that will be extracted rapidly by the biological environment, thereby leaving a solid implant after injection. The solvents usually utilized for such delivery systems are dimethylsulfoxide (DMSO) or N-methyl-2-pyrrolidone (NMP) (66). Studies conducted in vitro from spherical formulations which were formed when the polymer solutions were dropped into phosphate-buffered saline showed an initial burst of release of bovine serum albumin (BSA) from all formulations prepared from high molecular weight $PLA_{25}GA_{50}$ (M_n = 75,000–115,000), whether containing DMSO or NMP. However, the release of BSA from formulations of low molecular weight $PLA_{25}GA_{50}$ (M_n = 10,000–15,000) was nearly constant for formulations of 30, 35, and 40% polymer in NMP and 33.5% polymer in DMSO.

Other work by Shively and collaborators has combined in vitro analysis with in vivo studies and ternary phase diagrams to predict the rate of solidification of the injected implants and their subsequent drug delivery performance (67). This work has shown that DMSO-based systems require less water to initiate the precipitation process than NMP-based systems with all other factors being equivalent. Tests of these systems in vivo have shown that the DMSO-based implants have less of a burst of release, as would be expected from the solubility data.

V. MICROPARTICLE DRUG DELIVERY SYSTEMS

By far the largest research effort utilizing PLAGA in controlled drug delivery is in microparticulate systems. These formulations, whether designed to be administered subcutaneously, orally, or transmucosally, have the tremendous advantage of supplying a continuous amount of drug over a long period of time. The delivery time usually ranges from weeks to months, and once the dosage is administered it is nearly impossible to reverse. In this section we have divided this enormous field into three categories: preparation, characterization, and in vivo evaluation of PLAGA microparticles. The purpose of this section is to provide an overview of the current research and development activities related to PLAGA microparticles.

A. Preparation of Particulate Systems

1. Solvent Evaporation

The preparation methods for PLAGA biodegradable microparticles are varied, but most are based on solvent evaporation or extraction techniques (68). The simplest methods involve dissolving the polymer in an appropriate organic solvent and suspending this solution in an aqueous continuous phase that contains an appropriate surfactant. Continuous stirring then allows for evaporation of the organic solvent and hardening of the microparticles. The key factors in the size as well as the size distribution of these particles are the polymer concentration in the solvent, the amount and type of surfactant, and the stirring rate. This solvent evaporation method is most appropriate for incorporating drugs that are soluble in the same organic solvent as the PLAGA. In this case, the drug and polymer are dissolved together in the organic solvent and a molecular mixture of polymer and drug will exist in the resulting microparticles (69–72).

The solvents used with these techniques include dichloromethane, acetone, methanol, ethyl acetate, acetonitrile, chloroform, and carbon tetrachloride. Polymer concentrations of 125–1100 mg/mL will usually yield microparticles in the size range of 10–150 μm (69–71). A summary of the ICH guidelines for residual levels for many solvents used in biodegradable microparticle preparation are given in Table 3 (73). Decreasing the polymer concentration to 20 mg/mL can yield much smaller particles, in the size range of 1.2–7.4 μm (74). The surfactants most commonly used are poly(vinyl alcohol), methylcellulose, gelatin, poly(vinyl pyrrolidone), and Tween-20 in concentrations of 0.1–1.0 % w/v. Complete solvent evaporation can take 8–10 h in some cases. Methods used to hasten microparticle formation include application of vacuum, elevation of temperature, and solvent extraction techniques that will be described shortly. Although there has been some work on PLAGA microparticles in the size range of 100 μm and larger prepared using basic solvent evaporation, most of the more recent research has concentrated either on preparing smaller nanoparticles or on developing techniques that can successfully incorporate water-soluble compounds.

Variations on this basic solvent evaporation technique include (a) solvent extraction (74); (b) double emulsions (75–83); (c) oil-in-oil systems (76,84); (d) phase separation or coacervation (85–88); and (e) multiple emulsion potentiometric dispersion (89). Many of these variations are designed to incorporate water-soluble drugs such as peptides and proteins or to modify the typical release profile seen from biodegradable microparticles. The methods described

Table 3 Recommended ICH Residual Solvent Levels (73)

Solvent	Permitted daily exposure (mg/day)	Concentration limit (ppm)
Acetaldehyde	Not listed	
Acetone[c]	50.0	5000
Acetonitrile[b]	4.1	410
Carbon tetrachloride[a]		4
Chloroform[b]	0.6	60
Dichloromethane[b]	6.0	600
Diethyl ether	Not listed	
Dimethylacetal	Not listed	
Dimethylformamide	Not listed	
Dimethylsulfoxide	Not listed	
1,4-Dioxane[b]	3.8	380
Ethanol[c]	50.0	5000
Ethyl acetate[c]	50.0	5000
Ethyl ether[c]	50.0	5000
Heptane[c]	50.0	5000
Methanol[b]	30.0	3000
Nitromethane[b]	0.5	50
N-Methyl-2-pyrrolidone	Not listed	
Tetrahydrofuran[c]	50.0	5000
1,1,1-Trichloroethane[a]		1500
1,1,2-Trichloroethylene	Not listed	

[a]Class 1 solvent to be avoided, toxic and/or environmental hazard.
[b]Class 2 solvent to be limited.
[c]Class 3 solvent with low toxic potential.

here and the references are by no means an exhaustive list of the tremendous amount of research that has been conducted on microparticles of PLAGA. Instead, the focus here is on work that has been published in the last few years.

2. Encapsulation of Water-Soluble Compounds

In cases where the drug to be encapsulated is not soluble in the organic solvent used, there are two options. The drug may either be incorporated as solid submicrometer particles within the polymeric microparticles, or a tri- or multiphase preparation method may be used. This water-in-oil-in-water technique is extremely useful for incorporation of highly water-soluble drugs (80). In the basic version of this technique, an aqueous drug solution is dispersed within the initial polymer/solvent solution that then becomes the center core of the resulting microparticle or microcapsule. One of the limiting factors in using this technique is the solubility of the drug in the two aqueous phases of the microparticle preparation system. A high solubility in the internal aqueous phase is highly desirable as this will give microparticles with high final drug loadings. However, it is preferable to have a low drug solubility in the external, continuous aqueous phase so that the maximum amount of drug will remain in the microparticles and not dissolve in the continuous, external aqueous solution.

The most widely studied model protein for encapsulation into PLAGA microparticles is BSA (75–78). Some researchers have seen evidence that the encapsulation efficiency as well as the decrease or lack of the initial burst of release can be related to the molecular weight of the PLA$_{25}$GA$_{50}$, with lower molecular weights being the most desirable (75). Other laboratories have seen no such dependence on the polymer molecular weight but instead see differences in efficiency and release due to coencapsulation of various surfactants, with undesirable results (76). Some of the higher BSA loadings reported are approximately 8–11% w/w. However, while the actual loading of 8.02% was achieved with a theoretical loading of 10%, an actual loading of only 10.68% was achieved with a theoretical loading of 25% (77). These particular particles had an average size of 1–1.5 μm and showed release, with a 10–40% burst, of up to 240 h. Large particles of 6–8 μm with a lower drug loading of 1.2% showed extended and almost constant release for 900 h (75). Even larger particles of 18–46 μm, still with low drug loadings, had extended release for at least 30 days with an initial burst of 2–25% of the total BSA released.

Other active agents that have been encapsulated using water-in-oil-in-water techniques include human erythropoietin (79,80), glycoprotein gp120 for treatment of AIDS (81,82), and human growth hormone (83). The formulations containing human erythropoietin showed an initial burst of release with at least 15% of the encapsulated drug being released within the first 24 h from particles in the size range of 20–40 μm (79,80). Maintaining the protein stability and avoiding aggregation appeared to be significant challenges in successfully preparing formulations with high entrapment efficiencies and long delivery times (80). Encapsulation efficiencies were also found to increase to 100% by increasing the kinematic viscosity of the PLAGA solution, in this case PLAGA in dichloromethane, by increasing the PLAGA concentration from 0.1 to 0.6 g/mL and lowering the temperature of the first emulsion to 0°C (81). This change in the kinematic viscosity also helped to significantly reduce the initial burst of drug release. Additional factors such as drying method, organic solvent used, and molecular weight of the PLAGA have also been correlated to changes in release profiles and microparticle properties (81). The encapsulation efficiency of microparticles of less than 10 μm in diameter may be enhanced by modifying the pH of the internal and external aqueous phases or by adding stabilizing agents to the inner aqueous phase during their preparation (82). However, the stabilizing agent may cause additional side effects by increasing the initial burst of release by forming pores in the microsphere structure, as was seen when ovalbumin was added to the inner aqueous protein solution but not when Pluronic F-68 was added.

Formulations containing human growth hormone have been tested both in an in vitro cell model and in vivo in rhesus monkeys where a burst of release was seen in both studies (83). Release continued for up to 50 days in vivo and 20–60 days in vitro, depending on the method used. An evaluation was conducted of a variety of in vitro test systems, including a semicontinuous flow system and separation of particles using high-speed centrifugation. A semicontinuous flow method showed in vitro results that were the most comparable to the in vivo results (83).

Despite these ingenious modifications, most protein-containing biodegradable microparticles only achieve drug loadings on the order of 0.1–10 wt % protein. For some active agents, these loading rates are acceptable, but a great deal of work continues to find methods to increase the final protein loading rates and more importantly the encapsulation efficiency, while also avoiding a significant burst of release upon administration of the microparticle system.

Another variation of the solvent evaporation technique utilizes an oil-in-oil emulsion method to encapsulate cisplatin (84). The initial cosolvent in this technique was dimethylformamide (DMF) because it had the lowest boiling point of the common solvents of cisplatin and $PLA_{37.5}GA_{25}$. The cisplatin and PLAGA solution was added dropwise to liquid paraffin containing Span-80. The system was stirred at an initial temperature of 25°C which was then raised, at various rates, to 40°C and continued for 40 h to remove all of the DMF. Those particles that were uniformly spherical were prepared from a solution of 8 wt % PLAGA and 5 wt % cisplatin, where the paraffin contained 10 wt % Span-80 and the temperature rise was 0.2°C/min. The average particle size decreased as the PLAGA molecular weight decreased. All formulations showed an initial burst, ranging from 5% to 80%, with the lowest burst and most constant release for the spherical particles mentioned above as well as similar formulations with 3 wt % cisplatin.

3. Other Preparation Methods

Phase separation or coacervation differs from solvent evaporation in that the solvent to be removed is extracted into another solvent as opposed to being allowed to dissipate through evaporation alone. The extracting solvents used include heptane to extract dichloromethane or ethyl acetate (85,86), diethyl ether to extract dichloromethane (87), and silicone oil to extract dichloromethane (88). Using these methods, ovalbumin can be entrapped at levels up to 6.5 wt %. These formulations do not show a significant burst of release and have relatively constant release in vitro for up to 40 days (86). Particles prepared containing ciprofloxacin are quite porous and not uniformly spherical (87). Release in vitro from particles in the size range of 250–425 μm showed square root of time dependence with no initial burst. Studies by Nihant and collaborators have evaluated the various microencapsulation parameters and their effect on the characteristics of the final microparticles (88). This work has determined that the rate of addition of the coacervation promoter will determine how far out of equilibrium the system is at any time and as such it is the most critical processing parameter in coacervation. Other important factors are the ratio of the dispersed aqueous phase to the oil phase, the stirring rate during dispersion, and the drug being incorporated, as the drug can interact with the polymer and promote interfacial complexation.

Other research groups have expanded the principle behind preparing biodegradable microparticles using multiple emulsions to prepare water-in-oil-in-oil-in-oil formulations (89). These formulations began with water-soluble compounds dissolved in an aqueous phase which is emulsified in soybean oil to form a first stable emulsion. This emulsion is dispersed in a $PLA_{25}GA_{50}$/acetonitrile solution that is then dispersed in a hardening solution of light mineral oil. This method protects the water-soluble drug from exposure to organic solvents with a layer of oil. Microparticles have also been made using a potentiometric dispersion technique that resulted in more uniform particles and higher drug loadings (89). Higher drug loadings may also be achieved, especially with lower stirring rates which produce larger microparticles. The particles are all spherical and smooth, with cross-sections of these multiphase microspheres showing numerous internal spheres within the microparticles.

4. Removal of Solvents During Particle Preparation

One of the greatest challenges in all of these techniques is the removal of residual solvent from the microparticles. A number of research groups are investigating removal techniques including variations in drying time and drying temperature as well as reduced pressure (90). It was found that the lowest residual solvent levels, for dichloromethane, were obtained when the drying temperature was near the glass transition temperature of the polymer. Removal of the hardening agent was most strongly dependent on the affinity between solvent, polymer, and hardening agent. Changes that may be made during the earlier steps of the microparticle formation process include implementing a temperature gradient or diluting the continuous phase (91). For microparticles containing salmon calcitonin, raising the temperature during the solvent removal step from 15°C to 40°C consistently resulted in particles with a hollow core and a porous surface. Dilution of the emulsion into either 1.5 or 2.5 times the original volume of the continuous phase resulted in particles with a honeycomb matrix and a porous surface but no hollow core. For those particles prepared with a temperature gradient, the residual dichloromethane was less than 10 ppm in all but one case.

In order to better understand the process of forming microparticles through solvent evaporation and solvent extraction processes, DeLuca and collaborators have used a kinetic and thermodynamic model to describe this process and have compared their predictions with their actual results (92,93). The model expresses the microparticle formation process by coupling equations for mass transfer in the dispersed phase with first-order evaporation from the continuous phase. The model predicts the amount of residual solvent in the forming microparticles, as the dispersed phase, as a function of time and as a function of radial position in the forming microparticles. It also describes the amount of residual solvent in the continuous phase that matches experimental data very well (92). Factors that were evaluated theoretically and experimentally included the ratio of the dispersed to continuous phase and the temperature of the system during solvent removal (93).

5. Preparation of Particles Using Spray Drying and Related Methods

A different technique that is showing considerable potential for formulating biodegradable microparticles is spray drying and variations using cryogenic processes (94–99). Spray-drying is widely used in the pharmaceutical and biochemical fields and the final particle size is controlled by a number of factors including the size of the nozzle used in the processing. Another critical factor in such a process is the solvent used for the PLAGA. A variety of solvents that have similar toxicity levels but widely varying physicochemical characteristics were studied by Gander and Merkle: acetaldehyde, dimethyl acetal, acetone, dichloromethane, dioxane, ethyl acetate, ethyl vinyl ether, nitromethane, tetrahydrofuran, 1,1,1-trichloroethane, and 1,1,2-trichloroethylene (95). Multiple different characteristics contributed to the final performance of the microparticles so that no trend could be established for a single property such as boiling point, vapor pressure, or polymer–solvent affinity. It was found that the encapsulation efficiency could reach 100% for a 2.9% loading of BSA using dichloromethane, ethyl acetate, and nitromethane. The lowest bursts of release, at only 5%, were seen for particles prepared from both dichloromethane and nitromethane.

Another method of preparing biodegradable microparticles, usually of PLA_{100}, is using supercritical fluid extraction where the solvent used is usually carbon dioxide (96–98). These processes can significantly diminish the use of traditional organic solvents such as dichloromethane. The particles prepared by this method are usually an order of magnitude smaller than those prepared by solvent evaporation methods, with typical particle sizes on the nanoparticle scale at 0.1–10 μm (97), depending on the specific method used. One process is rapid expansion of a supercritical solution (RESS) whereby polymer and drug are dissolved in a supercritical fluid, and then the fluid expands rapidly to a state where the solubility is significantly lower. This change leads to supersaturation of the solvent, which causes the formation of small and uniform particles. A critical factor here is the solubility of the polymer and drug in the supercritical gas. Ideally, the polymer and drug are sufficiently soluble in the supercritical carbon dioxide, but this is rarely the case and the materials must be dissolved in dichloromethane before being added to the supercritical fluid. Another complication is that for those materials that are soluble in the supercritical carbon dioxide alone, the resulting particles are quite porous and would provide little control over the release of any incorporated drugs (98). Particle size, agglomeration, and polydispersity may be controlled by varying the spraying pressure, pulsation method, and other factors. Particles have been prepared, using supercritical carbon dioxide and minimal amounts of dichloromethane, that contain gentamicin, naloxone, rifampin, and naltrexone (97). The loading efficiencies varied from 10% to 100%. The in vitro drug delivery was linearly dependent on the square root of time and showed anywhere from 4% to 78% of the drug being released in the initial burst.

While many of these preparation techniques still exist at only a laboratory scale, some companies have been successful in scaling up their microparticle preparation techniques. These specific techniques include those used by Southern Research Institute, Alkermes (99), and others. A development scale process to encapsulate recombinant human growth hormone (rHGH) begins with a lyophilized complex of the hormone with zinc (99). Particles of zinc-rhGH and zinc carbonate are reduced in size to 1–3 μm and are suspended in a 50:50 PLAGA solution in dichloromethane. This suspension is sprayed through a sonicating nozzle into liquid ethanol at $-105°C$. The mixture is gradually warmed to $-40°C$ and the microspheres harden as the ethanol extracts the dichloromethane, a process that takes a few hours. The suspension is then filtered to collect the microparticles that are subsequently dried.

B. Characterization of Biodegradable Microparticles

In order to correctly evaluate biodegradable microparticles, the particles must be studied for both their physical and chemical behavior. The macroscopic properties of particle size, shape, and size distribution are as critical as the microscopic properties of the amorphous or crystalline nature of the polymer and the presence or absence of drug and polymer microdomains. These physical properties play a strong role in the chemical drug delivery behavior of these particles.

1. Analysis of Particle Size and Size Distribution

Within the microparticle size range, optical techniques as well as a variety of laser light scattering techniques may be used to evaluate the size and shape of a batch of biodegradable microparticles. When the microparticle size is less than 10 μm, then electron microscopy and other more indirect methods are necessary. Most size evaluation techniques provide either size and size distribution information (laser light scattering) or more specific shape information (optical techniques). Unfortunately, while electron microscopy can provide the greatest detail regarding the external and internal physical form of biodegradable microparticles, this technique ultimately destroys the microparticles being analyzed. One of the best, and nondestructive, techniques for macroscopic analysis of microparticles involves concurrent videomicroscopic and laser light scattering analysis, arranged perpendicular to one another (71,100). This type of analysis, using a Galai CIS-100 (Brookhaven Instruments, Holtsville, NY) allows nondestructive analysis of particle size and shape over long times, while concurrently evaluating their drug release performance. Using this sort of analysis, it is straightforward to show that the PLAGA particles degrade through a bulk degradation mechanism and to follow the degradation of a single group of particles through their entire lifetime. An example of the images collected using this method, the particle size distributions, and microscopic images of a single formulation batch of microparticles prepared from $PLA_{37.5}GA_{25}$ of molecular weight 50,900 are shown in Fig. 2–4. Figure 2 shows images of the microparticles before degradation and Fig. 3 shows their particle size distribution measured concurrently with the Galai image shown in Fig. 2a. While the optical micrographs obtained on the Galai are not as sharp as the microscopic images since the Galai images were taken when the particles were stirring in solution, the images provide qualitatively the same data on particle shape and porosity. The images in Fig. 4 show the particles at different times during their in vitro degradation in distilled, deionized water at 25°C. The degradation at 210 days (4a) shows evidence of both degraded and whole particles. By 350 days many of the particles had degraded into pieces of polymer with a loose association between the original parts of the microparticles where these associations still had sizes very close to those of the original particles, as shown in Fig. 4b. Although some particle fragments were still evident at day 511 (Fig. 4c), no particles or associations of particle fragments approaching the original microparticle size could be found.

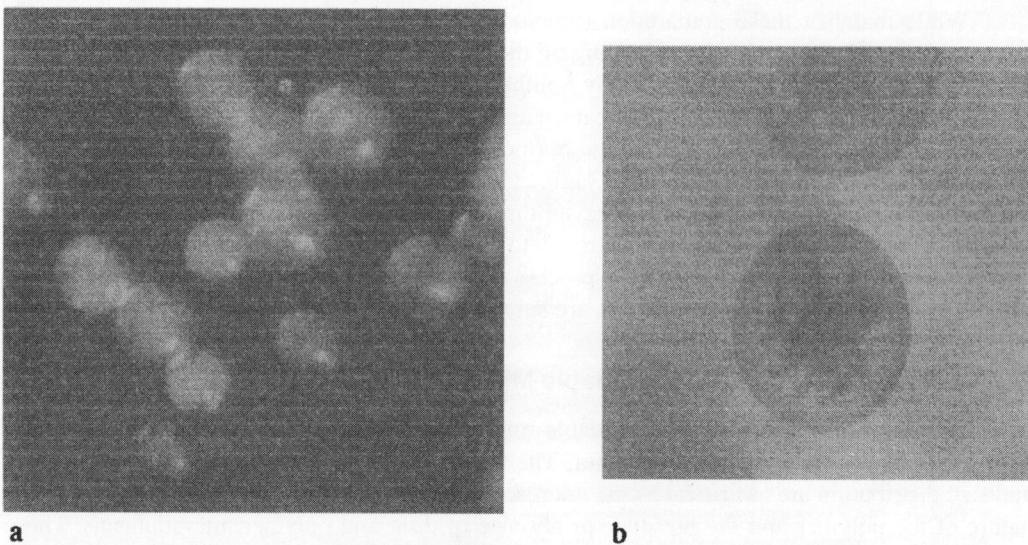

Figure 2 Microparticles of $PLA_{37.5}GA_{25}$, molecular weight 50,900, before degradation as seen using optical microscopy (a) and Galai CIS-100 imaging (b).

Many researchers will analyze the microparticle size and size distributions using equipment such as a Malvern particle size analyzer (101). Particle sizers coupled with scanning electron microscopy provide a full range of size and shape analysis, which can be used to determine both the external and internal particle structure (102–105). These studies can be done on the particles at any time during the degradation and release studies. A full analysis of the internal structure of microparticles is always desirable in order to determine not only their porosity but also if they are monolithic particles or, instead, microcapsules with a hollow core. In addition, Schugens and collaborators (103) have used mercury porosimetry to determine quantitatively the porosity and pore size distribution for PLA microparticles in the size range of 250–315 μm diameter.

2. Analysis of Particle Morphology

Differential scanning calorimetry (DSC) can be a very useful technique not only for determining the form of the polymer and drug in a microparticle formulation, but also for assessing potential interactions between the polymer and the drug (106). For microparticles prepared from only poly(L-lactic acid) or only poly(D-lactic acid), this technique may be used to determine the degree of crystallinity of the polymer in the microparticles. However, most formulations are prepared from poly(DL-lactic acid) or PLAGA so the measurements will be more useful in determining the glass transition temperature of the polymer. This glass transition temperature is dependent on the molecular weight of the polymer as well as on the presence of solvents or plasticizers such as water. As the PLAGA degrades and the molecular weight decreases throughout the bulk of the polymer, Park has found that the glass transition temperature of PLAGA microparticles undergoing in vitro hydrolysis and degradation, originally of 17,000 molecular weight, will drop from 41.7°C to 10°C over 33 days (107). As the glass transition temperature of the polymer approaches and passes the temperature of its environment, degradation and release behavior can change dramatically.

This technique is useful not only for evaluation of the polymer morphology but also of the drug morphology and possible polymer–drug interactions. Comparison of DSC thermograms

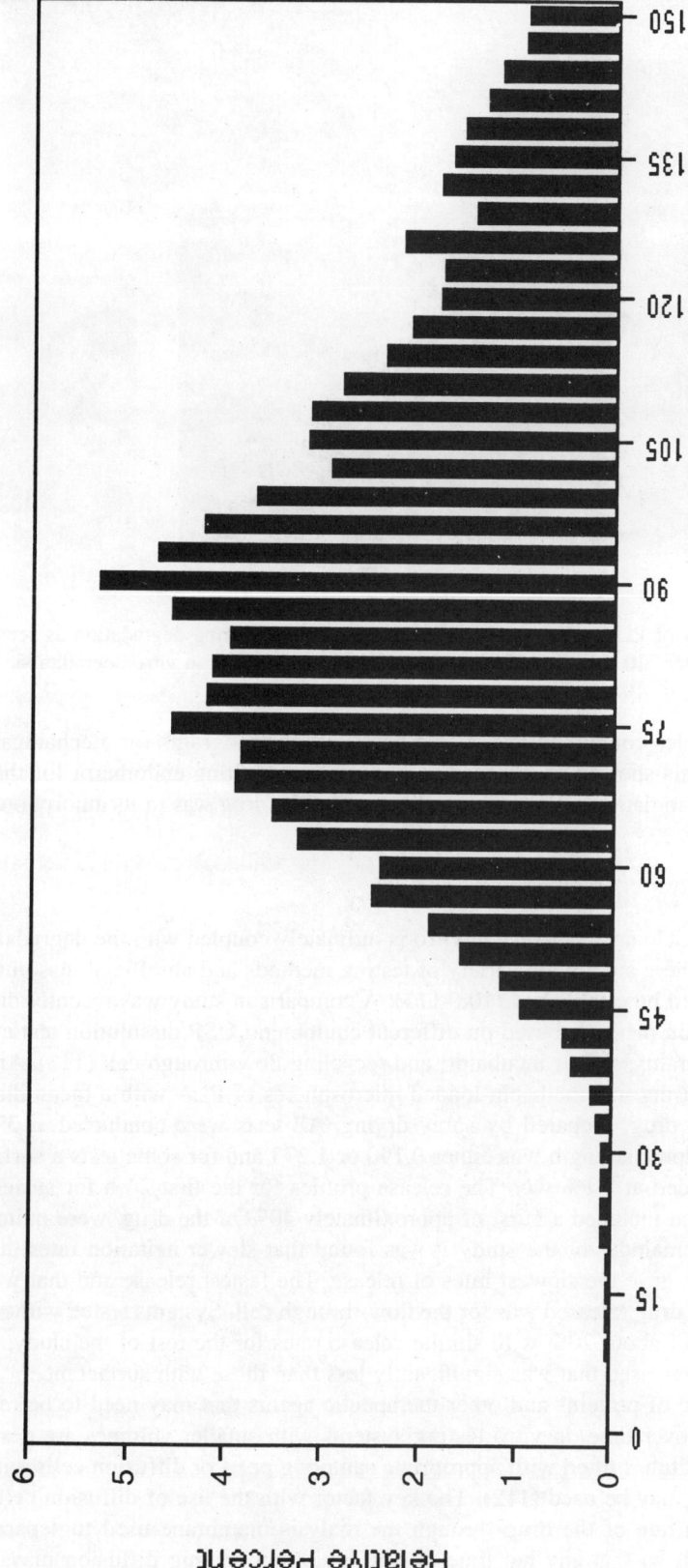

Figure 3 Volume average microparticles size distribution for microparticles of PLA$_{37.5}$GA$_{25}$, molecular weight 50,900, before degradation using Galai CIS-100 particle analysis system.

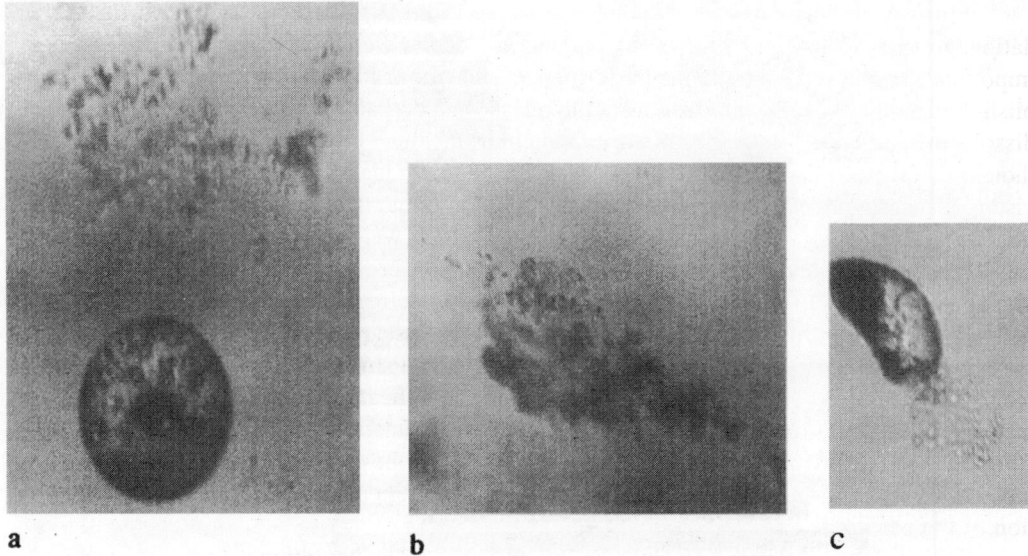

Figure 4 Microparticles of $PLA_{37.5}GA_{25}$, molecular weight 50,900, during degradation as seen using Galai CIS-100 imaging after 210 days (a), 350 days (b), and 511 days (c) of in vitro degradation.

for PLAGA microparticles containing levamisole base with thermograms for mechanical mixtures of the two materials showed an absence of a crystalline melting endotherm for the drug for the microparticle formulations (104). This indicates that the drug was in its amorphous state in the microparticles.

3. Analysis of Particle Degradation and Drug Delivery

The testing of microparticle drug delivery in vitro is intimately coupled with the degradation of the PLAGA polymer. There are a wide variety of testing methods and an official dissolution or related method has yet to be established (108–111). A comparison study was recently done on four of the most common methods based on different equipment: USP dissolution test apparatus; rotating bottle apparatus; shaker incubator; and recycling flow-through cell (111). An evaluation was performed using indomethacin-loaded microspheres of PLA with a mean diameter of 3.14 μm, at 31.25% drug, prepared by spray drying. All tests were conducted at 37°C in buffers of pH 7.4. The ionic strength was either 0.190 or 1.273 and for some tests a surfactant, polysorbate 20, was added at 0.1% w/v. The release profiles for the first 24 h for systems including surfactant, which included a burst of approximately 40% of the drug, were quite similar. However, for the remainder of the study it was found that slower agitation rates, as seen with a shaker incubator, gave the slowest rates of release. The fastest release and that with the greatest total amount of drug released was for the flow-through cell. Systems tested without surfactant showed a burst of about 20% with similar release rates for the rest of the study, giving a final amount of drug released that was significantly less than those with surfactant.

For testing release of proteins and other therapeutic agents that may need to be released in very small amounts over time, in vitro testing systems with smaller volumes are desirable. Here simple shaken test tubes fitted with appropriate sampling ports or diffusion cells with volumes as small as 1 mL may be used (112). The key factor with the use of diffusion cells is to determine the diffusion rate of the drug through the dialysis membrane used to separate the donor and receptor cells so that any lag time or rate limitation in drug diffusion may be accounted for in later calculations of the drug delivery from the particles.

Since the drug delivery from the microparticles is directly dependent on the polymer degradation, an analysis of the change in the polymer molecular weight during degradation is also an important factor in determining the performance behavior of PLAGA microparticles. To accomplish this, particles can be removed from the release and degradation media at specific times and dissolved in an appropriate solvent such as dichloromethane or chloroform (104,113,114). Although the average polymer molecular weight during degradation used to be determined using viscosity measurements, most studies now use SEC or gel permeation chromatography to obtain not only an average molecular weight but a full molecular weight distribution.

Because of the acidic nature of the biodegradation products of PLAGA, lactic acid and glycolic acid, the pH of the environment around such a delivery system as well as inside these delivery systems will decrease with time (113,115). The degradation solution for in vitro tests may be changed periodically, as is often done to simulate sink conditions and to remove samples for analysis. Nevertheless, studies have shown a significant drop in the pH of a degradation medium from 7.4 to just over 3 in 28 days for systems containing 20 mg of particles, prepared from 50:50 low molecular weight PLAGA, in 2 mL of phosphate-buffered saline (113). This more acidic environment surrounding the particles will often contribute to accelerated degradation of the particles.

Within the particles themselves, the increasingly acidic environment not only accelerates the particle degradation, but also poses a stability risk for proteins and other drugs which have been encapsulated and which should remain stable until release. Kissel and collaborators have used the nondestructive technique of electron paramagnetic resonance spectroscopy (EPR) to determine the pH within degrading $PLA_{25}GA_{50}$ microparticles that have been loaded with spin-labeled albumin (115). Although the readings could only be taken for the first 50 h for albumin within PLAGA microparticles, the pH has been shown to be as low as 3.5 within some particles during degradation.

4. Microparticle Behavior In Vivo

Most in vitro microparticle performance studies are intended to assist in predicting the ultimate in vivo behavior of a given microparticle formulation. While these correlations are still qualitative at best, many current efforts are bridging that gap with studies of the behavior of dispersed, as opposed to aggregated, particles (114) or direct comparison of in vitro and in vivo performance of the same formulations (116). Some of these studies by Tracy and collaborators at Alkermes (116) have shown that for six different formulations of $PLA_{25}GA_{50}$ containing 15% rHGH the rate of degradation as measured by changes in polymer molecular weight is 2–4 times faster in vivo than in vitro. The in vitro degradation was carried out in 50 mM HEPES buffer at pH 7.4 and 37°C. The in vivo degradation was studied by injecting microspheres subcutaneously into male Sprague-Dawley rats. The factor having the greatest effect on the degradation, both in vitro and in vivo, was whether the end groups of the polymer were capped (hydrophobic) or uncapped (hydrophilic). Microparticles prepared from PLAGA with uncapped end groups exhibited faster degradation times both in vitro (two fold) and in vivo (four fold) than the same particles prepared from polymer with capped end groups.

Many different formulation types have been studied in vivo for a wide variety of applications. One such system, in which the burst of release often seen from microparticle formulations would be an advantage, is in vaccine development. Researchers at Southern Research Institute and their collaborators have studied a number of delivery systems, including those that boost the IgG antistaphylococcal enterotoxin B toxin response for at least 90 days in mice with a single injection of encapsulated toxoid (117). Another study investigated the effects of injecting encapsulated ovalbumin (OVA) into the peritoneal cavity of mice. It was found that the production of anti-OVA IgG antibody could be seen in vivo for at least 14 weeks from particles whose in vitro delivery only lasted 35 days (118). In order to help develop a longlasting in vivo delivery system, PLA and PLAGA microspheres containing 12% leuprorelin acetate, a highly active agonist of luteinizing hormone–releasing hormone, were injected subcutaneously into rats. The resulting drug delivery profiles were highly dependent on the molecular weight and composition of the PLA or PLAGA polymers used in the formulations (119). The duration of drug delivery ranged from 4 weeks for formulations prepared from PLA of molecular weight 4700 and $PLA_{37.5}GA_{25}$ of molecular weight 15,800 to more than 16 weeks for formulations prepared from PLA with molecular weight 53,300. For a 3-month injection that would give the most constant release rate over that time, it was found that using PLA with a molecular weight of 11,800–17,300 provided linear sustained release in vivo for 3 months.

Many research groups are studying microparticle formulations that could be used to treat cancerous tissues. These include delivery of cisplatin from microparticles of $PLA_{12.5}GA_{75}$ where intraperitoneal injection of these particles in mice with murine tumors significantly increased their survival time (120). In fact, while the mean survival time for untreated animals was only 30 days, the mean survival time was greater than 120 days for mice that received more than 1000 μg of encapsulated cisplatin. All mice receiving this level of free cisplatin died within 4 days due to the toxicity of the drug. For the mice receiving 1770 μg of encapsulated cisplatin in a single injection, 40% died because of drug toxicity, but the remaining 60% showed no evidence of any tumor cells after 198 days. Another drug that is widely used in cancer treatment is 5-fluorouracil (5-FU). Intravenous administration of 3-6 μm microspheres containing 5-FU in mice showed that these particles concentrated in the liver, making them appropriate candidates for treatment of liver cancer (121). For treatment of brain tumors, similar microparticles may be implanted directly into the brain at the desired site of delivery (122). These microparticles, prepared from $PLA_{25}GA_{50}$ at either 19% or 30% 5-FU, increased survival time in rats, with only one animal receiving the 19% loaded microparticles showing evidence of a tumor at day 90.

While most microparticulate systems are designed to be administered subcutaneously, there are also other means and sites of delivery. A single intramuscular injection of 80 mg of $PLA_{45}GA_{10}$ encapsulated norethisterone has been shown to suppress estrus for up to 45 days in rats (123). Other formulations are designed for pulmonary delivery, which can be useful for systemic delivery, but are more important for targeting delivery to the lung (124,125). Utilizing particles under 5 μm in diameter, biodegradable particles can deliver agents to treat allergic and asthmatic diseases (124) or pulmonary infections (125) directly to the bronchoalveolar region of the lung. A comparison study was conducted by Poyner and collaborators to evaluate the delivery of tobramycin, an antibiotic, from liposomes and PLA_{100} microparticles administered both intravenously and endotracheally (125). They found that the microparticles, of average diameter 0.736 μm, were well retained in the lung for at least 24 h. Although the particle size was such that the microparticles were retained to some extent within the vasculature of the lungs after intravenous administration, endotrachael administration was preferable with nearly 50% of the drug still in the lung 24 h after endotracheal administration of microparticles, as opposed to just under 30% for particles administered intravenously.

In addition to the desired in vivo event of successful polymer degradation and drug delivery, reactions also occur to PLAGA on a cellular level, whether microparticles have been injected subcutaneously or administered by other routes. Injection site reaction to microparticles seems to be minimal, with little tissue reaction to the degradation byproducts or to the more acidic microenvironment that may exist near and in the microparticles during their degradation. There is also little evidence of encapsulation of microparticles as is seen with larger implantable systems. Usually, mild inflammation and normal wound healing are observed (126). However, some studies have shown that phagocytosed PLA_{100} particles can cause limited cell death (127). It is believed that this is primarily due to the degradation products from the microparticles and the effect will depend on the type of cell as well as the type of injection solution used. Analysis of the cellular and fibrotic events in tissue response to implanted microspheres of PLA_{50}, $PLA_{25}GA_{50}$ with blocked end groups, and $PLA_{25}GA_{50}$ with unblocked end groups showed cellular infiltration of all particles at 30 days, with the greatest cellular infiltration in the microparticles prepared from the unblocked PLAGA (128). A recent review by Anderson and Shive (129) provides a thorough analysis of the biocompatibility of PLA and PLAGA microparticles, including discussions of the variations in tissue response which are dependent on the drug incorporated in the biodegradable microparticles.

VI. COPOLYMERS OF PLA, PLAGA AND OTHER MATERIALS

While many research groups are working with blends of PLA, PGA, and PLAGA with other polymers and natural materials, here we will concentrate on novel polymers that are actually copolymers which include PLA, PGA, or PLAGA in the polymer structure. Most of this effort has focused on copolymers with poly(ethylene glycol), poly(ethylene oxide), or poly(ϵ-caprolactone).

A. Copolymers with Poly(ethylene glycol) and Poly(ethylene oxide)

Considerable research effort has focused on combining poly(ethylene glycol) (PEG) or poly(ethylene oxide) (PEO) with PLA or PLAGA. The structure of PEG and PEO are the same, with PEG usually referring to polymers of less than 20,000 molecular weight and PEO referring to polymers with larger molecular weights. The focus on this combination of materials is driven by a desire to combine the hydrophilic and biocompatible nature of PEG with the degradable properties of PLAGA to give a copolymer whose characteristics may be varied from hydrophilic to hydrophobic and from nondegradable to degradable, depending on its precise composition.

Some of the earliest work in developing block copolymers of PLA_{100} and poly(ethylene oxide) was presented by Cohn and Younes in 1988 (130). These copolymer matrices were characterized in a variety of ways, including infrared spectroscopy, differential scanning calorimetry, and nuclear magnetic resonance spectroscopy. By incorporating PEO chains within the polymer the equilibrium water content could reach more than 60%. For these particular copolymers, the lactic acid portion ranged from 20 to 84 mol% and the PEO chains were from 600 to 6000 molecular weight. Other work with random block copolymers of PLA and PEG has evaluated the degradation behavior of these materials (131) and their utility as microparticles for drug delivery (132). Degradation rates appear to be strongly dependent on the PEG content, with partially degraded PLA segments sometimes being solubilized by attached PEG before they would otherwise have been released from the bulk polymer.

One particular copolymer structure has received a great deal of attention, one with a PEG or PEO central block and PLA chains at either end (133–144). These polymers are usually prepared by starting with a PEG segment of a given length and then polymerizing the PLA while using the PEG as the initiator for the polymerization reaction. Studies have evaluated the effect of the length of the PEG block (135) as well as the length of the PLA_{100} blocks (136,137) on water absorption and degradation of these copolymers. A series of papers by Kissel (138–144) have explored the synthesis of these triblock materials, in vitro degradation, drug delivery, in vitro biocompatibility, in vivo biocompatibility, as well as the microenvironment of PLA-PEO-PLA microparticles during degradation. The biocompatibility studies have shown that PLA-PEO-PLA polymers show very similar and minimal adverse tissue reactions. Drug delivery studies that compared in vitro delivery of BSA from microparticles prepared from PLA_{100}-PEO-PLA_{100} and $PLA_{50}GA_{50}$-PEO-$PLA_{50}GA_{50}$ polymers showed that the PLAGA-containing polymers exhibited fairly continuous release while PLA-containing polymers had two phases of release more typical of PLAGA microparticles (139). Release studies of cytochrome c and FITC-dextran from $PLA_{50}GA_{50}$-PEO-$PLA_{50}GA_{50}$ microparticles also showed continuous release in vitro (141).

B. Copolymers with ϵ-Caprolactone

A number of research groups have also been investigating copolymers of PLA or PGA with ϵ-caprolactone (145–148). Sawhney and Hubbell evaluated a series of 66 different terpolymers of DL-lactide, glycolide, and ϵ-caprolactone to determine the degradation rates and other properties of cast films (145). They found that the longest degradation times were for polymers with a 2:1:7 ratio of glycolide lactide ϵ-caprolactone and the fastest degradation for polymers with a 6:3:1 ratio. The physical properties of copolymers of lactide and ϵ-caprolactone have been found to vary from hard to rubbery as the ϵ:-caprolactone content increased from 5 to 20 wt % (147). Porous copolymers with 50% ϵ-caprolactone content have been evaluated as implants for meniscal tissue regeneration in the knee joint (148). The polymers showed a bulk degradation behavior and, during degradation, separated into a crystalline phase containing mainly L-lactide and an amorphous phase composed mainly of ϵ-caprolactone.

C. Other Copolymer Systems

A few other copolymer combinations have also been investigated, including copolymers with glycine (149), p-hydroxybenzoic acid and p-hydroxycinnamic acid (150), and aspartic acid (151). All of these materials should still function as biodegradable materials, albeit with different degradation and release properties than PLA or PGA alone. Work on all of these copolymers is still at a stage where basic structural information is being gathered and detailed degradation and drug delivery information is not yet available.

VII. CONTROLLED DRUG DELIVERY PRODUCTS UTILIZING PLAGA

Although PLAGA polymers have been widely accepted as absorbable sutures and as orthopedic pins, screws, and anchors (152), they are still poised to significantly impact the market in controlled drug delivery formulations. The first implantable formulations, which have been available since 1989, are the Lupron Depot (TAP Pharmaceuticals and Takeda Chemical) and Zoladex (Zeneca). Both of these products have been designed to release a hormone for treatment of prostate cancer. In the form of a 1mm cylinder, Zoladex contains goserelin acetate (up to 15%), a synthetic decapeptide analogue of luteinizing hormone–releasing hormone, also known as gonadotropin-releasing hormone, dispersed in a matrix of PLAGA containing less than 2.5% acetic acid (153). The original implant formulation contained 3.6 mg of goserelin acetate and was designed for monthly use. The implant is administered by injection with a 16-gauge needle into the fat just below the skin of the abdomen. An additional formulation of Zoladex was approved in 1996 that contains 10.8 mg of goserelin acetate and is to be administered every 3 months.

The Lupron Depot, in contrast, is a microparticle-based delivery system. This formulation, designed to release leuprolide acetate, a synthetic nanopeptide analogue of naturally occurring gonadotropin-releasing hormone, in a controlled manner over 1 month's time following intramuscular injection (153). The formulation contains leuprolide acetate (7.5 mg) in microparticles of DL-lactic acid and glycolic acid copolymer (66.2 mg) and also includes purified gelatin (1.3 mg) and D-mannitol (13.2 mg). The injection vehicle contain carboxymethylcellulose sodium (7.5 mg), D-mannitol (75 mg), and polysorbate 80 (1.5 mg) in water. The Lupron Depot is designed to inhibit the growth of certain hormone-dependent tumors in adults and for treatment of central precocious puberty in children. Additional clearance was received from the FDA in July of 1997 for a 4-month delivery system containing 30 mg of leuprolide acetate.

Some recently published work from Takeda Chemical (154) describes additional work that has been done to develop 3-month delivery systems for leuprolide acetate in both subcutaneous and intramuscular injections. These formulations have shown reliable efficacy in treating patients with prostate cancer, mammary tumors, endometriosis, uterine fibroids, adenomyosis, and precocious puberty. A number of other research groups, associated with medical schools and hospitals, describe promising results of clinical trials for the use of these biodegradable microspheres in treatment of prostate cancer (155) as well as endometriosis and uterine leiomyomata (156).

Other work with Cetrorelix, a synthetic decapeptide that is structurally similar to gonadotropin-releasing hormone, has shown that this drug is suitable for cancer treatment as well as for in vitro fertilization for women with fertility problems. The mode of action of Cetrorelix differs from that of the LHRH agonists that have already been commercialized. An implantable formulation is currently being developed by Asta Medica Group.

Another company with a variety of implantable systems, based on PLAGA, is Atrix Laboratories. Their Atrigel formulations are based on a flowable, bioabsorbable formulation consisting of 36.7% poly(DL-lactide) dissolved in 63.3% NMP. By mixing this delivery vehicle with an active agent of 42.5 mg doxycycline hyclate, a viscous liquid is formed that may be injected into the subgingival area of the periodontal pocket. There it solidifies upon contact with the crevicular fluid and releases drug for up to a week for treatment of periodontal disease. This product, known as Atridox, was approved by the FDA in September 1998.

Some formulations based on PLAGA microparticles are in the final stages of study by Alkermes. Formulations using their ProLease delivery system containing PLAGA polymer, lyophilized drug to be delivered, and a release modifier are showing excellent promise. One formulation for growth hormone, in partnership with Genentech, has just finished successful phase III clinical trials. Formulations containing interferon and epoetin are in the preclinical stages of development.

VIII. FUTURE OPPORTUNITIES UTILIZING POLY(LACTIDE-CO-GLYCOLIDE)

With the recent drug approvals of a number of formulations, both implantable and injectable, the concept of using biodegradable polymers in nonoral drug products is finally gaining acceptance. Those companies with products currently on the market, as well as many other companies and researchers, have an outstanding opportunity to utilize the ability of PLAGA and other biodegradable polymers to provide control and duration that has never been possible in pharmaceutical formulations. Now that 4-month delivery systems have been approved, the only force holding back products of even longer duration is the technology and resources to develop them.

For injectable products containing fragile and expensive proteins and peptides, biodegradable systems may very well be the formulation of choice within the next 10 years. Most biodegradable formulations will be those that treat life-threatening diseases and conditions, however, because of the cost of developing such systems, the possibility of adverse reactions, and the difficulty of removing these formulations after administration.

Some of the most exciting opportunities will be found at the interface of drug delivery and tissue engineering, where PLAGA is the scaffold of choice to grow new tissues and organs. The three-dimensional biological architecture that must be achieved can be tremendously enhanced with judicious use of growth factors and other active agents being released from the tissue engineering scaffold concurrently with the cell and tissue growth into and around the degrading polymer. The techniques that must be developed as a means to control this desired cell growth in a synthetic tissue environment may also teach researchers new methods of halting cell growth in cancerous tissues within the body itself.

REFERENCES

1. Frazza, E. J. and Schmitt, E. E., 1971. A new absorbable suture. J. Biomed. Mater. Res. Symp., 1: 43–58.
2. Wasserman, D., 1971. US Patent 1,375,008.
3. Schmitt, E. E., Suen, T. J., and Updegraff, I. H., 1974. Water-degradable resins containing recurring, contiguous, polymerized glycolide units and process for preparing same, US Patent 3,784,585, Jan. 8, 1974, American Cyanamid.
4. Stricker, H., Entemann, G., Kern, O., Mikhail, M., and Zierenberg, B., 1988. Implantierbares, biologisch abbaubares Wirkstoffreigabesystem, European Patent 0311065A1, June 10, 1988, Boehringer Ingelheim.
5. Tanaka, M., Ogawa, Y., Miyagawa, T., and Watanabe, T., 1985. Polymer and its production, European Patent 0172636A1, March 7, 1985, Wako Pure Chemical Industries, Ltd., Takeda Chemical Industries, Ltd.
6. Brekke, J. H., 1989. Biodegradable, osteogenic, bone graft substitute, UK Patent 2215209A, Sept. 20, 1989, Osmed Inc.
7. Dunn, R. L., English, J. P., Strobel, J. D., Cowsar, D. R., and Tice, T. R., 1988. Preparation and evaluation of lactide/glycolide copolymers for drug delivery, In: C. Migliaresi (Ed.), Polymers in Medicine, Vol. 3, Amsterdam, Elsevier.
8. Vert, M., Li, S. M., Spenlehauer, G., and Guerin, P., 1992. Bioresorbability and biocompatibility of aliphatic polyesters. J. Mater. Sci. Mater. Med., 3: 432–446.
9. Kularni, R. K., Moore, E. G., Hegyeli, A. F., and Leonard, F., 1971. Biodegradable poly(lactic acid) polymers. J. Biomed. Mater. Res., 5: 169–181.
10. Holland, S. J., Tighe, B. J., and Gould, P. L., 1986. Polymers for biodegradable medical devices. 1. The potential of polyesters as controlled macromolecular release systems. J. Controlled Release, 4: 155–180.
11. Nieuwenhuis, J. and Mol, A. C., 1988. Polymer lactide, method for preparation of polymer lactide of this type and also composition which contains a polymer lactide of this type, European Patent 0314245A1, May 3, 1989, C. C. A. Biochem B. V.
12. Takayanagi, H., Kobayashi, T., Masuda, T., and Shinoda, H., 1988. Process of preparing DL-lactic acid-glycolic acid copolymer, European Patent 0299730A2, Janu. 18, 1989, Mitsui Toatsu Chemicals Inc.
13. Li, S. and Vert, M., 1995. Biodegradation of aliphatic polyesters, In: G. Scott and D. Gilead (Eds.), Biodegradable Polymers, Principles and Applications, London, Chapman & Hall, pp. 43–87.
14. Vert, M., Chabot, F., Leray, J., and Chrsitel, P., 1981. Bioresorbable polyesters for bone surgery. Makromol. Chem. Suppl., 5: 30.
15. Vert, M., Li, S. M., and Garreau, H., 1995. Recent advances in the field of lactic acid/glycolic acid polymer-based therapeutic systems. Macromol. Symp., 98: 633–642.

16. Schoberl, A. and Wiehler, C., 1955. Uber dis dehydratisierun von thioglykolsäure, deren kondensationspolymere und über dithioglykolid. Liebigs Ann. Chem., 595: 112–118.
17. Vert, M., Christel, P., Chabot, F., and Leray, J., 1984. Bioresorbable plastic materials for bone surgery, In: G. W. Hastings and P. Ducheyne (Eds.), Macromolecular Biomaterials, New York, CRC Press, p. 119.
18. Braud, C., Devarieux, R., Atlan, A., Ducos, C., and Vert, M., 1998. Capillary zone electrophoresis in normal or reverse separation modes for the analysis of hydroxy acid oligomers in neutral phosphate buffer. J. Chromatogr. B, 706: 73–82.
19. Buchholz, B., 1991. Verahren zur herstellung von polyesteren auf der basis von hydroycarbon saüren, EC Patent 0,443,542 A2, 1991.
20. Kleine, J. and Kleine, H., 1959. Makromol. Chem., 30: 23–38.
21. Chabot, F., Vert, M., Chapelle, S., and Granger, P., 1983. Configurational structures of lactic acid stereocopolymers as determined by 13C-^{1}H-NMR. Polymer, 24: 53–59.
22. Bero, M., Kasperczik, J., and Jedlinski, J., 1990. Coordination polymerization of lactides. I. Structure determination of obtained polymers. Makromol. Chem., 191: 2287–2296.
23. Coudane, J., Ustariz-Peyret, C., Schwach, G., and Vert, M., 1997. More about the stereodependence of DD- and LL-pair linkages during the ring opening polymerization of racemic lactide. J. Polym. Sci., Polym. Chem. Ed., 35: 1651–1658.
24. Vert, M., Schwach, G., and Engel, R., 1998. Something new in the field of PLA/GA bioresorbable polymers. J. Controlled Release, 53: 85–92.
25. Schwach, G., Coudane, J., Vert, M., and Huet-Olivier, J., 1996. Catalyseur et composition catalytique pour la fabrication d'un polymere biocompatible résorbable, et procédés les mettant en oeuvre, French Patent 96 02140.
26. Schwach, G., Coudane, J., Engel, R., and Vert, M., 1998. Ring opening polymerization of DL-lactide in the presence of zinc-metal and zinc-lactate. Polym. Interact., 46: 177–182.
27. Pitt, C. G., Gratzel, M. M., Kimmel, G. L., Surles, J., and Schindler, A., 1981. Aliphatic polyesters. 2. The degradation of poly(DL-lactide), poly (ϵ-caprolactone) and their complexes in vivo. Biomaterials, 2: 215–220.
28. Li, S. M., Garreau, H., and Vert, M., 1990. Structure-property relationships in the case of the degradation of massive aliphatic poly-(alphahydroxy acids) in aqueous media: Part 1: Poly(DL-lactic acid). J. Mater. Sci. Mater. Med., 1: 123–130.
29. Vert, M., 1998. Bioresorbable synthetic polymers and their operation field, In: G. Walenkamp (Ed.), Biomaterials in Surgery, Stuttgart, Georg Thieme, pp. 97–101.
30. Li, S., Garreau, H., and Vert, M., 1990. Structure-property relationships in the case of degradation of solid aliphatic poly (α-hydroxy acids) in aqueous media: 2. PLA37.5GA25 and PLA75GA25 copolymers. J. Mater. Sci. Mater. Med., 1: 131–139.
31. Li, S., Garreau, H., and Vert, M., 1990. Structure–property relationships in the case of degradation of solid aliphatic poly(α-hydroxy acids) in aqueous media: 3. Amorphous and semi-crystalline PLA 100. J. Mater. Sci. Mater. Med., 1: 198.
32. Vert, M., 1990. Degradation of polymeric biomaterials with respect to temporary applications, In: Degradable Materials, Boca Raton, CRC Press, pp. 11–37.
33. Visscher, E. G., Pearson, J. E., and Fong, J. W., 1988. Effects of particle size on the in vitro and in vivo degradation rates of poly(DL-lactide-co-glycolide) microcapsules. J. Biomed. Mater. Res., 22: 736–746.
34. Grizzi, I., Garreau, H., Li, S., and Vert, M., 1995. Biodegradation of devices based on poly(DL-lactic acid): Size dependence. Biomaterials, 16: 305–311.
35. Li, S. M., Girod-Holland, S., and Vert, M., 1996. Hydrolytic degradation of poly(DL-lactic acid) in the presence of caffeine base. J. Controlled Release, 40: 41–53.
36. Schwach, G., Engel, R., Coudane, J., and Vert, M., 1994. Stannous octoate versus zinc-initiated polymerization of racemic lactide: effect of configurational structures. Polym. Bull., 32: 617–623.
37. Schwach, G., Coudane, J., Engel, R., and Vert, M., 1997. More about the initiation mechanic of lactide polymerization in the presence of stannous octoate. J. Polym. Sci., Part A: Polym. Chem., 35: 3431–3440.

38. Agrawal, C. M., Niederauer, G. G., and Athanasiou, K. A., 1995. Fabrication and characterization of PLA-PGA orthopedic implants. Tissue Eng., 1: 241–252.
39. Smith, J. L., Jin, L., Parsons, T., Turek, T., Ron, E., Philbrook, C. M., Kenley, R. A., Marden, L., Hollinger, J., Bostrom, M. P. G., Tomin, E., and Lane, J. M., 1995. Osseous regeneration in preclinical models using bioabsorbable delivery technology for recombinant human bone morphogenetic protein 2 (rhBMP-2). J. Controlled Release, 36: 183–195.
40. Tunc, D. C., 1995. Orientruded polylactide based body-absorbable osteosynthesis devices: A short review. J. Biomater. Sci. Polym. Ed., 7: 375–380.
41. Mainil-Varlet, P., Rahn, B., and Gegolewski, S., 1997. Long-term in vivo degradation and bone reaction to various polylactides. Biomaterials, 18: 257–266.
42. Bostman, O., Hirvensalo, E., Vainionpaa, S., Vihtonen, K., Tormala, P., and Rokkanen, P., 1990. Degradable polyglycolide rods for the internal fixation of displaced bimalleolar fractures. Int. Orthop., 14: 1–8.
43. Dunnen, W. F. A. d., Lei, B. v. d., Robinson, P. H., Holwerda, A., Pennings, A. J., and Schakenraad, J. M., 1995. Biological performance of a degradable poly(lactic acid-ϵ-caprolactone) nerve guide: Influence of tube dimensions. J. Biomed. Mater. Res., 29: 757–766.
44. Schugens, C., Grandfils, C., Jerome, R., Teyssie, P., Delree, P., Martin, D., Malgrange, B., and Moonen, G., 1995. Preparation of macroporous biodegradable polylactide implant for neuronal transplantation. J. Biomed. Mater. Res., 29: 1349–1362.
45. Agrawal, C. M., Haas, K. F., Leopold, D. A., and Clark, H. G., 1992. Evaluation of poly(L-lactic acid) as a material for intravascular polymeric stents. Biomaterials, 13: 176–182.
46. Athanasiou, K. A., Schmitz, J. P., and Agrawal, C. M., 1998. The effects of porosity on in vitro degradation of polylactic acid-polyglycolic acid implants used in repair of articular cartilage. Tissue Eng., 4: 53–63.
47. Pegoretti, A., Fambri, L., and Migliaresi, C., 1997. In vitro degradation of poly(L-lactic acid) fibers produced by melt spinning. J. Appl. Polym. Sci., 64: 213–233.
48. Andriano, K. A., Pohjonen, T., and Törmälä, P., 1994. Processing and characterization of absorbable polylactide polymers for use in surgical implants. J. Appl. Biomater., 5: 133–140.
49. Eenink, M. J. D., Feijen, J., Olijslager, J., Albers, J. H. M., Rieke, J. C., and Greidanus, P. J., 1987. Biodegradable hollow fibers for the controlled release of hormones. J. Controlled Release, 6: 225–247.
50. Witte, P. v. d., Esselbrugge, H., Paters, A. M. P., Dijkstra, P. J., Feijen, J., Groeneweggen, R. J. J., Smid, J., Olijslager, J., Schakenraad, J. M., Eenink, M. J. D., and Sam, A. P., 1993. Formation of porous membranes for drug delivery. J. Controlled Release, 24: 61–78.
51. Bodmeier, R. and Chen, H., 1989. Evaluation of biodegradable poly(lactide) pellets prepared by direct compression. J. Pharm Sci., 78: 819–822.
52. Asano, M., Fukuzaki, H., Yoshida, M., Kumakura, M., Mashimo, T., Yuasa, H., Imai, K., and Yamanaka, H., 1989. In vivo characteristics of low molecular weight copoly(DL-lactic acid) formulations with controlled release of LH-RH agonist. Biomaterials, 10: 569–572.
53. Asano, M., Fukuzaki, H., Yoshida, M., Kumakura, M., Mashimo, T., Yuasa, H., Imai, K., Yamanaka, H., Kawaharada, U., and Suzuki, K., 1991. In vivo controlled release of a luteinizing hormone-releasing hormone agonist from poly(DL-lactic acid) formulations of varying degradation patterns. Int. J. Pharm., 67: 67–77.
54. Asano, M., Yoshida, M., Omichi, H., Mashimo, T., Okabe, K., Yuasa, H., Yamanaka, H., Morimoto, S., and Sakakibara, H., 1993. Biodegradable poly(DL-lactic acid) formulations in calcitonin delivery system. Biomaterials, 14: 797–799.
55. Yamakawa, I., Kawahara, M., Watanabe, S., and Miyake, Y., 1990. Sustained release of insulin by double-layered implant using poly(D,L-lactic acid). J. Pharm. Sci., 79(6): 505–509.
56. Zhang, X., Wyss, U. P., Pichors, D., Amsden, B., and Goosen, M. F. A., 1993. Controlled release of albumin from biodegradable poly(DL-lactide) cylinders. J. Controlled Release, 25: 61–69.
57. Zhang, X., McAuley, K. B., and Goosen, M. F. A., 1995. Towards prediction of release profiles of antibiotics from coated poly(DL-lactide) cylinders. J. Controlled Release, 34: 175–179.

58. Zhang, X., Wyss, U. P., Pichora, D., and Goosen, M. F. A., 1994. A mechanistic study of antibiotic release from biodegradable poly(DL-lactide) cylinders. J. Controlled Release, 31: 129–144.
59. Gangadharam, P. R. J., Ashtekar, D. R., Farhi, D. C., and Wise, D. L., 1991. Sustained release of isoniazid in vivo from a single implant of a biodegradable polymer. Tubercle, 72: 115–122.
60. Zhang, X., Wyss, U. P., Pichora, D., Goosen, M. F. A., Gonzal, A., and Marte, C. L., 1994. Controlled release of testosterone and estradiol-17β from biodegradable cylinders. J. Controlled Release, 29: 157–161.
61. Bhardwaj, R. and Blanchard, J., 1997. In vitro evaluation of poly(DL-lactide-co-glycolide) polymer-based implants containing the alpha-melanocyte stimulating hormone analog, Melanotan-I. J. Controlled Release, 45: 49–55.
62. Mauduit, J., Bukh, N., and Vert, M., 1993. Gentamycin/poly(lactic acid) blends aimed at sustained release local antibiotic therapy administered per-operatively. III. The case of gentamycin sulfate in films prepared from high and low molecular weight poly(DL-lactic acids). J. Controlled Release, 25: 43–49.
63. Mauduit, J., Perouse, E., and Vert, M., 1996. Hydrolytic degradation of films prepared from blends of high and low molecular weight poly(DL-lactic acid)s. J. Biomed. Mater. Res., 30: 201–207.
64. Lewis, K. J., Irwin, W. J., and Akhtar, S., 1995. Biodegradable poly(L-lactic acid) matrices for the sustained delivery of antisense oligonucleotides. J. Controlled Release, 37: 173–183.
65. Jimoh, A. G., Wise, D. L., Gresser, J. D., and Trantolo, D. J., 1995. Pulsed FSH release from an implantable capsule system. J. Controlled Release, 34: 87–95.
66. Lambert, W. J. and Peck, K. D., 1995. Development of an in situ forming biodegradable polylactide-co-glycolide system for the controlled release of proteins. J. Controlled Release, 33: 189–195.
67. Shively, M. L., Coonts, B. A., Renner, W. D., Southard, J. L., and Bennett, A. T., 1995. Physiochemical characterization of a polymeric injectable implant delivery system. J. Controlled Release, 33: 237–243.
68. Brannon-Peppas, L., 1995. Recent advances on the use of biodegradable microparticles and nanoparticles in controlled drug delivery. Int. J. Pharm., 116: 1–9.
69. Matsumoto, A., Matsukawa, Y., Suzuki, T., Yoshino, H., and Kobayashi, M., 1997. The polymer-alloys method as a new preparation method of biodegradable microspheres: principle and application to cisplatin-loaded microspheres. J. Controlled Release, 48: 19–27.
70. Shenderova, A., Burke, T. G., and Schwendeman, S. P., 1997. Stabilization of 10-hydroxycamptothecin in poly(lactide-co-glycolide) microsphere delivery vehicles. Pharm. Res., 14: 1406–1414.
71. Birnbaum, D. T., Kosmala, J. D., and Brannon-Peppas, L., 1997. Simultaneous analysis of particle size distribution, particle shape, and drug delivery from biodegradable microparticles. Polym. Prepr., 38: 600–601.
72. Denkbas, E. B., Kaitian, X., Tuncel, A., and Piskin, E., 1994. Rifampicin-carrying poly(D,L-lactide) microspheres: loading and release. J. Biomater. Sci., Polym. Ed., 6: 815–825.
73. European Agency for the Evaluation of Medicinal Products, 1997. ICH Topic Q3C, Impurities: residual solvents.
74. Kim, J. H., Kwon, I. C., Kim, Y. H., Sohn, Y. T., and Jeong, S. Y., 1997. The modified solvent extraction method on the preparation of poly(L-lactic acid) microspheres. Int. Symp. Control. Rel. Bioact. Mater., Vol. 24, pp. 549–550.
75. Boury, F., Marchais, H., Proust, J. E., and Benoit, J. P., 1997. Bovine serum albumin release from poly(alpha-hydroxy acid) microspheres: effects of polymer molecular weight and surface properties. J. Controlled Release, 45: 75–86.
76. Blanco, D. and Alanso, M. J., 1998. Protein encapsulation and release from poly(lactide-co-glycolide) microspheres: effect of the protein and polymer properties and of the co-encapsulation of surfactants. Eur. J. Pharm. Biopharm., 45: 285–294.
77. Conway, B. R. and Alpar, H. O., 1996. Double emulsion microencapsulation of proteins as model antigens using polymers: effect of emulsifier on the microsphere characteristics and release kinetics. Eur. J. Pharm. Biopharm., 42: 42–48.

78. Crotts, G. and Park, T. G., 1995. Preparation of porous and nonporous biodegradable polymeric hollow microspheres. J. Controlled Release, 35: 91–105.
79. Morlock, M., Koll, H., Winter, G., and Kissel, T., 1997. Microencapsulation of rh-erythropoietin, using biodegradable poly(D,L-lactide-co-glycolide): protein stability and the effects of stabilizing excipients. Eur. J. Pharm. Biopharm., 43: 29–36.
80. Bittner, B., Morlock, M., Koll, H., Winter, G., and Kissel, T., 1998. Recombinant human erythropoietin (rhEPO) loaded poly(lactide-co-glycolide) microspheres: influence of the encapsulation technique and polymer purity on microsphere characteristics. Eur. J. Pharm. Biopharm., 45: 295–305.
81. Cleland, J. L., Lim, A., Barron, L., Duenas, E. T., and Powell, M. F., 1997. Development of a single-shot subunit vaccine for HIV-1: Part 4. Optimizing microencapsulation and pulsatile release of MN rgp120 from biodegradable microspheres. J. Controlled Release, 47: 135–150.
82. Couvreur, P., Blanco-Prieto, M. J., Puisieux, F., Roques, B., and Fattal, E., 1997. Multiple emulsion technology for the design of microspheres containing peptides and oligopeptides. Adv. Drug Del. Rev., 28: 85–96.
83. Cleland, J. L., Johnson, O. L., Putney, S., and Jones, A. J. S., 1997. Recombinant human growth hormone poly(lactic-co-glycolic acid) microsphere formulation development. Adv. Drug Del. Rev., 28: 71–84.
84. Kyo, M., Hyon, S.-H., and Ikada, Y., 1995. Effects of preparation conditions of cisplatin-loaded microspheres on the in vitro release. J. Controlled Release, 35: 73–82.
85. McGee, J. P., Davis, S. S., and O'Hagan, D. T., 1994. The immunogenicity of a model protein entrapped in poly(lactide-co-glycolide) microparticles prepared by a novel phase separation technique. J. Controlled Release, 31: 55–60.
86. McGee, J. P., Davis, S. S., and O'Hagan, D. T., 1995. Zero order release of protein from poly(D,L-lactide-co-glycolide) microparticles prepared using a modified phase separation technique. J. Controlled Release, 34: 77–86.
87. Owusu-Ababio, G. and Rogers, J. A., 1996. Formulation and release of ciprofloxacin from poly(L-lactic acid) microparticles. Eur. J. Pharm. Biopharm., 42: 188–192.
88. Nihant, N., Grandfils, C., Jerome, R., and Teyssie, P., 1995. Microencapsulation by coacervation of poly(lactide-co-glycolide) IV. Effect of the processing parameters on coacervation and encapsulation. J. Controlled Release, 35: 117–125.
89. O'Donnell, P. B., Iwata, M., and McGinity, J. W., 1995. Properties of multiphase microspheres of poly(D,L-lactic-co-glycolic acid) prepared by a potentiometric dispersion technique. J. Microencapsulation, 12: 155–163.
90. Thomasin, C., Johansen, P., Alder, R., Bemsel, R., Hottinger, G., Altorfer, H., Wright, A. D., Wehrli, G., Merkle, H. P., and Gander, B., 1996. A contribution to overcoming the problem of residual solvents in biodegradable microspheres prepared by coacervation. Eur. J. Pharm. Biopharm., 42: 16–24.
91. Jeyanthi, R., Thanoo, B. C., Metha, R. C., and DeLuca, P. P., 1996. Effect of solvent removal technique on the matrix characteristics of polylactide/glycolide microspheres for peptide delivery. J. Controlled Release, 38: 235–244.
92. Li, W.-I., Anderson, K. W., and DeLuca, P. P., 1995. Kinetic and thermodynamic modeling of the formation of polymeric microspheres using solvent extraction/evaporation. J. Controlled Release, 37: 187–198.
93. Li, W.-I., Anderson, K. W., Mehta, R. C., and DeLuca, P. P., 1995. Prediction of solvent removal profile and effect on properties for peptide-loaded PLGA microspheres prepared by solvent extraction/evaporation method. J. Controlled Release, 37: 199–214.
94. Giunchedi, P. and Conte, U., 1995. Spray-drying as a preparation method of microparticluate drug delivery systems: an overview. STP Pharma Sci., 5: 276–290.
95. Gander, B., Wehrli, E., Alder, R., and Merkle, H. P., 1995. Quality improvement of spray-dried, protein-loaded D,L-PLA microspheres by appropriate polymer solvent selection. J. Microencapsulation, 12: 83–97.

96. Debenedetti, P. G., 1990. Homogeneous nucleation in supercritical fluids. AIChE J., 36: 1289–1298.
97. Falk, R., Randolph, T. W., Meyer, J. D., Kelly, R. M., and Manning, M. C., 1997. Controlled release of ionic compounds from poly(L-lactide) microspheres produced by precipitation with a compressed antisolvent. J. Controlled Release, 44: 77–85.
98. Thies, J. and Muller, B. W., 1998. Size controlled production of biodegradable microparticles with supercritical gases. Eur. J. Pharm. Biopharm., 45: 67–74.
99. Herbert,.P., Murphy, K., Johnson, O., Dong, N., Jaworowicz, W., Tracy, M. A., L. Cleland, J., and Putney, S. D., 1998. A large-scale process to produce microencapsulated proteins. Pharm. Res., 15: 357–361.
100. Chen, L., Apte, R. N., and Cohen, S., 1997. Characterization of PLGA microspheres for the controlled delivery of IL-1α for tumor immunotherapy. J. Controlled Release, 43: 261–272.
101. Pettit, D. K., Lawter, J. R., Huang, W. J., Pankey, S. C., Nightlinger, N. S., Lynch, D. H., Schuh, J. A. C. L., Morrissey, P. J., and Gombotz, W. R., 1997. Characterization of poly(glycolide-co-D,L-lactide)/poly(D,L-lactide) microspheres for controlled release of GM-CSF. Pharm. Res., 14: 1422–1430.
102. O'Donnell, P. B. and McGinity, J. W., 1997. Preparation of microspheres by the solvent evaporation technique. Adv. Drug Del. Rev., 28: 25–42.
103. Schugens, C., Laruelle, N., Nihant, N., Grandfils, C., Jerome, R., and Teyssie, P., 1994. Effect of the emulsion stability on the morphology and porosity of semicrystalline poly l-lactide microparticles prepared by w/o/w double emulsion-evaporation. J. Controlled Release, 32: 161–176.
104. Fitzgerald, J. F. and Corrigan, O. I., 1996. Investigation of the mechanisms governing the release of levamisole from poly(lactide-co-glycolide) delivery systems. J. Controlled Release, 42: 125–132.
105. Takahata, H., Lavelle, E. C., Coombes, A. G. A., and Davis, S. S., 1998. The distribution of protein associated with poly(DL-lactide co-glycolide) microparticles and its degradation in simulated body fluids. J. Controlled Release, 50: 237–246.
106. Rosilio, V., Deyme, M., Benoit, J. P., and Madelmont, G., 1998. Physical aging of progesterone-loaded poly(D,L-lactide-co-glycolide) microspheres. Pharm. Res., 15: 794–798.
107. Park, T. G., 1994. Degradation of poly(D,L-lactic acid) microspheres: effect of molecular weight. J. Controlled Release, 30: 161–173.
108. Park, T. G., Lu, W., and Crotts, G., 1995. Importance of in vitro experimental conditions on protein release kinetics, stability, and polymer degradation in protein encapsulated poly(D,L-lactic acid-co-glycolic acid) microspheres. J. Controlled Release, 33: 211–222.
109. Kamijo, A., Kamei, S., Saikawa, A., Igari, Y., and Ogawa, Y., 1996. In vitro release test system of (D,L-lactic-glycolic) acid copolymer microcapsules for sustained release of LHRH agonist (leuproprelin). J. Controlled Release, 40: 269–276.
110. Crotts, G. and Park, T. G., 1997. Stability and release of bovine serum albumin encapsulated within poly(D,L-lactide-co-glycolide) microparticles. J. Controlled Release, 44: 123–134.
111. Conti, B., Genta, I., Giunchedi, P., and Modena, T., 1995. Testing of in vitro dissolution behavior of microparticulate drug delivery systems. Drug Dev. Ind. Pharm., 21: 1223–1233.
112. Birnbaum, D. T., Kosmala, J. D., Henthorn, D. B., and Brannon-Peppas, L., 1999. Controlled release of β-estradiol from PLGA microparticles: the effect of organic phase solvent on encapsulation and release. J. Controlled Release, in press.
113. Witschi, C. and Doelker, E., 1998. Influence of the microencapsulation method and peptide loading on poly(lactic acid) and poly(lactic-co-glycolic acid) degradation during in vitro testing. J. Controlled Release, 51: 327–341.
114. Sansdrap, P. and Moes, A. J., 1997. In vitro evaluation of the hydrolytic degradation of the dispersed and aggregated poly(DL-lactide-co-glycolide) microspheres. J. Controlled Release, 43: 47–58.
115. Mäder, K., Bittner, B., Li, Y., Wohlauf, W., and Kissel, T., 1998. Monitoring microviscosity and microacidity of the albumin microenvironment inside degrading microparticles from poly(lactide-co-

glycolide) (PLG) or ABA-triblock polymers containing hydrophobic poly(lactide-co-glycolide) A blocks and hydrophilic poly(ethyleneoxide) B blocks. Pharm. Res., 15: 787–793.
116. Tracy, M. A., Zhang, Y., Verdon, S. L., Dong, N., and Riley, M. G. I., 1997. In vivo and in vitro degradation of poly(lactide-co-glycolide) microspheres. Int. Symp. Control. Rel. Bioact. Mater., Vol. 24: pp. 623–624.
117. Eldridge, J. H., Staas, J. K., Meulbroek, J. A., McGhee, J. R., Tice, T. R., and Gilley, R. M., 1991. Biodegradable microspheres as a vaccine delivery system. Mol. Immun., 28: 287–294.
118. Nakaoka, R., Tabata, Y., and Ikada, Y., 1995. Enhanced antibody production through sustained antigen release from biodegradable ganules. J. Controlled Release, 37: 215–224.
119. Okada, H., Doken, Y., Ogawa, Y., and Toguchi, H., 1994. Preparation of three-month depot injectable microspheres of leuprorelin acetate using biodegradable polymers. Pharm. Res., 11: 1143–1147.
120. Itoi, K., Tabata, C.-Y., Ike, O., Shimizu, Y., Kuwabara, M., Kyo, M., Hyon, S. H., and Ikada, Y., 1996. In vivo suppressive effects of copoly(glycolic/L-lactic acid) microspheres containing CDDP on murine tumor cells. J. Controlled Release, 42: 175–184.
121. Ciftci, K., Hincal, A. A., Kas, H. S., Ercan, T. M., Sungur, A., Guven, O., and Ruacan, S., 1997. Solid tumor chemotherapy and in vivo distribution of fluorouracil following administration in poly(L-lactic acid) microspheres. Pharm. Dev. Techn., 2: 151–160.
122. Menei, P., Boisdron-Celle, M., and Guy, G., 1996. Effect of stereotactic implantation of biodegradable 5-fluorouracil-loaded microspheres in healthy and C6 glioma–bearing rats. Neurosurgery, 39: 117–124.
123. Zhifang, Z., Mingxing, Z., Shenghao, W., Fang, L., and Wenzhao, S., 1993. Preparation and evaluation in vitro and in vivo of copoly(lactic/glycolic) acid microspheres containing norethisterone. Biomat. Art. Cells Immob. Biotech., 21: 71–84.
124. Wichert, B. and Rohdewald, P., 1993. Low molecular weight PLA: a suitable polymer for pulmonary administered microparticles? J. Microencapsulation, 10: 195–207.
125. Poyner, E. A., Alpar, H. O., Almeida, A. J., Gamble, M. D., and Brown, M. R. W., 1995. A comparative study on the pulmonary delivery of tobramycin encapsulated into liposomes and PLA microspheres following intravenous and endotracheal delivery. J. Controlled Release, 35: 41–48.
126. Yamaguchi, K. and Anderson, J. M., 1993. In vivo biocompatibility studies of Medisorb 65/35 D,L-lactide/glycolide copolymer microspheres. J. Controlled Release, 24: 81–93.
127. Lam, K. H., Schakenraad, J. M., Esselbrugge, H., Feijen, J., and Nieuwenhuis, P., 1993. The effect of phagocytosis of poly(L-lactic acid) fragments on cellular morphology and viability. J. Biomed. Mater. Res., 27: 1569–1577.
128. Daugherty, A. L., Cleland, J. L., Duenas, E. M., and Mrsny, R. J., 1997. Pharmacological modulation of the tissue response to implanted polylactic-co-glycolic acid microspheres. Eur. J. Pharm. Biopharm., 44: 89–102.
129. Anderson, J. M. and Shive, M. S., 1997. Biodegradation and biocompatability of PLA and PLGA microspheres. Adv. Drug Del. Rev., 28: 5–24.
130. Cohn, D. and Younes, H., 1988. Biodegradable PEO/PLA block copolymers. J. Biomed. Mater. Res., 22: 993–1009.
131. Penco, M., Marcioni, S., Ferruti, P., D'Antone, S., and Deghenghi, R., 1996. Degradation behaviour of block copolymers containing poly(lactic-glycolic acid) and poly(ethylene glycol) segments. Biomaterials, 17: 1583–1590.
132. Li, X., Xiao, J., Deng, X., Li, X., Wang, H., Jia, W., Zhang, W., Men, L., Yang, Y., and Zheng, Z., 1997. Preparation of biodegradable microspheres encapsulating proteins with micron sizes. J. Appl. Polym. Sci., 66: 583–590.
133. Zhu, K. J., Xiangzhou, L., and Shilin, Y., 1990. Preparation, characterization, and properties of polylactide (PLA)-poly(ethylene glycol) (PEG) copolymers: a potential drug carrier. J. Appl. Polym. Sci., 39: 1–9.
134. Shah, S. S., Zhu, K. J., and Pitt, C. G., 1994. Poly-DL-lactic acid: polyethylene glycol block copolymers. The influence of polyethylene glycol on the degradation of poly-DL-lactic acid. J. Biomater. Sci. Polym. Ed., 5: 421–431.

135. Mohammadi-Rovshandeh, J., Farnia, S. M. F., and Sarbolouki, M. N., 1998. Synthesis and thermal behavior of triblock copolymers from L-lactide and ethylene glycol with long center PEG block. J. Appl. Polym. Sci., 68: 1949–1954.
136. Rashkov, I., Manolova, N., Li, S. M., Espartero, J. L., and Vert, M., 1996. Synthesis, characterization, and hydrolytic degradation of PLA/PEO/PLA triblock copolymers with short poly(L-lactic acid) chains. Macromolecules, 29: 50–56.
137. Li, S. M., Rashkov, I., Espartero, J. L., Manolova, N., and Vert, M., 1996. Synthesis, characterization, and hydrolytic degradation of PLA/PEO/PLA triblock copolymers with long poly(L-lactic acid) blocks. Macromolecules, 29: 57–62.
138. Youxin, L. and Kissel, T., 1993. Synthesis and properties of biodegradable ABA triblock copolymers consisting of poly(L-lactic acid) or poly(L-lactic-co-glycolic acid) A-blocks attached to central poly(ethylene) B-blocks. J. Controlled Release, 27: 247–257.
139. Youxin, L., Volland, C., and Kissel, T., 1994. In vitro degradation and bovine serum albumin release of the ABA triblock copolymers consisting of poly(L-lactic acid) or poly(L-lactic acid-co-glycolic acid) A-blocks attached to central polyoxyethylene B-blocks. J. Controlled Release, 32: 121–128.
140. Ronneberger, B., Kao, W. J., Anderson, J. M., and Kissel, T., 1996. In vivo biocompatibility study of ABA triblock copolymers consisting of poly(L-lactic-co-glycolic acid) A blocks attached to central poly(oxyethylene) B blocks. J. Biomed. Mater. Res., 30: 31–40.
141. Kissel, T., Li, Y. X., Volland, C., Gorich, S., and Koneberg, R., 1996. Parenteral protein delivery systems using biodegradable polyesters of ABA block structure, containing hydrophobic poly(lactide-co-glycolide) A blocks and hydrophilic poly(ethylene glycol) B blocks. J. Controlled Release, 39: 315–326.
142. Zange, R., Li, Y., and Kissel, T., 1997. In vitro degradation study and in vitro biocompatability testing of PEO containing ABA triblock copolymers. Int. Symp. Control. Rel. Bioact. Mater., 24: 511–512.
143. Bittner, B., Mader, K., Li, Y. X., and Kissel, T., 1997. Evaluation of the microenvironment inside biodegradable microspheres from ABA triblock copolymers of poly(L-lactide-co-glycolide) and poly(ethylene oxide) prepared by spray drying. Int. Symp. Control. Rel. Bioact. Mater., 24: 535–536.
144. Ronneberger, B., Kissel, T., and Anderson, J. M., 1997. Biocompatibility of ABA triblock copolymer microparticles consisting of poly(L-lactic-co-glycolic acid) A-blocks attached to central poly(oxyethylene) B-blocks in rats after intramuscular injection. Eur. J. Pharm. Biopharm., 43: 19–28.
145. Sawhney, A. S. and Hubbell, J. A., 1990. Rapidly degraded terpolymers of dl-lactide, glycolide, and ϵ-caprolactone with increased hydrophilicity by copolymerization with polyethers. J. Biomed. Mater. Res., 24: 1397–1411.
146. Stevels, W. M., Bernard, A., Witte, P. v. d., Dijkstra, P. J., and Feijen, J., 1996. Block copolymers of poly(L-lactide) and poly(ϵ-caprolactone) or poly(ethylene glycol) prepared by reactive extrusion. J. Appl. Polym. Sci., 62: 1295–1301.
147. Hiljanen-Vainio, M. P., Orava, P. A., and Seppälä, J. V., 1997. Properties of ϵ-caprolactone/DL-lactide (ϵCL/DL-LA) copolymers with a minor ϵ-CL content. J. Biomed. Mater. Res., 34: 39–46.
148. deGroot, J. H., Zijlstra, F. M., Kulpers, H. W., Pennings, A. J., Klompmaker, J., Veth, R. P. H., and Jansen, H. W. B., 1997. Meniscal tissue regeneration in porous 50/50 copoly(L-lactide/ϵ-caprolactone) implants. Biomaterials, 18: 613–622.
149. Helder, J. and Feijen, J., 1986. Copolymers of DL-lactic acid and glycine. Makromol. Chem., Rapid Commun., 7: 193–198.
150. Jin, X., Carfagna, C., Nicolais, L., and Lanzetta, R., 1995. Synthesis, characterization and in vitro degradation of a novel thermotropic ternary and p-hydroxybenzoic acid, glycolic acid, and p-hydroxycinnamic acid. Macromolecules, 28: 4785–4794.
151. Elisseeff, J., Anseth, K., Langer, R., and Hrkach, J. S., 1997. Synthesis and characterization of photo-cross-linked polymers based on poly(L-lactic acid-co-L-aspartic acid). Macromolecules, 30: 2182–2184.

152. Perrin, D. E. and English, J. P., 1997. Polyglycolide and Polylactide, In: A. J. Domb, J. Kost, and D. W. Wiseman (Eds.), Handbook of Biodegradable Polymers, Amsterdam, Harwood, pp. 1–27.
153. Physicians' Desk Reference, 1994. Montvale, NJ, Medical Economics.
154. Okada, H., 1997. One- and three-month release injectable microspheres of the LH-RH superagonist leuprorelin acetate. Adv. Drug Del. Rev., 28: 43–70.
155. Sharifi, R., Ratanawong, C., Jung, A., Wu, Z., Browneller, R., and Lee, M., 1997. Therapeutic effects of leuproelin microspheres in prostate cancer. Adv. Drug Del. Rev., 28: 121–138.
156. Miller, J. D. and Anderson, M. G., 1997. Therapeutic effects of leuprorelin microspheres on endometriosis and uterine leiomyomata. Adv. Drug Del. Rev., 28: 139–155.

7
Use of Infrared and Raman Spectroscopy for Characterization of Controlled Release Systems

A. B. Scranton and B. Drescher
Michigan State University, East Lansing, Michigan

E. W. Nelson and J. L. Jacobs
3M Corporation, St. Paul, Minnesota

I. INTRODUCTION

Infrared (IR) and Raman spectroscopy are becoming increasingly important tools for the investigation of polymer systems (1). As sampling techniques, lasers, detection systems, computers, and software become more sophisticated, previous limitations of these techniques continue to be overcome. For example, it is now possible to examine a variety of polymer systems in situ (2), when previously off-line measurements were most common. Infrared spectroscopy is still used more extensively than Raman techniques. However, with the advent of inexpensive laser light sources, Raman spectroscopy has developed as a complementary technique (3). Once regarded solely as a laboratory technique, Raman spectroscopy can now be used for on-line process analysis and environmental monitoring. For example, there are now commercially available, portable, on-line Raman systems containing various novel lasers, fiberoptic sampling probes, charge couple device (CCD) detectors, and complete computer analysis systems.

The usefulness of IR and Raman spectroscopy ultimately lies in the variety of qualitative and quantitative information they can provide about the polymer under investigation. Information that can be obtained using these techniques includes the chemical nature (structural units, branching, end groups, additives, and impurities), steric order (isomerism and stereoregularity), conformational order (physical arrangement of the chain), state of aggregation (crystalline, mesomorphous, amorphous phases, number of chains per unit cell, etc.), and orientation of the polymer chain and side groups (3).

Infrared and Raman spectra provide complementary rather than duplicate information. For example, IR spectroscopy is generally better suited for the identification of polar groups, while Raman is especially good for the investigation of the homonuclear polymer backbone (3). In addition, Raman spectroscopy is well suited for the study of aqueous systems such as hydrogels since water exhibits very low Raman scattering. This is a distinct advantage over IR techniques since water absorbs strongly in the IR region and overwhelms the spectrum (4). Other advantages of Raman spectroscopy arise from the fact that Raman allows vibrational spectroscopy to be performed using visible light. In the visible region of the spectrum, optics can be made of relativity inexpensive and robust materials such as glass or quartz, and sensitive detectors with high signal-to-noise ratios are readily available (5). Indeed, the use of visible light for Raman spectroscopy allows remote sampling with fiberoptic probes, making the technique amenable to in situ and on-line measurements.

As discussed in detail later in this chapter, IR and Raman spectroscopy are based on distinctly different physical processes. Fundamentally, Raman is a scattering technique while IR spectroscopy is based on light absorption; therefore, the sampling techniques of the two methods are significantly different. In transmission IR spectroscopy the light is required to pass through the sample to reach the detector; therefore, severe constraints are imposed on the sample thickness (typically the thickness must be less than about 40 μm). Methods such as attenuated total reflectance (ATR) may be used with thick samples, but they present their own problems and limitations associated with the contact to the ATR crystal and the limited depth of penetration. In contrast, since Raman spectroscopy is based on light scattered by the sample, thick samples are not a problem since backscattered light may be collected and analyzed. Therefore, Raman spectroscopy generally requires very little if any sample preparation.

The advantages and capabilities or IR and Raman spectroscopy have led to their widespread use for the investigation and characterization of hydrogels. In this chapter we will provide a review of the literature on the use of these techniques for the study of hydrogels. For each of these techniques, we will begin with a discussion of the physical basis for the method, including an overview of the instrumentation, and the sampling considerations for the technique. Next we discuss the applications of each technique for the characterization of hydrogels, including investigations of controlled drug release delivery systems; identification of biocompatible polymers; and characterization of polymerization systems.

II. PHYSICAL BASIS FOR INFRARED SPECTROSCOPY

A brief introduction to the basic principles of IR spectroscopy is presented in this section. The IR region of the spectrum consists of light with wave numbers between 10,000 cm^{-1} and 10 cm^{-1} (wavelengths between 1.0 μm and 1,000 μm), with the range from 10,000 to 4000 cm^{-1} (1000–2.5 μm) referred to as the near-infrared; 4000 to 400 cm^{-1} (2.5–25 μm) the midinfrared; and 400 to 10 cm^{-1} (25–1000 μm) the far-infrared regions (5,6). When photons in the IR region of the spectrum are absorbed by matter, they lead to molecular vibrational transitions. Therefore, when infrared light is passed through a sample, certain frequencies are absorbed while others are transmitted, resulting in an absorption spectrum that is dependent on the molecular vibrational frequencies.

In an IR spectrometer, the sample under investigation is exposed to the light which spans the entire IR region [either simultaneously as in an Fourier transform IR (FTIR) or one wavelength at a time as in a dispersive IR]. The sample absorbs the light only at the specific frequencies that match the natural vibrational frequencies of its constituent molecules (7). In order for a molecular vibration to absorb in the IR region it must cause a change in the magnitude of the dipole moment (3,8,9). In fact, it has been shown that the intensity of an IR absorption band is proportional to the square of the change in its dipole moment (7–9). For this reason, if a molecule has a center of symmetry in its equilibrium configuration, then any vibrations for which this symmetry is retained will be IR-inactive (7).

The frequency of a photon, ν_p, is related to its energy, E_p, by the well-known Planck's equation:

$$E_p = h\nu_p \tag{1}$$

Quantum mechanical considerations dictate that molecular energy assumes only specific discrete values. The harmonic oscillator model is useful for providing qualitative insight into the vibrational transitions in molecules. According to this model, the values of the vibrational energy levels, E_{vib}, are given by the following equation:

$$E_{vib} = \left(n + \frac{1}{2}\right)h\nu \qquad (2)$$

where h is Planck's constant, ν is the classical vibrational frequency of the oscillator, and n is a quantum number. If this equation is applied to the infrared absorption of a photon where the vibrational energy of the molecule is E_m, and the frequency of the induced vibration is ν_m, then by substitution,

$$E_m = \left(n + \frac{1}{2}\right)h\nu_m \qquad (3)$$

The only variable in this equation is the quantum number, which can only have integer values. If the quantum number changes by $+1$ or -1, then the molecule gains or loses energy, respectively. For an unsymmetrical diatomic molecule this amount of energy is ΔE_m, which is equal to the difference between the energy of the n quantum level and the energy of the $n \mp 1$ level. This gives the result (7),

$$\Delta E_m = h\nu_m \qquad (4)$$

Since the change in energy, ΔE_m, is due to the transfer of energy from the photon to the molecule, $\Delta E_m = E_p$. Therefore $\nu_p = \nu_m$. This states that the frequency, ν_p, of a photon that has the proper energy to cause the vibrational quantum number to jump up one level is equal to the classical vibrational frequency of the molecule, ν_m (7). For harmonic vibration the vibrational quantum number may only change by ± 1; all other transitions are forbidden. This selection rule corresponds to conditions where the electric field of the photon causes the molecule to vibrate at the field's frequency and induces a molecular dipole moment. For an anharmonic quantum mechanical oscillator the selection rule allows for integer changes in the quantum number of ± 1, ± 2, ± 3, etc. In this case, the excited molecule vibrates at the corresponding integer multiple of the molecular frequency (7). At room temperatures most molecules are in the ground vibrational state; therefore, the allowed transition that dominates IR spectroscopy and is of most interest is from $n = 0$ to $n = 1$. This is referred to as the fundamental transition. The relative intensities of other allowed transitions are low since the populations of the higher energy levels are low compared to the ground state at room temperatures (7). Additional bands, known as overtones and combination bands, may result from anharmonic terms in the potential energy of the molecule (10). Since anharmonic oscillator energy levels are not equally spaced, the frequency is no longer completely independent of amplitude (7). The additive effect of the harmonic and anharmonic terms results in the appearance of absorption bands that are shifted from their characteristic absorption wavelength.

III. INSTRUMENTATION FOR INFRARED SPECTROSCOPY

The original IR spectrometers were dispersive instruments that consisted of prisms or gratings that separated or dispersed the IR radiation into its component wavelengths (10). Generally modern dispersive IR spectrometers are made using gratings rather than prisms with a series of diffraction gratings used to separate the entire IR region of the spectrum (7). A movable mirror allowed a progressive scanning of the individual wavelengths, which passed through a slit onto the sample. The distinctive feature of the dispersive spectrometers is that the spectrum is scanned continuously, one wavelength band at a time, and that the light absorbed by the sample is determined by comparing the transmitted light (as a function of wavelength) to the incident light. This scanning process is time consuming, and dispersive instruments are rarely used today.

In contrast to the traditional dispersive instruments, the modern FTIR spectrometers are not based on slits or monochromators. Instead, light containing all IR frequencies is passed through the sample simultaneously, and the IR absorption spectrum is resolved using a Michelson interferometer. In the Michelson interferometer, a beam splitter is used to transmit half of the source radiation to a movable mirror and to reflect the other half to a fixed mirror. The two beams are then reflected back to the beamsplitter and recombined either constructively or destructively depending on the position of the movable mirror (7). In an FTIR spectrometer, this recombined beam is then generally passed through the sample to a detector (3), where the interferogram is obtained. In the simplest case of a monochromatic radiation source the intensity (amplitude) of the detector signal is merely the cosine function of the mirror position (3,7). For polychromatic radiation, however, the interferogram is a summation of all of the constructive and destructive interferences resulting from the interactions between all of the wavelengths (7). The cosine Fourier transform provides the mathematical relationship between the detected interferogram intensity, I(x), which is a function of the mirror position, and the infrared absorption intensity, I(v), as a function of frequency (7,11):

$$I(x) = \int_{-\infty}^{\infty} I(\nu) \cos(2\pi x \nu) d\nu \tag{5}$$

In order to obtain the infrared spectrum from this interferogram quickly, a computer is required to calculate the following inverse transform (7,11):

$$I(\nu) = \int_{-\infty}^{\infty} I(x) \cos(2\pi x \nu) dx \tag{6}$$

The optical path difference, x, is a function of the position of the moveable mirror and is very accurately determined through the use of an internal standard (typically a helium-neon laser) (11).

When selecting an IR spectrometer, the choice of detector can be important. Infrared detectors consist of two general types: thermal and photon. Thermal detectors measure a change in a physical property of a material as it is heated, whereas photon detectors use changes in the electrical properties of a semiconductor caused by incoming photons to detect IR radiation (12). Thermal detectors tend to be nonselective detectors in that they have a response that is directly proportional to the incident energy and largely independent of the wavelength (7). Photon detectors, on the other hand, are much more selective detectors since they have a response curve that is strongly dependent on the wavelength of the incident radiation. Because of their relative wavelength independence (7) and versatility (12), nonselective thermal detectors have traditionally been the better choice for spectroscopy. However, these types of detectors tend to have slow response times and low relative sensitivity (12). With improvements in semiconductor technology and the increasing need for fast response times and better sensitivity, photon detectors are gaining favor. Thermal detectors include thermocouples, thermopiles, thermistors, bolometers, and pyroelectric detectors. Some examples of photon detectors include photoconductive and photovoltaic cells (12).

Thermocouples and bolometers are two common thermal detectors. The bolometers are based on the temperature-dependent electrical resistance of a material, offering the advantages over thermocouples of faster response times and greater sensitivities. The fast response requirements of the rapid-scanning interferometers in FTIR instruments, and the convenience of room temperature operation is often meet by the use of a pyroelectric detector (3). This detector's response is based on the temperature sensitivity of the residual electrical polarization that can be induced in pyroelectric crystals, such as triglycine sulfate (7). When this type of material is polarized by an electrical field a residual polarization is retained by the material after the field is removed. The voltage across this crystal is then temperature-dependent and is measured by electrodes placed on the crystal faces. This device is essentially independent of wavelength from the near-IR through the far-IR (7).

Photoconductive and photovoltaic detectors have the advantages of rapid response times and high sensitivity compared to thermal detectors. However, they have the disadvantage of being limited in their detection range, providing poor performance in the far-IR region (12). In addition, they often require liquid nitrogen or helium cooling. Both of these detectors depend on the quantum interaction between photons from the incident light and the semiconductor material in the detector (12).

Overall for the slower dispersive IR instruments, the cheaper thermal detectors are generally the best choice. For high-speed applications and especially rapid FTIR work, a photon detector is essential (12). More detailed information on the various types of detectors available for IR spectroscopy is presented by Colthup et al. in Ref. 7 and Ciurczak in Ref. 12.

IV. SAMPLING TECHNIQUES FOR INFRARED SPECTROSCOPY

The physical state (i.e., solid, optically dense) of most polymers makes careful sample preparation imperative since it is generally necessary for the IR beam to be transmitted through the sample. Therefore, at least some sample preparation is necessary before an IR spectrum can be obtained. In addition, the quality of the spectrum is often dependent on the care taken in preparing the sample. Poorly prepared samples that are too thick, nonuniform, or contain impurities can result in poor or misinterpreted data. There are a number of methods for polymer sample preparation available depending on the physical state of the sample. For solid polymers, IR samples may be prepared by dispersion into KBr pellets or mulls, casting into thin film, or microtoming (3,6,13). For liquid polymer samples, liquid films can be examined by placing several drops between two salt plates (6).

The method of dispersing the polymer into an IR-transparent matrix of KBr is common for the study of hydrogels. This technique involves grinding the polymer sample into a fine powder and then mixing a small amount with an IR transparent matrix, such as powdered potassium bromide. This mixture is then molded at high pressures in a special die. Often the die is evacuated (7) and pressures range up to 1000 N/mm^2 (3). A disadvantage of this technique is that many of the matrix materials (salts) absorb water and exhibit water absorbance peaks near 3450 cm^{-1} and 1635 cm^{-1} (3). A similar technique that is more useful for water-sensitive samples is the mull method. In this method the polymer is ground into a powder and dispersed into a liquid phase, commonly mineral oil (Nujol) (7), hexachlorobutadiene, or perfluorocarbon (3). This paste is squeezed between two IR-transparent plates. The major disadvantage of this method is the limitation of spectral regions that can be observed due to absorbance bands of the dispersion material (3). A table of transmission ranges and refractive indices for a number of common matrix materials is presented by Siesler in Ref. 3.

A second sample preparation technique often used for polymers, but with limited utility for hydrogels, is preparation of a film solvent casting, melt casting, or hot pressing. This method has the advantage of providing a means for studying polymers in their solid state. The dimensional requirements of the film are such that it is large enough to cover the entire cross-section of the light beam, and that it is thick enough to provide sufficiently intense bands for groups that are present in low concentrations but thin enough to allow beam penetration. Typical dimensions are on the order of 15 mm × 5 mm with thicknesses in the range of 0.001–1 mm (3). Solvent casting is useful for polymers that can be readily dissolved in a volatile solvent but is not appropriate for crosslinked hydrogels. While melt casting can be used for thermoplastics, some samples require hot pressing in which a hydraulic press is used to provide thinner sample films (3).

Two final sample preparation methods are microtoming and microsampling. Microtoming involves the use of a sharp glass or diamond knife to cut extremely thin samples with thicknesses down to the nanometer scale. The technique is rather tedious and requires considerable practice to master, but may be useful for highly crosslinked polymers and hydrogels which do not dissolve in any solvents. In order to be microtomed, a sample it must be suitably hard so as not to deform greatly under the knife pressure. Softer samples often must be microtomed under cryogenic conditions. Microsampling is a technique that is used to obtain IR spectra from very small specimens, such as a microtomed sample (3). This technique requires the attachment of an optical device that reduces the image of the monochromator slit at the sample position (3). This type of system can introduce several sources of error that need to be considered. As an example, diffraction phenomena or imperfections in the optical system can cause false radiation that will result in smaller intensities of the absorption bands (3).

Finally, for polymer samples for which satisfactory transmission spectra cannot be obtained by any of the above techniques it may be possible to use ATR to acquire an IR spectra (14,15). ATR is based on the phenomenon of total internal reflectance between two materials of different refractive indices. Experimentally, the sample under investigation with a refractive index of n_2 is placed in direct contact with the reflecting surface of a prism. The prism has a refractive index of n_1 that is larger than n_2. Total internal reflectance occurs at an angle above the critical angle of incidence, α_c, of the light beam. This angle is defined by the relation (3,7):

$$\sin \alpha_c = n_2/n_1 \qquad (n_1 > n_2) \tag{7}$$

The penetration depth of the light beam into the sample is generally on the order of several micrometers. This provides the absorption path without requiring transmission of the radiation through the entire thickness of the sample. The spectrum obtained is very similar to the transmission spectrum. The only difference is that the absorption bands observed with ATR at longer wavelengths have higher intensities compared to transmission spectra (3).

A second type of reflection spectroscopy is reflection-absorption (RA) spectroscopy. This technique makes use of external reflections. A thin film of the sample is placed on a reflecting metal surface and irradiated with a light beam having an angle of incidence usually between 70° and 89°. This technique has been used for the detection of thin polymer films on metal surfaces, and investigations of the adhesion between polymers and metals (16).

V. APPLICATION OF INFRARED SPECTROSCOPY TO HYDROGELS

Infrared spectroscopy, especially FTIR, has found widespread application for the characterization of hydrogels. IR spectroscopy has been used to characterize both the polymerization systems used to produce hydrogels and the resulting hydrogel polymers. In addition, IR spectroscopy has been used to characterize intermolecular interactions and diffusional processes in hydrogels. In this chapter we will divide the literature on the application of IR spectroscopy to hydrogels into the following two classifications: (a) papers that report the analysis of the polymerization process, including characterization of polymerization kinetics, network formation, and identification of functional groups; and (b) papers that report the investigation of molecular interactions (especially hydrogen bonding) and diffusion. We will summarize the literature in each of these areas, using representative rather than exhaustive references.

A. Characterization of Polymerization Processes

Infrared spectroscopy has been successfully used in the analysis of the polymerization process, including characterization of polymerization kinetics, network formation, and identification of functional groups. With the use of high-speed FTIR spectrometers, kinetic studies can often be performed in situ to determine reaction order and activation energy. IR spectra can also be used to identify the structural changes and the extent of crosslinking that occur in a polymerization reaction (10). For chain polymerizations of unsaturated monomers, the polymerization can often be monitored based on the decrease in the peak corresponding to double-bond stretching (which typically occurs at ~ 1640 cm^{-1}) (11).

Hasirci used IR spectroscopy to study crosslinking in controlled release hydrogels synthesized by copolymerizing 2-vinylpyridine with divinylbenzene or ethylbenzene monomers in reactions that were initiated with gamma radiation. Based upon these studies, this author concluded that the major source of crosslinks was the bifunctional divinylbenzene monomer (17). Earhart et al. used FTIR spectroscopy in their investigation of the effect of poly(vinyl alcohol) on the mechanism and kinetics of the copolymerization of vinyl acetate and butyl acrylate. These investigators used FTIR spectroscopy to monitor the increase in the concentration of acetate moieties on the polymer chains resulting from the grafting of vinyl acetate onto poly(vinyl alcohol) (18). Finally, Gulari et al. used FTIR spectroscopy to follow, in real time, the conversion of the bulk polymerization of both styrene and methyl methacrylate. By monitoring the integrated peak area for the IR absorbance of the carbon–carbon double bond (1643 cm^{-1}), they were able measure conversion with less error than methods involving the ring breathing mode of the aromatic ring at 1000 cm^{-1} as an internal reference (19).

Infrared spectroscopy often plays an important role in the preparation of hydrogels for controlled release applications by providing a convenient means of characterizing the final products. For example, Allcock and Kwon used IR spectroscopy to help characterize the structures of hydrogels formed from glyceryl phosphazenes. These authors were specifically interested in the crosslinking and binding ability of the hydroxyl units present on the glyceryl side groups. IR spectroscopy was used to help verify the synthesis of isopropylideneglycerol and to aid in the identification of the hydrolytic degradation products of glyceryl polyphosphazenes by measuring the IR absorbance of the O—H (3500–3200 cm^{-1}) and P=N (1250 cm^{-1}) groups (20). Edwards et al. used IR and Raman spectroscopy to characterize copolymers of methyl methacrylate with butadiene. They compiled a complete table of the wavenumbers and vibrational assignments for the 50:50 methyl methacrylate-1,3-butadiene copolymer (21,22).

Rose and co-workers (23,24) used IR spectroscopy to provide proof of grafting. Gelatin was graft copolymerized with poly(hydroxyethyl methacrylate and butyl acrylate) (HEMA-BA). Fibrin of bovine origin was incorporated into these polymers. Spectra of the gelatin–polymer–fibrin were compared to the spectra of its components, namely gelatin, fibrin, and HEMA-BA. The gelatin and fibrin proteins showed the characteristic amide absorption bands at 1600 cm^{-1}, 1550 cm^{-1}, 1250 cm^{-1}. The IR spectra for the HEMA-BA copolymer showed a characteristic ester-carbonyl band at 1720 cm^{-1}. The spectrum taken for the purified gelatin-grafted copolymer showed absorption bands for both amide and ester carbonyl groups, indicating grafting. In a second paper, written by Rose et al. (24), bovine serum albumin was copolymerized with poly(hydroxyethyl methacrylate). Analogously, the grafting was verified using IR specroscopy.

Huang et al. (25) reported an experimental study to investigate the effect of the crosslinking agent ethylene glycol dimethacrylate (EGDMA) on the curing kinetics of the polymerization of 2-hydroxyethyl methacrylate. FTIR spectroscopy was used to determine the conversion of the carbon double bonds. An IR absorption band characteristic of carbon double-bond stretching was compared before curing, after isothermal curing and after rescanning was compared. The influence of different curing temperatures and weight ratios of EGDMA/HEMA was studied. These studies revealed that the conversion decreases as the weight ratio of the EGDMA/HEMA increases and the reaction temperature decreases in an isothermal run.

Zhou et al. (26) reported that IR spectra of some novel superabsorbent copolymers prepared from acrylamide (AM), sodium methallylsulfonate (MSAS), sodium acrylate (AA), and the crosslinking agent methylenebisacrylamide (BisA). The authors assigned the absorption peaks at 3400 and 3196 cm^{-1} to NH_2 groups. In addition, they assigned adsorption peaks at 1664 and 1617 cm^{-1} to carbonyl stretching. Hennink et al. (27) investigated the performance of glycidyl methacrylate–derivatized dextran as a releasing agent for proteins. The conversion of the methacrylate groups was determined by FTIR spectroscopy using the peak height of the IR absorption at 813 cm^{-1} (double bond of glycidyl methacrylate) and 763 cm^{-1} (dextran).

Shah et al. (28) developed hydrogels of poly(vinyl alcohol) (PVA) crosslinked with glutaraldehyde. The authors used infrared spectroscopy to monitor crosslinking by comparing the IR spectra of the pure PVA with the correspond spectra from the crosslinked samples. The significant reduction in intensity of the broad hydroxyl group peak for the crosslinked compared to the pure polymer confirmed crosslinking. Park and co-workers (29) grafted poly(acrylic acid) (PAA) onto a porous glass filter using a silane-coupling compound. The untreated, silane-coupled, and PAA-grafted filter surfaces were subject of IR spectroscopy. While the spectra of the two first samples did not differ markedly, the carbonyl absorption peak at 1720 cm^{-1} confirmed the graft polymerization of PAA after a glow discharge treatment.

Gonzales et al. (30) used IR spectroscopy to investigate bond formation of PAA crosslinked with glycerol. These hydrogels were studied for comtrolled release of metoclopramide. The IR spectrum collected after polymerization of the hydrogel with the crosslinking agent showed a new bond at 1737 cm^{-1} corresponding to the ester formed between the polymer carbonyl groups and the hydroxy groups of glycerol. Noncrosslinked polymers only showed the carbonyl stretching of acrylic acid at 1712 cm^{-1} and of metoclopramide at 1651 cm^{-1}.

The polymerization of poly[N-vinylpyrrolidone–acrylic acid]–polyethylene glycol hydrogel networks was studied with the use of IR spectroscopy by Shanta et al. (31). In these studies, the disappearance of the vinyl bond at 1040 cm^{-1} was taken as an indication of successful polymerization. The carbonyl peak at 1652 cm^{-1} and the hydroxyl peak at 3400 cm^{-1} were cited to indicate a formation of an "interpolymer system." The same authors (32) applied the same technique to analyze the copolymerization of methacryloyloxyazobenzene (MAB) with hydroxyethyl methacrylate (HEMA). Characterizing bands of the azo group representing MAB and the hydroxy group representing HEMA were found in the copolymer poly(MAB-HEMA).

Kakoulides et al. (33) used IR spectroscopy to characterize the polymerization of acrylic acid crosslinked with 4,4'-divinylazobenzene (DVAB). Formation of the copolymer was indicated by the disappearance of the characteristic vinyl group absorptions of DVAB and acrylic acid and the emergence of new bonds characteristic of the aliphatic, —CH_2—CHR—, backbone. For comparison, the homopolymer of PAA was characterized by a broad band in the region of 3700–2500 cm^{-1}, due to hydrogen bonding and the carbonyl stretch at 1710 cm^{-1}. Incorporation of the crosslinking agent within the polymer matrix gives rise to characteristic absorption at 1598 and 840 cm^{-1} due to the aromatic nature of the DVAB molecule. The increase of relative intensities of these absorptions as compared to the carbonyl stretch at 1710 cm^{-1} for increasing amounts of the crosslinker present provided evidence for the complexation of the crosslinking reaction. In addition, as the crosslinking density increases, the broad hydrogen bonding absorption decreases in intensity, indicating that the incorporation of DVAB disrupts the hydrogen bonds of the network.

Bicak et al. (34) studied hydrogels prepared with the water-soluble crosslinker N,N'-diallylmalonamide. This crosslinking agent was synthesized using with equimolar amounts of allylamine and diethylmalonate in dioxane, and its structure was confirmed by FTIR spectroscopy. The crosslinking agent was copolymerized with the comonomer acrylamide, and FTIR was used to monitor the unreacted allyl groups by measuring areas of olefinic C—H stretching vibration peaks at 3080 cm^{-1}.

Heat-treated and crosslinked hydrogels (PVA-MA), consisting of poly(vinyl alcohol) esterificated with maleic anhydride, were studied by Liou and Wang (35). First, by comparing IR spectra of untreated, heat-treated, and photocrosslinked PVA-MA films, these authors characterized the crosslinking in the system. Strong absorption peaks at 1640 and 1720 cm^{-1} that were assigned to the stretching of carbon double-bond and carbonyl groups of the maleic ester were both found in the untreated and heat-treated samples. In contrast, the peak assigned to the vinyl stretching was absent in the spectrum for the crosslinked PVA-MA, suggesting that almost all vinyl groups have participated in the crosslinking reaction. Second, the authors used IR spectroscopy to investigate the dependence of pH-dependent swelling on the dissociation of the carboxylic groups in the gel. For crosslinked PVA-MA films, the absorption peak at around 1580 cm^{-1}, assigned to the carboxylate ions intensifies with increasing pH value from 2 to 7, indicating the dissociation of the carboxylic acid. Further titration to basic conditions did not further increase the intensity. However, for heat-treated hydrogels, raising the pH value continuously from pH 2 to pH 12 the peak intensity at 1580 cm^{-1} increased consecutively. Therefore, results from IR spectra analysis in combination with acid–base titration suggest that the ionization of carboxylic acid accounts for the 'pH-induced gel swelling and the differences in the swelling behavior.

The kinetics of photopolymerization was characterized using ATR/FT-IR (36). The polymerization of a precursor film consisting of the monomers poly(ethylene glycol) diacrylate and vinylferrocene and the photoinitiator 2-2'-dimethyxy-2-phenylacetophenone were spread out over the surface of the ATR crystal. The sample was covered by a borosilicate class plate and illuminated with a 365-nm UV-visible light at 20 W/cm^2. The infrared peak corresponding to the carbon double bond in the wavenumber range of 1630–1680 cm^{-1} was used as a measure for conversion.

B. Characterization of Molecular Interactions and Diffusion

The advent of modern personal computers and the ease with which IR spectra can be digitized and manipulated has enhanced the usefulness of FTIR spectroscopy for studying the interactions between hydrogels and aqueous phases. For example, the ability to quickly obtain a difference spectrum is important in the study of many biological and hydrogel systems since the large water absorption bands, which can obscure the spectra of interest, may be subtracted out (3,37,38). For example, Gendreau et al. have used FTIR/ATR to study the adsorption of blood plasma proteins onto various surfaces. The sensitivity and absorbance subtraction ability of FTIR spectroscopy was crucial in allowing them to construct a time-resolved picture of the proteins' rapid absorbance including changes that occurred in a small percentage of proteins. These investigators further used their FTIR/ATR technique in kinetic studies to determine total as well as relative protein absorbance by plotting individual IR band intensities vs. time (38).

In the synthesis of hydrogels, intermolecular hydrogen bonding can play a significant role in both the reactivity of the monomer and the structure of the resulting polymer. Several investigators have used IR spectroscopy to examine the effect of hydrogen bonding during polymerization of acrylic or methacrylic acid (39–42). For example, Saini et al. used IR spectroscopy to characterized the solvent-dependent composition of the copolymer of methacrylamide with methyl methacrylate (39). Other researchers found similar effects for the polymerization of acrylic (40–42), methacrylic (41,42), and itaconic (42) acids. Bajoras and Makuška used IR spectroscopy to examine hydrogen bonding during polymerization of acrylic acid in a solvent mixture of dimethylsulfoxide and water. The authors concluded that hydrogen bonding resulted in a marked decrease in the polymerization activity of the acid. They concluded that this decrease was the result a decreased probability for the formation of π complexes caused by an increase in the activity of the acid molecules in the hydrogen bond complexes when in the presence of water (42).

Monti and Simoni (43) studied the effect of hydrogen bonding on the molecular structure of poly(vinylpyrrolidone) (PVP) and 2-hydroxyethyl methacrylate (PHEMA), which are hydrogels commonly used for soft contact lens. The investigators used both FTIR and Raman spectroscopy to determine how the adsorbed water interacted with the hydrogels by comparing the spectra of dried and hydrated soft contact lenses. They found that the water interacts with the carbonyl groups by hydrogen bonding. Furthermore, they determined that the strength of this interaction is dependent on which hydrophilic group is involved and that for PVP lenses the water alters the conformation of the hydrophobic groups (43). Long and van Luyen (44) report that hydrogels formed from chitosan and carboxymethylcellulose (CMC) mixtures were obtained by simple complexation in the aqueous phase. IR spectroscopy was used to confirm complexation between the carboxylic groups in CMC and the amine in chitosan.

In an excellent paper by Perova et al. (45), IR spectroscopy of PHEMA with water has been studied as a function of water content in the range of 38–2.6 wt % water and in the temperature range of 300–373 K. The effect of water on the matrix of the PHEMA hydrogel was investigated by comparing the IR spectrum of the hydrogel with that of a dry sample. The authors found four absorption bands whose frequencies and intensities were affected by the quantity of water in the system. The carbonyl stretching band was found to lie in the region of 1540–1820 cm^{-1} for different water contents and to be centered at 1720 cm^{-1} for a dry sample. With an increase of water content a shoulder develops at 1650 cm^{-1} which is assigned to H—O—H bending vibrations of loosely bound water molecules. This phenomenon appears for a water content that exceeds 30%. Moreover, the carbonyl bond is itself deconvoluted into the non-hydrogen-bonded, hydrogen-bonded (due to self-association), and irregular hydrogen-bonded carbonyl bond involving a specific geometry. In addition, the H—O—H bonding was resolved into the contributions of loosely bound water molecules that are connected to each other by hydrogen bonding and those which are physically bound to the polymer. The O—H stretching vibration and a composite band were similarly discussed in that paper. The IR results show evidence that loosely bound water exists in systems with water amounts greater than 18% whereas tightly bound water exists for water concentrations below it.

Shojaei and Li (46) conducted ATR-IR studies of crosslinked copolymers consisting of a poly(acrylic acid) backbone with poly(ethylene glycol) (PEG) side chains or grafts. ATR-IR spectroscopy was used to evaluate the formation of hydrogen bonds in the presence of mucin and acetic acid. The spectra reveal that the stretching of C—O in the ethylene glycol unit is significantly perturbed in the presence of the hydrogen donor groups of mucin and acetic acid compared to pure crosslinked copolymers. The authors attribute that to the formation of hydrogen bonds between PEG as a hydrogen acceptor and the proton donor of mucin and acetic acid.

Mazumdar et al. (47) used FTIR spectroscopy to study the specific interaction between iodine and the copolymer of methyl methacrylate (MAA) and N-vinylpyrrolidone (NVP). Distinct absorption bands corresponding to the ester carbonyl group of MMA (1731 cm^{-1}) and the carbonyl group of NVP (1682 cm^{-1}) were observed without the iodine present. For the iodinated copolymer, the carbonyl ring adsorption was shifted to a weaker band at 1646 cm^{-1}; however, the ester carbonyl band remained unaffected. Hence, the results suggest the presence of specific interactions between the pyrrolidone repeating units and iodine.

FTIR spectroscopy has also been used to study the complexation of PEG in poly(methacrylic acid) (PMAA) hydrogels. Philippova and Starodubtzev (48) identified three bands arising from stretching vibrations of PMAA carboxy groups that were attributed to the hydrogen-bonded PMAA-PEG complexes, the intramolecular hydrogen bonded PMAA complexes, and the dehydrated uncomplexed hydroxy groups of PMAA. Based on this IR spectroscopy data, conclusions about the fraction of carboxylic groups that participate in the formation of the intermolecular complex could be drawn. In addition, distributions of PEG throughout the gel layers for different ratios of PEG/PMAA repeating unit ratios were studied by comparing the intensity of adsorption band of PEG at 1100 cm^{-1}. It has been found that for an excess of PMAA with respect to PEG the complex forms preferentially in the outer layer, while for excess of PEG, the complex distribution is even.

Ichikawa et al. (49) collected IR spectra for dry thin film samples of polyelectrolyte complexes composed of poly(ϵ-lysine) (PEL) and CMC. These authors varied the composition of the films and investigated CMC with various degrees of substitution and molecular weights. With increasing PEL content a new band at 1670 cm^{-1} was detected. This band was assigned to an amino group which differs from that of PEL alone at 1639 cm^{-1}. The authors attribute this IR band shift to a strong ionic interaction between the oppositely charged compounds.

Ozeki et al. (50) used IR spectroscopy to investigate the effect of pH on the intermolecular complex between poly(ethylene oxide) (PEO) and carboxyvinylpolymer (CP). Polymer solutions of PEO and CP were dissolved into a 50:50 (v/v) mixture of ethanol and water. Polymer films were prepared by solution casting and were used without modification for the IR measurements. It was observed that the magnitude of the carbonyl peak of CP at 1734 cm^{-1} decreased with increasing pH values from pH = 1.2–5.5. This peak is assigned to the carbonyl group shifted by hydrogen bonding between the ether groups of PEO and the hydroxyl group of the carboxylic acid. Under nearly neutral (pH 6.8) and basic conditions (pH 9.0), the peak disappeared. Furthermore, new peaks at about 1580 and 1400 cm^{-1} which were assigned to deionized carboxylic groups (COO$^-$) that emerged. Hence the authors demonstrate that IR spectroscopy is capable of monitoring the forming and breaking of hydrogen bonds in intermolecular complexes.

In a very interesting contribution, Zhang et al. (52) used infrared spectroscopy in combination with visible sum-frequency vibrational surface spectroscopy for a detailed characterization of the molecular rearrangement on a polymer surface. These techniques were used to monitor structural changes of a polyurethane surface when the polymer is transferred from air to water. Sahlin and Peppas (53) report that diffusion in polymer systems may be examined by near-field FTIP spectroscopy. In this investigation, the diffusion of PEG free chains across a PAA gel/gel interphase was investigated. Based on a concentration profile of the PEG in the PAA laminate obtained by collecting a series of IR spectra from sections excised of the gel laminate, a PEG diffusion coefficient was calculated.

Infrared spectroscopy studies were conducted by Bhatia and co-workers (54) to identify the effect of iontophorensis and chemical penetration enhancers on the transdermal delivery of a hormone. The IR spectra of a stratum cornum treated with different combinations of enhancers (oleic acid/propylene glycol and ethanol/propylene glycol) were analyzed. Absorbance bands in the region of 2850 cm^{-1} and 2920 cm^{-1} were assigned to symmetrical and antisymmetrical —CH— stretching of the lipids. An observed shift of these peaks to higher wavenumbers after treatment was attributed to an increase in the degree of disorder of the lipid in acryl chains. The authors concluded that iontophorensis, in combination with the enhancers, led to the fluidization of the lipid matrix and an increase in the hormone permeability. Similarly, Senels et al. (55) investigated the enhancing effect of sodium glycodeoxycholate (GDC) on penetration of morphine sulfate through bovine buccal mucosa. Tissues incubated with 100 mM GDC solution for up to 4 h were used for FTIR studies. Again, the peaks of interest arose from the C—H stretching bonds. An observed decrease in area of the integrated peaks for tissues treated for 4 h was attributed to the reduction of the long chain lipids due to solvent extraction.

Changes in the structure of the crystalline regions of poly(tetramethylene terephthalate) due to an applied stress were studied by Ward and Wilding using FTIR spectroscopy (56). These authors found that differences between the IR spectra for the stressed and unstressed states could be attributed to changes in the trans/gauche isomerism of the polymer chains. Under stress the conformation changed from a gauche–trans–gauche form (identified by C—H rocking bands at 917 cm^{-1} and 752 cm^{-1}) to an all-trans conformation (identified by C—H rocking bands at 962 cm^{-1} and 840 cm^{-1}) (56). Finally, IR spectroscopy has been used to characterize the conformation and stereoregularity of PMMA (57–59). For example, Dybal et al. used the IR spectra of PMMA to find that in a stereocomplex of isotactic and syndiotactic PMMA, the extended chain form of the syndiotactic PMMA is preferred (58).

VI. PHYSICAL BASIS FOR RAMAN SPECTROSCOPY

Raman spectroscopy involves the inelastic scattering of photons rather than their direct absorption or emission. When electromagnetic radiation interacts with matter, the incident radiation may be absorbed, transmitted, refracted, diffracted, or reflected. If we consider only the fraction of the light that is scattered, most of these photons will undergo elastic scattering, also known as Rayleigh scattering, and will be unchanged in energy. A smaller fraction of the radiation will be scattered inelastically, and will be shifted to higher or lower energy by an amount equal to the energy of a vibrational transition. The Raman scattering intensity is typically four orders of magnitude lower than the Rayleigh scattering intensity (8). In a classical picture, the Raman effect arises from the molecule undergoing a change in polarizability during one of its normal modes of vibration. As a result, the scattered waveform has three frequency components: one corresponds to the Rayleigh scattered radiation, the other two correspond to the Raman scattering and are shifted to higher and lower frequencies by an amount equal to the frequency of the vibration. Therefore, Raman scattering leads to two vibrational spectra that occur on either side of the Rayleigh scattering line.

The Raman spectrum of a compound may look very similar to the IR spectrum of the same compound because both techniques are ultimately based on vibration transitions. However, since the two techniques are based on completely different phenomena (IR arises from absorption of photons, while Raman arises form scattering), some bands that are very prominent in the IR spectrum may be very weak in the Raman spectrum. For example, water exhibits a broad and intense peak in the IR spectrum but leads to little Raman scattering. In addition, the Raman effect allows vibrational spectroscopy to be performed using visible or ultraviolet light (the investigator is free to choose the best wavelength for the experiment), and therefore allows faster and more sensitive detectors than are available at the infrared wavelengths.

The intensity of the molecular scattering is dependent on the frequency of the excitation source to the fourth power, as well as the polarizability of the scattering molecules as shown in Eq. 8 (1).

$$I_{mn} = \frac{2^7 \pi^5}{3^2 c^2} I_0 (\nu_0 + \nu_{mn})^4 \sum_{\rho\sigma} |(\alpha_{\rho\sigma})_{mn}|^2 \tag{8}$$

Here the subscripts m and n represent a transition from the m vibrational level to the n level. Alpha, α, is the $\rho\sigma$ component of the polarizability tensor, where $\rho\sigma$ assumes nine possible designations (xx, xy, xz, yz, etc.). The net result is a strong dependence of the Raman intensity on the excitation frequency with higher frequency excitation leading to a larger Raman scattering cross-section and higher intensity Raman signals.

The inelastic scattering of radiation results in two possible processes. In the quantum mechanical description of the process, molecules in the ground state give Raman scattering with energy $h(\nu_0 - \nu_1)$. These transitions result in a reduction of the energy and this is known as Stokes scattering. The second possibility results when vibrationally excited state molecules inelastically scatter back to the ground state, giving an energy $h(\nu_0 + \nu_1)$. These transitions result in an increase in energy and are known as anti-Stokes scattering. If the system is at thermal equilibrium, the ratio of the Stokes and anti-Stokes intensity is governed by the sample temperature in accordance with the Boltzmann distribution, as shown below:

$$\frac{\text{Anti-Stokes intensity}}{\text{Stokes intensity}} = \frac{(\nu + \nu_m)^4}{(\nu - \nu_m)^4} e^{-(h\nu_m/kT)} \tag{9}$$

Near room temperature most of the molecules exist in the ground state and therefore Stokes lines have greater intensities than anti-Stokes lines. It is therefore possible to use the ratio of Stokes and anti-Stokes to determine the temperature of a sample.

Near-IR Fourier transform (FT) Raman spectroscopy is designed to eliminate the fluorescence problem encountered in conventional Raman spectroscopy (60). If a sample is even slightly fluorescent, the intensity of the fluorescence emission will normally be much higher than the intensity of the Raman scattering. The use of an excitation frequency below the threshold for the fluorescence process, such as 1064 nm, circumvents many of the problems associated with fluorescence interference, although there is a tradeoff since the scattered intensity for this near-IR wavelength will be significantly lower than the scattered intensity for a higher energy photon from the UV or visible region of the spectrum. The Raman scattering from 1064 nm will occur in the near-IR region of the spectrum. Conventional FTIR instrumentation with added filters for rejection of the Rayleigh line can be used with little modification.

Fourier transform Raman spectroscopy holds significant yet untapped promise for bulk chemical characterization of biomaterials and drug delivery systems (61). In addition to the ability to circumvent the fluorescence problem, advantages of FT Raman spectroscopy include ease of sample preparation and rapid analysis time for most materials (61). These advantages of FT Raman are counterbalanced by the difficulties in the distinction between inherently weak Raman and strong Rayleigh scattering. In the Fourier transform process, the noise in the intense Rayleigh line is redistributed across the entire spectrum (60). Therefore, FT Raman spectroscopy must have an extremely effective means of removing stray light at the laser wavelength.

When the laser wavelength used to excite the Raman effect lies under an intense electronic absorption band of a chromophore, a resonance enhancement of the Raman signal by a factor of 10^3–10^6 may occur (60). The enhanced vibrational modes are generally totally symmetrical and are associated only with the electronic chromophore being excited. Accordingly, the enhancement can increase the Raman signal in certain cases. However, nonlinear variations in intensities that depend in a complex way on the proximity of the laser excitation wavelength to the electronic maximum of the sample can be seen in certain samples (62). Therefore, care must be exercised in quantitative analysis to account for this nonlinearity in peak intensity when resonance-enhanced Raman spectroscopy is used.

VII. INSTRUMENTATION FOR RAMAN SPECTROSCOPY

Before the advent of lasers in the 1960s, Raman spectroscopy saw little application for chemical analysis. Due to the inherent low signal intensity of Raman scattering, an intense light source is needed. In addition, to achieve adequate resolution of the Raman peaks the light source must be monochromatic. These requirements made it very difficult to perform Raman scattering experiments using mercury arc lamps as the incident light sources, and the early Raman experiments required high concentrations and high sample volumes. However, the advent of lasers solved this problem, and applications of Raman spectroscopy began to flourish (7). Today there are many different types of lasers available, covering a wide range of frequency and power output. Not only can high-power Ar^+ and Kr^+ lasers be used directly, but they can also be used for pumping dye lasers and tunable solid-state lasers in order to increase the range of possible excitation frequencies. This ability to choose nearly any excitation frequency provides the investigator with an important degree of flexibility when designing a Raman experiment. For example, problems associated with fluorescence and low detector sensitivity can be circumvented by choosing excitation wavelengths that do not exhibit these limitations.

Gratings used in early monochromators for Raman spectroscopy were mechanically ruled. Modern holographically ruled gratings are now commonly available, providing dramatic improvements in signal-to-noise ratios. Furthermore, the introduction of concave holographic gratings in place of the conventional planar gratings has led to increased throughput since concave gratings require no additional optical elements. In addition, since stray light rejection and throughput are of critical importance for the Raman experiment, improvements in double and triple monochromator design have also increased the signal-to-noise ratios. Finally, higher quality materials and improvements in the manufacture of optical components have increased the light collection of Raman spectrometers.

Recent advances in detector technology have also lead to significant improvements in the quality of Raman scattering data. Photomultiplier tubes and photodiode arrays are now being replaced in Raman spectrometers by charge couple devices (CCDs). The CCD detectors are a class of extremely low-noise devices that often consist of millions of pixels. CCD detectors can be cooled to liquid nitrogen temperatures giving remarkably low dark current levels, thereby allowing for long exposure time experiments. Although CCD technology has had more than 20 years to mature, advances are continually being made in CCD manufacturing technology and design techniques. New CCD devices can provide nearly photocounting performance in each pixel and simultaneously achieve dynamic ranges between 10^4 to 1 counts and 10^6 to 1 counts. CCD detectors also offer the possibility of two-dimensional imaging, which may be used to determine the homogeneity of samples and be coated to have high sensitivity in the UV, Vis, X-ray, and IR regions. The high sensitivity of CCDs in the 700- to 1000-nm region has reduced the problems caused by intense visible fluorescence of some samples.

Optical fiber–based devices for Raman spectroscopy are becoming more important in a variety of applications. Optical fiber technology allows the excitation and emitted light to be routed to and from the point of interest using a small sampling probe, thereby offering the advantages of flexibility and remote sampling. Small portable, fiberoptic Raman systems can now be purchased commercially from several sources.

The last major component of a Raman system is the data acquisition system. The improvements in speed and power of compact computers allow complete analysis systems to run on microcomputers. Collection of large numbers of data points, data manipulation, background removal, spectrum plotting, and analysis can now be accomplished with smaller and faster computers. For analysis of complex multicomponent data, new computer systems also include spectral identification programs based on growing spectral libraries.

Technological advances, such as those described above, allow high-quality Raman data to be obtained for systems and samples that would have been impossible to investigate a decade ago. Limitations of old techniques have been removed and new applications are being continually developed. Furthermore, as technology advances, Raman spectroscopy systems are becoming less expensive, thereby opening a wider variety of potential applications.

VIII. SAMPLING TECHNIQUES FOR RAMAN SPECTROSCOPY

One advantage of Raman over IR spectroscopy is the relative ease of sample preparation. If it is desired to perform Raman spectroscopy on a sample in solution, the polymer solution may simply be contained in a glass or quartz capillary tube and the scattered light viewed at a right angle to the excitation radiation. The laser beam excitation source is narrow, collimated, and unidirectional, so it can be manipulated in a variety of ways to access many sample configurations (10). As mentioned earlier, water has an extremely weak Raman spectrum and is an excellent solvent for Raman spectroscopy. Thus, solution studies on water-soluble or water-swellable polymers are increasing in importance (3,63).

Solid sampling techniques for Raman spectroscopy depend on the nature of the sample. Highly scattering and turbid samples are most often studied in a front surface geometry, while for clear samples, right angle scattering can be used. Powdered samples can be packed into glass tubes or cavities for a front surface or a transverse sampling geometry. Deformation caused by high temperatures or swelling processes in solid polymeric materials can be studied by Raman polarization measurements by varying the sample orientation. Microsampling in Raman can easily be obtained because the coherent visible light source can be tightly focused. In the micro-Raman experiment, microscopes are coupled to the Raman spectrometer allowing samples from 2 to 10 μm in size to be examined (5). The ability to examine small spot sizes allows micro-Raman to be employed in characterizing heterogeneities in solid polymer samples. Micro-Raman can also be used to study small volume gas and liquid samples down to the nanoliter range (5).

Surface-enhanced Raman scattering (SERS) spectroscopy has been established as a powerful method for elucidation of the structure of molecules adsorbed on specially prepared metal surfaces (64). The enhancement effect can increase Raman scattering by a factor of 10^3–10^6 (65). Furthermore, adsorption of molecules on the SERS active metal surface causes fluorescence quenching in some highly fluorescent compounds, thereby reducing the fluorescence interference. However, for this sampling technique, the overall theoretical approach to successfully explain these phenomena is not yet fully developed (5).

IX. APPLICATION OF RAMAN SPECTROSCOPY TO HYDROGELS

Although Raman spectroscopy is not as common as IR spectroscopy, its advantages have led to its application to the characterization of polymers and hydrogels. In this chapter we will divide the literature on the application of Raman spectroscopy for the characterization of hydrogels into the following three classifications: (a) papers that report the structural and compositional characterization of hydrogels; (b) papers that address the conformational and orientational characterization of polymer chains; and (c) papers that deal with characterization of the polymerization process. We will summarize the literature in each of these areas using representative rather than exhaustive references.

A. Structural and Compositional Characterization of Hydrogels

In the realm of structural and compositional characterization of polymers, Raman spectroscopy can be used for qualitative and quantitative studies. For example, Edwards et al. reported the application of Raman spectroscopy to the study of polymer systems. These authors used quantitative micro-Raman spectroscopy to characterize impurities in polymer systems. In these studies, the micro-Raman technique offered the ability to use small samples, therefore allowing analysis of localized impurities that were contaminating the polymers (21).

Davies et al. studied the role of additive–polymer interaction with drugs by monitoring shifts in Raman bands indicative of chemical changes at the molecular level (61). In this contribution, in situ solid-state analyses of excipients or additive molecules within a polymeric biomaterial were performed using Raman spectroscopy. An important feature of this study was the ability to detect quantitatively the molecular structures of a drug and polymer by Raman spectroscopy. The same authors report the use of micro-Raman and FT Raman to monitor the appearance or disappearance of specific functional groups within a polymer after hydrolysis or irradiation (61). This type of study is especially important for controlled release devices that are based on polymer hydrolysis or degradation. Again, Raman spectroscopy is especially attractive because it permits study of the degradation process in aqueous biological systems in situ (61). Moreover, the use of micro-Raman coupled with optical fibers for routing the excitation and scattered light may allow the studies to be performed in vivo (61).

In general, the Raman studies of films less than 5 μm thick are extremely challenging due to the small scattering volume of the sample (66). A technique known as waveguide Raman spectroscopy (WRS) was been developed to overcome this limitation. In this technique, the radiation is coupled into the polymer sample using a prism and the light propagates by total internal reflection. This technique has been used to study organic films, laminates, and orientation studies of isotactic PMMA (21). Furthermore, the partial orientation of small guest molecules in poly(vinyl alcohol) matrices has been analyzed by the WRS technique (67). Recently, near-infrared FT Raman spectroscopy applications of WRS have been demonstrated. For example, in a study reported by Zimba et al. (68), WRS using near-IR excitation and a Michelson interferometer WRS combined with the use of optical fibers for examination of submicrometer cellulose acetate and poly(vinyl alcohol) films. FT Raman spectra of films containing small-molecule chromophores embedded in polymer matrices were obtained. This technique seems to have potential for advancement in many areas.

Chao and Wu (69) used Raman spectroscopy to examine the function of crown ethers in the synthesis of faujasite zeolites. These authors reported that Raman spectra of the gel phase obtained during aging at ambient temperature indicated the formation of an aluminosilicate hydrogel. Raman spectra obtained after further reaction at 115°C were used to monitored the formation of tetrameric aluminosilicate and silicate anions. The formation of hexagonal faujasite was attributed to two characteristic bands that correspond to a low-frequency torsion mode from a cation–lattice interaction and a Si—O—Si or Al—O—Al vibration of four-membered aluminosilicate rings, thus providing structural information.

Raman and IR spectra of azoaromatic polyethers and corresponding model compounds were extensively analyzed by Tecklenburg et al. (70). These authors made peak assignments in the Raman and IR spectra based on vibrational and computational studies of substituted azobenzenes and azoxybenzenes in the 1650–900 cm^{-1} region of the spectrum. Analysis of the band arising from the N=N stretch illustrated that all of the compounds existed in the trans configuration. In addition, the polyethers exhibited a peak corresponding to an OH stretch that indicated a network of intermolecular hydrogen bonds among the polymer chains.

William and Wilcock (71–73) provide an excellent overview of new technological advancements of Raman spectroscopy and highlight their impact on applications for polymers. Newly developed Raman imaging microscope systems equipped with highly sensitive CCD detectors and dielectric radiation filters provide fast, high-throughput analysis. In addition, the advent of confocal Raman spectroscopy has opened new applications (73). Using this technique it is possible to discriminate effectively between the Raman signal coming from the focused laser spot and that coming from the out-of-focus region. Therefore, it is possible to restrict the analysis to specific layers beneath the surface of the sample providing that their Raman signal meets an acceptably detectable intensity. In this way, confocal Raman spectroscopy could be used to examine thin polymer multilayer laminates one layer at a time. For example, Hajatdoost et al. (73) applied confocal Raman microspectroscopy for depth profiling of PMAA, poly(vinyl alcohol) (PVA), and laminates. Observed changes of the bandwidth of the carbonyl stretching band was used as an indicator of hydrogen bonding in the interfacial region.

Wang et al. (74) used Raman spectroscopy to investigate the action of a plasticizing agent in polyacrylonitrile). The authors hypothesized that the plasticizing agent ethylene carbonate (EC) formed a complex with the host polyacrylonitrile. The authors compared the Raman spectra obtained for pure poly(acrylonitrile), pure ethylene carbonate, and various mixtures of the polymer and the plasticizer. The authors attributed observed changes in intensity and bandwidth of the bands related to the carbonyl group to the formation of a complex between the carbonyl and nitrile groups.

B. Conformational and Orientational Characterization of Polymer Chains

Raman spectroscopy has been used to characterize the conformations of polymer chain in both the solution state and in the solid state. The conformation of a hydrophilic polymer chain can change markedly upon dissolution or swelling, or in response to changes in pH, ionic strength, or salt concentration (75). For this reason it is important to have an experimental technique that can be used to characterize in polymer in situ in aqueous solutions. Since water exhibits very little inelastic light scattering, Raman spectroscopy is attractive for studying changes in polymer chain conformation in aqueous solutions. For example, Koenig et al. investigated the conformation of syndiotactic PMAA at various degrees of neutralization in aqueous solutions (76). These authors used Raman spectroscopy to characterize PMAA chains with degrees of neutralization ranging from 0.1 to 0.4. These authors also found that the Raman spectra of PMAA in the solid state and in aqueous solution were strikingly similar (76). The only observed frequency shifts were attributed to the difference in the state of hydrogen bonding in the solid and aqueous solution. The similarity in Raman spectra suggested that little, if any, detectable conformational changes in the PMAA structure occurs with dissolution. Koenig has also studied PEG in aqueous solutions (77). In this case, the Raman spectra suggested that the PEG molecules in aqueous solution have changed from a helical conformation to a less ordered conformation.

Raman spectroscopy has also been used to characterize the stereoregularity of polymers in both the solution and the solid state. For example, Tudor et al. used FT Raman spectroscopy to reveal the morphology of polyanhydride samples for use in drug release polymers (4). These authors illustrated that polymer morphology was a crucial factor in the hydrolysis rate of polymers used for the drug release systems (4). In addition, the stereoregularity of PMMA has been extensively studied using Raman spectroscopy (57,78,79). These studies show the promise of Raman techniques for nondestructive orientation and stereoregularity studies of polymers in solution and solid state.

Claybourn et al. (80) investigated the applicability of an expert system for the automatic interpretation of Raman spectra of complex acrylic and styrenated acrylic copolymers. These authors also provided a table of characteristic shift ranges and Raman intensities of common structural fragments.

Kister et al. (81) used Raman and IR spectroscopy to study poly(glycolic acid) polymers with different degrees of crystallinity. A number of bands were found whose intensities changed as the degree of crystallinity was altered. Based on these studies, the authors concluded that an inversion center was present in the crystal structure. Williams and Wilcock (71) also investigated the use of Raman spectroscopy to distinguish regions of differing polymer crystallinity. Regions of higher crystallinity exhibited sharpened Raman bands with lower bandwidth.

C. Characterization of Polymerization Processes

Raman spectroscopy has also been used to characterize the polymerization process. Raman may be used in situ to determine the extent of polymerization as a function of time, as well as structural information about the final polymer product. Raman spectroscopy offers some important advantages for kinetic studies of polymerization. Unlike physical techniques such as viscometry, Raman spectroscopy does not lose sensitivity at the gel point and can be used to characterize the entire reaction. In addition, since Raman allows vibrational spectroscopy to be performed using visible light, diode array and CCD detectors may be used to provide excellent time resolution and sensitivity. Finally, since Raman places few constraints on the sample geometry or configuration, it is relatively easy to maintain isothermal conditions in a thermostated sample cell. For monitoring chain polymerizations of unsaturated monomers, investigators typically analyze a Raman peak arising from the carbon double bond. This peak typically appears at a location near 1630 wavenumbers and is found to decrease in intensity as the polymerization progresses.

Chu et al. (82) reported the use of Raman spectroscopy for kinetic studies of polymerizations of styrene. These investigators found that the intensity of the aliphatic double bond peak located at 1632 cm^{-1} exhibited a linear dependence with conversion, and could therefore be used as a sensitive and convenient method to monitor the polymerization. These authors ratioed the 1632 cm^{-1} monomer peak to an internal standard to render the technique insensitive to laser power fluctuations or sample turbidity. Similarly, Gulari et al. (19) used Raman spectroscopy to study polymerizations of styrene and methyl methacrylate. Again these authors found that the intensity of the Raman peak at 1631 cm^{-1} corresponding to stretching of the carbon double bond varied linearly with conversion, and concluded that since their spectrometer was mechanically stable, there was no need to perform internal referencing.

Clarkson et al. (83) used Raman scattering of the vinyl moiety to study the kinetics of polymerizations of several commercial acrylates. In agreement with the previous authors, Clarkson et al. found that the peak intensity varied linearly with monomer concentration and that there was no need for normalization with an internal reference. Nelson and Scranton

(84,85) used Raman spectroscopy for kinetic studies of cationic photopolymerizations of hydrophilic divinyl ethers. In these studies, reaction profiles of the double-bond conversion vs. time were obtained by monitoring the Raman peaks at 1322 and 1622 cm^{-1} arising from the vinyl ether functionality. Similar reaction profiles were obtained using either of these peaks, while the intensity of a Raman signal at 1458 cm^{-1}, arising from an unreactive ethyl ether functionality, was found to be independent of conversion. Complete profiles of the reaction rate as a function of time were obtained, and the final limiting conversion was found to increase with increasing reaction temperature.

The advent of optical noninvasive fiber assemblies suitable for routing the excitation and the scattered light has led to the possibility of using Raman spectroscopy for remote sensing and process monitoring (86,87). For example, the near-infrared Fourier transform Raman technique described previously is well suited for fiberoptic assemblies (88). In these systems, problems associated with sample alignment and the generation of excessive temperatures can be alleviated using optical fibers due to the ease of positioning of the fiber probe and the lower laser power densities required for meaningful signal-to-noise ratios (88). Due to the lower power requirement, near-infrared FT Raman spectra of systems which contain highly absorbing or fluorescing molecules can be readily obtained without large temperature increases.

Claybourn et al. (89) reported the use of near-infrared FT Raman spectroscopy for the investigation of aqueous emulsion polymerizations of methyl methacrylate, butyl acrylate, and allyl methacrylate monomers. The authors found that the polymerizations could be easily monitored by following the Raman peak arising from symmetrical stretching of the carbon double bond and that this peak was affected by self-aborption due to water.

SYMBOLS

α_c	Critical angle of incidence
E_m	Vibrational energy of the molecule
E_p	Energy of a photon
E_{vi}	Value of the vibrational energy levels
h	Planck's constant
I(v)	Desired intensity of the frequency of the infrared radiation
I(x)	Detected interferogram intensity
J	Rotational quantum number
n	A quantum number
n_1	Refractive index of the prism
n_2	Refractive index of sample
ν	Classical vibrational frequency of the oscillator
ν_m	Frequency of vibration induced by absorption of a photon
ν_p	Frequency of a photon
x	Optical path difference

REFERENCES

1. Painter, P. C., Coleman, M. M. and Koenig J. L., 1982. The Theory of Vibrational Spectroscopy and Its Applications to Polymeric Materials. John Wiley & Sons, New York.
2. Ishida, H. (Ed.), 1987. Fourier Transform Infrared Characterization of Polymers. Polymer Science and Technology, Vol. 36, Plenum Press, New York.

3. Siesler, H. W. and Holland-Moritz, K., 1980. Infrared and Raman Spectroscopy of Polymers, Practical Spectroscopy Series, Vol. 4, Marcel Dekker, New York.
4. Tudor, A. M., Melia, C. D., Davies, M. C., Hendra, P. J., Church, S. Domb, A. J. and Langer. R., 1991. The application of Fourier transform Raman spectroscopy to the analysis of poly(anhydride) homo- and co-polymers. Spectrochim. Acta, 47A: 1335–1343.
5. Grasselli, J. G., Snavely, M. K. and Bulkin, B. J., 1981. Chemical Applications of Raman Spectroscopy. John Wiley & Sons, New York.
6. Rabek, J. F., 1980. Experimental Methods in Polymer Chemistry: Physical Principles and Applications. John Wiley & Sons, New York.
7. Colthup, N. B., Daly, L. H. and Wiberley, S. E., 1975. Introduction to Infrared and Raman Spectroscopy, 2nd ed., Academic Press, New York.
8. Hendra, P. J., 1974. Raman Spectroscopy. In: D. O. Hummel, Ed., Polymer Spectroscopy, Verlag Chemie, Weinheim, pp. 112–185.
9. Ingle, J. D. and Crouch, S. R., 1988. Spectrochemical Analysis. Prentice-Hall, Englewood Cliffs, NJ.
10. Koenig, J. L., 1992. Spectroscopy of Polymers. ACS Professional Reference Book, ACS, Washington, D.C.
11. Fanconi, B. M., 1984. Fourier transform infrared spectroscopy of polymers: synthesis and characterization. J. Test. Eval., 12: 33–39.
12. Ciurczak, E. W., 1993. Detectors in infrared spectroscopy. Spectroscopy, 8(8): 12.
13. Brown, S. C. and Harvey, A. B., 1977. Polymers, Infrared and Raman Spectroscopy, Part C. In: Brame, E. G. and Grasselli, J. G. (Eds.), Vol. 1, Practical Spectroscopy Series, Marcel Dekker, New York, pp. 873–932.
14. Polchlopek, S. E., 1966. Attenuated Total Reflectance, Applied Infrared Spectroscopy. D. N. Kendall, Ed., Reinhold, New York, p. 462.
15. Harris, R. L. and Svoboda, G. R., 1962. Determination of alkyd and monomer modified alkyd resins by attenuated total reflectance infrared spectrometry. Anal. Chem., 34(12): 1655–1657.
16. Tompkins, H. G., 1974. Infrared reflection–absorption spectroscopy. In: A. W. Czanderna (Ed.), Methods of Surface Analysis, Elsevier, Amsterdam, p. 447.
17. Hasirci., V. N., 1982. PVNO–DVB hydrogels: synthesis and characterization. J. Appl. Polym. Sci., 27: 33–41.
18. Earhart, N. J., Dimonie, V. L., El-Aasser, M. S. and Vanderhoff, J. W., 1990. Infrared studies on the grafting reactions of poly(vinyl alcohol), polymer characterization. In: C. D Craver and T. Provder (Eds.), Polymer Characterization: Physical Property, Spectroscopic, and Chromatographic Methods, Vol. 227, American Chemical Society, pp. 333–341.
19. Gulari, E., McKeigue, K. and Ng, K. Y. S., 1984. Raman and Fourier transform infrared Raman spectroscopy of polymerization: bulk polymerization of methyl methacrylate and styrene. Macromolecules, 17, 1822–1825.
20. Allcock, H. R. and Kwon, S., 1988. Glyceryl polyphosphazenes—Synthesis, properties and hydrolysis. Macromolecules, 21, 1980–1985.
21. Edwards, H. G. M. Johnson, A. F. and Lewis, I. R., 1993. Applications of Raman spectroscopy to the study of polymers and polymerization processes. J. Raman Spectrosc. 24: 475–483.
22. Edwards, H. G. M., Johnson, A. F., Lewis, I. R. and Wheelwright, S. J., 1993. Raman and FTIR spectroscopic studies of copolymers of methyl-methacrylate with butadiene. Spectrochim. Acta, 49A: 457–464.
23. Babu, P. R., Sastry, T. P., Rose C. and Rao N. M., 1997. Hydrogels based on gelatin poly(hydroxyethyl methacrylate) and poly(butyl acrylate) graft copolymer impregnated with fibrin. J. Appl. Polym. Sci., 65: 555–560.
24. Rose, C., Sastry, T. P., Madhavan, V. and Rao, N. M., 1998. Graft copolymerization of 2-hydroxyethyl methacrylate onto bovine serum albumin: preparation and characterization. Pure Appl. Chem., A35: 193–202.
25. Huang, C.-W., Sun, Y.-M. and Huang, W.-F., 1997. Curing Kinetics of the synthesis of poly(2-hydroxyethyl methacrylate) (PHEMA) with ethylene glycol dimethacrylate (EGDMA) as a crosslinking agent. J. Polym. Sci. A: Polym. Chem. 35: 1873–1889.

26. Zhou, W. J., Yao, K. J. and Kurth, M. J., 1997. Studies of crosslinked poly(AM-MSAS-AA) Gels. I. Synthesis and Characterization, J. Appl. Polym. Sci., 64: 1001–1007.
27. Hennink, W. E., Franssen, O., van Dijk-Wolthuis, W. N. E. and Talsma H., 1997. Dextran hydrogels for the controlled release of proteins. J. Controlled Release, 48: 107–114.
28. Shah, D., Shah, Y. and Pradhan, R., 1997. Development and evaluation of controlled-release diltiazem HCl microparticles using cross-linked poly(vinyl alcohol). Drug Dev. Ind. Pharm., 23: 567–574.
29. Park, Y. S.; Ito, Y. and Imanishi, Y., 1997. pH-Controlled gating of a porous glass filter by surface grafting of polyelectrolyte brushes. Chem. Mater., 9: 2755–2758.
30. García González, N. G., Kellaway, I. W., Blanco Fuente, H., Anguiano Igea, S., Delgado Charro, B., Otero Espinar F. J. and Blanco Méndez J., 1994. Influence of glyceral concentration and carbopol molecular weight on swelling and drug release characteristics of metoclopramide hydrogels. Int. J. Pharm., 104: 107–113.
31. Ravichandran, P., Shanta, K. L. and Rao, K. P., 1997. Preparation, swelling characteristics and evaluation of hydrogels for stomach specific drug delivery. Int. J. Pharm., 154: 89–94.
32. Shanta, K. L., Ravichandran, P. and Rao, P., 1995. Azo polymeric hydrogels for colon targeted drug delivery. Biomaterials, 16: 1313–1318.
33. Kakoulides, E., Smart, J. and Tsibouklis, J., 1998. Azocross-linked poly(acrylic acid) for colonic delivery and adhesion specificity: synthesis and characterisation. J. Controlled Release, 52: 291–300.
34. Bicak, N., Karaoglan, S. and Senkal, B. F., 1998. Synthesis of N,N'-diallylmalonamide and its copolymer gels with acrylic acid and acrylamide. Die Angewandte Makromolekulare Chemie, 255: 13–16.
35. Liou, F. J. and Wang, Y. J., 1996. Preparation and characterization of crosslinked and heat-treated PVA-MA films. J. Appl. Polym. Sci., 59: 1395–1403.
36. Sirkar, K. and Pishko, M. V., 1998. Amperometric biosensors based on oxidoreductases immobilized in photopolymerized poly(ethylene glycol) redox polymer hydrogels. Anal. Chem., 70: 2888–2894.
37. Gendreau, R. M. and Jakobsen, R. J., 1978. Fourier transform infrared technique for studying complex biological systems. Appl. Spectrosc., 32: 326–328.
38. Gendreau, R. M., Winters, S., Leininger, R. I., Fink, D., Hassler, C. R. and Jakobsen, R. J., 1981. Fourier transform infrared spectroscopy of protein absorption from whole blood: ex vivo dog studies. Appl. Spectrosc., 35: 353–357.
39. Saini, G., Leoni, A. and Simone, F., 1971. Solvent and effects in radical copolymerization. Die Makromolekulare Chemie, 147: 213–218.
40. Chapiro, A. and Dulieu, J., 1977. Influence of solvent on the molecular associations and on the radical initiated polymerization of acrylic acid. Eur. Polym. J., 13: 563–577.
41. Makushka, R. Y., Bayoras, G. I., Shulskus, Y. K., Bolotin, A. B., Roganova, Z. A. and Smolyanskii, A. L., 1985. Effect of complex formation on reactivity of acrylic and methacrylic acids in radical polymerization. Polym. Sci. USSR, 27(3): 634–641.
42. Bajoras, G. I. and Makuˇska, R. Y., 1986. Peculiarities of radical homopolymerization and copolymerization of acrylic, methacrylic and itaconic acids in complexing solutions. Polym. J., 18(12): 955–965.
43. Monti, P., and Simoni, R., 1992. The role of water in the molecular structure and properties of soft contact lenses and surface interactions. J. Mol. Struct., 269: 243–255.
44. Long D. D. and van Luyen, D., 1996. Chitosan-carboxymethylcellulose hydrogels as supports for cell immobilization, J. Macromol. Sci. Pure Appl. Chem., A33(12): 1875–1884.
45. Perova, T. S., Vij, J. K. and Xu, H., 1997. Fourier transform infrared study of poly(2-hydroxyethyl methacrylate) PHEMA. Colloid Polym. Sci., 275: 323–332.
46. Shojaei, A. H. and Li, X., 1997. Mechanism of buccal mucoadhesion of novel copolymers of acrylic acid and polyethylene glycol monomethylether monomethacrylate. J. Controlled Release, 47: 151–161.
47. Mazumdar, N. A., Vardarajan, R. and Singh, H., 1996. Iodine-incorporated copolymer of methyl methacrylate and N-vinylpyrrolidone. I. Synthesis and characterization. J. Pure Appl. Chem., A33: 353–370.

48. Philippova, O. E. and Starodubtzev S. G., 1995. Intermacromolecular complexation between poly(methacrylic acid) hydrogels and poly(ethylene glycol). J. Pure Appl. Chem., A32: 1893–1902.
49. Ichikawa, T., Mitsumura Y. and Nakajima T., 1994. Water-sorption properties of poly(ϵ-lysine): carboxymethyl cellulose (CMC) dietary complex films. J. Appl. Polym. Sci., 54: 105–112.
50. Ozeki, T., Yuasa, H. and Kanaya, Y., 1998. Mechanism of medicine release from solid dispersion composed of poly(ethylene oxide)–carboxyvinylpolymer interpolymer complex and pH effect on medicine release. Int. J. Pharm., 171: 123–132.
51. Lowe, T. L., Benhaddou, M. and Tenhu H., 1998. Partially Fluorinated Thermally Responsive Latices of Linear and Crosslinked Copolymers. J. Polym. Sci. Part B: Polym. Phys., 36: 2141–2152.
52. Zhang, D., Ward, R. S., Shen, Y. R. and Somorjai G. A., 1997. Environment-induced surface structural changes of a polymer: an in situ + IR + visible sum-frequency spectroscopic study. J. Phys. Chem. B, 101: 9060–9064.
53. Sahlin, J. J. and Peppas, N. A., 1996. An investigation of polymer diffusion in hydrogel laminates using near-field FTIR microscopy, Macromolecules, 29: 7124–7129.
54. Bhatia, K. S., Gao, S. and Singh, J., 1997. Effect of penetration enhancers and iontophoresis on the FT-IR spectroscopy and LHRH permeability through porcine skin. J. Controlled Release, 47: 81–89.
55. Senels, S., Capan, Y. et al., 1997. Enhancement of transbuccal permeation of morphine sulfate by sodium glycodeoxycholate in vitro. J. Controlled Release, 45: 153–162.
56. Ward, I. M. and Wilding, M. A., 1977. Infrared and Raman spectroscopy of poly (m-methylene terephthalate) polymers. Polymer, 18: 327–335.
57. Dybal, J. Spevácek, J. and Schneider, B., 1986. Ordered structures of syndiotactic poly (methyl methacrylates) studied by a combination of infrared, Raman, and NMR spectroscopy. J. Polym. Sci., Part B: Polym. Phys., 24: 657–674.
58. Dybal, J., Stokr, J. and Schneider, B., 1983. Vibrational spectra and structure of stereo regular poly (methyl methacrylates) and of the stereo complex. Polymer, 24: 971–980.
59. Dybal, J. and Krimm, S., 1990. Normal mode analysis of infrared and Raman spectra of crystalline isotactic poly(methyl methacrylate). Macromolecules, 23: 1301–1308.
60. Hirschfeld, T. and Chase, B., 1986. Fourier transform Raman spectroscopy: development and justification. Appl. Spectrosc. 40: 133.
61. Davies, M. C., Binns, J. S., Mellia, C. D. and Bourgois, D., 1990. Fourier transform Raman spectroscopy of polymeric biomaterials and drug delivery systems. Spectrochim. Acta, 46A: 277–283.
62. Asher, S. A. and Johnson, C. R., 1984. Raman Spectroscopy of a coal liquid shows that fluorescence interference is minimized with ultraviolet excitation. Science, 225, 311 (1984).
63. Peticolas, W. L., 1975. Biochimie, 57: 417.
64. Suh, J. S. and Michaelian, K. H., 1987. Surface-enhanced Raman-spectroscopy of acrylamide and polyacrylamide absorbed on silver colloid surfaces: polymerization of acrylamide on silver. J. Raman Spectrosc., 18: 409–414.
65. R. Chang, F. Furtak, Eds., Surface enhanced Raman scattering. Plenum Press, New York, 1982.
66. Howe, M. L. Watters, K. L. and Greenler, R. G., 1976. Investigation of thin surface films and absorbed molecules using Raman laser spectroscopy. J. Phys. Chem., 80: 382.
67. Schlotter, N. E. and Rabolt, J. F., 1984. Measurements of the optical anisotropy of trapped molecules in oriented polymer films by waveguide Raman spectroscopy (WRS). Appl. Spectrosc., 38(2): 208.
68. Zimba, C. G., Hallmark, V. M., Turrell, S., Swalen, J. D. and Rabolt J. F., 1990. Applications of Fourier-transform Raman spectroscopy to studies of thin polymer films. J. Phys. Chem., 94: 939–943.
69. Wu, C. N. and Chao, K. J., 1995. Synthesis of Faujasite zeolites with crown-ether templates. J. Chem. Soc. Faraday Trans., 91: 167–173.
70. Tecklenburg, M. M. J., Kosnak, D. J., Bhatnagar, A. and Mohanty, D. K., 1997. Vibrational characterization of azobenzenes, azoxybenzenes and azoaromatic and azoaromatic polyethers. J. Raman Spectrosc., 28: 755–763.
71. Williams, K. P. J. and Wilcock, I. C., 1997. Raman spectroscopy of polymers. Polymers Polym. Composites, 5: 443–449.

72. Williams, K. P. J., Pitt, G. D., Smith, B. J. E. and Whitley, A., 1994. Use of a rapid scanning stigmatic Raman imaging spectrograph in the industrial environment. J. Raman Spectrosc., 25: 131–138.
73. Hajatdoost, S. and Yarwood, J., 1996. Depth profiling of poly(methyl methacrylate), poly(vinyl alcohol) laminates by confocal Raman microspectroscopy. Appl. Spectrosc., 50: 558–564.
74. Wang, Z., Huang, B., Huang, H., Xue, R. and Chen, L., 1996. Experimental evidence of the interaction between polyacrylonitrile and ethylene carbonate plasticizer by Raman spectroscopy. J. Raman Spectrosc., 27: 609–613.
75. Koenig, J. L., 1971. Raman scattering of synthetic polymers: review. Appl. Spectrosc. Rev., 4(2): 233–306.
76. Koenig, J. L. Angood, A. C. Semen, J. and Lando, J. B., 1969. Laser-excited Raman studies of the conformational transition syndiotactic polymethacrylic acid in water. J. Am. Chem. Soc., 91: 7250.
77. Koenig, J. L. and Angood, A. C., 1970 Raman spectroscopy of polyethylene glycol in solution. J. Polym. Sci., 8: 1787–1796.
78. Purvis, J. and Bower, D. I., 1974. A study of molecular orientation in poly (methyl methacrylate) by means for laser Raman spectroscopy. Polymer, 15: 645–654.
79. Neppel, A. and Bulter, I. S. 1984. Raman spectra of fully deuterated syndiotactic and isotactic poly (methyl methacrylate). J. Raman Spectrosc. 15(4): 257–263.
80. Claybourn, M., Luinge, H. J. and Chalmers, J. M., 1994. Automated interpretation of Fourier transform Raman spectra of complex polymers using an expert system. J. Raman Spectrosc., 25: 115–122.
81. Kister, G., Cassanas G. and Vert, M., 1997. Morphology of poly(glycolic acid) by IR and Raman spectroscopies. Spectrochim. Acta Part A, 53: 1399–1403.
82. Chu, B., Fytas, G. and Zalczer, G., 1981. Study of thermal polymerization of styrene by Raman scattering. Macromolecules, 14: 395–397.
83. Clarkson, J. Mason, S. M. and Williams, K. P. J., 1991. Bulk radical homopolymerization studies of commercial acrylate monomers using near infrared Fourier transform Raman spectroscopy. Spectrochim. Acta, Part A, 47: 1345–1351.
84. Nelson, E. W. and Scranton, A. B., 1996. Kinetics of cationic photopolymerization of divinyl ethers characterized using in situ Raman spectroscopy. J. Polym. Sci., Part A, 34: 403–411
85. Nelson, E. W. and Scranton, A. B., 1996. In situ Raman spectroscopy for cure monitoring of cationic photopolymerizations of divinyl ethers. J. Raman Spectrosc., 27: 137–144.
86. Williams, K. P. J., 1990. Raman spectroscopy: Al^{3+} fibers in Raman spectroscopy. J. Raman Spectrosc., 21: 147.
87. Hendra, P. J., Ellis, G. and Cutler, D. J., 1988. J. Raman Spectrosc., 19: 413.
88. Lewis, E. N., Kalasinsky, V. F. and Levin, I. W., 1988. Near infrared Fourier transform Raman spectroscopy using fiber-optic assemblies. Anal. Chem., 60: 2658–2661.
89. Claybourn, M., Massey, T., Highcock, J. and Gogna, D., 1994. Analysis of processes in latex systems by Fourier transform Raman spectroscopy. J. Raman Spectrosc., 25: 123–129.

8
Accurate Models in Controlled Drug Delivery Systems

Balaji Narasimhan
Rutgers, The State University of New Jersey, Piscataway, New Jersey

I. INTRODUCTION

Controlled delivery of drugs, proteins, and other bioactive agents can be achieved by incorporating them, either in dissolved or dispersed form, in polymers (1,2). In the development of controlled release systems, mathematical modeling of the release process plays a significant role as it establishes the mechanism(s) of drug (solute) release and provides more general guidelines for the development of other systems. It is well accepted that numerous successful controlled delivery systems have been developed as a result of an almost arbitrary selection of components, configurations, and geometries. Yet development of advanced controlled release systems is increasingly dependent on judicious application of the fundamentals of solute diffusion through polymers.

From a mathematical modeling point of view, controlled release systems may be classified according to the controlling physical mechanism(s) of release of the incorporated drug. We use a convenient method (3) based on the mechanism of transport in these systems as diffusion-controlled, swelling-controlled, and chemically controlled systems.

The objectives of designing controlled drug delivery systems are to:

Predict drug release rates from and drug diffusion behavior through polymers, thus avoiding excessive experimentation
Elucidate the physical mechanisms of drug transport by simply comparing the release data to mathematical models
Design new drug delivery systems based on general release expressions, and
Optimize the release kinetics

Accurate mathematical models that take into account the mechanistic aspects of the transport processes in drug delivery systems and the structural characteristics of the polymer can help fulfill the above objectives. The model equations can be used to design new systems by selecting the optimal geometry, method of formulation, and size (4–10).

Modeling of such systems is complicated and relies on careful representation of the physical situation. For example, proposed models must interpret the numerous problems that arise in testing of the controlled release systems, e.g., in vitro or in vivo. The large drug loading and/or the solvent penetration into the polymer carrier could result in nonconstant diffusion coefficients. The polymer carrier could swell/deswell due to solvent transport. The occurrence of multicomponent transport instead of single drug diffusion and the (possible) presence of macromolecular relaxational phenomena complicate the analysis. Accurate mathematical models can overcome many of the above shortcomings; hence, mathematical models play a pivotal role in the design of systems for controlled drug delivery.

Here we present a critical review and evaluation of important mathematical models for the description of drug release from polymeric systems. In this analysis we have tried to incorporate only models that accurately depict the physical situation of the problems modeled. Unfortunately, the pharmaceutical literature includes a variety of inappropriately simplified, semiempirical, or pseudo-steady-state models. The validity of these models is questionable and their utility in analysis of drug diffusion data doubtful.

Mechanistic aspects of the diffusion phenomena observed in drug delivery systems are by necessity related to an accurate mathematical model and to the structural characteristics of the polymer under consideration. However, very few reviews address these two aspects of controlled release systems (3–6). Regrettably, lack of a systematic analysis and classification is responsible for the use of inappropriate models, not necessarily describing the experimental conditions of the work of many investigators.

II. MATHEMATICAL MODELING OF DIFFUSION PROCESSES

A. Fick's Law of Diffusion

The process of the transport of a drug or of a bioactive agent through a polymer or a controlled release device can be usually described by Fick's law of diffusion. Exceptions to this mechanism exist, such as in solute transport from swellable/soluble release systems, and these will be discussed later.

Written in its differential form in one dimension, Fick's law can be expressed as

$$J_1 = -D_{12} \frac{\partial c}{\partial z} \tag{1}$$

Here J_1 is the molar flux of the drug (in mol/cm^2 s), D_{12} is the mutual diffusion coefficient of the drug in the polymer (in cm^2/s), c_1 is the concentration of the drug (in mol/cm^3), and z is the position in the device (in centimeters).

Assuming that the molar flux of the drug and the mutual diffusion coefficient are constant, the above equation can be integrated to give the integrated form of Fick's law:

$$J_1 = D_{12} K \frac{\Delta c}{\delta} \tag{2}$$

Here K is a thermodynamic partition coefficient and δ is the device thickness. The partition coefficient K is the ratio between the drug concentration at the interface and the drug concentration in the bulk. Several misconceptions related to the partition coefficient, its definition and use are clarified by Lightfoot (11).

To determine the variation of the drug concentration (within the device) with time, i.e., in unsteady-state problems, Fick's second law is used. This is written as

$$\frac{\partial c_1}{\partial t} = D_{12} \frac{\partial^2 c_1}{\partial z^2} \tag{3}$$

The above equation is written in one dimension and assumes constant diffusion coefficients and constant boundaries.

B. Solutions to Fick's Law

Equations 1 and 3 can be solved to obtain drug concentration profiles for diffusion in polymer samples of various geometries. Crank (12) presents solutions of the diffusion equation for various initial and boundary conditions in infinite and semi-infinite media and for various geometries.

The most common analytical techniques for solving Eq. 3 used by most researchers working in the area of drug diffusion in polymers are separation of variables, Laplace transforms, and the method of reflection and superposition. For example, a solution of Eq. 3 can be obtained with the use of separation of variables by writing

$$c_1(x, t) = X(x)T(t) \tag{4}$$

The two resulting ordinary differential equations can be solved to obtain a general solution of the form:

$$c_1 = \sum_{n=0}^{\infty} (A_n \sin \lambda_n x + B_n \cos \lambda_n x) \exp(-\lambda_n^2 D_{12} t) \tag{5}$$

The parameters A_n, B_n, and λ_n can be determined from the initial and boundary conditions of the specific problem. Typical information obtained from the above solutions includes

- Fractional release of the drug, M_t/M_∞, where M_t is the mass of drug released at time t and M_∞ is the mass of drug released at time $t = \infty$; it is often assumed that M_∞ is the initial loading and that all of the drug is released.
- Mass of drug released at time t per unit cross-sectional area A of the device (in mol/cm^2 or g/cm^2).
- Drug release rate per unit cross sectional area, $dM_t/(A \cdot dt)$ (in mol/cm^2.s or g/cm^2.s).
- Drug concentration profiles in the polymer during release (obtained directly from the solution).

Usually, these profiles are reported in terms of the normalized concentration of drug $c_1/c_{1,0}$, where $c_{1,0}$ is the initial concentration of the drug, as a function of dimensionless position x/δ for various dimensionless times $D_{12}t/\delta^2$.

The above comments refer to analytical solutions of the Fickian equation. Such analytical solutions are often preferred in the pharmaceutical field because they provide a facile correlation between parameters. Yet in modeling of general transport phenomena, numerical solutions are equally helpful. Numerical solutions of Fick's law allow for an easy presentation of modeling results and for evaluation of changing design parameters.

III. INCORPORATION OF POLYMER STRUCTURE IN MODELING EQUATIONS

A. Concentration-Dependent Diffusion Coefficients

The assumption that the diffusion coefficient does not depend on the concentration of drug is unfortunately incorrect. The diffusion coefficient does not remain constant with concentration. Very rarely can the drug diffusion coefficient be assumed to be a constant value. This occurs in the case of very dilute solutions and in systems where quasi-equilibrium approximations are valid. Typical values of the drug diffusion coefficients in polymers range from 10^{-6} to 10^{-7} cm^2/s for diffusion in rubbery polymers and from 10^{-10} to 10^{-12} cm^2/s for diffusion in glassy polymers.

The concentration dependence of the drug diffusion coefficient modifies Eq. 3 as

$$\frac{\partial c_1}{\partial t} = \frac{\partial}{\partial z}\left[D_{12}(c_1)\frac{\partial c_1}{\partial z}\right] \tag{6}$$

Of interest is the exponential dependence of the drug diffusion coefficient on concentration proposed by Fujita (13) based on the free volume theory. This is represented in Eq. 7.

$$D_{12}(c_1) = D_{10} \exp[-\beta_1(c_1 - c_0)] \tag{7}$$

Here D_{10} and c_0 are surface diffusion coefficient and concentration, respectively, and β_1 is a constant that is system-dependent. A similar expression can be written for the diffusion coefficient to show the influence of solvent concentration, as expressed in Eq. 8.

$$D_{12}(c_1) = D_{10} \exp[-\beta_2(c_s - c_1)] \tag{8}$$

Here c_s is the concentration of the solvent and β_2 is a constant of the system.

B. Thermodynamic Considerations

Thermodynamic ideality is assumed when the flux J_1 in Eq. 1 is written in terms of the concentration gradient. For systems departing from ideality, Fick's law is expressed in terms of the chemical potential gradient. This can be written as

$$J_i = -cD_i \frac{x_i}{RT} \frac{\partial \mu_i}{\partial z} \tag{9}$$

Here μ_i is the chemical potential of species i, x_i is the mole fraction of species i, R is the universal gas constant, and T is the temperature. The chemical potential can be expressed in terms of the activity a_i as

$$\mu_i = RT \ln a_i + \mu_i^0 \tag{10}$$

Here μ_i^0 is the chemical potential of the pure species i. Relating the activity a_i to the activity coefficient γ_i, we can write

$$J_i = -cD_i\left[1 + \frac{\partial \ln \gamma_i}{\partial \ln x_i}\right]\frac{\partial x_i}{\partial z} \tag{11}$$

Comparing Eqs. 1 and 11, we can define an effective diffusion coefficient, D_{eff}, as

$$D_{eff} = D_i\left[1 + \frac{\partial \ln \gamma_i}{\partial \ln x_i}\right] \tag{12}$$

In the above analysis, D_i is an activity-based diffusion coefficient that is less dependent on concentration than D_{ij}.

C. Effect of Polymer Morphology

Proposed models must incorporate the influence of a number of structural parameters on D_{12}. These include degree of crystallinity and crystallite size (for drug diffusion through semicrystalline polymers), degree of swelling (for swollen matrices and membranes), the "mesh size" of crosslinked polymer networks, the porous structure and tortuosity for porous polymers, and the translational and relaxational behavior observed in swellable systems. All these will be discussed in detail in the forthcoming sections.

IV. MODELING OF CONTROLLED RELEASE DEVICES

In this section, specific models for controlled release systems will be discussed based on an understanding of the underlying diffusion mechanism(s). We adopt a classification first presented by Peppas and Langer (3) and later modified by others (4,14) and analyze diffusion-, swelling-, and chemically controlled systems.

A. Diffusion-Controlled Systems

1. Matrix (Monolithic) Devices

In matrix (monolithic) systems the bioactive agent is incorporated in the polymer phase either in dissolved or in dispersed form. Therefore, the solubility of the drug in the polymer becomes a controlling factor in the mathematical modeling of these systems. When the initial drug loading is below the solubility limit, release is achieved by simple diffusion through the polymer. However, when the drug loading is above the solubility limit, dissolution of the drug in the polymer becomes the limiting factor in the release process.

Solutions of the transient diffusion equation (Eq. 3) can be obtained for a variety of initial and boundary conditions (12), which represent appropriate experimental situations. Some of these solutions are presented here. However, the reader is cautioned that unusual experimental conditions of release will require solution of Eq. 3 under the boundary conditions that best describe the experimental situation.

It is also important to note that most mathematical models for controlled release kinetics presented in the literature have been derived with the assumption of an experimentally somewhat unattainable boundary condition of zero (and constant) drug concentration at the interface of the device. This condition requires complete elimination of boundary layer effects, probably by high agitation during the release experiment.

In this section we include, in addition to the conventional solutions of the diffusion equation (Eq. 3) widely used in controlled release technology, new models and mathematical solutions with boundary conditions affected by drug mass transfer from the surface of the polymer to the liquid phase. These models do not require that the concentration at the polymer interface be constant or zero, although previous determination of the mass transfer coefficient is needed. The mass transfer coefficient can be determined by a variety of expressions or experimental techniques discussed in standard monographs on mass transfer (15) if the flow characteristics of the release experiment are known.

2. Dispersed Drug, Nonporous Systems

In these systems the matrix consists of a drug that is dispersed in the polymer at a concentration, c_d, that is greater than the drug solubility in the polymer, c_s. The first modeling attempt to describe these systems invoked the pseudo-steady-state solution and was introduced by Higuchi (16). The Higuchi model assumes that the solute (dry) particle size is much smaller in comparison to the polymer film thickness and neglects boundary effects (Fig. 1). Fick's law is used in the form of Eq. 1, i.e., for thermodynamically ideal systems. The expression derived by Higuchi for the amount of drug released at time t, M_t, is

$$M_t = A \sqrt{Dc_s (2c_d - c_s) t} \qquad (13)$$

Here D is the diffusion coefficient of the drug in the polymer and A is the cross-sectional area of the polymer film. The Higuchi model predicts a square root of time dependence of the mass of drug released and an inverse square root of time dependence of the drug release rate.

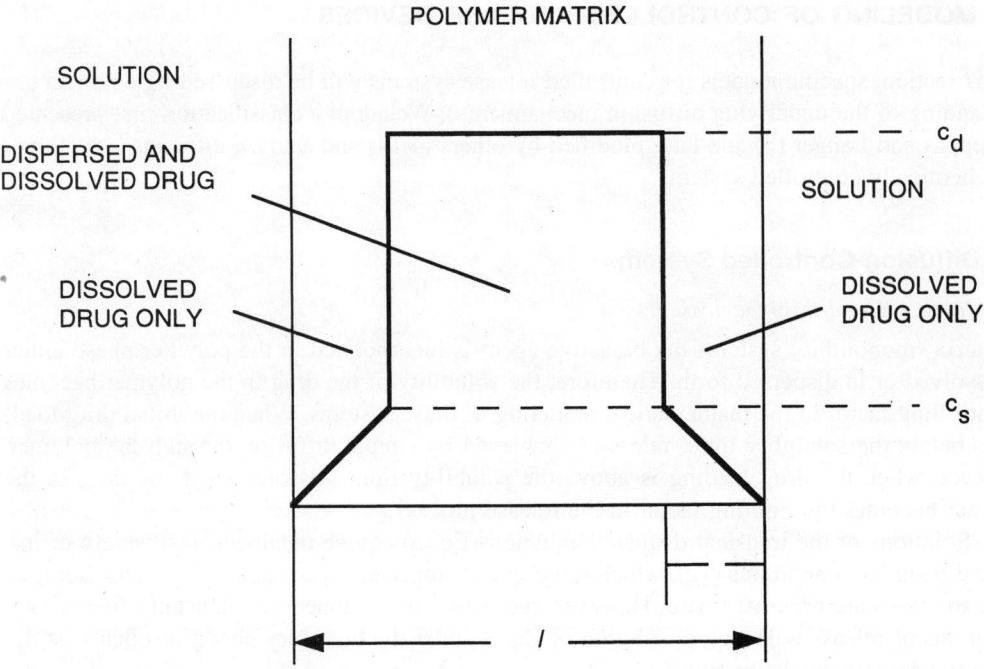

Figure 1 Parameter definition for the case of drug delivery in nonporous systems using the Higuchi model.

Paul and McSpadden (17) obtained exact solutions to the problem of drug diffusion from dispersed matrix systems. The exact solution for the amount of drug released at time t is

$$M_t = \frac{2c_s A}{\text{erf } \xi^*} \sqrt{\frac{Dt}{\pi}} \tag{14}$$

The term ξ^* is the polymer film thickness, given by Eq. 15, and can be calculated from the roots of the transcendental equation (Eq. 16).

$$\xi^* = \frac{x^*}{2\sqrt{Dt}} \tag{15}$$

$$\sqrt{\pi}\, \xi^* \exp(\xi^{*2})\, \text{erf } \xi^* = \frac{c_s}{c_d - c_s} \tag{16}$$

This solution predicts significant deviations from the Higuchi equation, especially at early times.

3. Dissolved Drug, Nonporous Systems

In this case, the drug is dissolved in the polymer below its solubility. For polymer films of thickness δ with initial drug concentration $c_{1,0}$ and negligible boundary effects, Eq. 3 can be solved for the drug concentration and integrated over the film thickness to give

Accurate Models in Controlled Delivery Systems

$$\frac{M_t}{M_\infty} = 1 - \sum_{n=0}^{\infty} \frac{8}{(2n+1)^2 \pi^2} \exp\left[-\frac{D(2n+1)^2 \pi^2}{\delta^2}\right] \tag{17}$$

For long periods the first term of the above equation (n = 0) is dominant and Eq. 17 reduces to

$$\frac{M_t}{M_\infty} = 1 - \frac{8}{\pi^2} \exp\left[-\frac{\pi^2 Dt}{\delta^2}\right] \qquad \text{for } \frac{M_t}{M_\infty} > 0.6 \tag{18}$$

For short times, the solution reduces to

$$\frac{M_t}{M_\infty} = 4\sqrt{\frac{Dt}{\pi\delta^2}} \qquad \text{for } \frac{M_t}{M_\infty} < 0.6 \tag{19}$$

In conclusion, matrix controlled release systems with dissolved drug (Fig. 2) give

$$M_t \alpha \sqrt{t}, \qquad \frac{dM_t}{dt} \alpha \frac{1}{\sqrt{t}} \tag{20}$$

Similar expressions for the amount of drug released and for the drug release rate can be obtained for cylinders and spheres (1). The type of release kinetics commonly known as zero-order release kinetics is characterized by constant drug release rates as opposed to the decreasing trend shown by Eq. 20. The design of zero-order release devices is very important for the development of sustained release systems, and we will present various examples of drug delivery systems that exhibit zero-order release.

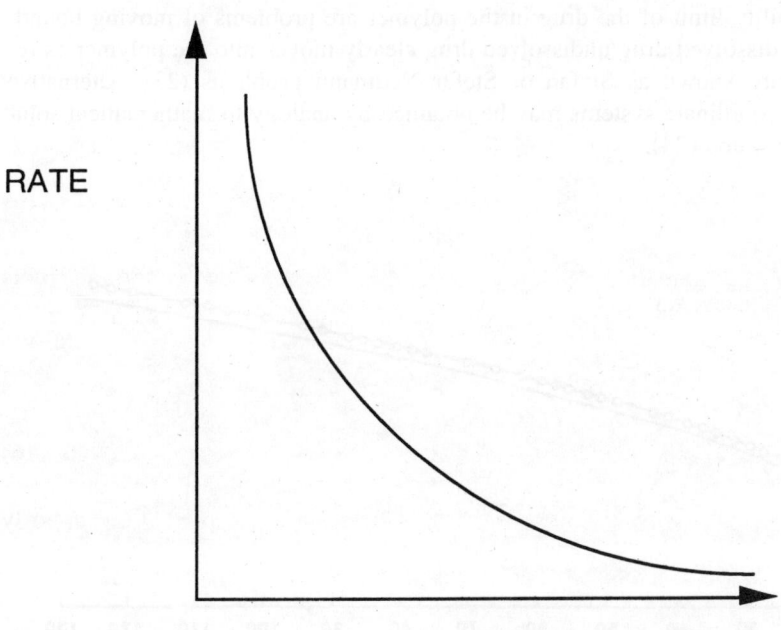

Figure 2 Drug release rates as a function of time for matrix systems with dissolved drug.

4. Drug Diffusion from Tablets

The model equation for drug release (18) from cylindrical tablets can be written as

$$\frac{\partial c_1}{\partial t} = D \left[\frac{\partial^2 c_1}{\partial r^2} + \frac{1}{r} \frac{\partial c_1}{\partial r} + \frac{\partial^2 c_1}{\partial z^2} \right] \quad (21)$$

The amount of drug released can be calculated as

$$\frac{M_t}{M_\infty} = 1 - \sum_{m=0}^{\infty} \frac{8}{\delta^2 R^2} \frac{\exp[-D\alpha_m^2 t]}{\alpha_m^2} \sum_{n=1}^{\infty} \frac{\exp\left[-\frac{D(2n+1)^2 \pi^2}{4\delta^2}\right]}{\beta_n^2} \quad (22)$$

Here α_m are the roots of $J_0(\alpha_m) = 0$ and

$$\beta_n = \frac{(2n+1)\pi}{2\delta} \quad (23)$$

The experimental and theoretical fractional drug releases from EVA-hydrocortisone tablets from the work of Fu et al. (18) are shown in Fig. 3. Very good agreement is observed between the model predictions and the experimental data.

The above analysis leads us to believe that it is not possible to achieve zero-order release of drugs using matrix systems and simple geometries. There exist exceptions, however (19–22). Geometries other than slabs, cylinders, or spheres can give zero-order release. For example, zero-order release is observed in the release of bovine serum albumin from EV Ac hemispheres as shown by Rhine et al. (19).

Mathematical problems of drug release from matrix systems initially loaded at concentrations above the solubility limit of the drug in the polymer are problems of moving boundaries, since the front of dissolved drug/undissolved drug clearly moves into the polymer as release proceeds. These are known as Stefan or Stefan-Neumann problems (23). Alternative solutions using moving coordinate systems may be obtained by analogy to mathematical solutions discussed by Danckwerts (24).

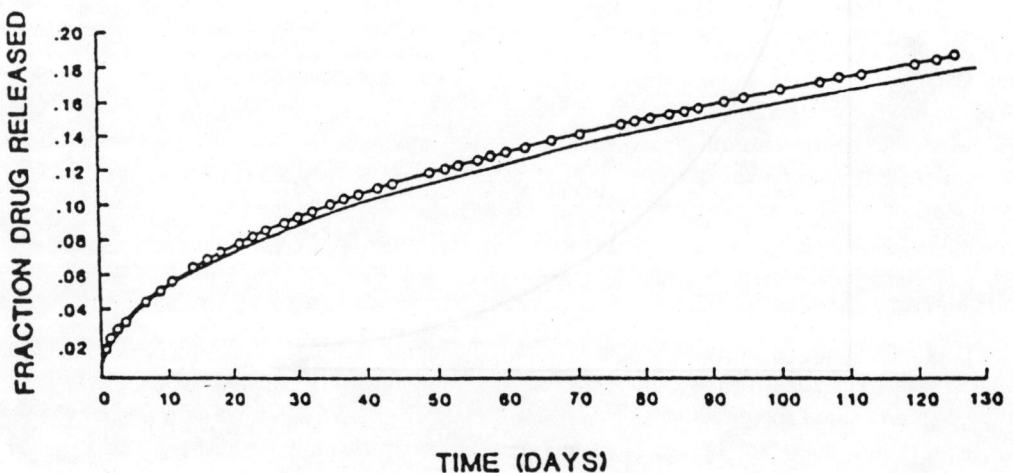

Figure 3 Experimental and theoretical drug release rate from EVA-hydrocortisone tablets. The points represent the data, and the line represents model predictions. (From Ref. 18.)

Certain problems require numerical or approximate solutions. For example, Lee (25) and Zhou and Wu (26) discuss a variety of diffusional release problems for slabs, spheres, and cylinders using Stefan-type analysis and offer approximate as well as numerical solutions.

5. Porous Systems

Considerable research has been performed on the analysis of porous systems (27). These systems are usually characterized in terms of the porosity and tortuosity factors. Porous systems are produced either by compression of microparticles of the polymer and the drug, or by dispersion of the drug in the polymer solution followed by subsequent evaporation of the solvent. The chaotic nature of the pore network and the continuous change of the pore structure during release render the mathematical modeling of the release kinetics quite difficult.

In semicrystalline polymers, drug diffusion is hindered due to the presence of crystallites. The volume fraction and the size of the crystallites affect the diffusion coefficient. The influence of these parameters is expressed in terms of tortuosity factors (28). Release from porous reservoir systems of hydrophobic polymers may be modeled by Eq. 24 where the diffusion coefficient is replaced by the effective diffusion coefficient, D_{eff}. This parameter describes diffusion through water-filled pores and incorporates the porosity (void fraction), ϵ, and tortuosity, τ, in the drug diffusion coefficient through water, D.

$$D_{eff} = D \frac{\epsilon}{\tau} \quad (24)$$

It is sometimes desirable to incorporate into this expression a partition coefficient, K_p, for possible adsorption of the drug on the walls of the pores, and a restriction coefficient, K_r, which accounts for hindered diffusion, and which is described according to Eq. 25, where λ is the ratio of the drug radius, r_s, to the pore average radius, r_p.

$$K_r = (1 - \lambda)^2 \quad \text{with } \lambda = r_s/r_p \quad (25)$$

Then, the effective diffusion coefficient of drug through the pores may be written as

$$D_{eff} = DK_pK_r \frac{\epsilon}{\tau} \quad (26)$$

The well-known theoretical analyses of Anderson and Quinn (29) and Colton et al. (30) are often used to predict the parameters K_p and K_r for drug release systems with fine pores. Very often, osmotic effects accompany diffusion through porous membranes as a result of which Eqs. 24–26 do not fully describe phenomena occurring in porous reservoir systems.

Modeling of the drug release kinetics of porous matrix systems is still at a rather primitive stage despite significant developments in recent years. Before using existing models one has to consider several aspects of the physics of this diffusion phenomenon.

If the polymer phase is hydrophobic, swelling is negligible and the problem can be treated as a constant volume diffusion problem. However, if the polymer phase is hydrophilic, two modeling routes may be considered. These approaches are discussed in this section.

> If the pores are large enough to be thought of as "channels" for diffusion (pore diameter greater than 150 Å), diffusion occurs predominantly through these water-filled pores and the effective diffusion coefficient D_{eff} of Eq. 24 must be used. However, if the pores are smaller than 100 Å, then the diffusion coefficient, D, through the swollen polymer can be used without corrections for porosity and tortuosity.
>
> Phenomena related to drug partition in the pore walls and hindered diffusion due to the relative size of the drug with respect to the pores can be addressed by including the

parameters K_p and K_r in the diffusion coefficient through water, and using the effective diffusion coefficient, D_{eff}, described by Eq. 26.

Phenomena related to elastically changing pore walls must be taken into consideration.

6. Dispersed Drug, Porous Systems

For drug diffusion through a porous polymer where the drug is dispersed throughout the polymer phase, Higuchi (31) developed a model that incorporates the void fraction ϵ and tortuosity τ of the polymer in the diffusion coefficient D_{eff}. The amount of drug released is

$$M_t = \sqrt{AD_{eff}c_s(2c_d - \epsilon c_s)t} \tag{27}$$

Similar models for other geometries have been developed by Roseman and Higuchi (32) and Fessi et al. (33). Drug binding and release have been treated by Desai et al. (34). The amount of drug released in this case is given by

$$M_t = \sqrt{AD_{eff}c_s [2c_d - c_s\{\epsilon + K(1 - \epsilon)\}]t} \tag{28}$$

Here K is a partition coefficient. However, these models may be unable to describe many experimental results with porous systems loaded with drug above its solubility limit in water.

7. Dissolved Drug, Porous Systems

The analysis for this case is similar to that of the case of dissolved drug in nonporous polymeric systems. The difference arises in the definition of the diffusion coefficient in Eqs. 13 and 14. In this case, an effective diffusion coefficient is defined by Eq. 24.

8. Diffusion/Dissolution Models

Two approaches have been proposed to explain the experimental results. In the first approach (35), the release of drugs from porous systems is treated as a dissolution-controlled phenomenon. To account for dissolution, a concentration term is added to the transport equation (Eq. 3) to give

$$\frac{\partial c_1}{\partial t} = D_{eff} \frac{\partial^2 c_1}{\partial z^2} + k(c_s - c_1) \tag{29}$$

The amount of drug released is given (34) as

$$\frac{M_t}{A} = \left[c_{is} \sqrt{D_{eff} k} \tanh\left(\frac{\delta}{2}\sqrt{\frac{k}{D_{eff}}}\right)\right]t - \frac{c_{is}D_{eff}}{\delta} \sum_{n=0}^{\infty} \frac{1 - \exp[-(D_{eff}\alpha_n^2 + k)t]}{(D_{eff}\alpha_n^2 + k)^2} \tag{30}$$

Here k is a dissolution constant and d is the half-thickness of the polymer slab. The term α_n is given by twice the value β_n (see Eq. 23).

The second modeling effort (20) assumes that solid drug fills completely the pores and dissolution occurs. This phenomenon can be modeled as an unsteady-state, moving-boundary (Stefan-type) problem. For this case, it can be shown that the released drug can be determined by Eq. 31.

$$M_t = \frac{2\epsilon^{2/3}c_s A}{\text{erf } \xi^*} \sqrt{\frac{D_{eff}t}{\pi}} \tag{31}$$

The term ξ^* is defined by Eq. 15 and the position of the front can be determined by Eq. 32.

$$\sqrt{\pi}\, \xi^* \exp(\xi^{*2})\, \text{erf } \xi^* = \frac{c_s}{\rho_1 M_1} \tag{32}$$

The diffusion coefficient D_{eff} is defined by Eq. 24, ρ_1 is the density of the drug, and M_i is its molecular weight. Due to the assumptions made, this model can be used to describe the unexpected release behavior of drugs from dense, hydrophobic matrix systems such as those studied by Langer and co-workers (19).

The release of drugs from nonswellable microparticles was studied by Harland et al. (36). For drug release from a spherical tablet of radius R, the transport equation is written as

$$\frac{\partial c_1}{\partial t} = D \left(\frac{\partial^2 c_1}{\partial r^2} + \frac{2}{r} \frac{\partial c_1}{\partial r} \right) + k \, (\epsilon c_s - c_1) \tag{31}$$

The diffusion coefficient D was given by a Fujita-based equation.

$$D = \frac{D_0}{\tau} \exp\left[-\alpha \, (\beta - c_1)\right] \tag{32}$$

Here α and β are constants of the system. The amount of drug released is given by

$$M_t = 8 \, \epsilon c_s \pi R^3 \sum f\left(\frac{kR^2}{D}, t\right) \tag{33}$$

The amount of drug released as a function of time for various values of the dissolution constant is shown in Fig. 4.

Chang and Himmelstein (37) proposed a model for dissolution-controlled drug delivery. They noted that previous models could not provide exact information about the duration of the zero-order release. They also pointed out that previous models treated the drug release as if it occurred in a homogeneous system. They proposed a model that corrected the previous discrepancies by setting diffusion equations for the solid and the dissolved drug phases.

The equation for the undissolved drug was written as

$$\frac{\partial c_{sd}}{\partial t} = -K(c_s - c_d) \tag{34}$$

Here K is the dissolution rate and c_s is the solubility of the drug. The equation for the dissolved drug was written as

$$\frac{\partial c_d}{\partial t} = \frac{\partial}{\partial z}\left[D\,(c_d)\,\frac{\partial c_d}{\partial z}\right] - \frac{\partial c_{sd}}{\partial t} \tag{35}$$

Here $D\,(c_d)$ is the diffusion coefficient of the drug in the polymer and is given by a free volume–based equation.

The model was solved numerically. Drug release profiles for various dissolution constants for the case of drug release from a polymer slab are shown in Fig. 5. These results agreed well with experimental data, thus providing another example of the usefulness of accurate mathematical models.

9. Membrane (Reservoir) Devices

In these systems, the drug or the bioactive agent is enclosed in relatively large quantities in a permeable synthetic membrane and is placed in contact with a fluid (usually water) at constant temperature. The drug may be present either in pure form or in solution. After an initial period of transient transport, steady states are reached. This enables determination of the drug release rates. Mathematical models can be formulated for membrane devices either with perfect sink conditions or with release in finite volumes.

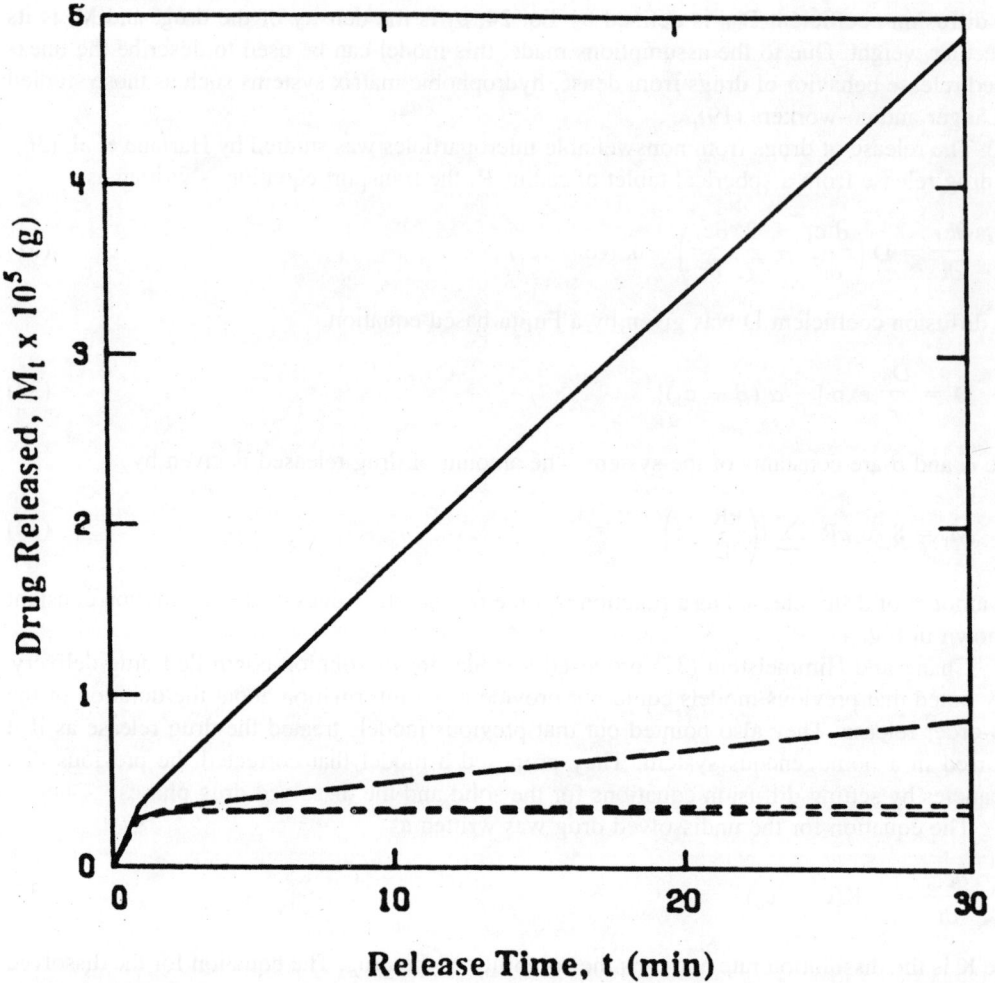

Figure 4 Amount of drug released as a function of release time. Drug diffusion coefficient $D = 1 \times 10^{-6}$ cm^2/s, ϵ. $c_s = 0.1$ g/cm^3, radius $R = 0.02$ cm. Curves from top to bottom are for drug dissolution constants of $k = 10^{-2}, 10^{-3}, 10^{-4},$ and 10^{-5}/s. (From Ref. 35.)

10. Perfect Sink Conditions

Modeling of these devices is done by applying Fick's law in its integrated form. The definition of the flux is invoked to obtain an expression for the drug release rate.

$$M_t = \frac{ADK \, \Delta c}{\delta} \tag{36}$$

Clearly drug release from these systems is zero-order, i.e., the release rate of drug does not depend on time. Similarly for cylindrical devices it is readily shown that

$$\frac{dM_t}{dt} = \frac{DKA}{\ln(r_e/r_i)} (c_{i2} - c_{i1}) \tag{37}$$

where r_e and r_i are the external and internal radii of the cylinder, respectively, and A is the length of the cylinder. In both situations of slabs and cylinders, one-dimensional diffusion is assumed. This as-

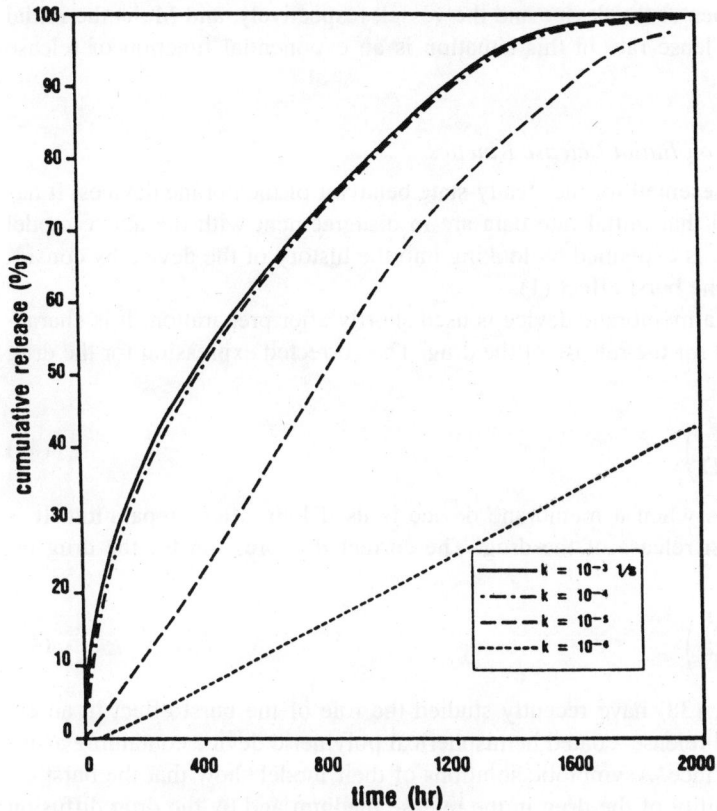

Figure 5 Drug release profile as a function of time from a slab device at various dissolution rates. Drug diffusion coefficient $D = 10^{-9}$ cm^2/s and slab half thickness = 0.1 cm. (From Ref. 36.)

sumption requires that these equations be applied only for analysis of release from thin membranes or long cylindrical systems. Corrections for edge effects due to violation of the one-dimensional diffusion assumption are available (30) if thick membranes are used. However, the preferable method of modeling would be numerical solution of the three-dimensional diffusion problem.

For spherical reservoir systems the corresponding equations for drug release are

$$\frac{dM_t}{dt} = \frac{4\pi DK}{(r_e - r_i)/r_e r_i} (c_{i2} - c_{i1}) \tag{38}$$

Therefore, drug release rates from conventional reservoir systems are time-independent. However, they depend on the concentration difference, geometry of the device, thermodynamic characteristics of the system (solubility, through the partition coefficient), and structure of the polymer (through the diffusion coefficient).

11. Finite Release Volumes

Situations of drug release from membrane systems at low initial drug concentration or to experimental vessels of finite volumes cannot be modeled with the equations given before. Instead, Eq. 39 has been derived (30) for the drug release rate from these systems.

$$\frac{dM_t}{dt} = \frac{M_\infty DKA}{V_1 \delta} \exp\left[\frac{-DKA(V_1 + V_2)}{\delta V_1 V_2} t\right] \tag{39}$$

12. Effect of System History on Initial Release Kinetics

The foregoing analysis was presented for the steady-state behavior of membrane devices. It has been experimentally observed that initial rate data are in disagreement with the above model predictions. This phenomenon is explained by looking into the history of the device by considering the time lag effect and the burst effect (1).

Time lag appears when a membrane device is used shortly after preparation. It is characterized by an induction period for the release of the drug. The corrected expression for the drug released is given by

$$M_t = \frac{ADK \Delta c}{\delta}\left(t - \frac{\delta^2}{6D}\right) \tag{40}$$

The burst effect appears when a membrane device is used long after preparation. It is characterized by a sudden fast release of the drug. The corrected expression for the drug released is given by

$$M_t = \frac{ADK \Delta c}{\delta}\left(t + \frac{\delta^2}{3D}\right) \tag{41}$$

Narasimhan and Langer (38) have recently studied the role of the burst effect in an essentially zero-order controlled release–coated hemispherical polymeric device containing a single, small orifice in its center face. Asymptotic solutions of their model show that the burst effect is controlled by the solubility of the drug in the release medium and by the drug diffusion coefficient. The rates of drug release during the burst effect ($t \to 0$) and the steady state ($t \to \infty$) are related by

$$\frac{[dM/dt]_{t \to 0}}{[dM/dt]_{t \to \infty}} = \frac{16}{B(6+B)} \tag{42}$$

Here B is given by c_s/c_0. The parameter c_0 is the initial drug loading and c_s is the solubility of the drug in the release medium. From the above equation, it can be concluded that the burst effect is significant for systems where $B \sim O(1)$. It was shown that as drug solubility increased, the drug released faster and the velocity of the interface between dissolved and dispersed drug was higher. The model solutions established that the burst behavior could be manipulated by using different initial drug distributions. Using the model, conditions under which the burst effect could be minimized/maximized were established. Figure 6 shows a plot of the fraction of bovine serum albumin released from an inwardly releasing ethylene vinyl acetate (EV Ac) hemisphere as a function of time, where the release as well as the burst period is zero order. This approach provides valuable guidelines to design drug delivery systems with pronounced burst effects and is yet another case study supporting the use of accurate models that account for the physics of the problem.

B. Swelling-Controlled Systems

Swelling-controlled released systems are rather difficult to model due to complex macromolecular changes occurring in the polymer during release. These systems consist of water-soluble drugs that are initially dispersed in solvent-free glassy polymers. If a slab is placed in contact

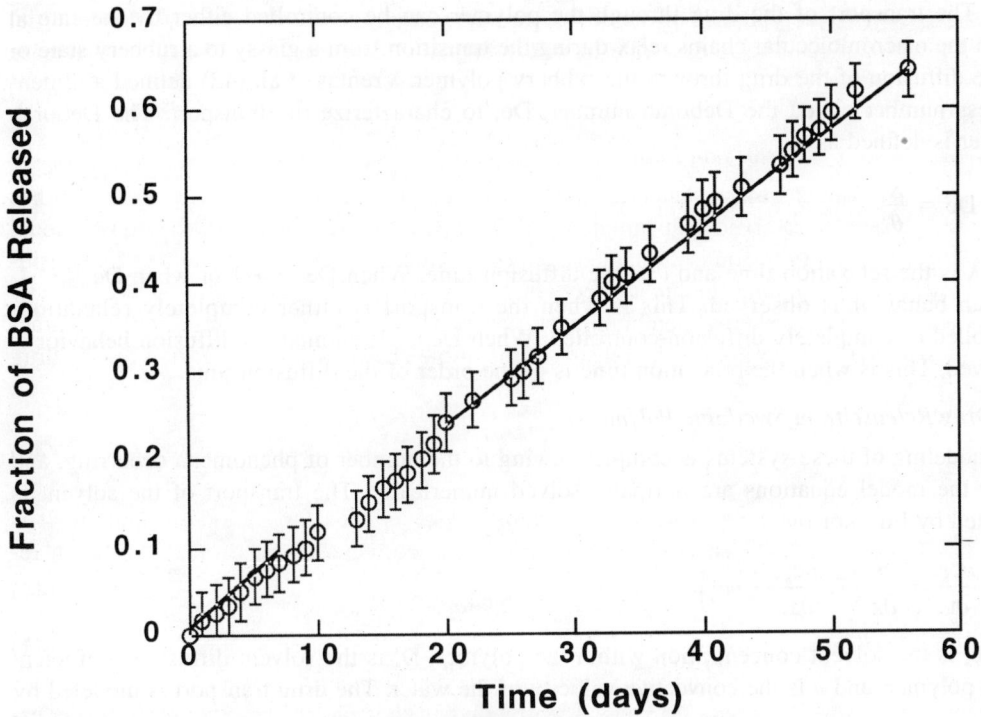

Figure 6 Fraction of bovine serum albumin released as a function of time from coated EVAc hemispheres. The open circles represent experimental data while the line represents model predictions. (From Ref. 37.)

with water, diffusion of water into the polymer will be observed depending on the thermodynamic interactions between the polymer and the solvent. This dynamic swelling phenomenon may lead to considerable volume expansion of the original slab. Two fronts (interfaces) are characteristic of the swelling behavior:

1. The swelling interface that separates the rubbery (swollen) state from the glassy state and which moves inward with velocity v; and
2. the polymer interface that separates the rubbery state from water and moves outward.

Swelling of glassy polymers is accompanied by macromolecular relaxation, which become important at the swelling interface (39). This relaxation in turn affects the drug diffusion through the polymer, so that Fickian or non-Fickian diffusion may be observed. In these systems, drug release is controlled by the velocity of the water penetration front, v, since drug diffusion through the glassy polymer is negligible.

Mathematical modeling of this type of diffusion behavior clearly belongs to a category of mathematical problems known as Stefan, or Stefan-Neumann, or moving-boundary problems. The Fickian diffusion equation (Eq. 2) is solved with concentration-dependent or independent drug diffusion coefficients and moving-boundary conditions (at the two fronts). If, in addition, one imposes problems of non-Fickian diffusion due to macromolecular relaxation, then the mathematical analysis becomes somewhat complicated (40). Some attempts to describe this behavior have been discussed by Peppas et al. (41), and a more complete literature review is given elsewhere (12).

The transport of the drug through the polymer can be controlled either by the rate at which the macromolecular chains relax during the transition from a glassy to a rubbery state or by the diffusion of the drug through the rubbery polymer. Vrentas et al. (42) defined a dimensionless number called the Deborah number, De, to characterize the transport. The Deborah number is defined as

$$De = \frac{\lambda}{\theta} \quad (43)$$

Here λ is the relaxation time and θ is the diffusion time. When De $\gg$ 1 or when De $\ll$ 1, Fickian behavior is observed. This is when the transport is either completely relaxation-controlled or completely diffusion-controlled. When De $\sim$ 1, anomalous diffusion behavior is observed. This is when the relaxation time is of the order of the diffusion time.

1. Drug Release from Swellable Polymers

The modeling of these systems is complex, owing to the number of phenomena occurring, and hence the model equations are normally solved numerically. The transport of the solvent is modeled by Eq. 6 or by

$$\frac{\partial c_s}{\partial t} = \frac{\partial}{\partial z}\left(D_s \frac{\partial c_s}{\partial z} - v c_s\right) \quad (44)$$

Here c_s is the solvent concentration within the polymer, D_s is the solvent diffusion coefficient in the polymer, and v is the convective velocity of the water. The drug transport is modeled by

$$\frac{\partial c_1}{\partial t} = \frac{\partial}{\partial z}\left(D \frac{\partial c_1}{\partial z}\right) \quad (45)$$

Here D_s and D are functions of c_s and sometimes c_1. These give rise to moving-boundary problems that are solved numerically.

An important contribution to the modeling aspects of drug delivery systems was made by Lee (43). The model formulated by Lee provided simple but accurate solutions for the problem of drug release from swellable matrices using a refined enthalpy balance method. It showed that swelling and erosion could be modeled within the same framework. The importance of the phenomenon of front synchronization was first recognized by Lee.

In order to obtain zero-order release from such devices, the drug distribution was studied. It was found that a sigmoidal type of initial drug distribution gave almost zero-order release (25,44). This effect is represented in Fig. 7. Other efforts to modify the initial drug distribution within the polymer have also resulted in zero-order release systems (45–47).

Lee (48) also considered the effect of time-dependent diffusion coefficients on the release process. A time-dependent drug diffusion coefficient was defined as

$$D(t) = D_i + (D_\infty - D_i)[1 - \exp(-kt)] \quad (46)$$

Here D_i is the drug diffusion coefficient initially, and D_∞ is that in the swollen polymer at long times. The model equations were exactly solved and the mass of drug released was obtained as

$$\frac{M_t}{M_\infty} = 1 - \sum_{n=0}^{\infty} \frac{8}{(2n+1)^2 \pi^2} \exp\left[-\pi^2(n+0.5)^2 \left\{\frac{D_\infty t}{\delta^2} + \frac{D_\infty}{k\delta^2}[1 - \exp(-kt)]\right\}\right] \quad (47)$$

A simple semiempirical equation to model the release kinetics was proposed by Peppas and co-workers (49). This is the power law equation given below.

$$\frac{M_t}{M_\infty} = kt^n \quad (48)$$

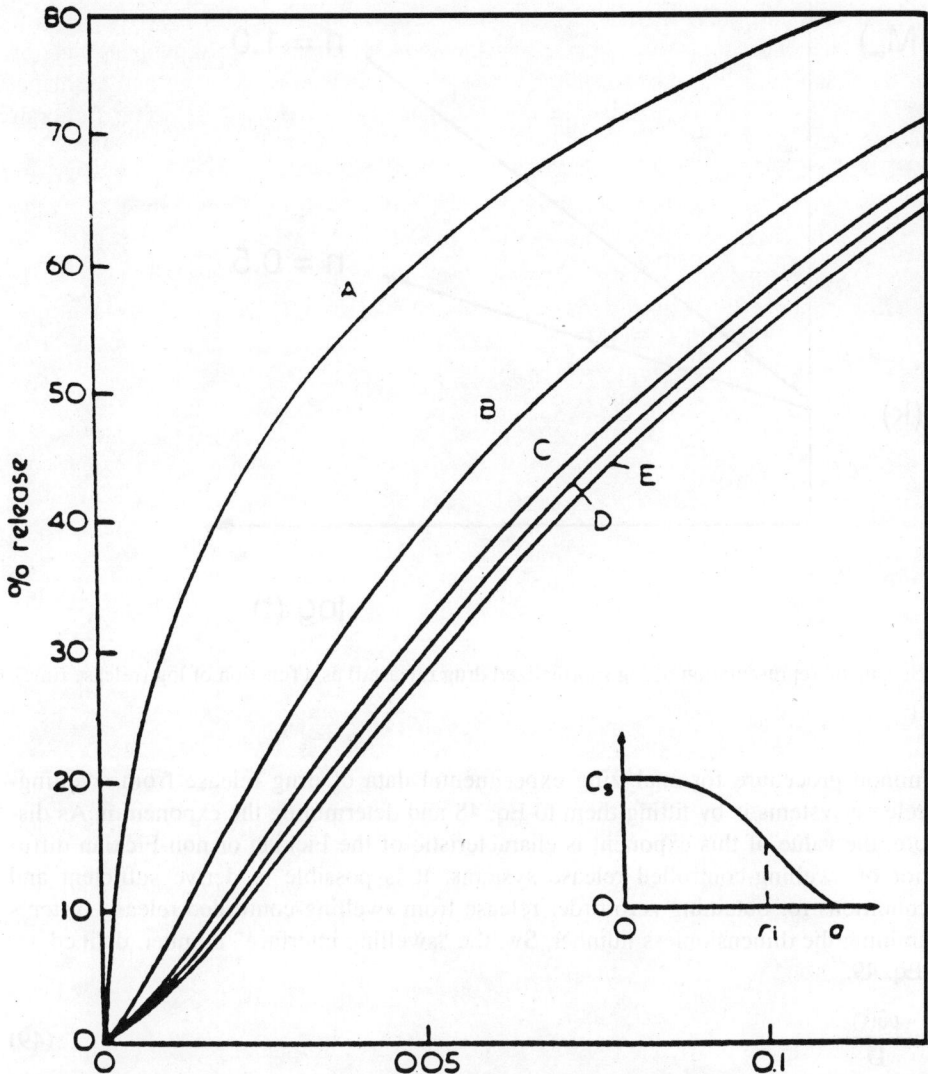

Figure 7 Effect of sigmoidal initial drug concentration distribution on the cumulative release from spherical matrices. Curves A through E represent different values of ξ_i. The term ξ_i is the initial position of the inflection point in the concentration profile. (From Ref. 43.) The distribution function is

$$f(\xi) = \frac{1 - \exp\left[-0.5\left(\frac{1-\xi}{1-\xi_i}\right)^2\right]}{1 - \exp\left[-0.5\left(\frac{1}{1-\xi_i}\right)^2\right]}$$

Here k and n are fitting parameters. The importance of this analysis is easily understood since most mathematical solutions of Eq. 2 for Fickian drug diffusion give release kinetics described by Eq. 48 with n = 0.5. Consequently, the release rate is proportional to $t^{-1/2}$. A special case of release kinetics with Eq. 48 occurs when n = 1. This of course describes zero-order release systems (Fig. 8).

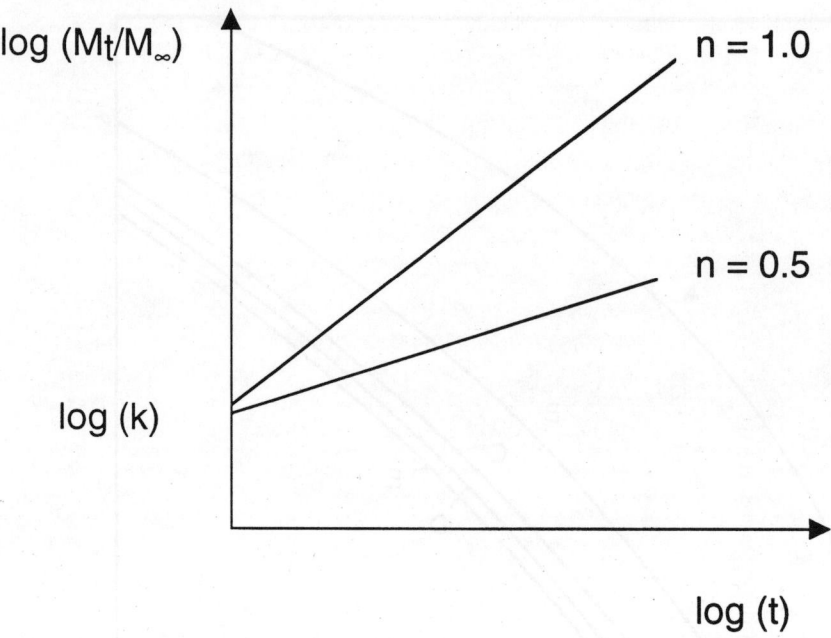

Figure 8 Schematic representation of log (normalized drug released) as a function of log (release time).

A common procedure for analyzing experimental data of drug release from swelling-controlled release systems is by fitting them to Eq. 48 and determining the exponent n. As discussed before, the value of this exponent is characteristic of the Fickian or non-Fickian diffusion behavior of swelling-controlled release systems. It is possible to derive sufficient and necessary conditions for obtaining zero-order release from swelling-controlled release systems (50) by examining the dimensionless number, Sw, the "swelling interface" number, defined according to Eq. 49.

$$Sw = \frac{v\delta(t)}{D} \qquad (49)$$

When Sw << 1, zero-order release should be expected, whereas for values of Sw >> 1, Fickian diffusion is observed.

Kou et al. (51) proposed a model for drug diffusion through swellable cylinders with Fickian equations and concentration-dependent diffusion coefficients. Cohen and Erneux (52,53) presented a treatment of free boundary problems that had fundamental ideas in solving drug delivery problems in swellable systems.

The first detailed model of drug transport with concentration-dependent diffusion coefficients and swelling was proposed by Korsmeyer et al. (54). Lustig and Peppas (55) proposed a free-volume-based model with three-dimensional swelling beyond the point where the fronts meet. Lustig et al. (56) proposed a mathematical model for drug release based on rational thermodynamics, containing a full viscoelastic description of the polymer and concentration-dependent transport of the drug, with three-dimensional swelling.

Drug release from environmentally responsive polymeric systems has also been studied in great detail. Peppas and Brannon-Peppas (57) studied the drug release rates in a system that responded to changes in temperature. The time-dependent response of the drug was also studied by Brannon-Peppas and Peppas (58) and by Bell and Peppas (59). Models for drug delivery from polymeric systems that responded to changes in the pH and ionic strength of the surrounding medium were proposed by Hariharan and Peppas (60,61).

In addition to these important modeling efforts, researchers have sought to analyze non-Fickian transport with relatively simple equations. One such effort relating the fractional release of the drug to time uses the so-called swelling area number, Sa (62). The swelling area number was defined as

$$Sa = \frac{1}{D}\frac{dA}{dt} \tag{50}$$

Here A is the area available for drug release and D is the drug diffusion coefficient. The swelling area number, Sa, has been used to describe systems with varying area due to swelling (specifically the Geomatrix systems).

C. Chemically Controlled Systems

Chemically controlled release systems include all polymeric formulations where drug diffusion is controlled by the disappearance of the polymer matrix. Modeling of these systems is similar to that followed for swelling-controlled release systems, since "mass erosion" replaces the "phase erosion" (moving front) observed in swelling-controlled systems. In this category there are systems where chemical reaction triggers the release. That reaction may be induced by hydrolysis, whether enzymatic or biochemical.

The difference between bioerosion and biodegradation is that the latter is the actual degradation, i.e., breaking down of the polymer due to chemical reaction that is taking place. The polymer will break down into small molecular weight materials. A matrix like that would be a polymeric material with the drug molecularly distributed throughout. In the case of biodegradable materials, the drug does not have to be molecularly dispersed; it can also be microscopically dispersed with large particles. The release process is controlled by a surface chemical reaction that will break down the polymer, giving oligomers and small molecular weight compounds. As time elapses, the geometry is unchanged but smaller, and the drug that was incorporated in the lost portion is free to dissolve and diffuse. That is why biodegradable systems, with a first-order biodegradation reaction with respect to the area, yield zero order release for a planar device where the area remains constant.

Bioerosion is a process whereby a phase of the carrier is lost, not by chemical reaction but by dissolution. When bioerodible polymers are brought in contact with physiological fluids, the fluids simply dissolve the polymer rather than break it down.

In most chemically controlled systems, the geometric shape of the device controls drug release. The controlling mechanism may be either polymer dissolution, or reaction and degradation at the polymer surface. Depending on the type of degradation reaction, these systems may be classified as chemically degradable (e.g., by hydrolysis) or biodegradable (e.g., by enzymatic reaction) controlled release systems.

Shrinking core models provide the most accurate description of this release. Cooney (63,64) developed simple expressions for drug release from spherical and cylindrical devices.

Hopfenberg (65) derived expressions for drug release from erodible slabs, cylinders, and spheres. The main argument used is that the erosion rate is proportional to the continuously changing area of the device. Solution of the model equation for various geometries gives the following general expression:

$$\frac{M_t}{M_\infty} = 1 - \left(1 - \frac{k_e t}{c_{io}L}\right)^n \tag{51}$$

Here n = 1 for a slab of thickness d = 2L, n = 2 for a cylinder of radius r = L, and n = 3 for a sphere of radius r = L.

Mathematical models of erodible systems where drug release from the surface is also important have been discussed by Lee (43) and further analyzed elsewhere (23).

Thombre and Himmelstein (66) developed models to describe drug release from poly(ortho esters). The diffusion–reaction model was solved in terms of typical Thiele moduli, ϕ_i, to describe the reaction/diffusion ratio and Biot numbers, Bi_i, to describe the mass transfer/diffusion ratio.

$$\phi_i = a \sqrt{\frac{k_i c_i}{D_i}}$$

$$Bi_i = \frac{k_i a}{D_i} \tag{52}$$

where k_i is the reaction constant of species i, D_i is the diffusion coefficient of the ith species, and a is the half-thickness of the polymer film.

Langer and co-workers used computer-aided methods (67,68) to model bioerosion. In these approaches, the polymer matrix is represented as the sum of individual matrix parts and the erosion of each part is regarded as a random event. Comparisons with experiment yielded good agreement. This analysis was later extended (69) to describe the release of a monomer from an eroding polymer. The model predicts parameters like the porosity of the eroding polymer, the matrix weight, and the amount of monomer released. The analysis could be extended to model drug release from such systems (70,71). The use of models that account for the governing physics (in this case, erosion of copolymers) has led to good understanding of the system behavior and has found good agreement with experimental data.

1. Pendant Chain Systems

Models have been proposed by Anderson and co-workers (72) to describe cortisol hydrolysis from bound PGA systems. The hydrolysis starts at the surface giving hydrophilic polymer. The rate of water permeation, R_w, in the hydrophobic zone and the rate of hydrolysis, R_h, are important parameters in tuning the release kinetics.

V. OTHER ASPECTS OF DRUG RELEASE MODELING

A. Osmotic Systems

Osmotic systems for drug delivery are designed by applying irreversible thermodynamics and the Kedem-Katchalsky (73) analysis. The total volume flow, J_u, and the total exchange flow, J_D, are respectively given by

$$J_u = L_p \Delta p + L_{pD} \Delta \pi_s$$
$$J_D = L_{Dp} \Delta p + L_D \Delta \pi_s \tag{53}$$

Here L_i (i = p, pD, Dp, D) represents Onsager coefficients, Δp the hydrostatic pressure, and $\Delta \pi_s$ the osmotic pressure of the solvent.

The systems under consideration may also be defined by the reflection coefficient, σ, and the permeability coefficient, L_p. The term σ is defined as

$$\sigma = -\frac{L_{pD}}{L_p} \tag{54}$$

The osmotic pressure is given by using a standard gas law. The volume flux dV/dt for a membrane of thickness δ and cross-sectional area A is given by

$$\frac{dV}{dt} = \frac{A}{\delta} (\sigma \Delta \pi_s - \Delta p) \tag{55}$$

The value $\sigma = 0$ represents a coarse filter and $\sigma = 1$ represents an impermeable drug. For large orifices, it can be assumed that $\Delta \pi_s \gg \Delta p$. Hence, dV/dt reduces to

$$\frac{dV}{dt} = \frac{A}{\delta} L_p \sigma \Delta \pi_s = \frac{A}{\delta} k \Delta \pi_s \tag{56}$$

Using $dM/dt = c\, dV/dt$, we have,

$$\frac{dM}{dt} = \frac{A}{\delta} kc \Delta \pi_s \tag{57}$$

Hence, the drug release rate in osmotically controlled systems can be tuned to achieve zero-order kinetics.

B. Dissolution-Controlled Systems

Dissolution-controlled systems have the additional characteristic that in addition to polymer swelling and drug diffusion through the continuously changing phase, they are accompanied by slow disentanglement of the polymer chains, leading to complete dissolution of the carrier. Obviously, this mechanism will occur only in uncrosslinked polymer carriers.

Harland et al. (74) formulated for a model for drug release in a dissolving polymer–solvent system. The transport was assumed to be Fickian and mass balances were written for the drug and the solvent at the glassy–rubbery interface and at the rubbery–solvent interface. The important parameters identified in the phenomenon were the polymer volume fraction c* at the glassy–rubbery transition, the polymer volume fraction c_d for disentanglement of the chains, and the dissolution/mass transfer coefficient, k. The expression for drug release as a function of time was obtained as

$$\frac{M_d}{M_{d,\infty}} = \frac{c_b}{a\, c_{cd}} \left(\sqrt{\frac{2[-D_s(c^* + c_s - c_d - c_b) + D_d(c_s - c_b) + D_d/c_b]^2 (1 - c^* - c_s)t}{D_s(2 - c^* - c_s)(c^* + c_s - c_d - c_b) + D_d(c^* + c_s)(c_s - c_b)}} + kc_b t \right) \tag{58}$$

Here D_s is the diffusion coefficient of the solvent in the polymer and D_d is the diffusion coefficient of the drug in the polymer. The parameter c_b is the volume fraction of the drug in the bulk. This model can predict both Fickian and non-Fickian behavior. It is to be noted that front synchronization leads to zero-order release in dissolution-controlled systems.

The above model was modified by Narasimhan and Peppas (75) by accounting for macromolecular chain disentanglement. This enabled a molecular understanding of the dissolution mechanism of the polymer. This information is important to design tailor-made drug delivery systems for specific applications. An expression for the fraction of the drug released (Fig. 9) was derived as

$$\frac{M_d}{M_{d,\infty}} = \frac{v_{d,eq} + v_d^*}{2L} (\sqrt{2At} + Bt) \tag{59}$$

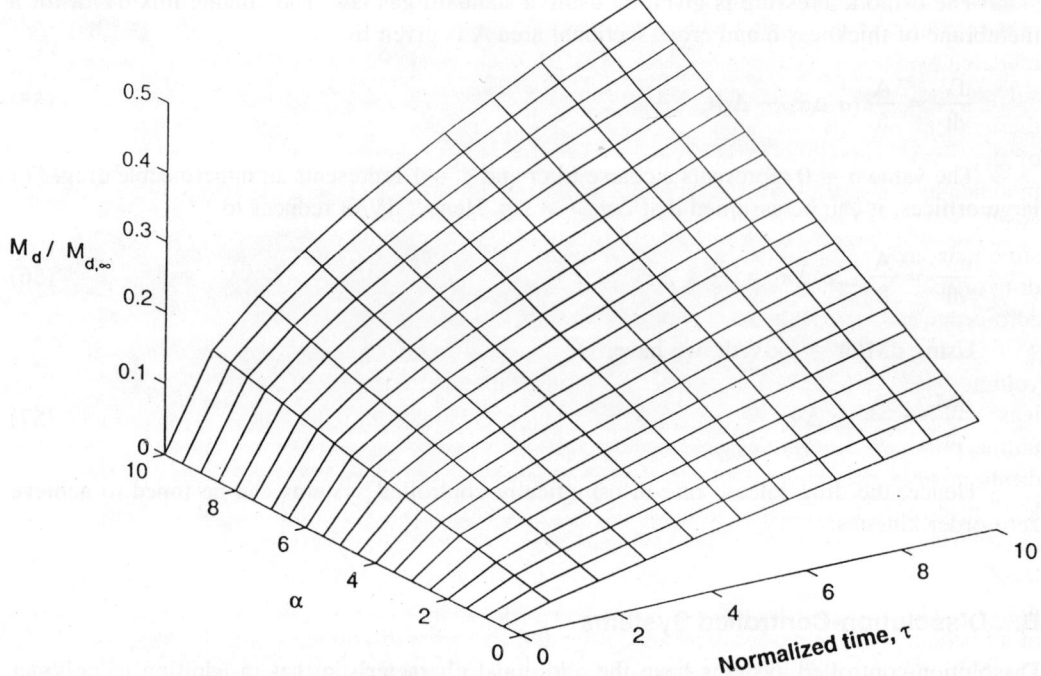

Figure 9 Predicted normalized drug released, $M_d/M_{d,\infty}$, as a function of normalized time, $\tau = Bt/\ell$, for different values of α ($\alpha = A/B$). (From Ref. 74.)

Here A and B are given as

$$A = D(v_{1,eq} - v_1^*)\left(\frac{v_{1,eq}}{v_{1,eq} + v_{d,eq}} + \frac{1}{v_1^* + v_d^*}\right) +$$
$$D_d(v_d^* - v_{d,eq})\left(\frac{v_{d,eq}}{v_{1,eq} + v_{d,eq}} + \frac{1}{v_1^* + v_d^*}\right) \quad (60)$$

$$B = \frac{k_d}{v_{1,eq} + v_{d,eq}} \quad (61)$$

Here L is the half-thickness of the polymer, D is the diffusion coefficient of the solvent and D_d is the diffusion coefficient of the drug, v_1^* and v_d^* are characteristic concentrations of solvent and drug, respectively, while $v_{1,eq}$ and $v_{d,eq}$ are equilibrium concentrations of solvent and drug, respectively. The parameter k_d is the disentanglement rate of the polymer chains and is calculated using reptation theory (76–78).

For the drug release rate to be zero-order (see Eq. 59), $B^2/A \gg 1$. Hence choosing a polymer–drug–solvent system such that the above inequality is satisfied would result in a zero-order drug release. This model also captures the transition between Fickian- and non-Fickian-type behavior. The acquisition of such broad insights from the mathematical model furthers the design and optimization of controlled drug delivery systems.

When the polymer carrier is semicrystalline, the process of carrier dissolution is preceded by a process of phase erosion of the crystalline region to an amorphous region. Under certain conditions, this transition may lead to relaxation-controlled conditions of drug transport. Drug release from a new class of such systems—crystal dissolution–controlled release systems—was modeled by Mallapragada and Peppas (79). In the presence of a thermodynamically compatible solvent, polymer crystals may start dissolving by crystal unfolding and disentanglement. In these dissolving phase erosion systems, the drug release rate is controlled by the transformation of the crystalline phase of the polymer to the amorphous phase. The crystalline regions are modeled as impermeable structures that do not permit drug diffusion. Therefore, as the polymer swells and drug is released, the concentration gradient for drug diffusion decreases; however, simultaneously disappearance of part of the crystalline phase causes an increase in the overall drug diffusion coefficient from the polymer. If these two effects compensate for each other, then zero-order drug release can be obtained.

A mathematical model was proposed by coupling crystal unfolding theories with free-volume-based drug diffusion theories (13) to predict conditions under which zero-order drug release can be obtained. Expressions were written for changes in the volume fractions of the crystalline polymer, amorphous polymer, and the drug as functions of time. The coupled partial differential equations were solved with the appropriate boundary conditions to yield drug release profiles as functions of time under various conditions (Fig. 10). Factors affecting the drug release rate were found to be the polymer degree of crystallinity, crystal size distribution, molecular weight of the polymer, the polymer–water interaction parameter, and the crystal unfolding rate. The release from these systems was found to be non-Fickian. This is the first instance of a mathematical model for controlled drug delivery from dissolving semicrystalline polymers. The modeling work helps enhancing the potential for materials such as poly(vinyl alcohol) as biomaterials.

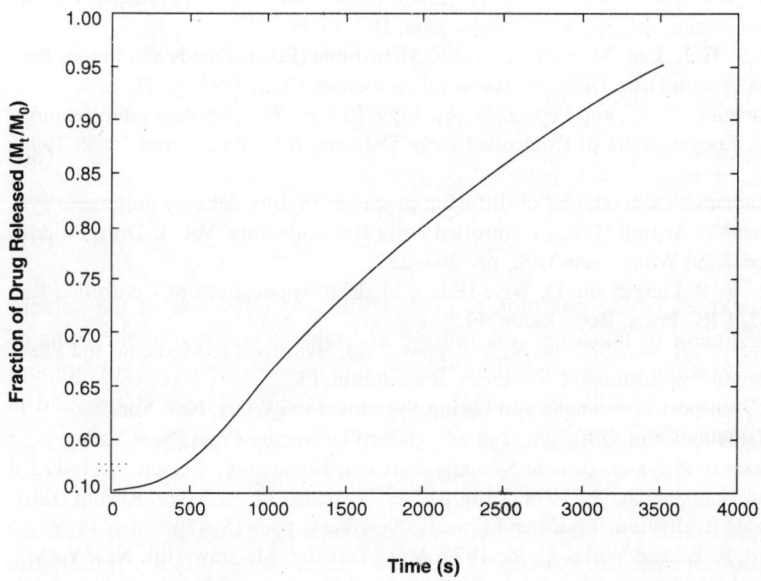

Figure 10 Predicted fraction of metronidazole released as a function of time from a poly(vinyl alcohol) sample with degree of crystallinity = 30% and drug loading of 2%. (From Ref. 78.)

VI. CONCLUSIONS AND FUTURE DIRECTIONS

Drug release through controlled delivery polymeric systems has been modeled predominantly by steady-state and transient description of drug diffusion by use of Fick's law. The correct interpretation of release kinetics from such drug release models depends on the mechanism of the release itself, the polymer microstructure, and the conditions of the experiment (in other words, the boundary conditions). More accurate mathematical descriptions are necessary in modeling drug release in swellable and porous polymeric systems. Consideration of aspects such as countercurrent solvent diffusion, chain disentanglement, polymer state transitions, polymer degree of crystallinity, phase-separated microstructures, and porous structure will enhance understanding and render models applicable to design a variety of sophisticated delivery devices. Advances in understanding interacting and noninteracting multicomponent diffusion phenomena are critical to the development of accurate models, and the next decade will hopefully provide much-needed solutions to rationally design controlled drug delivery devices.

REFERENCES

1. Baker, R. W. and Lonsdale, H. K., 1974. Controlled release: mechanisms and rates. In: A. C. Tanquary and R. E. Lacey (Eds.), Controlled Release of Biologically Active Agents, Plenum Press, New York, pp. 15–72.
2. Langer, R., 1990. New methods of drug delivery. Science, 249: 1527–1533.
3. Langer, R. and Peppas, N. A., 1983. Chemical and physical structure of polymers as carriers for controlled release of bioactive agents: a review. J. Macromol. Sci., Rev. Macromol. Chem. Phys., C23(1): 61–126.
4. Narasimhan, B. and Peppas, N. A., 1997. The role of modeling in the development of future controlled release devices. In: K. Park (Ed.), Controlled Drug Delivery, ACS, Washington, DC, pp. 529–557.
5. Rogers, C. E., 1976. In: D. R. Paul and F. W. Harris, (Eds.), Controlled Release Polymeric Formulations, ACS Symposium Series, Vol. 33, ACS, Washington, DC, 1976, p. 15.
6. Peppas, N. A., 1995. In: V. H. L. Lee, M. Hashida, and Y. Mizushima (Eds.), Trends and Future Perspectives in Peptide and Protein Drug Delivery, Harwood Academic, Chur, 1995, p. 23.
7. Narasimhan, B., Mallapragada, S. K., and Peppas, N. A., 1999. Release kinetics–data interpretation. In: E. Mathiowitz (Ed.), Encyclopedia of Controlled Drug Delivery, John Wiley, New York, 1999, pp. 921–935.
8. Peppas, N. A., 1984. Mathematical modeling of diffusion processes in drug delivery polymeric systems. In: V. F. Smolen and L. A. Ball (Eds.), Controlled Drug Bioavailability, Vol. 1, Drug Product Design and Performance, John Wiley, New York, pp. 203–237.
9. Peppas, N. A., 1984. In: R. S. Langer and D. Wise (Eds.), Medical Applications of Controlled Release Technology, Vol. 2, CRC Press, Boca Raton, FL.
10. Peppas, N. A. and Korsmeyer, R. W., 1987. In: N. A. Peppas (Ed.), Hydrogels in Medicine and Pharmacy, Vol. 3, Properties and Applications, CRC Press, Boca Raton, FL.
11. Lightfoot, E. N., 1974. Transport Phenomena and Living Systems, John Wiley, New York.
12. Crank, J., 1975. The Mathematics of Diffusion, 2nd ed., Oxford University Press, New York.
13. Fujita, H., 1961. Diffusion in Polymer–Diluent Systems. Fortschr. Hochpolym.-Forsch., 3: 1–47.
14. Mallapragada, S. K. and Narasimhan, B., 1998. Drug delivery systems. In: A. F. von Recum (Ed.), Handbook of Biomaterials Evaluation, Taylor and Francis, New York, pp. 415–426.
15. Sherwood, T. K, Pigford, R. L., and Wilke, C. R., 1975. Mass Transfer, McGraw-Hill, New York.
16. Higuchi, T., 1961. Rate of release of medicaments from ointment bases containing drugs in suspension. J. Pharm. Sci., 50: 874–875.
17. Paul, D. R. and McSpadden, S. K., 1976. Diffusional release of a solute from a polymer matrix. J. Membr. Sci., 1: 33–48.

18. Fu, J. C., Hagemeier, C., and Moyer, D. L., 1976. A unified mathematical model for diffusion from drug–polymer composite tablets. J. Biomed. Mater. Res., 10: 743–758.
19. Rhine, W. D., Sukhatme, V., Hseih, D. S. T., and Langer, R., 1980. A new approach to achieve zero-order release kinetics from diffusion-controlled polymer matrix systems. In: R. Baker (Ed.), Controlled Release of Bioactive Materials, Academic Press, New York, pp. 177–187.
20. Gurny, R., Doelker, E., and Peppas, N. A., 1982. Modeling of sustained release of water-soluble drugs from porous, hydrophobic polymers. Biomaterials, 3: 27–32.
21. Chandrasekaran, S. K. and Paul, D. R., 1982. Dissolution-controlled transport from dispersed matrices. J. Pharm. Sci., 71: 1399–1402.
22. Korsmeyer, R. W. and Peppas, N. A., 1983. Swelling-controlled delivery systems for pharmaceutical applications: macromolecular and modeling considerations. In: S. Z. Mansdorf and T. J. Roseman (Eds.), Controlled Release Delivery Systems, Marcel Dekker, New York, p. 77.
23. Crank, J., 1984. Free and Moving Boundary Problems, 2nd ed., Oxford University Press, New York.
24. Danckwerts, P. V., 1950. Trans. Faraday Soc., 46: 701.
25. Lee, P. I., 1980. Diffusional release of a solute from a polymeric matrix—approximate analytical solutions. J. Membr. Sci., 7: 255–275.
26. Zhou, Z. and Wu, X. Y., 1997. Finite element analysis of diffusional drug release from complex matrix systems. I. Complex geometries and composite structures. J. Contr. Rel., 49: 277–288.
27. Siegel, R. A., 1989. In: M. Rosoff (Ed.), Controlled Release of Drugs. VCH, New York, p. 1.
28. Harland, R. S. and Peppas, N. A., 1989. Solute diffusion in swollen networks. VII. Diffusion in semicrystalline networks. Coll. Polym. Sci., 267: 218–225.
29. Anderson, J. L. and Quinn, J. A., 1974. Biophys. J., 14: 130.
30. Colton, C. K., Smith, K. A., Merrill, E. W., and Farrell, P. C., 1971. Permeability studies with cellulosic membranes. J. Biomed. Mater. Res., 5: 459–488.
31. Higuchi, T., 1963. Mechanism of sustained-action medication—theoretical analysis of rate of release of solid drugs dispersed in solid matrices. J. Pharm. Sci., 52: 1145–1149.
32. Roseman, T. J. and Higuchi, W. I., 1970. Release of medroxyprogesterone acetate from a silicone polymer. J. Pharm. Sci., 59: 353–357.
33. Fessi, H., Marty, J. P., Puisieux, F., and Carstensen, J. T., 1978. Higuchi square root equation applied to matrices with high content of soluble drug substance. Int. J. Pharm., 1: 265–274.
34. Desai, S. J., Singh, P., Simonelli, A. P., and Higuchi, W. I., 1966. Investigation of factors influencing release of solid drug dispersed in inert matrices. II. Quantitation of procedures. J. Pharm. Sci., 55: 1224–1229.
35. Swan, E. A. and Peppas, N. A., 1981. Drug release kinetics from hydrophobic porous monolithic devices. Proc. Symp. Control. Rel. Bioact. Mater., 8: 18–19.
36. Harland, R. S., Dubernet, .C., Benoit, J.-P., and Peppas, N. A., 1988. A model of dissolution-controlled, diffusional drug release from non-swellable polymer microspheres. J. Contr. Rel., 7: 207–215.
37. Chang, N. J. and Himmelstein, K. J., 1990. Dissolution-diffusion controlled constant-rate release from heterogeneously loaded drug-containing materials. J. Contr. Rel., 12, 201–212.
38. Narasimhan, B. and Langer, R., 1997. Zero order release of micro- and macromolecules from polymeric devices: the role of the burst effect. J. Contr. Rel., 47: 13–20.
39. Peppas, N. A. and Korsmeyer, R., 1980. Polymers for sustained release of macromolecules. Polym. News, 6: 149–155.
40. Wu, J. C. and Peppas, N. A., 1993. Modeling of penetrant diffusion in glassy polymers with an integral sorption Deborah number. J. Polym. Sci. Polym. Phys. Ed., 31: 1503.
41. Peppas, N. A., Wu, J. C., and von Meerwall, E. D., 1994. Mathematical modeling and experimental characterization of polymer dissolution. Macromolecules, 27: 5626–5638.
42. Vrentas, J. M., Jarzebski, C. M., and Duda, J. L., 1975. A Deborah number for diffusion in polymer–solvent systems. AIChE J., 21: 894–900.
43. Lee, P. I., 1984. Effect of non-uniform initial drug concentration distribution on the kinetics of drug release from glassy hydrogel matrices. Polymer, 25: 973–978.
44. Lee, P. I., 1986. Initial concentration distribution as a mechanism for regulating drug release from diffusion-controlled and surface erosion–controlled matrix systems. J. Contr. Rel., 4: 1–11.

45. Bodmeier, R. and Paeratakul, O., 1990. Drug release from laminated polymeric films prepared from aqueous latexes. J. Pharm. Sci., 79: 32–36.
46. Conte, U., Maggi, L., Colombo, P., and La Manna, A., 1993. Multi-layered hydrophilic matrices as constant release devices (Geomatrix Systems). J. Contr. Rel., 26: 39–47.
47. Fassihi, R. A. and Ritschel, W. A., 1993. Multiple-layer, direct-compression, controlled-release system: in vitro and in vivo evaluation. J. Pharm. Sci., 82: 750–754.
48. Lee, P. I., 1987. Interpretation of drug release kinetics from hydrogel matrices in terms of time-dependent diffusion coefficients. In: P. I. Lee and W. Good (Eds.), Controlled Release Technology, ACS Symposium Series, ACS, Washington, DC, pp. 71–83.
49. Ritger, P. L. and Peppas, N. A., 1987. A simple equation for description of solute release. 1. Fickian and non-Fickian release from non-swellable devices in the form of slabs, spheres, cylinders or discs. J. Contr. Rel., 5: 23–36.
50. Peppas, N. A. and Franson, N. M., 1983. The swelling interface number as a criterion for prediction of diffusional solute release mechanisms in swellable polymers. J. Polym. Sci., Polym. Phys., 21: 983–997.
51. Kou, J. H., Fleisher, D., and Amidon, G. L., 1990. Modeling drug release from dynamically swelling poly(hydroxyethyl methacrylate-co-methacrylic acid) hydrogels. J. Contr. Rel., 12: 241–250.
52. Cohen, D. S. and Erneux, T., 1988. Free boundary problems in controlled release pharmaceuticals. 1. Diffusion in glassy polymers. SIAM J. Appl. Math., 48: 1451–1465.
53. Cohen, D. S. and Erneux, T., 1988. Free boundary problems in controlled release pharmaceuticals. 2. Swelling-controlled release. SIAM J. Appl. Math., 48: 1466–1474.
54. Korsmeyer, R. W., Lustig, S. R., and Peppas, N. A., 1986. Solute and penetrant diffusion in swellable polymers. 1. Mathematical modeling. J. Polym. Sci., Polym. Phys., 24: 395–408.
55. Lustig, S. R. and Peppas, N. A., 1987. Solute and penetrant diffusion in swellable polymers. J. Appl. Polym. Sci., 33: 533–549.
56. Lustig, S. R., Caruthers, J. M., and Peppas, N. A., 1992. Continuum thermodynamics and transport theory for polymer–fluid mixtures. Chem. Eng. Sci., 47: 3037–3057.
57. Peppas, N. A. and Brannon-Peppas, L., 1990. Hydrogels at critical conditions. 1. Thermodynamics and swelling behavior. J. Membr. Sci., 48: 281–290.
58. Brannon-Peppas, L. and Peppas, N. A., 1991. Time-dependent response of ionic polymer networks to pH and ionic strength changes. Int. J. Pharm., 70: 53–57.
59. Bell, C. L. and Peppas, N. A., 1993. Complexation in poly(ethylene glycol-methacrylic acid) hydrogels. Polym. Prepr., 34(1): 831–832.
60. Hariharan, D. and Peppas, N. A., 1993. Swelling of ionic and neutral polymer networks in ionic solutions. J. Membr. Sci., 78: 1–12.
61. Hariharan, D. and Peppas, N. A., 1993. Modeling of water transport and solute release in physiologically sensitive gels. J. Contr. Rel., 23: 123–136.
62. Colombo, P., Catellani, P. L., Peppas, N. A., Maggi, L., and Conte, U., 1992. Swelling characteristics of hydrophilic matrices for controlled release: new dimensionless number to describe the swelling and release behavior. Int. J. Pharm., 88: 99–109.
63. Cooney, D. O., 1971. Slow dissolution of implanted beds of spherical particles as a method for prolonged-release medication. AIChE J., 17: 754–756.
64. Cooney, D. O., 1971. Effect of geometry on the dissolution of pharmaceutical tablets and other solids: surface detachment kinetics controlling. AIChE J., 18:446–449.
65. Hopfenberg, H. B., 1976. Controlled release from erodible slabs, cylinders, and spheres. In: D. R. Paul and F. W. Harris (Eds.), Controlled Release Polymeric Formulations. ACS Symposium Series, Vol. 33, ACS, Washington, DC, p. 222.
66. Thombre, A. G. and Himmelstein, K. J., 1985. A simultaneous transport-reaction model for controlled drug delivery from catalyzed bioerodible polymer matrices. AIChE J., 31: 759–766.
67. Goepferich, A. and Langer, R., 1993. Modeling of polymer erosion. Macromolecules, 26: 4105–4112.
68. Goepferich, A. and Langer, R., 1995. Modeling monomer release from bioerodible polymers. J. Contr. Rel., 33: 55–69.

69. Goepferich, A., 1996. Mechanisms of polymer degradation and erosion. Biomaterials, 17: 103–114.
70. Goepferich, A., 1997. Polymer bulk erosion. Macromolecules, 30: 2598–2604.
71. Zygourakis, K. and Markenscoff, P. A., 1996. Computer-aided design of bioerodible devices with optimal release characteristics: a cellular automata approach. Biomaterials, 17: 125–135.
72. Tani, N., Van Dress, M., and Anderson, J. M., 1981. In: D. H. Lewis (Ed.), Controlled Release of Pesticides and Pharmaceuticals, Plenum Press, New York, p. 79.
73. Kedem, O. and Katchalsky, A., 1958. Thermodynamic analysis of the permeability of biological membranes to non-electrolytes. Biochem. Biophys. Acta, 27: 229–246.
74. Harland, R. S., Gazzaniga, A., Sangani, M. E., Colombo, P., and Peppas, N. A., 1988. Drug/polymer matrix swelling and dissolution. Pharm. Res., 5: 488–494.
75. Narasimhan, B. and Peppas, N. A., 1997. Molecular analysis of drug delivery systems controlled by dissolution of the polymer carrier. J. Pharm. Sci., 86(3): 297–304.
76. Narasimhan, B. and Peppas, N. A., 1996. Disentanglement and reptation during dissolution of rubbery polymers. J. Polym. Sci., Polym. Phys. Ed., 34: 947–961.
77. Narasimhan, B. and Peppas, N. A., 1996. On the importance of chain reptation in models of dissolution of glassy polymers. Macromolecules, 29: 3283–3291.
78. De Gennes, P.-G., 1979. Scaling Concepts in Polymer Physics, Cornell University Press, Ithaca, NY.
79. Mallapragada, S. K. and Peppas, N. A., 1997. Crystal dissolution–controlled release systems: I. Physical characteristics and modeling analysis. J. Contr. Rel., 45: 87–94.

9
Drug Release from Swelling-Controlled Systems

Paolo Colombo, Patrizia Santi, Ruggero Bettini, and Christopher S. Brazel
Parco Area delle Scienze, Parma, Italy

Nicholas A. Peppas
Purdue University, West Lafayette, Indiana

I. INTRODUCTION

Swelling and matrix are key systems in the field of drug delivery systems. However, these systems are differently identified in the pertinent literature. For instance, Peppas (1) used the term swelling-controlled release systems, Lee (2) named them as hydrogel matrices or polymeric matrices exhibiting moving boundaries. Lippold (3) adopted the physicochemical definition of hydrocolloid matrices, whereas Ford (4) proposed the pharmaceutical term hydrophilic matrix tablets. These systems can be appropriately referred to as swellable matrix tablets, considering that this definition contains the two key words of drug delivery systems, along with the indication of the pharmaceutical manufacturing procedure.

II. GENERAL ANALYSIS OF SOLVENT TRANSPORT IN POLYMER MATRICES

Penetrant uptake behavior into crosslinked polymers has been investigated over the past several decades, with several notable contributions made to the understanding of deviations from classical Fickian diffusion (5–8). Due to the viscoelastic properties of polymers, which are enhanced by the presence of a crosslinked network, anomalous penetrant transport can be observed. This behavior is bound by pure Fickian diffusion and case II transport. Case II, or constant rate, transport has been observed for several polymer/penetrant systems (8). Transport in all of these physical situations can generally be reduced to three types of driving forces: a penetrant concentration gradient, a polymer stress gradient, and osmotic forces. Osmotic behavior is observed as a result of the hydrophilicity of the polymer network; its magnitude is amplified when a hydrophilic drug is embedded in the matrix such as in the case of swelling-controlled release devices.

Swelling-controlled release systems are based on the above principles, where an appropriate polymer can counterbalance normal Fickian diffusion by hindering the release of an embedded drug, leading to an extended period of drug delivery, and possibly zero-order release (9). In addition, the presence of a polymer network surrounding a drug or protein molecule has also been shown (10) to act as a stabilizer, maintaining biological activity until the solute is released.

Despite significant work to accurately model transport in swelling-controlled release systems (11–14), simpler molecular models are needed which can relate the characteristics of specific polymer–drug systems to predicted drug release profiles, allowing a scientist to design an optimal drug delivery device. Here we investigate molecular mechanisms of water and drug transport in swellable systems. From knowledge of the polymer properties, including composition, crosslinking density and concentration during the crosslinking reaction, as well as solute size and shape, and initial loading concentration, drug release profiles can be predicted.

The use of swellable materials for drug delivery applications has followed experimental and theoretical investigations of solvent and solute transport in polymeric systems, with several important observations and mathematical models developed that describe transport behavior in polymeric systems.

A. Fickian, Case II and Anomalous Transport in Polymers

Unique sorption behavior when polymers were subjected to vapors and liquids was noted as early as 1953 (15). In nonswelling systems, or in cases where the relative relaxation time of the polymer is much shorter than the characteristic diffusion time for water transport, Fickian diffusion is observed, with water transport controlled by a concentration gradient. Once solvated, these polymers assume an equilibrium state almost immediately. In the case where polymer relaxation is the rate-limiting step to water transport, case II transport or time-independent diffusion is observed. However, in many systems the water uptake mechanism leads to transport behavior intermediate to Fickian and case II transport, termed anomalous transport. Specific polymeric systems exhibiting the limiting cases of Fickian and case II transport have been identified by Frisch et al. (13) and Thomas and Windle (16).

B. Structural and Compositional Factors in Swelling Polymer Systems

Many experimental parameters can affect the kinetic swelling behavior of polymers. The effects of sample geometry on penetrant uptake have been investigated by several investigators (17,18). The effects of crosslinking density (19), drug loading (20), and copolymer composition (10) on swelling kinetics have also been determined experimentally. Recently, Colombo et al. (21) determined that there is a strong correlation between front motion and drug release kinetics, with case II drug release resulting when water and degradation fronts are synchronised.

There have been many experimental investigations of diffusion in polymers, with results showing a range of transport behavior. In swelling polymer systems, stresses arising during the polymer swelling process have significant effects on penetrant (not only water) uptake behavior. Crazing phenomena have been noted in extreme systems, whereas in other systems, these stresses can cause anomalous or case II transport (12).

Alfrey et al. (12) identified case II transport with the existence of a sharp penetrant front advancing at a constant velocity. Their results indicated that a polymer placed in a thermodynamically compatible solvent will swell and rearrange to accommodate the solvent, leading to anomalous and possibly case II transport, whereas poor solvents will be restricted to diffusion in the pore space inside the polymer, leading to Fickian transport. The rate of penetrant uptake and compatibility of the polymer with a particular solvent leads to stresses occurring between the rubbery and glassy areas of the swelling polymer, which were noted to crack or craze in the presence of especially good solvents.

Similarly, Hopfenberg and Frisch (7) showed how the type of transport observed for the same polymer–solvent pair ranges from pure Fickian to case II with variations in the temperature and solvent activity. Thomas and Windle (16) studied classical case II absorption and showed that weight gain in these systems was linear with respect to time up to the point where two fronts in a thin-disc sample met. Penetrant concentration profiles inside the network were also determined; they show a very sharp front at the glassy/rubbery transition, with significantly higher, though not equilibrium, concentration of penetrant in the rubbery regions (22). Characteristic sharp changes in the thickness and area of thin-disc samples confirmed the presence of a glassy region remaining in the center of the material until the fronts met (23).

Osmotic pressure is also an important factor in penetrant uptake kinetics for polymer systems restrained by crosslinks (17,24). These investigators utilized an osmotic pressure driving force to account for penetrant uptake; however, they did not consider the increase in osmotic pressure for solute-loaded samples, which can be significant in a number of systems, leading to entirely different solvent uptake kinetics in the same polymeric material.

Gehrke et al. (25) investigated water uptake in poly(2-hydroxyethyl methacrylate), an important biomedical polymer used frequently in controlled drug delivery systems. They found that penetrant uptake as well as front velocities were dependent on the square root of time, indicating Fickian transport. It was theorized that this was a result of the small size of water molecules relative to the pore space in the network, thereby having no convective flux term. In cases where transport was facilitated by a concentration gradient and polymer relaxation occurred quickly, Fickian diffusion was expected.

There have been many experimental investigations to elucidate the state of a solvent (particularly water) in polymer networks (26–28). In hydrogels of certain compositions, water can bind with the polymer chains, creating a rigid area around the mesh that is not accessible to solute or solvent diffusion. This can greatly influence the type of transport observed, since the effective porosity of the material is decreased by bound water. Koda et al. (26) determined that the velocity of ultrasonic waves was decreased markedly in polyelectrolyte hydrogels, indicating the presence of bound water.

C. Dimensionless Parameters to Describe Water and Drug Transport

Water uptake and drug delivery from swelling-controlled release systems can be described sufficiently by two dimensionless parameters: the diffusional Deborah number, De, which relates net water motion to the rate of polymer relaxation, and the swelling Interface number, Sw, relating water penetration into a network to diffusion of a dispersed solute from the polymer. These parameters are sensitive to both polymer and drug properties.

The diffusional Deborah number is expressed as a ratio between the characteristic polymer relaxation time and a characteristic diffusion time:

$$\text{De} = \frac{\lambda}{\theta} = \frac{\lambda D_{1,2}}{[\delta(t)]^2} \tag{1}$$

where λ is the characteristic relaxation time for the polymer when subjected to swelling stresses, and θ is the characteristic penetrant diffusion time into a swelling sample (29,30). θ is defined as the square of the half-thickness of a thin-disc sample divided by the diffusion coefficient of water in the polymer ($\delta^2/D_{1,2}$). If either the relaxation time (De $\gg$ 1) or solvent diffusion (De << 1) dominates the swelling process, the time dependence is Fickian; however, if De is on the order of 1, the two processes will occur on the same time scale, leading to anomalous transport behavior.

The swelling interface number, Sw, is important in describing the balance between solvent penetration and solute diffusion (30).

$$Sw = \frac{v\delta_r}{D_{3,21}} \qquad (2)$$

where v is the velocity of the moving glassy/rubbery front, δ is the thickness of the swollen gel layer, and $D_{3,21}$ is the diffusion coefficient of solute in the polymer. Sw is sensitive to both the polymer structure (as it affects penetrant uptake) and drug properties through the solute diffusion coefficient. When Sw is significantly greater or smaller than 1, either water penetration or drug diffusion will control the release pattern, and the time dependence will be Fickian; however, when Sw is on the order of 1, anomalous behavior prevails.

Both dimensionless numbers, De and Sw, have been shown to vary with time, as the diffusion coefficients and swelling front velocity are not constant during the swelling process. Therefore, either the initial or equilibrium values of Sw and De were determined for experimental results in the referred work.

D. General Characteristics of Swelling-controlled Release Systems

Polymeric hydrogels have been utilized for the purpose of extended drug delivery, as well as drug targeting and patterned release profiles. Typical pharmaceutical formulations, such as tablets, include an active ingredient compressed in a powder, such as a cellulose derivative. However, these systems can only control drug release during the initial stages after the drug is placed in a body. Coated capsules can protect a drug for a period of time before releasing at an optimal site, thereby prolonging the active lifetime of the drug. However, these systems have limited applications for long-term drug delivery. Hydrogel delivery systems are capable of slow release of an embedded drug, with release controlled by the rate of swelling and relaxation of the polymer (31,32).

The major application of swelling-controlled release is in the delivery of drugs over an extended period. In the past two decades, much research in polymer diffusion has focused on the use of hydrogel materials for delivery of pharmaceutically active agents.

Hopfenberg and Hsu (33) studied Sudan red IV dye release from polystyrene, achieving a nearly constant release profile, without an initial burst effect, common to membrane reservoir systems. The effects of polymer type and loading concentration on drug release profiles can be very pronounced. Pham and Lee (34) investigated the motion of fronts in three grades of hydroxypropylmethylcellulose (HPMC) loaded with fluorescein as a model drug. It was observed that the effects of HPMC grade on the front velocity was minimal, but the loading of fluorescein into the network had a large influence.

In 1983, Korsmeyer et al. (35) found that solute size and polymer composition had profound effects on release profiles. There have been several contributions by our groups to understanding the swelling and relaxational behavior of hydrogels. These behaviors in poly(hydroxyethyl methacrylate-co-methyl methacrylate) [P(HEMA-co-MMA)] hydrogels were observed by Davidson and Peppas (20), with polymer relaxation times determined by mechanical stress relaxation experiments, and used in calculation of diffusional Deborah numbers, which decreased with an increase in hydrophobic network content. Korsmeyer et al. (5,6) showed dimensional changes in gel behavior with poly(hydroxyethyl methacrylate-co-N-vinylpyrrolidone) P(HEMA-co-NVP), monitored swelling fronts using polarized light, and studied the effect of polymer thickness and composition on theophylline release. They were also able to estimate diffusion coefficients through pulsed gradient spin-echo nuclear magnetic resonance (PGSE-NMR).

Davidson and Peppas (20), were able to couple Fickian diffusion to polymer relaxation and observe relaxational effects on dynamic behavior. Ritger and Peppas (18) proposed an equation to describe drug release kinetics from swelling-controlled drug delivery systems.

The equation is based on a power law dependence of the fraction released on time. The exponent n has values that can range between 0.43 and 1, according to the geometry and the prevalence of the Fickian or the case II (relaxation) transports. The equation has the following form:

$$\frac{M_t}{M_\infty} = kt^n \qquad (3)$$

where M_t is the drug released at time t, M_∞ is the amount of drug released at infinite time, k is a kinetics constant, and n is the diffusional exponent.

These authors (20) studied various sample geometries and determined appropriate n values for spherical, cylindrical, and slab geometries. In addition, they defined an aspect ratio that could be used to determine the appropriate exponent for a system. The values that the exponent n can assume and their meanings are reported in Table 1.

Franson and Peppas (10) observed front motion using polarized light to view stressed regions in P(HEMA-co-MMA) and P(HEMA-co-NVP) pyrrolidone) gels when exposed to water. Sorption experiments were fit to the power law expression. They also noted the importance of gel history on swelling behavior. After a sample is swollen to equilibrium, some macromolecular entanglements can be broken to yield a different structure and different swelling kinetics upon subsequent experimentation. They were also able to correlate diffusional exponent, n, values to polymer composition. They also introduced the swelling interface number, Sw, as an important dimensionless parameter to characterize the relative quantitative effects of solvent transport compared to solute release. They showed that Sw values correlated with the order of release, n, in an inverse logarithmic fashion.

Korsmeyer, von Meerwall, and Peppas (6) confirmed the existence of sharp fronts in P(HEMA-co-NVP) gels between rubbery and glassy regions, and noted a unique pattern of dynamic thickness observed in the swelling of disc-shaped hydrogels. They also studied the effects of sample thickness on swelling and release behavior, and determined the diffusivities of solvent and solute in hydrogels using PGSE-NMR techniques.

In two studies by Lustig and Peppas (37), penetrant uptake and the subsequent release of a solute from a hydrogel were modeled using Fickian expressions for each transient problem,

Table 1 Dependence of the Diffusional Exponent, n, on Sample Geometry (36)

Diffusional exponent mechanisms			
Plane sheet	Cylinder	Sphere	Transport
0.5	0.45	0.43	Fickian
>0.5	>0.45	>0.43	Anomalous
<1.0	<0.89	<0.85	Anomalous
1.0	0.89	0.85	Case II
>1.0	>0.89	>0.85	Super case II

with concentration-dependent diffusivities. They showed in tabular form what effects several of the model parameters would have on the uptake and release profiles. In 1988, Lustig and Peppas derived a scaling law to relate the diffusivity of drug in a gel, $D_{3,12}$, to its free solution diffusion coefficient, $D_{3,1}$:

$$D = \frac{D_{3,12}}{D_{3,1}} = \left(rQ^{-3/4}\right)^{\left(\frac{-Y}{Q-1}\right)} \quad (4)$$

Here r is the solute radius and Q is the volume swelling ratio. By determining the relative importance of these factors on the diffusion coefficient of the drug in a gel, optimization of carriers for drug delivery was more efficient.

The use of Eq. 3 for drug release kinetics description from hydroxypropylmethylcellulose matrices requires some statistical attention for a significant measure of the n value (38). A more interesting equation for the analysis of the drug release data was proposed by Peppas and Salhin (39). This is an equation in which the approximate contributions of the diffusional and relaxational (or erosion) mechanisms are estimated by the constants k_1 and k_2.

$$\frac{M_t}{M_\infty} = k_1 t^m + k_2 t^{2m} \quad (5)$$

Here M_t is the drug released at time t, M_∞ is the amount of drug released at infinite time, k_1 is the diffusional constant, k_2 the relaxational constant, and m the diffusional exponent.

Equation 5 allows the quantitative estimation of the mechanisms involved, by means of calculation of the ratio between the relaxation contribution, R, and the diffusional contribution, F, according to the following formula:

$$\frac{R}{F} = \frac{k_2}{k_1} t^m \quad (6)$$

In the above work, polymers were utilized that were amorphous. However, in many polymer systems, such as poly(vinyl alcohol) and polyethylene, high degrees of polymer crystallinity can influence transport behavior, as the crystalline regions function effectively as physical crosslinks, but they can also dissolve during the sorption and release process. To determine the effects of crystallinity on transport in polymers, Harland and Peppas (40) developed a model for diffusion in semicrystalline networks.

Drug/solute release from pH-sensitive materials can have additional factors influencing release profiles. Brannon-Peppas and Peppas (41) studied swelling and release behavior of pH-sensitive hydrogels, calculating Deborah and swelling interface numbers. am Ende et al. (42) described the factors influencing drug release from polyelectrolyte hydrogels, with special attention given to drug–polymer interactions, as examined by Fourier transform infrared (FTIR) spectroscopy.

III. DRUG RELEASE CONTROL AND MECHANISMS IN SWELLABLE MATRIX TABLETS

A. Water Penetration, Swelling of Matrix, and Gel Layer Formation Dynamics

Swellable matrix tablets are activated by water, and drug release control depends on the interactions between water, polymer, and drug. Water penetration into the matrix is the first step leading to polymer swelling and polymer and drug dissolution. The presence of water decreases the glassy-rubbery temperature (e.g., for HPMC from 184°C to lower than 37°C), giving rise to the transformation of glassy polymer in a rubbery phase (gel layer). The enhanced mobility of the polymeric chains favors the transport of dissolved drug. Polymer relaxation phenomena determine the swelling or volume increase of the matrix. The latter may add a convective contribution to the drug transport mechanism in drug delivery.

Depending on the polymer characteristics, the polymer amount in the rubbery phase, at the surface of the matrix, could reach the disentanglement concentration; therefore, the gel layer varies in thickness and the matrix dissolves or erodes. The concentration at which polymeric chains can be considered disentangled was demonstrated to correspond to an abrupt change in the rheological properties of the gel (43). This value has been measured for HPMC and has been found not to be significantly different from the one obtained by applying to drug release data a model equation describing gel layer and drug release behavior (44). More recently, Bonferoni et al. showed good parallel between the rheological behavior of HPMC gels and their erosion rate, confirming that the polymer–polymer and polymer–water interactions are responsible for the gel network structure and its sensitivity to erosion. In turn, they affect drug release rate in case of poorly soluble drugs (45).

The gel layer thickness depends on the relative contributions of water penetration, chain disentanglement, and mass (polymer and drug) transfer in the water. At the beginning, the water penetration is more rapid than chain disentanglement and a quick buildup of gel layer thickness takes place. But when the water penetrates slowly, due to the increase of the diffusional distance, little change in gel thickness is obtained because water penetration and polymer disentanglement rates are similar (46). Thus, the gel layer thickness dynamics in swellable matrix tablet shows three distinct regimes: it increases when the penetration of water is the fastest phenomenon (Fig. 1a, b), stays constant when the disentanglement rate is similar to the penetration (Fig. 1b, c), and decreases when all of the polymer is in the rubbery phase (Fig. 1c, d) (44).

Drug release kinetics is strictly associated with the dynamics of the gel layer. It ranges initially from Fickian to anomalous (non-Fickian), and subsequently from quasi-constant to constant, becoming first order at the end. Due to an insufficient external polymeric mass

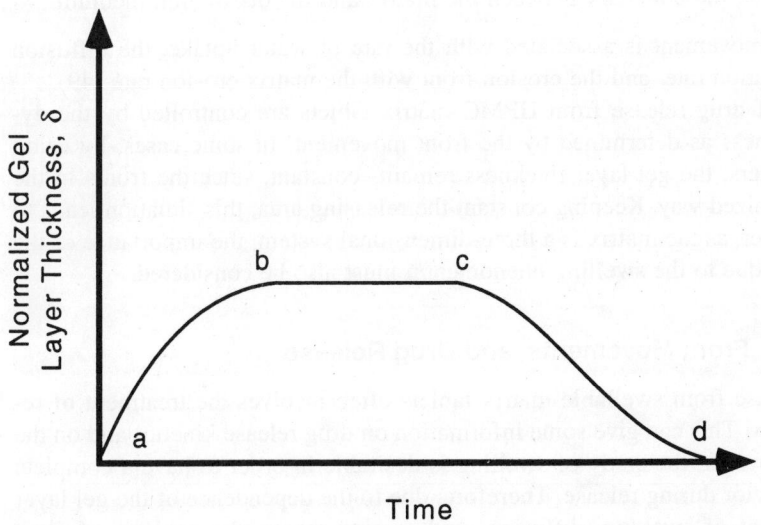

Figure 1 Time dependence of normalized gel layer thickness in presence of drug. (Modified from Ref. 44.)

transfer due to a low chain disentanglement rate, HPMC swellable matrices rarely show all three described regimes during the release time of the drug.

In summary, release mechanisms have the gel layer formed around the matrix in response to water penetration as a central element of their analysis. The gel must be capable of preventing matrix disintegration and controlling additional water penetration. Phenomena governing gel layer formation and, consequently, drug release rate are water penetration, polymer swelling, drug dissolution and diffusion, and matrix erosion. The drug release control is obtained by diffusion of molecules through the gel layer that can dissolve or erode. Recently, we showed the importance of a convective contribution to drug transport in the gel layer due to the extension of polymer chains (47).

B. Boundaries of Gel Layer and Relevant Fronts

Given the central role of the gel layer, it is fundamental to define its boundaries. These correspond to the fronts separating different matrix phases. Their movements determine the dynamics of gel layer formation. It is common knowledge that gel layer thickness is defined by the front separating the matrix from the dissolution medium, i.e., the erosion front, and by the front separating the glassy from the rubbery polymer, (i.e., the swelling front). Therefore, erosion and swelling front movements are the controllers of gel layer behavior.

The presence of a third front inside the gel layer was described by Lee in swellable matrices (48) containing diclofenac, as the consequence of precipitation in gel layer of this poorly soluble drug already molecularly dispersed in the glassy matrix. This front, named diffusion front, corresponds to the boundary between undissolved and dissolved drug. It was further shown that, depending on the function of drug solubility and loading (47), its presence is highly probable in swellable matrix tablets. Therefore, in swellable matrix tablets conditions exist under which the following three fronts can be present at the same time (Fig. 2):

a. The *swelling* front, the boundary between the still glassy polymer and its rubbery phase
b. The *diffusion* front, the boundary between the solid as yet undissolved drug and the dissolved drug in gel layer, and
c. The *erosion* front, the boundary between the matrix and the dissolution medium.

The swelling front movement is associated with the rate of water uptake, the diffusion front with the drug dissolution rate, and the erosion front with the matrix erosion rate (49).

Rate and kinetics of drug release from HPMC matrix tablets are controlled by the dynamics of gel layer thickness as determined by the front movement. In some cases, by using sufficiently soluble polymers, the gel layer thickness remains constant, since the fronts in the matrix move in a synchronized way. Keeping constant the releasing area, this situation leads to zero-order release. However, as the matrix is a three-dimensional system, the importance of the increase of releasing area due to the swelling phenomenon must also be considered.

C. Swelling Behavior, Front Movements, and Drug Release

The analysis of drug release from swellable matrix tablets often involves the treatment of release data with a power law. This can give some information on drug release kinetics and on the mechanisms involved. However, the study of swelling is desirable in order to have a complete picture of the matrix behavior during release. Therefore, due to the dependence of the gel layer thickness on the movement of swelling, diffusion, and erosion fronts, the analysis of front movement allows for interpreting drug release in relation to swelling.

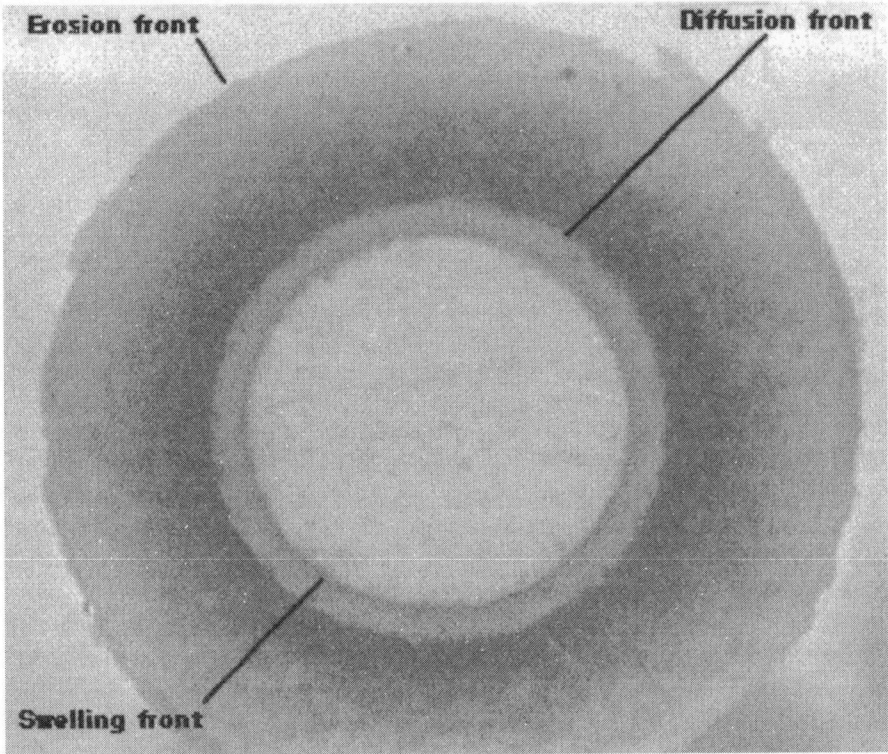

Figure 2 Picture of the top of a swellable matrix tablet during drug release showing the three fronts. (Modified from Ref. 49.)

The presence of a diffusion front necessitates reconsideration of the relevance of the swelling and erosion front positions on drug release control. Recent data have shown the importance of front movement, in particular diffusion front movement, on drug release kinetics. Figure 3 illustrates the typical movement of the fronts in HPMC matrix tablets (highly loaded with soluble drug) in which swelling and release were kept rigorously in radial direction (50). These data are part of experiments in which the viscosity of the polymer, the solubility of the drug, and the porosity of the matrix were varied. It was shown that drug release depended on the dynamics of gel layer thickness in the sense that the increase of thickness was inversely related to the release rate. However, with that HPMC grade matrices, synchronization of front movement is difficult to obtain. Thus, the kinetics of drug release depends on the relative position of the erosion and swelling or diffusion fronts.

These last two fronts, under certain conditions of drug solubility and loading, move separately making the distance between diffusion and erosion fronts decisive for the release kinetics. This leads to the new finding that, when the diffusion front is present, the *dissolved drug gel layer thickness* (distance between diffusion and erosion fronts) is the reference element for drug release, instead of the *whole gel layer thickness* (distance between swelling and erosion fronts).

The data mentioned previously also showed that the rate of drug delivery was dependent on the diffusion front velocity. In fact, when the swelling front accelerated (due to faster water penetration, as in the case of matrix porosity increase) but the diffusion front rate remained unchanged, drug flux remained unmodified (50). Additionally, when the drug solubility was

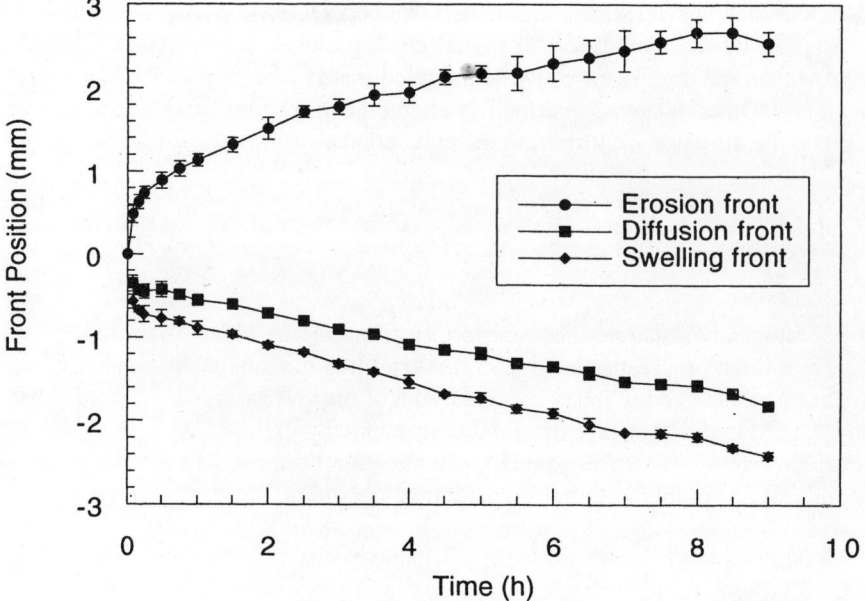

Figure 3 Position of fronts as a function of time. (Modified from Ref. 50.)

increased and the movement of the erosion front was not significantly affected, both the diffusion front movement and the release rate increased. It was also interesting to note that the drug release rate was inversely related to the dynamics of dissolved drug gel layer thickness. Since the movement of the diffusion front is almost linear, the dynamics of gel layer thickness follows the erosion front movement. As a consequence, in swellable matrix tablets the erosion front movement determines the kinetics and the diffusion front movement the rate of drug release.

In summary, the mechanisms of drug release from swellable matrix are diffusion of drug through the gel layer and drug transport due to the relaxation of the polymer. The rate of diffusion through the gel layer depends on drug dissolution and matrix erosion, both evidently affecting the drug concentration gradient in gel layer. Drug release from swellable matrix tablet is strictly linked to gel layer dynamics, also where the solubility of the drug is so low that the possibility exists for it to be released as solid particles from the dissolving layer of gel (51).

IV. SWELLABLE MATRIX TABLETS AS DRUG DELIVERY SYSTEMS

Swelling-controlled release systems for drug delivery are very often prepared as monoliths, i.e., matrices, formed by compression of hydrophilic microparticulate powders. They are typically composed of a drug and a hydrophilic swellable polymer, the amount of the latter usually ranging from 10% to 30% of the total weight of the matrix. Although many natural or synthetic polymers such as xanthan gum, guar gum, amylose starches, karaya gum, poly(ethylene oxide) (PEO), poly(vinyl alcohol) (PVA), and others have been studied, HPMC is certainly the most widely used class of polymers for their manufacture.

Different types of swellable matrix tablets can be prepared by the use of hydrophilic polymers. The most common are the *free swellable matrix tablets* (polymer and solid drug mixed and compressed), in which swelling is unhindered. In order to introduce additional elements for drug release control, the swelling of these matrix tablets can be affected by matrix surface modification, as, for instance, by the application of partial coatings. Their function is to alter the swelling behavior and then the drug release. These modified matrix tablets are called *swelling-restricted matrix tablets*. Other systems, in which swellable polymers are used as coating for delaying or controlling the diffusion of drug from the core, are the *swelling-controlled reservoir systems*.

A. Free Swellable Matrix Tablets

1. Drug Release Analysis

In the literature, several papers illustrate the manufacturing and the behavior of swellable matrix tablets that swell without any restriction (52–57). Very often the amount of drug released from these matrices can be analyzed in terms of square root of time (Higuchi's law). Yet the use of this relationship is not justified because the conditions applied by Higuchi to Fick's law are not valid for swellable systems. Moreover, the Higuchi equation does not take into consideration that the systems can be soluble and that relaxation of polymeric chains can contribute to drug transport.

Therefore, the analysis of drug release from swellable matrix could not be done with a model imposing the drug release dependence on square root of time. As mentioned before, an empirical equation was proposed by Ritger and Peppas (18) that rapidly gained popularity for the analysis of release data in these systems.

The analysis based on the use of the exponent n, done by different authors on various systems manufactured with HPMC or PEO, showed that the release was usually identified as anomalous transport, due to the contribution to drug transport of a second mechanism other than diffusion. In fact, published data for discs (58,59) showed that typical values of the exponent n were around 0.6 and 0.8 for HPMC and PEO matrices, respectively.

The relative contribution of drug diffusion, polymer relaxation, and matrix erosion to drug release from HPMC matrices in disc form originates n values ranging from 0.5 to 1.0. In order to shift release kinetics toward linearity, the matrix formulation can be built up to facilitate one of the previously described contributions. This was demonstrated by Catellani et al. (60) in swellable matrices formulated to increase the susceptibility of cylindrical matrix to relaxation or erosion by proper use of swellable excipients, including HPMC. Figure 4 shows that the introduction on an inert basic matrix of swellable and soluble polymers gave rise to a reduction of release rate variability, leading to a quasi-constant rate in the case of the use of 50% of swellable and soluble polymers.

Other attempts of improved formulations were made to shift the release kinetics of HPMC matrices toward constant rate. They consisted mainly of methods of modification of the drug diffusivity, or the proper use of soluble and/or insoluble fillers (61).

The improvement of linearity can also be obtained by mixing HPMC with other swellable polymers. HPMC matrices show an initial burst of drug release rate, due to the release from the surface and the time needed for the formation of an efficient gel layer capable of controlling water penetration and drug diffusion. This is particularly evident in the case of very soluble drugs. It was observed that, due to their swelling and dissolution properties, sodium carboxymethylcellulose (CMCNa) matrices did not show initial burst release (62). Using optimized mixtures of HPMC and CMC, Baveja et al. (63) obtained zero-order release of β-adrenergic blockers. The results were explained speculatively in terms of rate of advancement of swelling front into matrix and of erosion of the gel layer, so that diffusional pathlength for drug diffusion remained fairly constant. When the data were fitted to the previous Eq. 3, the exponent n reached the value of 0.89.

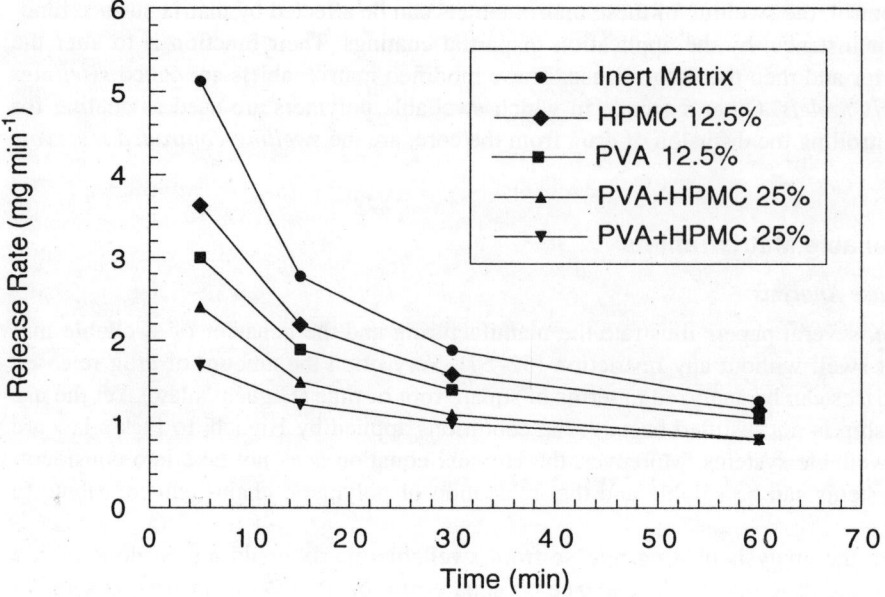

Figure 4 Variation of release rate as a function of time in matrices containing different amounts of swellable excipients. (Modified from Ref. 60.)

Kim and Fasshi (64–66) showed that a possibility exists to obtain zero-order release kinetics using a binary polymer matrix constituted by highly methoxylated pectin and HPMC in the case of either soluble or poorly soluble drugs. With these matrices drug release rate could be modulated according to the pectin HPMC ratio.

An additional possibility to limit the burst effect of HPMC matrices is the use of polymer powders with reduced particle size, thus allowing for quick hydration and gelation of the matrix (52,67).

2. Matrix Swelling Analysis and Relationship with Drug Release

Considering that the drug release from swellable matrix tablets is related to the swelling of the matrix, numerous studies on matrix swelling or water penetration have been published. Previous data obtained with optical methods in swellable matrix tablets having disc shape described a predominant axial swelling (68). In fact, at the beginning of the experiment, the matrix swells predominantly in the axial direction, showing an evident restriction to swelling on the lateral side due to the glassy core. However, very quickly the swelling of the matrix moves in both axial and radial directions. An example of axial and radial matrix increase is shown in Fig. 5.

The more pronounced axial swelling was related by Papadimitriou et al. (69) to the relief of the stresses induced during compaction of the matrix tablet. The swelling of HPMC matrices was also studied by NMR imaging (70). The technique allowed both the dimensional change of the core and the development of the gel layer to be studied. It was found that the gel layer developed at the same extent both in the axial and in the radial direction, independently on the HPMC type. A predominant axial swelling was reported as a result of expansion of ungelled tablet core in an axial direction. Similar results were reported by Gao and Meury, who applied an optical image analysis method to the dynamic swelling behavior of HPMC matrices containing lactose and adinazolam mesylate (71).

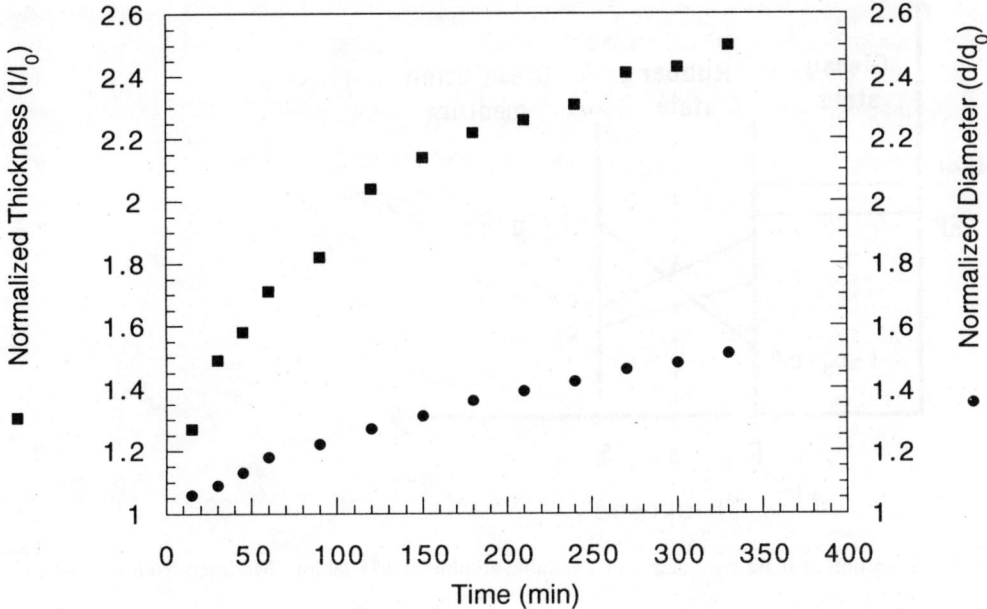

Figure 5 Increase of normalized diameter and thickness of a swellable matrix tablet as a function of time during drug release. (Modified from Ref. 68.)

The degree of swelling is typically expressed as the equilibrium volume swelling ratio, Q, defined as the volume of the equilibrium swollen gel divided by the volume of the same gel before swelling (68). The swelling ratio, Q, is expressed as:

$$Q = \frac{V_t}{V_0} = \left(\frac{R_t}{R_0}\right)^2 \left(\frac{l_t}{l_0}\right) \qquad (7)$$

where V_0 and V_t are volumes, R_t and R_0 radii, and l_t and l_0 thicknesses of the disc at time t and at time 0.

Usually, the change of Q is described as dependent on the square root of time, indicating a mechanism of dynamic swelling predominantly Fickian. However, non-Fickian conditions, indicating an important chain relaxation phenomenon, have also been observed (72).

Liquid penetration profiles in HPMC matrix tablets containing ibuprofen and propranolol HCl were studied (73). Liquid uptake was fitted to various models, including Eq. 5, described for drug release, which incorporates both the Fickian and case II transports. The results obtained showed that the increase of polymer content in the matrix shifted the ratio of the two contributions to the overall liquid uptake toward an increase of the Fickian diffusional component. The diffusional or relaxational water transport was also dependent on the type of filler mixed with HPMC. For instance, lactose improved Fickian uptake, whereas dicalcium phosphate reduced it. The influence of concentration and/or viscosity grade of HPMC on swelling ratio was also studied by the same authors (74).

As stated in the first part of this chapter, a successful mechanistic analysis of drug release in relation to matrix swelling can be done using the swelling interface number, Sw (30). This number is analogous to the Peclet number in that it compares a pseudo-convective process to a diffusional process. However, whereas the Peclet number defines these processes for the same diffusant, the swelling interface number relates transport phenomena of a penetrant and a solute.

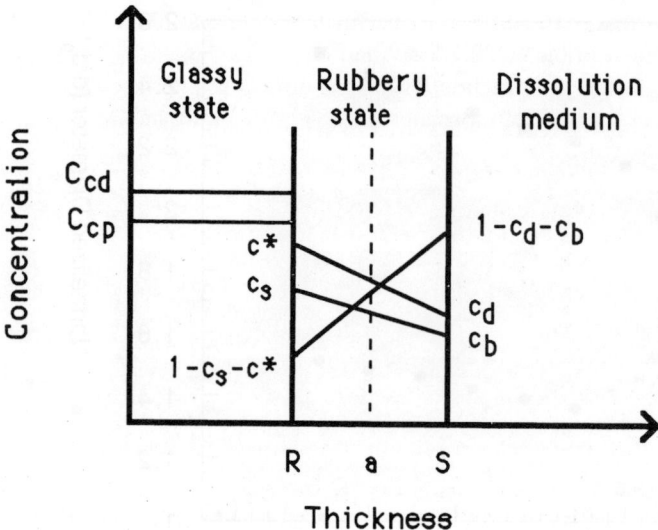

Figure 6 Definition of main parameters in swellable-soluble matrix tablet. (Modified from Ref. 44.)

As the term $v\,\delta(t)$ of Eq. (2) has units of area over time, a new dimensionless number, similar to Sw, describes the significant three-dimensional expansion of the matrix due to swelling and its associated influence on drug release. This is important because Sw is inherently related to one-dimensional transport (disc or films), whereas the improved dimensionless number can describe the behavior of truly three-dimensional matrices. As the swellable matrix tablet is characterized by a major change of surface area, the water front mobility is replaced in the new dimensionless number by a matrix swelling expansion characteristic. The increase of the releasing area produced by the matrix during swelling is used as a measure of the matrix expansion. Therefore the new number, the *swelling area number*, Sa, is defined as:

$$Sa = \frac{1}{D}\frac{dA}{dt} \tag{8}$$

where dA/dt is the expansion rate of the surface area of the swellable matrix. Data demonstrating the usefulness of this new dimensionless number for swellable matrix tablet analysis were reported by Colombo et al. (75).

The Sa number suggests a dependence of drug release on matrix releasing area. In fact, when the area increase and drug release during matrix swelling were compared directly, by plotting the fractional release vs. the corresponding area, linear relationships were obtained, indicating a direct dependence of drug release from the extent of releasing area produced by swelling. When swelling was affected by erosion (76), the relationship deviated from linearity.

A model capable of predicting the drug release and the water concentration profiles with simultaneous swelling was developed by Peppas et al. (77). In this model the phenomenon of polymer dissolution that frequently occurs with swellable matrices was not considered.

Successive models, accounting for concomitant swelling and dissolution of the polymer, were proposed by Lee and Peppas (78) and by Harland et al. (44). These models take into consideration the position of the relevant fronts and the pertinent parameters of drug and polymer. The considered fronts, i.e., the swelling front (R) and the erosion front (S), are illustrated in Fig. 6, together with the gradient involved in the analysis. The pertinent parameters are defined as follows:

D_s is the water diffusion coefficient in the drug–polymer matrix.
D_d is the drug diffusion coefficient in the swollen polymer.
c_s is the drug solubility (expressed as volume fraction) at the drug core interface (R).
c_b is the drug volume fraction at the gel–solution interface (S).
c^* is the polymer volume fraction at R.
c_d is the polymer volume fraction at S.
c_{cd} is the drug volume fraction in the glassy core.
c_{cp} is the polymer volume fraction in the glassy core.

For a cylindrical tablet having thickness a and surface area of one base A, from which the release is one-dimensional, the normalized gel layer thickness, δ, is given by the relative position of swelling and dissolution fronts, according to the expression:

$$\delta = \frac{(S - R)}{a} \tag{9}$$

The gel layer thickness varies with time, according to Fig. 1. The behavior of the gel layer thickness reveals two different types of drug quantity released in time. The first one is relative to the early swelling region where the thickness of gel layer increases. In this case, a very special approximate solution of the basic Fickian equations gives rise to a prediction of the amount of drug released, expressed as:

$$\frac{M_t}{M_\infty} = \frac{c_b}{c_{cd} a} \left\{ \left[\frac{2[-D_s(c_s + c^* - c_d - c_b) + D_d(c_s - c_b) + \left(\frac{D_d}{c_b}\right)(c_s - c_b)]^2 (1 - c^* - c_s) t}{[D_s(2 - c^* - c_s)(c^* + c_s - c_d - c_b) + D_d(c^* + c_s)(c_s - c_b)]} \right]^{\frac{1}{2}} + k c_d t \right\} \tag{10}$$

where t is the time and k is the mass transfer coefficient of the dissolved drug at S. It should be noted that Eq. 8 predicts that the amount of drug released is expressed as:

$$\frac{M_t}{M_\infty} = \alpha t^{1/2} + \gamma t \tag{11}$$

where α and γ are constants.

Equation 11 is similar to the empirical one (Eq. 5) proposed by Peppas and Sahlin (39) for the analysis of swellable systems, where the two mechanisms controlling the release, both relaxation and diffusion, occur. The equation predicts that the drug released is described by the addition of a relaxational term (with t dependence) to a diffusional term (with $t^{1/2}$ dependence).

The second type of drug quantity released in time is relative to the synchronization region, when the value of δ remains constant. The amount released in this situation is expressed as:

$$\frac{M_t}{M_\infty} = \zeta + \epsilon t \tag{12}$$

where ζ and ϵ are constants.

In this part of drug release, the delivery equation can be expressed as a zero-order equation. This indicates that in the synchronization region (gel layer thickness constant), drug release is a function of drug loading, c_{cd}, receiving solution concentration, c_b, and true dissolution parameter of polymer, c_d. No effect from drug solubility is predicted when the gel layer thickness stays constant. This result was experimentally anticipated in matrices containing drugs exhibiting different solubility: from swellable discs exposing a constant surface to dissolution fluid, diclofenac Na, diprophylline, and cimetidine HCl, three drugs having solubilities ranging from 3% to 100%, were released at the same rate. The synchronized gel layer showed constant thickness, increasing in value with the solubility of drug (62).

More recently, another model involving the polymer disentanglement concentration was developed by Ju et al. to describe the swelling dissolution behavior and drug release from hydrophilic matrices (79). According to this model, some important parameters, such as polymer disentanglement concentration $\rho_{p,dis}$, fractional polymer released, $M_{pt}/M_{p\infty}$, and fractional drug released, $M_{dt}/M_{d\infty}$, can be predicted simply on the base of polymer molecular weight, M. In fact, three scaling laws were established as in the following equations:

$$\rho_{p,dis} = M^{-0.8} \tag{13}$$

$$\frac{M_{pt}}{M_{p\infty}} = M^{-1.05} \tag{14}$$

$$\frac{M_{dt}}{M_{d\infty}} = M^{-0.24} \tag{15}$$

2. Swelling Restricted Matrix Tablet

The use of swellable matrix tablets in controlled release is of great interest due to their ease of preparation and low cost. Many attempts have been made to adapt the release rate to therapeutic needs. A number of papers focused on the modification of the matrix release rate using external surface interventions (80–89).

The partial coating of swellable matrix tablets containing soluble polymers with impermeable films created conditions for attainment of zero-order release. In fact, by covering one base and the lateral surface of the cylindrical matrix, a constant area for matrix swelling and drug release was obtained. The time needed for reaching constant drug release was related to the polymer solubility, which determined the matrix front synchronization. By using less soluble polymers, such as HPMC, front synchronization cannot be obtained during the release time. In this case, as showed by Conte et al. (62), the swelling of the matrix predominated over the erosion and polymer dissolution phenomena. Only when a low percentage (5% w/w) of HPMC was used for matrix formulation, an attempt of synchronization did appear, as seen by the trend of gel layer thickness values.

In addition, Shenouda et al. (90) presented data indicating the possibility of obtaining the linear release of diphylline from HPMC (Methocel K4M) matrix coated on the side wall and one base with the water-soluble poly(ethyloxazoline); however, in this case no data concerning front movement were given.

The possibility of modifying the kinetics of drug release from HPMC swellable matrix tablets has also been investigated by alteration of the swelling of the matrix. In order to achieve drug release modulation from swellable matrix, Colombo et al. (68,84) first described a new method for the manufacture of HPMC swelling restricted matrices by partially coating different portions of the external matrix surface with an impermeable film. The idea was to change the swelling rate of the matrix by reduction of the surface available for water uptake, leaving the diffusional characteristics of the drug practically unchanged. HPMC (Methocel K 100M) cylindrical matrix tablets containing diltiazem HCl were partially coated with an acetone solution of cellulose acetate propionate, in order to obtain impermeable film after water evaporation. The systems prepared were the uncoated matrix used as reference (case 0), the matrix coated on one base (case 1), the matrix coated on two bases (case 2), the matrix coated on the lateral surface (case 3), and the matrix coated on one base and the lateral surface (case 4).

The analysis of matrix swelling during drug release demonstrated that the presence on the surface of partial coatings strongly affected the changes in the matrix morphology. The swelling behavior of the five cases was quantified by measuring the releasing area (uncoated surface) vs.

time (Fig. 7). It was evident that the increase in the coated surface of the matrix determined a reduction of the rate of increase of area available for drug release, along with a modification of swelling kinetics. As a consequence, drug release kinetics varied. In particular, the release rate curves of cases 2 and 4 were close to linearity a short time after the beginning of release. The analysis of release data according to Eq. 1 revealed an anomalous transport for all of the systems exhibiting, for case 2–4 systems, n values of 0.79 and 0.76, respectively. It was concluded that the presence of the coating altered the relationship between swelling and drug transport, with respect to the uncoated matrix.

A more detailed analysis of these data was done by means of Eq. 5. In order to show the contribution to drug release of polymer relaxation and drug diffusion in the gel layer, drug release was described in terms of an R/F ratio (Eq. 6). Figure 8 shows that the presence of impermeable coating shifted the ratio of the two release mechanisms toward an increase of the relaxational contribution. Additionally, as anticipated for the uncoated matrix, a linear relationship between matrix swelling and drug release was found when the amount of drug released was plotted vs. the corresponding releasing area (Fig. 9). This confirmed the dependence of drug release from swelling area. In fact, after normalization of the different release rates of the five cases with the corresponding releasing areas, insignificantly different drug fluxes were observed. Therefore, in systems in which front synchronization cannot be achieved during the release time, the swelling kinetics, expressed as increase of releasing area, controls the release kinetics.

As the partially coated swellable matrices are characterized by a substantial change of release surface as a function of the extent of coating applied, the previously described swelling area numbers, Sa, for the five systems were compared at the same value of fraction release. Sa is particularly useful for the analysis of systems having the same composition, but exhibiting different rates of swelling. It was observed that, among the five cases, Sa values scaled in the same order as the corresponding drug release kinetics, which approached linearity when the

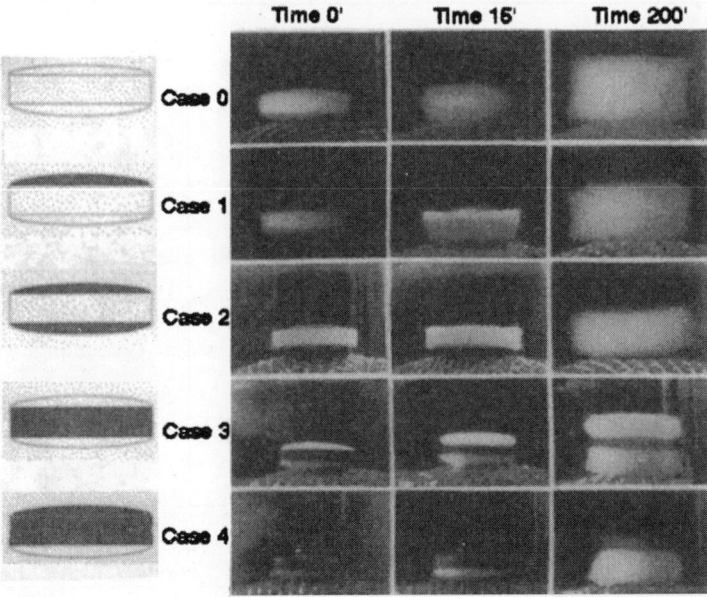

Figure 7 Swelling behavior of partially coated swelling matrix tablets at different times. (Modified from Ref. 75.)

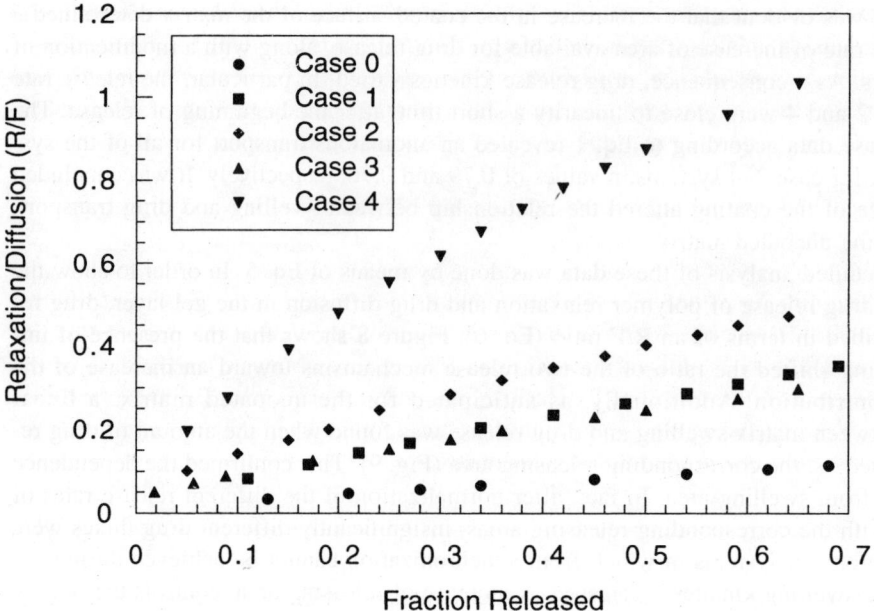

Figure 8 Ratio between relaxational and diffusional contribution to drug release vs. time of partially coated swellable matrix tablets at different times. (Modified from Ref. 75.)

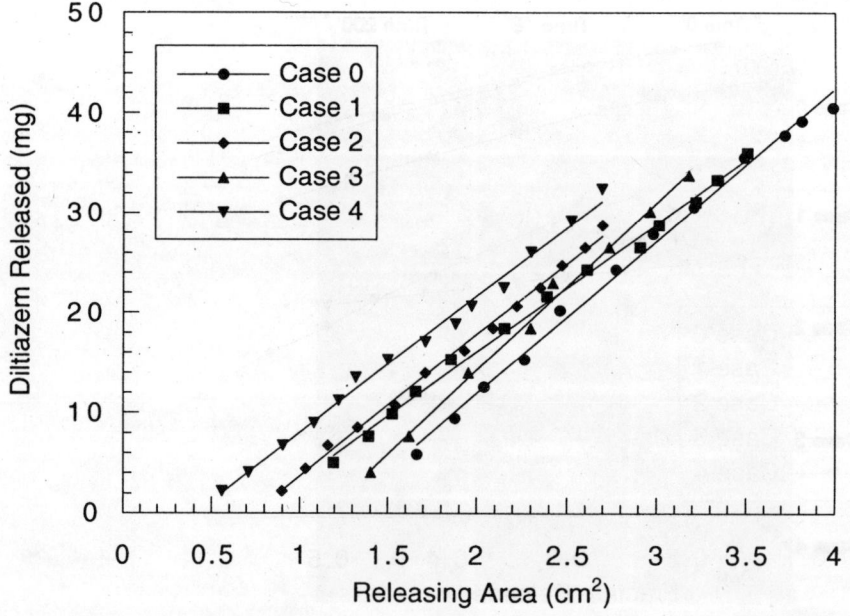

Figure 9 Relationship between drug released and releasing area for partially coated swelling matrix tablets at different times. (Modified from Ref. 75.)

Drug Release from Swelling-Controlled Systems

releasing area production rate decreased (Fig. 10). Once more, when the polymer dissolution is negligible, the releasing area increase is the variable controlling drug release.

Additional studies on swelling-restricted matrices were done by Bettini et al. (76) who measured the release of a very soluble drug, i.e., buflomedil pyridoxal phosphate, from matrices prepared with three different grades of HPMC (Methocel K 4M, K 15M, and K 100M) and coated as case 1 and case 2. The analysis of the swelling behavior, obtained by comparing the releasing area normalized over initial value, demonstrated that the location of coating on the two bases of the cylindrical matrix (case 2) strongly affected the swelling kinetics shown by the uncoated matrix (case 0) (Fig. 11). By plotting the fraction of drug released vs. the releasing area for the case 2 system made with the less viscous polymer, Methocel K 4M, an evident positive deviation from the linearity was observed, suggesting a certain liability to erosion.

A mathematical analysis of water transport and drug release from swellable matrix tablets coated with impermeable film was done by Hariharan et al. (91) for the case 0, case 1, and case 2 systems. According to this model, water and drug transport in swellable systems were described by Fick's second law in cylindrical coordinates:

$$\frac{\partial c_i}{\partial t} = \frac{D_d}{r} \frac{\partial}{\partial r}\left(\frac{1}{r} \frac{\partial c_i}{\partial r}\right) + D_i \frac{\partial^2 c_i}{\partial z^2} \tag{16}$$

where c_i is the concentration of the diffusing species (water or drug), D_i is the diffusion coefficient of the diffusing species, r is the radial coordinate, and z is the axial coordinate.

The model was solved numerically for the three mentioned cases, under fixed boundary conditions based on the type of system. The initial diameter-to-thickness ratio of tablet was selected as 7:5 or 2:1, to indicate special cases of interest. The most interesting result was that, although the overall water uptake vs. time for cases 0 and 1 systems could be fitted to the $t^{1/2}$ dependence, the case 2 system did not fit this relationship. As a consequence, a non-Fickian

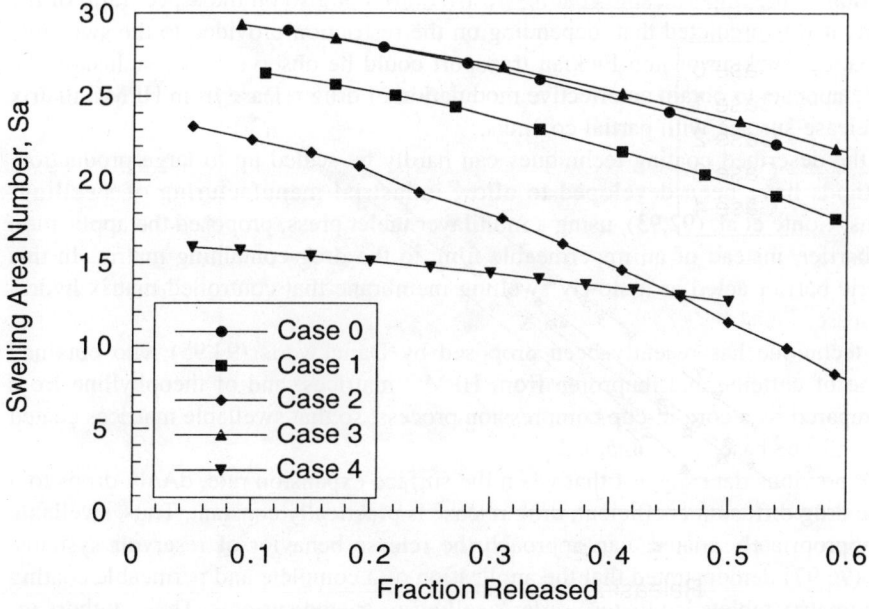

Figure 10 Calculated swelling area number as a function of drug released from partially coated swelling matrix tablets at different times. (Modified from Ref. 75.)

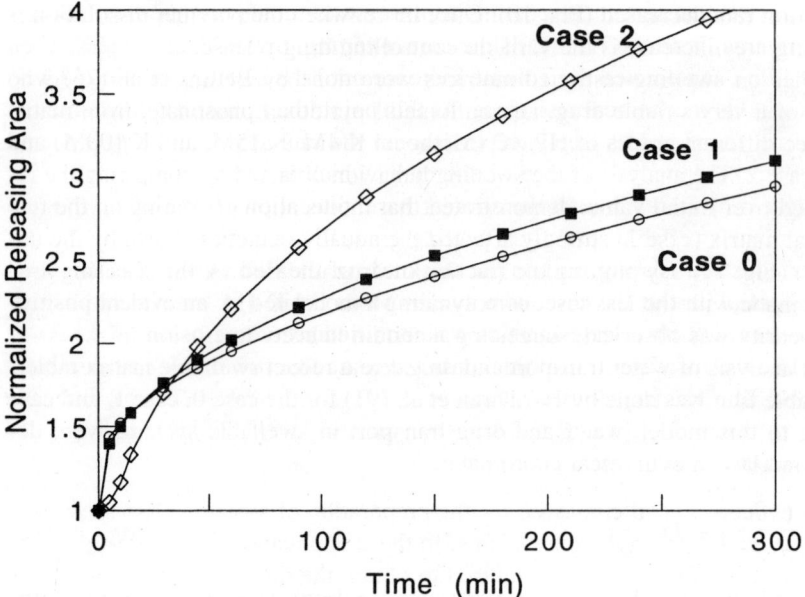

Figure 11 Area of release normalized over the initial value of three partially coated swelling matrix tablets at different times. (Modified from Ref. 76.)

behavior was expected in case 2 tablets with an aspect ratio of 7:5. The appreciable change in the relaxational behavior of the swellable system was attributed to the restrictions of swelling due to the coating. Moreover, dynamic swelling and drug release behavior were dependent not only on the position of the impermeable coating (restriction), but also on the aspect ratio of the matrix. Therefore, it was predicted that, depending on the restriction provided to the swellable matrix by the coating, Fickian or non-Fickian transport could be observed. In conclusion, the possibility clearly appears to obtain an effective modulation of drug release from HPMC matrix by altering the release surface with partial coatings.

However, the described coating techniques can hardly be scaled up to large production. Alternative methods have been developed to allow industrial manufacturing of swelling-restricted systems. Conte et al. (92,93), using a multilayer tablet press, proposed the application of a polymeric barrier, instead of an impermeable film, to the drug-containing matrix. In this way the polymeric barrier acted as a slowly swelling membrane that controlled matrix hydration and drug release.

A similar technique has recently been proposed by Danckwerts (94,95) who obtained zero-order release of caffeine and ibuprofen from HPMC matrices, and of theophylline from acacia matrix, prepared by a core-in-cup compression process, so that swellable matrices coated on the side wall and one base were obtained.

Finally, the previous data suggest that when the surface expansion rate, dA/dt, drops to a value close to the drug diffusion coefficient, drug release is practically constant. Thus, swellable matrix tablets, appropriately coated, can approach the release behavior of reservoir systems. Gazzaniga et al. (96,97) demonstrated that the application of a complete and permeable coating on swellable minimatrix tablets led to zero-order swelling-restricted systems. These authors investigated the in vitro release kinetics of verapamil HCl and dyprophylline from HPMC (Methocel K 15M) minimatrix tablets, pan-coated with a film obtained from a mixture of

Eudragit RL, RS, and E. Depending on the coating applied, water could more or less rapidly permeate the film and interact with the HPMC of the core, exerting, by swelling, a pressure on the covering film. The film counteracted the volume increase until the swelling pressure developed by the core overcame its mechanical resistance. At this point, the film broke down and the core increased its volume, more or less freely, depending on the rate at which the film peeled away. Usually the film broke down at an edge of the core, which is the weakest point of its structure, and the fracture propagated around the circular base, thus allowing the swelling pressure to be squeezed from the swellable core. Core peeling gradually occurred depending on the relative composition of core and coating, and on the thickness of the film. As long as the coating remained on a substantial part of the core, core swelling was limited by the residual adherent coating. As a consequence, drug release kinetics was modified according to the thickness of the applied film (Fig. 12); the increase in film thickness led to a reduction of drug release rate, along with an increased linearity of kinetics.

3. Swelling Controlled Reservoir Systems

Recently, HPMC polymers have been employed for the preparation of swellable membranes or barriers for drug delivery control in reservoir systems. In these applications, the complete transition of the barrier from glassy to rubbery is required to obtain the diffusion of the drug from the reservoir. Therefore, drug release is delayed for the period of time required for the hydration of the barrier.

After attainment of barrier hydration, drug release proceeds according to a constant rate, until the reservoir contains solid drug. The feasibility of the idea of applying a swellable barrier in order to manufacture delayed release forms was already demonstrated several years ago by using PVA polymers (98). In a similar way, Conte et al. (99) suggested the use of a dry coating technique using HPMC polymer for manufacturing press-coated systems capable of releasing a

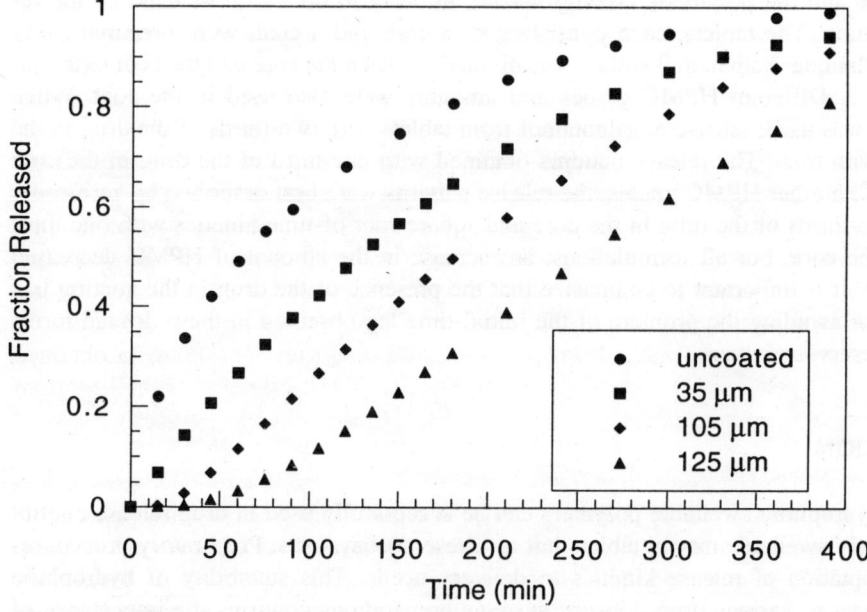

Figure 12 Drug release curves of swellable minimatrix tablets uncoated and coated with different film thickness. (Modified from Ref. 97.)

drug at a specific rate. In these systems the release starts after a well-defined period of time. The mechanism of release from such a system is based on the presence of the swellable polymeric barrier around the core that hydrates slowly, thus preventing drug release for a programmable period of time, depending on the swelling and/or dissolution characteristics of the polymer. After a silent phase, i.e., time necessary for polymeric barrier to swell, a constant drug release was obtained.

Further applications of this concept of delaying the system's release were done for the pulsatile delivery of ibuprofen (100). A partially coated three-layer cylindrical tablet with two drug-loaded layers was prepared. Each drug layer contained half a dose of ibuprofen and was separated by an intermediate polymeric swellable layer. An outer impermeable film, applied on the base and the side of the three-layer tablet, sealed half the dose of drug and the swellable layer. The systems worked in vitro according to the following steps: The uncoated part of the system disintegrated quickly after contact with water giving rise to the first pulse of the drug. Then the swellable layer, which remained exposed to the dissolution medium, started swelling. When sufficient water diffused through the swollen barrier, disintegration by the second drug layer destroyed the swollen barrier and gave rise to the second pulse of ibuprofen. In vivo data demonstrated good correlation with the measured in vitro behavior.

Gazzaniga et al. (101–103) proposed the use of a high-viscosity HPMC polymeric coating to delay the release of drug from either spray or press-coated fast disintegrating cores. The technique of HPMC application by spray coating can be of particular interest especially for time-programmed release or for site-specific delivery. A burst delivery of indomethacin or verapamil after a predetermined lag phase, based on the water/polymeric coating interaction, was obtained. A more advanced system based on this procedure was successively proposed by the same authors for the oral delayed release of ketoprofen for colonic-specific delivery (104,105).

The development and biopharmaceutical evaluation of press-coated matrices have been widely investigated also by Sirkia et al. (106–108). The in vitro release kinetics of salbutamol was studied from press-coated tablets in which the drug was distributed in different ratios between the core and the polymeric coating barrier, in order to obtain an increase of the release rate with time. The tablets, each consisting of a core and a coat, were prepared using press-coating technique. Salbutamol sulfate was divided between the core and the coat in the ratio of 2:1 or 1:2. Different HPMC grades and amounts were also used in the coat. When HPMC K M100 was used, release of salbutamol from tablets with two-thirds of the drug in the core increased with time. The release patterns obtained with one-third of the drug in the core were biphasic. With other HPMC grades, the release patterns were best described by zero-order kinetics with two-thirds of the drug in the core and square-root-of-time kinetics with one-third of the drug in the core. For all formulations, an increase in the amount of HPMC decreased drug release rate. It is important to emphasize that the presence of the drug in the coating is a necessary tool for avoiding the problem of the initial time lag observed in these dosage forms that behave as reservoir systems.

V. CONCLUSION

In conclusion, hydrophilic swellable polymers can be successfully used in drug release control to prepare not only swellable matrix tablets but also reservoir systems. Preparatory procedures easily allow adaptation of release kinetics to delivery needs. This suitability of hydrophilic swellable polymers to various drug delivery systems preparations confirms the importance of these specialized excipients in pharmaceutical applications. They certainly represent the choice solution for many oral delivery problems.

Moreover, the literature continuously provides new information on the factors that control drug release from these systems. Drug dissolution and diffusion in the gel layer, matrix erosion, and polymer swelling are the main mechanisms studied. Their combination results in the release kinetics observed. Much work remains to be done to clarify the relative importance of each mechanism, in order to provide to the formulator an easy tool for tailoring the desired drug release profile.

REFERENCES

1. Korsmeyer, R. W., and N. A. Peppas, (1983) Macromolecular and modelling aspects of swelling-controlled systems. In: T. J. Roseman and Z. F. Mansdorf (Eds.), Controlled Release Delivery Systems, Marcel Dekker, New York, pp. 77–89.
2. Lee, P. I. (1985) Kinetics of drug release from hydrogel matrices, J. Controlled Release, 2, 277–288.
3. Mockel, J. E., and B. C. Lippold (1993) Zero-order drug release from hydrocolloid matrices, Pharm. Res., 10, 1066–1070.
4. Ford, J. L. (1994) Fundamental aspects of drug release from hydrophilic matrix tablets. Proc. Colorcon Controlled Release Symposium, Vols. 1–26.
5. Korsmeyer, R. W., S. R. Lustig, and N. A. Peppas (1986) Solute and penetrant diffusion in swellable polymers. I. Mathematical modeling, J. Polym. Sci. B Polym. Phys., 24, 395–408.
6. Korsmeyer, R. W., E. von Meerwall, and N. A. Peppas (1986) Solute and penetrant diffusion in swellable polymers. II. Verification of theoretical models, J. Polym. Sci. B Polym. Phys., 24, 409–434.
7. Hopfenberg, H. B., and H. L. Frisch (1969) Transport of organic micromolecules in amorphous polymers, Polym. Lett. 7, 405–409.
8. Kwei, T. K., T. T. Wang, and H. M. Zupko (1972) Diffusion in glassy polymers. V. Combination of Fickian and case II mechanisms, Macromolecules, 5, 645–649.
9. Astarita, G., and G. C. Sarti (1978) A class of mathematical models for sorption of swelling solvents in glassy polymers, Polym. Eng. Sci., 18, 388–395.
10. Franson N. M., and N. A. Peppas (1983) Influence of copolymer composition on non-Fickian water transport through glassy copolymers, J. Appl. Polym. Sci., 28, 1299–1310.
11. Wu, J. C., and N. A. Peppas (1993) Modeling of penetrant diffusion in glassy polymers with an integral sorption Deborah number, J. Polym. Sci. B Polym. Phys., 31, 1503–1518.
12. Alfrey, T., Jr., E. F. Gurnee, and W. G. Lloyd (1966) Diffusion in glassy polymers, J. Polym. Sci. C, 12, 249–261.
13. Frisch, H. L., T. T. Wang, and T. K. Kwei (1969) Diffusion in glassy polymers. II., J. Polym. Sci., A2, 7 879–887.
14. Wang, T. T., T. K. Kwei, and H. L. Frisch, (1969) Diffusion in glassy polymers. III., J. Polym. Sci. A2, 7, 2019–2028.
15. Crank, J., (1953) A theoretical investigation of the influence of molecular relaxation and internal stress on diffusion in polymers, J. Polym. Sci., 11, 151–168.
16. Thomas, N., and A. H. Windle, (1978) Transport of methanol in poly(methyl methacrylate), Polymer, 19, 255–265.
17. Peterlin, A., (1979) Diffusion with discontinuous swelling. V. Type II diffusion into sheets and spheres, J. Polym. Sci. B Polym. Phys., 17, 1741–1756.
18. Ritger, P. L., and N. A. Peppas, (1987) A simple equation for description of solute release. II. Fickian and anomalous release from swellable devices, J. Controlled Release, 5, 37–42.
19. Orienti, I., E. Gianasi, V. Zecchi, and U. Conte, (1995) Release of ketoprofen from microspheres of poly(2-hydroxyethyl methacrylate) or poly(2-hydroxyethyl methacrylate-co-b methacryloyloxyethyl deoxycholate) crosslinked with ethylene glycol dimethacrylate and tetraethylene glycol dimethacrylate, Eur. J. Pharm. Biopharm., 41, 247–253.

20. Davidson, G. W. R. III, and N. A. Peppas, (1986) Solute and penetrant diffusion in swellable polymers V. Relaxation controlled transport in P(HEMA-co-MMA) copolymers, J. Controlled Release, 3 243–258.
21. Colombo, P., R. Bettini, P. Santi, A. De Ascentiis, and N. A. Peppas, (1996) Analysis of the swelling and release mechanisms from drug delivery systems with emphasis on drug solubility and water transport, J. Controlled Release, 39, 231–237.
22. Thomas, N. L., and A. H. Windle (1982) A theory of case II diffusion, Polymer, 23, 529–542.
23. Thomas, N. L., and A. H. Windle, (1981) Diffusion mechanics of the system PMMA-methanol, Polymer, 22, 627–639.
24. Windle, A. H., Case II Sorption. In: J. Cowyn (Ed.), Polymer Permeability, Elsevier, London, 1985, pp. 75–118.
25. Gehrke, S. H., N. Vaid, and L. Uhden. (1995) Enhanced loading and activity retention of proteins in hydrogel delivery systems, Proc. Int. Symp. Control. Rel. Bioact. Mater., 22, pp. 145–146.
26. Koda, S., K. Yamashita, S. Iwai, and H. Nomura, (1994) Ultrasonic investigation of the states of water in hydrogels, Polymer, 35, 5626–5629.
27. Xu, H., and J. Vij, (1994) Wide-band dielectric spectroscopy of hydrated poly(hydroxyethyl methacrylate), Polymer, 35, 227–234.
28. Roorda, W. (1994) Review: Do hydrogels contain different classes of water? J. Biomater. Sci. Polym. Edn., 5, 383–395.
29. Vrentas, J. S., C. M. Jarzebski, and J. L. Duda, (1975) A Deborah number for diffusion in polymer–solvent systems, AIChE J., 21, 894–901.
30. Peppas, N. A., and N. M. Franson (1983) The swelling interface number as a criterion for prediction of diffusional solute release mechanisms in swellable polymers, J. Polym. Sci. B Polym. Phys., 21, 983–997.
31. Peppas, N. A., and A. R. Khare, Preparation, structure and diffusional behavior of hydrogels in controlled release, Adv. Drug Deliv. Rev., 11, 1–35.
32. Klier, J., and N. A. Peppas (1988) Solute and penetrant diffusion in swellable polymers. VIII. Influence of the swelling interface number on solute concentration profiles and release, J. Controlled Release, 7, 61–68.
33. Hopfenberg, H. B., and K. C. Hsu (1978) Swelling-controlled, constant rate delivery systems, Polym. Eng. Sci., 18, 1186–1191.
34. Pham, A. T., and P. I. Lee, (1994) Probing the mechanisms of drug release from hydroxypropylmethyl cellulose matrices, Pharm. Res., 11, 1379–1384.
35. Korsmeyer, R. W., R. Gurny, E. Doelker, P. Buri, and N. A. Peppas, (1983) Mechanisms of solute release from porous hydrophilic polymers, Int. J. Pharm., 15, 25–35.
36. Peppas, N. A., and L. Brannon-Peppas (1994) Water diffusion and sorption in amorphous macromolecular systems and food, J. Food Eng., 22, 189–210.
37. Lustig, S. R., and N. A. Peppas (1987) Solute and penetrant diffusion in swellable polymers. VII. A free volume–based model with mechanical relaxation, J. Appl. Polym. Sci., 33, 533–549.
38. Peppas, N. A. (1985) Analysis of Fickian and non-Fickian drug release from polymers, Pharm. Acta Helv., 60, 101–111.
39. Peppas, N. A., and J. J. Sahlin (1989) A simple equation for the description of solute release. III. Coupling of diffusion and relaxation, Int. J. Pharm., 57, 169–172.
40. Harland, R. S., and N. A. Peppas (1989) Solute diffusion in swollen membranes. VII. Diffusion in semicrystalline networks, Colloid Polym. Sci., 267, 218–225.
41. Brannon-Peppas, L., and N. A. Peppas (1989) Solute and penetrant diffusion in swellable polymers. IX. The mechanisms of drug release from pH-sensitive swelling-controlled systems, J. Controlled Release, 8, 267–274.
42. am Ende, M. T., D. Hariharan, and N. A. Peppas (1995) Factors influencing drug and protein transport from ionic hydrogels, Reactive Polym., 25, 127–137.
43. Caramella, C., F. Ferrari, M. C. Bonferoni, M. Ronchi, and P. Colombo, (1989) Rheological properties and diffusion dissolution behaviour of hydrophilic polymers, Boll. Chim. Farmaceutico, 128, 298–301.

44. Harland, R. S., A. Gazzaniga, M. E. Sangalli, P. Colombo, and N. A. Peppas (1988) Drug/polymer matrix swelling and dissolution, Pharm. Res., 5, 488–494.
45. Bonferoni M. F., S. Rossi, F. Ferrari, M. Bertoni, R. Sinistri, and C. Caramella (1995) Characteization of three hydroxypropylmethyl-cellulose substitution types: rheological properties and dissolution behaviour, Eur J. Pharm. Biopharm., 41, 242–246.
46. Lee, P. I. (1981) Controlled drug release from polymeric matrices involving moving boundaries. In: D. H. Levis (Ed.), Controlled Release of Pesticides and Pharmaceuticals, Plenum Publishing, New York, pp. 39–48.
47. Bettini, R., N. A. Peppas, and P. Colombo (1998) Polymer relaxation in swellable matrices contributes to drug release, Proc. Int. Symp. Control. Rel. Bioact. Mater., 25, pp. 26–37.
48. Lee, P. I., and C. Kim (1991) Probing the mechanisms of drug release from hydrogels, J. Controlled Release, 16, 229–236.
49. Colombo, P., R. Bettini, G. Massimo, P. L. Catellani, P. Santi, and N. A. Peppas (1995) Drug diffusion front movement is important in drug release control from swellable matrix tablets, J. Pharm. Sci., 84, 991–997.
50. Bettini, R., P. Colombo, G. Massimo, P. Santi, P. L. Catellani, and N. A. Peppas (1994) Moving fronts and drug release from hydrogel matrices, Proc. Int. Symp. Control. Rel. Bioact. Mater., 21, pp. 19–20.
51. Colombo, P., A. Gazzaniga, C. Caramella, U. Conte, and A. La Manna, (1987) In vitro programmable zero-order release drug delivery system, Acta Pharm. Technol., 33, 15–20.
52. Alderman, D. A. (1984) A review of cellulose ethers in hydrophilic matrices for oral controlled-release dosage form, Int. J. Pharm. Tech. Prod. Mfr., 5, 1–9.
53. Ranga Rao, K. V., and K. Padmalatha Devi (1988) Swelling controlled-release systems: recent developments and applications, Int. J. Pharm., 48, 1–13.
54. Hogan, J. E. (1989) Hydroxypropylmethylcellulose sustained release technology, Drug Dev. Ind. Pharm., 15, 975–999.
55. Sung K. C., P. R. Nixon, J. W. Skoug, T. R. Ju, P. Gao, E. M. Topp, and M. V. Patel (1996) Effect of formulation variables on drug and polymer release from HPMC-based matrix tables, Int. J. Pharm., 142, 53–60.
56. Veiga F., T. Salsa, M. E. Pina (1998) Oral controlled release dosage forms. II. Glassy polymers in hydrophilic matrices, Drug. Dev. Ind. Pharm., 24, 1–9.
57. Altaf S. A., K. Yu, J. Parasrampuria, and D. R. Friend (1998) Guar gum–based sustained release diltiazem, Pharm. Res., 15, 1196–1201.
58. Skoug, J. W., M. V. Mikelsons, C. N. Vigneron, and N. L. Stemm (1993) Qualitative evaluation of the mechanism of release of matrix sustained release dosage forms by measurement of polymer release, J. Controlled Release, 27, 227–245.
59. C-J. Kim (1995) Drug release from compressed hydrophilic Polyox-WSR tables, J. Pharm. Sci., 84, 303–306.
60. Catellani, P., P. Colombo, T. Vitali, and C. Caramella (1988) Modified release tablet formulation, Polym. Med., 3, 169–174.
61. Feely, I. C., and S. S. Davis (1988) The influence of polymeric excipients on drug release from hydroxypropylmethylcellulose matrices, Int. J. Pharm., 4, 131–139.
62. Conte, U., P. Colombo, A. Gazzaniga, M. E. Sangalli, and A. La Manna (1988) Swelling-activated drug delivery systems, Biomaterials, 9, 489–493.
63. Baveja, S. K., K. V. Ranga Rao, and K. Padmalatha Devi, (1987) Zero-order release hydrophylic matrix tablets of β-adrenergic blockers, Int. J. Pharm., 39, 39–45.
64. Kim, H., and R. Fasshi (1996) Application of a binary polymer system in drug release rate modulation. 1. Characterisation of release mechanism, J. Pharm. Sci., 86, 316–322.
65. Kim, H., and R. Fasshi (1996) Application of a binary polymer system in drug release rate modulation. 2. Influence of formulation variables and hydrodynamic conditions on release kinetics, J. Pharm. Sci., 86, 323–328.
66. Kim, H., and R. Fasshi (1997) A new ternary polymeric matrix system for controlled drug delivery of highly soluble drugs: I. Diltiazem hydrocloride, Pharm. Res., 14, 1415–1421.

67. Kabanda, L., R. A. Lefevre, H. J. Van Bree, and J. P. Remon (1994) In vitro and in vivo evaluation in dogs and pigs of a hydrophilic matrix containing propylthiouracil, Pharm. Res., 11, 1663–1668.
68. Colombo, P., U. Conte, L. Maggi, M. E. Sangalli, N. A. Peppas, and A. La Manna (1990) Drug release modulation by physical restrictions of matrix swelling, Int. J. Pharm., 63, 43–48.
69. Papadimitriou, E., G. Buckton, and M. Efentakis (1993) Probing the mechanism of swelling of hydroxypropylmethylcellulose matrices, Int. J. Pharm., 98, 57–62.
70. Rajabi-Siahboomi, A. R., R. W. Bowtell, P. Mansfield, A. Henderson, M. C. Davis, and C. D. Melia (1994) Structure and behaviour in hydrophilic matrix sustained release dosage forms: 2. NMR-imaging studies of dimensional changes in the gel layer and core of HPMC tablets undergoing hydration, J. Controlled Relese, 31, 121–128.
71. Gao P., and R. H. Meury (1996) Swelling of hydroxipropyl methylcellulose matrix tablets. 1. Characterisation of swelling using a novel optical imaging method, J. Pharm. Sci., 85, 725–731.
72. Brannon-Peppas, L., and N. A. Peppas (1990) Dynamic and equilibrium swelling behaviour of pH-sensitive hydrogels containing 2-hydroxyethylmethacrylate, Biomaterials, 11, 635–644.
73. Wan, L. S. C., P. W. S. Heng, and L. F. Wong (1994) Effect of additives on liquid uptake into hydroxypropylmethylcellulose matrices, S.T.P. Pharma Sci., 4, 213–219.
74. Wan, L. S. C., P. W. S. Heng, and L. F. Wong (1992) Relationship between polymer viscosity and drug release from a matrix system, Pharm. Res., 9, 1510–1514.
75. Colombo, P., P. Catellani, N. A. Peppas, L. Maggi, and U. Conte (1992) Swelling characteristics of hydrophilic matrices for controlled release: new dimensionless number to describe the swelling and release behaviour, Int. J. Pharm., 88, 99–109.
76. Bettini, R., P. Colombo, G. Massimo, P. Catellani, and T. Vitali (1994) Swelling and drug release in hydrogel matrices: polymer viscosity and matrix porosity effects, Eur. J. Pharm. Sci., 2, 213–219.
77. Peppas, N. A., R. Gurny, E. Doelker, and P. Buri (1980) Modelling of drug diffusion through swellable polymeric systems, J. Membr. Sci., 7, 241–253.
78. Lee, P. I., and N. A. Peppas (1987) Prediction of polymer dissolution in swellable controlled-release systems, J. Controlled Release, 6, 207–215.
79. Ju, R. T. C., P. R. Nixon, M. V. Patel, and D. M. Tong (1995) Drug release from hydrophilic matrices. 2. A mathematical model based on the polymer disentanglement concentration and the diffusion layer, J. Pharm. Sci., 84, 1464–1477.
80. Vandelli, M. A., G. Coppi, and R. Cameroni (1993) Selective coating of cylindrical matrices with a central hole. II. An interpretation of the release process, Int J. Pharm., 100, 115–121.
81. Conte, U., L. Maggi, M. L. Torre, P. Giunchedi, and A. La Manna (1993) Press-coated tablets for time-programmed release of drugs, Biomaterials, 14, 1017–1023.
82. Gazzaniga, A., M. E. Sangalli, U. Conte, C. Caramella, P. Colombo, and A. La Manna, (1993) On the release mechanism from coated swellable minimatrices, Int. J. Pharm., 91, 167–171.
83. Santi, P., P. L. Catellani, A. Cassarà, and P. Colombo (1989) Alprenolol-HCl compressed matrices: discontinuous barrier for zero order release rate, Chimica Oggi, 21–23.
84. Colombo, P., L. Maggi, A. Gazzaniga, U. Conte, A. La Manna, and N. A. Peppas (1988) Drug release from sweallable matrices restricted by impermeable film coatings, Proc. Int. Symp. Control. Rel. Mater., 15, 40–41.
85. Bettini, R., G. Massimo, P. L. Catellani, N. A. Peppas, and P. Colombo (1995) Zero order release by partial coating of HPMC matrix tablets with permeable and semipermeable films, Proc. 1st World Meeting Pharmaceutics, Biopharm., Pharm. Technol., 288–289.
86. Chidambaram, N., W. Porter, K. Flood, and Y. Qiu (1998) Formulation and characterisation of new layered diffusional matrices for zero-order release, J. Controlled Release, 52, 149–158.
87. Munday, D. L. (1996) Bimodal in vitro release from polymeric matrix tablets containing centralised drug cores, S.T.P. Pharma Sci., 6, 182–187.
88. Yang L., and R. Fassihi (1997) Examination of drug solubility, polymer types, hydrodynamics and loading dose on drug release behavior from a triple-layer asymmetric configuration delivery system, Int. J. Pharm., 155, 219–229.

89. Catellani, P. L., P. Colombo, N. A. Peppas, P. Santi, and R. Bettini (1998) Partial permselective coating adds an osmotic contribution to drug release from swellable matrixes, J. Pharm. Sci, 87, 726–731.
90. Shenouda, L. S., K. A. Adams, and M. A. Zoglio (1990) A controlled release delivery system using two hydrophilic polymers, Int. J. Pharm., 61, 127–134.
91. Hariharan, D., N. A. Peppas, R. Bettini, and P. Colombo (1994) Mathematical analysis of drug delivery from swellable systems with partial physical restrictions or impermeable coatings, Int. J. Pharm., 112, 47–54.
92. Conte, U., L. Maggi, P. Colombo, and A. La Manna (1993) Multi-layered hydrophilic matrices as costant release devices (Geomatrix systems), J. Controlled Release, 26, 37–47.
93. Conte U., and L. Maggi (1988) Multy-layer tablets as drug delivery devices, Pharm. Tech. Eur.
94. Danckwerts, M. P. (1994) Development of a zero-order release oral compressed tablet with potential for commercial tabletting production, Int. J. Pharm., 112, 37–45.
95. Danckwerts, M. P., J. G. van der Watt, and I. Moodley (1998) Zero-order release of theophylline from a core-in-cup tablet in sequenced simulated gastric and intestinal fluid, Drug. Dev. Ind. Pharm., 24, 163–167.
96. Gazzaniga, A., M. E. Sangalli, U. Conte, C. Caramella, P. Colombo, and A. La Manna (1988) Swellable minimatrices for controlled release of drugs, Proc. Int. Symp. Control. Rel. Bioact. Mater., 15, 464–465.
97. Gazzaniga, A., P. Colombo, M. E. Sangalli, C. Caramella, and A. La Manna (1988) A multiple unit modified release system, Polym. Med., 3, 201–208.
98. Conte, U., P. Colombo, C. Caramella, and A. La Manna (1984) Press-coated, zero order drug delivery system, Il Farmaco, 39, 67–75.
99. Conte, U., L. Maggi, M. L. Torre, P. Giunchedi, and A. La Manna (1993) Press-coated tablets for time programmed release of drugs, Biomaterials, 14, 1017–1023.
100. Conte, U., P. Giunchedi, L. Maggi, M. E. Sangalli, A. Gazzaniga, P. Colombo, and A. La Manna (1992) Ibuprofen delayed release dosage forms: a proposal for the preparation of an in vitro-in vivo pulsatile system, Eur. J. Pharm. Biopharm., 38, 209–212.
101. Maffione, G., P. Iamartino, and A. Gazzaniga (1991) High-viscosity HPMC as a film-coating agent, Proc. 10th Pharm. Technol. Conf., 3, 66–73.
102. Maffione, G., P. Iamartino, G. Guglielmi, and A. Gazzaniga (1993) High-viscosity HPMC as a film-coating agent, Drug Dev. Ind. Pharm., 19, 2043–2053.
103. Gazzaniga, A., M. E. Sangalli, and F. Giordano (1994) Oral Chronotropic drug delivery systems: achievment of time and/or site specificity, Eur. J. Pharm. Biopharm., 40, 246–250.
104. Gazzaniga, A., P. Iamartino, G. Maffione, and M. E. Sangalli (1994) Oral delayed-release system for colonic specific delivery, Int. J. Pharm., 108, 77–83.
105. Gazzaniga, A., C. Busetti, L. Moro, M. E. Sangalli, and F. Giordano (1995) Time-dependent oral delivery systems for colon targeting, S.T.P. Pharma Sci., 5, 83–88.
106. Sirkia, T., J. Antila, M. Marvola, M. Kauppi, and I. Happonen (1993) Use of hydrophilic polymers to control drug release from press-coated oxybutynin hydrochloride tablets, S.T.P. Pharma Sci., 3, 453–458.
107. Sirkia, T., M. Makiimarti, S. Liukko-Sipi, and M. Marvola (1994) Developement and biopharmaceutical evaluation of a new press-coated prolonged-release salbutamol sulphate tablet in man, Eur. J. Pharm. Sci., 1, 195–201.
108. Sirkia, T., J. Niemi, T. Lindqvist, and I. Happonen (1994) Effect of potassium carbonate and viscosity grade of hydroxypropylmethylcellulose on the bioavailability of furosemide from press-coated prolonged-released tablets, S.T.P. Pharma Sci., 4, 257–263.

10
Superporous Hydrogels as a Platform for Oral Controlled Drug Delivery

Jun Chen, Haesun Park, and Kinam Park
Purdue University, West Lafayette, Indiana

I. INTRODUCTION

A. Importance of Gastric Retention Devices

The importance of controlled drug delivery systems that release bioactive components over an extended period of time has long been recognized in the pharmaceutical field. Of the many routes of drug delivery, oral administration remains the most convenient and commonly employed means for introducing drugs to the systemic circulation. Recent advances in controlled release technology have made it possible to release drugs at a constant rate for days to years. Application of such controlled release technology to oral drug delivery, however, has been limited because the actual time for effective drug delivery is restricted by the gastrointestinal transit time, which typically ranges from several hours to 12 h depending on various factors (1). Thus, unless a drug has a long half-life, it needs to be administered a few times a day.

Gastric retention devices are designed to prolong the gastric residence time of oral controlled release dosage forms. Thus, they result in increased contact time for drugs that act locally, such as pepsin inhibitor and gastric acid secretion inhibitor, increased absorption for drugs that have absorption windows, and better absorption for drugs less soluble in the intestinal fluid.

B. Physiology of Gastric Emptying

There are two distinct modes (i.e., fasted and fed) of gastrointestinal motility patterns that consume food in humans and animals. In the fed state, the stomach handles liquids and solid materials in different ways (2–4). Liquids are emptied first (usually within 30 min) by the slow and sustained contractions of the proximal stomach (5,6). The gastric emptying time of a solid meal depends on the type (7,8), nutrition density (9), quantity, and particle size (10) of the meal. It can be extended to over 14 h if fed state conditions are maintained (11). Particles less than 5 mm in diameter are known to be emptied by the contraction of the distal stomach following the emptying of liquids. Emptying of the solid digestible food particles larger than 5 mm is delayed until they are reduced in size by the grinding action of the stomach (12). Indigestible solids larger than 5 mm in diameter are retained within the stomach until the digestive process is complete. The gastric emptying time for a regular meal is about 2–6 h (13).

The emptying of large indigestible objects from the stomach is dependent on the contraction activity of the interdigestive migrating motor complex (IMMC) (12,14,15). The IMMC, which occurs only in the fasted state (i.e., the state in which the liquids and digestible solid foods been cleared from the stomach completely), is characterized by three phases of myoelectric and motor activity (12,15). Phase I, represented by a period of motor inactivity with only rare contraction, lasts about 45–60 min. Phase II, marked with random peristaltic activity with increased frequency and amplitude, lasts over a 30- to 45-min period. Phase III, the "active front," represents the intense burst of action potentials and contractions which continue for 5–10 min. This powerful electromechanical activity of phase III sweeps slowly from the stomach to the ileum and is responsible for emptying of indigestible debris left over from a meal. (This is called the "housekeeper" wave of the gastrointestinal tract) (6). The gastric emptying time for the conventional nondisintegrating dosage forms is mainly determined by the onset of phase III activity of IMMC. On an average, this cyclical pattern occurs every 120 min in fasted humans. Under the fasted condition, the gastric empty time of insoluble drug formulation is usually 1–2 h. Consequently, for once-a-day oral drug delivery to be feasible, the gastric retention device must be constructed to overcome the peristaltic contraction associated with phase III of the IMMC.

C. Previous Studies on Gastric Retention Devices

Several different approaches have been developed to achieve extended gastric residence time of the oral drug delivery systems. This particular topic was recently reviewed by Hwang et al. (16).

1. Food Excipient Method

Incorporation of passage-delaying food excipients, especially fatty acids, can extend the gastric emptying time (17,18). More than 2 h gastric residence time was achieved in the fasted state when triethanolamine myristate was used as excipient (17).

2. Floating Devices

Floating dosage forms have a bulk density lower than that of gastric fluids and therefore, are expected to remain buoyant on the stomach contents to prolong the gastric retention time (19–21). For the floating dosage forms to be effective, however, large amounts of water have to be present in the stomach all the time. Since, as mentioned before, the stomach empties liquids very quickly (within 30 min), these floating devices will not be effective without continuous drinking of large quantities of water. Davis et al. (22) studied floating capsules and tablets and found that their gastric retention had little or no advantage over the traditional dosage forms.

3. High-Density Dosage Forms

Bechgaard and Ladefoged (23) attempted to prolong the gastric retention time by the use of high-density pellets. They reported that for ileostomy subjects the average transit time for light and heavy pellets (density = 1.0 g/cm^3 and 1.6 g/cm^3, respectively) from mouth to ileostomy bag were 7 and 25 h, respectively. However, more recent studies by the same group showed that such differences did not exist (24).

4. Mucoadhesive Dosage Forms

These dosage forms are based on the adhesive capacities of some polymers with mucins covering the surface epithelium of the stomach. For examples, polycarbophil or crosslinked poly(acrylic acid) (25,26) and a hydrophobic protein called zein (27) were used to design formulations that can adhere to the stomach lining for the extended gastric retention. The main weakness of this approach is that the mucoadhesives can be easily contaminated by the soluble mucins and other proteins present in the gastric juice. This leads to loss of their adhesive capacity to the stomach lining.

5. Dosage Forms with Special Shapes

Cargill et al. reported certain shape elastomers or plastics made from polyethylene or nylon could increase the gastric retention time (28). Tetrahedrons (each leg 2 cm in length) and rings (3.6 cm in diameter) provided gastric retention longer than 24 h. These dosage forms, however, were neither digestible nor easy to load and release drugs.

6. Magnetic Dosage Forms

"Magnetic tablets" were made by mixing ferrite powder with other excipients (29,30). After administration, these tablets were retained in the stomach by an externally applied strong magnetic field. The strong external magnetic field, however, is not readily available in practical use.

7. Balloon Devices

Michaels et al. (31) developed a device that comprised a collapsed envelope containing a liquid, such as n-pentane, converting to a gas at body temperature. The device can expand to a size larger than the pyloric canal for retention in the stomach. Instead of low-boiling-point organic solvents, osmotic agents can be used to inflate the envelope (32). This approach, while effective, is not easy to implement.

8. Highly Swelling Hydrogel Dosage Forms

Hydrogels can be retained in the stomach by swelling to a size larger than that of the pyloric canal (33–35). Although a hydrogel can swell to hundreds of times its dried size, its swelling is very slow. It takes several hours before it reaches a size large enough to be retained in the stomach. Because the cyclic IMMC movement occurs every 2 h, the hydrogel is most likely to be expelled from the stomach before it swells to a required size. Thus, hydrogels should possess a fast swelling property to be useful as a gastric retention device.

For the last several years, we have focused on preparation of hydrogels that quickly swell to equilibrium size regardless of size. Recently, we synthesized superporous hydrogels with fast swelling and superabsorbent properties.

II. PRINCIPLE AND REQUIREMENTS FOR THE GASTRIC RETENTION OF SUPERPOROUS HYDROGELS

A. Principle of the Gastric Retention of Superporous Hydrogels

The gastric retention of superporous hydrogels is based on their fast swelling property. The idea of the approach is described in Fig. 1. A superporous hydrogel is enclosed in a capsule so that the initial volume is small for easy swallowing (Fig. 1A). After oral administration, it swells quickly in the gastric juice to a large size, so that its emptying into the intestine is prevented. When the gastric contraction reaches the hydrogel, the gastric tissues slide over the hydrogel (Fig. 1B–D), since it is elastic and slippery. While a drug is released from this dosage form, it slowly undergoes degradation in the stomach by either mechanical force or chemical/enzymatic

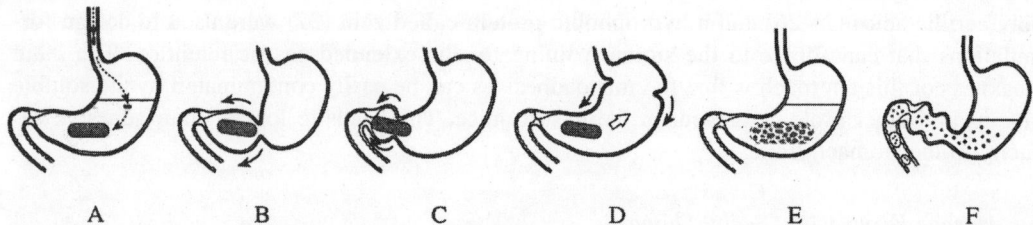

Figure 1 Schematic description of gastric retention and subsequent emptying of a superporous hydrogel.

hydrolysis of the polymer chains constituting the hydrogel (Fig. 1E). Eventually, the degraded superporous hydrogel dosage form is eliminated from the stomach (Fig. 1F). The sequence shown in Fig. 1 is based on animal studies conducted on gastric retention of hydrogels (33,34,36).

B. Requirements for Gastric Retention of Superporous Hydrogels for Drug Delivery

For practical use in oral drug delivery the superporous hydrogels must possess the following properties. First, the size is small enough for easy swallowing. In our study, hard gelatin capsules with size 000 were used to house the superporous hydrogel dosage form. Second, swelling is fast enough to overcome the gastric emptying by IMMC. Third, the size of the swollen gel is large enough to be retained in the stomach. The diameter of the pyloric sphincter is about 2 cm in humans. Under normal conditions, the pylorus sphincter is closed. However, it could be stretched and pass an object larger than 2 cm. Fourth, the swollen gel should be strong enough to withstand the peristaltic contraction. The maximal stomach contraction pressure in humans is about 50–70 cm water pressure (37). This number, however, reflects only the direct compression pressure. Abrasion and shear forces are also present in the stomach. Therefore, to maintain the superporous hydrogel as an integral dosage form, it must be able to withstand much higher pressure than the 50–70 cm water pressure.

To be applicable in humans as a drug delivery vehicle, a superporous hydrogel dosage form should be emptied from the stomach after drugs are released. This could be achieved by either mechanical degradation to break the dosage form into small pieces or by chemical/enzymatic degradation by incorporating biodegradable crosslinkers, such as glycidyl acrylate–modified albumin (36).

III. SYNTHESIS AND CHARACTERIZATION OF SUPERPOROUS HYDROGELS

A. Preparation of Superporous Hydrogels for Gastric Retention Study

1. Synthesis of Superporous Hydrogels

Synthesis of superporous hydrogels is similar to the synthesis of ordinary hydrogels except that a foaming agent is added to make superporous hydrogels. The timing of the polymerization has to be matched with the timing of foam formation. If the kinetics of the two processes are different, then superporous hydrogels with interconnected pores will not be formed (38). Figure 2 describes the foaming process for the preparation of superporous hydrogels. The key to this process is to use acid to control the polymerization kinetics. Addition of $NaHCO_3$ results in

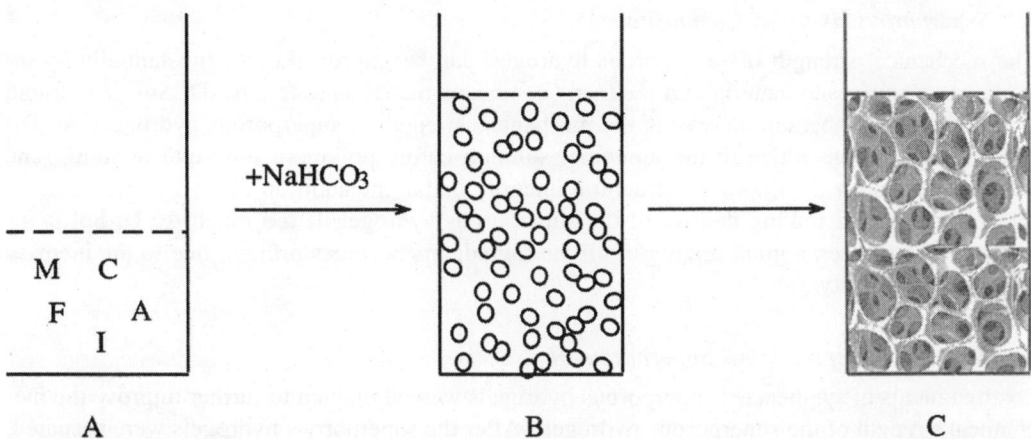

Figure 2 Schematic representation of the superporous hydrogel preparation. The pH of the monomer mixture is low due to the addition of acid (A), and this makes polymerization very slow. The addition of $NaHCO_3$ results in foaming and at the same time the pH of the solution increases (B). The pH increase accelerates the polymerization process, which is completed before the foam subsides. This leads to the superporous hydrogel formation (C). A, acid; C, crosslinker; F, foaming agent; I, initiator; and M, monomer.

foam formation as well as increase in pH, which accelerates the polymerization process. Within a few minutes after the addition of $NaHCO_3$, polymerization becomes complete.

2. Superporous Hydrogels for Gastric Retention Experiments

Any vinyl monomer can be used to make superporous hydrogels using the process shown in Fig. 2 (38). The type of monomer used in the superporous hydrogel preparation significantly affects the overall properties of the superporous hydrogels. One of the important properties is the mechanical property for the reasons described above. When acrylamide (AM) was used as the only monomer, the superporous hydrogels show neither large swelling volume nor good mechanical strength. When sulfopropylacrylamide potassium salt (SPAK) was used alone, the superporous hydrogels swelled to a large size in the simulated gastric fluid (SGF) but were not strong. When AM and SPAK were copolymerized, however, superporous hydrogels showed good swelling and also good mechanical properties. In this study, SPAK-containing superporous hydrogels were made using the following procedure.

Poly(AM-co-SPAK) superporous hydrogel was prepared in a glass test tube (outer diameter 22 mm, inner diameter 19 mm, and height 175 mm). The following components were added sequentially to the test tube: 1200 µL of 50% AM; 900 µL of 50% SPAK; 450 µL of 2.5% N,N'-methylenebisacrylamide (Bis); 90 µL of 10% Pluronic F127; 30 µL of 50% (v/v) acrylic acid; 45 µL of 20% ammonium persulfate. The test tube was shaken to mix the solution after each ingredient was added. Then 270 mg Ac-Di-Sol powder was added to the mixture and stirred using a spatula for uniform distribution. After this, 45 µL of 20% N,N,N',N'-tetramethylethylenediamine (TEMED) was added to the mixture and the test tube was shaken again to mix it. Finally, 100 mg of $NaHCO_3$ powder was added and the mixture was immediately stirred vigorously using a spatula for 10 s. The superporous hydrogel was cured at room temperature for 10 min. Then the superporous hydrogel was retrieved from the test tube and washed in a 1-L beaker containing 400 mL of SGF (pH 1.2 based on USP) for 24 h. This step was called acidification. After this, the superporous hydrogel was dried at room temperature for 5 days.

3. Superporous Hydrogel Composites

The mechanical strength of superporous hydrogels can be improved quite substantially by introducing a composite material. Of the many composite materials tested, Ac-Di-Sol® was found to be superior to others in increasing the mechanical strength of superporous hydrogels. Ac-Di-Sol particles can be added to the monomer solution before polymerization and foaming. The possible reason for the improved structural integrity is that the addition of Ac-Di-Sol increases the (physical) crosslinking density of the superporous hydrogel. If too much Ac-Di-Sol is incorporated, however, a good mixing of all the ingredients becomes difficult due to the increase of solution viscosity.

4. Acidification of the SPAK Superporous Hydrogels

Posttreatments of synthesized superporous hydrogels were attempted to further improve the mechanical strength of the superporous hydrogels. After the superporous hydrogels were prepared, they were washed in the SGF (pH 1.2) for 24 h. Then they were dried in 60°C oven or air-dried at room temperature. The dried superporous hydrogels were allowed to swell in SGF and their mechanical properties were tested using a bench comparator.

The ultimate compression pressure (UCP) was used to measure the mechanical strength of superporous hydrogels. UCP was determined by applying increasing amounts of weights until a point when the superporous hydrogel started cracking. The pressure at that point was defined as UCP. Figure 3 shows the values of UCP of three types of superporous hydrogels: superporous hydrogels without any treatment after synthesis; superporous hydrogels that were washed in SGF after synthesis and then oven dried at 60°C for 24 h; and superporous hydrogels that were washed in SGF after synthesis and then air-dried at room temperature for 5 days. The

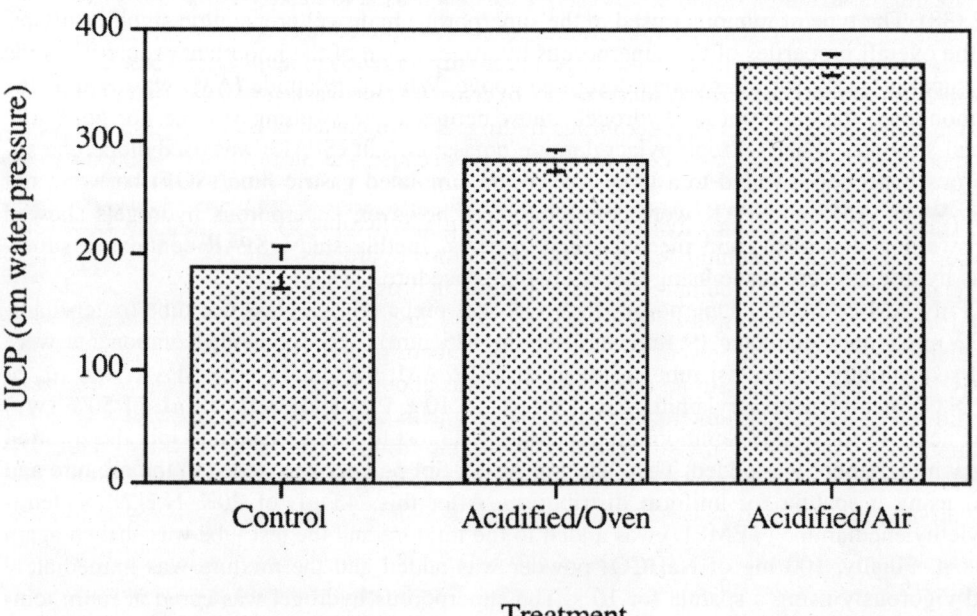

Figure 3 The effect of acidification on the UCP of the SPAK superporous hydrogels. The UCP of superporous hydrogels was measured without any treatment (control), after acidification and dried in a 60°C oven (acidified/oven), or after acidification and dried in air at 24°C (acidified/air).

washing step partially acidified the anionic SO_3^- group into SO_3H group (acidification) and substantially changed the properties of the superporous hydrogels. The UCP value for the three samples were 189, 284, and 368 cm water pressure, respectively. The acidification of the superporous hydrogels made them much stronger than the superporous hydrogels without acidification. Moreover, the UCP of the acidified superporous hydrogels that were dried at room temperature were even stronger than those dried in a 60°C oven. The reason is not clear at this point, but it shows that further treatment of the synthesized superporous hydrogels, such as acidification, provides significant improvement in mechanical properties.

B. Surface Slipperiness of Superporous Hydrogels

The slippery property of a hydrogel is an important factor for gastric retention (36). The slippery surface is believed to help the smooth migration of the peristaltic contraction over a hydrogel (Fig. 1). Thus, making the surface of the acidified SPAK superporous hydrogels slippery is expected to be important for gastric retention.

1. Mucin Coating on the Surface of Superporous Hydrogels

Mucin is responsible for the slippery nature of many biological surfaces. Mucin from porcine stomach was coated on the surface of the superporous hydrogel in an attempt to increase surface slipperiness. Mucin solution (10% w/v, Sigma Chemical Company, type II, crude, from porcine stomach) was applied to the surface of the acidified superporous hydrogels using a cotton swab. The exact amount of the applied mucin was not measured. Rather, the effect of mucin coating on the surface slipperiness was measured (see below). The mucin-coated superporous hydrogels were heated in a 130°C oven for 40 min. The coating and heating processes were repeated twice.

Heating albumin emulsion at 100–160°C has been used to make crosslinked albumin microspheres (39). At high temperature, protein forms crosslinked networks. In this study, mucin was crosslinked on the surface of the superporous hydrogels at 130°C. The slipperiness was maintained even after the coated superporous hydrogels were washed in SGF for more than 2 days. On the other hand, if the superporous hydrogels were coated but dried at room temperature, then the slipperiness was kept for only 1 h because the surface-adsorbed mucin was washed away in SGF.

The coated superporous hydrogels were then made flexible by incubating in a moisture chamber of well-defined humidity. The soft superporous hydrogels were squeezed into the 000 size gelatin capsules. The compressed superporous hydrogels with mucin coating swelled in about 10 min to equilibrium at 37°C in SGF. (It took an additional 3–5 min for dissolution of the gelatin capsules). The swelling time of the mucin-grafted superporous hydrogels was slightly longer than those with no coating (which was about 5–6 min). The swelling size, however, did not change. It was interesting to note that mucin coating by heating at 130°C resulted in reduction of the UCP of the superporous hydrogels from 368 to 280 cm water pressure. A possible reason for this decrease is that the repetitive heating at 130°C might partially destroy the hydrogel networks and cause the decease of UCP.

2. In Vitro Test of Slipperiness

A simple device was used to test the slipperiness (Fig. 4). A slope made of a glass plate 30 cm long was supported by a lab jack. The swollen superporous hydrogel (cylindrical) was placed longitudinally on the glass surface to prevent it from rolling. The height, H, was adjusted by a lab jack. The height was gradually increased until a point when the superporous hydrogel

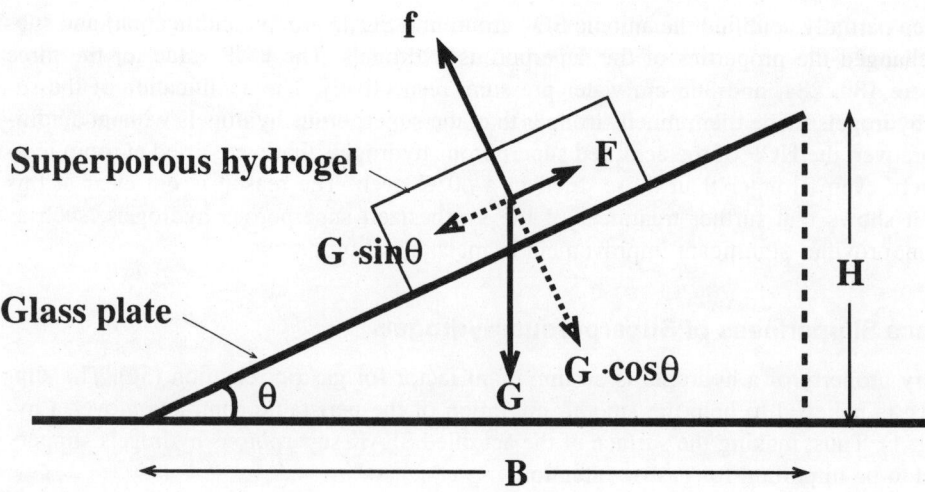

Figure 4 Schematic description of the device used to measure the surface slipperiness of superporous hydrogels. A superporous hydrogel is placed longitudinally on a glass slope to prevent it from rolling. The height of the slope (H) is adjusted by a lab jack. B is the length of the base. θ is the angle between the slope and the base. G is the gravity of the superporous hydrogel. f is the supporting force exerted by the slope. F is the static friction force. H is increased gradually from 0 to a point at which the superporous hydrogel starts to slide. H and B are used to calculate the static friction coefficient.

started to slide. Since only the sliding friction coefficient was measured in this experiment, data were discarded whenever rolling of a superporous hydrogel occurred.

When a superporous hydrogel just started to slide, the forces parallel to the slope surface were balanced:

$$F = G \sin \theta$$

where F is the static friction force, G is the gravity of the superporous hydrogel, and θ is the angle of the slope. $G \sin \theta$ is the vector of the gravity parallel to the slope. At the same time, the force perpendicular to the slope is also balanced:

$$f = G \cos \theta$$

where f is the supporting force exerted by the slope and $G \cos \theta$ is the vector of the gravity perpendicular to the slope. By definition:

$$F = \mu f$$

where μ is the static friction coefficient. Combining the above three equations leads to:

$$\mu = \sin \theta / \cos \theta = H/B$$

where H is the height of the slope and B is the base length of the slope. Both values can be accurately measured by ruler.

In this study, the slipperiness of a superporous hydrogel was represented by the static friction coefficient (μ) between the superporous hydrogel and a glass surface. The lower static friction coefficient indicates the more slippery superporous hydrogel. This is of course only an approximation of the actual slipperiness that a superporous hydrogel may have with the stomach surface, but it will provide comparative values for increased slipperiness by mucin coating.

The static friction coefficients of the control, acidified, and acidified as well as mucin-coated superporous hydrogels were 0.37 ± 0.06, 0.63 ± 0.05, and 0.24 ± 0.03, respectively. This result shows that acidification substantially decreased the slipperiness of a superporous hydrogel, and mucin coating significantly increased the slipperiness.

IV. IN VIVO STUDY IN A CANINE MODEL

A. Radiopaque Marker and Image Analysis

In previous studies in our laboratory, gastrografin (Solvay Animal Health, Inc.), an x-ray opaque material, was incorporated in hydrogels as radiopaque marker (34). In the beginning of this study, gastrografin was mixed with the monomer solution and incorporated into the superporous hydrogels. However, a few hours after a superporous hydrogel was swollen, the x-ray marker became too pale to be seen from the x-ray pictures. For this reason, small hydrogel pellets containing $BaSO_4$ were used as the x-ray marker in later studies.

The $BaSO_4$-containing hydrogel pellets were prepared in a plastic tube (inner diameter of 3.35 mm). First, the following components were sequentially mixed in a glass vial: 1300 μL of 50% AM; 800 μL of 2.5% Bis; 150 μL of 20% ammonium persulfate (APS); 1300 μL of 40% $BaSO_4$ suspension (E-Z-Paque $BaSO_4$ suspension, E-Z-EM, Inc., Westbury, NY); and 80 μL of 20% TEMED. The vial was swirled to mix the ingredients after each component was added. The mixture was then injected into the plastic tube. The gelling of the mixture started within 5 min after the addition of TEMED. After curing for 1 h at room temperature, the gel strand was retrieved from the plastic tube, cut into small segments, and dried in a 60°C oven for 5 h. The dried gel pellets were white and had a diameter of 2 mm and a length of 2 mm. These pellets were used as markers for x-ray image analysis.

To incorporate the $BaSO_4$ hydrogel pellets into a superporous hydrogel, two to six pellets were placed in the monomer solution before the addition of APS. After the addition of $NaHCO_3$, the mixture was mechanically stirred for 5–10 s to distribute the pellets evenly. The $BaSO_4$ particles or suspension can be considered as drug particles or suspension, and the same method can be used to load the drugs.

There are a few advantages to use of the $BaSO_4$ hydrogel pellets. First, they provide very high contrast over the background and therefore are easy to monitor even after they are swollen for several days. Second, the dried hydrogel pellets are kept very small so that the pellets do not affect the packing of a superporous hydrogel into a capsule. Third, several pellets can be incorporated in a superporous hydrogel, so that the fragmentation of the superporous hydrogel can be easily monitored.

B. In Vivo Study in Dogs

For all in vivo experiments of the gastric retention in dogs, the superporous hydrogels were dried, moistened, and then squeezed to load into the size 000 gelatin capsules. Superporous hydrogels with different properties were tested under fasted or fed conditions. The dogs used in all experiments weighed about 50 pounds. The fasted condition was achieved by withholding a dog from food for 36 h but allowing free access to water before the experiment. The fed condition was achieved by giving a dog 450 g canned food right before the oral administration of the capsule. In each experiment (fasted state or fed state), the dog was given 300 mL water by stomach tube right before the oral administration of the capsule. Then the capsule containing the superporous hydrogel was swallowed by the dog with no water. X-ray pictures were taken

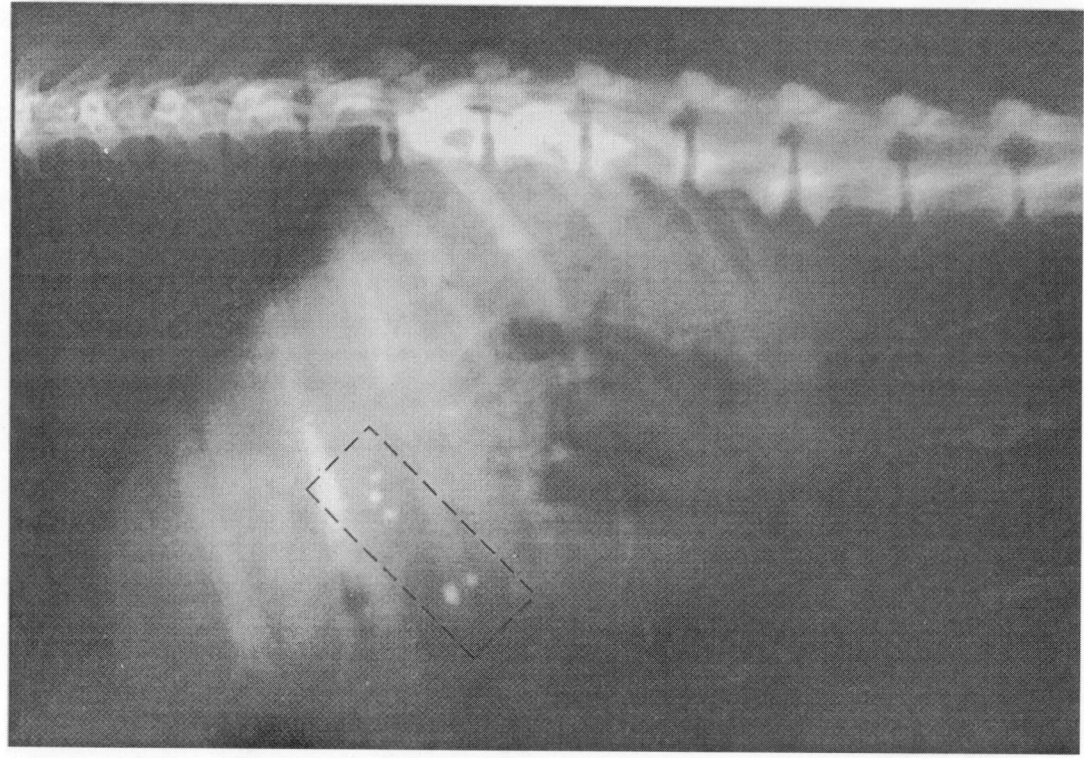

Figure 5 An x-ray of a stomach of a dog after administration of a superporous hydrogel containing several opaque hydrogel particles. The dotted rectangle around the small opaque (white) hydrogel particles represents the superporous hydrogel in the stomach. The intactness of the superporous hydrogel can be assessed from the relative position of the opaque hydrogel particles.

at timed intervals after the administration of the capsule. Figure 5 shows an example of x-ray pictures showing $BaSO_4$ hydrogel pellets inside a superporous hydrogel in the stomach.

Table 1 lists properties of superporous hydrogels used in the animal experiments. Synthesis of poly(AM-co-SPAK) superporous hydrogels was described above. In experiment 1, the superporous hydrogel was used without the acidification step. X-ray pictures were taken at t = 0, 0.5 h, 1 h, 2.5 h, 3 h, and 4 h. At 2.5 h, all six markers were seen in the stomach, but one $BaSO_4$ pellet was a little bit apart from the others. This means that the superporous hydrogel remained in the stomach but the fragmentation of the superporous hydrogel just started. At 3 h, two pellets were seen in the small bowel while the other four remained in the stomach. At 4 h, all six pellets were found in the small bowel. The superporous hydrogel used apparently had a size large enough to be retained in the stomach in the beginning, but its mechanical strength was not high enough to withstand several hours of repetitive gastric contraction. Even though the UCP of the tested superporous hydrogel (170 cm water pressure) was significantly higher than the maximum gastric pressure reported in the literature (50–70 cm water pressure), the superporous hydrogel still broke apart. It is possible that the local pressure exerted to the superporous hydrogel by gastric tissues is much higher than the average pressure reported in the literature.

In experiment 2, the superporous hydrogel was made using a test tube with a smaller diameter (20 mm of outer diameter rather than 22 mm). All other experimental conditions for the

Table 1 In Vitro Properties and Gastric Retention of Superporous Hydrogels Used in Animal Experiments

Exp. No.	Swelling time[a] (min)	Size of swollen gel[b] (diam. × length)	UCP[c] (cm H_2O)	Initial state[d]	Gastric retention time[e] (h)
1	10	3.3 cm × 4.0 cm	170	Fasted	< 4
2	6	2.1 cm × 3.9 cm	370	Fasted	< 3
3	(A) 6	2.4 cm × 3.4 cm	370	Fasted	< 3.8
	(B) 10	2.4 cm × 3.5 cm	280	Fasted	< 5
4	6	2.4 cm × 3.5 cm	370	Fed	> 27

[a]In 37°C SGF. Superporous hydrogels were not encapsulated in a gelatin capsule.
[b]In 37°C SGF.
[c]Ultimate compression pressure on the swollen superporous hydrogels.
[d]In the fed state, the food was given only in the beginning of the experiment.
[e]Determined from the x-ray pictures taken at timed intervals.

synthesis of superporous hydrogel were the same. The superporous hydrogel was acidified to change the anionic SO_3^- groups into the protonated form of SO_3H. Consequently, the swollen size of the superporous hydrogel decreased but the UCP increased significantly. X-ray pictures taken at 1 h and at 2 h showed the x-ray markers maintaining their relative positions in the stomach. At time 3 h, however, all three markers were found in the colon but still maintained their relative positions, i.e., the superporous hydrogel was emptied from the stomach as an intact whole piece. It suggested that the mechanical strength of the superporous hydrogel was strong enough to keep its structural integrity, but it was not large enough.

In experiment 3, two acidified superporous hydrogels were administered into the dog's stomach at a 30-min interval. The superporous hydrogels A and B were the same except that the superporous hydrogel B was coated with mucin to impart slipperiness. The mucin coating resulted in reduction of the UCP value from 370 to 280 cm water pressure as described above. The static friction coefficients of superporous hydrogels A and B against glass were 0.63 and 0.24, respectively. Superporous hydrogel B was given to the dog at time 0, and superporous hydrogel A was given to the dog at time 0.5 h. To distinguish the two hydrogels, different numbers of x-ray markers were used. The superporous hydrogel A remained in the stomach for 3 h. During the next 50 min, the dog threw up only the superporous hydrogel A. The vomited superporous hydrogel was still intact with diameter of 2.4 cm and length of 3.4 cm. The superporous hydrogel B remained intact in the stomach as shown by the picture taken at time 4.3 h. At time 5 h, the x-ray markers in the superporous hydrogel B were found far apart in the intestine, indicating that the superporous hydrogel B was fragmented and then emptied from the stomach by time 5 h. The main difference between the superporous hydrogels A and B is that the surface of the gel B was coated and thus was much more slippery than gel A. The fact that gel B remained in the stomach even after gel A was vomited suggests that the surface slipperiness is an important factor in maintaining the gel in the stomach without any discomfort. However, confirmation of this will require more study. Were the mucin-coated superporous hydrogel (B) mechanically stronger, it could have stayed in the stomach for a longer time.

In experiment 4, food was given to the dog in the beginning of the study to achieve the fed state. The fed state was maintained for the first 6 h according to the x-ray pictures. Since then no food was found in the stomach and the dog was in the fasted state until the end of the experiment. The dog had free access to water throughout the experiment. X-ray pictures taken at timed intervals until 27 h showed the presence of the $BaSO_4$ hydrogel x-ray markers maintaining their relative positions in the stomach. The image taken at time 32 h shows that one of the markers was emptied into the small bowel while the other two remained in the stomach. Fragmentation of the superporous hydrogel started between 27 h and 32 h. The superporous hydrogels stayed in the stomach even after the dog maintained the fasted state. It appears that improved mechanical strength can prolong the gastric retention time to more than 27 h under certain conditions. The superporous hydrogel in this experiment was large enough to be retained in the stomach, and the mechanical strength was high enough to withstand the gastric contraction force. The presence of food in the beginning of the experiment may have helped to make the surface of the superporous hydrogel smooth. Even the superporous hydrogels with high mechanical strength can become fragmented after repetitive gastric contractions.

Our study indicates that the UCP of 370 cm water pressure is more than enough to withstand the pressure exerted on the superporous hydrogels. It also indicates that the presence of food in the beginning somehow results in long-term gastric retention, extending beyond the fed state. The fed state ended after several hours of food intake, but the superporous hydrogels remained for more than 27 h. While more experiments are required to reach clear conclusions, our study thus far shows that the superporous hydrogels with high mechanical strength can be used as a long-term gastric retention device, especially when given in the fed state.

REFERENCES

1. Khosla, R., and Davis, S. S.: Gastric emptying and small and large bowel transit of non-disintegrating tablets in fasted subjects, Int. J. Pharm., 52: 1–10, 1989.
2. Hinder, R. and Kelly, K.: Canine gastric emptying of solids and liquids, Am. J. Physiol., 233: E335–E340, 1977.
3. Siegal, J., Urbain, J., Adler, L., Charkes, N., Maurer, A., Krevsky, B., Knight, L., Fisher, R., and Malmud, L.: Biphasic nature of gastric emptying, Gut, 29: 85–89, 1988.
4. Horowitz, M., Maddox, A., Bochner, M., Wishart, J., Krevsky, B., Collins, P., and Shearman, D.: Relationship between gastric emptying of solid and caloric liquid meals and alcohol absorption, Am. J. Physiol., 257: G291–G298, 1989.
5. Gupta, P. K., and Robinson, J. R.: Gastric emptying of liquids in the fasted dog, Int. J. Pharm., 43: 45–52, 1988.
6. Mojaverian, P., Reynolds, J. C., Ouyang, A., Wirth, F., Kellner, P. E., and Vlasses, P. H.: Mechanism of gastric emptying of a nondisintegrating radiotelemetry capsule in man, Pharm. Res., 8: 97–100, 1991.
7. Weiner, K., Graham, L., Reedy, T., Elashoff, J., and Meyer, J.: Simultaneous gastric emptying of two solid foods, Gastroenterology, 81: 257–266, 1981.
8. Lin, H. C., Doty, J., Reedy, T., and Meyer, J.: Inhibition of gastric emptying by sodium oleate depends on length of intestine exposed to nutrient, Am. J. Physiol., 259: G1031–G1036, 1990.
9. Hunt, J., and Stubbs, D.: The volume and energy content of meal as determinants of gastric emptying, J. Physiol., 245: 209–225, 1975.
10. Davis, S. S., Hardy, J. G., Taylor, M. J., Whalley, D. R., and Wilson, C. G.: Effect of food on the gastrointestinal transit of pellets and an osmotic device (Osmet), Int. J. Pharm., 21: 331–340, 1984.
11. Mojaverian, P., Ferguson, R., Vlasses, P., Rocci, M., Oren, A., Fix, J., Caldwell, L., and Gardner, C.: Estimation of gastric residence time of the Heidelberg capsule in humans: effect on varying food composition, Gastroenterology, 89: 392–397, 1985.
12. Kelly, K. A.: Motility of the stomach and gastroduodenal junction, in Physiology of the Gastrointestinal Tract, L. R. Johnson, ed., Raven Press, New York, 1981, pp. 393–410.
13. Chien, Y. W. Novel Drug Delivery Systems, Marcel Dekker, Inc., New York, 1992, p. 162.

14. Minami, H., and McCallum, R. W.: The physiology and pathophysiology of gastric emptying in humans, Gastoenterology, 86: 1592–1610, 1984.
15. Itoh, T., Higuchi, T., Gardner, C. R., and Caldwell, L.: Effect of particle size and food on gastric residence time of non-disintegrating solids in beagle dogs, J. Pharm. Pharmacol, 38: 801–806, 1986.
16. Hwang, S. J., Park, H., and Park, K.: Gastric retentive drug delivery systems, Crit. Rev. Ther. Drug Carrier Syst., 15: 243–284, 1998.
17. Gröning, R. and Heun, G.: Oral dosage forms with controlled gastrointestinal transit, Drug Dev. Ind. Pharm., 10: 527–539, 1984.
18. Palin, K. J., Whalley, D. R., Wilson, C. G., Davis, S. S., and Philips, A. J.: Determination of gastric-emptying in the rat: influence of oil structure and volume, Int. J. Pharm., 12: 315–322, 1982.
19. Sheth, P. R., and Tossounlan, J.: The hydrodynamically balanced system (HBS): a novel drug delivery system for oral use, Drug Dev. Ind. Pharm., 10: 313–339, 1984.
20. Thanoo, B. C., Sunny, M. C., and Jayakrishnan, A.: Oral sustained-release drug delivery systems using polycarbonate microspheres capable of floating on the gastric fluid, J. Pharm. Pharmacol., 45: 21–24, 1993.
21. Bolton, S., and Desai, S.: Floating sustained release therapeutic compositions, U.S. Patent, 4,814,179: 1989.
22. Davis, S. S., Stockwell, A. F., Taylor, M. J., Hardy, J. G., Whalley, D. R., Wilson, C. G., Bechgaard, H., and Christensen, F. N.: The effect of density on the gastric emptying of single- and multiple-unit dosage forms, Pharm. Res., 3: 208–213, 1986.
23. Bechgaard, H. and Ladefoged, K.: Distribution of pellets in the gastrointestinal tract. The influence on transit time exerted by the density or diameter of pellets, J. Pharm. Pharmacol., 30: 690–692, 1978.
24. Bechgaard, H., Christensen, F. N., Davis, S. S., Hardy, J. G., Taylor, M. J., Whalley, D. R., and Wilson, C. G.: Gastrointestinal transit of pellet systems in ileostomy subjects and the effect of density, J. Pharm. Pharmacol., 37: 718–721, 1985.
25. Park, K., and Robinson, J. R.: Bioadhesive polymers as platforms for oral-controlled drug delivery: method to study bioadhesion, Int. J. Pharm., 19: 107–127, 1984.
26. Park, H., and Robinson, J. R.: Physico-chemical properties of water insoluble polymers important to mucin/epithelial adhesion,, J. Controlled Rel., 2: 45–57, 1985.
27. Mathiowitz, E., Chickering, D., Jacob, J., Dibiase, M., Bernstein, H., Gunn, K., and Sherman, M.: GI transit studies of hydrophobic protein microspheres, Proc. Int. Symp. Contr. Rel. Bioact. Mater., 21: 27–28, 1994.
28. Cargill, R., Caldwell, L. J., Engle, K., Fix, J. A., Porter, P. A., and Gardner, C. R.: Controlled gastric emptying. 1. Effects of physical properties on gastric residence times of nondisintegrating geometric shapes in beagle dogs, Pharm. Res., 5: 533–536, 1988.
29. Fujimori, J., Machida, Y., and Nagai, T.: Preparation of magnetically responsive tablet and confirmation of its gastric residence in beagle dogs, STP Pharm. Sci., 4: 425–430, 1994.
30. Fujimori, J., Machida, Y., Tanaka, S., and Nagai, T.: Effect of magnetically controlled gastric residence of sustained release tablets on bioavailability of acetaminophen, Int. J. Pharm., 119: 47–55, 1995.
31. Michaels, A. S., Bashwa, J. D., and Zaffaroni, A.: Integrated device for administering beneficial drug at programmed rate, U.S. Patent, 3,901,232, 1975.
32. Mamajek, R. C., and Moyer, E. S.: Drug-dispensing device and method, U.S. Patent, 4,207,890, 1980.
33. Shalaby, W. S. W., Blevins, W. E., and Park, K.: In vitro and in vivo studies of enzyme-digestible hydrogels for oral drug delivery, J. Controlled Rel., 19: 131–144, 1992.
34. Shalaby, W. S. W., Blevins, W. E., and Park, K.: Use of ultrasound imaging and fluoroscopic imaging to study gastric retention of enzyme-digestible hydrogels, Biomaterials, 13: 289–296, 1992.
35. Urquhart, J., and Theeuwes, F.: Drug delivery system comprising a reservoir containing a plurality of tiny pills, U.S. Patent, 4,434,153, 1984.
36. Shalaby, W. S.-W.: Enzyme-digestible hydrogels for oral drug delivery, Doctoral dissertation, Purdue University, West Lafayette, IN, 1992.

37. Guyton, A. C. Basic Human Physiology: Normal Function and Mechanisms of Disease, 2nd Ed., W. B. Saunders, Philadelphia, 1977, pp. 662–664.
38. Chen, J., Park, H., and Park, K.: Synthesis of superporous hydrogels: hydrogels with fast swelling and superabsorbent properties, J. Biomed. Mater. Res., 44: 53–62, 1999.
39. Arshady, R.: Albumin microspheres and microcapsules: methodology of manufacturing techniques, J. Controlled Rel., 14: 111–131, 1990.

11
Osmotic Implantable Delivery Systems

Cynthia L. Stevenson, Felix Theeuwes, and Jeremy C. Wright
ALZA Corporation, Palo Alto, California

I. INTRODUCTION

Implantable drug delivery systems offer benefits over repetitive administration of conventional drug therapy by providing unattended continuous delivery within the therapeutic window. Controlled implantable drug delivery avoids the highly variable peak and trough concentrations often seen after immediate-release dosing. Alleviation of this peak and trough serum profile by maintenance of a continuous drug concentration can result in enhanced drug efficacy and minimized side effects. Patient compliance is also a benefit of continuous dosing with these implants.

Compliance is often conceptualized as an issue for patients and physicians, but it is also a problem in preclinical research in that laboratory animals may not ingest the desired quantity of an investigational agent dispersed in food or water. The compound may also have a short half-life and poor bioavailability, restricting the range of possible experiments. Additionally, many researchers lack an adequate system for investigating the benefits of controlled delivery. Researchers in pharmacology were the first to recognize the value of continuous drug delivery with osmotic delivery systems to solve these inherent problems (1). Design principles for subsequent osmotic systems were then developed; the Alzet, Duros, and Oros technologies are based on these early design principles (2,3). In this chapter, the Alzet pump and the Duros implant will be discussed; Oros systems are described in other sources (4).

The Alzet pump and the Duros implant were designed for the delivery of pharmaceutically active compounds in laboratory animals and in humans, respectively. These implantable osmotic pumps are also a viable alternative for delivering therapeutic doses of macromolecules continuously over an extended period.

Proteins and peptides are often poorly bioavailable when given orally, due to rapid degradation and poor absorption in the gastrointestinal tract. Biomolecular therapies can be delivered continuously via parenteral administration of sustained release and controlled release systems. Depot injections of proteins circumvent bioavailability issues and provide sustained release; however, poor drug stability and high variability in drug delivery are often an issue.

Conversely, ambulatory pumps can offer improved drug stability and controlled delivery; however, patient compliance and convenience may not be optimal. Ambulatory pumps have been used in hospital and home care settings for the delivery of analgesics and chemotherapeutics (5), and for the treatment of spasticity and diabetes.

Following the successful application of the Alzet osmotic pump in research settings, Duros osmotic implants were developed for human use. The Duros implants are a family of drug-dedicated, osmotic, controlled release systems for the delivery of therapeutic agents, especially macromolecules that are difficult to deliver by other techniques.

There are few implantable pumps for human use. Implantable pumps are typically peristaltic, solenoid, or freon-driven (5). Peristaltic pumps are usually programmable, have 10- to 20-mL drug reservoirs, deliver 100 μL/day to 1 mL/h, and weigh approximately 175 g unfilled. Freon-driven pumps deliver drug from a restrictive tube and weigh approximately 200 g when empty. The drug reservoir volumes for these pumps average 20 to 60 mL and can deliver 250 μL to 4 mL/day (6). In contrast, a Duros implant weighs 1.2 g, delivers 0.5–5 μL/day, and contains 150 μL of formulation. Alzet Model 2004 and 2ML2 pumps, for example, weigh 1.1 and 5.1 g, have drug reservoir volumes of 200 and 2000 μL, deliver 0.25 and 5 μL/h, and last 4 and 2 weeks, respectively.

Osmotic delivery systems tend to be unaffected by in vivo variables and to exhibit excellent correlation between in vivo and in vitro release (6,7). They offer a precise delivery rate and are not dependent on the physical or chemical properties of the drug substance. Therefore, these systems can be designed to provide a variety of release profiles for targeted or systemic delivery, such as increasing or decreasing in dosage rate or zero order (8–11). The systems can also be engineered to control the site of drug action. Depending on the design of the osmotic pump, the desired site of delivery may be a targeted organ, the central nervous system, or the systemic circulation.

II. OSMOTIC SYSTEM THEORY

Osmotic systems release a therapeutic agent at a predetermined, typically zero-order, delivery rate based on the principle of osmosis (1–3,12,13). Osmosis is the natural movement of a solvent through a semipermeable membrane into a solution of higher solute concentration, leading to equal concentrations of the solute on both sides of the membrane. Osmotic systems imbibe water from the body through a semipermeable membrane into an osmotic material, which swells, resulting in slow and even delivery of drug formulation.

A semipermeable membrane is defined as a membrane that is permeable to a solvent (e.g., water), but impermeable to ionic compounds and higher molecular weight compounds. The semipermeable membrane (A) is permeable to water (compartment C) but impermeable to the solute in compartment B (Fig. 1) (14). When the pressure is equal between compartments B and C ($P^0 = P$), water (solvent) will permeate through the semipermeable membrane from compartment C to compartment B, reflecting the gradient in chemical potential of the solvent between the two compartments. As the pressure is increased in compartment B, the chemical potential of the solvent in that compartment increases. When the pressure in compartment B reaches the osmotic pressure of the solution in compartment B, the chemical potential of the solvent in the two compartments becomes equalized, and net transport of the solvent through the membrane ceases. The osmotic pressure (π) of the solution in compartment B is given by the following:

$$\pi = (\mu_C - \mu_B)/\underline{v} \qquad (1)$$

where μ is the chemical potential of the water and $\underline{v}$ is the partial molar volume of the water. When the chemical potential is written in terms of activity, a, of the solvent in compartment B, then

$$\pi = -RT (\ln a)/\underline{v} \qquad (2)$$

Osmotic Implantable Delivery Systems

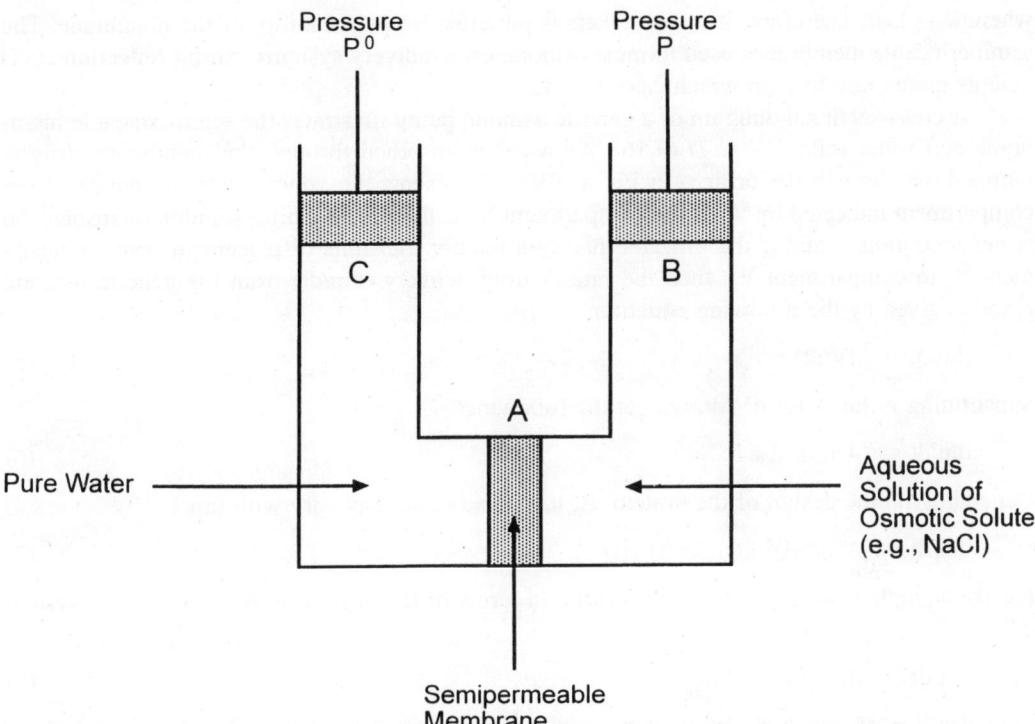

Figure 1 Diagram of a semipermeable membrane (A) separating an aqueous solution of an osmotic solute (B) from pure water (C).

The osmotic pressure is the driving force for fluid transport through the semipermeable membrane. The greater the gradient in osmotic pressure, the greater will be the rate of transport of solvent through the membrane. From nonequilibrium thermodynamics, the rate of water transport through the membrane can be written as follows (2):

$$dV/dt = (A/h) \, L_p \, (\sigma \Delta \pi - \Delta p) \qquad (3)$$

where dV/dt is the volume flow of solvent through the membrane, A is the cross-sectional area for transport, h is the membrane thickness, L_p is the hydraulic permeability of the membrane, σ is the reflection coefficient, $\Delta \pi$ is the osmotic pressure difference across the membrane, and Δp is the hydrostatic pressure difference across the membrane.

Hydrostatic pressure inside most osmotic drug delivery systems is generally less than 1 atm, although some systems may attain pressures as high as several atmospheres. The osmotic pressure of saturated solutions of sodium chloride, sucrose, potassium sulfate, and mannitol are 356, 150, 39, and 38 atm, respectively (15). Hence, in comparison with the osmotic pressures of saturated solutions of most pharmaceutical solutes, the hydrostatic pressure differential is negligible (2,3):

$$\Delta \pi \gg \Delta p$$

Equation 3 can then be written as follows:

$$dV/dt = (A/h) \, k \, \Delta \pi \qquad (4)$$

where $k = L_p \sigma$. Therefore, k can be taken as the effective permeability of the membrane. The semipermeable membranes used in most osmotic drug delivery systems exhibit reflection coefficients quite close to 1, in which case, $k \sim L_p$.

A cross-sectional diagram of a generic osmotic pump illustrates the semipermeable membrane and water influx (Fig. 2) (3,16). As water is absorbed through the membrane, drug is pumped out through the orifice. In Eq. 4, dV/dt represents the volume rate of change of the compartment indicated by V_s. If the compartment V_d is filled with a drug solution or suspension at concentration c, and if the movable partition readily transmits displacement from compartment V_s to compartment V_d, then the rate of drug delivery (dm/dt) from the generic osmotic pump is given by the following equation:

$$dm/dt = (dV/dt) \, c \qquad (5)$$

Substituting in Eq. 4 for dV/dt, we get the following:

$$dm/dt = (A/h) \, k \, \Delta\pi \, c \qquad (6)$$

Depending on the design of the system, A, h, k, $\Delta\pi$, and c may vary with time:

$$dm/dt = [A(t)/h(t)] \, k(t) \, \Delta\pi(t) \, c(t) \qquad (7)$$

For some applications, Eq. 7 can be written in terms of the degree of hydration of the system (H):

$$dm/dt = (A_H/h) \, k \, \Delta\pi_H \, c \qquad (8)$$

Consideration of Eqs. 6–8 reveals that a variety of delivery rate profiles (increasing over time, decreasing over time, or zero-order) are possible depending on the specific design of the osmotic system.

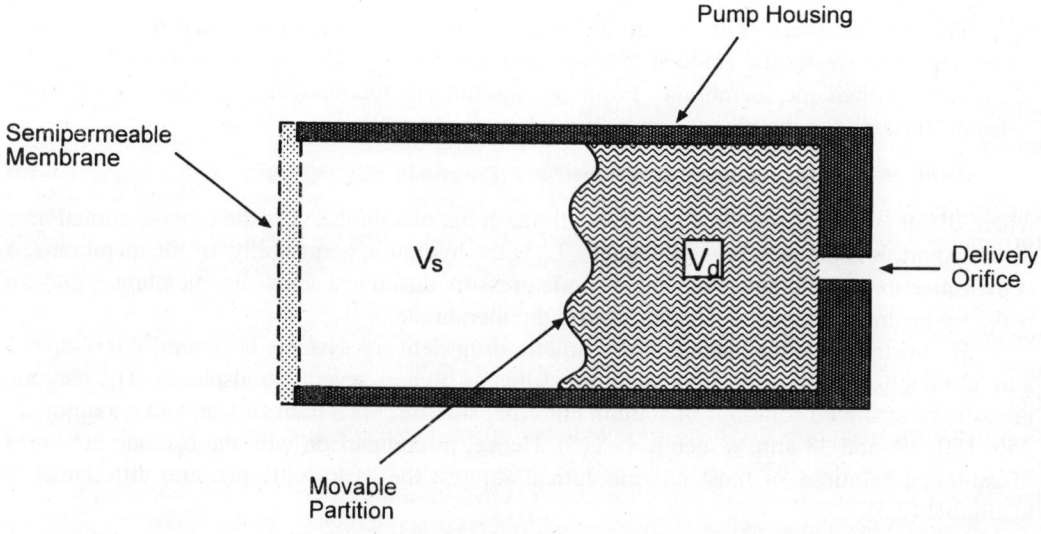

V_s Volume of Osmotic Driving Agent (e.g., Salt) Compartment

V_d Volume of Drug Compartment

Figure 2 Schematic representation of a generic osmotic pump.

Osmotic Implantable Delivery Systems

Osmotic drug delivery technology is primarily based on semipermeable membranes. These membranes are permeable to water but impermeable to ionic or higher molecular weight compounds. Cellulosic ester and polyurethane semipermeable membranes have been used in the applications discussed in this chapter. The permeability of the membrane is controlled by a number of factors, including the polymer chemistry and processing variables. For example, the water content in cellulosic ester membranes varies linearly with acetyl content, and the hydraulic permeability varies exponentially with acetyl content (17). Typical membrane permeabilities range from 10^{-7} to 10^{-6} g/cm s; permeabilities can be altered by incorporating additives during processing (11). For most pharmaceutical applications, the osmotic agent of choice is sodium chloride. This is primarily due to the ubiquitous presence of sodium chloride in the body and the availability of high-purity pharmaceutical grade material. Usually the system design provides for sufficient sodium chloride to maintain a saturated solution throughout the delivery period.

The delivery orifice of an osmotic system is designed within a critical range, i.e., small enough to minimize diffusional fluxes and large enough to prevent pressure buildup. If the effective cross-sectional area of the orifice is too large and the orifice length too short, then the diffusional fluxes can be of the same order of magnitude as the osmotic delivery rate (2). For improperly designed orifices, diffusional contributions can be erratic, with convective alteration of boundary layer thickness and a resulting erratic drug delivery rate. Generally, the diffusional contributions to the overall delivery rate can be minimized by decreasing the effective orifice cross-section and increasing the effective orifice length.

Nevertheless, the orifice must be sufficiently large to prevent pressure buildup in the system, especially for delivery of suspensions. Because of the relatively high viscosities of suspension formulations, diffusional fluxes are usually negligible. However, the increased viscosity of the suspension can result in significant pressure buildup inside the system during operation. The delivery orifice must be properly sized to prevent internal pressures from exceeding the mechanical design limits of system components, which could potentially result in system failure.

Suspensions represent a specialized subclass of formulations that can be delivered from osmotic systems. Suspension formulations have been successfully delivered by several osmotic pump technologies (18,19). As noted above, Eq. 6–8 also describe the delivery of suspensions, where c is the concentration of the suspended drug (mg of drug per mL of formulation).

Suspensions that appear stable under static conditions may exhibit instabilities under flow conditions. Suspending particles in a vehicle increases the effective viscosity of the resulting formulation. At low concentrations, this effect can be estimated by the Einstein equation:

$$\eta = \eta_0 (1 + 2.5 \phi) \tag{9}$$

where η = effective viscosity of the suspension, η_0 = viscosity of the vehicle, and ϕ = the volume fraction of the particles in the suspension. This equation contains the following assumptions: $\phi < 0.10$ and particles have approximately the same density as the vehicle. Formulation of a suspension requires a vehicle with sufficient viscosity to keep the particles suspended over the shelf storage and implanted delivery period. The suspension and delivery of microparticulate formulations are often aided by using a vehicle with a measurable yield stress.

Macromolecular suspensions (e.g., peptides and proteins) pose special challenges because particles of these compounds can readily aggregate and sediment, especially at system surfaces. Classical oral and topical formulations often rely on suspensions that settle but are easily resuspended on agitation and do not form an irreversible cake. However, for physical stability in an implantable system, the drug particles must remain suspended. Furthermore, care must be taken to formulate biomolecules so that the drug molecule does not separate from the excipient and a homogeneous dose is delivered over time. Sieving excipients under extremely low flow rates and preferential delivery of excipient must also be avoided.

Since suspensions are subject to aggregation and sedimentation, formulating suspensions for implants requires a fundamental understanding of particle charge, size distribution, surface area, wetting, electrostatic double-layer formation, ζ potential, and flocculation profile (20). To minimize sedimentation, controlled flocculation is often utilized to obtain a homogeneous suspension; titration of electrolytes, surfactants, and polymers is used to achieve this. For example, polymers can be added to the formulation to provide sufficient viscosity to keep the particles suspended over the shelf storage and implanted delivery lifetime.

III. ALZET PUMPS

A. System Design

Alzet osmotic pumps are miniature, implantable, research drug delivery systems for laboratory animals. The pumps are designed to deliver homogeneous solutions or suspensions continuously at a controlled rate for extended periods. Alzet pumps were first introduced in 1977 as an alternative to dosing animals orally or with heavy infusion pumps (3,6). The pumps are capsule-shaped and range from 1.5 to 5.1 cm in length and 0.6 to 1.4 cm in diameter.

Alzet osmotic pumps are composed of three concentric layers: the drug reservoir, the osmotic sleeve, and the rate-controlling, semipermeable membrane (Fig. 3). The drug reservoir is a cylindrical cavity molded from a synthetic hydrocarbon elastomer with an orifice for drug delivery. The reservoir walls are impermeable to water and thus prevent migration of chemical moieties between the drug reservoir and the osmotic sleeve. An osmotic sleeve containing sodium chloride surrounds the drug reservoir. The outermost layer is composed of a rigid semipermeable membrane made of a cellulose ester blend. At the orifice end, a flow moderator with a 21-gage stainless steel tube is inserted into the body of the osmotic pump after filling. The flow moderator minimizes passive diffusion and convective losses, and reduces the effect of air bubbles trapped in the drug solution. A catheter can be attached to the flow moderator.

When the pump is placed in an aqueous environment, water is transported across the semipermeable membrane into the osmotic sleeve. As the osmotic sleeve imbibes water, it swells, generating pressure to collapse the flexible drug reservoir. Therefore, the delivery rate of an Alzet pump is determined by the rate at which water crosses the semipermeable membrane and enters the osmotic sleeve (Eq. 4). The rate of water influx into the osmotic sleeve is in turn dependent on the permeability and dimensions of the semipermeable membrane; this rate is also affected by the temperature and osmotic pressure difference across the membrane. The difference in osmotic pressure between the osmotic sleeve and the surrounding interstitial fluid (on implantation) constitutes the osmotic gradient. The osmotic driving agent (NaCl) maintains a constant osmotic gradient for the duration of drug delivery. In turn, the osmotic gradient drives water through the membrane, swelling the osmotic sleeve, collapsing the reservoir, and delivering drug from the reservoir at a controlled rate. Therefore, the characteristics of the drug formulation do not affect the delivery profile (except in viscous or nonhomogeneous suspensions, as discussed above). Using Alzet pumps in most mammalian species (37°C and osmolality 310 mOsm/L) is simple, although these values may change for heterothermic animals (6).

B. System Configurations

Alzet pumps deliver at fixed rates between 0.25 and 10 μL/h for 1 day to 4 weeks (Fig. 4) (6,21,22). For example, Alzet Model 1002 has a reservoir volume of 100 μL, a pumping rate of

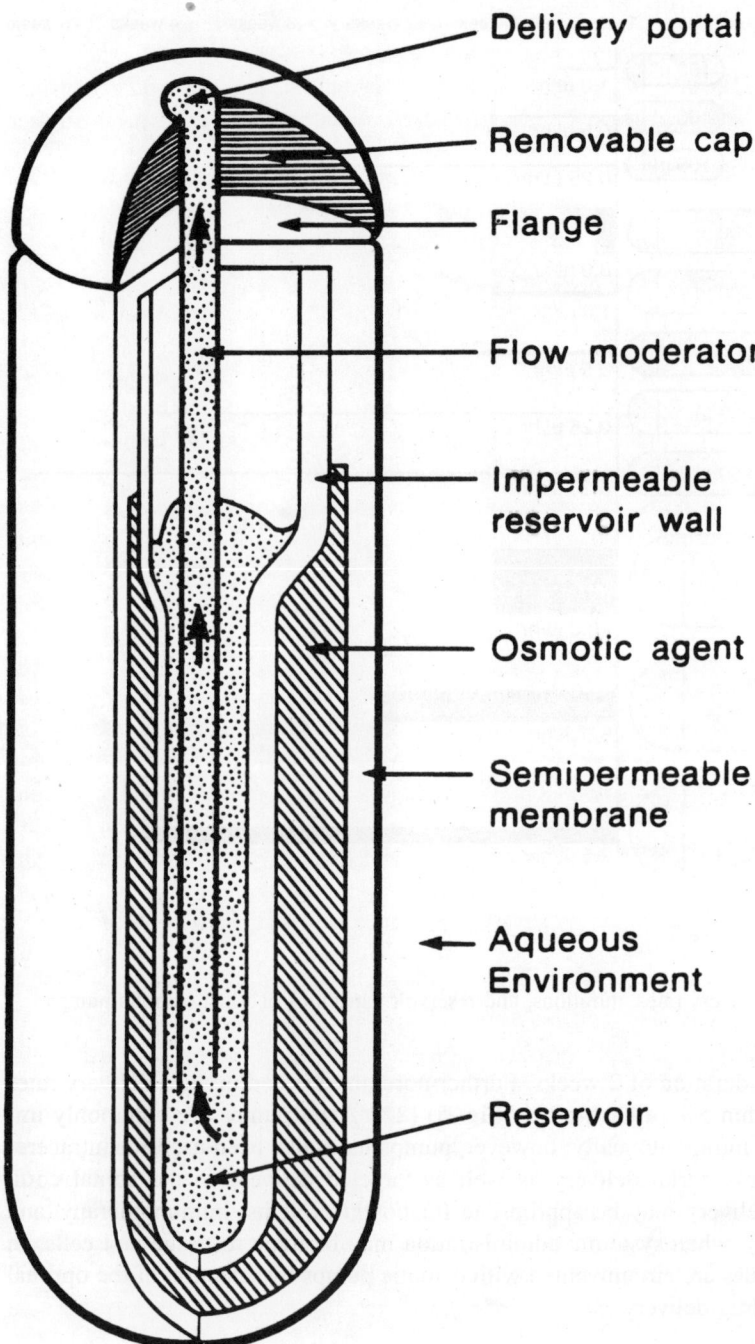

Figure 3 Cross-section of a functioning Alzet osmotic pump.

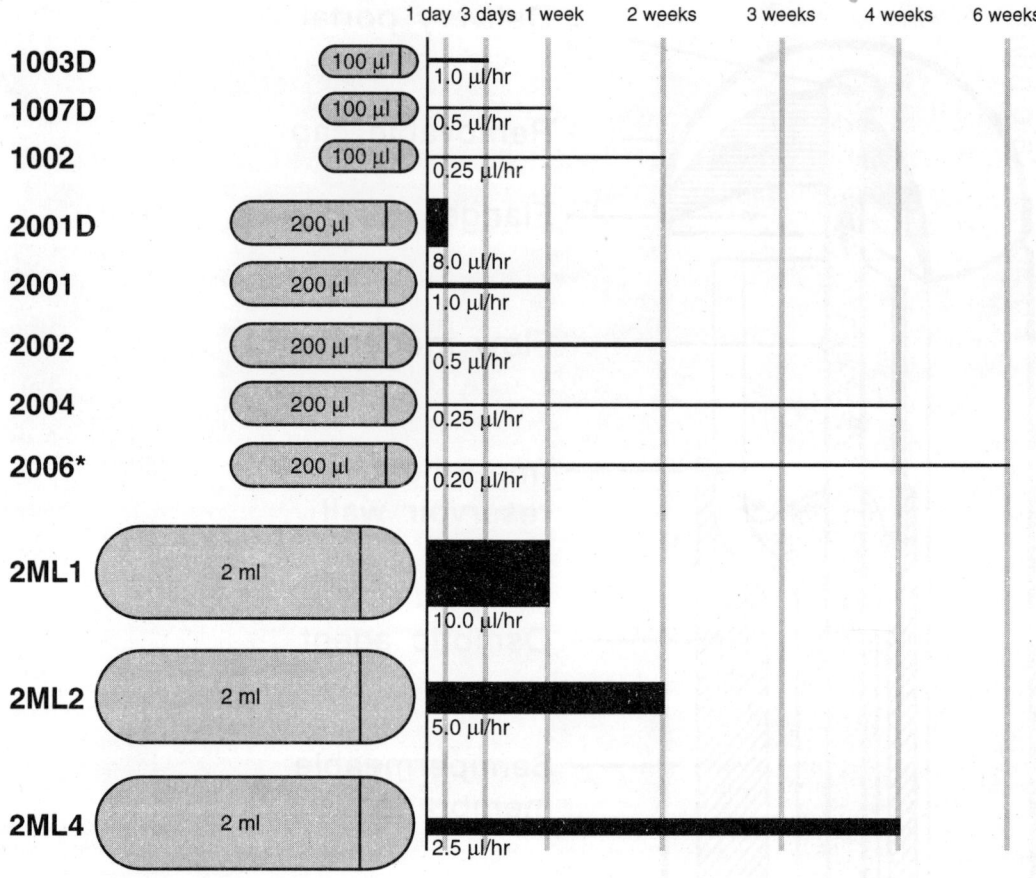

*Planned availability in 1999.

Figure 4 Comparison of delivery rates, durations, and reservoir capacities of Alzet osmotic pumps.

0.25 µL/h, and a pumping duration of 2 weeks. Furthermore, in vivo and in vitro delivery rates from Alzet pumps are within 5% of each other (Fig. 5) (22). Alzet pumps are commonly implanted subcutaneously or intraperitoneally; however, pumps have also been used for intracerebral, intravenous, and intra-arterial delivery as well as targeted delivery to the spinal cord, spleen, and liver. Local delivery may be appropriate for potent proteins, immunotherapy, and antisense and gene therapy, when systemic administration may be toxic to tissue and cells. In general, bioavailability issues are circumvented with osmotic pumps by selection of the optimal delivery site for targeted drug delivery.

C. Formulation Parameters

Optimal formulations for Alzet pumps must be compatible with the drug, the pump reservoir, and the site of administration. Alzet pump reservoirs are compatible with buffers, acidic and basic aqueous solutions, 2% Tween, and cosolvent mixtures containing dimethylsulfoxide (DMSO), ethanol, glycerol, propylene glycol, or poly(ethylene glycol) (PEG) 300, but they are not compatible with most natural oils. The solution formulations should be at room temperature

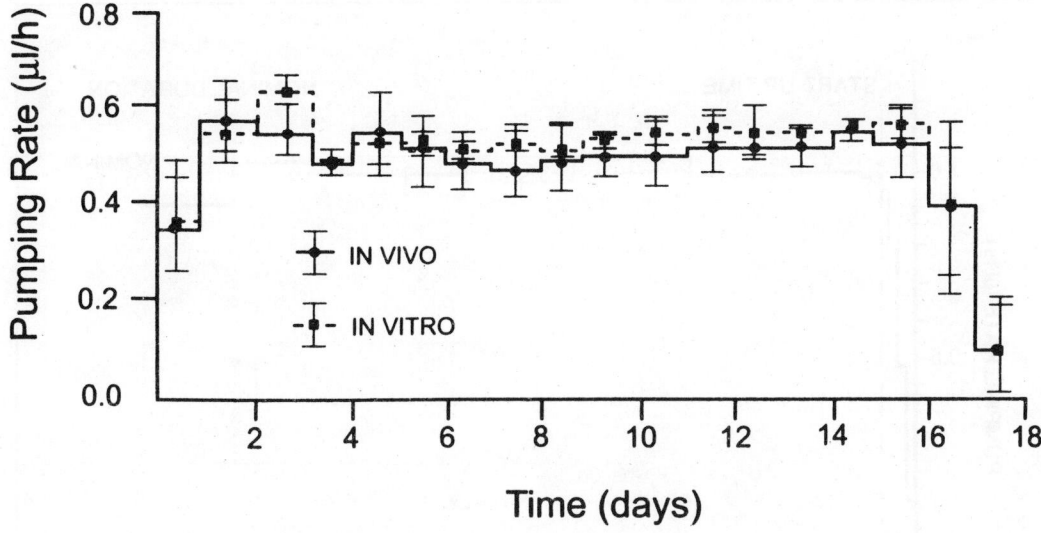

Figure 5 In vitro and in vivo pumping rates of a Model 2002 Alzet osmotic pump designed to deliver 0.5 μL/h of an agent for 14 days.

so that pumps can be filled without generating trapped air bubbles. Viscous drug solutions and homogeneous suspensions can be administered. Care should be taken to ensure drug stability, sterility, and isotonicity so that degradation, microbial contamination, and inflammation do not occur.

D. Implantation

Most filled Alzet pumps reach steady-state delivery in 4 to 6 h (Fig. 6). In order to obtain a more rapid startup, prefilled pumps can be stored in a sterile saline solution at 37°C for 4–6 h (preferably overnight) before implantation. This prehydration procedure is highly recommended for pumps used with catheters and highly viscous solutions.

Osmotic pumps have been used to explore the physiological and pharmacological characteristics of proteins and peptides in laboratory animals, as well as to deliver small-molecule therapeutics. The Alzet pump has been used in nearly 6000 studies to deliver 1600 compounds in 40 animal species. Animals weighing at least 10 g tolerate subcutaneous (but not intraperitoneal) implantation with 100-μL pumps. Animals weighing at least 20 g can tolerate subcutaneous implantation of either 100- or 200-μL pumps, but can only tolerate intraperitoneal implantation of pumps up to 100 μL.

Renal rat arteries perfused at 0.5–1.0 μL/h showed no damage or edema (23). Researchers using pumps with catheters determined that intrarenal infusion of prednisolone via the suprarenal or testicular artery prolonged graft survival time to 26 days compared with an intraperitoneal infusion–sustained graft of 9 days (24). The use of a catheter also allows direct access to the central nervous system, bypassing the blood–brain barrier (21).

The widespread use of Alzet pumps for the delivery of anesthetics, antibacterials, antibiotics, antibodies, barbiturates, benzodiazepines, catecholamines, cytokines, growth factors, hormones, neurotransmitters, antisense oligonucleotides, opiates, prostaglandins, and steroids has been demonstrated. Alzet pumps have also proved useful in biotechnology for characterizing novel proteins and peptides, and have been utilized for basic research on antisense

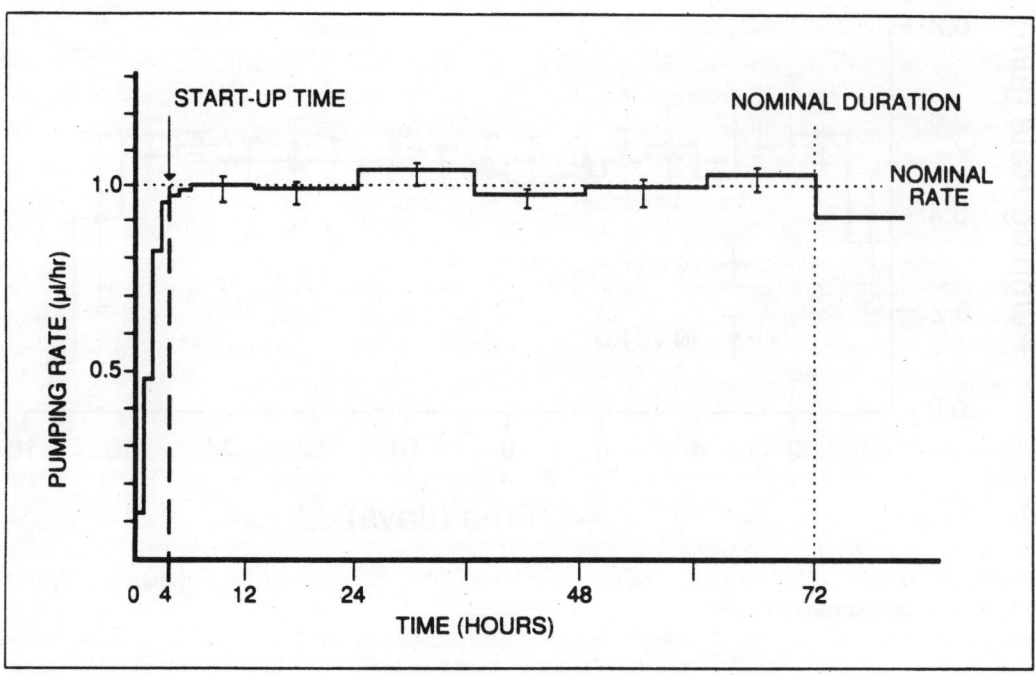

Figure 6 The pumping rate of the model 1003D Alzet osmotic pump in 0.9% NaCl at 37°C (±0.5°C).

oligonucleotide and gene therapy. Although Alzet pumps are frequently used in preclinical research, they have also been used in other specialized applications. For example, they have been used to dispense fresh medium in a prototype study of a cell cultivation instrument for Spacelab (25), to test the delivery of recombinant human growth hormone (rhGH) in rats on board the space shuttle *Discovery* (25), and to test the effects of rhGH on the atrophic response of the soleus muscle in space (26). Alzet pumps have also been used in endangered species: Green iguanas and cheetahs have both been bred in captivity by infusing gonadotropin-releasing hormone (GnRH) to induce ovulation (27).

E. Selected Applications

Alzet pumps have been used to deliver a range of small and large molecules in a wide variety of animal species (6,22). This section highlights pharmaceutically relevant biomolecular applications, such as the application of Alzet pumps for extended zero-order delivery, tumor site targeting, delivery of molecules with the aid of a catheter to the central nervous system, and formulation strategies to extend stability of the drug moiety for longer durations.

Alzet pumps have been used to deliver human growth hormone, insulin, enkephalin, melanocyte-stimulating hormone, bombesin, parathyroid hormone, and γ-interferon (6,22). For example, recombinant human granulocyte colony-stimulating factor (rhG-CSF) has been delivered intravenously to hamsters, causing increased granulocyte and leukocyte counts (28). Glucagon-like peptide (GLP-1) has been administered to diabetic rats for up to 1 month with a glucose-dependent increase in insulin secretion (29). Several additional examples are provided below.

1. Antisense Oligonucleotides

Treatment of malignancies with antisense oligonucleotides can downregulate gene expression and retard tumor growth. Administration of oligonucleotides via an osmotic pump provides zero-order release, thus counteracting the rapid degradation and clearance of these molecules in biological systems. N-myc-expressing human neuroectodermal tumors were grown as subcutaneous xenografts in athymic mice (30). Antisense and sense phosphodiester oligodeoxynucleotides directed against N-myc were delivered to the tumor area by a subcutaneously implanted pump (Alzet Model 1007D). Pumps were filled with 5 mM aqueous solutions of oligonucleotide with a perfusion rate of 0.5 μg/h; flow was directed to the tumor site for 2 weeks. The mean tumor mass was 50% smaller in the antisense-treated animals than in the animals treated with sense oligonucleotides. Therefore, local perfusion of antisense oligonucleotides can downregulate gene expression in human tumor xenografts.

Other researchers have pursued antisense treatment to the c-myb gene to control leukemia cell growth (31). Mice were subcutaneously implanted with Alzet pumps after detection of overt leukemia. The sense and antisense oligonucleotides were diluted in water and dosed to animals at 1 μL/h (100 μg/day). Untreated human leukemia-scid mouse chimeras survived approximately 2–6 days after circulating leukemia blast cells were detected. However, animals treated with antisense phosphorothioate oligonucleotides survived approximately 17 days, resulting in a three-to-eight-fold longer survival rate (Fig. 7) (31). In addition, animals receiving antisense c-myb oligonucleotides had less disease at the two sites most frequently manifesting leukemic cell infiltration (central nervous system and ovaries).

Antisense therapy has also been targeted to cell adhesion molecules, resulting in tumor regression (32). Inhibition of NF-κB transcription factor function retards cell adhesion in a wide variety of cell types. Antisense and sense phosphorothioate oligonucleotides of p65 (a protein composing NF-κB) were delivered to mice over 2 weeks. Mice were injected with either fibrosarcoma or melanoma cell lines that grew aggressively in control animals. Seventy percent of the antisense-treated animals showed a reduction in tumor size.

2. Nerve Growth Factor

Nerve growth factor (NGF) is critical for the normal development and maintenance of the peripheral sympathetic and sensory ganglia. Continuous administration of NGF to the central nervous system significantly reduced retrograde neuronal death of septal cholinergic neurons after injury (33). NGF (250 μg/mL 2.5S) was dissolved in saline and continuously infused into the lateral ventrical of rats for 2 weeks at 0.5 μL/h (Alzet Model 2002) with the aid of an infusion cannula. After pump explantation at the end of the study, the remaining NGF was assayed and was found to have retained activity. Following a 2-week infusion of NGF, identification of cholinergic neurons revealed a 350% increase in the survival of axotomized septal cholinergic neurons (33).

Similar results were observed in aged rodents with learning and memory impairments associated with a decline in cholinergic function (34). This decline in neuronal function is similar to Alzheimer-type dementia in humans. Continuous intracerebral infusion of 22 μg/mL 7S NGF with a cannula for 1 month partially reversed the cholinergic atrophy and improved retention of spatial memory tasks in impaired rats. When 7S NGF was reconstituted at 11 μg/mL in artificial cerebrospinal fluid with rat serum and incubated at 37°C for 14 days, biological activity was maintained (35). Finally, 180 μg/mL 2.5S mouse NGF was infused into primates at 2.5 μL/h (Alzet Model 2ML4) for 1 month. The NGF substantially reduced lesion-induced cholinergic neuronal degeneration (36).

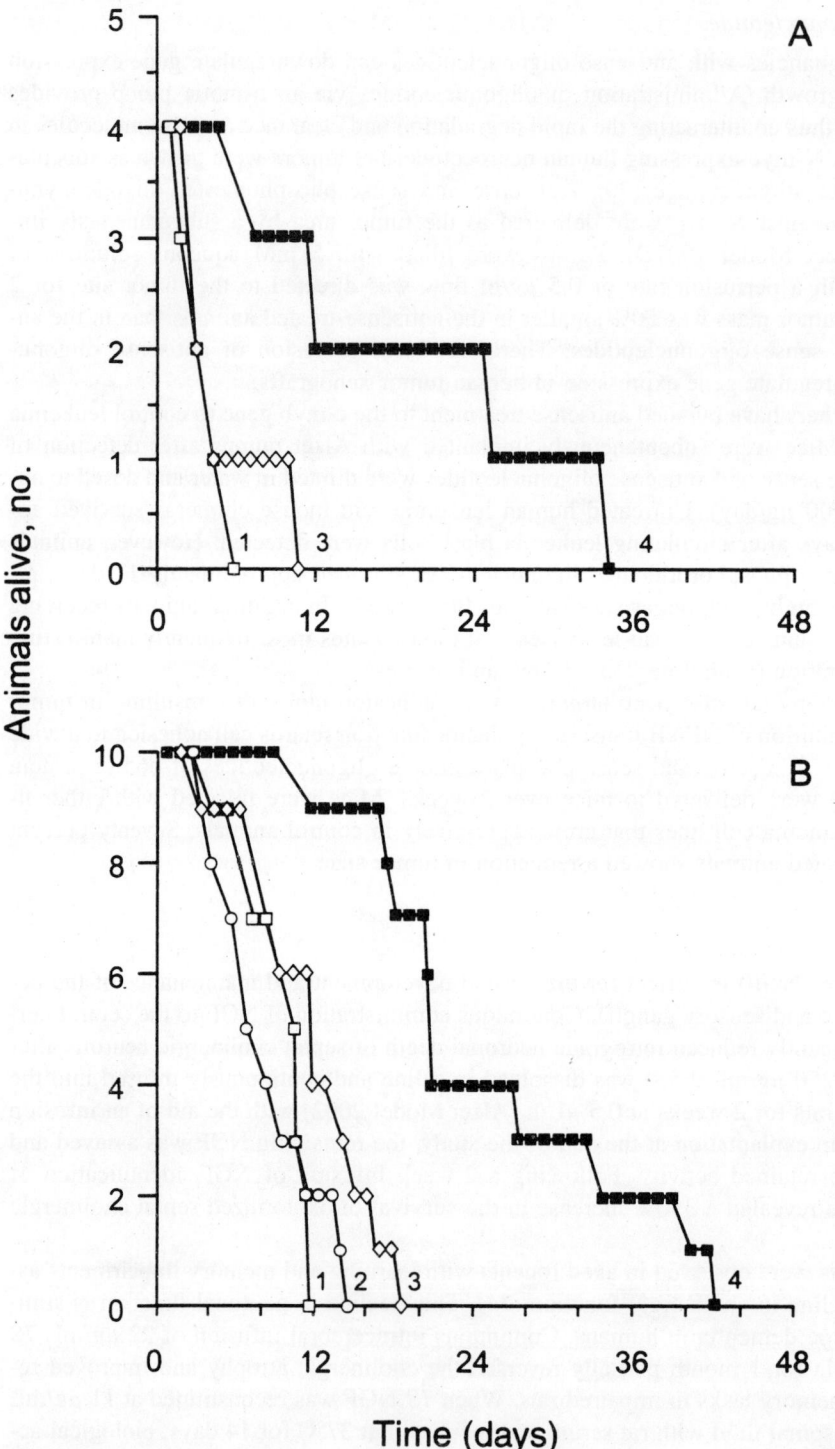

Figure 7 Survival curves of scid–human chimeric animals transplanted with K562 chronic myelogenous leukemia cells. Animals received an infusion of oligomers at 100 μg/day for 7 (A) or 14 (B) days. Curves: 1, control; 2, scrambled; 3, sense; 4, antisense.

3. Interleukins

Interleukin-6 (IL-6) is a multifunctional cytokine that acts as a signal for lymphocyte activation and host defense mechanisms for the immune system. It was administered subcutaneously to rats for 1 month (Alzet Models 2ML2 and 2ML4) after an adjuvant injection was given to induce arthritis (37). Continuous infusion of IL-6 significantly ($p < 0.05$) reduced adjuvant arthritis (Fig. 8) (37). For example, IL-6-treated animals demonstrated a mean arthritis score of 2, while control animals scored 8–10.

Interleukin-2 receptors are also important targets for immunosuppressive therapy. IL-2 can be fused with *Pseudomonas exotoxin* (PE40) to form a chimera targeted to activated lymphocytes (38). Activated lymphocytes express high-affinity IL-2 receptors and are believed to play a crucial role in rheumatoid arthritis. Since the in vivo half-life of IL-2–PE40 is 1–2 h, continual delivery is required to maintain elevated blood levels. Two pumps were implanted in each rat, delivering 1 µL/h (0.5 µl/g/day). When stability of the chimera was assessed at 37°C, biological activity was found to be lost within a few hours. The loss of activity was attributed to enzyme activity of the exotoxin. Therefore, 40–100 ng/mL IL-2–PE40 was formulated in 1% human serum albumin (HSA) and 1 mM β-nicotinamide

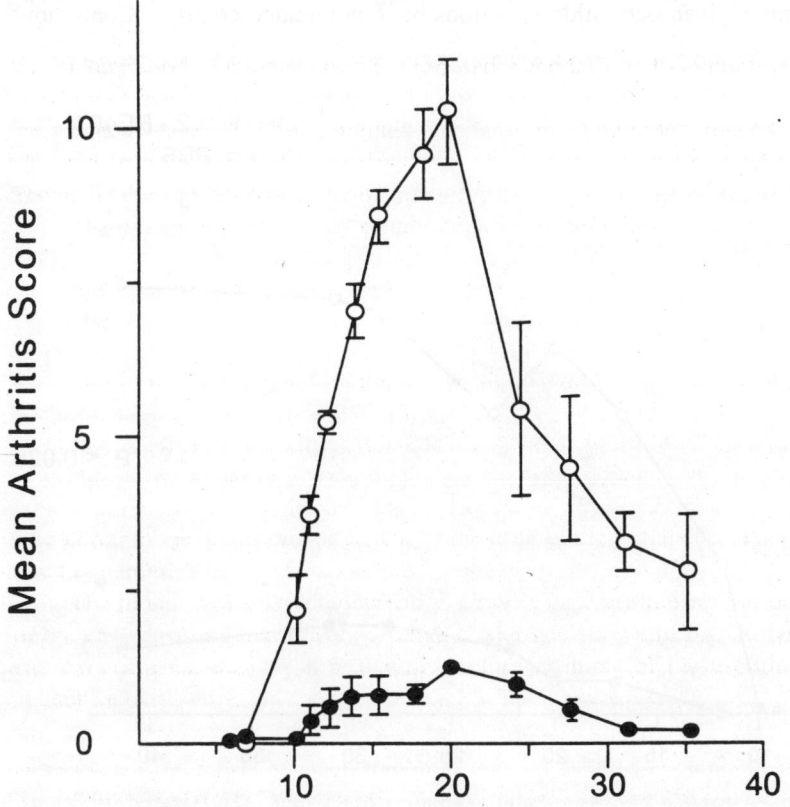

Figure 8 Time course of adjuvant arthritis development after IL-6 treatment (mean ± SE). Following injection, rats (n = 4) were treated for 4 weeks with IL-6 (●) 10.5 µg/day or with HSA as a control (○).

adenine dinucleotide (NAD) to stabilize and provide a substrate for the exotoxin portion of the chimera, respectively. Rats were infused with the IL-2–PE40 chimera for 7–8 days (Alzet Model 2001), and biological activity was observed in serum on days 2 and 6. Dosing rats with IL-2–PE40 prevented adjuvant-induced arthritis. Animals followed for 40 days had five to six times less severe arthritis than control animals (Fig. 9) (38). Continual delivery via pumps demonstrated a dose–savings effect over injections, and rats had fewer and less severe side effects (ascites) during treatments.

Conversely, IL-1 plays a role in the pathogenesis of osteoarthritis by stimulating the release of collagenase, which degrades cartilage. IL-1 (200 U/mL) infused intra-articularly into rabbit knees for 7 days (Alzet Model 2ML1) induced lesions in the knee cartilage. This system can be used as a model for osteoarthritis (39). IL-1 was prepared in sterile saline with 0.1% rabbit serum albumin and showed no loss of biological activity after 7 days at 37°C.

4. Octreotide

Expression of somatostatin receptors on human tumors, including neuroendocrine, lung, and breast malignancies, has been documented (40). Alzet pumps (Model 2002) were implanted subcutaneously in mice and delivered 0.5 µL/h octreotide, an analog of somatostatin, for 2 weeks (41). Growth of human breast tumors was significantly inhibited in mice with pumps compared with that in mice given octreotide injections or in nontreated controls. Continuous

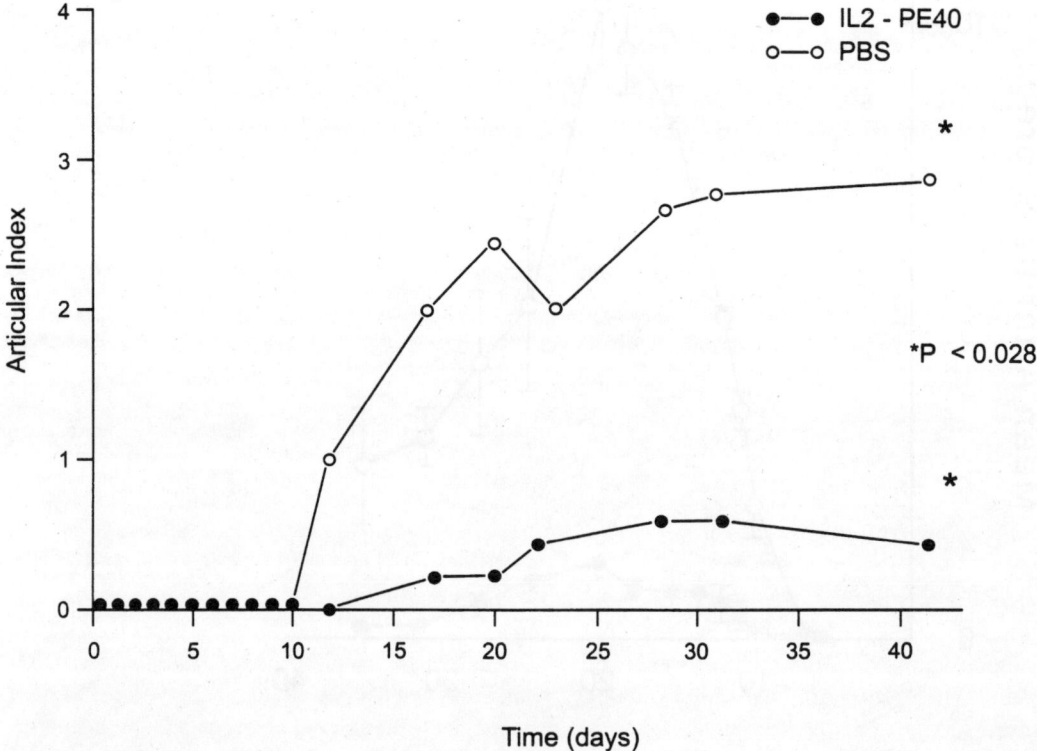

Figure 9 Arthritis index for IL-2–PE40-treated (●) and phosphate-buffered saline (PBS)-treated (○) rats. Data represent one of three trials (n = 5 in each trial).

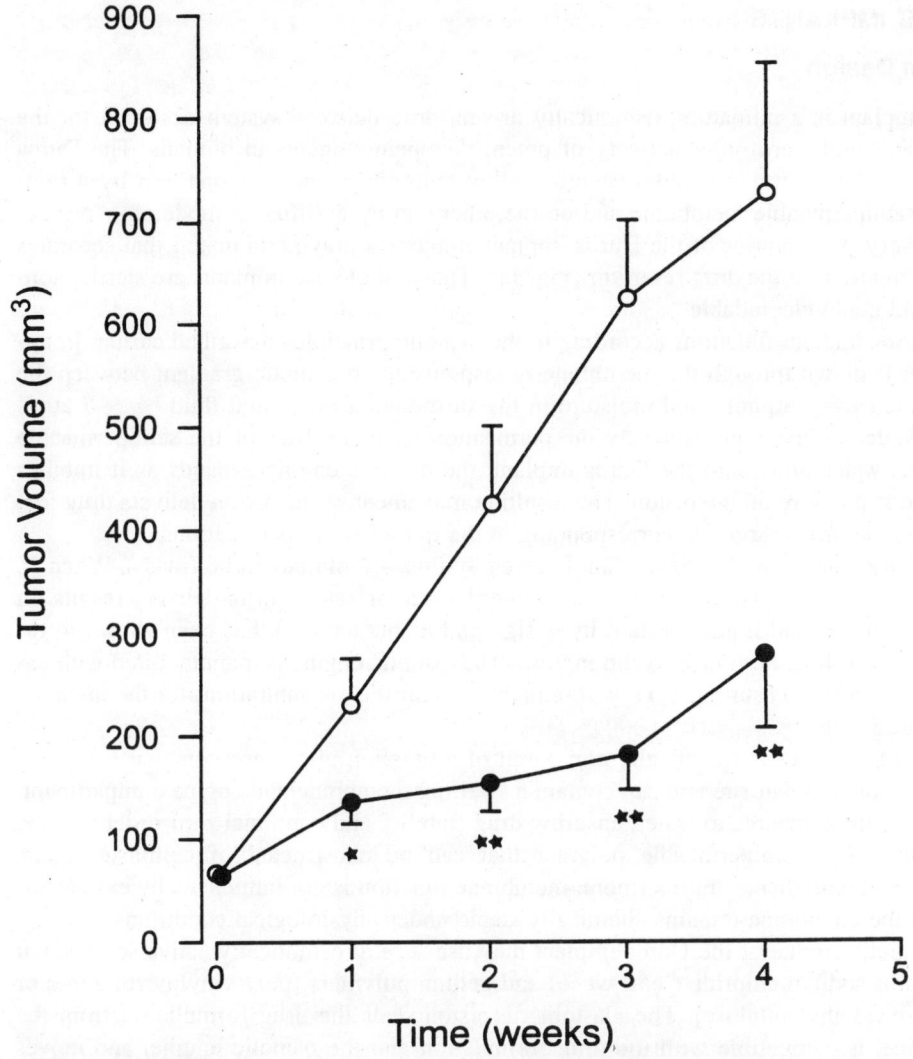

Figure 10 Antiproliferative action of continuously infused octreotide in nude mice bearing solid ZR-75-1 tumors (mean ± SE). Mice received octreotide (●) (n = 14) or saline control (○) (n = 12). *P < 0.01, **P < 0.001.

infusion of 10 μg/kg/h octreotide yielded plasma levels of 5.7 ng/mL, with a mean tumor volume 37% of that of the control animals at 1 month (Fig. 10) (40).

Further studies in rats with 7, 12-dimethylbenz(a)anthracene (DMBA)–induced mammary tumors were given 10 μg/kg/h octreotide for 6 weeks. After 6 weeks, tumor growth was significantly suppressed and the mean number of tumors per rat was reduced by 50%, when compared with control animals. Octreotide has been shown to enhance the antineoplastic effects of tamoxifen in rat mammary carcinomas (42). The antiproliferative effects of octreotide have also been demonstrated on gastroenteropancreatic tumors with good results (41).

The applicability of Alzet pumps to many laboratory studies further highlighted the need and potential clinical utility of a comparable human implantable pump.

IV. DUROS IMPLANTS

A. System Design

The Duros implant is a miniature, osmotically driven, drug delivery system designed for the long-term, parenteral, zero-order delivery of potent therapeutic agents in humans. The Duros implant consists of an impermeable, titanium alloy cylinder capped on one end by a rate-controlling, semipermeable membrane and on the other end by a diffusion moderator (orifice) for drug delivery. The interior of the Duros implant contains a polymeric piston that separates the osmotic engine from the drug reservoir (Fig. 11). These single-use implants are sterile, nonpyrogenic, and nonbiodegradable.

The Duros implant functions according to the osmotic principles described earlier. In operation, water is drawn through the membrane in response to an osmotic gradient between the osmotic engine ($\pi = 356$ atm) and moisture in the surrounding interstitial fluid ($\pi \sim 7$ atm). The rate of water influx is governed by the permeation characteristics of the semipermeable membrane. As water flows into the Duros implant, the osmotic engine expands as it imbibes water and exerts pressure on the piston. The resulting movement of the piston delivers drug formulation from the orifice at a rate corresponding to the rate of water permeation.

The release rate of the Duros implant is given by Eqs. 4 (volume) and 6 (mass). When A, h, k, and $\Delta\pi$ are held constant, a continuous zero-order release rate of drug delivery results. In the Duros implant, A and h are constant by design and manufacture; k has been shown to remain constant over time, both in vivo and in vitro. The osmotic engine is manufactured with excess sodium chloride to ensure that $\Delta\pi$ will remain constant (i.e., at saturation) for the intended duration of drug delivery.

The Duros implant is specifically composed of a titanium alloy reservoir that can withstand impact at the implant site and can contain a swelling membrane and engine compartment. The reservoir is impermeable to water, ensuring drug stability and continual zero-order release. The membrane is a semipermeable polymer that can be constructed of cellulose esters, polyamides, or polyurethanes. Furthermore, membrane function is not influenced by extracellular fluid, and the membrane remains chemically stable under physiological conditions.

The osmotic engine of the Duros implant may use several osmotically active solutes, but usually contains sodium chloride (>50 wt %) and gelling polymers [poly(vinylpyrrolidone) or sodium carboxymethylcellulose]. The elastomeric piston seals the drug formulation from the osmotic engine, is compatible with the drug formulation and the osmotic engine, and moves with relatively little resistance.

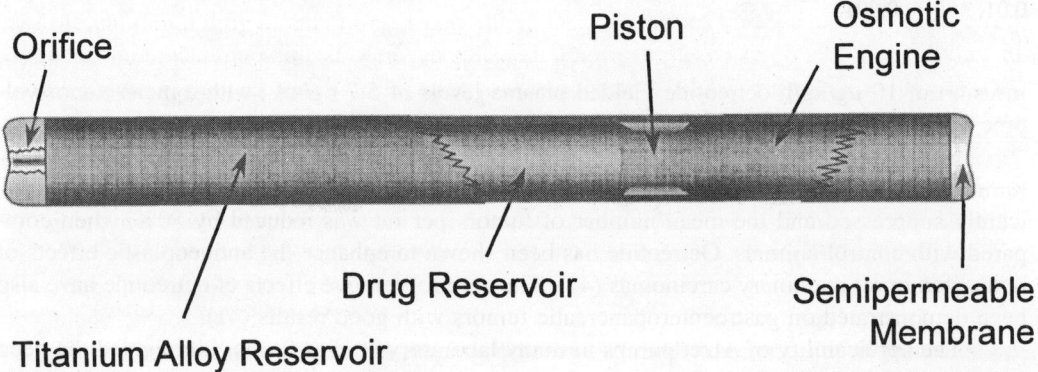

Figure 11 Schematic of a Duros implant.

The orifice was designed with a small inner diameter and a suitable length so that the diffusional contribution to the release rate is minimized at low delivery rates. These features also help to prevent back-diffusion of extracellular components when the system is implanted, preventing exposure of the drug formulation to the surrounding tissue prior to release.

B. System Configurations

The release rate and duration of a Duros implant depend on the drug concentration, the overall system and reservoir size, and the membrane and osmotic engine design. Altering the membrane permeability can change the release rate and system duration. For example, the 4-mm diameter by 45-mm length Duros implant has been developed to achieve 1-, 2-, 3-, 5-, and 12-month duration systems (Fig. 12). Further membrane alterations can result in tailored implants with longer system pumping durations. Higher release rates also shorten the duration of the 4-mm by 45-mm implant since the drug reservoir volume is fixed (150 μL). Assuming a drug concentration and an implant duration, the release rate can be calculated (Table 1). For example, in a 150-μL drug reservoir, a 2-month system would deliver 2.5 μL/day. With a 400 mg/mL solution drug formulation, the implant would deliver 1.0 mg/day (60 mg/implant).

To accommodate less potent molecules and their higher therapeutic doses, implants with larger drug reservoir volumes can be designed (Table 2). In order to obtain a 500-μL drug reservoir, the Duros implant length remains essentially unchanged; however, the diameter increases slightly. For example, a larger implant lasting 12 months could deliver 1.4 μL/day of a 100 mg/mL drug formulation. Similarly, a drug formulation at 400 mg/mL could deliver 560 μg/day (200 mg/implant).

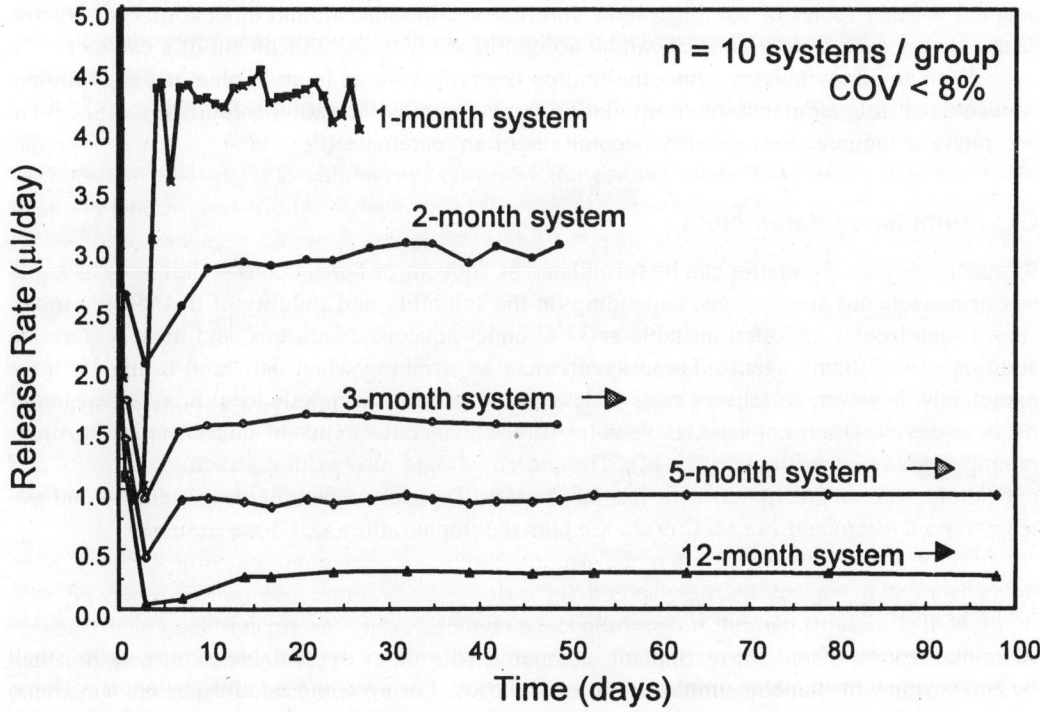

Figure 12 Comparison of release rates in Duros implants as a function of system duration.

Table 1 Duros Implant Dose Delivery (mg/day) Based on a 150-μL Drug Reservoir

Pump		Protein loading		
Duration (days)	Rate (μL/day)	5% w/v 7.5 mg	20% w/v 30.0 mg	40% w/v 60.0 mg
7	21.43	1.07	4.29	8.57
180 (6 mo)	0.83	0.04	0.17	0.33
360 (12 mo)	0.42	0.02	0.08	0.17

Table 2 Duros Implant Dose Delivery (mg/day) Based on a Theoretical 500-μL Drug Reservoir

Pump		Protein loading		
Duration (days)	Rate (μl/day)	5% w/v 25.0 mg	20% w/v 100.0 mg	40% w/v 200.0 mg
7	71.43	3.57	14.29	28.57
180 (6 mo)	2.78	0.14	0.56	1.11
360 (12 mo)	1.39	0.07	0.28	0.56

The Duros implant is most often implanted subcutaneously; however, the implant can be adapted to other routes of administration. Intravenous, intrathecal, and other forms of targeted drug delivery such as intratumoral can be accomplished with the attachment of a catheter.

With any drug delivery route, the limited reservoir volume in an implant usually requires concentrated drug formulations. Formulation issues such as saturation solubility and chemical and physical (aggregation) stability become important parameters.

C. Formulation Parameters

Biotechnology drug moieties can be formulated as aqueous or nonaqueous solutions or as aqueous or nonaqueous suspensions, depending on the solubility and stability of the specific molecule. Biomolecules are often unstable at 37°C under aqueous conditions, and most require the addition of stabilizing agents. These agents may be irritating when delivered in high-volume parenterals; however, at delivery rates of less than 1 μL/day, very little local or systemic toxicity is observed. Often nonaqueous vehicles offer enhanced stability of biomolecules by minimizing degradation pathways (43,44). The protein should also exhibit structural stability and not unfold, gel, or precipitate with loss of activity. Typically, adequate drug stability and potency for a 2-year shelf life (4°C or 25°C) plus the implant life (37°C) are desired.

D. Implantation

A unique feature of the Duros implant, compared with other implantable pumps, is its small size, allowing subcutaneous implantation in the body. For systemic administration, the Duros system is implanted subcutaneously in an outpatient setting with local anesthesia. Removal at the end of the delivery period is accomplished by an outpatient procedure. The implant is also adaptable to other sites of administration.

E. Selected Applications

1. Duros Leuprolide Implant

The Duros leuprolide implant has been designed to provide an alternative to periodic depot injections of leuprolide for the palliative treatment of advanced prostate cancer. It is implanted subcutaneously in the inner aspect of the upper arm. After a year, it is removed and replaced with a new system. The Duros leuprolide implant delivers leuprolide continuously over 1 year at approximately 120 μg/day (0.4 μL/day) from a 150-μL drug reservoir volume.

Testicular androgen ablation (decrease of serum testosterone levels to castrate levels) has been the standard for primary therapy of advanced prostate cancer for more than 50 years (45). The progress of prostate cancer is dependent on circulating androgen levels. Continuous administration of leuprolide results in the saturation and downregulation of pituitary receptors (46–48), resulting in a decrease in serum testosterone to castrate levels and retardation of tumor growth.

Preliminary formulation screening in water, propylene glycol, and poly(ethylene glycol) produced gelled formulations with less chemical stability (49). Both aqueous and nonaqueous solution formulations demonstrated 80–95% leuprolide remaining after 12 months at 37°C, when assayed by reverse-phase high-performance liquid chromatography (RP-HPLC) and size exclusion chromatography (SEC) (43,44). Leuprolide was formulated as a stable nonaqueous solution at 37 wt % free base in DMSO. This highly concentrated solution of leuprolide forms a viscous liquid with a saturation solubility of approximately 500 mg/mL. The formulation demonstrated good stability in Duros implants at 25°C and 37°C (Fig. 13) (50,51). The leuprolide formulation in DMSO used for clinical trials provided 92% stability for 3 years at 37°C.

In vitro release rate studies on Duros implants were performed by placing implants in test tubes containing phosphate-buffered saline (PBS) at 37°C. Constant zero-order delivery was

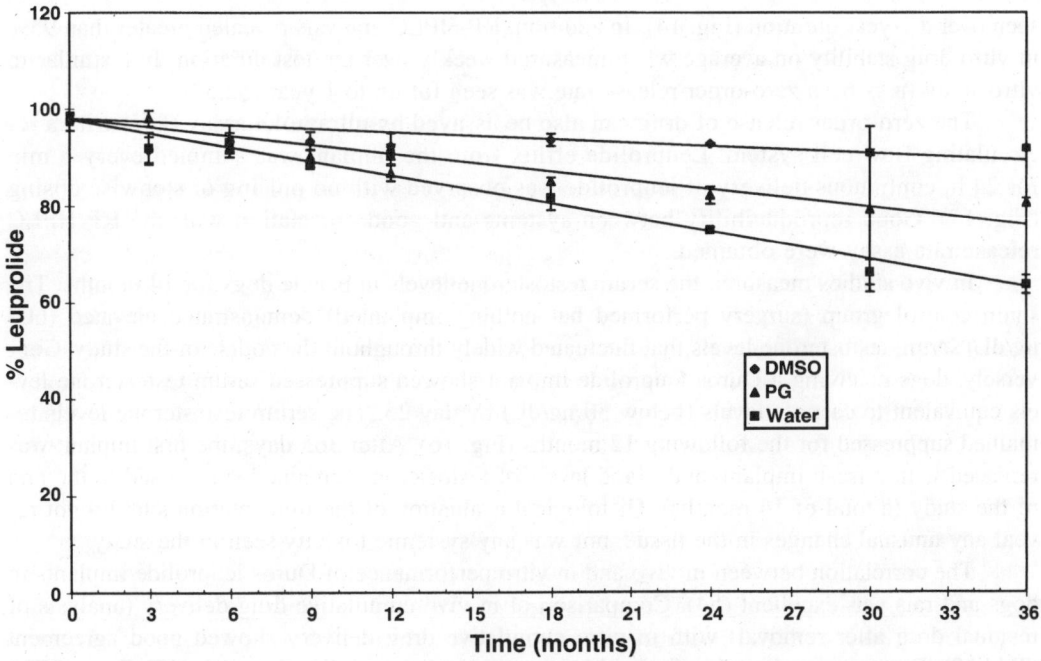

Figure 13 In vitro leuprolide (370 mg/ml) stability in Duros implants over 36 months at 37°C (n=3).

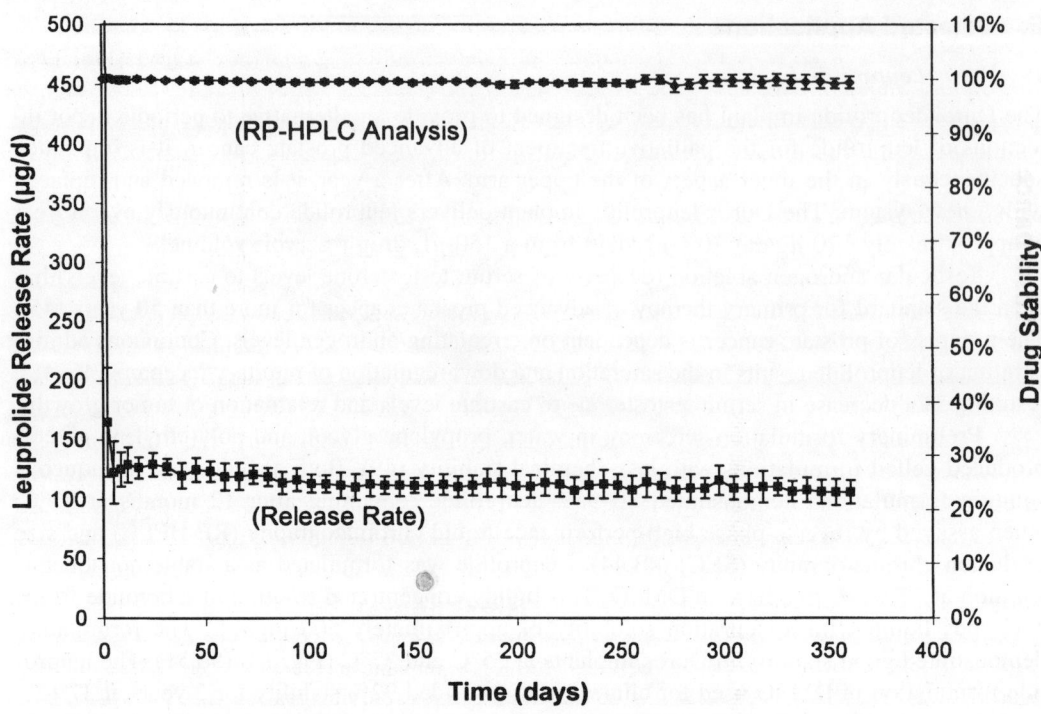

Figure 14 In vitro release rate and formulation stability (at 37°C) of the Duros leuprolide implant (n = 24) over 1 year.

seen over a 1-year duration (Fig. 14). In addition, RP-HPLC analysis revealed greater than 95% in vitro drug stability on average when measured weekly over the test duration. In a similar in vitro study (n = 6), a zero-order release rate was seen for up to 1 year (52,53).

The zero-order release of drug can also be assayed by ultraviolet assay (UV) with a recirculating flow cell system. Leuprolide efflux from the implant was sampled every 6 min for 24 h; continuous delivery of leuprolide was observed with no pulsing or stepwise dosing (Fig. 15). Good reproducibility between systems and good correlation with the RP-HPLC release rate assay were obtained.

In vivo studies measured the serum testosterone levels in beagle dogs for 14 months. The sham control group (surgery performed but nothing implanted) demonstrated elevated (600 ng/dL) serum testosterone levels that fluctuated widely throughout the course of the study. Conversely, dogs receiving a Duros leuprolide implant showed suppressed serum testosterone levels equivalent to castrate levels (below 50 ng/dL) by day 25. The serum testosterone levels remained suppressed for the following 12 months (Fig. 16). After 365 days, the first implant was replaced with a fresh implant, and blood levels of testosterone remained suppressed to the end of the study (a total of 14 months). Histological evaluation of the implantation site did not reveal any unusual changes in the tissue, nor was any systemic toxicity seen in the study.

The correlation between in vivo and in vitro performance of Duros leuprolide implants in dogs and rats was excellent (54). Comparison of in vivo cumulative drug delivery (analysis of residual drug after removal) with in vitro cumulative drug delivery showed good agreement (Table 3). Furthermore, both in vivo and in vitro leuprolide stability data (RP-HPLC and SEC) showed over 96% leuprolide remaining after 52 weeks (53).

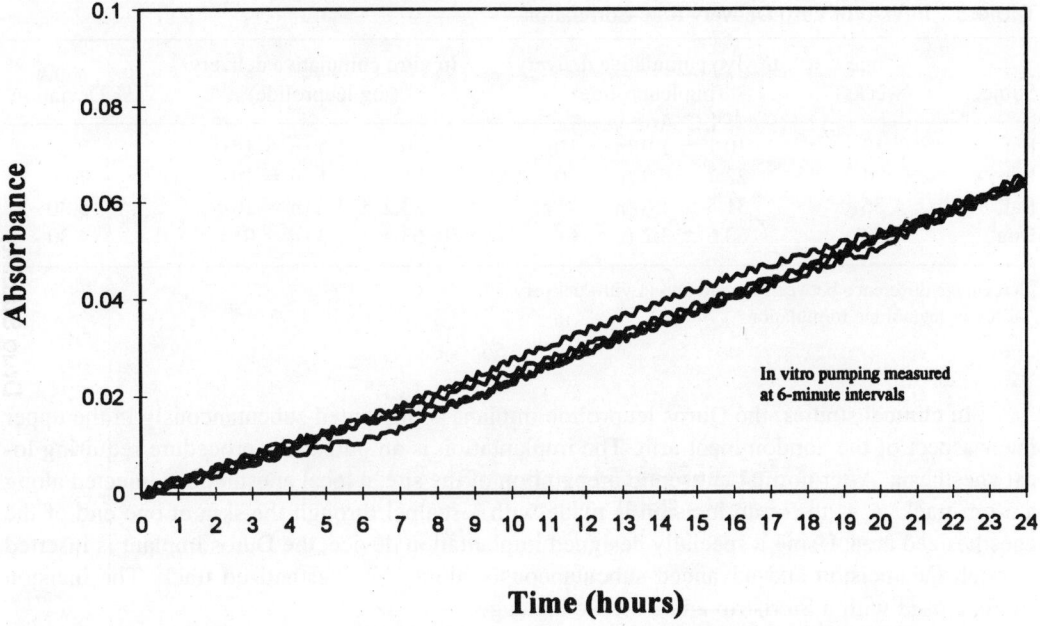

Figure 15 In vitro release rate in the Duros leuprolide implant, measured by UV absorbance at 6-min intervals. The Duros leuprolide implant had been pumping in vitro for several months before this experiment.

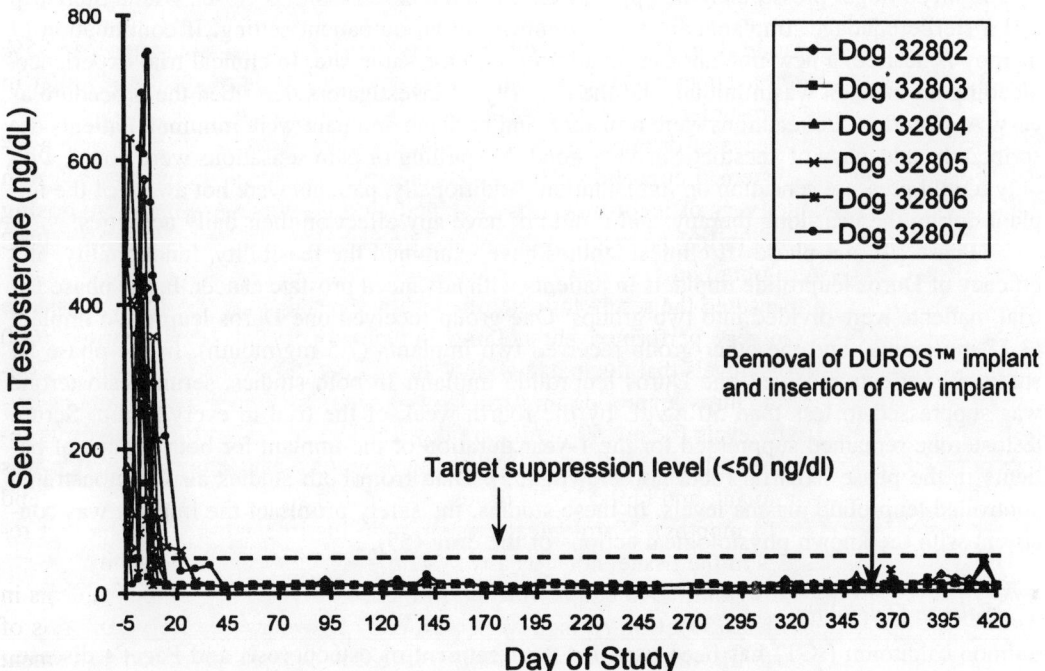

Figure 16 Serum testosterone concentration in dogs with the Duros leuprolide implant.

Table 3 In Vivo/In Vitro Delivery Rate Correlation

Subject	Time (weeks)	In vivo cumulative delivery (mg leuprolide)	In vitro cumulative delivery (mg leuprolide)	% Deviation[a]
Rat	12	10.1 ± 1.9 (n = 10)	9.3 ± 1.4 (n = 10)	8.20
Rat	24	22.7 ± 0.9 (n = 10)	24.5 ± 1.1 (n = 10)	7.60
Rat	36	31.5 ± 1.6 (n = 9)	33.2 ± 1.2 (n = 10)	5.30
Dog[b]	52	60.6 ± 3.2 (n = 6)[b]	63.5 ± 2.3 (n = 9)	4.80

[a]Percentage difference between in vivo and in vitro delivery.
[b]Different membrane formulation.

In clinical studies, the Duros leuprolide implant is implanted subcutaneously in the upper inner aspect of the nondominant arm. The implantation is an outpatient procedure requiring local anesthesia. After normal antiseptic preparation of the site, a local anesthetic is injected along a 5-cm track. A 4- to 5-mm incision is made with a scalpel through the skin at one end of the anesthesized area. Using a specially designed implantation device, the Duros implant is inserted through the incision and advanced subcutaneously along the anesthetized track. The incision site is closed with a Steristrip and a sterile bandage.

Removal is accomplished by external palpation and localization of the implant followed by incision and explantation. After normal antiseptic preparation of the site, local anesthetic is injected at one end of the implant, and a 4- to 5-mm incision is made over the previous incision, perpendicular to the implant. Finger pressure is applied to the other end of the implant to elevate the removal end of the implant (Fig. 18). A small slit is then made through any surrounding nonvascularized fibrotic tissue to expose the implant. The implant is then pushed out by continued finger pressure on the opposite end, and the incision site is closed with a Steristrip and a sterile bandage. Implants are easily removed in an outpatient setting. If continuation of therapy is desired, a new implant can be inserted into the same site. In clinical trial experience, bleeding on incision was minimal, and the majority of investigators described the procedure as easy. Application site reactions were transient, and bruising and pain were minimal. Patients described the adequacy of anesthetic as very good. No pulling or pain sensations were noted, with only a mild pressure sensation on implantation. Additionally, patients were not aware of the implant during the year-long therapy, and it did not have any effect on their daily activities.

Phase I/II and phase III clinical studies have examined the feasibility, functionality, and efficacy of Duros leuprolide implants in patients with advanced prostate cancer. In the phase I/II trial, patients were divided into two groups: One group received one Duros leuprolide implant (3.75 mg/month) and the other group received two implants (7.5 mg/month). In the phase III study, all patients received one Duros leuprolide implant. In both studies, serum testosterone was suppressed to less than 50 ng/dL by the fourth week of the trial in every group. Serum testosterone remained suppressed for the 1-year duration of the implant for both groups of patients in the phase I/II trial (data not shown) (55). Data from both studies also demonstrated controlled leuprolide plasma levels. In these studies, the safety profile of the implant was consistent with the known physiological actions of the drug (55).

2. Salmon Calcitonin

Salmon calcitonin (sCT) has been used for the treatment of osteoporosis and Paget's disease, where calcitonin inhibits osteoclastic bone resorption and induces calcium uptake (56). Standard doses range from 12 to 25 μg/day (57). Therefore, assuming a 12-month implant duration

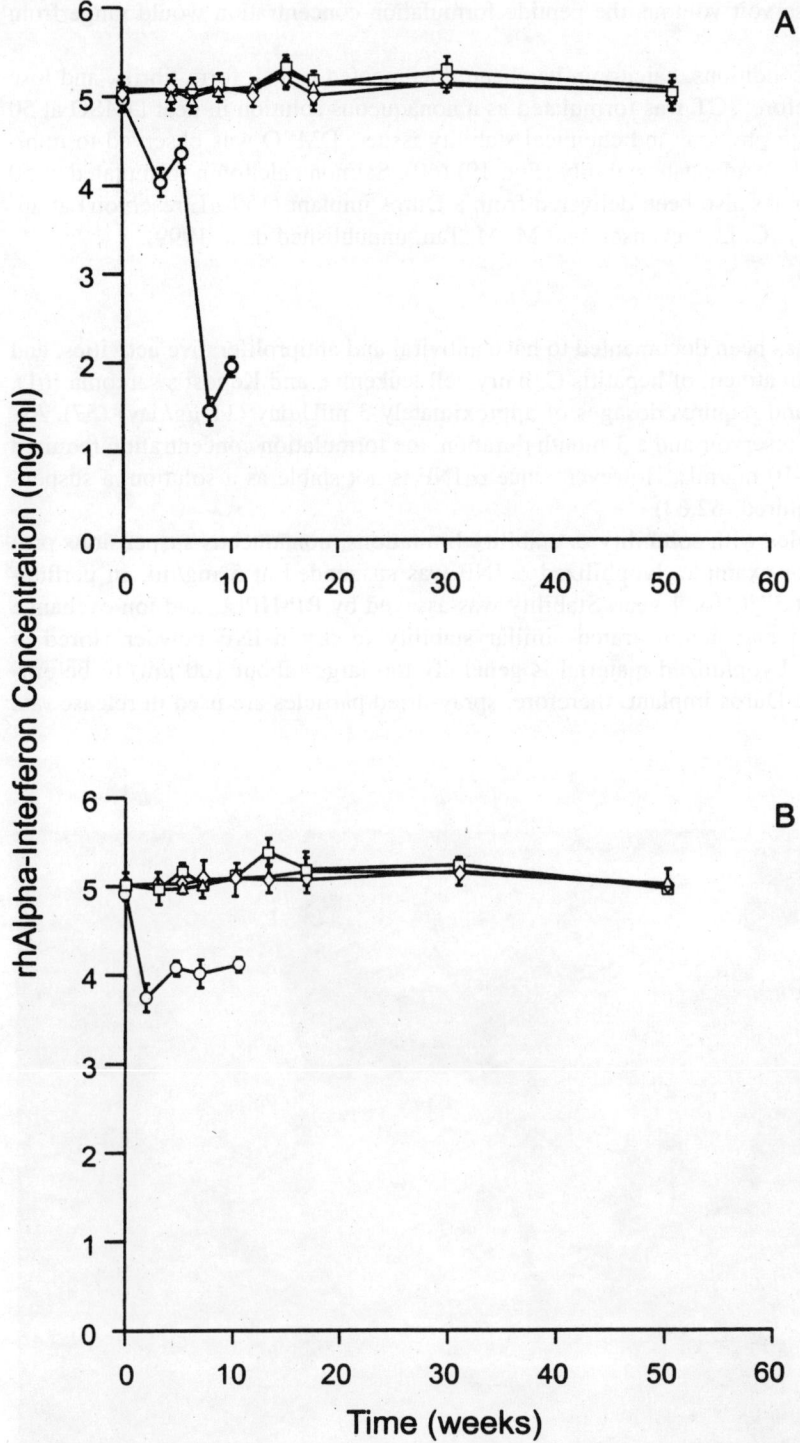

Figure 17 Stability of rhα-IFN powder measured by RP-HPLC (A) or IEX (B). Key: (◊) lyophilized powder stored at −80°C; (□) lyophilized powder stored at 37°C; (△) perfluorodecalin suspension stored at 37°C; (○) methoxyflurane suspension stored at 37°C. Mean ± SD of three individual samples taken from three separate vials.

and a 150-μL drug reservoir volume, the peptide formulation concentration would range from 30 to 60 mg/mL.

Under aqueous conditions, calcitonin has been documented to gel, form fibrils, and lose potency (58,59). Therefore, sCT was formulated as a nonaqueous solution in neat DMSO at 50 mg/mL to alleviate both physical and chemical stability issues. DMSO was observed to minimize gelation and produce adequate stability (Fig. 19) (60). Salmon calcitonin formulated at 50 mg/mL in neat DMSO has also been delivered from a Duros implant (150-μL reservoir) at approximately 0.4 μL/day (C. L. Stevenson and M. M. Tan, unpublished data, 1999).

3. α-Interferon

α-Interferon (α-INF) has been documented to have antiviral and antiproliferative activities, and has been used for the treatment of hepatitis C, hairy cell leukemia, and Kaposi's sarcoma (61). α-INF is very potent and requires dosages of approximately 3 mIU/day (11 μg/day) (57). Assuming a 150-μL drug reservoir and a 3-month duration, the formulation concentration required for a potent dose is 5–10 mg/mL. However, since α-INF is not stable as a solution, a suspension formulation is required (62,63).

For drug molecules with solubility or stability limitations, nonaqueous suspensions provide an alternative. For example, lyophilized α-INF was suspended at 5 mg/mL in perfluorodecalin and stored at 37°C for 1 year. Stability was assayed by RP-HPLC and ion exchange chromatography (IEX) and demonstrated similar stability to dry α-INF powder stored at −80°C (Fig. 17) (62). Lyophilized material is generally too large (about 100 μm) to be efficiently pumped from a Duros implant; therefore, spray-dried particles are used in release rate studies.

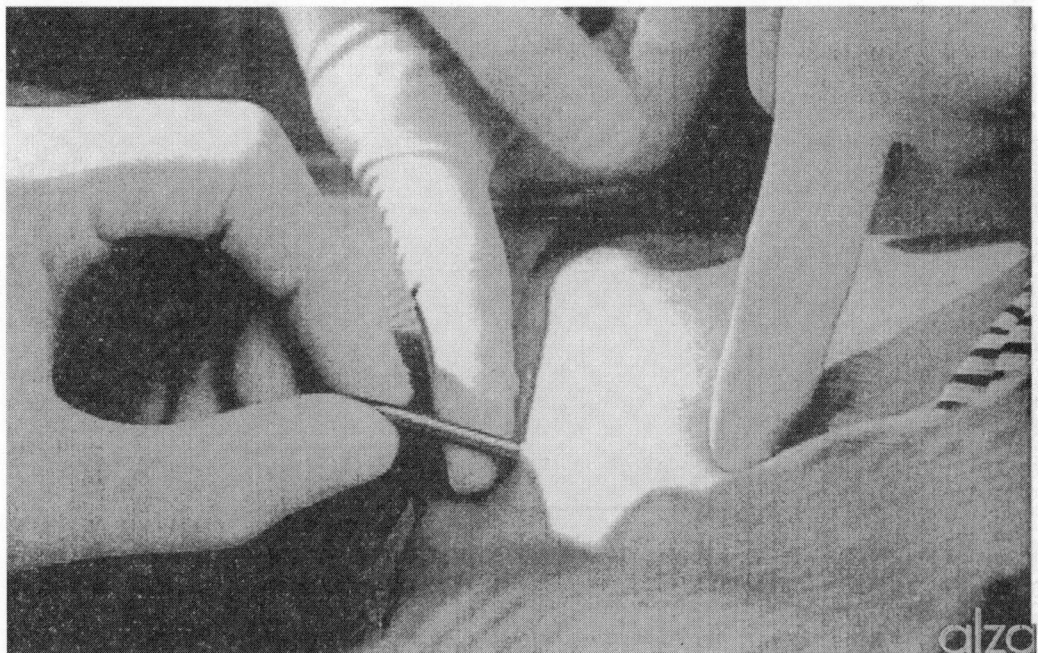

Figure 18 Removal of Duros leuprolide implant.

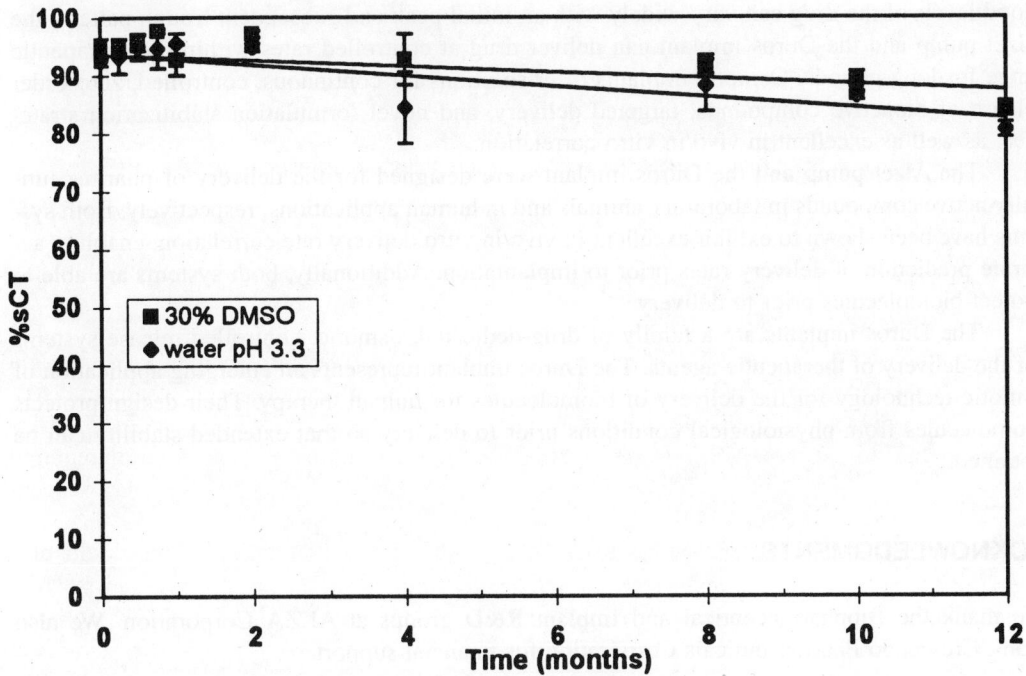

Figure 19 Effect of 30% DMSO on sCT (50 mg/mL) stability at 37°C for 1 year.

4. Factor IX

Factor IX (FIX) is a serine protease in the clotting cascade that is used in the treatment of hemophilia B (64,65). Factor IX is given as a maintenance dose of 10–20 IU/kg/day (57). An implantable dosage of factor IX would be of most benefit in pediatric cases, resulting in a maximum of 500 IU/day (about 2 mg/day). Assuming a 3-month duration and a larger system design, a suspension formulation requires at most 360 mg/mL factor IX. Because factor IX is administered intravenously, a catheter would be needed.

Preliminary factor IX (FIX) suspension stability was performed by suspending 1 mg/mL FIX in PEG-400, soybean oil, or perfluorodecalin for 6 months at 37°C (62). Soybean oil and PEG-400 gave poor stability; however, perfluorodecalin yielded promising stability. Stability in perfluorodecalin was similar to that of lyophilized dry powders stored at 37°C when analyzed by SEC and clotting bioassay.

V. CONCLUSIONS

Continuous zero-order release allows the therapeutic potential of drugs with short half-lives, such as proteins and peptides, to be fully realized. Use of a continuous drug delivery system, such as the Alzet pump and the Duros implant, offers a relatively smooth pharmacokinetic profile as compared with traditional bolus dosing methods. Unlike dosing by injection, where blood levels of the drug can vary widely with an initial peak and subsequent trough pattern, the Alzet pump and the Duros implant can deliver drug at controlled rates within the therapeutic range for long periods. Osmotic implants offer solutions for continuous, controlled, zero-order release of bioactive compounds, targeted delivery, and novel formulation stabilization strategies, as well as excellent in vivo/in vitro correlation.

The Alzet pump and the Duros implant were designed for the delivery of pharmaceutically active compounds in laboratory animals and in human applications, respectively. Both systems have been shown to exhibit excellent in vivo/in vitro delivery rate correlation, enabling accurate prediction of delivery rates prior to implantation. Additionally, both systems are able to protect biomolecules prior to delivery.

The Duros implants are a family of drug-dedicated, osmotic, controlled release systems for the delivery of therapeutic agents. The Duros implant represents an emerging application of osmotic technology for the delivery of biomolecules for human therapy. Their design protects biomolecules from physiological conditions prior to delivery so that extended stability can be obtained.

ACKNOWLEDGMENTS

We thank the Biopharmaceutical and Implant R&D groups at ALZA Corporation. We also thank Crescendo Pharmaceuticals Corporation for financial support.

REFERENCES

1. Rose, S., and Nelson, J. F., 1955. A continuous long-term injector. Aust. J. Exp. Biol., 33: 415–420.
2. Theeuwes F. 1975. Elementary osmotic pump. J. Pharm. Sci., 64: 1987–1991.
3. Theeuwes, F., and Yum, S. E., 1976. Principles of the design and operation of generic osmotic pumps for the delivery of semisolid or liquid drug formulations. Ann. Biomed. Eng., 4: 343–353.
4. Theeuwes, F., Wong, P. S. L., and Yum, S. E., 1991. Drug delivery and therapeutic systems. In: J. Swarbrick and J. C. Boylan (Eds.), Encyclopedia of Pharmaceutical Technology, Vol. 4, Marcel Dekker, New York, pp. 303–348.
5. Rhode, T. D., Buchwald, H., and Blackshear, P. J., 1988. Osmotic pumps. In: T. Praveen (Ed.), Drug Delivery Devices, Marcel Dekker, New York, pp. 235–260.
6. Fara, J. W. and Ray, N., 1988. Osmotic pumps. In: T. Praveen (Ed.), Drug Delivery Devices, Marcel Dekker, New York, pp. 137–176.
7. Chien, Y. W., 1987. Implantable therapeutic systems. In: Controlled Drug Delivery, Marcel Dekker, New York, pp. 481–522.
8. Siegel, R. A., and Firestone, B. A., 1990. Mechanochemical approaches to self-regulating insulin pump design. J. Controlled Release, 11: 181–192.
9. U.S. Pat. 4,723,958 (Feb. 9, 1988), D. G. Pope and A. E. Royce (to Merck & Co., Inc.).
10. U.S. Pat. 5,017,381 (May 21, 1991), F. Maruyama and R. Cortese (to Alza Corp.).
11. U.S. Pat. 4,160,020 (July 3, 1979), A. D. Ayer and F. Theeuwes (to Alza Corp.).
12. Baker, R., 1987. Osmotic and mechanical devices. In: R. Baker (Ed.), Controlled Release of Biologically Active Agents, John Wiley and Sons, New York, pp. 132–155.
13. U.S. Pat. 3,732,865 (May 15, 1973) T. Higuchi and H. Leeper (to Alza Corp.).
14. Heilman, K., 1984. Therapeutic Systems, Rate-Controlled Drug Delivery: Concept and Development, 2nd ed., Thieme-Stratton, New York, p. 29.
15. U.S. Pat. 4,077,407 (March 7, 1978), F. Theeuwes and A. D. Ayer (to Alza Corp.).
16. Eckenhoff, B., Theeuwes, F. and Urquhart, F., 1987. Osmotically actuated dosage forms for rate-controlled drug delivery. Pharm. Technol., 11: 96–105.

17. Lonsdale, H. K., 1966. Properties of cellulose acetate membranes. In: U. Mertens (Ed.), Desalination by Reverse Osmosis. MIT Press, Cambridge, pp. 93–160.
18. Eckenhoff, B., 1981. Osmotically driven pumps for rate-controlled delivery of solutions and viscous suspensions. In: S. K. Chandrasekaran (Ed.), AIChE Symposium Series, 77, 1–9.
19. Zingerman, J. R., Cardinal, J. R., Chern, R. T., Holste, J., Williams, J. B., Eckenhoff, B. and Wright, J. 1997. The in vitro and in vivo performance of an osmotically controlled delivery system-IVOMEC SR bolus. J. Controlled Release, 47: 1–11.
20. Martin, A; Swarbrick, J., and Cammarata, A., 1983. Physical Pharmacy. Lea & Febiger, Philadelphia, pp. 544–553.
21. Alza Corporation, Technical Information Manual, Alzet Osmotic Pumps, March 1996.
22. Amkraut, A., Eckenhoff, J. B. and Nichols, K., 1990. Osmotic delivery of peptides and macromolecules. Adv. Drug Deliv. Rev., 4: 255–276.
23. Davison, T. F., Freeman, B. M., and Rea, J., 1983. Chronic local infusion into the renal artery of unrestrained rates. Am. J. Physiol., 244: H304–H307.
24. Ruers, T. J. M., Buurman, W. A., Smits, J. F. M., van der Linder, C. J., van Dongen, J. J., Struyker-Boudier, H. A. J., and Kootstra, G., 1986. Local treatment of renal allografts, a promising way to reduce the dosage of immunosuppressive drugs. Transplantation, 41: 156–161.
25. Gmunder, F. K., Nordau, C-G., Tschopp, A., Huber, B., and Cogoli, A., 1988. Dynamic cell culture system: a new cell cultivation instrument for biological experiments in space. J. Biotechnol., 7: 217–228.
26. Cronin M., Battersby, J., Hancock, W., Schwall, R., and Clark, R. 1992. Delivery of recombinant human growth hormone to rats during exposure to microgravity on NASA space shuttle discovery. Physiologist, 35(1): S51–S52.
27. Alza Corporation, Special Delivery, March 1986, p. 2.
28. Cohen, A. M., Zsebo, K. M., Inoue, H., Hines, D., Boone, T. C., Chazin, V. R., Tsai, L., Ritch, T., and Souza, L. M. 1987. In vivo stimulation of granulopoiesis by recombinant human granulocyte colony-stimulating factor. Proc. Natl. Acad. Sci. USA, 84: 2484–2488.
29. Kawai, K., and Ohashi, S., 1993. Long-term (1-month) administration of GLP-1(7-36) amide to normal and diabetic rats. Digestion, 54: 359–360.
30. Whitesell, L., Rosolen, A., and Neckers, L. M., 1991. In vivo modulation of N-myc expression by continuous perfusion with an antisense oligonucleotide. Antisense Res. Dev., 1: 343–350.
31. Ratajczak, M. Z., Kant, J. A., Luger, S. M., Hijiya, N., Zhang, J., Zon, G., and Gewirtz, A. M., 1992. In vivo treatment of human leukemia in a scid mouse model with c-myb antisense oligonucleotides. Proc. Natl. Acad. Sci. USA, 89: 11823–11827.
32. Higgins, K. A., Perez, J. R., Coleman, T. A., Dorshkind, K., McComas, W. A., Sarmiento, U. M., Rosen, C. A., and Narayanan, R., 1993. Antisense inhibition of the p65 subunit of NF-κB blocks tumorigenicity and causes tumor regression. Proc. Natl. Acad. Sci. USA, 90: 9901–9905.
33. Kromer, L. F., 1986. Nerve growth factor treatment after brain injury prevents neuronal death. Science, 235: 214–216.
34. Fischer, W., Wictorin, K., Bjorklund, A., Williams, L. R., Varon, S., and Gage, F. H., 1987. Amelioration of cholinergic neuron atrophy and spatial memory impairment in aged rats by nerve growth factor. Nature, 329: 65–68.
35. Williams, L. R., Varon, S., Peterson, G. M., Wictorin, K., Fischer, W., Bjorklund, A., and Gage, F. H., 1986. Continuous infusion of nerve growth factor prevents basal forebrain neuronal death after fimbria fornix transection. Proc. Natl. Acad. Sci. USA, 83: 9231–9235.
36. Tuszynski, M. H., U, H. S., Amaral, D. G., and Gage, F. H., 1990. Nerve growth factor infusion in the primate brain reduces lesion-induced cholinergic neuronal degeneration. J. Neurosci., 10: 3604–3614.
37. Mihara, M., Ikuta, M., Koishihara, Y., and Ohsugi, Y., 1991. Interleukin 6 inhibits delayed-type hypersensitivity and the development of adjuvant arthritis. Eur. J. Immunol., 21: 2327–2331.
38. Lorberboum-Lalski, H., Lafyatis, R., Case, J. P., Fitzgerald, D., Wilder, R. L., and Pastan, I., 1991. Administration of IL-2-PE40 via osmotic pumps prevents adjuvant arthritis in rats. Int. J. Immunopharmacol., 13: 305–315.

39. Borella, L., Eng, C. P., DiJoseph, J., Wells, C., Ward, J., Caccese, R., and Baeder, W. L. 1991. Rapid induction of early osteoarthritic-like lesions in the rabbit knee by continuous intra-articular infusion of mammalian collagenase or interleukin-1. Agents Actions, 34: 220–222.
40. Weckenbecker, G., Liu, R., Tolcsvai, L., and Bruns, C., 1992. Antiproliferative effects of the somatostatin analogue octreotide (SMS 210-995) in ZR-75-1 human breast cancer cells in vivo and in vitro. Cancer Res., 52: 4973–4978.
41. Weckenbecker, G., Tolcsvai, L., Liu, R., and Bruns, C., 1992. Preclinical studies on the anticancer activity of the somatostatin analogue octreotide (SMS 201-995). Metabolism, 41: 99–103.
42. Weckenbecker, G., Tolcsvai, L., Stolz, B., Pollack, M., and Bruns, C., 1994. Somatostatin analogue octreotide enhances the antineoplastic effects of tamoxifen and ovariectomy on 7,12-dimethylbenz(a)-anthracene-induced rat mammary carcinomas. Cancer Res., 54: 6334–6337.
43. Hall, S. H., Leonard, J. J., and Stevenson, C. L. 1999. Characterization and comparison of leuprolide degradation profiles in water and dimethyl sulfoxide. J. Peptide Res., 53, 432–441 (1999).
44. Stevenson C. L., Corley C. A., Cukierski M., Falender C. A., Hall S. C., Johnson P., Leonard J. J., Tan M. M., and Wright J. C., Characterization of a stable leuprolide formulation for one year in an implantable device. Program and Abstracts, The 1997 American Peptide Symposium; 14–19 June 1997; Nashville, Tennessee.
45. Crawford, E., DeAntonio, E. P., Labrie, F., Schroder, F. H., and Geller, J., 1995. Endocrine therapy of prostate: optimal form and appropriate timing. J. Clin. Endocrinol. Metab., 80: 1062–1078.
46. Kaisary, A., Tyrell, C. J., and Peeling, W. B., 1991. Comparison of LHRH analogue (Zoladex) with orchiectomy in patients with metastatic prostatic carcinoma. Br. J. Urol., 67: 502–508.
47. Huben, R. P., and Murphy, G. P., 1988. A comparison of diethylstilbestrol or orchiectomy with buserelin and with methotrexate plus diethylstilbestrol or orchiectomy in newly diagnosed patients with clinical stage D2 cancer of the prostate. Cancer, 62: 1881–1887.
48. Soloway, M. S., Chodak, G., and Vogelzang, N. J., 1991. Zoladex versus orchiectomy in treatment of advanced prostate cancer: a randomized trial. Urology, 37: 46–51.
49. Tan, M. M., Corley, C. C., and Stevenson, C. L. 1998. Effect of gelation on the chemical stability and conformation of leuprolide. Pharm. Res. 15: 1442–1447.
50. Stevenson, C. L., Leonard, J. J., Corley, C. A., Tan, M. M., Ryan, D. A., and Prestrelski, S. J. 1996. Solution stability and arrhenius kinetics of an LHRH agonist, leuprolide, at high peptide concentration. Pharm. Res., 13: S–110.
51. Stevenson, C. L., Leonard, J. J., Falender, C. A., Tao, S. A., Corley, C. A., Tan, M. M., Dionne, K. E., Wright, J. C., and Prestrelski, S. J., 1996. Formulation stability and continuous release of a peptide delivered from an osmotically driven implantable device. Proc. 23rd Int. Symp. Control. Rel. Bioact. Mater., 23: 837–838.
52. Wright, J. C., Magruder, J., Skowronski, R., Dionne, K., Stevenson, C., Leonard, J., Prestrelski S., Tao S., Falender C., Cukierski M., Johnson P., and Brown J., 1997. A one-year implantable, osmotic delivery system (Duros Leuprolide Implant) for the treatment of advanced prostate cancer. Proc. 24th Int. Symp. Control. Rel. Bioact. Mater., 24: 59–60.
53. Wright, J., Chen, G., Cukierski, M., Falender, C. Mabanglo, D., Peery, J., Ponnekanti, L., Skowronski, R., Stevenson, C., Tao, S., and Brown, J., 1998. DUROS® leuprolide implant for continuous one-year treatment of prostate cancer, Proceed. 25th Intl. Symp. Control. Rel. Bioact. Mater., 25: 516–517.
54. Wright, J. C., Stevenson, C. L., and Stewart, G. R., 1999. Duros osmotic implant. In: E. Mathiowitz (Ed.), Encyclopedia of Controlled Drug Delivery, 1st ed. John Wiley and Sons, New York 909–915.
55. Fowler, J. E., Gottesman, J. E., Bardot, S. F., Reid, C. F., Bernhard, P. H., Rivera-Ramirez, I., Libertino, J. A. and Soloway, M. S., 1998. A Phase I/II dose ranging study of the Duros (leuprolide) implantable therapeutic system in patients with advanced prostate cancer. J. Urol., 159 (5 Suppl.): 335.
56. Lee, K. C., Lee, Y. J., Song, H. M., Chun, C. J., and DeLuca, P. P., 1992. Degradation of synthetic salmon calcitonin in aqueous solution. Pharm. Res., 9: 1521–1523.
57. Physicians Desk Reference. 1998. Medical Economics, Montvale, NJ.
58. Cudd, A., Arvinte, T., Gaines Das, R. E., Chinni, C., and MacIntyre, I., 1995. Enhanced potency of human calcitonin when fibrillation is avoided. J. Pharm. Sci., 84: 717–719.

59. Arvinte, T., Cudd, A., and Drake, A. F., 1993. The structure and mechanism of formation of human calcitonin fibrils. J. Biol. Chem., 268: 6415–6422.
60. Tan, M. and Stevenson, C., 1997. Salmon calcitonin gel formulations: chemical, physical and structural stability at 37°C by FTIR and HPLC. Pharm. Res. 14: S–227.
61. Johnson, H. M., Bazer, F. W., Szente, B. E. and Jarpe, M. A., 1994. How interferons fight disease. Sci. Am., May, 68–75.
62. Knepp, V. M., Muchnik, A., Oldmark, S., and Kalashnikova, L., 1998. Stability of nonaqueous suspension formulations of plasma derived factor IX and recombinant human alpha interferon at elevated temperatures. Pharm. Res. 15: 1090–1095.
63. Ip, A. Y., Arakawa, T., Silvers, H., Ransone, C. M. and Niven, R. W., 1995. Stability of recombinant consensus interferon to air-jet and ultrasonic nebulization. J. Pharm. Sci., 84: 1210–1214.
64. Lawn, R. M., 1985. The molecular genetics of hemophilia: blood clotting factors VIII and IX. Cell, 42: 405–406.
65. Smith, K. L., 1992. Factor IX concentrates: the new products and their properties. Transfus. Med. Rev., 6: 124–136.

12
Bioadhesive Controlled Release Systems

Nicholas A. Peppas, Monica D. Little,* and Yanbin Huang
Purdue University West Lafayette, Indiana

I. MUCOADHESIVE CONTROLLED DRUG DELIVERY

Mucoadhesion, or the attachment of a natural or synthetic polymer to a biological substrate, is a practical method of drug immobilization or localization and an important new aspect of controlled drug delivery. While the subject of mucoadhesion is not new, there has been increased interest in recent years in using mucoadhesive polymers for drug delivery (1,2). Therefore, the study and alteration of the adhesion of bioadhesive materials, as well as the diffusion of various drugs from bioadhesive devices, is of significance.

The motivation for controlled drug release is the necessity to maintain a constant effective drug concentration in the body for an extended time period. For optimal performance, drug concentrations in the body should be maintained above the effective level and below the toxic level. However, when a drug is administered to a patient, the initial concentration of the drug in the body will peak above a toxic level before gradually diminishing to an ineffective level due to excretion. Furthermore, dilution of the drug in the body fluids will impede its absorption by tissues and its transport into the bloodstream.

A mucoadhesive controlled release device can improve the effectiveness of a drug by helping to maintain the drug concentration between the effective and toxic levels, inhibiting the dilution of the drug in the body fluids, and allowing targeting and localization of a drug at a specific site. A drug can be incorporated into a crosslinked polymeric device that would adhere to a mucous substrate in the body. The drug can then diffuse from the device directly into the tissues.

Mucoadhesion also increases the intimacy and duration of contact between a drug-containing polymer and a mucous surface. It is believed that the mucoadhesive nature of the device can increase the residence time of the drug in the body. The combined effects of the direct drug absorption and the decrease in excretion rate allow for an increased bioavailability of the drug with a smaller dosage and less frequent administration. Another advantage of using a polymer carrier for drug delivery is the prevention of first-pass metabolism of certain protein drugs by the liver through the introduction of the drug via a route bypassing the digestive tract. Drugs that are absorbed through the mucosal lining of tissues can enter directly into the bloodstream and not be inactivated by enzymatic degradation in the gastrointestinal (GI) tract (3). A polymeric device also allows for slow, controlled, and predictable drug release over time and

---

*Current affiliation: 3M Company, St. Paul, Minnesota

reduces the initial drug loading concentration needed. This reduction also decreases the toxicity and waste of expensive drugs (3) as well as improves patient compliance because the drug would not have to be administered as often.

Several polymeric bioadhesive drug delivery systems have been fabricated and studied in the past. Several such devices are currently used in clinical applications involving dental, orthopedic, ophthalmological, and surgical uses. Viable application sites include the mouth, intestine, nose, eye, and vagina. Acrylic-based hydrogels have been used extensively for bioadhesive devices. Hydrogels are crosslinked hydrophilic polymer matrices that are glassy when dry but become rubbery when water is incorporated. Acrylic-based hydrogels are well suited for bioadhesion due to their flexibility and nonabrasive characteristics in the partially swollen state, which reduce damage-causing attrition to the tissues in contact (4). Furthermore, their high permeability in the swollen state allows unreacted monomer, uncrosslinked polymer chains, and the initiator to be washed out of the matrix after polymerization. This washing step is essential, as the monomer may be toxic and the linear polymer may cause tissue irritation. Acrylic-based polymer devices also exhibit a very high adhesive bond strength (4). However, the adhesive and drug delivery capabilities of these devices can continue to be improved as presently known bioadhesive materials are modified and more bioadhesive materials are discovered (5–16).

II. STRUCTURE AND PHYSIOLOGY OF MUCIN

Mucus is the general term used for the heterogeneous secretion found on epithelial cells (1). Mucus is produced at several sites in the body, including the ear, eye, nose, mouth, and the GI, reproductive, and respiratory tracts. The principal role of the mucus is to protect and lubricate the epithelial tissue beneath it. At some sites, the mucus has been known to perform other functions. For example, the human cervical mucus is involved in both conception and contraception (2). In addition to lubricating the corneal epithelium, ocular mucin helps to hydrate, clean, and remove cell debris from the eye. These mucins also serve to defend against pathogens. Due to their strong repulsion to the corneal epithelium, they form a barrier against nonpolar tear film lipids and hydrophilic bacteria (17). Human respiratory mucus is an important factor in the removal of inhaled particles and microorganisms, while the surface mucosal gel of the stomach and duodenum has a bicarbonate barrier that supports neutralization of luminal acid and acts as a diffusion barrier to pepsin. The cervical mucus separates the uterus from the vagina, and facilitates or hinders the passage of sperm, depending on the concentrations of hormones that regulate the mucus viscosity.

The mucous layer is a highly viscous product secreted by the goblet cells that coat the epithelial cell surface (18–20). The secretion may be either an intermittent or a continuous process. Although the amount of mucin secreted depends on the age, sex, location in the body, and state of health of the individual, the average mucin turnover rate is typically about 6 hours (2). Mucus is primarily composed of approximately 95% water, 1% electrolytes, 0.5–1% proteins, and 0.5–1% lipids and glycoproteins. This composition or turnover rate may be altered slightly depending on the mucin source (18) and pathological conditions (19). For example, intestinal ulceration and inflammation may result in a thinning of the mucin layer, while patients with cystic fibrosis may have a thicker and denser intestinal mucin layer (21). It is important to note that the placement of an adhesive polymer device on the mucosal surface decreases the rate of mucin turnover, which can result in the mucoadhesive remaining on the mucus for up to 15 hours (22). Therefore, the location of application and any presence of disease should be considered when designing a mucoadhesive device.

The principal biochemical component of mucus is the mucous glycoprotein, a large molecular weight molecule that is highly glycosylated (1). The glycoprotein portion of the mucus is responsible for its gel-like characteristic (2). A mucous glycoprotein consists of a protein core with carbohydrate side chains attached over 63% of its length (2). The attachments are made predominantly by O-glycosidic linkages through the serine and threonine amino acids (18).

The molecular weight of a glycoprotein chain may exceed 45×10^6, though the average molecular weight (2) is approximately 1.8×10^6. The glycoproteins may be seen via electron microscopy as flexible, thread-like, polydisperse structures. Mucin peptide precursors with repeating unit molecular weights between 200,000 and 400,000 have been identified through the use of antibodies directed against them. The amino acid sequence and the various oligosaccharide groups connected to the backbone will determine the protein chain conformation and thus the manner and types of interactions the glycoproteins will have with other molecules (2). There is general agreement that the glycoprotein is a polymeric structure, the predominant unit being a relatively high molecular weight glycopeptide, or subunit, known to be covalently bound to other subunits through disulfide bonds located in nonglycosylated sections of the protein core. This subunit also interacts, probably intermolecularly, with the other subunits through ionic bonds and entanglements (18). The cohesive nature of the mucous gel is due to entanglements, that is, disulfide and secondary bonds. The disulfide bonds are believed to be intrachain in nature, whereas interchain hydrogen bonds are thought to stabilize other physical junctions. Other non-covalent interactions may exist between carbohydrate side chains or between these chains and the peptide backbone of the glycoprotein (18).

The glycoprotein is a highly expanded random coil, 1 g of which would occupy a 40 mL volume in solution (2). The glycoprotein monomer varies in size, depending on the location in the body. For the stomach and small intestine, the monomer molecular weights are 5.5×10^5 and 2.4×10^5, respectively. The unglycosylated portion of the protein core consists of terminal regions, but subunits of chains are joined through peptide linkages and intramolecular cysteine–cysteine disulfide bridges.

About 800 amino acid residues compose the protein core of the glycoprotein chain. Threonine, serine, and proline are the predominant amino acid components in the glycosylated region of the core. O-Glycosidic linkages of the oligosaccharide side chains occur at about one of every three residues in this region. Between 70 and 90 wt % of the glycoprotein consists of carbohydrates. A fundamental function of the carbohydrates is to make the glycoprotein chain more compatible with water, so that they may act as a shield against proteolytic degradation. There are five main carbohydrate side chain components—N-acetyl galactosamine (galNAc), where the sugars connect to hydroxyl groups on the serine and threonine residues of the main protein chain; galactose (gal); N-acetyl glucosamine; fucose; and N-acetyl neruaminic (sialic) acid (23,24). Although the range is from 2 to 20 residues, each side chain averages (8) amino acid residues in length (1), and is composed of alternating gal and glcNAc residues with fucose and sialic acid as the terminal sugars (2). The side chains may be either linear or branched (18,19). Ester sulfate residues, which can occur at intermediate positions in the side chain, and sialic acid residues each have pK_a values (18) of approximately 2. Hence, dissociation occurs at pH values above 3 and a net negative charge is imparted on the glycoprotein molecule (2).

Subunits of the glycoprotein macromolecule are joined by peptide linkages and intramolecular cysteine–cysteine disulfide bridges. The mucus glycoprotein subunit has been isolated from mucus secretions at various sites of many species. Included are the rat small intestine; pig stomach, intestine, and colon; human airway, stomach, and cervix. The repeating unit molecular weight is estimated to be between 380,000 and 720,000 depending on its source (1). Rat goblet cell mucin, which has a molecular weight of 2×10^6, has subunits connected by 34 disulfide bridges (25). Reduction of these bridges releases a negative protein fraction from the glycoprotein, representing about 3.7% by weight of the glycoprotein. This fraction has a high cysteine content; has very little serine, threonine, or proline; and is reported to have a molecular weight of 70,000, 90,000, and 118,000. Proteolytic digestion also cleaves about 5% by weight of protein from glycoprotein (23).

The mucous coating on the epithelial surface is uneven, with thickness varying between 5 and 200 μm in the gastric and duodenal regions of the rat, to about twice this variation in the human (24). Glycoprotein concentrations determine the cohesion of the mucous gel. A gel forms only after attaining a critical concentration at which the hydrodynamic volumes of the molecules begin to overlap. Above this concentration, entanglements of the carbohydrate side chains and the formation of secondary bonds are induced. For gastric glycoprotein, the gel formation occurs at a concentration of 30–40 mg/mL.

When pathological conditions occur, hypersecretion of mucus is more common than hyposecretion. Upon exposure to an irritant, the acidic side chains of the glycoprotein increase from 50% to 80%, due to an increase in sialic acid terminal sugars as well as an increase in sulfonation. The result is a more negatively charged molecule. The submucosal gland layer depth increases as the number of goblet cells increases. These increases lead to mucus hypersecretion. The pH and total nondialyzable solids content also increase. In the GI tract, the addition of DNA and albumin thickens the mucus. Hypersecretion in the GI tract is linked to malabsorption syndromes, whereas hyposecretion is associated with ulcerative states (2).

The amount and type of mucus secretion depends on several factors, including age, sex, location, and pathological conditions. The presence of a mucoadhesive device may alter the mucin turnover rate or thickness. The transit time of a GI mucoadhesive may be reduced due to hypersecretion of mucus in this region. Therefore, the design of an effective mucoadhesive device will be challenging because it must take these factors into consideration.

III. INTERACTION MECHANISMS OF BIOADHESION

Adhesion of a polymer to a tissue involves contributions from three main regions: the surface of the bioadhesive material, the first layer of the natural tissue, and the interfacial region between the two layers. The development of a successful bioadhesive device is dependent on an understanding of how these components interact so that the properties of the bioadhesive may be modified to optimize the adhesion.

Adhesion between a polymer and a tissue is primarily due to three types of interactions: physical or mechanical bonds; secondary chemical bonds; or ionic, primary, or covalent chemical bonds. These same types of interactions are also important in the adhesion between two polymers (18,19,26).

A physical or mechanical bond may be formed when the polymer material is deposited on and included in the crevices of the tissue (27,28). This inclusion is necessary for the establishment of intimate contact between the polymer and the tissue, which is critical to the occurrence of a good bioadhesive bond (18). The surface roughness of the substrate becomes important under such conditions (29). The microscopic characteristics of the surface roughness in tissues has been discussed by Merrill (30). The ratio of the maximum depth, d, to the width, h, may be used to define the surface roughness, as shown in Fig. 1. A d/h value less than 1/20 may be considered negligible in terms of surface roughness.

When the aspect ratio exceeds this value, only highly fluid materials or suspensions can be used on these substrates for successful bioadhesion. Therefore, a negligible surface roughness is needed to form intimate contact between a solid polymer device and a tissue surface, and hence a successful bioadhesive bond.

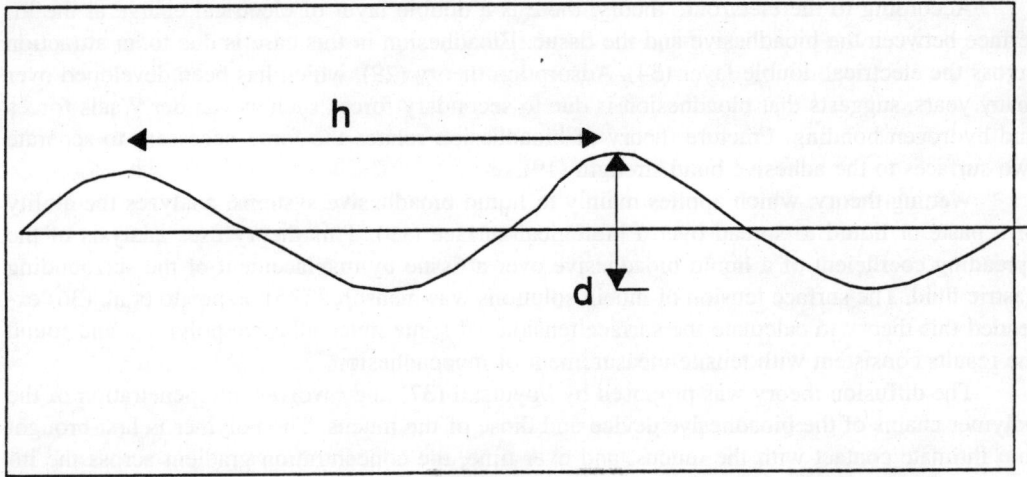

Figure 1 Schematic representation of the roughness of tissue surfaces. The surface roughness is measured as the ratio of the maximum depth, d, to the width, h.

Secondary chemical bonds, including hydrogen bonding and van der Waals forces, can contribute to bioadhesion. The van der Waals forces are a combination of two different effects: dispersion forces due to movement of the internal electrons, and polar forces due to the orientation of the permanent electric dipoles. The polar forces are more significant than the dispersion forces (31,32). Hydrogen bonding between certain groups on the polymer and the tissue can also contribute to a bioadhesive bond when a hydrophilic polymer is used. Some functional groups that form hydrogen bonds contributing to adhesion include hydroxyl, carboxyl, sulfate, and amino groups on both the bioadhesive material and on the glycoproteins of the mucus.

Primary bonds are formed by chemically reacting the polymer and the substrate. This type of bonding is only desirable when the connection between the substrate and the adhesive is to be permanent, such as in dental or orthopedic applications (29). For this reason, most bioadhesive bonds are achieved through physical bonds, hydrogen bonds, or other secondary bonds.

Hydrogen bonding is the most important secondary bond in bioadhesion (18). Thus, polymers containing hydroxyls and carboxyls, such as poly(vinyl alcohol), poly(acrylic acid), poly(hydroxyalkyl methacrylate), and their respective copolymers are ideal candidates for bioadhesion (19).

IV. GENERAL THEORIES OF BIOADHESION

The theories of polymer–polymer adhesion can be adapted to polymer–tissue adhesion or bioadhesion by recognizing that bioadhesion is different only because of the differing properties of the tissue as opposed to those of the polymer (19). It should be noted that many theories have been developed to explain the phenomenon of bioadhesion. No individual theory has been universally accepted as the singular mechanism by which bioadhesion occurs, though a combination of theories may be used to describe the phenomenon. This section discusses some of the predominant theories, i.e., the electronic, adsorption, fracture, wetting, and diffusion theories (29,33).

According to the electronic theory, there is a double layer of electrical charge at the interface between the bioadhesive and the tissue. Bioadhesion in this case is due to an attraction across the electrical double layer (34). Adsorption theory (29), which has been developed over many years, suggests that bioadhesion is due to secondary forces such as van der Waals forces and hydrogen bonding. Fracture theory of bioadhesion relates the force necessary to separate two surfaces to the adhesive bond strength (19).

Wetting theory, which applies mainly to liquid bioadhesive systems, analyzes the ability of a paste or liquid to spread over a biological surface (19). This theory uses analysis of the spreading coefficient of a liquid bioadhesive over a tissue by displacement of the surrounding gastric fluid. The surface tension of mucin solutions was measured (35). Esposito et al. (36) extended this theory to calculate the surface tensions of some mucoadhesive polymers and found the results consistent with tensile measurement of mucoadhesion.

The diffusion theory was proposed by Voyutskii (37) and involves interpenetration of the polymer chains of the bioadhesive device and those of the mucus. The polymer is first brought into intimate contact with the mucus, and over time, the concentration gradient across the interface causes the diffusion of the chains of the bioadhesive into the mucus layer and also the diffusion of the glycoprotein chains of the mucus into the bioadhesive polymer, as illustrated in Fig. 2. In the case of a crosslinked polymer, it is the chain ends and smaller molecular weight chains that contribute to the interpenetration process. The rate of the diffusion is dependent on the chemical potential gradient and the diffusion coefficient of a macromolecule through a crosslinked network. The chains that have diffused across the interface serve as anchors to aid in securing the bioadhesive device in place semipermanently. The interpenetration distance necessary for good bioadhesion is approximately equal to the end-to-end distance of the macromolecular chains (18).

Adequate solubility of the bioadhesive in the mucus is essential for good bioadhesion. Consequently, the solubility parameters of each substance must be similar, which can be achieved by creating a bioadhesive device that is of similar chemical structure as mucus. Thus,

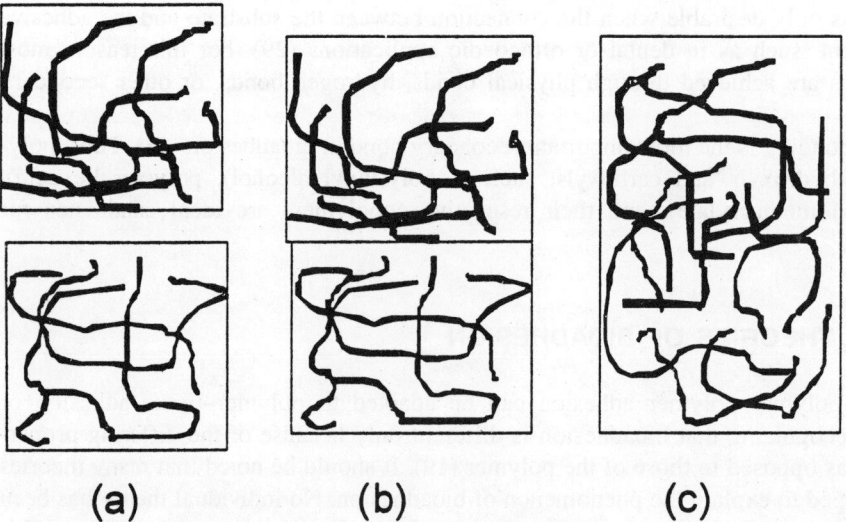

Figure 2 Schematic representation of diffusion theory of adhesion. (a) Top polymer layer and bottom layer before contact. (b) Right after contact. (c) The interface become diffuse after contact for a period of time.

polymers containing hydroxyl, carboxyl, and some amines and sulfates make good bioadhesive devices. Other structural aspects found to favor good mucoadhesion are good diffusion and entanglement between the bioadhesive device and the mucus, and a polymer molecular weight that is high but does not exceed a certain value. If the polymer chains are too long, their ability to diffuse is limited.

V. MOLECULAR MODELING OF BIOADHESION PROCESSES

It is important to understand the bioadhesion process in the molecular level in order to optimize the design of novel bioadhesive controlled release systems. In the last decade, our group (38–42) proposed a list of theoretical models for hydrogel bioadhesion based on the diffusion theory of adhesion.

According to the diffusion theory of adhesion, the hydrogel bioadhesion can be enhanced by two kinds of *adhesion promoters* (43): (a) the free polymer chains (sol fraction) in the interface region; and (b) grafted polymer chains on the gel surface. In bioadhesion, these polymer chains penetrate into the mucous layer and bridge the base hydrogel and the mucous gel.

For the case of *free chain adhesion promoters*, as shown in Fig. 3, the driving potential for the free chains to be transported across the hydrogel–mucus interface is their chemical potential gradient. This consists of three contributions: (a) the concentration gradient of free chains across the interface, i.e., the translational entropy contribution; (b) the physical structure and environment difference between hydrogel and mucus, i.e., the configurational contribution; and (c) the chemical structure difference between hydrogel and mucus, i.e., the interaction energy contribution. A chain transport process occurs if the sum of these three chemical potential contributions is favorable.

Using scaling concept, Mikos and Peppas (39,40) presented the kinetic analysis for the diffusion of free polymer chains across hydrogel–mucus interfaces. According to their analysis,

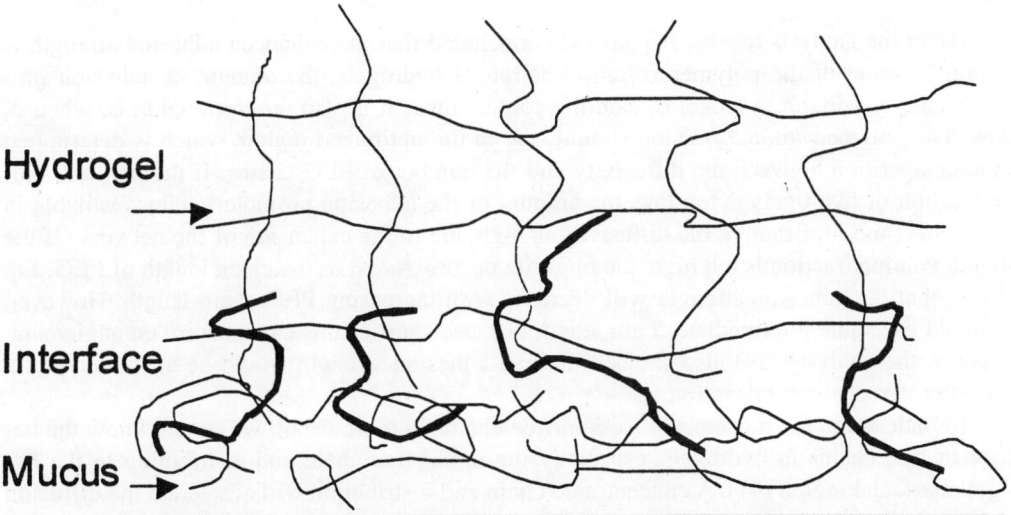

Figure 3 The free polymers across the hydrogel–mucus interface act as adhesion promoters. The free chains are initially in the networks. When placed in contact, the chemical potential gradient causes mutual diffusion of chains across the interface.

the fracture energy of adhesion at contact time t, $G_F(t)$, turned out to be proportional to the number of effective polymer chains crossing per unit area $N_{eff}(t)$. A polymer chain crossing is considered effective if the chain crosses the interface and is entangled about it. Then,

$$G_F(t) \sim N_{eff}(t) \tag{1}$$

Furthermore, the following scaling law was derived for the number of effective chain crossings:

$$N_{eff}(t) \sim v_2 \phi_f g_b^{1/2} D_b^{1/2} N^{-2/3} t^{1/2} \tag{2}$$

Here v_2 is the equilibrium polymer volume fraction of the hydrogel, ϕ_f is the volume fraction of the adhesion promoter chains initially trapped in the hydrogel on a dry basis, g_b is the number of repeating units between hydrogel crosslinks, D_b is the diffusion coefficient of the adhesion promoter chains in the hydrogel, N is the degree of polymerization of the adhesion promoter chains, and t is the contact time. In their analysis, it was assumed that the hydrogel and mucus have the same chemical and physical structure, and hence the only contribution to the chemical potential gradient is the concentration gradient.

Recently, Peppas (41) extended the above general analysis to a particular case: poly(ethylene glycol) (PEG) chains transport across a swollen poly(acrylic acid) (PAA)–mucus interface, using PEG as an adhesion promoter. He expressed the diffusion coefficient D_b as a function of size of the PEG chains and the equilibrium polymer volume fraction of the PAA hydrogel. Finally, the following scaling expression for the enhanced adhesion strength was obtained:

$$A(t) \sim v_2 \phi_f g_b^{1/2} \left(\frac{M_{PEG}}{44}\right)^{-3/2} t^{1/2} \sqrt{k_1 \exp\left[\frac{3\left(\frac{M_{PEG}}{44}\right) k_2 \alpha^2 C_n l^2 v_2}{1 - v_2}\right]} \tag{3}$$

Here M_{PEG} is the PEG molecular weight, α is the swollen PEG expression factor which can be calculated (44), C_n is the characteristics ratio of PEG in water and can be taken as 4, ℓ is C–C bond length, k_1 and k_2 are constants. All the other parameters are the same as those in Eq. 2.

Using the analysis results, Peppas (41) concluded that the enhanced adhesion strength is a strong function of the polymer volume fraction of hydrogels, the amount of adhesion promoter chains inside the hydrogel ϕ_f, and the contact time. It is also proportional to ϕ_f when ϕ_f is low. The polymer volume fraction should stay in the optimized region, which is determined by the competition between the diffusivity and the number of PEG chains. If the polymer volume fraction of hydrogels is too low, the amount of the adhesion promoter chains available in the system is too low, though the diffusivity is high due to the expansion of the network. If the polymer volume fraction is too high, the opposite occurs. As far as the chain length of PEG, Eq. 3 shows that the adhesion strength will decrease with increasing PEG chain length. However, we should use some intermediate chain length because short chains cannot form entanglement. Moreover, the analysis (24) also showed that the adhesion strength would be at its maximum value after the terminal relaxation τ_r.

To understand the transport process of free chains in more detail, we should know the behavior of free chains in hydrogels, especially the initial free chain end distribution in the hydrogel interfacial region (41). A concentrated chain end distribution will accelerate the diffusion process.

Besides the free chains, polymer chains tethered on hydrogel surfaces are also able to act as adhesion promoters, as shown in Fig. 4. The *tethered chain adhesion promoters* can be the dangling chains formed in the polymerization process, or polymer chains grafted after the

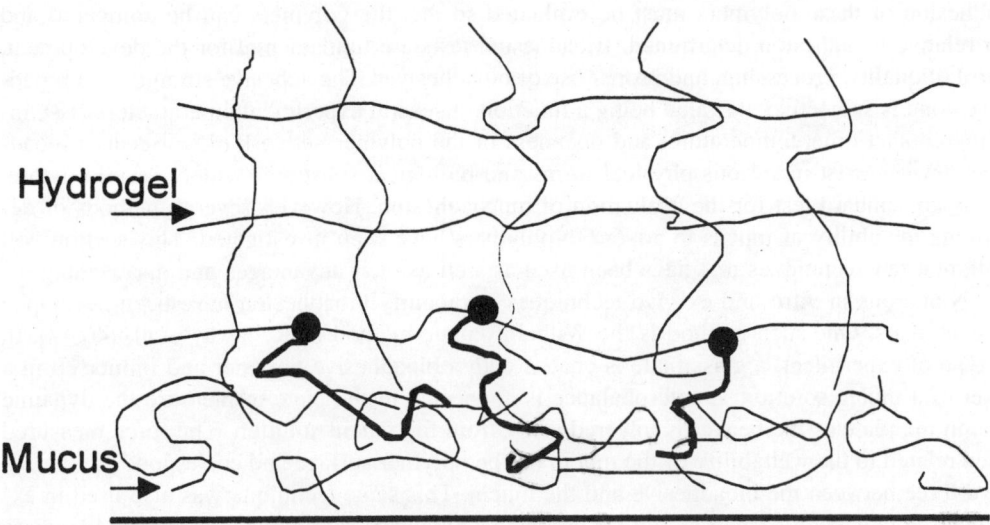

Figure 4 The polymer chains tethered on hydrogel surfaces act as adhesion promoters. When the hydrogel is placed in contact with mucus, tethered chains penetrate into the mucous layer and bridge the two gels.

formation of hydrogels. Tethered chains have one of their ends attached on the hydrogel surface and leave the other free. Although their diffusivity is lower than that of the free chains, tethered chains still have a significant ability to penetrate into mucus.

Huang et al. (43) presented a molecular analysis of polymer chains tethered on hydrogel surfaces and their effect on hydrogel bioadhesion. At normal physical conditions, tethered polymer chains have most of their segments outside the hydrogel and there is a concentrated distribution of their free ends in the outer tethered structure layers. The tethered layer structure is the function of the following factors: (a) the polymer volume fraction of hydrogels; (b) the interaction among tethered polymer, hydrogel polymer, and solvent molecules; (c) the graft density; and (d) tethered chain length.

More important is the fact that tethered polymer chains will introduce repulsion between the base hydrogel and the mucus if there is no strong attractive interaction between tethered polymer and mucus gel. This repulsion is mainly due to the configurational entropy decrease of tethered chains when they penetrate into the mucous layer, so it is a nonspecific interaction. The magnitude of this energy barrier depends on the same parameters affecting the tethered structure. On the other hand, a hydrogel with tethered chains strongly attractive to the mucous polymer will be attractive to mucus. This attraction is specific because it depends on the chemical structures of local mucus and tethered polymer. These results, along with the fact that local mucus properties depend on the their location and pathology conditions, suggest that the desirable site-specific bioadhesive controlled release system could be designed by suitably designing the tethered structure on hydrogel carriers.

VI. EXPERIMENTAL TECHNIQUES IN MUCOADHESION ANALYSIS

Several acrylic-based polymer devices, as well as other polymers, exhibit a very high adhesive bond strength. Furthermore, the adhesive capabilities of these devices can be improved as current bioadhesive materials are modified and more bioadhesive materials are discovered. The bioadhesion of these polymers must be evaluated so that the polymers can be compared and their relative bioadhesion determined. Bioadhesion tests are fundamental for the development, control of quality, processing, and proper use of bioadhesives. The adhesive strength of a bioadhesive bond is subjective, its value being a function of several experimental parameters (18), including contact time, temperature, and openness of the polymer network (45). Because bioadhesive devices exist in various physical forms and biological substrates widely vary in nature, there is no standard test for the evaluation of mucoadhesion. However, several methods of determining the ability of mucus to adhere to polymers have been investigated. This section will highlight a few techniques that have been used as well as their advantages and disadvantages.

Numerous in vitro and ex vivo techniques to quantify bioadhesion have been developed in recent years. One such method is the Wilhelmy plate method of Kellaway et al. (46,47). In this type of experiment, a glass plate is coated with a bioadhesive polymer and immersed in a beaker of a mucin solution. A microbalance is connected to the plate to measure the dynamic force on the plate as the beaker is lowered away from the mucin solution. The force measured is then related to the wettability of the mucin on the polymer surface and corresponds to the adhesive force between the bioadhesive and the mucin. This same technique was also used in experiments conducted by Smart et al. (47) in which a bioadhesive polymer was coated on a glass plate and immersed in a purified glycoprotein. The force on the glass plate was measured as it was removed from the glycoprotein, and this force for removing a clean glass plate from the same solution. This technique has the advantage of being inexpensive and rapid, although disadvantages include possible errors resulting from capillary forces, hysteresis, and polymer dissolution in the mucin solution.

Table 1 lists several polymers tested in our laboratory (48) using this method and their relative mean adhesive forces. The qualitative bioadhesive property is also listed. Robinson and associates (49) developed an ex vivo fluorescence method of measuring bioadhesion in which human epithelial cells are labeled with the fluorescent probes pyrene or fluorescein isothiocyanate. These cells are then combined with bioadhesive polymers. When a photoexcited moiety combines with an unexcited moiety, an excimer is formed. The ratio of excimers to monomers is monitored as a function of time in order to assess the affinity of the cells for the mucin. While the inventors of this technique feel it is promising for screening potential bioadhesives, there are some minor problems associated with it. Migration of pyrene from the cells may act to reduce excimer formation, showing an underestimated value for the affinity of the cells for the mucin. The relation of this technique to in vivo bioadhesion is unclear.

Mikos and Peppas (50) developed a flow channel technique in which a bioadhesive spherical polymer particle was placed on a mucus surface inside a Plexiglas channel. A laminar flow

Table 1 Relative Mucoadhesive Performances of Water-Soluble Polymers (48)

Polymer	Relative bioadhesive capacity	Qualitative bioadhesive property
Sodium Alginate	4.75 ± 0.32	Excellent
Sodium Carboxymethylcellulose	3.83	Excellent
Alginic Acid	2.11	Very Good
Poly(acrylic acid)	1.91	Very Good
Poly(methacrylic acid)	1.13	Satisfactory
Poly(2-hydroxy ethyl methacrylate)	1.11	Satisfactory
Poly(N-vinyl-2-pyrrolidone)	1.01	Poor

of air or a viscoelastic solution was directed over the particle while photographs were taken to determine the static and dynamic bioadhesive behavior of the particle (51–54).

Ho et al. (55) developed the falling film for measuring the ability of a polymer in a flowing fluid to adhere to mucus. Using this method, small spherical latex particles are coated with a bioadhesive polymer and combined with a buffer solution to create a suspension of particles with a known concentration. The solution with the contained microspheres is then pumped over a rat small intestine that has been cut lengthwise and placed in a semicylindrical trough. The eluted solution and particles are collected in a beaker and the collected particles are counted using an electronic particle counter. The fraction of particles that adhered to the mucus during the flow experiment is then related to the bioadhesion of the polymer.

Numerous tensiometric techniques of measuring mucoadhesive ability have been invented. In these techniques, the tensile strength needed to separate a bioadhesive from tissues is measured. Several combinations of bioadhesive polymers and tissues can be used. One such technique is that of Ponchel and Peppas (56–58) in which an animal tissue is placed on a clamp of a tissue device and brought into contact with a bioadhesive polymer tablet. Swelling of the tablet occurs at the interface over time while it is in contact with the mucus. A vertical force is applied until the tablet and mucus separate, and this force is used to calculate the work of adhesion. If a good bioadhesive material is used, the adhesion of the mucus to the polymer is stronger than the cohesion of the mucous gel, causing mucin molecules to part from the mucous gel upon separation.

An in vivo technique has been developed by based on γ-scintigraphy (59). Using this method, a bioadhesive device is labeled with ^{99}Tc or ^{111}In, and administered to an animal while the residence time of the device in the body is monitored with a gamma camera. The length of time the device spends in the gastric area is related to the mucoadhesive ability of the device. This technique is advantageous because it is noninvasive.

VII. RECENT DEVELOPMENTS

Recent work in the area of bioadhesion shows promising evidence to support the diffusion theory of adhesion for both crosslinked and uncrosslinked polymers (60). Although the tie points present in crosslinked polymers limit the diffusion of chains, the mobility is sufficient to form an adequate bioadhesive bond to mucus (61). Grafting mucophilic copolymers onto the backbone of a crosslinked polymer has been found to increase the mucoadhesive capacity of some polymers (43,61,62). The grafted polymer chains are able to diffuse from the network and into the mucus layer to aid in the bioadhesion process (42). The addition of a nongrafted mucophilic polymer in the network can increase the bioadhesive capacity to a greater extent due to the enhanced diffusion ability of the polymer.

When the hydrogel system comes into contact with mucus, over time the concentration gradient across the interface is expected to cause the free mucophilic chains of the mucoadhesive device to diffuse from the network into the mucous layer, while the glycoprotein chains of the mucus diffuse into the polymer. This phenomenon acts to reinforce the attachment of the device to the mucus. Polyethylene glycol can be used as a typical mucophilic component. It can adhere to the surface of the polymer. In addition, the dangling ends of the crosslinked network can be readily available for interpenetration.

The observed mucoadhesion of the swollen particles can be decreased from that of the dry particles. These effects are time-dependent and may be diminished when mucoadhesion is measured after a shorter particle swelling time. A shorter swelling time will allow the network to expand sufficiently to facilitate PEG diffusion from the PAA into the mucous layer without eliminating the entanglement in the PAA, which secures the particles to the mucus.

When these microparticles are used in a drug delivery device, it is necessary to enclose the dry particles in a capsule of a substance that dissolves only at the pH of the intestinal fluid. Assuming that the dissolution of the coating is rapid, the particles would not be swollen to a large extent when they came into contact with the mucus that lines the GI tract. Thus, there would not be a significant amount of PEG lost from the polymer network before this contact occurs, which would allow interpenetration of PEG into the mucus to take place. In this case, the mucoadhesion would be expected to follow the trend exhibited in the studies done using initially dry polymers.

The adhesion-promoting characteristics of PEG are associated with the chain penetration and diffusion of free PEG chains from the swelling or equilibrium-swollen polymer microparticles to the mucosa or mucin solution. This process is a standard diffusion phenomenon that can be analyzed by simple application of diffusion theories, the molecular analysis of de Ascentiis et al. (61), and the early modeling work of Mikos and Peppas (39–41).

Several different methods of preparing the polymers have been investigated (43,61,63) in order to limit the amount of unreacted and uncrosslinked monomer that remained in the networks following polymerization. Polymer films prepared by thermal initiation from 10 mol % acrylic acid solutions were ground into particles with sizes between 150 and 425 μm. These particles were swollen in 2, 5, 10, and 20 wt % aqueous PEG solutions of molecular weights 1000, 8000, and 18,500 for several days and then dried in air to incorporate free PEG chains in the PAA networks. In a typical study, about 30 mg of particles was dispersed over a 30 wt % mucin solution, and after a 20-min interaction time the mucoadhesive capacity was calculated as the percentage of particles that remained on the mucus after the experiment. It was found that for the particles that were swollen in the 5% PEG solution and were initially dry when dispersed on the mucin, the mucoadhesive capacity generally increased with increasing molecular weight of the incorporated PEG. This increase was related to the increase in the maximum possible interpenetration distance, which aids in securing the particles on the mucous surface. There appears to be an optimum PEG molecular weight above which the mucoadhesive capabilities are limited for the contact time used in these studies. This limitation is due to the decreased diffusion of the PEG in the polymer network and the shorter interpenetration distance that results.

For both the swollen and unswollen particles, the more highly crosslinked PAA polymers exhibited an increased mucoadhesive capacity, believed to be due to the increased concentration of chain ends at the interface that resulted from a decrease in the amount of swelling undergone by the particles. The addition of PEG to these particles may result in an increase in mucoadhesion due to the decreased amount of swelling that the particles could undergo and the decreased amount of dilution of bioadhesive chains at the polymer–tissue interface. However, this increase in adhesion with an increase in crosslinking ratio could only exist up to the point where a limitation of PEG diffusion results from the small mesh size of the PAA network. Also, with a small mesh size and limited PEG diffusion there is a limited diffusion of any drug that is present in the network. If the drug diffusion is hindered, the particles are no longer useful as drug delivery devices. Therefore, it may be important to investigate how the mucoadhesive capacity of PAA–PEG polymers is affected when PEG is added to more highly crosslinked PAA networks.

ACKNOWLEDGMENTS

This work was supported by grants from the National Science Foundation and the National Institutes of Health GM56231.

REFERENCES

1. Marriott, C. and Gregory, N. P., 1990, Mucus physiology and pathology. In: V. Lenaerts and R. Gurny (Eds.), Bioadhesive Drug Delivery Systems, CRC Press, Boca Raton, FL, pp. 1–24.
2. Marriott, C. and Hughes, D. R. L., 1990, Mucus physiology and pathology. In: R. Gurny and H. E. Junginger (Eds.), Bioadhesion—Possibilities and Future Trends, Wissenschaftliche Verlagsgesellschaft mbH, Stuttgart, pp. 29–43.
3. Langer, R. S. and Peppas, N. A., 1992, New drug delivery systems. BMES Bull., 16: 3–7.
4. Duchene, D., Touchard, F. and Peppas, N. A., 1988. Pharmaceutical and medical aspects of bioadhesive systems for drug administration. Drug Dev. Ind. Pharm., 14: 283–318.
5. Gurny, R., Meyer, J. M. and Peppas, N. A., 1984. Bioadhesive intraoral release systems; design, testing and analysis. Biomaterials, 5: 336–340.
6. Duchene, D., Ponchel, G., Wouessidjewe, D., Lejoyeux, F. and Peppas, N. A., 1988. Methodes d' evaluation de la bioadhesion et facteurs influants. STP Phama, 4: 688–697.
7. Lejoyeux, F., Ponchel, G., Wouessidjewe, D., Peppas, N. A. and Duchene, D., 1989. Bioadhesive tablets: Influence of the testing medium composition on bioadhesion. Drug Dev. Ind. Pham., 15: 2037–2048.
8. Gursoy, A., Sohtorik, I., Uyanik, N. and Peppas, N. A., 1989. Bioadhesive controlled release systems for vaginal delivery. STP Pharm., 5: 886–892.
9. Achar, L. and Peppas, N. A., 1994, Preparation, characterization and mucoadhesive interactions of poly(methacrylic acid) copolymers with rat mucosa. J. Controlled Release, 31: 271–276.
10. Peppas, N. A. and Lowman, A. M., 1998. Protein delivery from novel bioaheisve complexation hydrogels. In: S. Frokjaer, L. Christrup and P. Krogsgaard-Larsen (Eds.), Peptide and Protein Delivery, Munksgaard, Copenhagen, pp. 206–216.
11. Peppas, N. A., Moniga, N. and Luttrell, 1995. Bioadhesive poly(vinyl alcohol) as a carrier for controlled release of growth factors and proteins. Proc. World Meeting APGI/APV, 1: 817–818.
12. Peppas, N. A. and Moniga, N. K., 1997. Ultrapure poly(vinyl alcohol) hydrogels with mucoadhesive drug delivery characteristics. Eur. J. Pharm. Biopharm., 43: 51–58.115.
13. Moniga, N. K., Anseth, K. S. and Peppas, N. A., 1996. Mucoadhesive poly(vinyl alcohol) hydrogels produced by freezing/thawing processes; application in the development of wound healing systems. J. Biomater. Sci. Polym. Ed., 7: 1055–1064.
14. De Ascentiis, A., Colombo, P. and Peppas, N. A., 1995. Screening of potentially mucoadhesive polymer microparticles in contact with rat intestinal mucosa. Eur. J. Pharm. Biopharm. 41: 229–234.
15. Hoffman, A. S., Chen, G., Wu, X., Ding, Z., Kabra, B., Randeri, K., Schiller, M., Ron, E. and Peppas, N. A., 1997. Graft copolymers of PEO-PPO-PEO triblock polyethers on bioadhesive polymer backbones: synthesis and properties. Polym. Prepr., 38: 524–525.
16. Hoffman, A. S., Chen, G., Wu, X., Ding, Z., Kabra, B., Randeri, K., Schiller, M., Ron, E., Peppas, N. A. and Brazel, C., 1997. Graft copolymers of PEO-PPO-PEO triblock polyethers on bioadhesive polymer backbones as drug delivery carriers. Polym. Mater. Sci. Eng. Proc., 76: 271–272.
17. Peppas, N. A. and Robinson, J. R., 1995. Bioadhesives for optimization of drug delivery. J. Drug Target., 3: 183–184.
18. Peppas, N. A. and Buri, P. A., 1985. Surface, interfacial and molecular aspects of polymer bioadhesion on soft tissues. J. Controlled Release, 2: 257–275.
19. Mikos, A. G. and Peppas, N. A., 1986. Systems for controlled release of drugs. V. Bioadhesive systems. STP Pharma. 2: 705–716.
20. Puchelle, E., 1987. Inaugural address at Inserm Seminar. Biorheology, 24: 411–412.
21. Gupta, P. K., Leung, S. S. and Robinson, J. R., 1990. Bioadhesives/mucoadhesives in drug delivery to the gastrointestinal tract. In: V. Lenaerts and R. Gurny (Eds.), Bioadhesive Drug Delivery Systems, CRC Press, Boca Raton, FL, pp. 105–136.
22. Yang, X. and Robinson, J. R., 1998. Bioadhesion in mucosal drug delivery. In: T. Okano (Ed.), Biorelated Polymers and Gels, Academic Press, San Diego, pp. 135–192.

23. Peppas, N. A., 1993. Novel Developments in Bioadhesive Systems for Transdermal and Oral Applications. In: Preceedings of the Third TDS Technology Symposium, Nihon Toshi Center, Bunkashoin, Tokyo, Japan, pp. 19–45.
24. Allen, A., Hutton, D. A., Pearson, J. P. and Sellars, L. A., 1984. Mucus glycoprotein structure, gel formation and gastrointestinal mucus function. In: Mucus and Mucosa, Ciba Foundation Symposium, 109: 137–156.
25. Forstner, J. F., Jabbal, I. and Forstner, G. G., 1973. Goblet cell mucin of rat small intestine. Can. J. Biochem., 51: 1154–1166.
26. Feijen, J., Beugeling, T., Bantjes, A. and Smit-Sibinga, C. T., 1979. Biomaterials and interfacial phenomena. In: D. N. Ghista (Eds.), Advances in Cardiovascular Physics, Vol. 3, Karger, Basel, pp. 100–132.
27. Hench, L. L. and Ethridge, E. C., 1982. Biomaterials: An Interfacial Approach. Academic Press, New York.
28. Gurny, R. and Peppas, N. A., 1990. Semisolid dosage forms as buccal bioadhesives. In: V. Lenaerts and R. Gurny (Eds.), Bioadhesive Drug Delivery Systems, CRC Press, Boca Raton, FL, pp. 153–168.
29. Kinloch, A. J., 1980. The science of adhesion I: Surface and interfacial aspects. J. Mater. Sci., 15: 2141–2166.
30. Merrill, E. W. 1977, Properties of materials affection the behavior of blood at their surfaces. Ann. N. Y. Acad. Sci., 283: 6–16.
31. Kaelbe, D. H. and Moacanin, J., 1977. A surface energy analysis of bioadhesion. Polymer, 18: 475–481.
32. Kaelbe, D. H., 1971. Physical Chemistry of Adhesion, Wiley, New York.
33. Kammer, H. W., 1983. Adhesion between polymers. Acta Polym., 34: 112–118.
34. Derjaguin, B. V. and Smilga, V. P., 1969. Adhesion: Fundamentals and Practices. McLaren, London.
35. Mikos, A. G. and Peppas, N. A., 1989. Measurement of the surface tension of mucin solutions. Int. J. Pharm., 53: 1–5.
36. Esposito, P., Colombo, I. and Loverecich, 1994. Investigation of surface properties of some polymers by a thermodynamic and mechanical approach: possibility of prediction mucoadhesion and biocompatibility. Biomaterials, 15: 177–182.
37. Voyutskii, S. S., 1963. Autohesion and Adhesion of High Polymers. Wiley, New York, NY.
38. Peppas, N. A., Hansen, P. J. and Buri, P. A., 1984. A theory of molecular diffusion in the intestinal mucus. Int. J. Pharm., 20: 107–118.
39. Mikos, A. G. and Peppas, N. A., 1990. Kinetics of mucus-polymer interactions. In: R. Gurny and H. E. Junginger (Eds.), Bioadhesion—Possibilities and Future Trends, Wissenschaftliche Verlagsgesellschaft mbH, Stuttgart, pp. 65–85.
40. Mikos, A. G. and Peppas, N. A., 1990. Scaling concepts and molecular theories of adhesion of synthetic polymers to glycoproteinic networks. In: V. Lenaerts and R. Gurny (Eds.), Bioadhesive Drug Delivery Systems, CRC Press, Boca Raton, FL, pp. 25–42.
41. Peppas, N. A., 1998. Molecular calculations of poly(ethylene glycol) transport across a swollen poly(acrylic acid)/mucin interface. J. Biomater. Sci. Polym. Ed., 9: 535–542.
42. Huang, Y., Szleifer, I. and Peppas, N. A., 2000. Gel-gel adhesion by polymer chains tethered on gel surfaces. J. Chem. Phys. (submitted).
43. Sahlin, J. J. and Peppas, N. A., 1997. Enhanced hydrogel adhesion by polymer interdiffusion: Use of linear poly(ethylene glycol) as an adhesion promoter. J. Biomater. Sci., Polym. Ed., 8: 421–436.
44. Merrill, E. W., Dennison, K. A. and Sung C., 1993. Partitioning and diffusion of solutes in hydrogels of poly(ethylene oxide). Biomaterials, 14: 1117–1126.
45. Leung, S. S. and Robinson, J. R., 1990. Polymer structure features contributing to mucoadhesion. II. J. Controlled Release, 12: 187–194.
46. Smart, J. D. and Kellaway, I. W., 1982. In-vitro techniques for measuring mucoadhesion. J. Pharm. Pharmacol. (Suppl.) 34: 70P.
47. Smart, J. D., Kellaway, I. W. and Worthington, H. E. C., 1984. An in-vitro investigation of mucosaadhesive materials for use in controlled drug delivery. J. Pharm. Pharmacol., 36: 295–299.

48. Robert, C., Buri, P. and Peppas, N. A., 1988. Experimental methods for bioadhesive testing of various polymers. Acta Pharm. Technol., 34: 95–98.
49. Park, K., Ch'ng, H. S. and Robinson, J. R., 1984. Alternative approaches to oral controlled drug delivery: Bioadhesive and in-situ systems. In: J. M. Anderson and S. W. Kim (Eds.), Recent Advances in Drug Delivery, Plenum Press, New York, pp. 163–183.
50. Mikos, A. G. and Peppas, N. A., 1990. Bioadhesive analysis of controlled-release systems. IV. An experimental method for testing the adhesion of microparticles with mucus. J. Controlled Release, 12: 31–37.
51. Mikos, A. G. and Peppas, N. A., 1989. Experiment methods for determination of bioadhesive bond strength of polymers with mucus. STP Pharma., 5: 187–191.
52. Mikos, A. G. and Peppas, N. A., 1990. Bioadhesive analysis of controlled release systems. IV. An experimental method for testing the adhesion of microparticles with mucus. J. Controlled Release, 12: 31–37.
53. De Ascentiis, A., Bettini, R., Colombo, P. and Peppas, N. A., 1996. Mucoadhesive properties of hydrophilic polymeric microparticles. Boll. Chim. Farm., 135: 101–103.
54. Mikos, A. G., Mathiowitz, E., Langer, R. S. and Peppas, N. A., 1991. The interaction of polymer microparticles with mucin gels as a means of characterizing polymer retention on mucus. J. Colloid Interf. Sci., 143: 366–373.
55. Teng, C. L. C. and Ho, N. F. L., 1987. Mechanistic studies in the simultaneous flow and absorption of polymer-coated latex particles on intestinal mucus. I. Methods and physical model development. J. Controlled Release, 6: 133–149.
56. Ponchel, G., Touchard, F., Duchene, D. and Peppas, N. A., 1987. Bioadhesive analysis of controlled release systems. I. Fracture and interpenetration analysis in poly(acrylic acid)–containing systems. J. Controlled Release, 5: 129–141.
57. Peppas, N. A., Ponchel, G. and Duchene, D., 1987. Bioadhesive analysis of controlled release systems. II. Time-dependent bioadhesive stress in poly(acrylic acid)–containing systems. J. Controlled Release, 5: 143–149.
58. Ponchel, G., Touchard, F., Wouessidjewe, D., Duchene, D. and Peppas, N. A., 1987. Bioadhesive analysis of controlled-release systems. III. Bioadhesive and release behavior of metronidazole-containing poly(acrylic acid)–hydroxypropyl methylcellulose systems. Int. J. Pharm., 38: 65–70.
59. Willson, C. G., 1990. In vivo testing of bioadhesion. In: R. Gurny and H. E. Junginger (Eds.), Bioadhesion—Possibilities and Future Trends, Wissenschaftliche Verlagsgesellschaft mbH, Stuttgart, pp. 93–108.
60. Jabbari, E., Wisniewski, N. and Peppas, N. A., 1993. Evidence of mucoadhesion by chain interpenetration at a poly(acrylic acid)/mucin interface using ATR-FTIR spectroscopy. J. Controlled Release, 26: 99–108.
61. De Ascentiis, A., deGrazia, J. L., Bowman, C. N., Colombo, P. and Peppas N. A., 1995. Mucoadhesion of poly(2-hydroxyethyl methacrylate) is improved when linear poly(ethylene oxide) chains are added to the polymer network. J. Controlled Release, 33: 197–201.
62. Sahlin, J. J. and Peppas, N. A., 1996. Hydrogels as mucoadhesive and bioadhesive materials: a review. Biomaterials, 17: 1553–1561.
63. Little, M. D., 1997. M. S. thesis, School of Chemical Engineering, Purdue University.

13
Microencapsulation Technology:
Interfacial Polymerization Method

A. Atilla Hıncal and H. Süheyla Kaş
Hacettepe University, Ankara, Turkey

I. INTRODUCTION

Microencapsules, which are small particles of solids or small droplets of liquids surrounded by a wall of natural and synthetic polymer films of varying thickness and degree of permeability, are prepared by several processes. These processes are divided into physical, physicochemical, and mechanical systems, or are classified as mechanical and chemical processes (1,2).

Interfacial polymerization technique is one in which two monomers, one oil-soluble and the other water-soluble, are employed and a polymer is formed on the droplet surface. The interfacial polymerization method is classified under physicochemical and chemical processes by Kondo and Thies, respectively (1,2). Interfacial polymerization method have been considered and reviewed with medical and biotechnological applications by several authors (1–15). The application of these microcapsules mainly depends on their size, morphology, and membrane properties. The first patent on this process was granted to the International Business Machines Corporation in 1961 (1).

The scope of this chapter is to describe the preparation procedures, state the monomers and solvents employed, and discuss the pharmaceutical and biotechnological applications of this commercialized encapsulation process.

II. MONOMERS AND SOLVENTS USED

The production of polyamides (nylon-6,10, polyphthalamides, sulfated and carboxylated polyphthalamides), polyesters (polyphenyl esters), and polyurethanes is realized with various combinations of water- and oil-soluble monomers and solvents. some of these are shown in Tables 1 and 2, respectively.

III. PREPARATION OF MICROCAPSULES BY INTERFACIAL POLYMERIZATION

It is possible to encapsulate a wide range of products, including aqueous solutions, water-immiscible liquids, and solids, by this approach (2). However, Kondo states that interfacial polymerization technique is suitable for encapsulating liquids rather than solids due to the fact

Table 1 Combination of Monomers for Preparing Microcapsules by Interfacial Polymerization

Water-soluble monomer	Oil-soluble monomer	Polymer formed	Ref.
I. Polyamine	**I. Polybasic acid halide**	**I. Polyamide**	
1. -1,6-hexamethylene diamine	-sebacoyl chloride	-nylon-6,10 or polyamide	3, 4, 9, 16, 17, 20, 28, 30, 36, 37, 49, 53–54, 61
	-terephtaloyl chloride	-polyterephthalamide	3, 16, 49
	-p-phthaloyl chloride	-polyphthalamide	30, 49
-diethylene diamine	-p-phthaloyl dichloride	-polyphthalamide	59
-p-phenylene diamine	-p-phthaloyl dichloride	-polyphenylene phthalamide	30
2. -L-lysine	-terephthaloyl chloride	-polyterephthalamide L-lysine	3, 9
	-p-phthaloyl dichloride	-poly-L-lysine phthalamide	34, 46
3. -piperazine	-p-phthaloyl dichloride	-polyphthaloyl piperzaine or polyphthalamide	18, 20, 30, 40, 49, 55, 61
	-terephthaloyl dichloride	-polyterephthalamide or polyphthalamide	16, 33
	-sebacoyl chloride	-poly sebacoyl piperazine or polysebacamide	16
-2,5-dimethylpiperazine	-p-phthaloyl dichloride	-polyphthaloyl 2,5-dimethylpiperazine	30
II. Polyamine	**II. Bischloroformate**	**II. Polyurethane**	
1. -piperazine	-2,2¹-dichlorodiethyl ether	-polyurethane or polyether	20
-1,6-hexamethylenediamine	-2,2¹-dichlorodiethyl ether	-polyurethane	20
III. Polyphenol	**III. Polybasic acid halide**	**III. Polyester**	
1. -2,2-bis (4-hydroxyphenyl) propane	-sebacoyl chloride	-polyphenyl ester	3, 4, 9
	-p-phthaloyl dichloride	-polyphenyl ester	19
-4,4¹ dihydroxydiphenyl sulfone	-p-phthaloyl dichloride	-polyphenyl ester	19
	-sebacoyl chloride	-polyphenyl ester	19

Source: Data from Refs. 6 and 22.

that penetration of reactants into the polymerization zone is much more easily accomplished from a liquid than a solid state (1). A unique feature of this film-forming technique is the polymerization of a monomer at the interface of two immiscible substances. Problems associated with this process are the reaction of the active substance with the reagents used to form the wall as well as the solubility of the active ingredients (14). The limitations of this method stated by Deasy

Table 2 Solvents Employed in the Interfacial Polymerization Method

Solvents	Ref.
Carbon tetrachloride	9, 36, 53, 54
Chloroform	16, 18–20, 32, 36, 46, 48, 49, 53, 61
Cyclohexane	16, 18–20, 32, 36, 46, 48, 49, 53, 61
Dichloroethane	9, 36, 53
Dimethylformamide	9, 36, 53
Dimethylsulfoxide	63
Methanol	9, 36, 53
Methylene chloride	63
Water	9
Xylene	9, 36, 53

are toxicity associated with the unreacted monomers, degradation caused by monomer reaction, high permeability of the coating, and fragility of the microcapsules (6).

The types of microcapsules produced by this process can have semipermeable or nonpermeable lipid membrane with aqueous core, or release controlling coating with a solid core. The preparation methods for both types have much in common (3). However, aqueous core with semipermeable membranes has pharmaceutical and biomedical applications. The pioneers in this area are Chang and Kondo. These scientists and their co-workers have used interfacial polymerization method to encapsulate oils, dye precursors, proteins, peptides, enzymes, antibodies, and cells (3–6).

A. Water-Immiscible Liquid Core

When the core material is a water-immiscible liquid, the monomer is dissolved in the liquid core. Generally isocyanate, acid chloride, or a combination is used as monomer. Later this solution, dispersed in an aqueous phase containing a dispersing agent and a coreactant, is added to the aqueous phase. This produces polymerization at the interface, which later forms the capsule wall.

B. Water-Miscible Liquid Core

An aqueous solution of a water-soluble liquid is dispersed into an organic phase with the aid of an emulsifier to form a water-in-oil emulsion. Formation of polymer membrane on the surface of liquid droplets is initiated by water-insoluble reactant added to the water-in-oil emulsion. Later the microcapsules are separated from water. The basic flow diagram of the method is illustrated in Fig. 1 (3).

C. Solid Core

Solid cores are either encapsulated by vinyl monomers that polymerize by free radical reactions or by polymerization of p-xylene at a gas–solid interface. In this system, polymerization takes place on the solid surface spontaneously.

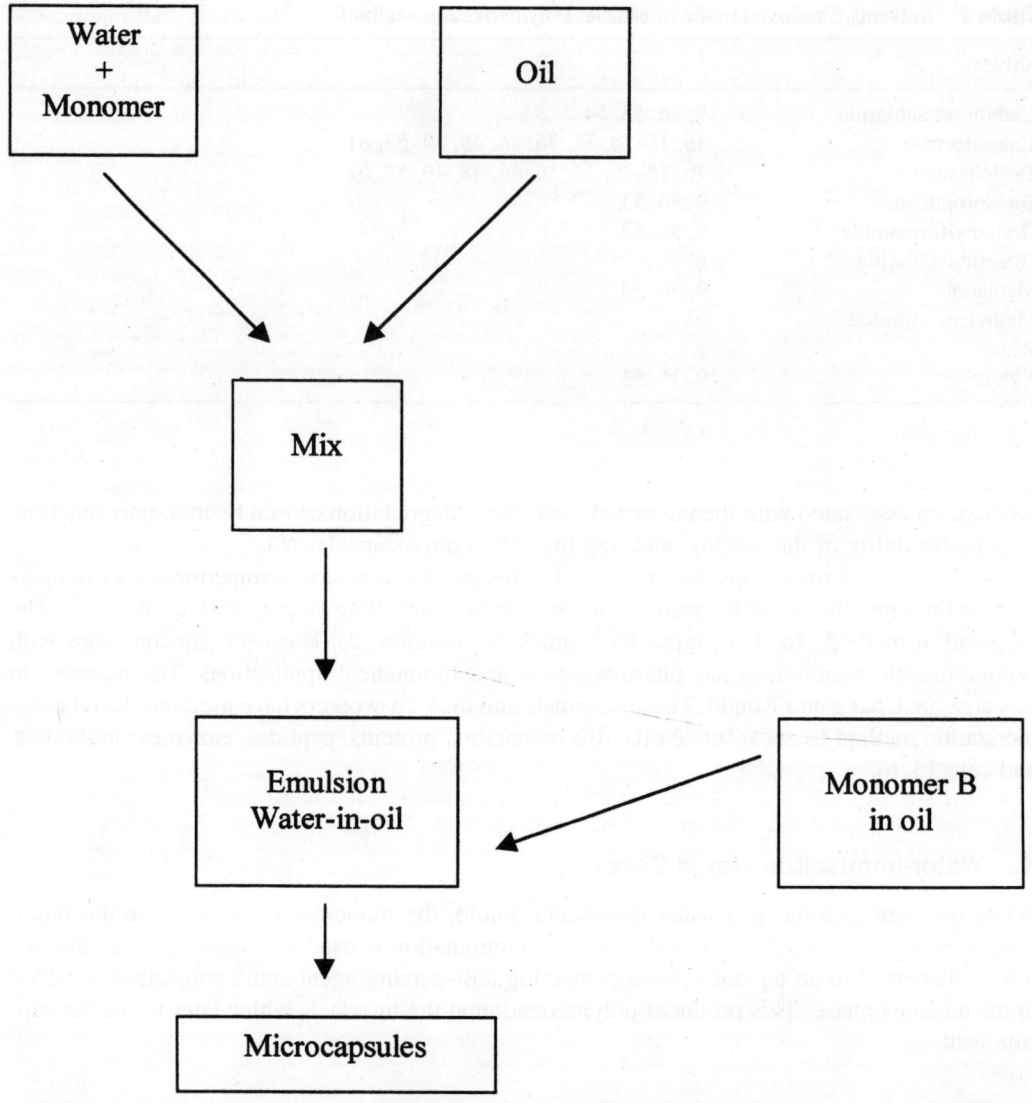

Figure 1 Basic flow diagram of interfacial polymerization method (3).

IV. FACTORS AFFECTING INTERFACIAL POLYMERIZATION REACTIONS

The factors affecting interfacial polymerization reactions were classified and discussed in detail by Whateley as reaction rate, precipitation of polymer, impurities, diamine partition coefficient, interfacial transfer rates, concentration ratio of reactants, stirring rate, hydrolysis of diacid chlorides, transfer rates of salts, solvent polarity, density, toxicity, surfactants, and temperature (3). The interfacial film formation rate of different polymers may differ. The reaction rate of aliphatic glycols is slow, whereas the reaction rates of nylon-6,10 and piperazine–terephthaloyl chloride are fast. The site of the reaction—either the water or the organic side of the interface—also affects the precipitation of the polymer. Concentration ratios of the monomers are also important when high molecular weight polymer is desired. Generally, the monomer soluble in the outer phase is used in excess. Stirring rate is a critical factor that affects the molecular weight of the polymer formed. The polarity and density of the solvent affects the stability of the emulsion system. Toxicity of the solvent is another important parameter in encapsulating pharmaceuticals. Surfactants play an important role in the formation of an emulsion in the transfer of the diamines to the organic phase. The main requirements of the surfactants is their low impurity. Although the interfacial polymerization reactions are carried out at room temperature, 4°C is preferred for proteins, peptides, and enzymes. High temperature is not favorable in interfacial polymerization. These are some of the important points of these factors. For detailed information and examples of factors affecting interfacial polymerization reactions, refer to Whateley (3).

V. PROPERTIES OF MICROCAPSULES PREPARED BY INTERFACIAL POLYMERIZATION

Surface morphology, size and size distribution, membrane properties (thickness, permeability, and stability), ζ potential, and flow properties of microcapsules prepared by this technique will be discussed with examples in the following section.

A. Surface Morphology

Microcapsules prepared by the interfacial polymerization method have spherical geometry with a continuous core: wall structure. The interior surface of these microcapsules is generally irregular, whereas the exterior surface is uniform and smooth (2). Figure 2 shows the smooth surface of hemoglobin microcapsules (16). However, Jenkins and Florence showed through

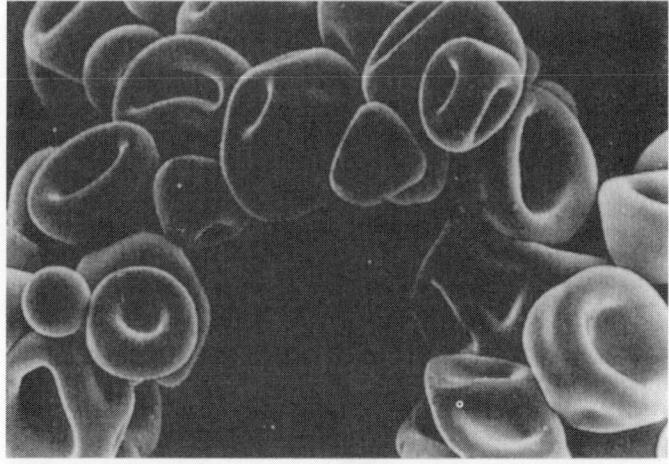

Figure 2 Scanning electron micrograph of hemoglobin microcapsules (terephthaloyl chloride) (16).

electron microscopy that the spherical microcapsules have a rough porous surface with deep splits penetrating to the center of the capsule (17).

B. Size and Size Distribution

In general, the interfacial polymerization method can be used to produce large microcapsules of around 20–30 μm diameter. However, microcapsules of 3–6 μm can also be produced by this method. The size of the microcapsules varied with the chemical structure of the reactants used in the polymerization step. Kondo forwarded an hypothesis which emphasized the importance of emulsion droplet sizes at an early stage of the polymerization when the membrane has insufficient strength (1).

Shigeri et al. investigated the effect of some organic salts with short alkyl chain on microcapsule size. They concluded that the presence of salts in the aqueous phase was found to increase the microcapsule size. This phenomenon was interpreted in terms of the ability of salts to facilitate the coalescence of droplets (18). Wakamatsu et al. stated size distribution to depend strongly on chemical structure of the reactants used (19). The effect of variations in polymerization conditions (such as variations in temperature and monomer concentration) on the size of microcapsules was studied by Shigeru et al. (20). Decrease in temperature and monomer concentration was found to increase microcapsule size. Etuk et al. also investigated the effect of process variables such as, nozzle size, flow rate of dispersed phase, interelectrode distance, and presence of an acid acceptor on the size distribution of nylon-6,10 microcapsules prepared in a high-voltage electric field (21). Increase in nozzle diameter and decrease in interelectrode distance was found to decrease the microcapsule size, whereas addition of an acid acceptor and a thickening agent resulted in an increase in the average capsule size. Zhang et al. demonstated that the diameter of the microcapsules decreased and their distribution became narrower as the emulsifying time was increased within the initial period of 45 s (22). Zhang et al. showed that raising the volume fraction of the dispersed phase led to a larger diameter and a wider distribution of the microcapsules. Both the diameter and the ζ potential of the microcapsules decreased in the order of ortho-, meta-, para-phthaloyl dichloride, indicating that the steric effect of the monomers play an important role in the microencapsulation process.

Cuff and co-workers studied the effect of agitation speed on particle size and found that as the agitation speed was increased, particle size decreased (23,24). Tan et al. also obtained decreased D_{50} values as the homogenizer speed and emulsifier concentration was increased (24,25). The addition of a co-surfactant significantly reduced the mean droplet size of the initial emulsion leading to the formation of microcapsules in the submicrometer range (26).

A novel emulsification technique, which employs microporous glass membranes, was adopted by Muramatsu et al. (27) to prepare polyamide microcapsules of narrow size distribution. This method also seemed promising to get various sizes of microcapsules by selecting the pore size of the glass membranes (27).

C. Membrane Properties

The thickness, permeability, and stability of the membranes are important parameters of the microcapsules prepared by interfacial polymerization method.

1. Membrane Thickness

The membrane thickness of microcapsules depends on the method of preparation. Microcapsules prepared by interfacial polymerization possess a thickness in the monometer range because the membrane thickening is restricted by the limited solubility of the reactants in the phase to be encapsulated (1). Jenkins and Florence also reported that the rapid equilibration of sodium and hydroxyl ions between the core of the capsules and the bathing solvent resulted in "thin membranes" several hundred angstroms thick (17). Table 3 shows the membrane thickness of some of the polyamide microcapsules.

2. Membrane Permeability

Information on the permeability characteristics of microcapsule membranes is very important in the design of drug delivery and artificial organs using microcapsules. The permeability characteristics of the microcapsules provide us with useful information for sustained/controlled release properties of the encapsulated drugs. Permeability is one of the most important properties when microcapsules are used in the medical and pharmaceutical fields. Nonantigenic surface, permeability to small molecules, and difficulty in achieving biodegradability are some of the important features of the semipermeable encapsulating membranes.

Membrane permeability is defined by the thickness, pore size, and chemical composition of the polymer shell. Membrane permeability defines the rate of substrate mass transfer from the surrounding solution into the microcapsule. The permeability of large poly(hexamethylene-sebacamide) microcapsules with a mean diameter of 211 μm and a membrane thickness of 20 nm has been determined by Chang and Poznansky (28). The authors determined the permeability coefficients for several organic solutes. The permeability coefficients for polyhexamethylene sebacamide microcapsules were in the range of 10^4 cm/s, whereas the permeability coefficients of polyphthaloylpiperazine microcapsules were in the order of 10^8 cm/s. These differences in permeability coefficients between two different polymer walls suggested the necessity to investigate the microcapsule permeability as a function of capsule size, membrane thickness, temperature, molecular size of solute, and concentration gradient (1). Miyauchi et al. studied the permeation of electrolyte ions through poly (L-lysine-alt-terephthalic acid) microcapsule membranes as a function of medium pH (29). The authors concluded that the permeation rate of electrolyte ions through microcapsule membranes was pH-dependent and exhibited a sudden jump at pH 4–6 where microcapsule size showed an abrupt increase. Takamura et al. investigated the permeation rate of various electrolytes through the membrane of poly(phthaloylpiperazine) microcapsules 2.26 μm in diameter with a membrane thickness of 13 nm (30).

3. Membrane Stability

Dufour et al. studied the stability of microcapsule membranes by varying the total ratio polymer, ratios of amines to acid chlorides, concentration of surfactants, and stirring speed (31). They obtained stable capsule membranes by increasing the ratio of amines to acid chlorides and with low concentration of total polymer.

Table 3 Membrane Thickness of Some of the Polyamide Microcapsules

Microcapsule	Membrane thickness (Å)	Ref.
Poly(phenylene phthalamide)	123	30
Poly(phthaloylpiperazine)	133	30
Poly(phthaloyldimethylpiperazine)	166	30
Poly(hexamethylene phthalamide)	167	30
Poly(hexamethylene sebacamide)	224	30
Poly(hexamethylene sebacamide)	200	54

Source: Data from Ref. 1.

Table 4 Examples of Substances Encapsulated by Interfacial Polymerization

Core material	Polymer formed	Ref.
Adsorbants		
Activated charcoal (immunoadsorbant)	Polyvinyl	63
Antibodies		
17-Hydroxyprogesterone antibody	Polyphthalamide	61
Antithyroxine antibody	Polyphthalamide	61
Enzymes		
Arginase	Polyphthalamide	40
Catalase	Polyamide	37
Chymotripsin	Polyamide	41
Glucose oxidase	Polyurea	42
Invertase	Polyamide	16
Histidase	Polyphthalamide	43
L-Asparaginase	Polyamide	36
Trypsin	Polyamide	41
Trypsinogene	Polyamide	41
Urease	Polyamide	38, 39
Hormones		
β-Estradiol	Polyacetal	60
Oils		
Oily liquids	Polyphthalamide	26, 36
	Polyurea	24
Pharmaceuticals		
Potassium chloride	Polyacetal	60
Calcium sulfate	Polyamide	23
Calcium alginate	Polyamide	23
Pericyazine emborate	Polyamide	55
	Polyphthalamide	55
Phenothiazine	Polyamide	55
Sodium pentobarbital	Polyamide	56
Sodium sulfathiazole	Polyamide	57
Trifluoperazine embonate	Polyamide	55
	Polyphthalamide	55

D. ζ Potential

Microcapsules prepared by the interfacial polymerization technique have a microcapsule membrane that does not bear any electric charge. However, when suspended in an aqueous medium, they migrate either to anode or cathode, depending on the sign of electric charge on the encapsulated polyelectrolyte (1,32–34). The effects of ionic strength and pH of the medium, addition of various dichlorides, concentration of polyelectrolytes, and addition of an emulsifier on the ζ potentials of the microcapsules were investigated by several authors (22,32–35).

Shiba et al. showed that the mobilities were decreased with increasing ionic strength of the medium. pH of the dispersing medium also affected the electrophoretic mobility. Microcapsules moved either to anode or cathode depending on the pH of the medium showing

Table 4 Continued

Core material	Polymer formed	Ref.
Pigments		
Pigment	Polyvinyl	25, 62
Polyelectrolytes		
Sodium heparinate	Polyphthalamide	32
Sodium acetate	Polyphthalamide	32
Sodium alginate	Polyphthalamide	18
Sodium methyl sulfonate	Polyphthalamide	18
Sodium methyl sulfate	Polyphthalamide	18
Sodium ethyl sulfate	Polyphthalamide	18
Sodium propyl sulfate	Polyphthalamide	18
Sodium sulfate	Polyphthalamide	18
Lithium chloride	Polyphthalamide	59
Sodium chloride	Polyphthalamide	59
Potassium chloride	Polyphthalamide	59
Cesium chloride	Polyphthalamide	59
Sodium bromide	Polyphthalamide	59
Sodium nitrate	Polyphthalamide	59
Sodium thiocyanate	Polyphthalamide	59
Sodium chromate	Polyphthalamide	59
Ammonium chloride	Polyphthalamide	59
Proteins		
Bovine fibrinogen	Polyphthalamide	24, 25
Bovine serum albumin	Polyamide	33, 49
	Polyphthalamide	46
Hemoglobin	Polyamide	40, 46
	Polyphthalamide	48
Human serum albumin	Polyphthalamide	24
Ovalbumin	Polyphthalamide	24

Source: Data from Ref. 22.

the existence of an isoelectric point (32,33). Other investigators demonstrated the decrease of the absolute value of the ζ potential in negatively charged microcapsules by increasing the concentration of the polyelectrolytes. The authors stated that this may be due to the increase in the concentration of counterions liberated from the encapsulated polyelectrolyte molecules (34). The decrease of microcapsule potentials when ortho-, meta-, or para-phthaloyl dichloride (in the order stated) were added to the oil-soluble monomer was shown by Zhang and co-workers (22). These results indicated the role of the steric effect of the monomers on microcapsule ζ potential values. Addition of an emulsifier to the aqueous phase also resulted in a decrease in the ζ potential of the microcapsules. This is demonstrated by Yan et al. (35).

E. Flow Properties

The flow properties of aqueous microcapsule suspensions have been studied with the aim of modeling blood flow in living vessels (1).

VI. APPLICATIONS

Interfacial polymerization is a promising immobilization technique widely used in a variety of commercial applications in the fields of agriculture, medicine, pharmacy, and biotechnology. Carbonless copy paper, encapsulated pesticides, and perfumes are among the commercial microencapsulated products. Recently, several investigators expanded this method into the area of drug delivery. In this section, examples to encapsulation of artificial cells, proteins, peptides, enzymes, hormones, antibodies, pharmaceuticals, pigments, oily liquids, polyelectrolytes, and adsorbants will be given from literature (Table 4).

A. Enzymes

Microencapsulation greatly extended the stability and duration of action of the enzymes. Microcapsules containing *asparaginase* prepared by interfacial polymerization exhibited membranes that were resistant to mechanical shock or attack of chymotripsin, and no leakage of asparaginase from microcapsules was observed (36). Chang and Poznansky encapsulated *catalase* enzyme with semipermeable coat to protect leakage and immunological reaction (37). Activity and distribution of *urease* following microencapsulation within polyamide membranes were studied by Monshipouri et al. (38). Chang reported that nylon microcapsules loaded with *urease* when injected intraperitoneally converted blood urea to ammonia efficiently (39). Microcapsules containing *arginase* were prepared by polyphthaloyl dichloride and piperazine. The authors reported that the reduction in the activity of encapsulated arginase was mainly due to contact with organic solvent and chemical incorporation into the membrane during microencapsulation (40). Microcapsules containing aqueous solutions of enzymes are artificial analogs of biological cells. Microencapsulation of *chymotripsin, trypsin,* and *trypsinogen* into nylon shells was performed by the method of Chang with some modifications (41). The authors reported the interactions inside the microcapsules also. Other investigators encapsulated *glucose oxidase, invertase,* and *histidase* into polyamide membranes (16,42,43).

B. Proteins

Hettler et al. prepared microcapsules of *human serum albumin, bovine fibrinogen,* and *ovalbumin* by an interfacial crosslinking process using terephthaloyl chloride (44). They were treated with alkaline hydroxylamine, which later resulted in attachment of hydroxamide groups to the membrane, making the microcapsules capable of iron binding. Lower amounts of iron were found to be complexed by human serum albumin as compared with fibrinogen and ovalbumin microcapsules. Interactions of poly (L-lysine-alt-terephthalic acid) microcapsules with fibrinogen were investigated by Kidonoro et al. by measuring the degree of microcapsule disintegration, fibrinogen adsorption to microcapsules, and the ζ potential of microcapsules as a function of fibrinogen concentration at different ionic strengths buffer solutions (45). The authors showed that increase in the ionic strength of the medium and the surface hydrophobicity of the microcapsules produced an increase in the degree of microcapsule disintegration by fibrinogen. Kondo et al. prepared poly (phthaloyl L-lysine) microcapsules containing *hemoglobin* solution to resemble artificial red blood cells. These microcapsules had negative charges and size and deformability similar to those of red blood cells. The authors investigated the ζ potential, flow properties, and oxygen absorption abilities of these microcapsules (46). Chang prepared the first modified hemoglobin as artificial red blood cells microencapsulating hemoglobin. The circulating time after infusion was extended by modification of surface properties and diameter (47). Hemoglobin microcapsules were prepared by Levy et al. through crosslinking of hemoglobin with various acyldichlorides (48). **Bovine serum albumin** is also encapsulated by interfacial polymerization (33,49).

C. Artificial Cells

Chang and co-workers investigated the use of microcapsules prepared by interfacial polymerization as artificial cells because of their semipermeable properties. Membranes of artificial cells are impermeable to macromolecules or suspensions but they are extemely permeable to solutes present in the biological fluid. This high permeability is a result of thin membrane, small particle size, and large surface area. Typical examples include their use in the treatment of chronic renal failure, acute intoxication, liver failure, enzyme and erythrocyte replacement. Chang and Poznansky prepared nylon microcapsules with diameter of 210 μm to study the permeability characteristics of semipermeable aqueous microcapsules, which they named as *artificial cells* (28). Urea, creatinine, uric acid, glucose, and salicylic acid equilibrated accross nylon microcapsule membranes with a pore radius of 1.8 nm. These semipermeable microcapsules have been prepared in an attempt to take advantage of some of the important properties of biological cells.

Chang and co-workers have been studying extensively on artificial cells since 1957. Chang has reviewed the preparation and clinical applications of these microcapsules as artificial cells in series of articles (47,50–54).

D. Pharmaceuticals

Florence and Jenkins incorporated **trifluoperazine embonate** and **pericyazine embonate** both in nylon-6,10 and piperazine–phthalamide microcapsules (55). **Phenothiazine, sodium pentobarbital,** and **sodium sulfathiazole** were other pharmaceuticals that were encapsulated by polyamide membranes (56,57). **Benzalkonium chloride**–loaded microcapsules were prepared by interfacial polymerization of methylene diisocyanate (58). The polymerization of the isocyanate took place at the interface between the oil and the aqueous phase by the hydrolysis of the isocyanate and the reaction of the amine formed with other isocyanate monomer molecules. Cuff et al. used **calcium sulfate** and **calcium alginate** as a model core substance in investigating the effect of formulation factors on the matrix pH of nylon microcapsules (23).

E. Oily Liquids

The production of *oil*-containing polyterephthalamide microcapsules formed by the reaction of terephthaloyl dichloride disolved in a water-immiscible solvent, with an aqueous solution of diethylenetriamine, was investigated by Alexandridou and Kiparissides (26). Yan et al. investigated the influence of operating variables on properties of oil-containing polyurea microcapsules with toluene 2,4-isocyanate and diethylene triamine as monomers (24). Yan et al. in their other work encapsulated *oily liquids* with polyphthalamide membranes (35). They have received information on the size distribution and ζ potential of oil-containing microcapsules. Still more information is necessary on oil-containing microcapsules because there has been little research in this area.

F. Polyelectrolytes

Shiba et al. studied the electrophoretic behavior of polyphthalamide microcapsules containing polyelectrolytes (32). Polyelectrolytes used in this work were **sodium heparinate** and **sodium** *alginate* as anionic; *methyl glycol chitosan* as cationic polyelectrolytes. Organic salts, *sodium acetate, sodium methyl sulfonate, sodium methyl sulfate, sodium ethyl sulfate, sodium propyl sulfate,* and *sodium sulfate* were also incorporated in polyphthalamide microcapsules (18). Takamura et al. studied the permeability of polyphthalamide microcapsules to various electrolytes like *chlorides, bromides, nitrates of sodium, potassium, lithium, ammonium, and cesium* (56).

G. Hormones and Antibodies

β-*Estradiol* was incorporated in semipermeable membranes (60). *17-Hydroxyprogesterone* antibody and *antithyroxine* antibody were encapsulated in terephthaloylamide microcapsules for use in immunoassays of clinically important hormones (39).

H. Pigments

A viscous organic phase containing up to 65% solid pigment was encapsulated by interfacial polymerization (25,62).

I. Adsorbants

Morishita et al. encapsulated *activated charcoal* and measured the adsorption capacity (63). Their objective in encapsulation was to apply this product to purification, decolorization, and extraction.

VII. CONCLUSION

Microencapsulation by interfacial polymerization, which is one of the commercialized encapsulation processes, is the most optimal method of immobilizing proteins, enzymes, antibodies, cells, and some pharmaceuticals. By this method, it is possible to obtain microcapsules with controllable size and wall thickness by using a variety of monomers. The thickness and the permeability of the semipermeable membrane are important parameters that define the rate of mass transfer. One of the main disadvantages of the method is the remainder if the nonpolymerized monomers.

ACKNOWLEDGMENTS

The authors are grateful to research associate Dr. Betül Arıca for her assistance in compiling the references. They also thank Ms. Özge Kaş for her valuable assistance during the preparation of tables and figures.

REFERENCES

1. Kondo, T., 1978. Microcapsules: their preparation and properties. In: Surface and Colloid Science, E. Matijevic (Ed.), Plenum Publ. Co., New York, pp. 1–22.
2. Thies, C., 1996. A survey of microencapsulation process. In: Microencapsulation Methods and Industrial Applications, S. Benita (Ed.), Marcel Dekker, New York, pp. 1–19.

3. Whateley, T. L., 1996. Microcapsules: preparation by interfacial polymerization and interfacial complexation and their applications. In: Microencapsulation Methods and Industrial Applications, S. Benita (Ed.), Marcel Dekker, New York, pp. 349–375.
4. Luzzi, L. A., 1976. Encapsulation techniques for pharmaceuticals: considerations for the microencapsulation of drugs. In: Microencapsulation, J. R. Nixon (Ed.), Marcel Dekker, New York, pp. 193–206.
5. Nack, H., 1970. Microencapsulation techniques: applications and problems. J. Soc. Cosmet. Chem., 21:85–98.
6. Deasy, P. B., Ed., 1984. Microencapsulation and Related Drug Processess, Marcel Dekker, New York, pp. 119–143.
7. Bakan, J. A., and Anderson, J. L., 1970. Microencapsulation. In: The Theory and Practice of Industrial Pharmacy, L. Lachman and J. L. Kanig (Eds.), Lea and Febiger, Philadelphia, pp. 420–437.
8. Fanger, G. O., 1974. Microencapsulation: a brief history and introduction. In: Microencapsulation: Process and Applications, J. E. Vandegaer (Ed.), Plenum Press, New York, pp. 1–19.
9. Arshady, R., 1989. Preparation of microspheres and microcapsules by interfacial polycondensation technique. J. Microencap., 6: 13–28.
10. Whateley, T. L., Ed., 1992, Microencapsulation of Drugs, Harwood Academic, Switzerland.
11. Donbrow, M., Ed., 1992. Microcapsules and Nanoparticles in Medicine and Pharmacology, CRC Press, Boca Raton, FL.
12. Chang, T. M. S., 1992. Recent advances in artificial cells with emphasis on biotechnological and medical approaches based on microencapsulation. In: Microcapsules and Nanoparticles in Medicine and Pharmacology, M. Donbrow (Ed.), CRC Press, Boca Raton, FL, pp. 323–339.
13. Arshady, R., 1988, Preparation of polymer nano-microspheres by vinyl polymerization techniques. J. Microencap., 5: 101–114.
14. Thies, C., 1987. Microencapsulation. In: Encyclopedia of Polymer and Engineering, J. I. Kroschwitz, H. F. Mark, N. M. Bikales, C. G. Overberger, G. Menges (Eds.), John Wiley and Sons, New York, pp. 724–745.
15. Watanabe, A., and Hayashi, T., 1976. Microencapsulation techniques of Fuji photo film and their applications. In: Microencapsulation, J. R. Nixon (Ed.), Marcel Dekker, New York, pp. 13–38.
16. Rambourg, P., Levy, J., and Levy, M.-C., 1982. Microencapsulation III. Preparation of invertase microcapsules. J. Pharm. Sci., 71: 753–758.
17. Jenkins, A. W. and Florence, A. T., 1973. Scanning electron microscopy of nylon microcapsules, J. Pharm. Pharmacol., 25, Suppl., 57P–61P.
18. Shigeri, Y., Koishi, M., Kondo, T., Shiba, M., and Tomioka, S., 1971. Studies on microcapsules. VIII: Effect of some organic salts with short alkyl chain on microcapsule size. Kolloid-Z.u.Z. Polymere, 249: 1051–1055.
19. Wakamatsu, Y., Koishi, M., and Kondo, T., 1974. Studies on microcapsules. XVII: Effect of chemical structure of acid dichlorides and bisphenols on the formation of polyphenyl ester microcapsules. Chem. Pharm. Bull., 22: 1319–1325.
20. Shigeri, Y., Koishi, M., and Kondo, T., 1970. Studies on microcapsules. VI. Effect of variations in polymerization condition on microcapsule size. Can. J. Chem., 48: 2047–2051.
21. Etuk, B. R., Weatherley, L. R., and Murray, K. R., 1995. Some factors affecting the size of nylon 6-10 microcapsules prepared by interfacial polymerization in a high voltage electric field. J. Microencap., 12: 173–183.
22. Zhang, M., Ni, P., and Yan, N., 1995. Effect of operation variables and monomers on the properties of polyamide microcapsules., J. Microencap., 12: 425–435.
23. Cuff, G. W., Combs, A. B., McGinity, J. W., 1984. Effect of formulation factors on the matrix pH of nylon microcapsules. J. Microencap., 1: 27–32.
24. Yan, N., Ni, P., and Zhang, M., 1993. Preparation and properties of polyurea microcapsules with non-ionic surfactant as emulsifier., J. Microencap., 10: 375–383.
25. Tan, H. S., Hwee, T. N. G., and Mahabadi, H. K., 1991. Interfacial polymerization encapsulation of a viscous pigment mix: emulsification conditions and particle size distributions. J. Microencap., 8: 525–536.

26. Alexandridou, S., and Kiparissides, C., 1994. Production of oil-containing polyterephthalamide microcapsules by interfacial polymerization. An experimental investigation of the effect of process variables on the microcapsule size distribution. J. Microencap., 11: 603–614.
27. Muramatsu, N., Shiga, K., and Kondo, T., 1994. Preparation of polyamide microcapsules having narrow size distribution. J. Microencap., 11: 171–178.
28. Chang, T. M. S., and Poznansky, M. J., 1968. Semipermeable aqueous microcapsules (artificial cells). V. Permeability characteristics. J. Biomed. Mater. Res., 2: 187–199.
29. Miyauchi, E., Togawa, Y., Makino, K., Ohshima, H., and Kondo, T., 1992. Dependence on pH of permeability towards electrolyte ions of poly (L-lysine-alt-terephthalic acid) microcapsule membranes. J. Microencap., 9: 329–333.
30. Takamura, K., Koishi, M., and Kondo, T., 1973. Microcapsules. XIV: Effects of membrane materials and viscosity of aqueous phase on permeability of polyamide microcapsules toward electrolytes., J. Pharm. Sci., 62: 610–612.
31. Dufour, P., Brun, H., Chapelon, R., and Pouyet, B., 1992. Improvement of a microencapsulation with aqueous core by factorial design. J. Microencap., 9: 465–468.
32. Shiba, M., Kawano, Y., Tomioka, S., Koishi, M., and Kondo, T., 1971. Studies on microcapsules: X. Electrophoretic behavior of polyphthalamide microcapsules containing aqueous solutions of polyelectrolytes., Kolloid-Z.Z. Polymere. 249: 1056–1060.
33. Shiba, M., Kawano, Y., Tomioka, S., Koishi, M., and Kondo, T., 1971. Studies on microcapsules. XI. Electrophoretic behavior of polyphthalamide microcapsules containing aqueous solutions of bovine serum albumin., Bull. Chem. Soc. Jpn., 44: 2911–2915.
34. Shiba, M., Tomioka, S., and Kondo, T., 1973. Studies on microcapsules. XV. Electrophoretic behavior of carboxylated polyphthalamide microcapsules containing aqueous solutions of polyelectrolytes., Bull. Chem. Soc. Jpn., 46: 2584–2586.
35. Yan, N., Zhang, M., and Ni, P., 1994. Study on polyamide microcapsules containing oily liquids., J. Microencap., 11: 365–372.
36. Mori, T., Sato, T., Matuo, Y., Tosa, T., and Chibata, I., 1972. Preparation and characteristics of microcapsules containing asparaginase. Biotech. Bioeng., 14: 663–673.
37. Chang, T. M. S., and Poznansky, M. J., 1968. Semipermeable microcapsules containing catalase for enzyme replacement in acatalasaemic mice. Nature., 218: 243–245.
38. Monshipouri, M., Neufeld, R. J., 1991. Activity and distribution of urease following microencapsulation within polyamide membranes. Enzyme Microb. Technol., 13: 309–313.
39. Chang, T. M. S., 1966. Semipermeable aqueous microcapsules (artificial cells): with emphasis on experiments in an extracorporeal shunt system., Trans. Am. Soc. Artif. Int. Organs, 12: 13–19.
40. Kondo, T., and Muramatsu, N., 1976. Enzyme inactivation in microencapsulation. In: Microencapsulation, J. R. Nixon (Ed.), Marcel Dekker, New York, pp. 67–75.
41. Aisina, R. B., 1992. Effect of microencapsulated enzymes. In: Microencapsulation of Drugs, T. L. Whateley (Ed.), Harwood Academic, Switzerland, pp. 215–231.
42. Hoshino, K., Muramatsu, N., and Kondo, T., 1989. A study on the thermostability of microencapsulated glucose oxidase. J. Microencap., 6: 205–211.
43. Wood, D. A., Whateley, T. L., and Florence, A. T., 1979. Microencapsulation of histidase for enzyme replacement therapy. J. Pharm. Pharmacol., 31: 79.
44. Hettler, D., Andry, M.-C., and Levy, M.-C., 1994. Polyhydroxamic microcapsules prepared from proteins: a novel type of chelating microcapsules. J. Microencap., 11: 213–224.
45. Kidokoro, M., Ohshima, H., and Kondo, T., 1991. Interaction of poly(L-lysine-alt-terephthalic acid) microcapsules with fibrinogen. J. Microencap., 8: 63–70.
46. Kondo, T., Arakawa, M., and Tamamushi, B., 1976. Poly (phthaloyl-L-lysine) Microcapsules containing hemoglobin solution: artificial red blood cells. In: Microencapsulation, J. R. Nixon (Ed.), Marcel Dekker, New York, pp. 163–172.
47. Chang, T. M. S., 1976. Semipermeable microcapsules as artificial cells: clinical applications and perspectives. In: Microencapsulation, J. R. Nixon (Ed.), Marcel Dekker, New York, pp. 57–66.
48. Levy, M.-C., Rambourg, P., Levy, J., and Potron, G., Microencapsulation IV: Cross-linked hemoglobin microcapsules. J. Pharm. Sci., 71: 759–763.

49. Shiba, M., Tomioka, S., Koishi, M., and Kondo, T., 1970. Studies on microcapsules. V. Preparation of polyamide microcapsules containing aqueous protein solution. Chem. Pharm. Bull., 18: 803–809.
50. Chang, T. M. S., 1967. Microcapsules as artificial cells. Science Journal, July: 62–66
51. Chang, T. M. S., Johnson, L. J., and Ransome, O. J., 1967. Semipermeable aqueous microcapsules. IV. Nonthrombogenic microcapsules with heparin-complexed membranes. Can. J. Physiol. Pharmacol., 45: 705–715.
52. Chang, T. M. S., 1995. Artificial cells with emphasis on bioencapsulation in biotechnology. In: Biotechnology Annual Review, Vol. 1, M. R. El-Gewely (Ed.), Elsevier Science B. V., pp. 267–295.
53. Chang, T. M. S., 1964. Semipermeable microcapsules. Science, 146: 524–525.
54. Chang, T. M. S., Macintosh, F. C., and Mason, S. G., 1966. Semipermeable aqueous microcapsules. I. Preparation and properties., Can. J. Physiol. Pharmacol., 44: 115–128.
55. Florence, A. T., and Jenkins, A. W., 1976. In vitro assessment of microencapsulated drug systems as sustained release parenteral dosage forms. In: Microencapsulation, J. R. Nixon (Ed.), Marcel Dekker, New York, pp. 40–55.
56. Luzzi, L. A., Zoglio, M. A., and Moulding, H. V., 1970. Preparation and evaluation of prolonged release properties of nylon microcapsules. J. Pharm. Sci., 59: 338–341.
57. Cuff, G. W., and McGinity, J. W., 1984. Expanded versatility of microcapsules prepared by interfacial polymerization. J. Microencap., 1: 343–347.
58. Pense, A. M., Vauthier-Holtzscherer, C., and Benoit, J.-P., 1992. Microencapsulation of benzalkonium chloride. In: Microencapsulation of Drugs, T. L. Whateley (Ed.), Harwood Academic, Switzerland, pp. 1–5.
59. Takamura, K., Koishi, M., and Kondo, T., 1971. Studies on microcapsules. IX: Permeability of polyphthalamide microcapsule membranes to electrolytes. Kolloid-Z.Z. Polymere, 248: 929–933.
60. Graham, N. B., and Amer, L. I., 1992, Surface polymerisation as an encapsulation technique. In: Microencapsulation of Drugs, T. L. Whateley (Ed.), Harwood Academic, Switzerland, pp. 123–137.
61. Wallace, A. M., 1992. Novel immunoassays for clinically important hormones based on microencapsulated antibodies. In: Microencapsulation of Drugs, T. L. Whateley (Ed.), Harwood Academic, Switzerland, pp. 243–253.
62. Mahabadi, H. K., Ng, T. H., and Tan, H. S., 1996. Interfacial/free radical polymerization microencapsulation: kinetics of particle formation., J. Microencap., 13: 559–573.
63. Morishita, M., Fukushima, M., and Inaba, Y., 1973. Microencapsulation of activated charcoal and its biochemical applications., Am. Chem. Soc. Div. Org. Coat. Plast. Chem. Pap., 33: 603–610.

14
Nanoparticulate Controlled Release Systems for Cancer Therapy

C. Dubernet, E. Fattal, and P. Couvreur
Centre d'Études Pharmaceutiques, Chatenay-Malabry, France

I. INTRODUCTION

Significant advances have already taken place in the treatment of some malignancies. However, there has been little progress in the treatment of most common solid tumors such as those of breast, lung, colorectum and brain. In the past decade, research works have shown that the lack of sensitivity of most tumors to treatment lies in the hindrance of drug penetration in the tumor interstitium (1,2). Indeed, to be effective, drugs need to reach a given concentration close to the tumor cells, which is far from being the case everywhere in the tumor.

The poor efficiency of conventional anticancer drugs can be explained by the special structure of solid tumors. First, the stromal component may represent as much as 90% of the tumor mass, depending on the tumor type. Of course, this interstitial space may play the role of reservoir for some drugs, but it also increases the distances between most of the tumor cells and the blood vessels, increasing the distances the drugs have to cross. Secondly, vasculature within the tumor is not homogeneous and in some areas, tumor cells are not available to blood supply. In addition, increased vessel tortuosity within the neovasculature causes high flow resistance, which leads in turn to reduced drug supply. Thirdly, the absence of well-defined lymphatic network is responsible for high pressure gradients in the interstitium, which hinders convective flow. Diffusion remains the only transport available for the drugs which considerably limits the interest of macromolecules. Endly, vessels are in some areas highly permeable and in others not, leading to regions either well or poorly accessible to therapy.

In addition to such a constitutive resistance to treatments due to physiological considerations, the emergence of multidrug resistance is often an additional problem to be solved, including overexpression of the transmembrane glycoprotein Pgp, multidrug resistance protein (MRP), and glutathione-S-transferase or topoisomerase modifications (2).

Because of this situation, the doses of anticancer drug have to be increased. However, toxicity is a very limiting factor for most of the chemotherapeutic agents, such as cardiotoxicity and myelosuppression for example.

Therefore, there is a need for a new therapy, that would be able to concentrate the drugs closely to the tumor site, and avoid their too large distribution. Some work has already been carried out in this direction, and alternative therapies include for example the local administration of polymeric implants for either interstitial sustained release or chemoembolization (3) and the use of soluble drug/polymer conjugates (4).

Because drug targeting can modulate drug distribution, the use of colloidal carriers has been proposed as a promising way of increasing the efficacy of chemotherapy while reducing adverse effects. In the following, the literature concerning the use of nanoparticles will be discussed. After some pharmacokinetics background, we will focus on several remarkable results successively dealing with *in vivo* models, multidrug resistance, oligonucleotide targeting, and tumor imaging.

II. EFFICACY OF NANOPARTICULATE SYSTEMS IN TUMOR MODELS

Among the various chemotherapeutic agents that are candidates for encapsulation, doxorubicin has been the focus of a great number of investigations. Liposomal formulations of doxorubicin are now marketed, and polyalkylcyanoacrylate nanoparticles entered clinical trials in the past decade (5). Various reviews are focused on the description of the preparation of nanoparticles (6–8), and this point will not be discussed in the present chapter. In the literature concerning tumor therapy, two major types of systems are most frequently encountered: polyalkylcyanoacrylate (PACA) and polylactide nanoparticles, the former being obtained by a polymerization process, and the latter by a solvent evaporation or a nanodeposition precipitation procedure.

The first and main interest of nanoparticulate carriers for chemotherapeutic agents was to avoid drug distribution in organs such as the heart and the kidneys where a toxic effect could be observed (9). Indeed, after IV administration, colloidal particles concentrate rapidly in the liver (70% of the injected dose) due to the opsonization process, increasing the liver concentration of the drug itself, whereas only traces can be found in the kidneys and the heart. The use of larger particles (generally larger than 5 μm) leads to accumulation in the lung, due to a capillary filtration effect (10).

Because bone marrow presents a sinusoidal endothelium, nanoparticles can also accumulate in this organ. Except in the case where the particle surface has been modified to target the bone marrow (11), the amount of drug concentrated in this organ remains low. Nevertheless, comparing polyisobutylcyanoacrylate (PIBCA) and polyisohexylcyanoacrylate (PIHCA) nanoparticles loaded with doxorubicin, Gibaud et al. (12,13) found a higher amount of drug in the bone marrow when PIHCA nanoparticles were used, possibly because of the lower bioerosion rate of this polymer compared to PIBCA. As far as doxorubicin is concerned, PIBCA has then to be preferred over PIHCA for myelosuppression considerations.

In the past 10 years, drug targeting has considerably progressed with the concept of long-circulating carriers, mainly peggylated carriers. Because increasing the circulation time in a tissue may increase total drug uptake, a number of authors have investigated the interest of this strategy in the field of cancer (14). Surprisingly, only Stealth liposomes have been developed in this aim. The results show an increased tumor uptake in almost every case even if, compared to conventional liposomes, peggylation decreases the blood/tumor ratio. Why are peggylated nanoparticles not investigated in solid tumors too? Perhaps convenient, biodegradable, peggylated nanoparticles are still not ready for use, although some development has been completed in this regard (15,16).

Considering the main results obtained with nanoparticulate carriers *in vivo*, the models used can be separated into two classes: the intramuscularty or intraperitoneally implanted tumors on one hand, and the liver metastases, on the other hand, which is the most relevant model for the investigation of nanoparticles for passive targeting.

A. Efficacy of Nanoparticles in Intramuscularly and Intraperitoneally Implanted Tumor Models

Mitoxantrone is an anthracenedione derivative that is particularly effective in the treatment of breast cancer, acute leukemia, and lymphoma. Even if this drug is less cardiotoxic than its parent doxorubicin, it remains toxic against the bone marrow, which limits its use. The interest of polybutylcyanoacrylate (PBCA) nanoparticles in reducing this adverse effect has been investigated by Beck et al. and Reska et al. (17,18) in two tumor models: P388 leukemia and B16 melanoma.

P388 cells were transplanted intraperitoneally in mice, whereas the drugs were administered intravenously. Nanoparticles were very disappointing in this model since they were found less effective than the free drug in terms of the mean survival time. In comparison, small unilamellar vesicles (SUV) liposomes increased the mean survival time of mice twofold compared to free mitoxantrone.

B16 melanoma was implanted intramuscularly and drugs injected intravenously as previously. Whereas SUV showed no advantage over the free drug in this model, the use of nanoparticles led to the important reduction of the tumor size. Mean survival time was not increased due to premature death of some animals just after the nanoparticles injection. The occurrence of embolism due to the likely presence of aggregates pointed out the need for sonication of the suspensions before injection. These results were, however, encouraging since the encapsulation efficiency of mitoxantrone in nanoparticles was only 8–15%. When pharmacokinetic data were obtained (18), it could be verified that only a part of the drug was colocalized with the ^{14}C polymer in the liver, for example, corresponding to the really encapsulated drug. Despite this fact, significantly higher amounts of drug were found in the tumor in the case of nanoparticles compared to the free drug, which might explain the improved efficacy of this formulation. In comparison, SUV liposomes considerably increased mitoxantrone concentration in the blood, even 24 hours after administration, without any significant consequence on the concentration of the drug located in the heart or in the tumor tissue. On the opposite, due to the low encapsulation efficiencies, nanoparticles were not effective in decreasing the heart concentration of mitoxantrone.

These overall results clearly showed the potential of PBCA nanoparticles in B16 melanoma if improved encapsulation efficiencies could be achieved. The results simultaneously obtained with SUV tend to indicate that a prolonged circulation time was not required for efficacy in B16 melanoma, whereas it was probably beneficial in the case of P388 leukemia, as explained before.

The association of actinomycin D with polymethylcyanoacrylate nanoparticles led to greater encapsulation efficiencies than previously found with mitoxantrone and PBCA. Experimented in a subcutaneous sarcoma in mice (19), these nanoparticles were found particularly effective.

Pharmacokinetic data obtained after IV administration of radiolabeled PIBCA nanoparticles in mice bearing a subcutaneously implanted Lewis lung carcinoma (20) confirmed that the carrier was able to concentrate in the tumor. The concentration in the tumor reached its maximum when nanoparticles disappeared from the bloodstream, suggesting that prolonged circulation time might have still allowed an increase in tumor uptake. The pharmacokinetic data also showed that a significant number of nanoparticles could be found in the lungs of tumor bearing mice, whereas they were totally absent in healthy animals. This finding has to be related to the presence of lung metastases and is a valuable argument to justify the further use of such nanoparticles in the treatment of pulmonary metastases.

Another example of a chemotherapeutic agent whose efficacy could be improved by encapsulation into nanoparticles is taxol. Indeed, its administration in clinics requires the use of solubilization adjuvant such as Cremophor (polyoxyethylated castor oil), which is rather poorly tolerated. Generally, such lipophilic drugs find interest to be encapsulated in nanoparticulate systems consisting of an oily core surrounded by a polymer shell, nanocapsules. Hence, Bartoli et al. (21) formulated polylactide nanocapsules and compared their efficacy to free and liposomal taxol in L1210 and P388 cell lines *in vitro*, and P388 leukemia transplanted intraperitoneally in mice.

Concerning *in vitro* results, nanocapsules were found to be as effective as the commercial solution of taxol in P388 but less cytotoxic in L1210. The low efficiency of nanocapsules in L1210 could be explained by the lower sensitivity to taxol of this cell line compared to P388, and to the existence of a lag period of release delaying the effect of nanocapsules compared to the free drug. It might be that the release rate of taxol from these nanocapsules was too slow because of the low water solubility of the drug.

Concerning in vivo results, nanocapsules were injected intraperitoneally in mice bearing P388. Results were expressed as increased life span. There was observed an increased mortality of mice receiving nanocapsules, presumably because of the toxicity of the formulation used containing benzylbenzoate. Consequently, no conclusion could be clearly drawn from these experiments concerning the efficacy of the encapsulation of taxol in colloidal particles. Comparatively, liposomal taxol was found as effective as free taxol, but complete toxicology studies would be required to claim the superiority of the encapsulated form over the commercial one.

Sharma et al. (22) also investigated the interest of nanoparticulate systems for the delivery of taxol. In this case, nanoparticles consisting of polyvinylpyrrolidone were prepared and were evaluated in B16F10 melanoma–bearing mice. B16F10 is a variant of the parent B16 melanoma, which after intramuscular transplantation gives rise to pulmonary metastases. The results showed a significantly greater efficacy of the nanoparticle-bound taxol in terms of reduction of the tumor volume and increase of the mean survival time compared to the free drug. Considering the very low size of the nanoparticles used (50–60 nm), one can wonder whether the greater efficacy of this formulation could be attributed to a prolonged circulation time in the blood.

B. Efficacy of Nanoparticles in a Liver Metastasis Model

Two studies will be reported in this section, both dealing with the M5076 tumor model. M5076 is a reticulum cell carcinoma grown in mice subcutaneously. It gives a reproducible number of hepatic metastases within 15 days after the intravenous injection of the tumor cells in suspension.

Chiannilkulchai et al. (23) first investigated the interest of doxorubicin-loaded PIHCA nanoparticles in different therapeutic schemes following intravenous injection. The efficacy of the targeted formulation was found in every case considerably greater than the free drug, especially at lower doses when free doxorubicin was inefficient. When administered once at day 7 or twice at days 7 and 9 in fractionated doses, nanoparticles reduced the number of metastases in the same way. However, when administered twice at days 11 and 13, the superiority of the nanoparticles was fully confirmed. Indeed, this therapeutic scheme corresponds to a very late treatment, when a great number of metastases were already formed. Free doxorubicin had no effect in this case even at the highest dose tested, whereas doxorubicin-loaded nanoparticles were still effective (Fig. 1).

The efficacy of the nanoparticulate formulation could be explained by a tissue targeting, doxorubicin being concentrated in the liver after the phagocytosis of nanoparticles by Kupffer cells. The macrophage were then assumed to play the role of reservoir, allowing the drug to diffuse toward the neoplastic cells. The determination of the intracellular concentrations of doxorubicin confirmed this hypothesis, since nanoparticles were shown to lead to a higher doxorubicin concentration in the neoplastic cells compared to the free drug, but to an even higher increase in Kupffer cells (24).

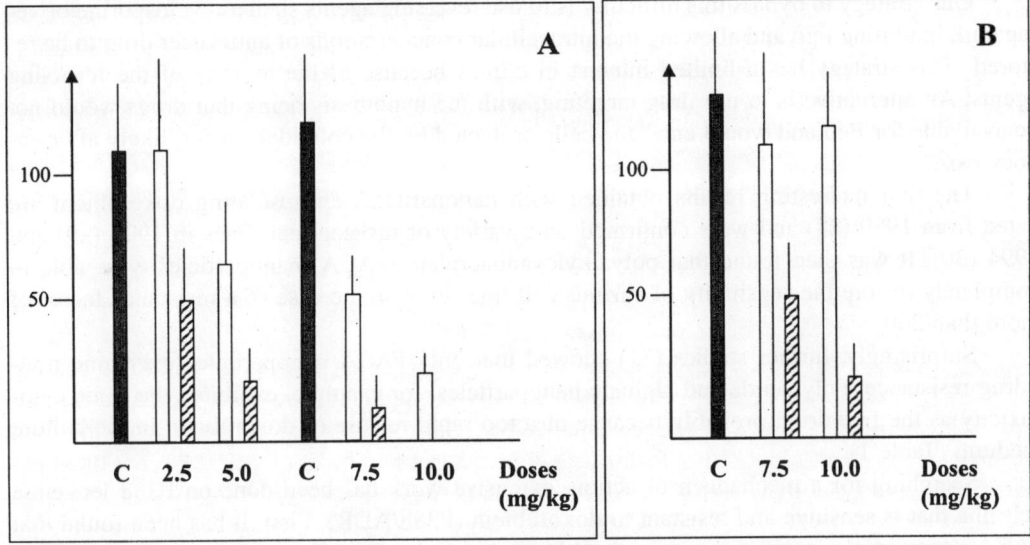

Figure 1 Number of hepatic metastases at day 15 in mice inoculated with M5076 cells and treated with free doxorubicin (white bars) or doxorubicin-loaded PIHCA nanoparticles (hatched bars) in two different therapeutic schedules: (A) two injections at days 7 and 9; (B) two injections at days 11 and 13. T are the untreated control groups.

Kupffer cells, together with pit cells (liver-associated lymphocytes), are considered to play a key role in controlling hepatic metastases (25). This control involves the release by Kupffer cells of cytolytic cytokines and opens interesting perspectives for immunotherapy. Immunomodulators are indeed able to activate macrophages and increase their cytolytic activity. The targeting of immunomodulators such as muramyl peptides directly to Kupffer cells in the treatment of liver metastases is then a very promising approach in therapeutics. A great number of studies concern the encapsulation of immunomodulators into liposomes, but Barratt et al. and Yu et al. (26,27) have also investigated nanocapsules to target the lipophilic derivative MDP-L-alanylcholesterol (MTP-Chol) toward the macrophages. First, MTP-Chol-loaded nanocapsules were shown to activate alveolar macrophages *in vitro* to tumor cytotoxicity in the same way that liposomes do. In a second step, the formulation was investigated in the M5076 hepatic metastases model. Injected before the administration of tumor cells in the animal, MTP-Chol nanocapsules were able to hinder the development of metastases. However, no effect could be observed when therapy was started after tumor cell inoculation. In consequence, these results indicate that such nanocapsules would not be useful to treat established liver metastases in patients. However, since the surgical removal of solid tumors are considered to increase the risk of metastases development, encapsulated immunomodulators could be proposed as a preventive treatment on the day after tumor removal.

III. EFFICACY OF NANOPARTICLES IN MULTIDRUG RESISTANCE

One of the main mechanism involved in multidrug resistance (MDR) is the overexpression of the transmembrane glycoprotein Pgp, acting as a pump and decreasing the intracellular concentration of a variety of drugs. To remain cytotoxic against resistant cells, the doses of chemotherapeutic agents have to be increased considerably, far above the tolerated doses in clinics.

One strategy to bypass this difficulty is to use reversing agents such as cyclosporine or verapamil, inhibiting Pgp and allowing the intracellular concentrations of anticancer drug to be restored. This strategy has a limited interest in clinics because of the toxicity of the reversing agents. An alternative is to use drug targeting, with the hypothesis being that drugs would not be available for Pgp and would enter the cells protected by the colloidal carrier, likely after endocytosis.

The first interesting results obtained with nanoparticles encapsulating doxorubicin are dated from 1989 (28) and were confirmed on a variety of resistant cell lines in 1992 (29) and 1994 (30). It was then found that polyalkylcyanoacrylate (PACA) nanoparticles were able to completely restore the sensitivity of various cell lines even in the case of a resistance factor of more than 200.

Surprisingly, further studies (31) showed that only PACA nanoparticles overcame multidrug resistance. Polylactide and alginate nanoparticles, for example, exhibited the same cytotoxicity as the free drug, probably because of a too rapid release of doxorubicin in the culture medium (Table 1).

Searching for a mechanism of action, extensive work has been done on P388 leukemia cell line that is sensitive and resistant to doxorubicin (P388/ADR). First, it has been found that PACA nanoparticles were not endocytosed by the tumor cells (32) but that direct contact between the nanoparticles and the tumor cells was essential to observe the reversion of the resistance (33). The most likely hypothesis was that nanoparticles adsorb onto the cell surface, leading to locally increased drug concentration gradient favoring in turn cellular penetration (Fig. 2). PACA nanoparticles release doxorubicin along with their bioerosion due to esterases and lead to the formation of soluble polycyanoacrylic acid. Colin de Verdière et al. (33) showed that the presence of this soluble polymer coming from the bioerosion of nanoparticles was able to increase both doxorubicin cytotoxicity and drug uptake by the resistant cells. Nevertheless, Hu et al. (34) found that PACA was unable to inhibit Pgp. The role of polycyanoacrylic acid must then be sought elsewhere.

Finally, the overall results clearly suggested the formation of a complex between doxorubicin and polycyanoacrylic acid, leading to a potentiation of doxorubicin efficacy. The drug being cationic and polycyanoacrylic acid anionic, ion pairs can form, leading to an uncharged and more hydrophobic compound than the original drug. Diffusion through cell membranes is then favored and intracellular concentrations can be increased (Fig. 3). The existence of such an ion

Table 1 P388 and P388/ADR Growth Inhibition Data[a]

Drug sample	IC_{50} (ng/mL)	
	P388-sensitive cells,	P388/ADR-resistant cells
Doxorubicin	30	1500
NS Dox PIBCA	30	100
NS Dox PIHCA	30	100
NS Dox PLA	50	1500
NS Dox PLGA	50	1500
NS Dox Alginate	50	1500

[a]Obtained when cells are incubated with different types of doxorubicin-loaded nanoparticles (polyisobutylcyanoacrylate, PIBCA; polyisohexylcyanoacrylate, PIHCA; poly(lactic acid), PLA; poly(lactic-co-glycolic acid, PLGA; and alginate) compared to free doxorubicin. Results are expressed in terms of IC_{50}, which corresponds to the concentration inhibiting 50% of cell growth.
Source: Data from Ref. 26.

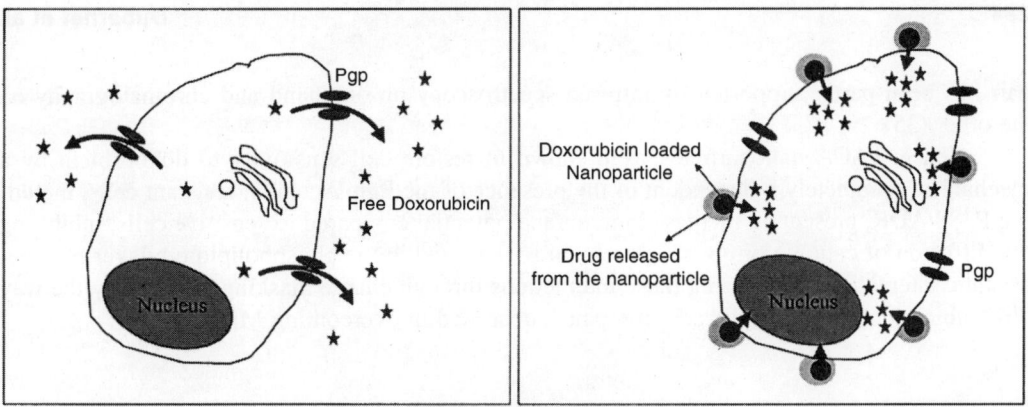

Figure 2 Schematic representations of the interaction of doxorubicin with resistant cells when incubated in solution (left), pumped out of the cell by Pgp, or in polyalkylcyanoacrylate nanoparticles (right). In this last case, nanoparticles adsorb onto the tumor cell and progressively release the encapsulated drug along with the polymer bioerosion. The high local drug concentration gradient favors the intracellular penetration of doxorubicin.

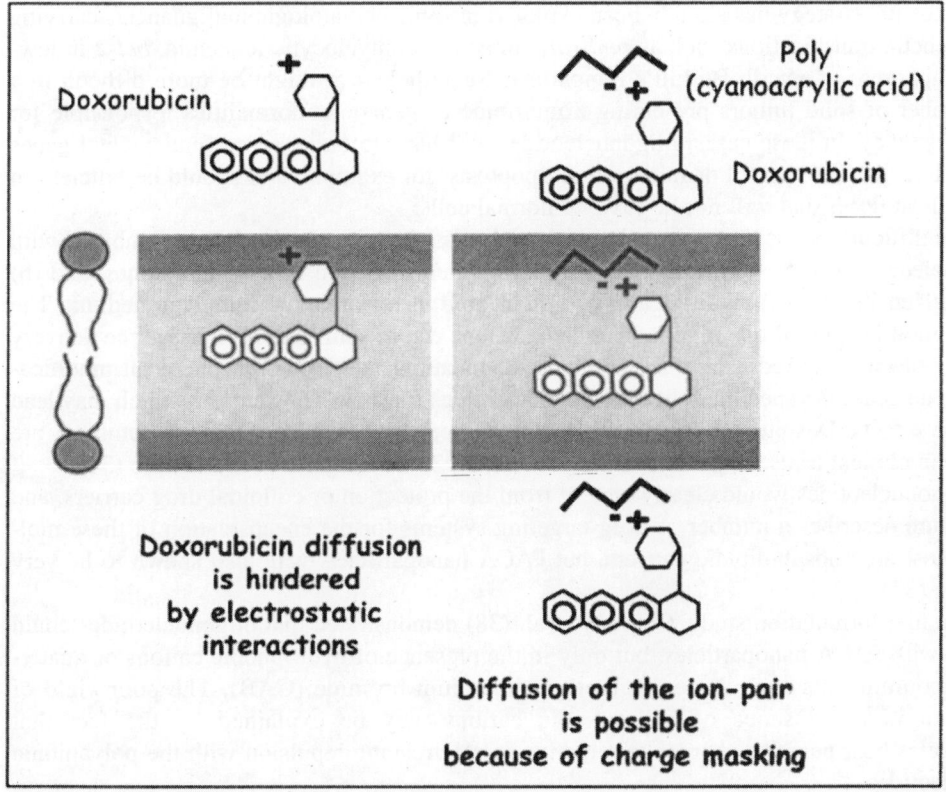

Figure 3 According to the hypothesis proposed in (33), doxorubicin molecules do not diffuse easily across the cell membranes because of electrostatic interactions with the polar head groups of phospholipids. When mixed with poly(cyanoacrylic acid) coming from the bioerosion of polyalkylcyanoacrylate nanoparticles, ion pairs can form and favor doxorubicin diffusion through the cell membranes, thus restoring tumor cell sensitivity.

pair has been partly supported by infrared spectroscopy on one hand and chromatography on the other (35).

Hence, PACA nanoparticles were shown to restore cell sensitivity to doxorubicin by a mechanism completely independent of the presence of the Pgp. Actually, resistant cells, including P388/ADR, present an increased membrane potential compared to sensitive cells, inhibiting the diffusion of cationic drugs which remain sequestered in the phospholipidic bilayer by electrostatic interactions. Bypassing these interactions through charge masking is probably the way doxorubicin/polycyanoacrylic acid ion pairs succeeded in overcoming MDR.

IV. NANOPARTICLES AND OLIGONUCLEOTIDE THERAPY OF CANCER

Conventional chemotherapeutic agents are cytotoxic drugs with limited specificity for tumor cells compared to host tissue. In addition, they are preferably effective against rapidly proliferating tumors. It would then be interesting to develop new therapeutic strategies taking benefit from the latest discoveries in cancer biology (36) which have identified specific molecular and biochemical targets implicated in tumor progression.

In this aim, oligonucleotides could be particularly useful to inhibit expression of oncogenes or other appropriate molecular targets in tumor tissues in a sequence-specific manner. This therapeutic strategy has already been explored in some hematologic malignancies carrying unique genetic translocations such as *pml-rara* in acute promyelocytic leukemia, *bcl-2* in low-grade lymphoma, or *myc* in Burkitt's lymphoma. Nevertheless, it might be more difficult in a wide number of solid tumors presenting a multitude of genetic abnormalities responsible for their malignancy. In these cases, oligonucleotides will have to target some fundamental genes involved in cell cycle control or initiation of apoptosis, for example, and should be efficient in tumor cells at doses that will not be toxic to normal cells.

The difficulty associated with oligonucleotides is (a) their anionic charge combined with a high molecular weight, which considerably limits their diffusion across membranes, and (b) their great sensitivity to enzymes, leading to their rapid inactivation in biological medium. The chemical modification of the oligonucleotide backbone can to some extent improve the delivery of these molecules by reducing the enzymatic degradation rate. However, chemical modifications also decrease the specificity of the oligonucleotides for their RNA targets, which may lead to adverse effects. Despite these problems, some compounds, especially phosphorothiates, are currently in clinical trials, targeting $PKC\alpha$, Ha-*ras*, *bcl2*, or *p53* genes, for example (36).

Oligonucleotides would clearly benefit from the protection of colloidal drug carriers, and the literature describes a number of drug targeting systems for the encapsulation of these molecules. Most are phospholipidic carriers, but PACA nanoparticles were also shown to be very promising (37).

In a first formulation study, Chavany et al. (38) demonstrated that oligonucleotides could associate with PACA nanoparticles, but only in the presence of hydrophobic cations or quaternary ammonium salts such as cetyltrimethylammonium bromide (CAB). The poor yield of association in the absence of hydrophobic cations may be explained by the fact that nanoparticles bear negative charges that induce an electrostatic repulsion with the polyanionic oligonucleotides.

The overall results suggested that adsorption took place via the formation of ion pairs (Fig. 4), more lipophilic than the original oligonucleotide molecules. The yield of oligonucleotide adsorption was correlated with the hydrophobicity of the cation serving as counterion. It was also found to be highly dependent on the oligonucleotide chain length, together with the concentration of the adsorbed cation, suggesting a cooperative character of the adsorption

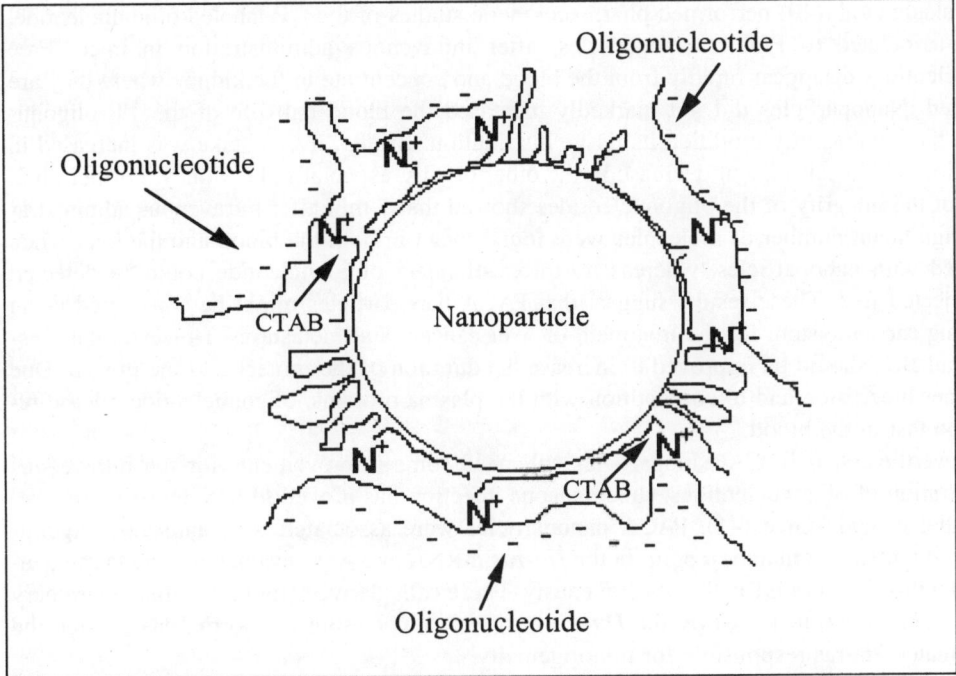

Figure 4 Schematic representation of oligonucleotide adsorption at the surface of polyalkylcyanoacrylate nanoparticles coated with a hydrophobic cation.

process. Finally, because electrostatic interactions were involved in the association of oligonucleotides with nanoparticles, adsorption decreased when ionic strength in the medium increased.

Despite the fact that oligonucleotides were only associated onto the nanoparticle surface, they could be efficiently protected against nucleases. The single ion pair complexes were also found partly protected against enzymatic degradation, but at phosphodiesterase concentrations leading to complete digestion of CTAB–oligonucleotide complexes, efficient protection of oligonucleotides adsorbed onto nanoparticles was achieved. This last result clearly demonstrates the interest of the oligonucleotide adsorption onto nanoparticles.

When incubated with U937 cells, a macrophage-like cell line, nanoparticles cytotoxicity was found to be exactly correlated with the CTAB concentration associated with the particles (39). Hence, the cation-mediating oligonucleotide association limits the concentration of particles that can be incubated with the cells, i.e., the maximum oligonucleotide concentration incubated.

When added in association with nanoparticles, oligonucleotides were shown to enter the U937 cells by an endocytotic-phagocytotic process. The extent of cellular uptake was increased compared to oligonucleotides in solution. In addition, intact oligonucleotides could be found in both the nuclear and extranuclear fractions even after 24 h of incubation in the case of nanoparticles, whereas no additional intact molecules could be found in the extranuclear fractions after 6 h incubation in the case of free oligonucleotides. This finding suggests that nanoparticles contribute greatly to the protection of oligonucleotides in the cells, even if this type of colloidal carrier is known to be finally digested by lysosomes where oligonucleotides will be degraded too. It is not out of the question for nanoparticles to escape from the endosomal compartment due to the presence of the adsorbed CTAB, which tends to exert a lytic action against the endosomal membranes.

Nakada et al. (40) performed pharmacokinetic studies of the ^{33}P-labeled oligonucleotide, free or associated to PACA nanoparticles, after intravenous administration in mice. Free oligonucleotides disappear rapidly from the blood and concentrate in the kidney where they are eliminated. Nanoparticles did not markedly increased the blood half-life of the ^{33}P oligonucleotide but significantly modified its tissue distribution. Briefly, liver uptake was increased in association with a subsequent decrease in the other organs, especially the kidney. Furthermore, control of the integrity of the oligonucleotides showed that 5 min after intravenous administration, a significant number of molecules were found intact in both the blood and the liver when associated with nanoparticles, whereas no traces of intact oligonucleotide could be detected when injected free. These results suggest that PACA nanoparticles might be considered as an interesting carrier system for the treatment of liver cancers and metastases. However, the present formulation should be improved to increase the duration of the protection time *in vivo*. Due to polymer bioerosion and to competition with the plasma proteins, oligonucleotide release remains too fast in the blood.

Nevertheless, if PACA nanoparticles still need some improvements for the intravenous administration of oligonucleotides, subcutaneous injection has proved to be interesting in a tumor model in nude mice (41). PACA nanoparticles were associated with antisense oligonucleotides directed to a mutation point in the *Ha-ras* mRNA and were evaluated in nude mice inoculated with HBL100ras1 cells subcutaneously. These cells derived from the human mammary HBL100 and were transfected by the *Ha-ras* oncogene, expressing the normal Ha-ras and the point-mutated Ha-ras responsible for tumorigenicity.

The model consisted of administring the oligonucleotides either 1 day before and 2 days after the inoculation of tumor cells in mice, in the area where the cells were implanted, or in established tumor, days 1, 4, 6, 8, and 11 after tumor inoculation. Tumor growth could be inhibited in a sequence-specific manner in every case with nanoparticles at a much lower oligonucleotide dose than when administered free.

This result can be explained by the local reservoir of intact oligonucleotides mediated by the nanoparticles at the injection site. This strategy offers a promising route to inhibit the growth of *ras*-dependent tumors, with a specific effect on cells expressing the mutant gene and with no or reduced effects on normal cells.

V. DRUG TARGETING TO LYMPH NODES

Some tumors, especially metastases, develop in the lymphatic system and, more precisely, in lymph nodes (peripheral lymphoid organs). In the search for more specific therapies, it would be useful to have a means of drug targeting in this area. Colloidal carriers are able to concentrate in the lymphatic system in given situations, depending on both the route of administration and the particles properties (42).

The site of administration must be an interstitial space such as that in intradermal, subcutaneous, or intramuscular injections. It is important to understand the physiology of the lymphatic vessels in order to optimize the lymphatic delivery with colloidal carriers such as nanoparticles. The main role of the lymphatic system is the absorption of proteins and particulate cellular matter from the interstitial fluid through thin endothelium of lymphatic vessels and their return to the blood. Lymph is then propelled via the lymphatic capillaries into larger collecting ducts that empty into lymph nodes.

To enter the lymph, colloidal carriers have, first, to be drained through the interstitium and, second, to cross the endothelium of lymphatic vessels. Both phenomena are tightly controlled by the particle size. Because of the viscous nature of the interstitium, particle progression is only possible in narrow aqueous tissue channels of approximately 100 nm diameter. The endothelial wall of lymphatic capillaries varies in thickness, with regions of discontinuous or even absent basement membrane. Because of the presence of proteins in the lymph, colloidal particles will be opsonized and then recognized by macrophages present in the lymph nodes, and finally phagocytosed.

As a consequence, after subcutaneous injection, for example, particles of less than a few nanometers will be exchanged through the blood capillaries, whereas particles with diameters up to few tens of nanometers will gain access to the lymph. Larger particles (over a few hundred nanometers), will be trapped in the interstitial space for a prolonged time (42). It must be noted, however, that size become less important after intraperitonel injection because drainage is simply from a cavity into the initial lymphatic without any diffusion through interstitial space. The adsorption of hydrophilic polymer on the surface of nanoparticles such as poloxamines enhances the drainage from the injection site and increases the lymphatic uptake after subcutaneous injection.

Finally, it must be pointed out that, after administration by interstitial routes, nanoparticles quite exclusively concentrate in the macrophages within the lymph nodes and very small amounts are found in the liver, spleen, and bone marrow.

The targeting of nanoparticles to the lymphatic system is done for either diagnostic or therapeutic purposes. Actually, very few works can be found in the field of chemotherapy. In his review on targeting to lymph nodes (42), Hawley only reports a couple of examples with somewhat deceptive results. The absence of real efficacy could be explained by the large size of the particles used, between 500 nm and 5 μm, whereas the optimal sizes for lymph nodes targeting range between 10 and 50 nm.

Conversely, much attention has been paid to the administration of contrast agents, and in the following, the main recent papers in this field will be briefly discussed.

Concerning magnetic resonance imaging, Weissleder et al. (43) investigated the utility of iron oxide nanoparticles as a contrast agent. Particles were injected either by the intravenous, subcutaneous, or intra-arterial routes for pharmacokinetic studies. The authors verified that extravasation of the nanoparticles was the limiting step allowing further nodal accumulation, with the trapping by lymph node macrophages occurring rapidly thereafter. Consequently, to allow the use of systemic administration, the authors suggested modifications of injection technique that would increase capillary permeability. The efficiency of these nanoparticles in differentiation of malignant and benign adenopathies was then demonstrated in two models: lymph node metastasis in rabbits and lymph node hyperplasia in rats.

Searching for higher tumor specificity in magnetic resonance imaging, Tiefenauer et al. (44) developed superparamagnetic particles of uniform size (9–10 nm) stabilized with a polypeptide coat and covalently bound to a monoclonal antibody specific to carcinoembryonic antigen (CEA). The resulting particles had a hydrodynamic radius of less than 50 nm and were shown to specifically bind to CEA *in vitro*. For further *in vivo* investigation, strategies to reduce the antigenicity and blood clearance rate of the particles needed to be developed.

In the field of x-ray contrast agents for computed tomography, iodinated nanoparticles were shown to efficiently enhance the imaging of lung-draining lymph nodes after pulmonary instillation (45). Particles of insoluble contrast agent were stabilized by poly(ethylene oxide/polypropylene oxide) block copolymers (Pluronics) and were 150–200 nm in size. The administration of small volumes of iodinated nanoparticles suspension was demonstrated to be safe and could be successfully used to aid staging of lung cancer. The authors mention that further studies are in progress, investigating both the colloid size and the type of polymer coating upon the translocation of the nanoparticles to lung lymph nodes.

Again in the development of contrast agents for computed tomography lymphography, Wisner et al. investigated varying administration routes for the imaging of varying lymph node locations (46,47). For example, they demonstrated that craniocervical and thoracic lymph nodes could be efficiently opacified from interstitial (subcutaneous) or intraperitoneal delivery of iodinated nanoparticles. The authors also showed that contrast increased in the first 12 h following subcutaneous and submucosal injections, and was dependent on the dose of iodinated nanoparticles administered (48). Finally, they underlined the ability to visualize architectural details in opacified lymph nodes. This last point is of particular interest when cancerous lymph nodes are explored. Experimental evidence was given in a cutaneous melanoma model in Sinclair miniature swine (49).

VI. CONCLUSION

Nanoparticulate carriers for cancer therapy have been successfully investigated in various fields, including chemotherapy of solid tumors, reversion of multidrug resistance, oligonucleotides targeting, and even tumor imaging. Because nanoparticles as well as liposomes have a pharmacokinetic profile specific to colloidal carriers, both systems are often compared. Liposomes are clearly ahead of nanoparticles when considering their marketing or even the formulation of long circulating systems, but this has to be related to their older development. One can guess that the near future will yield arguments to convince industry of the therapeutic potential of nanoparticulate carriers.

REFERENCES

1. R. K. Jain (1987) Transport of molecules in the tumor interstitium: a review. Cancer Res. 47, 3039–3051.
2. J. C. Murray, J. Carmichael (1995) Targeting solid tumours: challenges, disappointments, and opportunities. Adv. Drug Deliv. Rev. 17, 117–127.
3. L. K. Fung, W. M. Qaltzman (1997) Polymeric implants for cancer chemotherapy. Adv. Drug Deliv. Rev. 26, 209–230.
4. R. Duncan (1997) Polymer therapeutics for tumor specific delivery. Chem. Ind. 7 April 1997.
5. J. Kattan, J. P. Droz, P. Couvreur, J. P. Marino, A. Boutan-Laroze, P. Rougier, P. Brault, H. Vranckx, J. M. Grognet, X. Morge, H. Sancho-Garnier (1992) Phase I clinical trial and pharmacokinetic evaluation of doxorubicin carried by polyisohexylcyanoacrylate nanoparticles. Invest New Drugs 10, 191–199.
6. S. J. Douglas, S. S. Davis, L. Illum (1987) Nanoparticles in drug delivery. Crit. Rev. Drug Carrier Syst. 3(3), 233–261.
7. Alleman E., Gurny R., Doelker E. (1993) Drug loaded nanoparticles—Preparation methods and drug targeting tissues. Eur. J. Pharm. Biopharm. 39(5), 173–191.
8. P. Couvreur, C. Dubernet, F. Puisieux (1995) Controlled drug delivery with nanoparticles: current possibilities and future trends, Eur. J. Pharm. Biopharm 41(1), 2–13.
9. C. Verdun, F. Brasseur, H. Vrancks, P. Couvreur, M. Roland (1990) Tissue distribution of doxorubicin associated with polyisohexylcyanoacrylate nanoparticles. Cancer Chemother. Pharmacol. 26, 13–18.
10. H. Sato, Y. M. Wang, I. Adachi, I Horikoshi (1996) Pharmacokinetic study of taxolloaded poly(lactic-co-glycolic acid) microspheres containing isopropyl myristate after targeted delivery to the lung in mice. Biol. Pharm. Bull. 19(12), 1596–1601.
11. L. Illum, S. S. Davis (1984) The organ uptake of intravenously administered colllloidal particles can be altered using a non ionic surfactant (poloxamer 338). FEBS Lett. 167, 79–83.
12. S. Gibaud, J. P. Andreux, C. Weingarten, M. Renard, P. Couvreur (1994) Increased Bone marrow toxicity of doxorubicin bound to nanoparticles. Eur. J. Cancer 30A(6), 820–826.

13. S. Gibaud, M. Demoy, J. P. Andreux, C. Weingarten, B. Gouritin, P. Couvreur (1994) Cells involved in the capture of nanoparticles in hematopoietic organs. J. Pharm. Sci. 85(9), 944–950.
14. G. E. Francis, C. Delgado, D. Fisher, F. Malik, A. K. Agrawal (1996) Polyethylene glycol modification: relevance of improved methodology to tumor targeting. J. Drug Target. 3, 321–340.
15. D. Bazile, C. Prudhomme, M. T. Bassoulet, M. Marlard, G. Spenlehauer, M. Veillard (1995) Stealth MePEG-PLA nanoparticles avoid uptake by the mononuclear phagocytes system. J. Pharm. Sci. 84, 493–498.
16. M. T. Perrachia, D. Desmaele, P. Couvreur, J. D'Angelo (1997) Synthesis of a novel poly (PEG cyanoacrylate-co-alkyl cyanonacrylate) amphiphilic copolymer for nanoparticle technology. Macrommolecules 30, 846–851.
17. P. Beck, J. Kreuter, R. Reska, I. Fichtner (1993) Influence of polybutylcyanoacrylate nanoparticles and liposomes on the efficacy and toxicity of the anticancer drug mitoxantrone in murine tumor models. J. Microencaps. 10(1), 101–114.
18. R. Reska, P. Beck, I. Fichtner, M. Hentschel, J. Richter, J. Kreuter (1997) Body distribution of free, liposomal and nanoparticle-associated mitoxantrone in B16 melanoma bearing mice. J. Pharmacol. Exp. Therapeut. 280(1), 232–237.
19. F. Brasseur, P. Couvreur, B. Kante, L. Deckers-Passau, M. Roland, C. Deckers, P. Speiser (1978) Actinomycin D adsorbed on polymethylcyanoacrylate nanoparticles. Eur. J. Cancer 16(2), 1441–1445.
20. L. Grislain, P. Couvreur, V. Lenaerts, M. Roland, D. Deprez-Decampeneere, P. Speiser (1983) Pharmacokinetics and distribution of a biodegradable drug carrier. Int. J. Pharm. 15(2), 335–345.
21. M. H. Bartoli, M. Boitard, H. Fessi, H. Bériel, J. P. Devissaguet, F. Picot, F. Puisieux (1990) In vitro and in vivo antitumoral activity of free and encapsulated taxol. J. microencaps. 7(2), 191–197.
22. D. Sharma, T. P. Chelvi, J. Kaur, K. Chakravorty, T. K. De, A. Maitra, P. Ralhan (1996) Novel taxol formulation: polyvinylpyrrolidone nanoparticle–encapsulated taxol for drug delivery in cancer therapy. Oncol Res 8 (7–8), 281–286.
23. N. Chiannilkulchai, Z. Driouich, J. P. Benoit, A. L. Parodi, P. Couvreur (1989) Doxorubicin-loaded nanoparticles: increased efficiency in murine hepatic metastases. Selective Cancer Therapeut. 5(1), 1–11.
24. N. Chiannilkulchai, N. Ammoury, B. Caillou, J. P. Devissaguet, P. Couvreur (1990) Hepatic tissue distribution of doxorubicin-loaded nanoparticles after i.v. administration in reticulosarcoma M5076 metastasis-bearing mice. Cancer Chemother. Pharmacol. 26, 122–126.
25. T. Daemen, R. Hoedemakers, G. Storm, G. L. Scherpof (1995) Opportunities in targeted drug delivery to Kupffer cells: delivery of immunomodulators to Kupffer cells—activation of tumoricidal properties. Adv. Drug Deliv. Rev. 17, 21–30.
26. G. M. Barratt, W. P. Yu, H. Fessi, J. P. Devissaguet, J. F. Tenu, L. Israel, J. F. Morere, F. Puisieux (1990) Delivery of MDP-L-alanyl-cholesterol to macrophages: comparison of liposomes and nanocapsules. Cancer J. 2, 439–443.
27. W. P. Yu, G. M. Barratt, J. P. Devissaguet, F. Puisieux (1991) Antimetastatic activity in vivo of MDP-L-alanyl-cholesterol entrapped in nanocapsules. Int. J. Immunopharmacol. 13, 167–173.
28. C. Kubiak, P. Couvreur, L. Manil, B. Clausse (1989) Increased cytotoxicity of nanoparticle carried adriamycin in vitro and potentiation by verapamil and amiodarone. Biomaterials 10(10), 553–556.
29. C. Cuvier, L. Roblot treupel, J. M. Millot, G. Lizard, S. Chevillard, M. Manfait, P. Couvreur, M. F. Poupon (1992) Doxorubicin loaded nanospheres bypass tumor cell multidrug resistance. Biochem. Pharmacol. 44(3), 509–517.
30. S. Bennis, C. Chapey, P. Couvreur, J. Robert (1994) Enhanced cytotoxicity of doxorubicin encapsulated in polyosohexylcyanoacrylate nanospheres against multidrug resistant tumor cells in culture. Eur. J. Cancer 30A, 89–93.
31. F. Némati, C. Dubernet, H. Fessi, A. Colin de Verdière, F. Puisieux, P. Couvreur (1996) Reversion of the multidrug resistance using nanoparticles in vitro: influence of the nature of the polymer. Int. J. Pharmaceut. 138, 237–246.
32. A. Colin de Verdière, C. Dubernet, F. Némati, M. F. Poupon, F. Puisieux, P. Couvreur (1994) Uptake of doxorubicin from loaded nanoparticles in multidrug resistant leukemic murine cells. Cancer Chemother. Pharmacol. 33, 504–508.

33. A. Colin de Verdière, C. Dubernet, F. Némati, E. Soma, M. Appel, J. Ferté, S. Bernard, F. Puisieux, P. Couvreur (1997) Reversion of the multidrug resistance with polyalkylcyanoacrylate nanoparticles: towards a mechanism of action. Br. J. Cancer, 76(2), 198–205.
34. Y. P. Hu, S. Jarillon, C. Dubernet, P. Couvreur, J. Robert (1996) On the mechanism of action of doxorubicin encapsulation in nanospheres for the reversal of multidrug resistance. Cancer Chemother. Pharmacol. 37, 556–560.
35. C. Dubernet, E. Soma, P. Couvreur, X. Pépin, L. Attali, C. Dombrault, S. Gallet, J. M. Metreau, Y. Renault, M. Imalalen, P. Cardot (1997) On the use of chromatographic ion pairing elution mode to elucidate doxorubicin release mechanism from polyalkylcyanoacrylate nanoparticles at the cellular level. J. Chromatogr., Biol. Appl. 702, 181–191.
36. A. L. Boral, S. Dessain, B. A. Chabner (1998) Clinical evaluation of biologically targeted drugs: obstacles and opportunities. Cancer Chemother. Pharmacol. 42 (Suppl), S3–S21.
37. E. Fattal, C. Vauthier, I. Aynié, Y. Nakada, G. Lambert, C. Malvy, P. Couvreur (1998) Biodegradable polyalkylcyanoacrylate nanoparticles for the delivery of oligonucleotides. J. Controlled Release 53, 137–143.
38. C. Chavany, T. Le Doan, P. Couvreur, F. Puisieux, C. Helene (1992) Polyalkylcyanoacrylate nanoparticles as polymeric carriers for antisense oligonucleotides. Pharmaceuet. Res. 9(4), 441–449.
39. C. Chavany, T. Saison-Behmoaras, T. Le Doan, F. Puisieux, P. Couvreur, C. Helene (1994) Adsorption of oligonucleotides onto polyisohexylcyanoacrylate nanoparticles protects them against nucleases and increases cellular uptake. Pharmaceuet. Res. 11(9), 1370–1378.
40. Y. Nakada, E. Fattal, M. Foulquier, P. Couvreur (1996) Pharmacokinetics and biodistribution of oligonucleotides adsorbed onto polyisohexylcyanoacrylate nanoparticles after intravenous administration in mice. Pharmaceuet. Res. 13(1), 38–43.
41. G. Schwab, C. Chavany, I. Duroux, G. Goubin, J. Lebeau, C. Helene, T. Saison-Behmoaras (1994) Antisense oligonucleotides adsorbed to polyalkylcyanoacrylate nanoparticles specifically inhibit mutated Ha-ras mediated cell proliferation and tumorigenicity in nude mice. Proc. Natl. Acad. Sci. USA 91, 10460–10464.
42. A. E. Hawleys, S. S. Davis, L. Illum (1995) Targeting of colloids to lymph nodes: influence of lymphatic physiology and colloidal characteristics. Adv. Drug Deliv. Rev. 17, 129–148.
43. R. Weissleder, J. F. Heautot, B. K. Schaffer, N. Nossiff, M. I. Papisov, A. Jr Bogdanov, T. J. Brady (1994) MR lymphography: study of a high efficiency lymphotropic agent. Radiology 191(1), 225–230.
44. L. X. Tiefenauer, G. Kuhne, R. Y. Andres (1993) Antibody-magnetite nanoparticles: in vitro characterization of a potential tumor-specific contrast agent for magnetic resonance imaging. Bioconjug. Chem. 4(5), 347–352.
45. G. L. McIntire, E. R. Bacon, J. L. Toner, J. B. Cornacoff, P. E. Losco, K. J. Illig, K. J. Nikula, B. A. Muggenburg, L. Ketaï (1998) Pulmonary delivery of nanoparticles of insoluble, iodinated CT X-ray contrast agents to lung draining lymph nodes in dogs. J. Pharm Sci 87(11), 1466–1470.
46. E. R. Wisner, R. W. Katzberg, P. D. Koblik, D. K. Shelton, P. E. Fisher, S. M. Griffey, C. Drake, P. P. Harnish, A. R. Vessey, P. J. Haley (1994) Iodinated nanoparticles for indirect computed tomography lymphography of the craniocervical and thoracic lymph nodes in normal dogs. Acad. Radiol 1(4), 377–384.
47. E. R. Wisner, R. W. Katzberg, P. D. Koblik, J. P. McGahan, S. M. Griffey, C. Drake, P. P. Harnish, A. R. Vessey, P. J. Haley (1995) Indirect computed tomography lymphography of subdiaphragmatic lymph nodes using iodinated nanoparticles in normal dogs. Acad. Radiol. 2(5), 405–412.
48. E. R. Wisner, R. W. Katzberg, S. M. Griffey, C. Drake, P. J. Haley, A. R. Vessey (1995) Indirect computed tomography lymphography using iodinated nanoparticles: time and dose response in normal canine lymph nodes. Acad Radiol 2(11), 985–993.
49. E. R. Wisner, R. W. Katzberg, D. P. Link, S. M. Griffey, C. Drake, A. R. Vessey, D. Johnson, P. J. Haley (1996) Indirect computed tomography lymphography using iodinated nanoparticles to detect cancerous lymph nodes in a cutaneous melanoma model. Acad. Radiol. 3(1), 40–48.

15
Microencapsulation Using Coacervation/Phase Separation:
An Overview of the Technique and Applications

H. Süheyla Kaş and Levent Öner
University of Hacettepe, Ankara, Turkey

I. INTRODUCTION

Microcapsules are small particles (liquids, solids, solutions, or dispersions) that contain an active substance coated by synthetic or natural polymers of varying thickness. Generally the active substance is called *core* and the coating is called *wall* material. Different configurations of microcapsules are shown in Fig. 1.

Microencapsulation is a method of wrapping small entities in individual coatings designed to protect, separate, or aid in storage. The reasons for microencapsulation are environmental protection, gastric irritation reduction, liquid–solid conversion, taste–odor masking, separation of incompatibilities, controlling and sustaining the action of active substances, and minimizing or eliminating side effects. Microencapsulation provides many possibilities for producing improved forms of pharmaceuticals and diagnostic aids. As Fanger (1) stated in his brief history on microencapsulation, creation of a living cell is the beginning of microencapsulation. Most of the one-celled animals are living examples of microencapsulation. Even a chicken egg has been engineered with a protective wall thick enough to provide protection and thin enough to allow breakage at hatching (1).

There are number of books and reviews on microencapsulation (1–34). It is not the scope of this chapter to give a complete review on the large number of microencapsulation processes. The purpose of this chapter is to provide information on coacervation/phase separation methodology with emphasis on the effects of selected variables, additives, and formulation techniques and phase relationships. Applications of coacervated microcapsules will also be stated with examples from literature.

II. COACERVATION

The term *coacervation* was suggested for the first time by two Dutch scientists, Bungenburg de Jong and Kruyt, to describe the phenomenon of phase separation in colloidal systems (17). They realized that this phase separation, which they called coacervation, was related to the precipitation or flocculation of the colloidal material from solution and that coacervation was a step taking place just before precipitation from solution. This separated phase in the form of

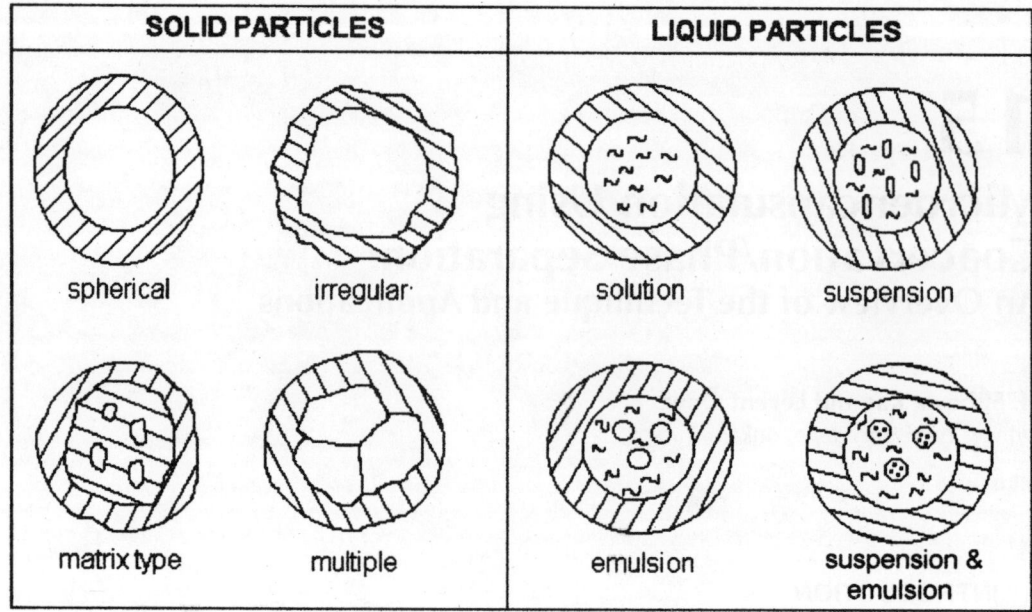

Figure 1 Different configurations of microcapsules (9,21).

amorphous, liquid droplets constituted the coacervate, which was the colloid-rich solution. The difference between the two phases is a difference in concentration of solute species. The word *coacervation* comes from the latin *acervus*, meaning aggregation, and the prefix *co*, signifying the preceding union of the colloidal particles.

Deposition of this coacervate around individual minute insoluble particles dispersed in the equilibrium liquid formed the embryonic capsules, and appropriate gelling of the coacervate deposit resulted in microcapsules (1,2,17,21,25,30–42). The unique property of the coacervation systems lies in the solvent components of the two phases being the same. This is the basic difference of a coacervate from two-phase systems involving two immiscible liquids (37).

III. CORE MATERIALS

The core represents a wide range of possible configurations. The core can be a liquid, solid, gas, liquid slurry, suspension, emulsion droplets, or spheronized solids (Fig. 1). Pharmaceuticals from different pharmacological classes have been microencapsulated, in particular analgesics, antibiotics, antihistamines, cardiovascular drugs, tranquilizers, iron salts, and vitamins. Appendix 1 lists some of the drugs that have been microencapsulated (9,21,43).

IV. WALL MATERIALS

The coating material can be selected from a wide variety of natural and synthetic polymers depending on the core material to be encapsulated and the desired characteristics. The amount of coating material used ranges from 3% to 30% of the total weight, which corresponds to a dry film thickness of less than 1–200 μm, depending on the surface to be coated. It may be more or less difficult to coat uniformly the core materials whose surfaces possess sharp peaks and depressions, whereas spherical particles could be uniformly encapsulated.

Natural or synthetic hydrophilic colloids are large molecules that are soluble or dispersible in aqueous solutions. Table 1 gives some examples of natural and synthetic hydrophilic colloids (21,25,44). Here the capsule wall presents a good barrier to oily and hydrophobic materials, but it is usually a poor barrier to hydrophilic substances. Hydrophobic colloids are realized in encapsulating water-soluble drugs. Ethylcellulose is a good example of this group (Table 1).

Table 1 Hydrophilic and Hydrophobic Colloids Used for Microencapsulation

Natural	Synthetic
Agar	Acrylic polymers
Albumin	■ Polyacrylamide
Alginates	■ Polyacrylic acid
Casein	→ Poly(ethyl-α–cynoacrylate)
Chitosan	→ Poly(batyl-α–cynoacrylate)
Collagen	■ Polyacrylcyanoacrylates
Dextran	■ Polymethyl methacrylate
Gelatin	■ Aliphatic polyesters
Gluten	■ Poly(lactic acid)
Gum arabic	■ Poly(lactic-co-glycolide)
Pectin	■ Poly(glycolic acid)
Starch	■ Poly(ϵ–caprolactone)
Waxes	■ Polyhydroxybutyrate
Beeswax	■ Poly(hydroxy butyrate-co-valerate)
Carnauba wax	Cellulose derivatives
Paraffin wax	■ Cellulose acetate
Spermaceti	■ Cellulose acetate butyrate
Zein	■ Cellulose acetate phthalate
	■ Cellulose acetate succinate
	■ Nitrate
	■ Ethylcellulose
	■ Hydroxyethylcellulose
	■ Hydroxypropylcellulose
	■ Hydroxypropylmethylcellulose
	■ Hydroxypropylmethylcellulose phthalate
	■ Methyl cellulose
	■ Sodium carboxymethylcellulose
	Poly(ortho esters)
	Polyurethanes
	Polyamides
	■ Nylon-6, 10
	■ Nylon-6
	Polylysine
	Polystyrene
	Poly(ethylene glycol)
	Poly(ethylene vinyl acetate)
	Polydimethylsiloxane
	Poly(vinyl acetate phthalate)
	Polyvinylalcohol
	Polyvinylpyrrollidone
	Shellac

Source: Data from Refs. 21 and 32.

V. PHASE BOUNDARY TRIANGULAR DIAGRAMS

As a preliminary to microencapsulation by coacervation/phase separation, phase boundary triangular diagrams must be prepared in order to obtain optimum composition within the coacervate region (2,9,35,36,41,43–51). Coacervation/phase separation can be obtained by temperature change, nonsolvent or salt addition, incompatible polymer addition, and polymer–polymer interaction.

A. Temperature Change

A general phase diagram where coacervation is induced thermally is shown in Fig. 2a (2,9). Phase separation of the dissolved polymer takes place in the form of immiscible liquid droplets. If a core substance is placed into the system, these droplets surround the core and form the microcapsules. As the solvent of the polymer-rich phase evaporates, gelation and solidification takes place. A system that utilizes ethylcellulose and cyclohexane at high temperature is an example of this thermally induced microencapsulation (45,47,48,52–68).

B. Salt Addition

Soluble inorganic salts can be added to aqueous solutions of water-soluble polymers to cause phase separation (Fig. 2b) (2,9). A gelatin–water–sodium sulfate system is an example. In this system, phase separation/coacervation is induced by adding dropwise 20% solutions of sodium sulfate (43–49,69–74).

C. Nonsolvent Addition

A liquid that does not dissolve the given polymer can be added to a solution of the polymer to cause phase separation (Fig. 2c) (2,9). This immiscible liquid polymer can be utilized to encapsulate an immiscible core (45,47,48,75–80).

D. Incompatible Polymer Addition

Microencapsulation can be accomplished by using the incompatibility of dissimilar polymers present in a common solvent (Fig. 2d) (2,9). Methylene blue–ethylcellulose–liquid polybutadiene is an example of microencapsulation by incompatible polymer addition (45,81–84).

E. Polymer–Polymer Interaction

The interaction of oppositely charged polyelectrolytes can result in the formation of a complex having such reduced solubility that phase separation occurs (Fig. 2e) (2,9). Gelatin and acacia are examples of oppositely charged polyelectrolytes because gelatin has a positive charge whereas acacia possesses a negative charge. Gelatin–gelatin, gelatin–carboxymethylcellulose (CMC), gelatin–Gantrez, and Carbopol–CMC are examples of other oppositely charged polyelectrolytes used in microencapsulation (74,85,91–93). When temperature, concentration, and pH of the two polymers are utilized according to the points obtained in the phase diagram, they interact through their opposite charges and exhibit phase separation/coacervation (85–94).

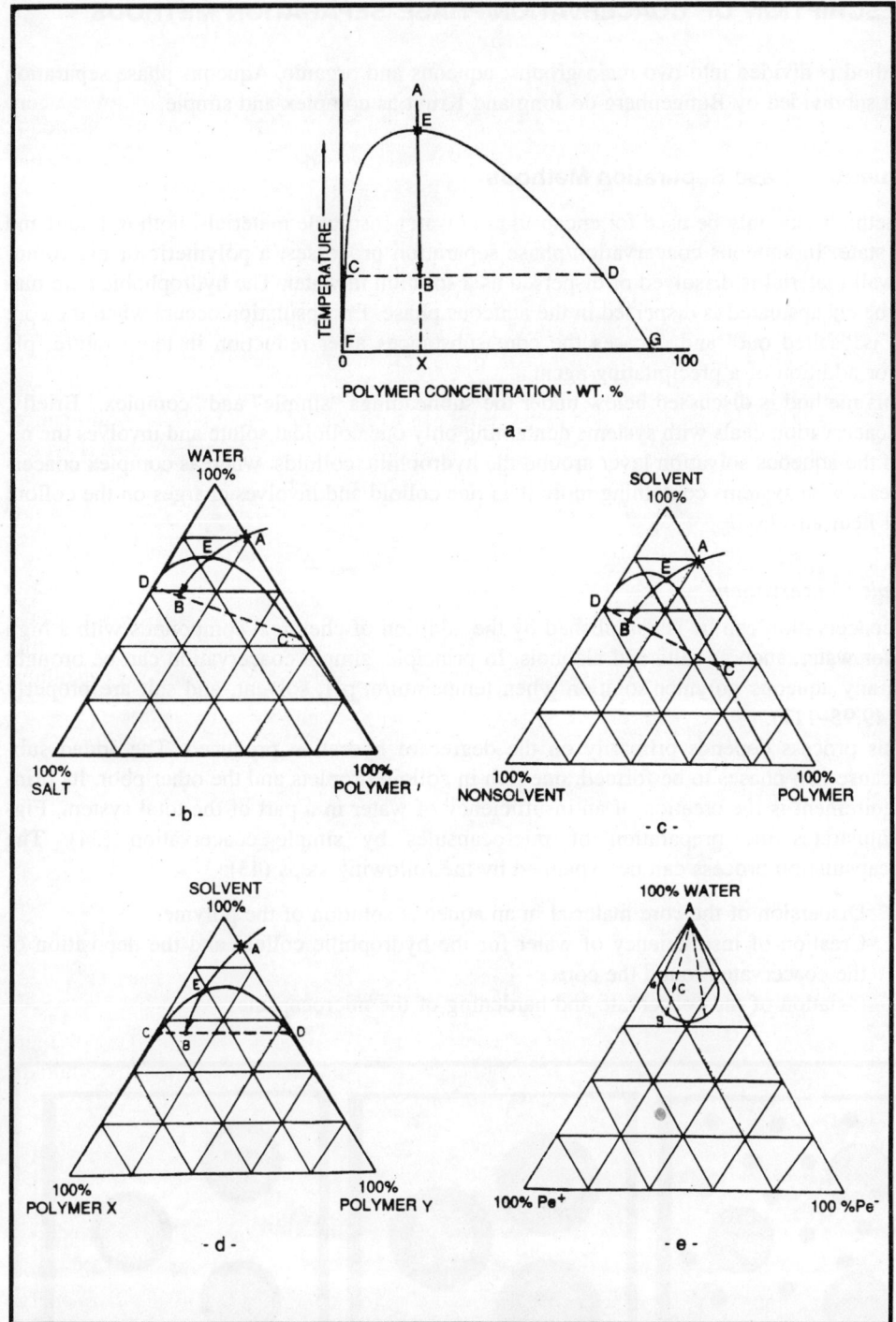

Figure 2 General phase diagrams of coacervation/phase separation techniques (2,9): (a) General phase diagram where coacervation is induced thermally. (b) General phase diagram obtained by salt addition. (c) General phase diagram induced by the addition of a nonsolvent. (d) General phase diagram obtained by the addition of an incompatible polymer. (e) General phase diagram by polymer interaction.

VI. DESCRIPTION OF COACERVATION/PHASE SEPARATION METHODS

This method is divided into two main groups: aqueous and organic. Aqueous phase separation has been subdivided by Bungenberg de Jong and Kruyt as complex and simple.

A. Aqueous Phase Separation Methods

These methods can only be used for encapsulating water-insoluble materials, both in liquid and in solid state. In aqueous coacervation/phase separation processes, a polymeric or macromolecular wall material is dissolved or dispersed as a solution in water. The hydrophobic core material to be encapsulated is dispersed in the aqueous phase. Encapsulation occurs when the core material is "salted out" and encases the core substances after reduction in temperature, pH change, or addition of a precipitating agent.

This method is discussed below under the subheadings "simple" and "complex." Briefly, simple coacervation deals with systems containing only one colloidal solute and involves the removal of the aqueous solvation layer around the hydrophilic colloids, whereas complex coacervation deals with systems containing more than one colloid and involves charges on the colloid and their neutralization.

1. Simple Coacervation

Simple coacervation can be accomplished by the addition of chemical compounds with a high affinity for water, such as salts and alcohols. In principle, simple coacervation can be brought about in any aqueous polymer solution when temperature, pH, solvent, and salt are properly chosen (49,95–117).

This process depends primarily on the degree of hydration produced. The added substances cause two phases to be formed, one rich in colloid droplets and the other poor. Its principal requirement is the creation of an insufficiency of water in a part of the total system. Figure 3 illustrates the preparation of microcapsules by simple coacervation (34). The microencapsulation process can be explained by the following steps (43):

1. Dispersion of the core material in an aqueous solution of the polymer
2. Creation of insufficiency of water for the hydrophilic colloid and the deposition of the coacervate around the core
3. Gelation of the coacervate and hardening of the microcapsules

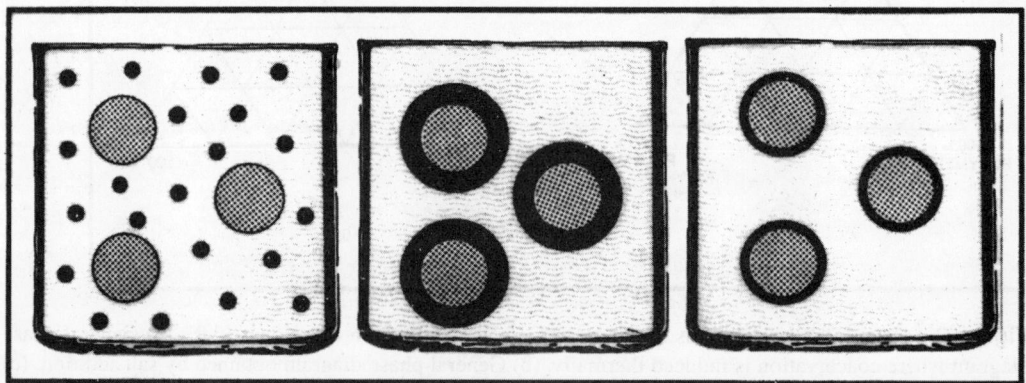

Figure 3 Schematic diagram of simple coacervation process (43).

The influence of the molecular weight of gelatin on simple coacervation has been studied by Nixon et al. (49). The results showed that as the molecular weight of gelatin increased, the required concentration of ethanol decreased. Nixon and Walker examined the effect of pH, temperature, drug content, and hardening on the in vitro release profile (100). In their other work, the authors studied the effect of gelatin type (101). They showed that pH has to be adjusted to a value in the vicinity of gelatin's isoelectric point before encapsulation with ethanol when acid-processed gelatin was employed, whereas no pH adjustment was required with sodium sulfate under the same conditions.

2. Complex Coacervation

Complex coacervation involves neutralization of the charges on the colloids and depends primarily on pH. This is accomplished by mixing two colloids of opposite charges together (54,55,58,70,71,92–94,96,118–144). The encapsulation process in complex coacervation consists of four steps:

1. Preparation of a hydrophilic colloid solution
2. Addition of a second hydrophilic colloid solution of opposite charge to induce coacervation
3. Deposition around the core
4. Gelation of the coacervate and hardening of the microcapsules.

A combination of gelatin and acacia at neutral pH (below the isoelectric point of gelatin) fulfills this condition (Fig. 4). At that pH gelatin carries a positive charge because of protonation of basic groups, whereas acacia carries a negative charge because of the ionization of the

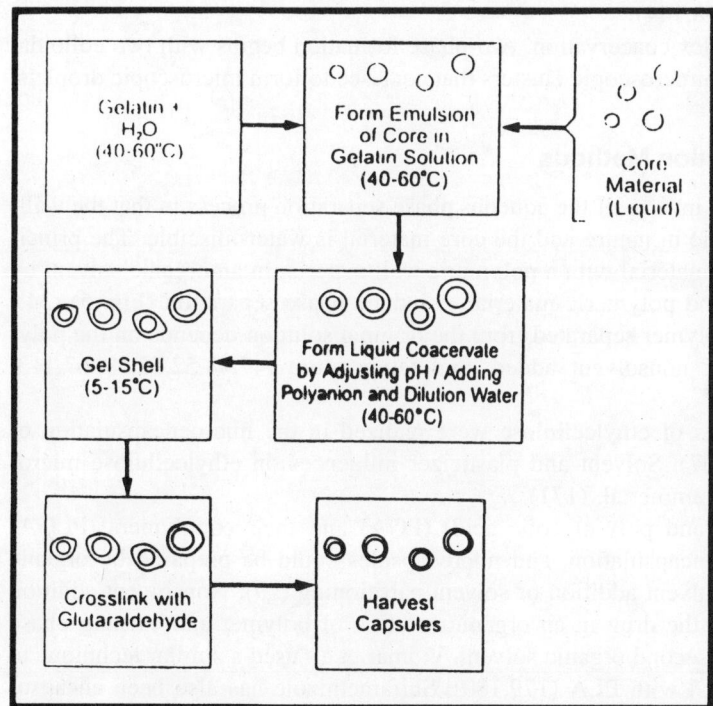

Figure 4 Flow diagram of microencapsulation by complex coacervation (34).

glucoronic acid groups. These two colloids attract each other and separate into a distinct liquid phase called "coacervate." Gelatin–acacia gels can be stabilized by chemical crosslinking. This technique of complex coacervation was first described by Phares and Sperandio (35,36). The method was developed by Madan et al. (39,73), who examined the effects of varying initial pH, temperature, the ratio of solid to encapsulating material, and final pH. Their results showed that all variables effected some degree of change in microcapsules as follows (73): There was little difference in the solid extracted when the starting pH was the variable; the amount extracted decreased as the starting temperature increased; the smaller the ratio, the greater the retaining power due to the thickness of the wall; as the final pH was increased, the quantity extracted increased.

Besides gelatin–acacia combinations, gelatin–gelatin, gelatin–CMC, gelatin–Gantrez, and Carbopol–CMC coacervations were also employed (74,85,91–93). Aqueous solutions containing gelatins of different isoionic points when mixed at a pH between the isoionic points of the gelatins caused a phase separation in which two phases were formed. As Veis et al. pointed out, both phases are rich in the same solvent and gelatin in this liquid–liquid complex coacervation (85). Burgess and Carless used acid- and alkali-processed gelatin to predict the optimum pH and ionic strength requirements for complex coacervation (70,71,91). The authors concluded that electrophoretic mobility profiles of the polyions could be used to determine the optimum coacervation pH and salt tolerance. Burgess and Carless also showed that the presence of salt could suppress complex coacervation depending on the nature and concentration of the salt (70,71). They also observed the influence of neutral salts on complex coacervation. Mordata et al. evaluated factors affecting the coacervation process between type A gelatin and Gantrez-AN polymer (polyvinylmethylether–maleic anhydride), such as polymer concentration, molecular weight, and pH of the gelatin solution (90,94).

The effect of surfactants and polyelectrolytes on the release of drugs from microcapsules was also investigated (72,73,118,144).

In both simple and complex coacervation, two-phase formation begins with two colloidal species aggregating to form submicroscopic clusters that coalesce to form microscopic droplets.

B. Organic Phase Separation Methods

Organic phase separation is the inverse of the aqueous phase separation process in that the wall-containing phase is hydrophobic in nature and the core material is water-miscible. The principle is to enclose water-soluble material with a polymeric wall material in an organic solvent by adding a nonsolvent or a second polymeric material to induce phase separation (Fig. 5) (34). The amount and the state of polymer separated from the original solution depends on the polymer concentration, amount of nonsolvent added, and temperature (47,48,52,53,59–67,113, 145–185).

Different viscosity grades of ethylcellulose were realized in the microencapsulation of pharmaceuticals (48,60,62,66,67). Solvent and plasticizer influences on ethylcellulose microcapsules were discussed by Palamo et al. (171).

Poly(lactic acid) (PLA) and poly(glycolic acid) (PGA) and their copolymers (PLGA) were also employed in microencapsulation, and microcapsules could be prepared by organic phase separation through nonsolvent addition or solvent partitioning (79). Nonsolvent addition technique involves suspending the drug in an organic solution of polymer and causing phase separation by the addition of a second organic solvent. Vidmar et al. used a similar technique to encapsulate oxytetracycline HCl with PLA (179,180). Sulfamethizole has also been encapsulated by this method using PLA and carboxyethylcellulose (181). Phase separation by solvent partitioning technique has been employed in encapsulating hydrocortisone (182). In this

Microencapsulation Using Coacervation

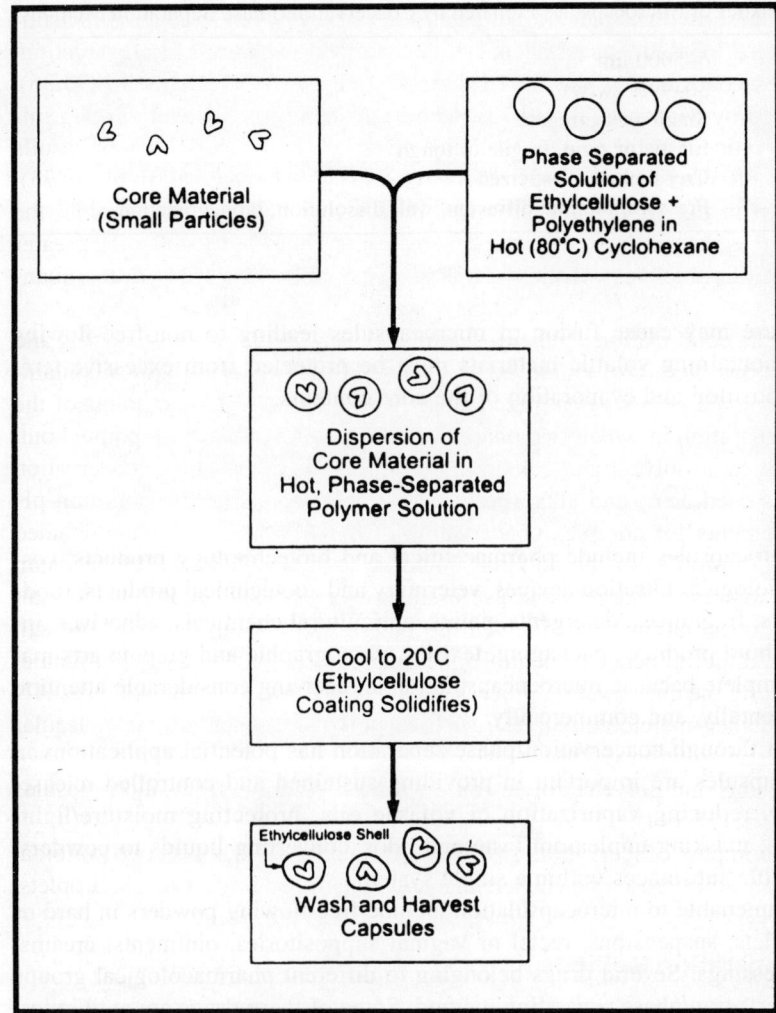

Figure 5 Flow diagram of microencapsulation by organic phase separation (34).

method, hydrocortisone suspended in PLA–methylene chloride solution is injected into a mineral oil, resulting in precipitation of polymer around the solid hydrocortisone. The authors claimed that this technique could produce microcapsules of desired size independent of drug loading. Recently, Thomasin et al. analyzed in detail the process of phase separation of various types of PLA/PLGA by establishing phase diagrams and by characterizing the coacervate and continuous phases in terms of volume, composition, polymer molecular weight, and rheological behavior (183–185).

VII. STORAGE CONDITIONS

The typical characteristics of microcapsules prepared by the coacervation/phase separation method are shown in Table 2. The conditions under which these microcapsules are stored vary widely. Factors of concern include pressure, temperature, humidity, light, radiation, and air

Table 2 Typical Characteristics of Microcapsules Prepared by Coacervation/Phase Separation Methods

Particle size	5–5000 μm
Capsule content	30–99% (w/w)
Capsule structure	Single or aggregate
Coating properties	Elastic or rigid, fragile or tough
Coating modification	Crosslinked, plasticized
Release mechanism	Pressure, thermal diffusion, wall dissolution, biodegradation

Source: Data from Ref. 17.

pollutants. Excess pressure may cause fusion of microcapsules leading to non-free-flowing product. Microcapsules containing volatile materials must be protected from excessive temperature to avoid decomposition and evaporation of the core contents.

VIII. APPLICATIONS

Application areas of microcapsules include pharmaceutical and biotechnology products, cosmetics, diagnostic aids, biological filtration devices, veterinary and zootechnical products, foods and food additives, flavors, fragrances, detergents, paints, agricultural chemicals, adhesives, industrial chemicals, household products, packaging, textiles, photographic and graphic arts materials. This list is not complete because microencapsulation is receiving considerable attention fundamentally, developmentally, and commercially.

Microencapsulation through coacervation/phase separation has potential applications in pharmacy. These microcapsules are important in providing sustained and controlled release, improving drug stability, reducing vaporization of volatile oils, protecting moisture/light/oxidation–sensitive drugs, masking unpleasant taste and odor, converting liquids to powders, and separating incompatible substances within a single system.

The dosage forms amenable to microcapsulation include free-flowing powders in hard or soft gelatin capsules, tablets, suspensions, rectal or vaginal suppositories, ointments, creams, aerosols, plasters, and dressings. Several drugs belonging to different pharmacological groups are encapsulated by coacervation/phase separation method. Some of these drugs are antibiotics, anti-inflammatory agents, bronchodilators, sulfa drugs, diuretics, antibacterials, metal salts, antiepileptics, analgesics, antihypertensives, anticancerogens, and vitamins (21,43,186,187). The purpose of this section is to focus on the pharmaceutical applications of microcapsules with examples taken from the literature.

A. Antibiotics

Amoxicillin, ampicillin, bacampicillin, cephalexin, cephradine, chloramphenicol, clarithromycin, eryithromycin, potassium pheneticillin, ofloxacin, and ciprofloxacin are some examples of the encapsulated antibiotics (52,53,76,88,106,163,168,188–197).

Goto et al. (106) encapsulated *amoxicillin* by organic phase separation using ethylcellulose to sustain the release and improve patient compliance. They observed a zero-order release pattern of amoxicillin from microcapsules. However, Ertan et al. (88) encapsulated amoxicillin by complex coacervation using CMC and gelatin at different core-to-wall ratios. The authors were able to sustain the release of amoxicillin. *Ampicillin* was also encapsulated by Ertan et al. (88) through complex coacervation to sustain the release of the drug. *Bacampicillin* (190), *cephradine* (189), and *cephalexin* (53) were encapsulated by ethylcellulose and ethylcellulose-

Eudragit mixtures, respectively. ***Cephalexin*** and ***chloramphenicol*** coacervations were accomplished by temperature elevation. Salib et al. showed that ethylcellulose is a potential sustained release coating for oral dosage forms (52). Friend (76) employed a nonsolvent coacervation technique where by gelatin microcapsules were suspended in a solution of Eudragit. The taste of ***clarithromycin*** was masked and its release was sustained by simple coacervation of gelatin and sodium sulfate. The unpleasant taste of ***clarithromycin*** and ***erythromycin*** was also masked by hydroxypropylmethylcellulose (HPMC) and Carbopol (188). Using ethylcellulose, ***potassium pheneticillin*** microcapsules have been prepared and tableted by direct compression (163,168). The dissolution profiles were found to be governed by the core-to-wall ratio of the microcapsules and to some extent by the compression pressure, and showed sustained release effect. ***Ofloxacin, ciprofloxacin, enoxacin,*** and ***oxytetracyline*** are other members of this group that are encapsulated by coacervation/phase separation technique (179,191–193,196,197).

B. Anti-inflammatory Drugs

Anti-inflammatory drugs are another group in which microencapsulation is employed. Diclofenac sodium, flufenamic acid, glaphenine, hydrocortisone, ibuprofen, indomethacin, naproxen, oxyphenbutasone, and prednisone are examples of encapsulated drugs in this group (54,55,91,127,128,164–166,169,171,195,198–203).

Bhatnagar and Nakhare (164) encapsulated ***diclofenac sodium*** (DS) using three-ply-wall (gelatin–acacia/polyvinylalcohol/sodium alginate) for controlled delivery, whereas Palamo et al. (171) microencapsulated DS to reduce gastric irritation and investigated the effect of solvent on DS-ethylcellulose microcapsules. The authors experimented with cellulose acetate phthalate by nonsolvent addition and simple coacervation; PVA by salt coacervation. Microcapsules of ***naproxen*** were prepared by complex coacervation of two oppositely charged gelatins (91). Meshali et al. encapsulated ***oxyphenbutazone*** and ***glaphenine*** by cellulose derivatives (HPMC and CMC) through coacervation/phase separation (165). The authors showed a decrease in the gastric ulcerogenic activity. In their earlier studies, the authors encapsulated ***flufenamic acid*** and ***indomethacin*** (166,203). Indomethacin microcapsules were prepared by complex coacervation using gelatin–acacia complex (54,127,128) and by organic phase separation using ethylcellulose at elevated temperature (55,169). The authors have studied the efficiency of encapsulation, particle size, as well as the release of indomethacin. Daniels and Mittermaler (198) investigated the effect of five different acids (HCl, HNO_3, H_2SO_4, acetic acid, and citric acid) used to adjust the coacervation pH on the obtained microcapsules. The dissolution profiles were found to be similar when different acids were used. Leelarasamee et al. employed poly(lactic acid) for encapsulating ***hydrocortisone*** (182). Other anti-inflammatory drugs, ***ibuprofen*** and ***ketoprofen***, were encapsulated by coacervation process using Eudragits (200–202).

C. Bronchodilators

Theophylline was encapsulated by ethylcellulose or ethylcellulose–cellulose triacetate through simple organic phase separation by nonsolvent addition or temperature elevation. Encapsulation process is employed to sustain the release, extend absorption, decrease gastric irritation, and mask bitter taste (45,75,77,105,148,160,167,175,177,204–210). Lin and Young prepared theophylline ethylcellulose microcapsules by ethylene–vinyl acetate copolymer as a coacervating agent (204). Lin et al. tableted ethylcellulose microcapsules by compression and showed that reduced surface area and porosity resulted in prolongation of the release (160). Donbrow et al. deposited Eudragit on theophylline particles by a phase separation process and regulated release rates (167). Microcapsules of theophylline were also prepared by the nonsolvent technique in the presence of silicon dioxide (75). Nixon and Wong evaluated the permeation of theophylline through ethylcellulose membranes as a model for release and interpreted the thermodynamics of phase separation of polymer solutions for film formation and microencapsulation (148). Terbutaline sulfate microcapsules were prepared by coacervation/phase separation method using ethylcellulose as the coating material to prolong its release. Phase separation was induced by increasing the temperature (57,211).

D. Sulfa Drugs

Sulfadiazine, sulfamethizole, sulfamethoxazole, sulfamerazine, and sulfisoxazole are some representatives of sulfa drugs that are encapsulated (46,78,82–84,99–103,123,157,181).

Sulfadiazine microcapsules were prepared employing a phase separation/coacervation method by means of thermal changes, nonsolvent addition, or by incompatible polymers (78,83,84,103). While Das investigated the coacervation effect of polybutadiene (78), Cameroni et al. used polyisobutylene as a protective colloid to prolong its release (156). Nixon and Walker have prepared sulfadiazine microcapsules by simple gelatin coacervation using sodium sulfate as coacervating agent (100). The effects of pH, temperature, drug content, and hardening on in vitro release profile have been examined (99). Sulfadiazine was successfully encapsulated by cellulose acetate phthalate (157). *Sulfamethizole* microcapsules were prepared by coacervation/phase separation by inducing polymer addition (82,181). *Sulfamethoxazole* was encapsulated by gelatin–acacia coacervate (123). The authors suggested that coacervation occurred on the surface of the drug particle with adsorbed acacia due to the fact that the ζ potential–pH profile of gelatin coincided with that of the coacervate. Nixon et al. examined the effect of gelatin type in the preparation of *sulfamerazine* microcapsules using simple coacervation technique (101,102). The authors were able to encapsulate sulfamerazine using alkaline gelatin–water–ethanol without pH adjustment. However, pH had to be adjusted when acid-processed gelatin was employed. İzgü and Doğanay encapsulated *sulfisoxazole* by coacervation and determined the microencapsulation conditions of gelatin succinate (46).

E. Diuretics

Furosemide, chlorothiazide, and sulfonamide were encapsulated in order to prepare sustained release formulations that would offer the advantage of avoiding short periods of peak diuresis observed with the conventional formulations (95,96,158,193,206). *Sulfonamide* and *chlorothiazide* microcapsules were prepared by simple coacervation (95,96). The release of the drug from microcapsules and tableted microcapsules of chlorothiazide were characterized by a rapid release followed by a more sustained release.

F. Urinary Antiseptics

Sustained release microcapsules of *nitrofurantoin* were prepared by complex coacervation technique. Gelatin–Gantrez (90), gelatin–peptone (212), gelatin–CMC (88), CMC–Carbopol (86), and CMC–aluminum sulfate (69) were employed during the microencapsulation process. Hashim et al. (150) used ethylcellulose to encapsulate nitrofurantoin and *nalidixic acid.*

G. Antiepileptic Drugs

Phenytoin sodium and beclamide could be stated as examples of this pharmacological group. Microcapsules of *phenytoin sodium* were formulated by organic phase separation method. Ethylcellulose and Eudragits were used with different core-to-wall ratios. The authors employed phase diagrams by changing the concentration of the nonsolvent and the temperature. The purpose of this microencapsulation was to sustain the release and to increase patient compliance. (47,48). Özer et al. encapsulated *beclamide* by simple coacervation using gelatin and sodium sulfate to mask the unpleasant taste (97). The microcapsules of beclamide were compressed into chewable and effervescent tablets.

H. Analgesics

Ethylcellulose is a coating material used to encapsulate *acetyl salicylic acid* (aspirin) to mask the bitter taste and to sustain the release of the drug by several authors (67,170,174,187). Paradissis and Parrot (99) employed gelatin coacervate to encapsulate aspirin. *Sodium salicylate* was encapsulated by ethylcellulose through temperature reduction using polyisobutylene as a protective colloid (68). The authors showed that addition of a protective colloid favored the formation of smooth-walled microcapsules, which is called "film type." *Acetaminophen* (paracetamol) microcapsules were prepared by Baykara and Karataş; and Ataberk using the coacervation/phase separation technique (175,213). Others encapsulated paracetamol using poylacrylic resins through phase separation from chloroform with polyisobutylene in cyclohexane (161). *Dextropropoxiphen HCl* was another encapsulated analgesic (214–216).

I. Antihypertensives

Isosorbide-5-mononitrate (IS-5-MN), dihydralazine sulfate, piretanide and propranolol HCl, captopril, nicardipin, and dipyridamole are examples of microencapsulated antihypertensives. *IS-5-MN* microcapsules were optimized and formulated to sustain the action and to overcome the tolerance developed in conventional preparations (65,66). Ethylcellulose with two different viscosities was employed and microcapsules were prepared by organic phase separation. *Dihydralazine sulfate* was also encapsulated using ethylcellulose as the coating material by the organic phase separation method (59,60,63). Core-to-wall ratios of 1:1 and 1:2 were employed and tablets of 2-kg hardness were prepared from microcapsules to sustain the release of the drug. Goto et al. encapsulated *piretanide* to maintain suitable blood levels for a long time with minimal frequency of administration (116). *Propranolol HCl* was encapsulated by ethylcellulose (187,217). *Captopril, nicardipin,* and *dipyridamole,* other antihypertensive drugs, were encapsulated by coacervation technique to sustain the release (218–220).

J. Anticancerogens

Carboquone was encapsulated by simple coacervation of gelatin (103), whereas *5-FU, doxorubicin, mitomycin C, bleomycin, 6-mercaptopurine,* and *cisplatin* were encapsulated by organic phase separation/coacervation using ethylcellulose to obtain prolonged drug release with minimal systemic side effects (103,115,159,221–223).

K. Tranquilizers

Oxazepam, diazepam, and tofizepam are examples from this group. *Oxazepam* was encapsulated by ethylcellulose through coacervation/phase separation (152,153,155). Core-to-wall ratios of 1:1 and 1:2 were employed and diffusion-controlled process was found to be responsible for the drug release. Microcapsules of *diazepam* were prepared using ethylcellulose and gelatin to sustain the action of the drug (122). Devay and Racz described the production of microcapsules containing *tofizepam* (170).

L. Sedative Hypnotics

Luzzi and Gerraughty encapsulated *pentabarbituric acid* by complex coacervation and studied the effect of surfactants on microencapsulation. Their results showed that polysorbate-20 enhanced the release rate of the active substance (73). Microcapsules of *sodium phenobarbitone* with a wall of ethylcellulose have been prepared by Jalsenjak et al. (86). These microcapsules behaved like plastic matrices during the dissolution experiments.

M. Electrolyte Replenisher

Harris encapsulated *potassium chloride* through gelatin–acacia coacervate systems. The encapsulated potassium chloride offered better controlled release when compared to standard tablet and powder forms (132). *Sodium chloride* was also encapsulated by deposition of Eudragits through the phase separation process (143). *Magnesium aluminum hydroxide hydrate* was also encapsulated (200).

N. Vitamins

Vitamins A, B_1, B_2, B_6, B_{12}, C, D, and *PP* were encapsulated by the coacervation/phase separation method (21,35,36,43,103,172,173,224). The role and effect of coacervation-inducing agents in microencapsulation of ascorbic acid were investigated by using phase preparation from cyclohexane solution with change of temperature. The formation of smooth- and thick-walled microcapsules largely prevented the aggregation of microcapsules and showed low dissolution rate (173).

O. Metal Salts

Öner and Öner et al. encapsulated *zinc sulfate* by the organic phase separation method to prolong the duration of action (61,62,64). The authors applied factorial design for optimization of the formulation and investigated in vitro and in vivo behavior of the microcapsules.

P. Converting Liquids to Free-Flowing Powders

Citrus essential oil, cod liver oil, benzaldehyde, carbon tetrachloride, and *oil droplets* were coated and recovered as fine powders (110,111,122,138,178). The authors have stated that the bulk droplet size of the encapsulated material appeared to be a factor in the strong capsule wall, which protects against vaporization and oxidation.

Q. Others

The tuberculostatic agent *isoniazid* (176,225), sympathomimetic agents *salbutamol sulfate* (226) and *phenylpropanolamine HCl* (227,228), antitussive *oxolamine* (229), antimalarial *chloroquine diphosphate* (230), cholinergic *pilocarpine HCl,* bronchodilator *bitolterol mesylate* (231), and the drugs listed in Appendix 1 are some other examples of microencapsulated drugs. This list is not by any means complete due to the large number of encapsulated drugs in this growing field.

Microencapsulation Using Coacervation

Appendix 1 Some Microencapsulated Drugs

Drugs	Reasons for microencapsulation	Ref.
Acetaminophen	MUT/RGI/SR/SIS	43, 130, 174, 175, 161, 213
Acetylspiramycin	SR	43
Acetylsalicylic acid	SR/SIS/RGI/MUT	43, 67, 99, 130, 170, 187
Aminophylline	SR/MUT	43, 130
Ammonium chloride	SR	43
Amobarbital	SR	43
Amoxicillin	SR	88, 106, 194
Amphetamine sulfate	SR	43
Ampicillin	MUT/RGI/SIS	43, 88, 130, 194
Attapulgit	SIS	21, 88
Bacampicillin	SR	190
Bacitracin	SR	43
Barium sulfate	MUT	43
Beclamide	SIS/MUT	97
Benzaldehyde	EP/CLP	122
Benzperoxide	CLP	130
Bitolterol mesylate	SR	231
Bleomycin HCl	SR	222
Butobarbitone	MUT	21
Caffeine	MUT/RGI/SIS	43, 130
Camphor	SIS	21
Captopril	SR	218
Carbon tetrachloride	CLP	138
Carboquone	SR	103
Castor oil	CLP/MUO/MUT	21, 43, 138
Cephalexin	SR	53
Cephradine	SR	130, 189
Chloramphenicol	SIS/PR	21, 43, 52
Chloroquine diphosphate	SR	230
Chlorothiazide	SR	96
Chlorpheniramine maleate	SR	21, 43, 130
Chlorpromazine HCl	SR	21
Choline tartrate	EP/SIS	43
Ciprofloxacin	SR	192, 197
Cisplatin	SR/IT	103, 159
Citric acid	EP/SIS/MUT	21, 43
Citrus essential oil	CLP	178
Clarithromycin	MUT/SR	76, 130, 188
Clofibrate	CLP	21, 43, 130
Cloxacillin	MUT	21, 43
Cod liver oil	CLP/MUO/MUT	38, 43, 122, 130, 138, 222
Codeine phosphate	SR	21, 43, 130
Cyclandelate	MUT	21
Cysteine	MUO/SIS/MUT	21, 43
Dextromethorphan HBr	SR	43, 130
Dextropropoxyphene HCl	SIS/EP/MUT	43, 214–216
Dextrose	SR	43
Diazepam	SR	21, 122
Diclofenac sodium	SR/RGI	164, 171
Dicloxacillin	MUT	21

Appendix 1 Continued

Drugs	Reasons for microencapsulation	Ref.
Dihydralazine sulfate	SR	59, 60, 63
Dimethicone fluid	CLP	21, 43
Diphenhydramine HCl	SR	21
Disulfiram	MUT	21, 43
Dithiazanine iodide	SR	43
Dipyridamole	SR/BF	220
Doxorubicin	SR/IT	103, 117
Doxycycline HCl	MUT	21
Enoxacin	SR	191, 196
Ephedrine HCl	MUT	43
Eprazinone	CLP	21
Erythromycin HCl	SR/MUT	43, 188
Fenfluramine	SR	21
Ferrous citrate	EP/SIS	21, 43
Ferrous fumarate	SIS/SR/MUT	21, 43, 130
Ferrous sulfate	SR/EP/RGI/MUT/SIS	21, 43
Flufenamic acid	SR	166
5-Fluorouracil	SR/IT	103
Furosemide	SR	158, 193, 206
Glaphenine	RGI	165, 166
Glycerol guaiacolate	SR	43
Glyceryl trinitrate	SR	21
Homocysteine	MUT	43
Hydrocortisone	SR	126
Hyoscine methonitrate	SIS/MUT	21
Ibuprofen	SR	200, 201
Indomethacin	RGI/SR	21, 54, 55, 127, 128, 166, 169, 198, 199, 203
Isoniazid	SR	176, 225
Isosorbite 5-mononitrate	SR/IT	65, 66
Ketoprofen	SR	202
Ketorolac tromethamide	SR	195
Levodopa	EP/MUT	21, 43
Lithium carbonate	SR/MUT	21, 43
Lobeline sulfate	SR	43
Magnesium aluminum hydroxide hydrate	SR	200
Meclofenoxate HCl	EP/MUT	21
Menthol	CLP	2, 21, 43
Meprobamate	SR/MUT	21, 43
Mercaptopurine	SR	221
Methaqualone	MUT	21, 43
Methenamine mandelate	SR	43
Methionine	MUO/MUT	21, 43
Methyl salicylate	RV	21, 43
Methylamphetamine HCl	SR/MUT	21, 43
Methylene blue HCl	SR	43
Mitomycin C	SR/IT	223
N-Acetyl-p-Aminophenol	RGI	21, 43, 213
Nalidixic acid	SR	150

Appendix 1 Continued

Drugs	Reasons for microencapsulation	Ref.
Naproxen	RGI/SR/MUT	91
Nicardipine HCl	SR	174, 219
Nitrofurantoin	SR	21, 48, 69, 86, 88, 150, 194, 212
Nortriptyline	PR/MUT	21
Noscapine	SR	21, 43
Ofloxacin	SR	193
Oxazepam	SR	152, 153
Oxolamine citrate	SR	229
Oxyphenbutazone	RGI	165, 166
Oxytetracycline	MUT	21, 43, 179
p-Aminosalicylic acid	MUT/SR	43
p-Aminobenzoic acid	SR	43
Papaverine HCl	SR	21, 130
Paraffin oil	CLP	43
Penicillin V acid	SR	43
Penicillin V potassium	SR	43
Pentabarbituric acid	SR	73
Pentaerythritol tetranitrate	SR	21
Phenacetin	EP/SIS	21, 43
Phenaglycodol	SR	43
Phenformin HCl	SR/MUT	21
Phenytoin sodium	SR	47, 48
Phenobarbitone Na	SR/MUT	43, 86
Phenylbutazone	RGI/MUT	21, 43
Phenylephrine HCl	SR/MUT	21, 43
Phenylpropanolamine HCl	SR/MUT	21, 43, 227, 228
Phenylephrine HCl	SR	43
Phosphorylcholine	EP/SIS	43
Pilocarpin HCl	SR	180
Piretanide	SR	116
Potassium chloride	SR/IT/RGI/SIS	43, 56, 130, 132
Potassium phenethicilline	SR	163, 168
Potassium iodide	SR	43
Prednisolone	MUT	21
Prednisone	SR	126
Procainamide HCl	EP/SR	21
Procaine penicillin	SR	130
Procaine penicillin G	SR	130
Propantheline Br	SR/MUT	21
Propranolol HCl	SR	21, 187, 217
Quinidine sulfate	MUT	21, 43
Reserpine	EP	21
Salbutamol sulfate	SR	226
Salicylamide	SR	43
Sodium bicarbonate	SIS	43
Streptomycin sulfate	SR	130
Sodium chloride	SR	143
Sodium salicylate	SR	43, 68
Sodium thiosulfate	SR	43

Appendix 1 Continued

Drugs	Reasons for microencapsulation	Ref.
Succinimide	MUT	21
Sulfadiazine	SR	46, 78, 83, 84, 99, 100, 103, 156, 157
Sulfamerazine	SR	43, 101, 102
Sulfamethizole	SR	82, 181
Sulfamethoxydiazine	SIS/MUT	21
Sulfisoxazole	SR	43, 46
Sulfamethoxazole	SR	123
Sulfonamide	SR	95
Tartaric acid	EP/MUT	21, 43
Terbutaline sulfate	SR	57, 211
Tetracycline HCl	MUT/RGI/SIS	43, 130
Theophylline	SR/RGI/MUT	43, 45, 75, 77, 148, 149, 156, 160, 162, 167, 175, 177, 183, 195, 204–206, 208, 210
Thiabendazole	SR	131, 140
Tofizepam	SR	170
Tolnaftate	SR	184
Trifluperazine embonate	SR	21
Trimeprazine tartrate	SR/MUT	21
Vitamin A palmitate	SIS	224
Vitamin B factor (nicotinamide)	EP/MUT	21
Vitamin B_1 thiamin HCl	EP/MUT/SIS	21, 43
Vitamin B_2 (riboflavin)	EP/MUT/SIS	21, 43
Vitamin B_6 (pyridoxine HCl)	EP/MUT/SIS	21, 43
Vitamin B_{12} (cyanocobalamin)	EP/SIS/RGI/MUT	21, 43, 130,
Vitamin C (ascorbic acid)	EP/MUT/SIS	21, 43, 173
Vitamin D	EP	130
Vitamin PP (nicotinamide)	MUT	43
Zinc sulfate	SR	61, 62, 64

SR, sustained release; MUT, masking unpleasant taste; MUO, masking unpleasant odor; SIS, separating incompatible substances; CLP, converting liquid to powders; EP, environmental protection; RGI, reducing gastric irritation; IT, improved tolerability; BF, better flow; RV, reducing volatility.
Source: Data from Refs. 21, 43, 130, and 187.

IX. CONCLUSION

Microencapsulation by coacervation/phase separation is one of the methods used in commercially available products. As can be seen from the examples listed, drugs belonging to different pharmacological groups have been encapsulated. Antibiotics, anti-inflammatory agents, analgesics, and antihypertensives are some of these groups. Microencapsulation provided improved forms of pharmaceuticals such as sustained release drugs and free-flowing powders, masked unpleasant tastes and odors, reduced gastric irritation, and provided protection from environmental conditions.

ACKNOWLEDGMENTS

The authors are grateful to the research associates H. Eroğlu, M. S. Kaynak, and E. Kaynarca for their assistance in compiling the references and to M. Kafalı for the figures. We also thank Özge Kaş for her valuable assistance during the preparation of tables.

REFERENCES

1. Fanger, G. O., 1974. Microencapsulation: a brief history and introduction. In: Microencapsulation Process and Applications, J. E. Vandegaer (Ed.), Plenum Press, New York, pp. 1–19.
2. Bakan, J. A. and Anderson, J. L., 1970. Microencapsulation. In: The Theory and Practice of Industrial Pharmacy. L. Lachman and J. L. Kanig (Eds.), Lea and Febiger, Philadelphia, pp. 420–437.
3. Nack, H., 1970. Microencapsulation techniques, application and problems. J. Soc. Cosmet. Chemists, 21: 85–98.
4. Luzzi, A. L., 1970. Microencapsulation. J. Pharm. Sci., 59: 1367–1376.
5. Serajuddin, A. T. M., 1972. Microencapsulation of pharmaceuticals. Bangladesh Pharm. J., 1: 6–11.
6. Bakan, J. A. and Sloan, F. D., 1972. Microencapsulation of drugs. Drug Cosmet. Ind., 110: 34–38.
7. Fanger, G. O., 1974. What good are microcapsules?. Chemtech., July: 397–405.
8. Racz, I., Gyarmati, L., 1974. Microencapsulated drugs. Gyogyszereszet., 18: 125–130.
9. Doelker, P. E. and Buri, P., 1975. Une tecnique récente en pharmacie galénique, le micro-encapsulage. Pharm. Acta. Helv., 50: 73–87.
10. Kondo, T., 1975. Techniques of microencapsulation. Gyogyszereszet., 19: 401–407.
11. Luzzi, L. A., 1976. Encapsulation Tecniques for Pharmaceuticals: Considerations for the Microencapsulation of Drugs. In: Microencapsulation. J. R. Nixon (Ed.), Marcel Dekker, New York, pp. 193–206.
12. Calanchi, M., 1976. New Dosage Forms. In: Microencapsulation. J. R. Nixon (Ed.), Marcel Dekker, New York, pp. 93–102.
13. J. R. Nixon (Ed.), Microencapsulation, 1976. Marcel Dekker, New York.
14. Salib, N. N., 1977. A review of microencapsulation. Pharm. Ind., 39: 506–516.
15. Parshotam, L. M., 1977. Microencapsulation: an overview. Pharm. Tech., Dec.: 29–32.
16. Jalsenjak, I., 1978. Microencapsulation of drugs. Farm. Glas., 34: 407–414.
17. Kondo, T., 1978. Microcapsules: their preparation and properties. In: Surface and Colloid Science, E. Matijevic (Ed.), Plenum Press, New York, pp. 1–22
18. Madan, P. L., 1978. Microencapsulation: interfacial reactions. Drug Dev. Ind. Pharm., 4: 289–304.
19. D'Onafrio, G. P., Openheim R. C. and Bateman N. H., 1979. Encapsulated microcapsules. Int. J. Pharm., 2: 91–99.
20. Deasy, P. B., 1980. Microencapsulation of pharmaceuticals. Int. Pharm. J., 58: 98–99.
21. Deasy, P. B., 1984. Microencapsulation and Related Drug Processes. Marcel Dekker, New York.
22. Merkle, H. P., 1984. Does microencapsulation have a future in drug formulation? Pharm. Int., 5: 88–91.
23. Arshady, R., 1992, Naming microcapsules. J. Microencap., 9: 187–190.
24. Chemtob, C., Chamucil J. C., and N'Dongo, M., 1986. Microencapsulation by ethylcellulose phase separation: microcapsule characteristics. Int. J. Pharm., 29: 1–7.
25. Thies, C. 1987. Microencapsulation. In: Encyclopedia of Polymer and Engineering, J. I. Kroschwitz, H. F. Mark, N. M. Bikales, C. G. Overberger, G. Menges (Eds.), John Wiley and Sons, New York, pp. 724–745.
26. Bogatay, M., Kristyl, A., Mrhar, A. and Kozjek, F., 1988. Microcapsules: preparations and control. Farm. Vestn. Ljubljana, 39: 239–252.
27. Arshady, R., 1988. Preparation of polymer nano and microspheres by vinyl polymerisation techniques. J. Microencap., 5: 101–114.

28. Arshady, R., 1989. Preparation of nano and microspheres by polycondensation technique, J. Microencap., 6: 1–12.
29. Arshady, R., 1989. Preparation of microspheres and microcapsules by interfacial polycondensation technique. J. Microencap., 6: 13–28.
30. Arshady, R., 1989. Microspheres and microcapsules—survey of manufacturing techniques: Part I: Suspension crosslinking. Polym. Eng. Sci., 29: 1746–1758.
31. Arshady, R., 1990. Microspheres and microcapsules—a survey of manufacturing techniques: Part II: Coacervation. Polym. Eng. Sci., 30: 905–914.
32. Whateley, T. L., 1992. Microencapsulation of Drugs. Harwood Academic, Switzerland.
33. Benita, S., 1996. Microencapsulation—Methods and Industrial Applications, Marcel Dekker, New York.
34. Thies, C., 1996. A survey of microencapsulation processes. In: Microencapsulation Methods and Industrial Applications, S. Benita (Ed.), Marcel Dekker, New York, pp. 1–19.
35. Russell, E., Phares, J. R. and Sperandio, G. J., 1964. Coating pharmaceuticals by coacervation. J. Pharm. Sci., 53: 515–518.
36. Russell, E., Phares, J. R. and Sperandio, G. J., 1964. Preparation of a phase diagram for coacervation. J. Pharm. Sci., 53: 518–521.
37. Vandegar, J. E., 1974. Encapsulation by coacervation. In: Microencapsulation—Process and Applications. American Chemical Soc. Symp. on Microencapsulation, Chicago, J. E. Vandegaer (Ed.), Plenum Press, New York, pp. 21–37.
38. Spieser, P., 1976. Microencapsulation by coacervation, spray encapsulation and nanoencapsulation. In: Microencapsulation, J. R. Nixon (Ed.), Marcel Dekker, New York, pp. 1–12.
39. Madan, P. L., 1978. Microencapsulation. I. Phase separation or coacervation. Drug Dev. Ind. Pharm., 4: 95–101.
40. Flinn, J. E., Nack, H., 1967. What is happening in microencapsulation. Chem. Eng., 4: 171–178.
41. Spittler, J., Mathis, C., and Stamm, A., 1977. Microencapsulation de cyclohexane par coacervation, First Int. Conf. on Pharm. Tech., France, pp. 119–125.
42. Speiser, P., 1978. La microencapsulation par coacervation et nébulasation. Labo- Pharma- Problemes et Techniques, 277: 547–552.
43. NCR Microencapsulation-Pharmaceuticals, 1971. National Cash Register Co., Dayton, OH, pp. 1–19.
44. Jalil, R. and Nixon, J., 1992. Microencapsulation with biodegradable materials. In: Microencapsulation of Drugs, T. L. Whateley (Ed.), Harwood Academic, Switzerland, pp. 177–188.
45. Nixon, J. R. and Meleka M. R., 1984. The preparation and characterisation of ethylcellulose-walled theophylline microcapsules, J. Microencap., 1: 53–64.
46. İzgü, E. and Doğanay, T., 1976. Determination of microencapsulation conditions of gelatine succinate by coacervation and dissolution rate of sulfisaxoazole from these microcapsules, J. Fac. Pharm., 6: 54–87.
47. Yazıcı, E., 1994. Investigations on the optimisation and in vitro release kinetics of phenytoin sodium microparticles, biopharmaceutics and pharmacokinetics M.Sc. Program, Institute of Health Sciences, Hacettepe University, Ankara, Turkey.
48. Yazıcı, E., Öner, L., Kaş, H. S. and Hıncal A. A., 1996. Phenytoin sodium microparticles: process optimisation and in vitro release kinetics. Pharm. Dev. Tech., 1: 175–183.
49. Nixon, J. R., Khalil, A. H. and Carless, J. E., 1966. Phase relationship in the simple coacervating system isoelectric gelatine:ethanol:water. J. Pharm. Pharmacol., 18: 409–416.
50. Beyger, J. W. and Nairn, J. G., 1986. Some factors affecting the microencapsulation of pharmaceuticals with cellulose acetate phthalate. J. Pharm. Sci., 75: 573–578.
51. Lavasanifar, A., Ghalandari, R., Ataei, Z., Zolfaghari, M. E. and Mortazavi, S. A., 1997. Microencapsulation of theophylline using ethylcellulose: in vitro drug release and kinetic modelling. J. Microencap., 14: 91–100.
52. Salib, N. N., El-Menshawy, M. E. and Ismail, A. A., 1976. Ethyl cellulose as a potential sustained release coating for oral pharmaceuticals. Pharmazie, 31: 721–723.
53. Nimmannit, U. and Suwanpatra, N., 1996. Microencapsulation of drugs by the coacervation technique using ethylcellulose and acrylate-methacrylate-copolymer as wall material. J. Microencap., 13: 643–649.

54. Tirkkonen, S., Turokka, L. and Paronen, P., 1994. Microencapsulation of indomethacin by gelatin–acacia complex coacervation in the presence of surfactants. J. Microencap., 11: 615–626.
55. Tirkkonen, S. and Paronen, P., 1993. Release of indomethacin tabletted ethylcellulose microcapsules. Int. J. Pharm., 92: 55–62.
56. Vitkova, M., Chalabala, M., Rak, J. and Prochazka, R., 1994. Ethylcellulose to prepare a matrix system of a hydrophilic drug by the microencapsulation process. STP Pharma. Sci., 4: 486–491.
57. Manekar, N. C., Puranik, P. K. and Joshi, S. B., 1991. Prolonged release of terbutaline sulphate microcapsules. J. Microencap., 8: 521–523.
58. Dhruv, A. B., Needham, T. E. and Luzzi, L. A., 1975. Effect of variables on gelatin-acacia coacervate volume. Can. J. Pharm. Sci., 10: 33–36.
59. Öner, L., 1983. Investigations in the microencapsulation and dissolution rate studies of long acting dihydralazine sulphate microcapsules, pharmaceutical technology M.Sc. Program, Institute of Health Sciences, Hacettepe University, Ankara Turkey.
60. Öner, L., Yalabık-Kaş, H. S., Cave, G. and Hıncal, A. A., 1985. Microencapsulation and in vitro dissolution kinetics of dihydralazine sulphate. Labo-Pharma., 32: 690–693.
61. Öner, L., 1987. Investigations on the formulation and bioavailability of zinc sulphate preparations, Pharmaceutical Technology Ph.D. Program, Institute of Health Sciences, Hacettepe University, Ankara, Turkey.
62. Öner, L., Kaş, H. S. and Hıncal, A. A., 1988. Studies on zinc sulphate microcapsules, 2: application of factorial design. J. Microencap., 5: 225–229.
63. Öner, L., Yalabık-Kaş, H. S. and Hıncal, A. A., 1984. Formulation and release of dihydralazine sulphate from tabletted microcapsules. J. Microencap., 1: 123–130.
64. Öner, L., Kaş, H. S. and Hıncal, A. A., 1988. Studies on zinc sulphate microcapsules, 1: microencapsulation and in vitro dissolution kinetics. J. Microencap., 5: 219–223.
65. Farivar, M., 1991. Investigations on the formulation and release rate studies of isosorbite-5-mononitrate microcapsules, Pharmaceutical Technology M.Sc. Program, Institute of Health Sciences, Hacettepe University, Ankara, Turkey.
66. Farivar M., Kaş, H. S., Öner, L. and Hıncal, A. A., 1993. Factorial design based optimisation of the formulation of isosorbite-5-mononitrate microcapsules. J. Microencap., 10: 309–317.
67. Khadjei, R., 1991. Investigations on the optimisation of acetylsalicylic acid containing ethylcellulose microcapsules, pharmaceutical technology M.Sc. Program, Institute of Health Sciences, Hacettepe University, Ankara, Turkey.
68. Deasy, P. B., Brophy, M. R., Ecanow, R. and Joy, M. M., 1980. Effect of ethylcellulose grade and sealant treatments on the production and in vitro release of microencapsulated sodium salicylate. J. Pharm. Pharmacol., 32: 15–20.
69. Ertan, G., Sarıgüllü, I., Karasulu, Y., Erçakır, E. and Güneri T., 1994. Sustained release dosage form of nitrofurantoin. Part I. preparation of microcapsules and in vitro release kinetics. J. Microencap., 11: 129–135.
70. Burgess, D. J. and Carless, J. E., 1984. Microelectrophoretic studies of gelatine and acacia for the prediction of complex coacervation J. Colloid Interf. Sci., 98:1–8.
71. Burgess, D. J., 1986. Complex coacervate formation between acid and alkaline processed gelatins. Coulombic Interact. macromol. Syst., 21:251–260.
72. Rozenblat, J., Magdassi, S., and Garti, N., 1989. Effect of elecrolytes, stirring and surfactants in the coacervation and microencapsulation processes in the presence of gelatine. J. Microencap., 6: 515–526.
73. Luzzi, L. A. and Gerraughty, R. J., 1967. Effect of additives and formulation techniques on controlled release of drugs from microcapsules. J. Pharm. Sci., 56: 1174–1177.
74. Yoshida, N. and Thies, C., 1967. The effect of neutral salts on gelatin–gum arabic complexes. J. Colloid. Interf. Sci., 24: 29–40.
75. Badavi, A. A., Shoukri, R. A. and El-Zainy, A. A., 1992. Optimisation of microencapsulation of theophylline with Eudragits. Part 2: Effect of additives on microencapsulation of theophylline with Eudragits, Egypt J. Pharm. Sci., 33: 651–666.
76. Friend, D. R., 1992. Polyacrylate resin microcapsules for taste masking of antibiotics. J. Microencap., 9: 469–480.

77. Wu, J. C., Chen, H. Y. and Chen, H., 1994. Studies on the properties of ethylcellulose microcapsules prepared by emulsion non-solvent addition method in the presence of nonsolvent in polymer solution. J. Microencap., 11: 519–529.
78. Das, S. K., 1993. Effect of polybutadiene on the encapsulation efficiency of ethylcellulose microcapsules of sulphadiazine. J. Microencap., 10: 437–447.
79. Jalil, R. and Nixon, J. R., 1990. Biodegradable poly(lactic acid) and poly(lactide-co-glycolide) microcapsules: problems associated with preparative techniques and release properties, J. Microencap., 7: 297–325.
80. Donbrow, M., Hoffman, A. and Benita, S., 1990. Phase seperation modulation and aggregation prevention: mechanism of the non-solvent addition method in the presence and absence of polyisobutylene as an additive. J. Microencap., 7: 1–15.
81. Wu, J. C., Jean, W. J. and Chen H., 1994. Evaluation of the properties of ethyl cellulose–cellulose acetate microcapsules containing theopyhlline prepared by different microencapsulation techniques. J. Microencap., 11: 507–518.
82. Itoh, M., Nakano, M., Juni, K. and Sekikawa, H., 1980. Sustained release of sulfamethizole, 5-fluorouracil, and doxorubicin from ethyl cellulose–polylactic acid microcapsules. Chem. Pharm. Bull., 28: 1051–1055.
83. Sheorey, D. S., Sai, M. S. and Dorle, H. K., 1991. A new technique for the encapsulation of water insoluble drugs using ethyl cellulose. J. Microencap., 8: 359–368.
84. Donbrow, M. and Benita S., 1977. The effect of polyisobutylene on the coacervation of ethyl cellulose and the formation of microcapsules. J. Pharm. Pharmacol. (Suppl), 29.
85. Veis, A., Bodor, E. and Mussel, S., 1967. Molecular weight fractionation and the self-suppression of complex coacervation. Biopolymers, 5: 37–59.
86. Jalsenyak, I., Nicolandou, C. F. and Nixon, J. R., 1976. The in-vitro dissolution of phenobarbitone sodium from ethylcellulose microcapsules. J. Pharm. Pharmacol., 28: 912–914.
87. Ertan, G., Sarıgüllü, I., Karasulu, Y., Aşıkoğlu, M. and Kantarcı, G., 1994. In-vitro dissolution studies on sustained release dosage forms of ampicillin and amoxicillin, Acta Pharm. Turcica, 36: 128–134.
88. Ertan, G., Özer, Ö., Baloğlu, E. and Güneri, T., 1997. Sustained release microcapsules of nitrofurantion and amoxicillin preparation, in-vitro release rate kinetics and micrometric studies. J. Microencap., 14: 379–388.
89. Koh, G. L. and Tucker I. G., 1988. Characterisation of carboxymethylcellulose gelatine complex coacervation by viscosity, turbidity, and coacervate wet weight and volume measurements. J. Pharm. Pharmacol., 40: 233–236.
90. Mordata, S. A. M., Egaky, A. M. E., Motawi, A. M. and Khodery K. A. E., 1987. Preparation of microcapsules from complex coacervation of Gantrez gelatine. II. In vitro dissolution of nitrofurantoin microcapsules. J. Microencap., 4: 23–37.
91. Burgess, D. J. and Carless, J. E., 1985. Manufacture of gelatine/gelatine coacervate microcapsules, Int. J. Pharm., 27: 61–70.
92. Veis, A., 1961. Phase separation in polyelectrolyte solutions, II. Interaction effects. J. Phys. Chem. 65: 1798–1803.
93. Veis, A. and Aranyi C., 1960. Phase separation in polyelectrolyte systems I. Complex coacervates of gelatine. J. Phys. Chem. 64: 1203–1210.
94. Mordata, S. A. M., Egaky, A. M. E., Motawi, A. M. and Khodery K. A. E., 1987. Preparation of microcapsules from complex coacervation of Gantrez gelatine, I. Development of technique, J. Microencap., 4: 11–21.
95. Mathews, B. R. and Nixon, J. R., 1974. Surface characteristics of gelatine microcapsules by scanning electron microscopy. J. Pharm. Pharmacol., 26: 383–384.
96. Nixon, J. R., 1981. In vitro and in vivo release of microencapsulated chlorothiazide, Proc. 4th Int. Symp. Microencap., Miami, FL, pp. 26–28.
97. Özer, A. Y. and Hıncal, A. A., 1990. Studies on the masking of unpleasant taste of beclamide microencapsulation and tabletting, J. Microencap., 7: 327–339.
98. Madan, P. L., Madan, D. K. and Price, L. C., 1976. The effect of pH on the fractionation of gelatine, Can. J. Pharm. Sci., 11: 21–25.

99. Paradissis, G. N. and Parrot, E. L., 1968. Gelatin encapsulation of pharmaceuticals. J. Clin. Pharmacol., January–February, 54–59.
100. Nixon, J. R. and Walker, S. E., 1971. The in vitro evaluation of gelatine coacervate microcapsules. J. Pharm. Pharmacol., 23 (Suppl.): 147S–154S.
101. Nixon, J. R., Khalil, S. A. H. and Carless, J. E., 1968. Gelatin coacervate microcapsules containing sulphamerazine: their preparation and the in vitro release of drug. J. Pharm. Pharmacol., 20: 528–538.
102. Khalil, S. A. H, Nixon, J. R. and Carless, J. E., 1968. Role of pH in the coacervation of the systems: gelatine–water–ethanol and gelatine–water–sodium sulphate. J. Pharm. Pharmacol., 20: 215–225.
103. Okada, J., Kusai A. and Ueda, S., 1985. Factors effecting microcapsule solubility in simple gelatine coacervation method. J. Microencap., 2: 163–173.
104. Komatsu, M., Tagawa, K., Kawata, M. and Goto, S., 1983. Biopharmaceutical evaluation of gelatine microcapsules of sulfonamides. Chem. Pharm. Bull., 31: 262–268.
105. Nixon, J. R. and Meleka, M. R., 1984. The in vivo performance of theophylline microcapsules, J. Microencap., 1: 65–72.
106. Goto, S., Moriya, F., Kawata, M. and Kimura, T., 1984. Preparation and biopharmaceutical evaluation of microcapsules of amoxicillin, J. Microencap., 1: 137–155.
107. Siddiqui, O. and Taylor, H., 1983. Physical factors affecting microencapsulation by simple coacervation of gelatine. J. Pharm. Pharmacol., 35: 70–73.
108. Tagawa, K., Kawata, M. and Goto, S., 1983. Biopharmaceutical evaluation of gelatine microcapsules of several antibiotics. Chem. Pharm. Bull., 31: 269–273.
109. Goto, S., Komatsu, M. Tagawa, K. and Kawata M., 1983. Preparation and evaluation of gelatine microcapsules of sulfonamides. Chem. Pharm. Bull., 31: 256–261.
110. Green, B. K., US Patent 2,800,458, July 23, 1957.
111. Green, B. K. and Schleicher, L., US Patent 2,800,457, July 23, 1957.
112. Madan, P. L., Jani, R. K. and Bartilucci, A. J., 1978. New method of preparing gelatine microcapsules of soluble pharmaceuticals. J. Pharm. Sci., 67: 409–411.
113. Veis, A., 1963. Phase separation in polyelectrolyte systems, III. Effect of aggregation and molecular weight heterogeneity. J. Phys. Chem., 67: 1960–1964.
114. Goto, S., Tsujiyama, T., Kawata, M. and Nobuo, S., 1985. Preparation and biopharmaceutical evaluation of gelatine microcapsules of pretanide. J. Contr. Rel., 1: 291–300.
115. Okamoto, Y., Konno, A., Togawa, K., Kato, T., Tamakawa, Y. and Amano, Y., 1986. Arterial chemoembolization with cisplatin microcapsules. Br. J. Cancer, 53: 369–375.
116. Dhupark. C., 1987. A method of preparing gelatine microcapsules, Drug Dev. Ind. Pharm., 13: 1023–1030.
117. Kawashima, Y., Lin, S. Y., Kasai, A., Takenaka, H., Matsunami, K., Nochida, Y. and Hirose H., 1984. Drug release properties of the microcapsules of the adriamycin hydrochlamide with ethylcellulose prepared by a phase separation technique. Drug Dev. Ind. Pharm., 10: 467–479.
118. Tirkkonen, S., Paronnen, P., Tillanen, J. and Turakka, L., 1990. Effect of surfactants on microencapsulation of indomethacin by gelatine acacia complex coacervation. Proc. 9th Pharm. Tech. Cong., Veldhovenn, The Netherlands, pp. 466–476.
119. Peters, H. J. W., Van Bommel, E. M. G. and Fokkens, J. G., 1992. Effects of different properties of gelatine and acacia on the microencapsulation of theobromine. Drug Dev. Ind. Pharm., 18: 123–134.
120. Burgess, D. J. and Carless, J. E., 1984. Microelectrophoretic studies of gelatine and acacia for the prediction of complex coacervation. J. Colloid. Interf. Sci., 98: 1–8.
121. Newton, D. W., McMullen, J. N. and Becker, C. H., 1977. Characterisation of medicated and unmedicated microglobules recovered from complex coacervation of gelatine-acacia, J. Pharm. Sci., 66: 1327–1330.
122. Nixon, J. R. and Nouh, A., 1978. The effect of microcapsule size on the oxidative decomposition of core material. J. Pharm. Pharmacol., 30: 533–537.
123. Takenaka, H., Kawashima, T. and Lin, S. Y., 1981. Electrophoretic properties of sulfamethoxazole microcapsules and gelatin-acacia coacervates. J. Pharm. Sci., 70: 302–305.

124. Palmieri, A., 1979. Microencapsulation and dissolution parameters of undecenovanillylamide: a potential coyote deterrent. J. Pharm. Sci., 68: 1561–1562.
125. Takenaka, M., Kawashima, Y. and Lin, S. Y., 1980. Micromeritic properties of sulfamethoxazol microcapsules and gelatin-acacia coacervates. J. Pharm. Sci., 69: 513–516.
126. Jizomoto, H., Kanaoka, E., Sugita, K., and Hirano, K., 1993. Gelatin-acacia microcapsules for trapping micro oil droplets containing lipophilic drugs and ready disintegration in the gastrointestinal tract. Pharm. Res., 10: 1115–1122.
127. Burgess, D. J. and Carless, J. E., 1986. Microelectrophoretic behaviour of gelatine and acacia complex coacervates and indomethacin microcapsules. Int. J. Pharm., 32: 207–212.
128. Rowe, J. S. and Carless, J. E., 1983. The influence of the microcapsule wall on the assay of indomethacine microcapsules in the presence of antacids: implications for product stability. Int J. Pharm., 13: 313–320.
129. Singh, O. N. and Burgess, F. D. J., 1989. Characterisation of albumin–alginic acid complex coacervation. J. Pharm. Pharmacol., 41: 670–673.
130. Maggi, G. C., Coppi, G., Calanchi, M. and Valducci, R., 1977. Presentation de quelques avantages de la microencapsulation appliquee aux medicaments. Proc. 1st Int. Cong. Pharm. Tech., France, pp. 132–143.
131. Nixon, J. R. and Hassan, M., 1980. The effect of preparative technique on the particle size of thiabendazole microcapsules. J. Pharm. Pharmacol., 32: 856–859.
132. Harris, M. S., 1981. Preparation and release characteristics potassium chloride microcapsules, Proc. 4th Int. Symp. Microencap., Miami, FL, pp. 41–44.
133. Madan, P. L., Luzzi, L. A. and Price, J. C., 1972. Factors influencing microencapsulation of a waxy solid by complex coacervation. J. Pharm. Sci., 61: 1586–1588.
134. Luzzi, L. A. and Gerraughty, R. J., 1964. Effects of selected variables on the extractability of oils from coacervate capsules. J. Pharm. Sci., 53: 429–431.
135. Ismail, N., Harris M. S. and Nixon J. R., 1984. Particle size analysis of gelatin-acacia coacervate and ethylcellulose walled microcapsules. J. Microencap., 1: 9–19.
136. Luzzi, L. A. and Gerraughty, R. J., 1967. Effects of selected variables on the microencapsulation of solids, J. Pharm. Sci., 56: 634–638.
137. Madan P. L., Luzzi, L. A. and Price J. C., 1974. Microencapsulation of a waxy solid: wall thickness and surface appearance studies. J. Pharm. Sci., 63: 280–284.
138. McMullen, J. N., Newton, D. W. and Becker C. H., 1982. Pectin–gelatin complex coacervates, I. Determination of microglobile size morphology and recovery as water dispersible powders. J. Pharm. Sci., 71: 628–633.
139. Nixon, J. R. and Nouh, A., 1978. The effect of microcapsule size on the oxidative decomposition of core material. J. Pharm. Pharmacol., 30: 533–537.
140. Nixon, J. R. and Hassan, M., 1981. The effect of pH on the release characteristics of thiabendazole microcapsules. Drug Dev. Ind. Pharm., 7: 305–316.
141. Zigmoto, H., 1984. Phase separation induced in gelatin-base coacervate systems by addition of water soluble non-ionic polymer. J. Pharm. Sci., 73: 879–882.
142. Takenaka, M., Kawashimo, Y. and Lin, S. Y., 1981. Electrophoretic properties of sulfamethoxal microcapsules and gelatin-acacia coacervates. J. Pharm. Sci., 70: 302–305.
143. Jalsenjak, I. and Kondo, T., 1981. Effect of capsule size on the permeability of gelatine acacia microcapsules toward sodium chloride. J. Pharm. Sci., 70: 456–457.
144. Duquemni, S. J. and Nixon, J. R., 1985. Effect of sodium lauryl sulphate, cetrimide and polysorbate surfactants on complex coacervate volume and droplet size. J. Pharm. Pharmacol., 37: 698–702.
145. Benita, S. and Danbrow, M., 1980. Coacervatizm of of ethyl cellulose; the role of polyisobutylene and the effect of its concentration. J. Colloid. Interf. Sci., 77: 102–109.
146. Smith, J., 1983. Discrete coated particles as drug delivery modules: microencapsulation and beyond. Pharm. Tech., 7: 26.
147. Suryakusuma, H. and Jun, H. W., 1984. Formation of encapsulated hydrophilic polymer beads by combined techniques of bead polymerisation and phase separation. J. Pharm. Pharmacol., 36: 493–496.

148. Nixon, J. R. and Wong, K. T., 1990. Evaluation of drug permeation through polymeric membranes as a model for release. Part 2. Ethyl cellulose walled microcapsules. Int. J. Pharm., 58: 31–40.
149. Sa, B., Bandyopadhyay, A. K. and Gupta B. K., 1990. Development and in vitro evaluation of ethylcellulose micropellets as a controlled release dosage form for theophyllin. Drug Dev. Ind. Pharm., 16: 1153–1169.
150. Hashim, F., Sakr, F. M. and Zeineldin, E., 1987. In vitro release and in vivo adsorption of nitrofurantoin and nalidixic acid from ethylcellulose microcapsules. Pharmazie, 315–317.
151. Benita, S. and Donbrow, M., 1982. Effect of polyisobuthylene on ethylcellulose walled microcapsules: wall structure and thickness of salicylamide and theophylline microcapsules. J. Pharm. Sci., 71: 205–210.
152. Kaş, H. S., 1981. Studies on microencapsulation and bioavailability of oxazepam. Pharmaceutical Technology Department, Faculty of Pharmacy, University of Hacettepe, Ankara, Turkey.
153. Yalabık-Kaş, H. S., 1983. Microencapsulation and in vitro dissolution of oxazepam from ethylcellulose microcapsules. Drug Dev. Ind. Pharm., 9: 1047–1060.
154. Devay, A. and Racz, I., 1988. Examination of parameters determining particle size distribution: acetylsalicylic acid microcapsules. J. Microencap., 5: 21–25.
155. Yalabık-Kaş, H. S., 1983. Gas chromatographic determination of oxazepam from tablets and microcapsules in urine. Drug Dev. Ind. Pharm., 9: 1541–1549.
156. Cameroni, R., Coppi, G., Formi, F., Iannucelli, V. and Barnebei, M. T., 1985. Sulfadiazine: studies on its release from microcapsules. Boll. Chim. Farm., 124: 393–400.
157. Milovanovic, D. and Naim, J. G., 1986. Microencapsulation of sulfadiazine with cellulose acetate phthalate. Drug Dev. Ind. Pharm., 12: 1249–1258.
158. El-Shattawy, H., Kassem, A. and El-Razzaz, M., 1991. Controlled release furosemide microcapsules: preformulation studies. Drug Dev. Ind. Pharm., 17: 2529–2537.
159. Hecquet, B., Fourier, C., Depadt, G. and Cappelaere, P., 1984. Preparation and release kinetics of microencapsulated cisplatin with ethylcellulose. J. Pharm. Pharmacol., 36: 803–807.
160. Lin, S. Y., 1988. Effect of excipients on tablet properties and dissolution behaviour of theophylline-tabletted microcapsules under different compression forces. J. Pharm. Sci., 77: 229–232.
161. Benita, S., Hoffman, A. and Donbrow, M., 1985. Microencapsulation of paracetamol using polyaciyllate reseins (Eudragit-Retard), kinetics of drug release and evaluation of kinetic model. J. Pharm. Pharmacol., 37: 391–395.
162. Lavasanifar, A., Ghalandari, R., Ataei, Z., Zolfaghari, M. E. and Mortazavi, S. A. 1997. Microencapsulation of theophylline using ethylcellulose: in vitro drug release and kinetic modelling. J. Microencap., 14: 91–100.
163. Alpar, O. H. and Walter, V., 1981. Prolongation of the in vitro dissolution of a soluble drug (phenethicillin potassium) by microencapsulation with ethylcellulose. J. Pharm. Pharmacol., 33: 419–422.
164. Bhatnagar, S., Nakhare, S. and Vyas, S. P., 1995. Poloaxamer-coated three-ply-walled microcapsules for controlled delivery of diclofenac sodium. J. Microencap., 12: 13–22.
165. Meshali, M. M., El-Dien, E. Z., Omar, S. A. and Luzzi, L. A., 1989. A new approach to encapsulating nonsteroidal anti-inflammatory drugs. III. Coating acidic as well as basic nonsteroidal anti-inflammatory drugs with cellulose derivatives having different functional groups. J. Microencap., 6: 339–353.
166. Meshali, M. M., El-Dien, E. Z., Omar, S. A. and Luzzi, L. A., 1989. A new approach to encapsulating nonsteroidal anti-inflammatory drugs. IV. Effect of cellulose derivatives with different functional groups on the bioavailability and gastric ulcerogenic activity of acidic as well as basic nonsteroidal anti-inflammatory drugs. J. Microencap., 6: 355–360.
167. Donbrow, M., Hoffman, A. and Benita, S., 1995. Gradation of microcapsule wall porosity by depositiom of polymer mixture. Phase separation of polymer mixtures and effects of external media and conditions of release. J. Microencap., 12: 273–285.
168. Alpar, O. H., 1980. Sustained-release characteristics of tablets of ethylcellulose microcapsules containing potassium phenethicillin. Il. Pharmaco-Ed. Pr., 36: 366–373.

169. Zour, E. and Lausier, J. M., 1984. Dissolution studies of microcapsulated indomethacin, effect of method and medium on dissolution. J. Microencap., 1, 47–51.
170. Dvay, A., and Racz, I., 1984. Production of microcapsules containing tofizepam. Acta Pharm. Hung., 54: 84–89.
171. Palamo, M. E., Ballesteros, M. P. and Frutos, P., 1996. Solvent and plasticizer influences on ethlcellulose microcapsules. J. Microencap., 13: 307–318.
172. Gupta, R. G. and Rao, B. C., 1985. Microencapsulation of vitamin B_{12} by emulsion technique. Drug Dev. Ind. Pharm., 11: 41–53.
173. Smejima, M., Hirata, G. and Koida, Y., 1982. Studies on microcapsules, Part I. Role and effect of coacervation inducing agents in the microcapsulation of ascorbic acid by phase seperation method. Chem. Pharm. Bull., 30: 2894–2899.
174. Özyazıcı, M. and Sevgi, F., 1993. Preparation of nicardipine hydrochloride microcapsules by 2^3 factorial design. Proc. 9th Int. Symp. Microencap., Ankara, Turkey, p. 48.
175. Baykara, T. and Karataş, A., 1993. Preparation of acetaminophen microcapsules by coacervation-phase seperation method. Drug Dev. Ind. Pharm., 19: 587–601.
176. Senjikovic, R. and Jalsenjak, I., 1981. Surface topography of microcapsules and drug release. J. Pharm. Pharmacol., 33: 665–666.
177. Robinson, D. H., 1989. Ethylcellulose solvent evaporation phase separation relationships relevant to coacervation microencapsulation processes. Drug Dev. Ind. Pharm., 15: 2597–2620.
178. Arnedo, C., Benoit, J. P. and Thies, C., 1986. Preliminary study of microencapsulation of essential oils by complex coacervation. STP Pharma 2: 303–306.
179. Vidmar, V., Smolcic-Bubalo, A. and Jalsenyak, I., 1984. Poly(lactic acid) microencapsulated oxytetracycline: in vitro and in vivo evaluation. J. Microencap., 1: 131–136.
180. Vidmar, V., Pepeljnjak, S. and Jalsenyak, I., 1985. The in vivo evaluation of poly(lactic acid) microcapsules of pilocarpine hydrochloride. J. Microencap., 2: 289–292.
181. Nakan, M., Itoh, M., Juni, K., Serikawa, H. and Arita, T., 1980. Sustained urinary excretion of sulfamethizole following oral administration of enteric coated microcapsules in humans. Int. J. Pharm. 4: 291–298.
182. Leelarasamee, N., Howard, S. A., Malanca, C. J. and Ma, J. K. H., 1988. A method for the preparation of poly(lactic acid) microcapsules of controlled particle size and drug loading. J. Microencap., 52: 147–157.
183. Thomasin, C., Merkle, H. P. and Gander, B., 1998. Drug microencapsulation by PLA/PLGA coacervation in the light of thermodynamics. 2. Parameters determining microsphere formation. J. Pharm. Sci., 87: 269–275.
184. Thomasin, C., Nam-Tran, H., Merkle, H. P. and Gander, B., 1998. Drug microencapsulation by PLA/PLGA coacervation in the light of thermodynamics. 1. Overview and theoretical considerations. J. Pharm. Sci., 87: 259–268.
185. Nihant, N., Grandfils, C., Jerome, R. and Teyssie, P., 1995. Microencapsulation by coacervation of poly(lactide-co-glycolide). 4. Effect of the processing parameters on coacervation and encapsulation. J. Contr. Rel., 35: 117–125.
186. Deasy, P. B., 1994. Evaluation of drug containing microcapsules. J. Microencap., 11: 487–505.
187. Gutcho, M. H., Ed., 1979. Microcapsules and Other Capsules: Advances Since 1975, Noyes Data Corp., New Jersey.
188. Lu, M. F., Borodkin, S., Woodward, L. and Vadnere, M., 1991. Polymer carrier system for taste masking of macrolide antibiotics. Pharm. Res., 8: 706–712.
189. Tunçel, T., Bergisadi, N., Akın, L., Otuk, G. and Kuşcu, I., 1996. In vitro and in vivo studies on microcapsules and tabletted microcapsules of cephradine. Pharmacie, 51: 168–171.
190. Kristi, A., Bógataj, M., Mrhar, A. and Kozjeli, F., 1991. Preparation and evaluation of ethylcellulose microencapsules with bacampicillin. Drug Dev. Ind. Pharm., 17: 1109–1130.
191. Ueda, M., Nakamura, Y., Makita, H. and Kawashimo, Y., 1993. One continuous process of agglomeration and microencapsulation for enoxacin. Preparation method and mechanism of microencapsulation. J. Microencap., 10: 25–34.
192. Aşıcı, S., Özer, Ö. and Baloğlu, E., 1993. Microcapsules of ciprofloxacin: formulation and in vitro release kinetics. Proc. 9th Int. Symp. on Microencapsulation., Ankara, Turkey, p. 34.

193. Aşıcı, S., Baloğlu, E. and Özer, Ö., 1993. Studies on ofloxacin microcapsules: microencapsulation and in vitro dissolution kinetics. Proc. 9th Int. Symp. on Microencapsulation., Ankara, Turkey, p. 32.
194. Ertan, G., Sarıgüllü, I, Karasulu, Y., Kantarcı, G. and Aşıkoğlu, M., 1993. A new microcapsule form of ampicillin and amoxycillin. Proc. 9th Int. Symp. on Microencapsulation., Ankara, Turkey, p. 56.
195. Genç, L., Demirel, M., Güler, E. and Megazy, N., 1998. Microencapsulation of ketorolac tromethamine by means of a coacervation phase separation technique induced by the addition of non-solvent. J. Microencap., 15: 45–54.
196. Ueda, M., Nakamura, Y., Makita, H. and Kawashima, Y., 1993. Preparation of microcapsules masking the bitter taste of enoxacin by using one continuous process technique of agglomeration and microencapsulation. J. Microencap., 10: 461–473.
197. Yu, W. P., Wong, J. P., and Chang, T. M., 1998. Preparation of polylactic acid microcapsules containing ciprofloxacin. J. Microencap., 15: 515–523.
198. Daniels, R. and Mittermaler, E. M., 1995. Influence of pH adjustment on microencapsules obtained from complex coacervation of gelatine and acacia. J. Microencap., 12: 591–599.
199. Jani, G. K., Chawhan, G. M., Gohel, M. and Patel, J., 1992. Microencapsulation of indomethacin by complex emulsification. Indian Drugs, 29: 450–452.
200. Kasai, S. and Koishi, M., 1977. Studies on the preparation of ethylcellulose microcapsules containing magnesium aluminum hydroxide hydrate. Chem. Pharm. Bull., 25: 314–320.
201. Weiss, G., Knoch, A., Laicher, A., Stanislaus, F., and Daniels, R., 1995. Simple coacervation of hydroxypropyl methylcellulose phthalate (HPMCP). 2. Microencapsulation of buprofen. Int. J. Pharm. 124: 97–105.
202. Palmieri, G. F., Martell, S., Lauri, D., and Wehrle, P., 1996. Gelatin–acacia complex coacervation as a method for ketoprofen microencapsulation. Drug Dev. Ind. Pharm., 22: 951–957.
203. Tirkkonen, S., Urtti, A. and Paronen, P., 1995. Buffer controlled release of indomethacin from ethylcellulose microcapsules. Int. J. Pharm., 124: 219–229.
204. Lin, S. Y. and Yang, J. C., 1987. Bioavailability studies of theophylline ethylcellulose microcapsules prepared by using ethylene vinyl acetate copolymer as a coacervation inducing agent. J. Pharm. Sci., 76: 219–223.
205. Chattaraj, S. C., Das, S. K., Karthiksyan, M., Ghiosal, S. K. and Gupta, B. K., 1991. Controlled theophylline release from microcapsules of acrylic and metacrylic acid ester copolymer. Drug Dev. Ind. Pharm., 17: 551–560.
206. Gohary, O. A. and Gamal, S. E., 1991. Release of furosemide from sustained release microcapsules prepared by phase separation technique. Drug Dev. Ind. Pharm., 17: 443–444.
207. Antal, I., Zelko, R., Roczey, N., Plachy, J. and Racz, I., 1997. Dissolution and diffuse reflectance characteristics of coated theophylline particles. Int. J. Pharm., 155: 83–89.
208. Moldenhauer, M. G. and Nairin, J. G., 1990. Formulation parameters affecting the preparation and properties of microencapsulated ion-exchange resin containing theophylline. J. Pharm. Sci., 79: 659–666.
209. Asker, A. F. and Ferdous, A. J., 1997. Effect of ultraviolet light on the release of theophylline from ethylcellulose-based sustained release microcapsules. PDA J. Pharm. Sci. Technol. 51: 125–129.
210. Bandyopadhyay, A. K. and Gupta, B. K., 1996. Effect of microcapsule size and polyisobutylene concentration on the release of theophylline from ethylcellulose microcapsules. J. Microencap., 13: 207–218.
211. Manekar, N. C., Puranik, P. K. and Joshi, S. B., 1992. Microencapsulation of terbutalinesulphate by the solvent evaporation technique. J. Microencap., 9: 481–487.
212. Chowdary, K. P. R., and Ranana-Murthy, K. V., 1985, Study of nitrofurantoin release from gelatine-peptine microcapsules. Ind. J. Pharm. Sci., July–August, 158–159.
213. Ataberk, P., 1992. Microencapsulation by phase separation using ethylcellulose. Ph.D. Program, Institute of Health Sciences, Gazi University, Ankara, Turkey.
214. Güler, E., Şumnu, M. and Yazan, Y., 1989. Studies on the microencapsulation of dextropropoxiphene hydrochloride. Part 2. The in vivo urinary excretion in man. Drug Dev. Ind. Pharm., 15: 295–301.

215. Yazan, Y., 1987. Studies on the microencapsulation of dextropropoxphene hydrochloride. Pharmaceutical Technology Ph. D. Program, Anadolu University, Eski ehir, Turkey.
216. Güler, E., Şumnu, M., Yazan, Y. and Öner, L., 1989. Studies on the microencapsulation of dextropropoxphene hydrochloride I. Preparation by coacervation and the in vitro evaluation. Drug Dev. Ind. Pharm., 15: 238–293.
217. Manekar, N. C., Puranik, P. K. and Joshi, S. B., 1992. Microencapsulation of propranolol hydrochloride by the solvent evaporation technique. Coacervation-phase separation induced by solvent evaporation. J. Microencap., 9: 63–66.
218. Singh, J. and Robinson, D. H., 1988. Controlled release captopril microcapsules: effect of non ionic surfactants on release from ethylcellulose microcapsules. J. Microencap., 5: 129–137.
219. Özyazıcı, M., Sevgi, F. and Ertan, G., 1997. Sustained release dosage form of nicardipine HCl: application of factorial design and effect of surfactant on release kinetics. Drug Dev. Ind. Pharm., 23: 761–770.
220. Türkoğlu, M. and Gürsoy, A., 1993. Is microencapsulation a good way of tabletting dipyridamole? A comparative study. Proc. 9th Int. Symp. on Microencapsulation., Ankara, Turkey, p. 63.
221. Mi, F. L., Tseng, Y. C., Chen, C. T. and Shya, S. S., 1997. Preparation and release properties of biodegradable chitin microspheres. I. Preparation of 6-mercaptopurine microcapsules by phase separation methods. J. Microencap., 14: 15–25.
222. Lin, S. Y., 1985. Influence of coacervation-inducing agents and cooling rates on the preparation and in vitro release of bleomycin HCl microcapsules. J. Microencap., 2: 91–95.
223. Eley, J. G., Whateley, T. L., Goldberg, J. A., Kerr, D. J., McArdle, C. S., Anderson, J. and Kato, T., 1992. Microencapsulation of mitomycin C using ethylcellulose and its evaluation in patients with liver metastases. In: Microencapsulation of Drugs, T. L. Whateley (Ed.), Harwood Academic, Switzerland, pp. 293–303.
224. Markus, A. and Pelah, Z., 1989. Encapsulation of vitamin A. J. Microencap., 6: 389–394.
225. Muhuri, G. and Pal, T. K., 1991. Computation of release kinetics of isoniasid microcapsules. Boll. Chim. Farm., 130: 167–171.
226. Yazan, Y., Demirel, M. and Güler, E., 1995. Preparation and in vitro dissolution of salbutamol sulphate microcapsules and tabletted microcapsules. J. Microencap., 12: 601–612.
227. Sevgi, F., Özyazıcı, M. and Güneri, T., 1994. Sustained release dosage forms of phenylpropanolamine hydrochloride, Part I: Microencapsulation and in vitro release kinetics. J. Microencap., 11: 327–334.
228. Sevgi, F., Özyazıcı, M. and Güneri, T., 1994. Sustained release dosage forms of phenylpropanolamine hydrochloride, Part II: Formulation and in vitro release kinetics from tabletted microcapsules. J. Microencap., 11: 335–344.
229. Kırılmaz, L., Kendirci, A. and Güneri, T., 1992. Sustained release dosage forms of oxolamine citrate: preparation and release kinetics. J. Microencap. 9: 167–172.
230. Ndesendo, V. M., Meixner, W., Korsatko, W. and Korsatko-Wabnegy, B., 1996. Microencapsulation of chloroquine diphosphate by Eudragit RS 100. J. Microencap., 13: 1–8.
231. John, P. M., Minatoya, H. and Rosenberg, F. J., 1979. Microencapsulation of bitolterol for controlled release and its effect on bronchodilator and heart rate activities in dogs. J. Pharm. Sci., 68: 475–481.

16
Microsphere Preparation by Solvent Evaporation Method

A. Atilla Hıncal and Sema Çalış
Hacettepe University, Ankara, Turkey

I. INTRODUCTION

Controlled/targeted drug delivery using biodegradable polymeric carriers has gained increasing interest in the last two decades. In a majority of studies the lactide/glycolide homo- and copolymers have been used for drug delivery applications because they can be fabricated into a variety of morphologies, including films, rods, and microparticles, by compression molding, solvent casting, and solvent evaporation techniques (1–6). For employment in the body, biodegradable polymers have an obvious advantage that after performing their function they degrade into nontoxic monomers, i.e., lactic and glycolic acids, thus avoiding the need for surgical removal. So, the risk of long-term toxicity or a probable immunological reaction when compared with nondegradable systems is also minimized. The release rate of an incorporated drug can be modulated by variation of the copolymer ratio and molecular weight. Göpferich reviewed polymer degradation mechanisms and mechanical properties extensively (7–9). An intelligent approach to therapeutics using drug carrier technology requires a detailed understanding of drug–carrier interactions with critical cellular and organ systems as well as an understanding of the limitations of the system with respect to formulation procedures and stability.

Microspheres are defined as homogeneous, monolithic particles in the size range of about 0.1–1000 μm and are widely used as drug carriers for controlled release. These systems have significant importance in biomedical applications. Administration of drugs in the form of microspheres usually improves the treatment by providing the localization of the active substance at the site of action and by prolonging release of drugs. Furthermore, sensitive drugs such as peptides and proteins may be protected against chemical and enzymatic degradation when entrapped in microspheres (10,11). In drug delivery applications, poly(DL-lactide-co-glycolide) microspheres are being considered as the pharmaceutical products of the future.

A wide range of microencapsulation techniques have been developed to date (12). The selection of the technique depends on the nature of the polymer, the drug, and the intended use. When preparing controlled release microspheres, the choice of the optimal method has utmost importance for the efficient entrapment of the active substance. Pharmaceutically acceptable microencapsulation techniques using hydrophobic biodegradable polymers such as poly(lactide-co-glycolide) and poly(lactic acid) as matrix materials are divided into four categories (10):

1. Emulsion–solvent evaporation (o/w, w/o, w/o/w)
2. Phase separation (nonsolvent addition and solvent partitioning)

3. Interfacial polymerization
4. Spray drying

The solvent evaporation method involves the emulsification of an organic solvent (usually methylene chloride) containing dissolved polymer and dissolved/dispersed drug in an excess amount of aqueous continuous phase, with the aid of an agitator. The concentration of the emulsifier present in the aqueous phase affects the particle size and shape. When the desired emulsion droplet size is formed, the stirring rate is reduced and evaporation of the organic solvent is realized under atmospheric or reduced pressure at an appropriate temperature. Subsequent evaporation of the dispersed phase solvent yields solid polymeric microparticles entrapping the drug. The solid microparticles are recovered from the suspension by filtration, centrifugation, or lyophilization (13). Phase separation is a nonaqueous method that is suitable for encapsulation of both water-soluble and water-insoluble drugs, generally used for the encapsulation of peptides and proteins (14). In interfacial polymerization a capsule shell is formed at or on the surface of a droplet or particle by polymerization (12). Spray drying is used to protect sensitive substances from oxidation based on the atomization of a solution by compressed air and drying across a current of warm air (14).

II. BIODEGRADABLE POLYMERS FOR MICROSPHERE PREPARATION

Polymers used as matrices for drug delivery can be classified under three basic types: water-soluble polymers, biodegradable polymers, and nonbiodegradable polymers (15). Both natural and synthethic polymers are used as matrix materials in the preparation of biodegradable microspheres. Biopolymers used for drug delivery purposes are shown in Table 1 (10). A discussion about water-soluble and nonbiodegradable polymers will not be included in this chapter as the scope is to cover preparation of microspheres by solvent evaporation technique in which lactic/glycolic acid polymers are the most widely used type.

Lactic/Glycolic Acid Polymers

Over the past 20 years, there has been an explosion in the field of controlled drug delivery using biodegradable polymeric carriers. Among these, aliphatic polyesters, such as poly(lactic acid) (PLA), poly(glycolic acid) (PGA), and poly(lactide-co-glycolide) (PLGA) (Fig. 1) have attracted the most attention and have been evaluated extensively for controlled release of a variety of therapeutic substances like anticancer agents (16–19), antibiotics (20–23), hormone

Table 1 Examples of Biodegradable Polymers Used in Drug Delivery Systems

	I. Animal proteins	II. Animal polysaccharides	III. Plant polysaccharides
Natural polymers	Albumin	Chitin	Starch
	Collagen	Chitosan	Dextrin
	Gelatin	Hyaluronic acid	Dextran
	Fibrinogen		Alginic acid
	Casein		
	Fibrin		
	Poly(lactic acid)	Poly(β-hydroxybutyric acid)	Poly(ortho esters)
Synthetic polymers	Poly(lactic/glycolic acid)	Poly(ϵ-caprolactone)	Polyalkylcyanoacrylate
		Polyanhydrides	

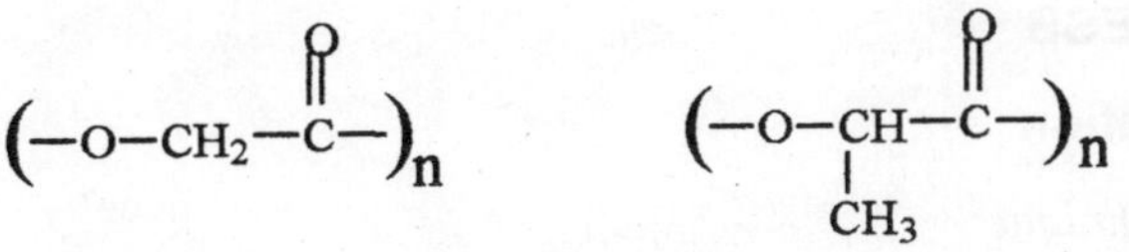

$$(-O-CH_2-\overset{\overset{\displaystyle O}{\|}}{C}-)_n \qquad (-O-\underset{\underset{\displaystyle CH_3}{|}}{CH}-\overset{\overset{\displaystyle O}{\|}}{C}-)_n$$

Figure 1 Structural formulae of (left) poly(lactic acid) and (right) poly(glycolic acid).

agonists and antagonists (24–26), nonsteroidal anti-inflammatory drugs (NSAIDs) (27–29), local anesthetics (30), contraceptives (31,32), and bioactive macromolecules (33–36). Various polymeric devices, including microspheres, microcapsules, nanoparticles, pellets, implants, and films, have been fabricated using these polymers for drug delivery. Biomaterial applications of biodegradable polyesters can be stated in brief as ligament reconstruction, vascular grafts, dental and fracture repairs, and surgical dressings (37,38). The medical uses of PLGA systems have been reviewed by Wise et al. (39).

Poly(glycolic acid) is the most hydrophilic member of the poly(α-ester) series and insoluble in organic solvents. It has a disadvantage of being too crystalline to be used for drug release (4). Another component of the PLGA polymer, i.e., PLA, has three forms due to the presence of a chiral center D(−), L(+), and racemic (DL) forms (40,41). PLA (lactic acid) is amorphous and is more hydrophobic than PGA, which is provided by the extra methyl group. PLA is a good candidate for drug matrix release. PLGA is a water-insoluble polymer; strength, hydrophobicity, and pliability are the significant physical advantages (42). As a polymeric vehicle, biocompability, biodegradability, predictability of degradation, ease of fabrication, and regulatory approval are features that make PLGA desirable for medical applications (43–46). A broad spectrum of performance characteristics can be reached by a careful manipulation of four key variables, including monomer stereochemistry, comonomer ratio, polymer chain linearity, and polymer molecular weight. PLGA polymers can be prepared in different molar ratios of lactic to glycolic acids as the proportion is critical in determining in vivo degradation rates (47) (Table 2).

Designing a sustained release parenteral dosage form requires an understanding of the physicochemical and biological properties of the related polymer, whereas successful microencapsulation depends on the selection of an appropriate preparative technique. In the past, several methods of microencapsulation have been employed for aliphatic polyesters. The most promising results were obtained by the emulsification solvent evaporation technique (48–51).

Table 2 In Vivo Biodegradation Times of Lactide/Glycolide Polymers

Polymer	Approx. biodegradation time (month)
Poly(L-lactide)	18–24
Poly(DL-lactide)	12–16
Poly(glycolide)	2–4
50:50 (DL-lactide-co-glycolide)	2
85:15 (DL-lactide-co-glycolide)	5

Source: Adapted from Ref. 47.

III. SOLVENT EVAPORATION PROCESS

A. Single-Emulsion Solvent Evaporation

1. O/W Emulsion Solvent Evaporation Technique

For emulsion solvent evaporation, there are basically two systems from which to choose: oil-in-water (o/w) or water-in-oil (w/o). Oil-in-water emulsions are more widely used than w/o emulsions due to the simplicity of the process and easy clean-up requirements for the final product (52). In this process, both the drug and the polymer should be insoluble in water, while a water-immiscible solvent is required for the polymer. A schematic representation of o/w emulsification–solvent evaporation technique is shown in Fig. 2 (53).

Problems relating to the efficient incorporation of water-soluble active substances into biodegradable polymer matrices using simple o/w emulsification with solvent evaporation is originating to a great extent from the separation and/or removal of water-soluble material into the aqueous continuous phase (54–56). Originally this technique was used by Beck et al. (57,58) to encapsulate progesterone. Afterward lipid-soluble drugs such as steroids (59), local anesthetics (60,61), bleomycin sulfate (62), doxorubicin (63), chlorpromazine (64), naltrexone, promethazine (65), 5-fluorouracil (15), HoAcAc, therapeutic radionuclide (66), nifedipine (67,68), and bovine serum albumin (69) were encapsulated successfully. In this process, methylene chloride (MC) and chloroform are the most common used solvents, whereas poly(vinyl alcohol) (PVA), gelatin, hydroxypropylmethylcellulose (HMPC), methylcellulose (MeC), and sodium oleate (SO) are widely used as emulsifiers. In the recent literature, active substances including testoesterone (70), β-estradiol (71), clonazepam (72), cisplatin (73), dexamethasone (74), salmon calcitonin (75,76) NSAIDs (27–29), and tumor necrosis factor–α (TNF-α) (77) have been reported as being encapsulated by the single-emulsion (o/w) technique. Details of dispersed phase polymer, dispersed phase solvent, emulsifier (type and concentration) concerning this technique for the above-mentioned drugs are given in Table 3.

Even MC is commonly used as a solvent for PLGA in the preparation of microparticles. Recently, ethyl acetate has seemed more favorable as it is considerably less toxic than MC and hence more likely to receive approval from regulatory bodies. MC is listed among class 2 solvents (solvents to be limited) in the first draft of the ICH guidelines, whereas ethyl acetate is a class 4 solvent (i.e., less toxic) (78,79).

In a study in which the effect of preparation solvent on the microencapsulation of β-estradiol was investigated, it was reported that encapsulation of β-estradiol is most efficient when the hormone is dissolved in ethyl acetate along with the PLGA prior to the formation of the o/w emulsion (71).

In general, solvent evaporation method is particularly suitable for the microencapsulation of lipophilic drugs that can be either dispersed or dissolved in the the dispersed phase of a volatile solvent. Clonazepam represents an interesting example of a lipophilic drug whose solubility properties make it difficult to form drug-loaded microspheres by the solvent evaporation process. A study by Benelli et al. (72) has demonstrated that during the manufacturing process clonazepam is drawn from MC into the continuous phase and there is crystallized more rapidly than the microspheres are formed and hardened. Hence crystals of drug were found outside of the microspheres due to the poor solubility of the drug in MC. Spray drying was found to be more suitable for the preparation of clonazepam-loaded PLGA microspheres. Kobayashi et al. (70) prepared poly(DL-lactide acid) microspheres containing testesterone by simple solvent evaporation process (o/w) and concluded that the effect of dispersed phase solvent on the surface morphology and drug loading was significant. Only 28% testosterone was incorporated in the case of MC (b.p. 39.95°C), whereas this value increased to 38% with chloroform (b.p. 61.15°C). Also, microscopic examination of the surface structure showed (Fig. 3) that a number

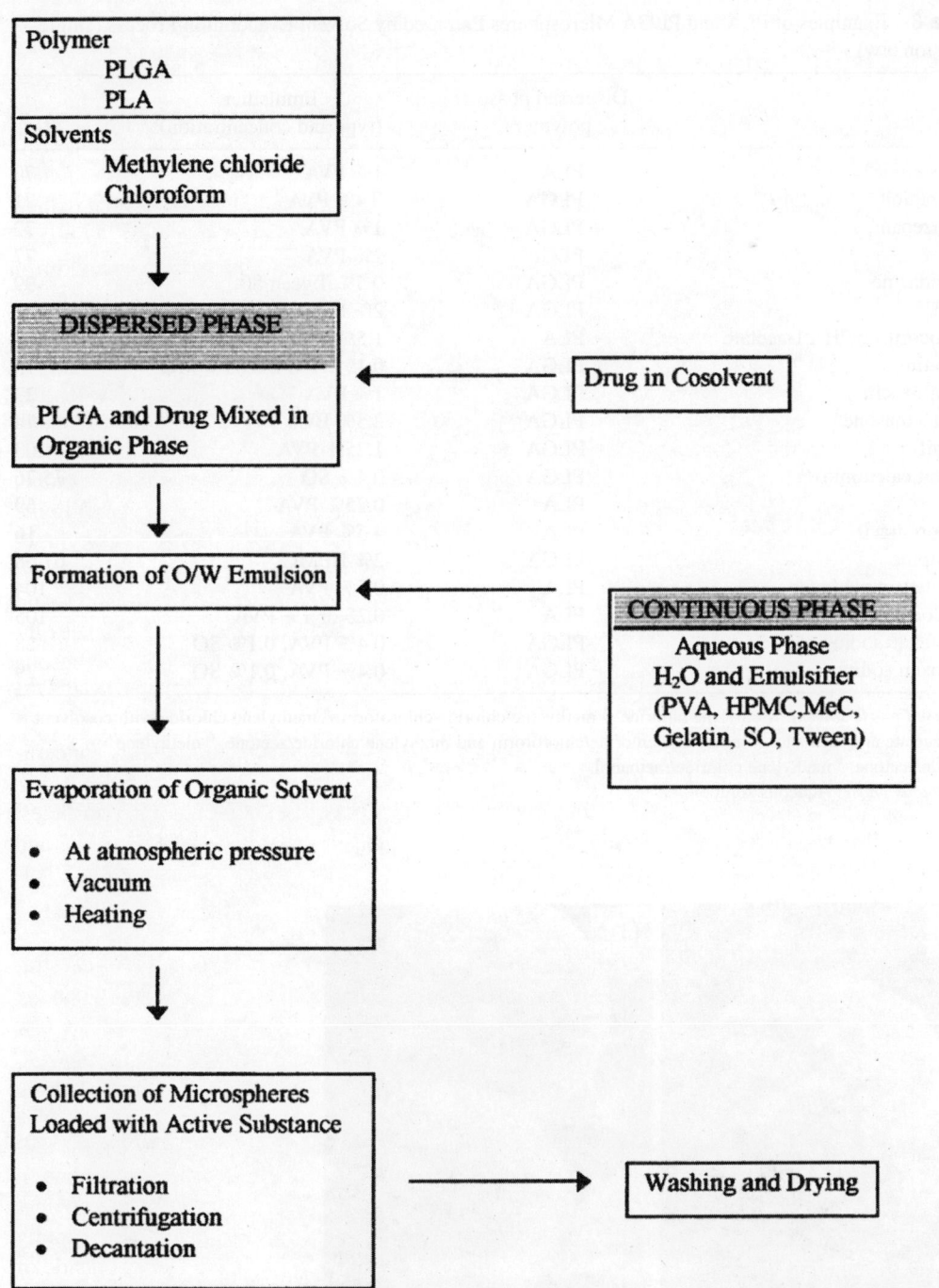

Figure 2 Schematic representation of the preparation of PLGA microspheres by o/w emulsification/solvent evaporation technique. (Adapted from Ref. 53.)

Table 3 Examples of PLA and PLGA Microspheres Prepared by Solvent Evaporation Process (single-emulsion o/w)

Drug	Dispersed phase polymer	Emulsifier (type and concentration)	Ref.
Testosterone[a]	PLA	1% PVA	70
β-Estradiol[b]	PLGA	0.4% PVA	71
Clonazepam[c]	PLGA	1% PVA	72
TNF-α	PLGA	2% PVA	77
Thioridazine	PLGA	0.5% Tween 80	99
BCNU	PLGA	2% PVA	102
Hydrocortisone/H-21-acetate	PLA	1.5% PVA	101
Cisplatin	PLGA	0.15% PVA, 0.05% MC	73
Ciprofloxacin	PLGA	1% PVA	23
Dexamethasone[d]	PLGA	2.5% PVA	74
Olvenil	PLGA	1.25% PVA	103
Salmon calcitonin	PLGA	0.4% SO	75,76
BSA	PLA	0.25% PVA	69
5-Fluorouracil	PLA	4.5% PVA	16
Nifedipine	PLGA	2% HPMC	67,68
Neurotensin analogue	PLA	0.5% PVA	104
Pseudoephedrine[e] HCl	PLA	0.25 or 1% PVA	105
Diclofenac sodium	PLGA	0.4% PVA, 0.1% SO	28
Naproxen sodium	PLGA	0.4% PVA, 0.1% SO	29

Dispersed phase solvent: Methylene chloride. [a] methylene chloride/chloroform, [b] methylene chloride/with cosolvent ethyl acetate and methanol, [c] methylene chloride/chloroform and methylene chloride/acetone, [d] methylene chloride/acetone, [e] methylene chloride/methanol.
Continuous phase: Aqueous solution.

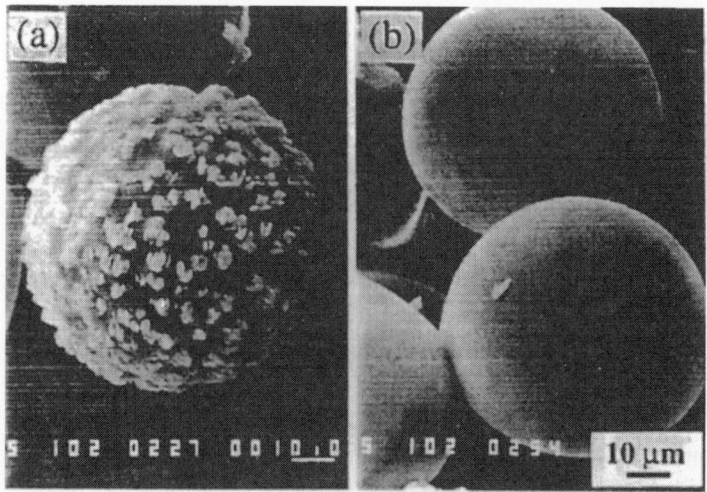

Figure 3 Microscopic view of drug-loaded PLA microspheres obtained with (a) methylene chloride and (b) chloroform.

of small drug crystals were deposited on the surface when the solvent was MC. In contrast, the drug-loaded PLA microspheres obtained with chloroform showed a highly homogeneous molecular dispersion of testosterone. Similar to this, Atkins et al. (20) also reported that high-percentage loading resulted in the initial deposition of vancomycin crystals in the surface layer of microspheres.

Although the solvent evaporation method seems to involve a relatively simple process, final product characteristics depend mainly on the formulation and process variables (Table 4). Garcia-Contreras et al. (73) prepared biodegradable cisplatin microspheres using PLGA (50:50) as the matrix polymer with the o/w solvent evaporation technique in which results revealed that mean particle size of the microspheres was inversely related to the stirring speed and emulsifier (PVA and MeC) concentration. Similar data were obtained by Jalil and Nixon (49) for PLA microspheres. Previous studies have shown that MeC results in stabilization of the initial emulsion when used at low concentration. Furthermore, formulations including MeC resulted in microspheres with a narrow particle size distribution as well as good sphericity as a result of good droplet formation during the evaporation process. Sansdrap and Moës (68) suggested that in order to obtain batches of microspheres with reproducible sizes, manufacturing factors such as emulsifier concentration, stirring rate, and organic phase volume should be under control. During the manufacturing process of nifedipine by an o/w single-emulsion process it was observed that for low HPMC amounts spherical microparticles for higher levels larger particles were obtained. For avoiding polymer aggregates, HPMC should be used in minimal (0.4%) concentration. It was also concluded that both dispersing agent and stirring rate were parameters of primary importance in the emulsification step.

2. Oil-in-Oil Emulsification–Solvent Evaporation Technique

The major problem of the o/w emulsification technique is the low encapsulation efficiency of moderately water-soluble and water-insoluble compounds (80). The drug can diffuse from the organic dispersed phase into the aqueous continuous phase, which results in poor entrapping. Water-soluble drugs such as theophylline, caffeine, and salicylic acid could not be loaded efficiently using an o/w emulsion method, whereas drugs with low water solubility such as diazepam, hydrocortisone, and progesterone were successfully entrapped in microspheres (81,82).

Oil-in-oil (sometimes referred as water-in-oil) emulsification process was developed for the encapsulation of highly water-soluble drugs. In this technique, polymer and drug, contained in a polar solvent such as acetonitrile, are emulsified into an immiscible lipophilic phase, with

Table 4 Various Formulation Factors Affecting Microencapsulation Process and Final Product

1. Polymer	Concentration, composition (hydrophilicity/hydrophobicity, amorphous crystalline), molecular weight, uncapped and capped terminal end group
2. Drug	Nature and solubility
3. Solvent	Nature (aqueous or nonaqueous)
4. Emulsifier	Nature and concentration
5. Emulsification process	Temperature, stirring/agitation speed, dispersed phase composition, continuous phase composition, dispersed phase/continuous phase ratio
6. Drug/polymer ratio	
7. Mode of solvent removal	

light mineral oil commonly being used, in the presence of an oil-soluble surfactant such as Span. However, an important drawback of using an oil external phase is cleaning up the final product. The oil has to be removed using organic solvents such as n-hexane (54). Diphenylhydramine hydrochloride (52), mitomycin C (83), adriamycin (18), cephradine and cefadroxil (84), phenobarbitone (85), and timolol maleate (86) are some examples of drugs that have been encapsulated by this procedure.

Atkins et al. (20) prepared spherical monolithic microspheres containing a range of vancomycin loadings with a honeycomb-like internal structure composed of PLGA 50:50 and 75:25 using an o/o (w/o) emulsification with solvent evaporation in which acetonitrile was used as dispersed phase solvent, with light mineral oil containing Span 40 at 2% concentration constructing the continuous phase. Authors reported that too rapid solvent evaporation resulted in a macroporous honeycomb-like matrix with a compressed periphery. Mean diameters of vancomycin-loaded PLGA 75:25 microspheres were larger than that PLGA 50:50 copolymer, indicating that mean microsphere diameter increased directly with fabrication polymer molecular weight and increased polymer viscosity. In the preparation of timolol maleate biodegradable microspheres by PLGA 50:50 copolymer by o/o emulsion technique (86), continuous phase consisted of sesame oil containing 2% Span-80 as emulsifier. By varying the PLGA concentration in the preparation procedure different particle sizes were obtained. Hydrophilic compounds, as well as glycine and its homopeptides diglycine, triglycine, tetraglycine, and homoglycine, were successfully entrapped using o/o emulsion and solvent evaporation technique (87). The inner phase consisted of micronized model compound suspended in DL-PLA solution in acetone while the external phase consisted of mineral oil including dissolved emulsifier (sorbitan sesquioleate). The authors reported that surface aggregation was minimum and yields were good.

Wang et al. (36) investigated the influence of formulation methods on the release of BSA containing PLGA 50:50 microspheres using o/o, o/w, and w/o/w emulsion methods. They reported that particles prepared by the o/o emulsion method were irregularly shaped, but complete entrapment of BSA was only achieved with this technique.

Hermann and Bodmeier (55,88,89) carried out a series of studies to evaluate various aqueous solvent evaporation methods. Somatostatin-containing microspheres were prepared using three aqueous and one nonaqueous methods based on the concept of solvent. The preparation conditions are summarized in Table 2 (55). Acceptable encapsulation efficiencies were obtained with all methods, regardless of physical state of drug and polymer type. The total volume of organic solvent and cosolvent content were found to be important preparation factors of the o/w cosolvent method. Replacing MC with ethyl acetate resulted in lower drug loadings. The preparation method affected the morphology and drug release of microspheres. A similar study realized with chlorpheniramine maleate (90) and various hydrophobic polymers could be successfully prepared with a nonaqueous solvent evaporation method.

B. Multiple-Emulsion Technique (w/o/w)

Multiple-emulsion or double-emulsion technique is appropriate for the efficient incorporation of water-soluble peptides, proteins, and other macromolecules (1,11,91–95). This method allows the encapsulation of water-soluble drugs with an external aqueous phase when compared to nonaqueous methods as the o/o solvent evaporation or organic phase separation. In brief (96), the polymers are dissolved in an organic solvent and emulsified into an aqueous drug solution to form a w/o emulsion. This primary emulsion is reemulsified into an aqueous solution containing an emulsifier to produce a multiple w/o/w dispersion. The organic phase acts as a barrier between the two aqueous compartments, preventing the diffusion of the active material toward the external aqueous phase. Microspheres manufactured by the (w/o/w method exhibit various morphologies such as porous or nonporous external polymer shell layers (97,98) enclosing hollow, macroporous, or microporous internal structures, depending on different parameters.

Hermann and Bodmeier (56) attempted to encapsulate the water-soluble peptide somatostatin acetate by classical solvent evaporation method (o/w) in which they could not obtain acceptable encapsulation efficiencies. Because of its high water solubility somatostatin acetate diffused into the external phase during microsphere preparation. Therefore they utilized w/o/w technique; micronized drug or an aqueous solution is dispersed in the organic polymer solution followed by emulsification into the external phase. Partitioning of the drug into the external phase was reported to be prevented.

In a recent study, O'Donnell and McGinity (99) prepared biodegradable microspheres of poly(DL-lactic-co-glycolic acid) containing thioridazine HCl using four types of emulsion solvent evaporation methods, including o/w, o/o, w/o/w, and w/o/o/o single-emulsion techniques and multiple-emulsion techniques, in order to investigate the effect of chemical interaction or hydrolytic degradation induced by encapsulated compounds. It was concluded that multiphase microspheres of the w/o/o/o type successfully prevent hydrolytic degradation of PLGA. Even the reactive substance thioridazine HCl was encapsulated; in addition, no change in release characteristics during storage was observed. Selection of the suitable solvent system for successful incorporation of active substances has a priority importance. Iwata et al. (77) reported that multiphase microspheres prepared by an anhydrous multiple-emulsion process had a significantly higher loading efficiency of intact TNF-α. In the w/o/w system the MC phase containing PLGA had a denaturing effect on TNF due to an interfacial interaction between the internal aqueous phase and the organic phase. The microencapsulation system for which acetonitrile and mineral oil were used as polymer solvent and evaporation medium TNF-α were incorporated into microspheres at approximately 80% or higher loading. The presence of sodium chloride in the continuous phase enabled the production of high-insulin-loaded

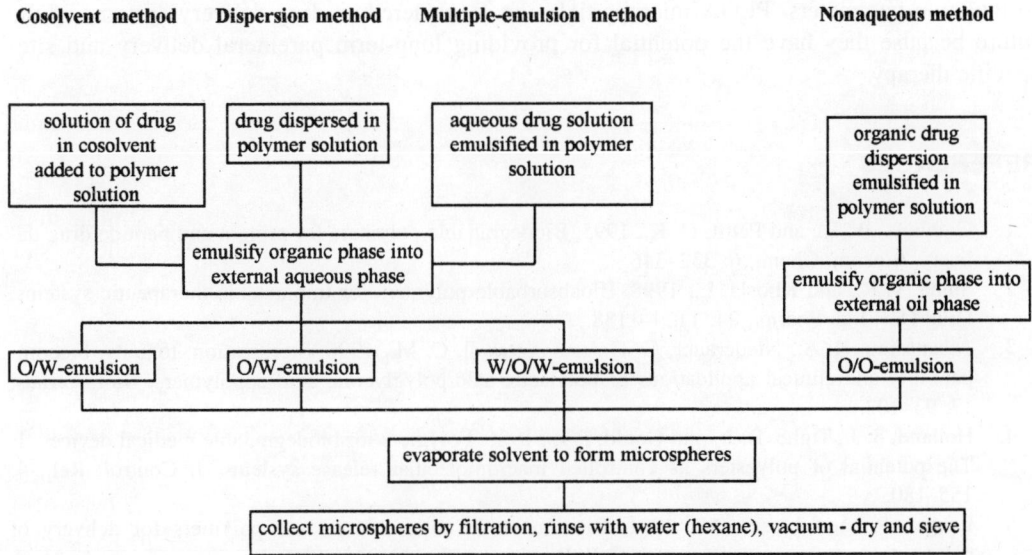

Figure 4 Schematic diagram of the preparation of somatostatin microspheres with various types of solvent evaporation methods. (Adapted from Ref. 56.)

microparticles in w/o/w emulsion solvent evaporation technique. Authors also reported that sizes of the microparticles were increased with increasing sodium chloride content. When employing the w/o/w solvent evaporation method, changing the pH of the external aqueous phase might modulate the entrapment and delivery from PLGA microspheres. Leo et al. (100) microencapsulated the milk protein β-betaglobulin into microspheres by a multiple emulsion/solvent evaporation of the pH of the outer aqueous phase on protein encapsulation and release. The investigators suggested that reducing the solubility of a protein in the external aqueous phase allowed the product of microspheres with a better encapsulation efficiency.

In some of the recently reported work, the spray-drying technique was suggested to have a number of advantages over the w/o/w technique. Bittner et al. (34) found that recombinant human erythropoietin (rhEPO) microparticles prepared by spray drying yielded higher entrapment of protein, lower content of high molecular weight EPO aggregates, and lower residual amounts of MC than those prepared by the w/o/w technique.

Giunchedi et al. (101) prepared PLA microspheres containing steroids using spray drying, o/w, and w/o/w emulsifications as preparation methods. They found that in the case of hydrocortisone, spray drying produced the highest loading and encapsulation efficiency compared to both single- and double-emulsion methods.

IV. CONCLUSION

Emulsification/solvent evaporation techniques offer a versatile, easy, and practical method for the manufacture of biodegradable microspheres. This technique makes possible the entrapment of a wide range of drugs having different physical properties and solubility characteristics. PLGA polymers emerged as the most promising synthetic biodegradable polymeric carriers because of their excellent biocompability and biodegradability. Its approval by the U.S. Food and Drug Administration for drug delivery applications makes it very attractive from a pharmaceutical perspective. It is possible to achieve various drug release profiles by the regulation of copolymer ratio, molecular weight, size of the microspheres, drug loading, porosity, and other formulation parameters. PLGA microparticles are considered as drug delivery systems of the future because they have the potential for providing long-term parenteral delivery and site-specific therapy.

REFERENCES

1. Gombotz, W. R., and Pettit, D. K., 1995. Biodegradable polymers for protein and peptide delivery. Bioconj. Chem., 6: 332–346.
2. Sinha, V. R., and Khosla, L., 1998. Bioabsorbable polymers for implantable therapeutic systems. Drug Dev. Ind. Pharm., 24: 1129–1138.
3. Athanasiou, K. A., Niederauer, G. G., and Agrawal, C. M., 1996. Sterilization, toxicity, biocompatibility and clinical applications of polylactic acid/polyglycolic acid copolymers. Biomaterials, 17: 93–102.
4. Holland, S. J., Tighe, B. J., and Gould, P. L., 1986. Polymers for biodegradable medical devices. 1. The potential of polyesters as controlled macromolecular release systems. J. Control. Rel., 4: 155–180.
5. Langer, R., and Moses, M., 1991. Biocompatible controlled release polymers for delivery of polypeptides and growth factors. J. Cell. Biochem., 45: 340–345.
6. Rafler, G., and Jobmann, M., 1994. Controlled release systems of biodegradable polymers. Pharm. Ind., 56: 565–570.

7. Göpferich, A., 1996. Mechanism of polymer degradation and erosion. Biomaterials, 17: 103–114.
8. Göpferich, A., 1997. Erosion of composite polymer matrices. Biomaterials, 18: 397–403.
9. Göpferich, A., 1996. Polymer degradation and erosion: mechanisms and applications, Eur. J. Pharm. Biopharm., 42: 1–11.
10. Okada, H., and Toguchi, H., 1995. Biodegradable microspheres in drug delivery. Crit. Rev. Ther. Drug Carrier. Syst., 12: 1–99.
11. Crotts, G., and Park, T. G., 1998. Protein delivery from poly(lactic-co-glycolic acid) biodegradable microspheres: release kinetics and stability issues. J. Microencap., 15: 699–713.
12. Thies, C., 1996. A survey of microencapsulation processes In: S. Benita (Ed.), Microencapsulation, Marcel Dekker, New York, pp. 1–21.
13. Watts, P. J., Davies, M. C., and Melia, C. D., 1990. Microencapsulation using emulsification/solvent evaporation: an overview of techniques and applications. Crit. Rev. Ther. Drug Carrier Syst., 7: 235–258.
14. Benoit, J. P., Marchais, H., Rolland, H., and Velde, V. V., 1996. Biodegradable microspheres: advances in production technology. In: S. Benita (Ed.), Microencapsulation, Marcel Dekker, New York, pp. 35–72.
15. Dunn, R. L., 1991. Polymeric Matrices. In: R. L. Dunn and R. M. Ottenbrite (Eds.), Polymeric Drugs and Drug Delivery Systems, American Chemical Society, Washington, DC, pp. 11–23.
16. Çiftçi, K., Kaş, H. S., Hıncal, A. A., Ercan, M. T., Güven, O., and Ruacan, Ş., 1996. In vitro and in vivo evaluation of PLAGA (50:50) microspheres containing 5-fluorouracil prepared by a solvent evaporation method. Int. J. Pharm. 131: 73–82.
17. Sakakura, C., Takahashi, T., Hagiwara, A., Itoh, M., Sasabet, T., Lee, M., and Shobayashi, S., 1992. Controlled release of cisplatin from lactic acid oligomer microspheres incorporating cisplatin: in vitro studies. J. Control. Rel., 22: 69–74.
18. Wada, R., Hyon, S. H., Ike, O., Watenaba, S., Shimizo, Y., and Ikada, Y., 1988. Preparation of lactic acid oligomer microspheres containing anticancer drugs by o/o type solvent evaporation process. Polym. Mater. Sci. Eng., 59: 803–806.
19. Kyo, M., Hyon, S.-H., and Ikada, Y., 1995. Effects of preparation conditions of cisplatin-loaded microspheres on the in vitro release. J. Control. Rel., 35: 73–82.
20. Atkins, T. W., Peacock, S. J., and Yates, D. J., 1998. Incorporation and release of vancomycin from poly(D,L-lactide-co-glycolide) microspheres. J. Microencap., 15: 31–44.
21. Jeyanthi, R., Akiyama, A., Roberts, F. D., Van Hamont, J., and Friden, P., 1997. One-month controlled release of antimicrobial peptide from biodegradable poly(lactide/glycolide) microspheres for the treatment of periodontitis. Proc. Int. Symp. Control. Rel. Bioact. Mater., 24: 883–884.
22. Van Hamont, J. E., Madden, E. F., Wood, B. A., Jacob, E., and Setterstrom, J. A., 1996. Evaluation of solvent extraction and solvent evaporation procedures for production of tobramycin-releasing microspheres. Proc. Int. Symp. Control. Rel. Bioact. Mater., 23: 365–366.
23. Martinez, B., Lairion, F., Pena, P. B., Di Rocco, P., and Nacucch o, M. C., 1997. In vitro ciprofloxacin release from poly(lactide-co-glycolide)microspheres. J. Microencap., 14: 155–161.
24. Cleland, J. L., Duenas, J. Y., Chu, H., Mukku, V., Mac, A., Roussakis, M., Yeung, D., Brooks, D., Maa, Y.-F., Hsu, C., and Jones, A. J. S., 1995. One month continuous release recombinant human growth hormone-PLGA formulations. Proc. Int. Symp. Control. Rel. Bioact. Mater., 22: 149.
25. Cleland, J. L., and Jones, A. J. S., 1996. Stable formulations of recombinant human growth hormone and interferon-γ for microencapsulation in biodegradable microspheres. Pharm. Res., 13: 1464–1475.
26. Cleland, J. L., Mac, A., Boyd, B., Yang, J., Duenas, E. T., Yeung, D., Brooks, D., Hsu, C., Chu, H., Mukku, V., and Jones, A. J. S., 1997. The stability of recombinant human growth hormone in poly(lactic-co-glycolic acid) (PLGA) microspheres. Pharm Res., 14: 420–425.
27. Guiziou, B., Armstrong, D. J., Elliot, P. N. C., Ford, J. L., and Rostron, C., 1996. Investigation of in vitro release characteristics of NSAID-loaded polylactic acid microspheres. J. Microencap., 13: 701–708.
28. Tunçay, M., Çalış, S., Kaş, S., Ercan, M. T., Ertürk, H., and Hıncal, A. A., 1998. Diclonefac sodium incorporated biodegradable microspheres. II: Antiinflammatory activity in the knee

joints of rabbits. Conference on Challenges for Drug Delivery and Pharmaceutical Technology, 9–11 June, Tokyo, pp. 188.
29. Bozdağ, S., Çalış, S., Kaş, S., Çapan, Y., Ercan, M. T., Ertürk, H., Hıncal, A. A., 1998. Intraarticular administration of biodegradable microspheres containing naproxen sodium. AAPS Annual Meeting, 15–19 November, San Fransisco.
30. Le Corre, P., Rytting, J. H., Gajan, V., Chevanne, F., and Le Verge, R., 1997. In vitro controlled kinetics of local anaesthetics from poly(D,L-lactide) and poly(lactide-co-glycolide) microspheres. J. Microencap., 14: 243–255.
31. Okada, H., 1997. One- and three-month release injectable microspheres of the LH-RH superagonist leuprorelin acetate. Adv. Drug Del. Rev., 28: 43–70.
32. Ogawa, Y., Yamamoto, M., Okado, H., Yashiki, T., and Shimamoto, T., 1988. A new technique to efficiently entrap leuprolide acetate into microcapsules of polylactic acid or copoly(lactic/glycolic) acid. Chem. Pharm. Bull., 36: 1095–1103.
33. Chen, l., Apte, R. N., and Cohen, S., 1997. Characterization of PLGA microspheres for the controlled delivery of IL-1α for tumor immunotherapy. J. Control. Rel., 43: 261–272.
34. Bittner, B., Morlock, M., Koll, H., Winter, G., and Kissel, T., 1998. Recombinant human erythropoietin (rhEPO) loaded poly(lactide-co-glycolide) microspheres: influence of the encapsulation technique and polymer purity on microsphere characteristics. Eur. J. Pharm. Biopharm., 45: 295–305.
35. Jeyanthi, R., Thanoo, B. C., Mehta, R. C., and DeLuca, P. P., 1996. Effect of solvent removal technique on the matrix characteristics of poly lactide/glycolide microspheres for peptide delivery. J. Control. Rel., 38: 235–244.
36. Wang, H. T., Schmitt, E., Flanagan, D. R., and Linhardt, R. J., 1991. Influence of formulation methods on the in vitro controlled release of protein from poly(ester) microspheres. J. Control. Rel., 17: 23–32.
37. Athanasiou, K. A., Niederauer, G. G., Agrawal, C. M., and Landsman, S., 1995. Applications of biodegradable lactides and glycolides in podiatry. Imp. Biomater., 12: 475–495.
38. Tanzawa, H., Biomedical polymers: current status and overview. 1993. In: T. Tsuruta, T. Hayashi, K. Kataoka, K. Ishihara, and Y. Kimura (Eds.), Biomedical Applications of Polymeric Materials, CRC Press, Boca Raton, FL, pp. 1–15.
39. Wise, D. L., Fellman, T. D., Sanderson, J. E., and Wentworth, W. L., 1979. Lactic/glycolic acid polymers. In: G. Gregoriadis (Ed.), Drug Carriers in Biology and Medicine. Academic Press, New York, pp. 237–270.
40. Gogolewski, S., and Mainil-Varlet, P., The effect of thermal treatment on sterility, molecular and mechanical properties of various polylactides. 1. Poly(L-lactide). Biomaterials, 17: 523–528.
41. Kitchell, J. P., and Wise, D. L., 1985, Poly(lactic/glycolic acid) biodegradable drug polymer matrix systems. In: K. J. Widder and R. Green (Eds.), Methods in Enzymology, Vol. 112. Academic Press, New York, pp. 436–448.
42. Gogolewski, S., and Mainil-Varlet, P., 1997. Effect of thermal treatment on sterility molecular and mechanical properties of various polylactides.2. Poly(D/L lactide) and poly(L/DL-lactide), Biomaterials, 18:251–255.
43. Zignani, M., Merkli, A., Sintzel, M. B., Bernatchez, S. F., Kloeti, W., Heller, J., Tabatabay, C., and Gurny, R., 1997. New generation of poly(ortho esters): synthesis, characterization, kinetics, sterilization and biocompatibility. J. Control. Rel., 48: 115–129.
44. Spenlehauer, G., Vert, M., Benoit, J. P., and Boddaert, A., 1989. In vitro and in vivo degradation of poly (D,L lactic/glycolic acid) type microspheres made by solvent evaporation methods. Biomaterials, 10: 557–563.
45. Heller, J., 1993. Polymers for controlled parenteral delivery of peptides and proteins. Adv. Drug Del. Rev. 10:163–204.
46. Vert, M., Mauduit, J., and Li, S., 1994. Biodegradation of PLA/GA polymers: increasing complexity. Biomaterials, 15: 1209–1213.
47. Lewis, D. H., 1990. Controlled release of bioactive agents from lactide/glycolide polymers. In: M. Chasin and R. Langer (Eds.), Biodegradable Polymers as Drug Delivery Systems, Marcel Dekker, New York, pp. 1–41.

48. Jalil, R., 1990. Biodegradable poly(lactic acid) and poly(lactide-co-glycolide) polymers in sustained drug delivery. Drug Dev. Ind. Pharm., 16: 2353–2367.
49. Jalil, R., and Nixon, J. R., 1989. Microencapsulation using poly(L-lactic acid). I: Microcapsule properties affected by the preparative technique. J. Microencap., 6: 473–484.
50. Jalil, R., and Nixon, J. R., 1990. Microencapsulation using poly(L-lactic acid) II: Preparative variables affecting microcapsule properties. J. Microencap., 7: 25–39.
51. Sprockel, O. L., and Prapaitrakul, W., 1990. A comparison of microencapsulation by various emulsion techniques. Int. J. Pharm., 58: 123–127.
52. Huang, H.-P., and Ghebre-Sellassie, I., 1989. Preparation of microspheres of water-soluble pharmaceuticals. J. Microencap., 6: 219–225.
53. Jalil, R. and Nixon, J. R., 1990. Biodegradable poly(lactic acid) and poly(lactide-co-glycolide) microcapsules: problems associated with preparative techniques and release properties. J. Microencap., 7: 297–325.
54. Arshady, R., 1990. Microspheres and microcapsules, a survey of manufacturing techniques. III. Solvent evaporation. Polym. Eng. Sci. 30: 915–924.
55. Bodmeier, R., and McGinity, J. W., 1988. Solvent selection in the preparation of poly(DL-lactide) microspheres prepared by the solvent evaporation method. Int. J. Pharm., 43: 179–186.
56. Hermann, J., and Bodmeier, R., 1998. Biodegradable, somatostatin acetate containing microspheres prepared by various aqueous and non-aqueous solvent evaporation methods. Eur. J. Pharm. Biopharm., 45: 75–82.
57. Beck, L. R., Cowsar, D. R., Lewis, D. H., Cosgrove, R. J., Ridel, C. T., Lowry, S., and Epperly, T., 1979. A new long acting injectable microcapsule system for administration of progesterone. Fertil. Steril., 31: 545.
58. Beck, L. R., Cowsar, D. R., Lewis, D. H., Gibson, J. W., and Flowers, C. E., 1979. New long acting injectable microcapsule contraceptive system. Am. J. Obstet. Gynecol., 135: 419.
59. Cavalier, M., Benoit, J. P., and Thies, C., 1986. The formulation and characterization of hydrocortisone loaded poly(D,L-lactide) microspheres. J. Pharm. Pharmacol., 38: 249–253.
60. Wakiyama, N., Juni, K., and Nakano, M., 1982. Influence of physicochemical properties of poly(lactic acid) on the characterization and in vitro release patterns of poly(lactic acid) microspheres containing local anaesthetics. Chem. Pharm. Bull., 30: 2621–2628.
61. Wakiyama, N., Juni, K., and Nakano, M., 1982. Preparation and evaluation in vitro and in vivo of poly(lactic acid) microspheres containing dibucaine. Chem. Pharm. Bull., 30: 3719–3727.
62. Juni, K., Ogata, J., Matsui, N., Kubota, M., and Nakano, M., 1985. Control of release rate of bleomycin from poly(lactic acid) microspheres by additives. Chem. Pharm. Bull., 33: 1609–1614.
63. Juni, K., Ogata, J., Nakano, M., Ichihara, T., Mori, K., and Akagi, M., 1985. Preparation and evaluation in vitro and in vivo of poly(lactic acid) microspheres containing doxorubicin. Chem. Pharm. Bull., 33: 313–318.
64. Suzuki, K., and Price, J. C., 1985. Microencapsulation and dissolution properties of neuroleptic in a biodegradable polymer, poly (D,L-lactide). J. Pharm. Sci., 74: 21–24.
65. Cha, Y., and Pitt, C. G., 1989. The acceleration of degradation-controlled drug delivery from polyester microspheres. J. Control. Rel., 8: 259–265.
66. Mumper, R. J., and Jay, M., 1992. Biodegradable radiotherapeutic polyester microspheres: optimization and in-vitro/in-vivo evaluation. J. Control. Rel., 18: 193–204.
67. Sansdrap, P., and Moës A. J., 1998. Influence of additives on the release profile of nifedipine from poly(DL-lactide-co-glycolide) microspheres. J. Microencap., 15: 545–553.
68. Sansdrap, P. and Moës A. J., 1993. Influence of manufacturing parameters on the size characteristics and the release profiles of nifedipine from poly (DL-lactide-co-glycolide) microspheres. Int. J. Pharm., 98: 157–164.
69. Guo, J. H., 1994. Preparation methods of biodegradable microspheres on bovine serum albumin loading efficiency and release profiles. Drug Dev. Ind. Pharm., 20: 2535–2545.
70. Kobayashi, D., Tsubuku, S., Yamanaka, H., Asano, M., Miyajima, M., and Yoshida, M., 1998. In vivo characteristics of injectable poly(DL-Lactic Acid) microspheres for long-acting drug delivery. Drug Dev. Ind. Pharm., 24: 819–825.

71. Birnbaum, B. T., Kosmala, D. J., and Brannon-Peppas, L., 1998. Effect of preparation solvent on the encapsulation and release of β-estradiol from PLGA microparticles. Proc. Int. Symp. Control. Rel. Bioact. Mater., 25: 152–153.
72. Benelli, P., Conti, B., Genta, I., Costantini, M., and Montarani, L., 1998. Clonazepam microencapsulation in poly-D,L-lactide-co-glycolide microspheres. J. Microencap., 15: 431–443.
73. Garcia-Contreras, L., Abu-Izza, K., and Robert Lu, D., 1997. Biodegradable cisplatin microspheres for direct brain injection: preparation and characterization. Pharm. Dev. Technol., 2: 53–65.
74. Song, C. X., Labhasetwar, V., Murphy, H., Qu, X., Humphrey, W. R., Shebuski, R. J., and Levy, R. J., 1997. Formulation and characterization of biodegradable nanoparticles for intravascular local drug delivery. J. Control. Rel., 43: 197–212.
75. Mehta, R. C., Jeyanthi, R. Calis, S. Thanoo, B. C., Burton, K. W., and DeLuca, P. P., 1994. Biodegradable microspheres as depot system for parenteral delivery of peptide drugs. J. Control. Rel., 29: 375–384.
76. Jeyanthi, R., Mehta, R. C., Thanoo, B. C., and DeLuca, P. P., 1997. Effect of processing parameters on the properties of peptide-containing PLGA microspheres. J. Microencap., 14: 163–174.
77. Iwata, M., Tanaka, T., Nakamura, Y., Mc Ginity, J. W., 1998. Selection of the solvent system for the preparation of poly(D,L-lactic-co-glycolic acid) microspheres containing tumor necrosis factor-alpha (TNF-α). Int. J. Pharm., 160: 145–156.
78. International Conference on Harmonization of Technical Requirements for Human Use (ICH) Residual Solvents, first draft (1995).
79. Witschi, C., Doelker, E., 1997. Residual solvents in pharmaceutical products: acceptable limits, influences on physicochemical properties, analytical methods and documented values. Eur. J. Pharm. Biopharm., 43: 215–242.
80. Jain, R., Shah, N. H., Malick, A. W., and Rhodes, C. T., 1998. Controlled drug delivery by biodegradable poly (ester) devices: different preparative approaches. Drug Dev. Ind. Pharm., 24: 703–727.
81. Fong, J. W., Nazarena, J. P., Pearson, J., and Maulding, H. V., 1986. Evaluation of biodegradable microcapsules prepared by solvent evaporation process using sodium oleate as emulsifier. J. Control. Rel., 3: 119–130.
82. Bodmeier, R., and McGinity, J. W., 1987. The preparation and evaluation of drug containing poly(D,L-lactide) microspheres formed by the solvent evaporation, Pharm. Res., 4: 465–471.
83. Tsai, D. C., Howard, S. A., Hogan, T. F., Malanga, C. J., Kandzari, S. J., and Ma, J. K. H., 1986. Preparation and in vitro evaluation of poly(lactic acid) mitomycin-C microcapsules. J. Microencap., 3: 181–193.
84. Uchida, T., and Goto, S., 1988. Biopharmaceutical evaluation of sustained-release ethyl cellulose microcapsules containing cefadroxil and cephradine using beagle dogs. Chem. Pharm. Bull., 36: 2135.
85. Jalil, R., and Nixon, J. R., 1990. Microencapsulation using poly(L-lactic acid). IV. Release properties of microcapsules containing phenobarbitone. J. Microencap., 7: 41–52.
86. Sturesson, C., Carlfors, J., Edsman, K., and Andersson M., 1993. Preparation of biodegradable poly(lactic-co-glycolic) acid microspheres and their in vitro release of timolol maleate. Int. J. Pharm., 89: 235–244.
87. Pradhan, R. S., and Vasavada, R. C., 1994. Formulation and in vitro release study on poly(DL-lactide) microspheres containing hydrophilic compounds: glycine homopeptides. J. Control. Rel., 30: 143–154.
88. Hermann, J., and Bodmeier, R., 1995. Somatostatin containing biodegradable microspheres prepared by a modified solvent evaporation method based on w/o/w multiple emulsions. Int. J. Pharm. 126: 129–138.
89. Hermann, J., and Bodmeier, R., 1995. The effect of particle microstructure on the somatostatin release from poly(lactide) microspheres prepared by a w/o/w solvent evaporation method. J. Control. Rel., 36: 63–71.
90. Bodmeier, R., Wang, H., and Herrmann, J., 1994. Microencapsulation of chlorpheniramine maleate, a drug with intermediate solubility properties, by a non-aqueous solvent evaporation technique. STP Pharma Sci., 4: 275–281.

91. Blanco, D., and Alonso, M. J., 1998. Protein encapsulation and release from poly(lactide-co-glycolide) microspheres: effect of the protein and polymer properties and of the co-encapsulation of surfactants. Eur. J. Pharm. Biopharm., 45: 285–294.
92. Okada, H., Yamamota, M., Heya, T., Inoue, Y., Kamei, S., Ogawa, Y., and Toguchi, H., 1994. Drug delivery using biodegradable microspheres. J. Control. Rel., 28: 121–129.
93. Park, T. G., Lu, W., and Crotts, G., 1995. Importance of in vitro experimental conditions on protein release kinetics, stability and polymer degradation in protein encapsulated poly(D,L-lactic acid-co-glycolic acid) microspheres. J. Control. Rel., 33: 211–222.
94. Bodmer, D., Kissel, T., and Traechslin, E., 1992. Factors influencing the release of peptides and proteins from biodegradable parenteral depot systems. J. Control. Rel., 21: 129–138.
95. Couvreur, P., Prieto, M. J., Puisieux, F., Raques, B., and Fattal, E., 1997. Multiple emulsion technology for the design of microspheres containing peptides and oligopeptides. Adv. Drug Del. Rev., 28: 85–96.
96. Sah, H. K., Toddywala, R., and Chien, Y. W., 1995. Biodegradable microcapsules prepared by a w/o/w technique: effects of shear force to make a primary w/o emulsion on their morphology and protein release. J. Microencap., 12: 59–69.
97. Crotts, G., and Park, T. G., 1995. Preparation of porous and nonporous biodegradable polymeric hollow microspheres. J. Control. Rel., 35: 91–105.
98. Crotts, G., Sah, H., and Park, T. G., 1997. Adsorption determines in-vitro protein release rate from biodegradable microspheres: quantitative analysis of surface area during degradation. J. Control. Rel., 47: 101–111.
99. O'Donnell, P. B., and McGinity J. W., 1998. Influence of processing on the stability and release properties of biodegradable microspheres containing thioridazine hydrochloride. Eur. J. Pharm. Biopharm., 45: 83–94.
100. Leo, E., Pecquet, S., Rojas, J., Couvreur, P., and Fattal, E., 1998. Changing the pH of the external aqueous phase may modulate protein entrapment and delivery from poly(lactide-co-glycolide) microspheres prepared by a w/o/w solvent evaporation method. J. Microencap., 15: 421–430.
101. Giunchedi, P., Alpar, H. O., and Conte U., 1998. PDLLA microspheres containing steroids: spray-drying, o/w and w/o/w emulsifications as preparation methods. J. Microencap., 15: 185–195.
102. Painbeni, T., Venier-Julienne, M. C., and Benoit, J. P., 1998. Internal morphology of poly(D,L-lactide-co-glycolide) BCNU-loaded microspheres. Influence on drug stability. Eur. J. Pharm. Biopharm., 45: 31–39.
103. Pak, S. J., Duong, H., Galloway, R., Wood, B. A., Vook, N., and Van Hamont, J. E., 1997. Microencapsulation of olvanil using 50:50 DL-poly(lactide-co-glycolide) using solvent evaporation processes. Proc. Int. Symp. Control. Rel. Bioact. Mater., 24: 639–640.
104. Yamakawa, I., Tsushima, Y., Machida, R. and Watanabe, S., 1992. Preparation of neurotensin analogue-containing poly(DL-lactic acid) microspheres formed by oil-in-water solvent evaporation. J. Pharm Sci., 81: 899–903.
105. Bodmeier, R., Chen, H., Tyle, P., and Jarosz, P., 1991. Pseudoephedrine HCl microspheres formulated into an oral suspension dosage form. J. Control. Rel., 15: 65–77.

17

Nanosuspensions: A Formulation Approach for Poorly Soluble and Poorly Bioavailable Drugs

R. H. Müller, B. H. L. Böhm, and M. J. Grau
Free University of Berlin, Berlin, Germany

I. INTRODUCTION: BASIC PROBLEM OF POORLY SOLUBLE DRUGS

Poor solubility is a major obstacle in the development of drug formulations. In many cases the poor solubility is associated with poor bioavailability. In addition, low-solubility drugs possess a low dissolution velocity. The challenge is to circumvent this problem by designing sophisticated delivery systems. Basically, drugs can be poorly soluble in:

1. Water and aqueous media,
2. Aqueous and (simultaneously) organic media

In the case of drugs being poorly soluble in aqueous media, a range of formulation approaches are available (1) such as the use of solubilizing solutions, complexing agents such as cyclodextrins, and mixtures of water with organic media (e.g., water–ethanol, water–propylene glycol). However, for many drugs these approaches do not lead to a sufficiently high increase in solubility, dissolution velocity, and subsequent bioavailability. Especially for drugs that are simultaneously poorly soluble in water and organic media, these approaches are of limited success (e.g., solubilizing solutions) or cannot be used at all (e.g., mixture of water and organic media). The traditional formulation for such drugs is micronization by a jet mill or using wet milling. Micronization leads to an increase in surface area and subsequently, according to the Noyes–Whitney equation, to an increase in the dissolution velocity. However, micronization is only an efficient tool in case the dissolution velocity is the rate-limiting factor for absorption, i.e., the factor limiting the bioavailability. It does not work in case the poor saturation solubility itself is the rate-limiting factor.

II. NANOPARTICLES MADE FROM POORLY SOLUBLE DRUGS

The transfer of drug microparticles to drug nanoparticles was the next step for further improvement of the bioavailability of poorly soluble drugs. There are basically three formulation principles:

Hydrosols,
NanoCrystals, and
Nanosuspensions (DissoCubes)

These systems differ in their method of production and in their physicochemical properties.

A. Hydrosols

Hydrosols are prepared by precipitation, i. e., addition of solvent to the nonsolvent or fast mixing of both (2–5). Of course, the necessity of dissolving the drug at least in one solvent limits the applicability of this approach. Drugs that are simultaneously poorly soluble in all solvents cannot be processed.

Production of hydrosols on lab scale is performed by mixing solvent and nonsolvent in a static blender (e.g., type SMV, Sulzer & Co., CH-Winterthur; mixing capacity: 3 L/h). Fast mixing is essential to pass the Ostwald–Mier region in the precipitation process, quickly leading to a highly dispersed product. A priori, the precipitation process needs to be well controlled to ensure the formation of nanoparticles. Typically, a normal precipitation leads to particles being in the lower micrometer range (6). A basic problem is the physical stabilization of the obtained suspension to avoid particle aggregation and crystal growth due to Ostwald ripening. A convenient method of stabilization is the immediate spray drying of the produced hydrosol. Before spray drying, 10% lactose or 5% mannitol is added to the hydrosol; the dry product can be stored for several years (2). In contrast to micronized products, the hydrosols can be injected intravenously. Due to the large surface area of the particles and large dissolution volume (blood in the body) a fast dissolution of the drug takes place. Intravenous administration of ciclosporine hydrosol compared to the trade product Sandimmun KZI (concentrate for infusion) showed that the hydrosol behaved as a micellar solution. No difference in the body distribution of the drug was found between the formulations (2,3).

Critical or potentially critical when formulating drugs as hydrosol is the need to control the precipitation conditions, possible simultaneous formation of microparticles, the need to use surfactants which are able to sufficiently stabilize the suspension but are not necessarily accepted for, say, intravenous use, and the necessity to use organic solvents (solvent residues).

B. NanoCrystals

An alternative is the reduction in drug particle size by a milling process. Milling instruments to be used are:

1. Jet mill
2. Colloid mill (wet milling)
3. Pearl mill

A basic problem when applying milling techniques is that the product contains not only nanoparticles but also a fraction of particles in the micrometer range. Jet milling—typically used for micronization—leads to relatively broad particle size distributions ranging from approximately a few hundred nanometers to about 25 μm, which means only a few percent of the product are nanoparticles (Fig. 1). Erosion of materials from the balls has been reported when using a pearl mill (7). Ball mill materials used are zircon oxide and glass. Erosion of these low-toxicity materials is considered as not critical when preparing nanoparticles for oral and peroral administration (e.g., NanoCrystals in pellets or tablets). Depending on the mill type and batch volume, the milling process itself can last up to a few days or a week, which means that it can be time consuming.

The company NanoSystems (Collegeville, PA, USA) produces drug nanoparticles by using pearl mills (8–10). The registered trade name for their product is NanoCrystals. Intensive in

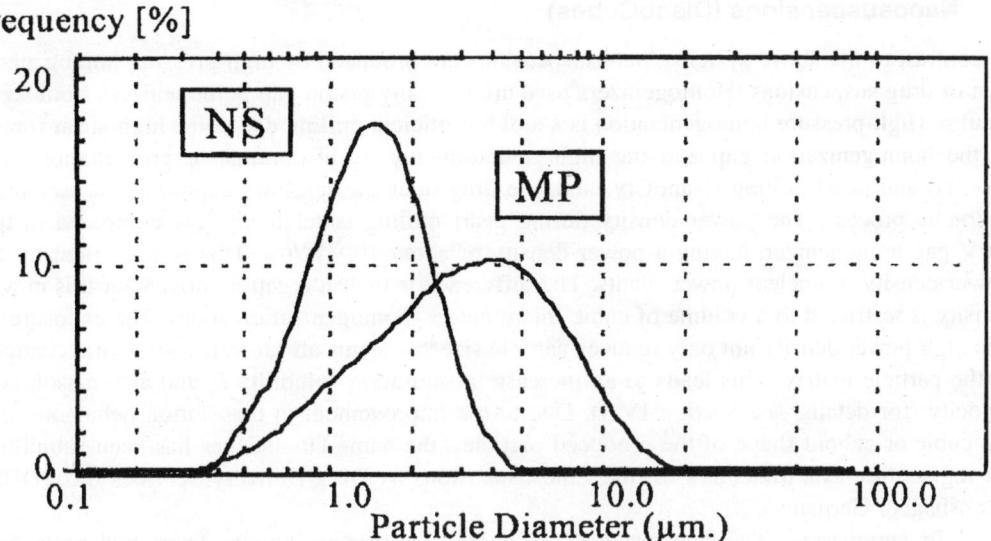

Figure 1 Size distribution of the microparticles obtained by air milling (MP) and after high-pressure homogenization leading to a nanosuspension (NS). Laser diffractometry (LD) data. (Modified from Ref. 6.)

vivo studies have been performed by NanoSystems, especially after peroral administration of the drug nanoparticles. According to Liversidge (11), the results can be summarized as follows: Nanosuspensions

1. Improve bioavailability,
2. Improve dose proportionality,
3. Reduce fed/fasted variability,
4. Reduce intersubject variability, and
5. Enhance the absorption rate.

The improved in vivo performance of NanoCrystals therefore is mainly attributed to

1. An increase in dissolution velocity due to the increase in surface area.
2. Adherence of nanoparticles to the GIT-wall after peroral administration due to generally adhesive properties of small particles.
3. Changed pharmacokinetics and organ distribution after intravenous administration of NanoCrystals compared to solutions (e.g., Paclitaxel NanoCrystals vs. Taxol).

There seems to be a contradiction between the i.v. administered cyclosporine hydrosol behaving like a solution (2) and the intravenously administered paclitaxel NanoCrystals behaving different from a paclitaxel solution (Taxol). A possible explanation for this apparent contradiction is the compound specificity of the dissolution velocity. The dissolution velocity does not depend solely on the surface area but also on the saturation solubility of the compound (Noyes–Whitney equation) and the dissolution pressure (Kelvin equation, see below). When the dissolution velocity is sufficiently low, drug nanoparticles will behave very differently from a drug solution.

C. Nanosuspensions (DissoCubes)

In contrast to the above systems, nanosuspensions are produced by high-pressure homogenization of drug suspensions. Homogenizers used are typically piston gap homogenizers from APV Gaulin. High-pressure homogenization is a tool for efficient milling due to the high-shear forces in the homogenization gap and the high cavitation forces. In contrast to precipitation (hydrosols) and pearl milling (NanoCrystals), the drug microparticles are exposed to a very high energetic process. The power density during pearl milling is relatively low compared to the APV gap homogenizer, having a power density of about 10^{13} W/m^3. This is equivalent to the power density in nuclear power plants. The difference is that in a gap homogenizer this power density is restricted to a volume of cubic micrometers (homogenization zone). The exposure to this high-power density not only reduces particle size but seems also to cause structural changes in the particle matrix. This leads to an increase in saturation solubility c_s and also dissolution velocity (for details, see Section IV.B). Due to the improvement in dissolution behaviour and the cubic or cuboid shape of the produced particles, the name DissoCubes has been submitted for registration as a trademark for the nanosuspensions by Drug Delivery Services Ltd. (DDS, Kronshagen, Germany).

To summarize: The nanosuspensions possess properties known from hydrosols and NanoCrystals in combination with the special feature of the increase of saturation solubility. This increase in c_s is above the increase due to the reduction of particle size and reduction of diffusional distance h.

III. PRODUCTION OF NANOSUSPENSIONS

Nanosuspensions are produced by high-pressure homogenization of drug microparticle suspensions (12). The powdered drug is dispersed in an aqueous surfactant solution by stirring or by use of a colloid mill. Generally it is beneficial to start with a micronized drug powder because it reduces the number of homogenization cycles. Depending on the hardness of the drug and the starting size of the drug microparticles, homogenization is performed at pressures between 200 and 1500 bar (approx. 2800–21,300 psi) applying typically between 3 and 10 homogenization cycles.

Figure 2 shows the decrease in mean particle size as a function of the number of homogenization cycles. One homogenization cycle is sufficient to produce a nanosuspension with a mean diameter of 800 nm; the mean particle size drops to about 600 nm at homogenization cycle 3. Further decrease is observed when increasing the cycle number, indicating that the limiting dispersivity at a given power density for this drug has been reached. Figure 3 shows the reduction in the diameter 99% as determined by laser diffractometry (volume distribution). The diameter 99% of the volume distribution is a highly sensitive parameter for detection of micrometer particles. A continuous reduction in the diameter 99% can be observed up to homogenization cycle 9; then the diameter remains practically unchanged (Fig. 3). It demonstrates that the "contamination" of the nanosuspension by microparticles can be efficiently reduced by multiple cycling until a low level has been reached which is acceptable for the envisaged administration route. The absolute number of microparticles per volume unit nanosuspension depends very much on the route of administration. For peroral administration (e.g., nanosuspension incorporated in a tablet), a production with one cycle is considered sufficient; for intravenous administration, multiple cycling is sensible. The acceptable number of microparticles per volume unit in intravenous products depends on the concentration of the nanosuspension (wt % solid), the dissolution velocity of micrometer particles in the blood and the administration volume.

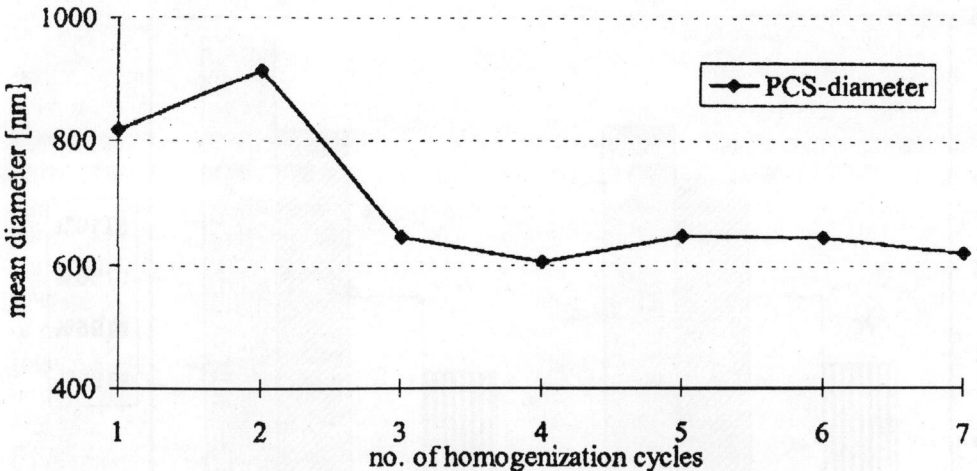

Figure 2 Decrease of nanosuspension particle size (PCS mean diameter) with increasing number of homogenization cycles (high-pressure homogenization). (Modified from Ref. 12.)

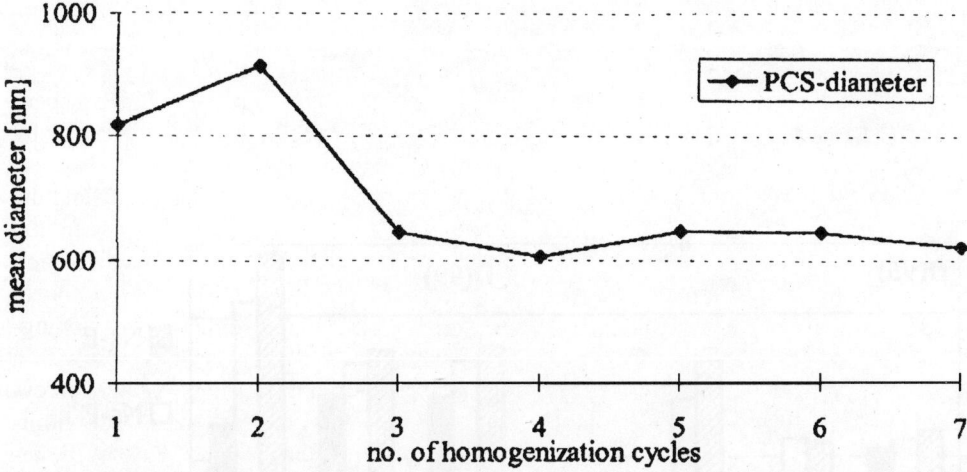

Figure 3 Decrease of nanosuspension particle size (LD diameter 99%) with increasing number of homogenization cycles (high-pressure homogenization). (Modified from Ref. 12.)

Typically the administration volumes are only a few milliliters (e.g., one dose of paclitaxel 10% nanosuspension: 3.5 mL), that means the microparticle content per volume unit is less critical.

Nanosuspensions can be freeze-dried or, alternatively, spray-dried; the latter is more cost-effective. The lyophilization of nanosuspensions is relatively unproblematic. With one drug a lyophilized product could be obtained that had good redispersibility even without using any cryoprotectant in the freeze-drying process (Fig. 4).

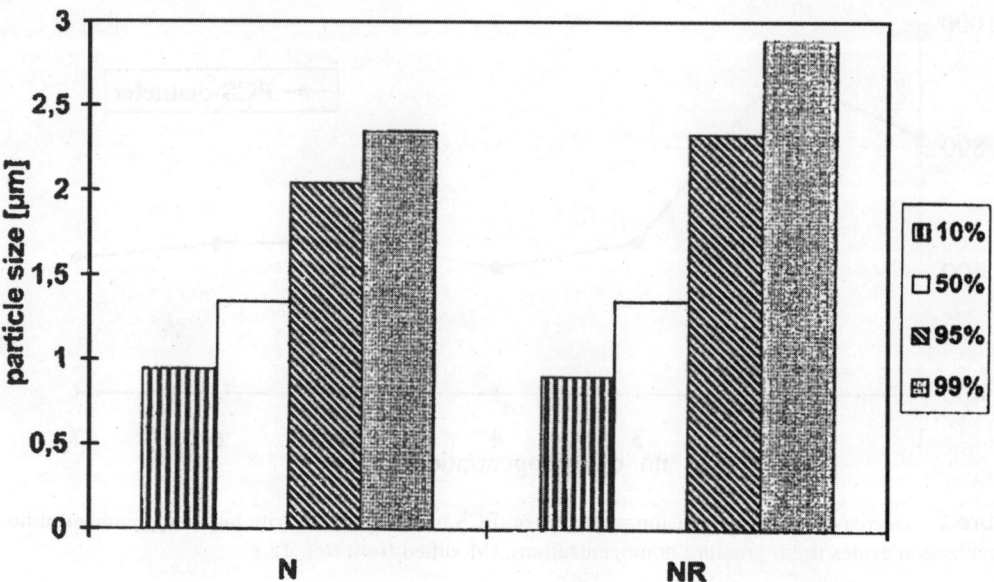

Figure 4 Particle size distribution of a model drug as nanosuspension (N) and after freeze drying and reconstitution with distilled water (NR). Diameters 10%, 50%, 95%, and 99%. LD data, volume distribution. (Modified from Ref. 13.)

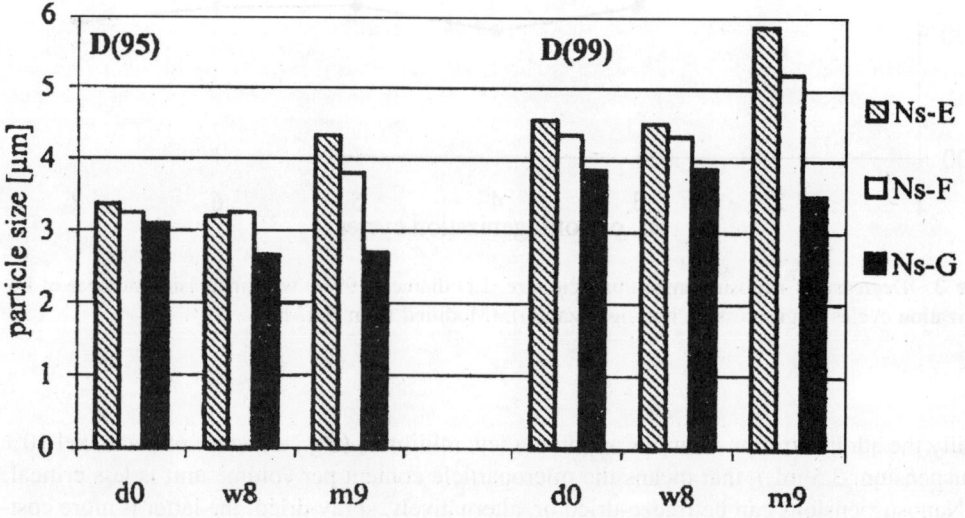

Figure 5 Diameter 95% [D(95), left] and 99% [D(99), right] of the nanosuspensions NS-E, NS-F, and NS-G at the day of production (d0), and after 8 weeks (w8) and 9 months (m9) of storage. LD data. (Modified from Ref. 6.)

IV. PROPERTIES OF NANOSUSPENSIONS

A. Physical Long-Term Stability

Nanosuspensions are a highly dispersed system; therefore, physical instability due to Ostwald ripening would be expected. According to the Ostwald–Freundlich equation, the saturation solubility increases with decreasing particle size (14). However, this effect is only pronounced for particles below approximately 2 µm, especially below 1 µm. It does not occur for powders of size normally processed in pharmacy. The differences in the concentrations of the saturated solutions around a small and a large particle leads to the diffusion of dissolved drug from the outer area of the small particles to the outer area of the large particles. As a result the solution around the large particles is super saturated leading to drug crystallization and growth of the large crystals. In turn, the solution around the small particles is no longer saturated, leading to dissolution of drug from the small particles and finally to disappearance of the small particles. Surprisingly, such particle growth did not occur in the aqueous nanosuspensions. The aqueous suspensions were stable at 4°C for months (Fig. 5, investigated periods by now) up to a few years (13). A priori Ostwald ripening is reduced to the extremely low solubility of the drugs formulated as nanosuspensions. An additional explanation for the absence of Ostwald ripening is that the homogenized particles are very homogeneous. There are no large differences in particle size, leading to the absence of differences in solubility sufficiently high to cause Ostwald ripening.

B. Saturation Solubility of Nanosuspensions

According to the Kelvin equation (15), the vapor pressure above curved surface is increased compared to a flat surface. The vapor pressure increases further with increasing curvature of the surface, which means decreasing particle size. The Kelvin principle is exploited in the spray-drying process, in which increase in surface area and increase in vapor pressure lead to a rapid evaporation of the sprayed liquid. The transition of a molecule from the liquid phase (droplet) to the surrounding gas phase is comparable to the transition of molecules from a solid phase (particle) to the surrounding liquid phase. Analogously to the vapor pressure, the dissolution pressure of a substance increases with decreasing particle size. The saturation solubility around a particle depends on the tendency of the molecule to move from the solid to the liquid phase (vapor pressure) and the tendency to recrystallize, i.e., the saturation solubility increases with reduction in particle size (Fig. 6, top).

According to the Prandtl equation (14), for small particles the diffusional distance h decreases with decreasing particle size (Fig. 6, bottom). The decrease in h and the simultaneous increase in c_s leads to an increase of the gradient $(c_s - c_x)/dh$ and, according to Noyes-Whitney, to an increase in the dissolution velocity.

Bearing these theoretical considerations in mind, particle size analysis of nanosuspensions by Coulter counter was performed in drug saturated 0.9% sodium chloride-solution to avoid dissolution effects. Saturation was performed using jet-milled drug with a mean particle diameter of 2.4 µm (laser diffractometer, volume distribution). This should avoid or minimize dissolution of the nanosuspension due to the size effect on the saturation solubility. Surprisingly, the nanosuspensions dissolved very quickly within the subsequent measurements in the Coulter counter Multisizer II (Fig. 7). Determination of the saturation solubility revealed an approximately twofold increase for the nanosuspensions compared to the 2.4-µm drug particles (Fig. 8).

For some other drugs, even higher increases in saturation solubility were found. These increases were not only attributed to the relatively small difference in size but to other factors as well. Possible reasons are the creation of higniy energetic surfaces during the disintegration of

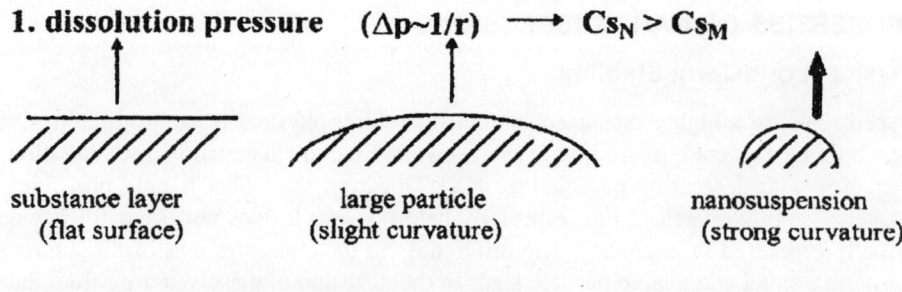

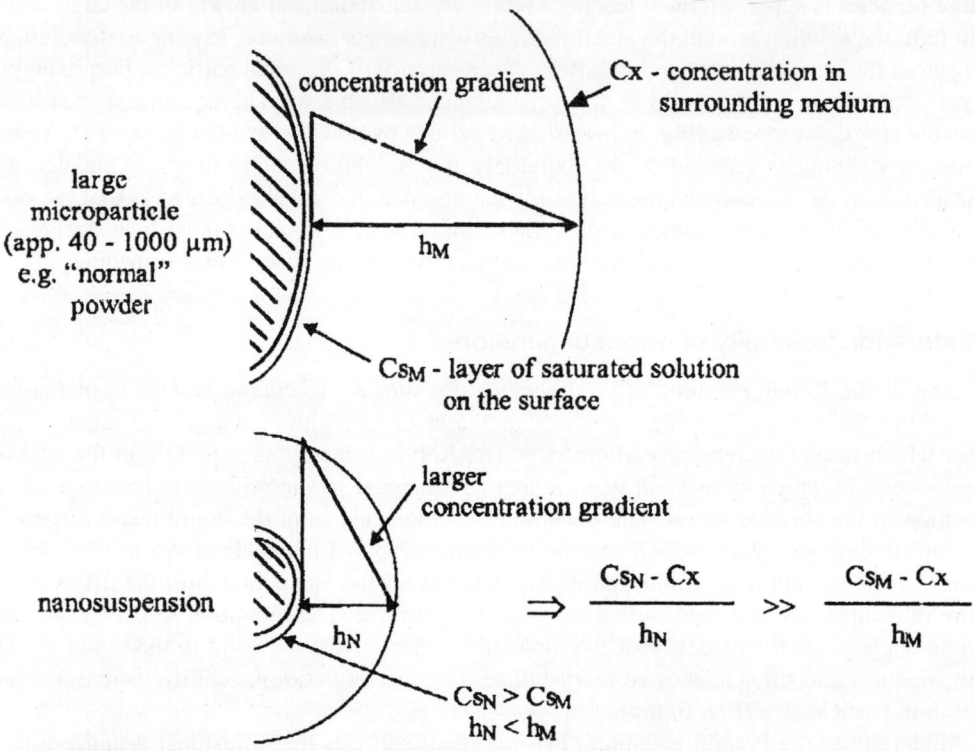

Figure 6 Mechanisms of increasing saturation solubility c_s and dissolution velocity in nanosuspensions. (Δp, dissolution pressure; Cs_N, saturation solubility nanoparticles; Cs_M, saturation solubility microparticles; h_M, diffusional distance microparticles; h_N, diffusional distance nanoparticles). (Ref. 22.)

the microparticles to nanoparticles and changes in the internal structure of the particle matrix (cf. internal structure of nanosuspensions). Breaking off the particles reveals new surfaces from the inside of the drug crystals. Such surfaces can be higher energetic (higher interfacial tension γ). The saturation solubility is also a function of the energy content of a drug crystal (e.g., different energetic modifications of polymorphs). According to the Ostwald–Freundlich equation, the saturation solubility is also affected by the interfacial tension of the particle surface. Consequently, creation of highly energetic surfaces by breaking of particles can contribute to the increase in saturation solubility.

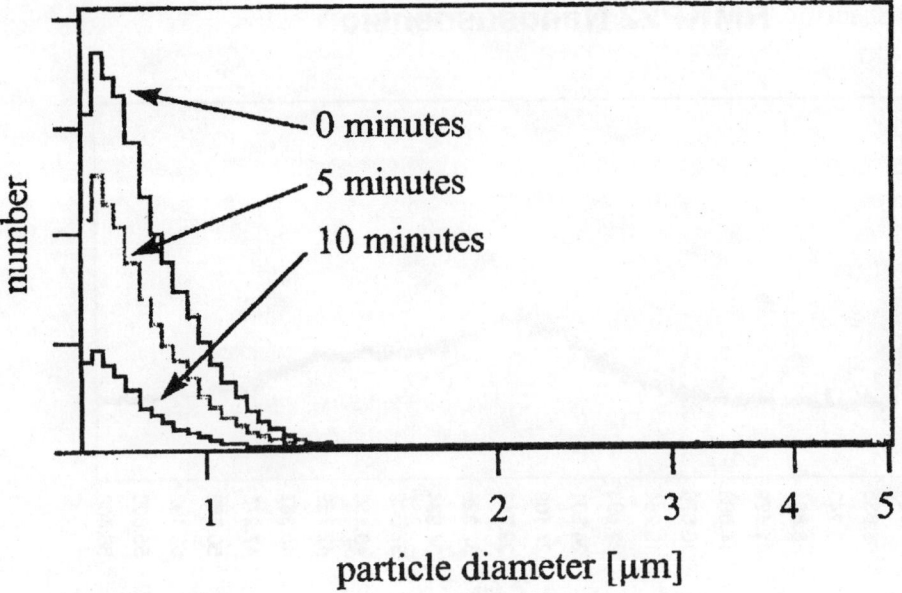

Figure 7 Three successive measurements of RMKP 22 nanosuspension in 0.9% NaCl solution saturated with RMKP 22 jet milled microparticles, measurements at 0/5/10 min (12).

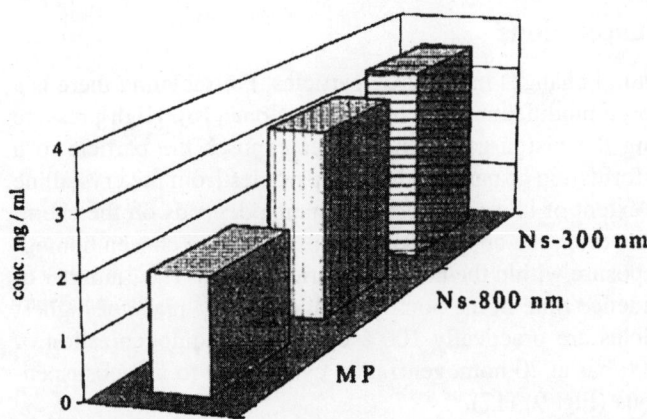

Figure 8 Solubility C_s of RMKP 22 microparticles (MP) with a mean diameter of 2400 nm and of two RMKP 22 nanosuspensions with diameters of 800 and 300 nm (Ns-800, Ns-300). (Modified from Ref. 12.)

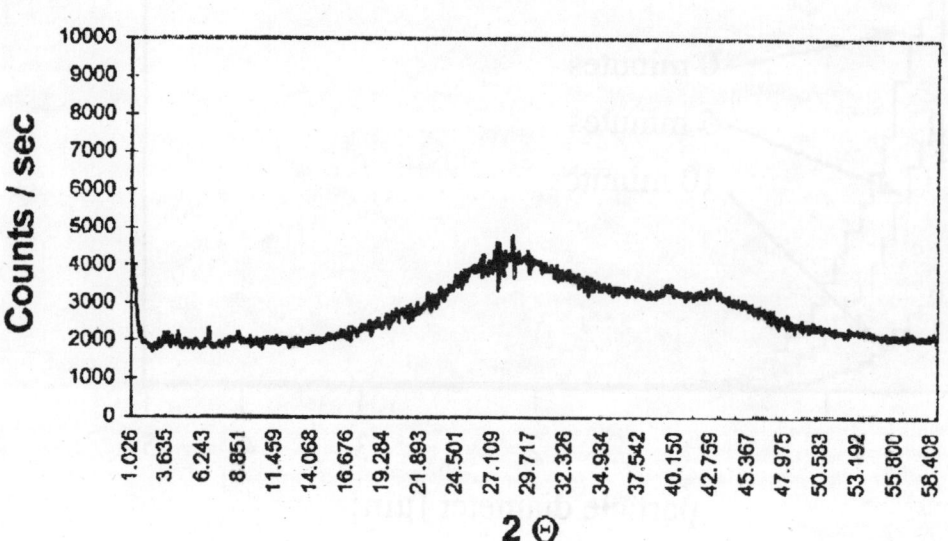

Figure 9 X-ray diffraction pattern of RMKP 22 nanosuspension after 20 cycles of high-pressure homogenization at 1500 bar (17).

C. Internal Structure of Nanosuspensions

The input of energy can lead to structural changes inside drug particles. For tableting there is a report of the transition of one polymorph modification to a high-energy one (16). High-pressure homogenization of the particles using the piston-gap homogenizer exposes the particle to a high-power density, leading to a transformation of parts of the nanoparticles from the crystalline state to an amorphous structure. The extent of internal structural change depends on the chemical nature and physical hardness of the drug, the applied power density via the chosen homogenization pressure, and the time of exposure within the homogenization process (i.e., number of homogenization cycles, i.e., total residence time in the homogenization gap as place of highest power density). RMKP22 microparticles are practically 100% crystalline; homogenization of the aqueous particle dispersion at 1000 bar at 20 homogenization cycles lead to a nanosuspension being practically 100% amorphous (Fig. 9) (17).

V. NANOSUSPENSION-BASED FORMULATIONS FOR DRUG DELIVERY

A. Topical Formulations

Incorporation of nanosuspensions into topical formulations (cremes, ointments, emulsions, gels) can be performed to create supersaturated systems. The increase in saturation solubility will lead to an increased diffusion pressure of drug into the skin. It might also be advantageous to combine nanosuspensions with solid lipid nanoparticles (SLN) (18–21). SLN in topical formulation has an occlusive effect. Due to the adhesive properties, the result is a thin layer of densely packed nanoparticles. The dimensions of the spaces between the particles are very small, obstructing air circulation in these spaces and minimizing evaporation of water from the skin. Increased diffusion pressure and occlusive effect should distinctly enhance drug concentration in the skin or even drug penetration and systemic absorption.

B. Oral Formulations

Oral formulations or application in the mouth (buccal, gingival, lingual, sublingual) might be efficient for a range of drugs, especially drugs that did not yet have a sufficiently high availability in traditional oral formulations. The nanosuspensions could be applied in the form of the aqueous dispersion (if necessary with enhanced viscosity of the water phase), gel, paste, or as an ointment or creme. Patches also appear possible. Due to the generally adhesive properties of small particles, these formulations could show an increased adhesion and prolonged residence time.

C. Peroral Formulations

Peroral administration of nanosuspensions features the advantages discussed in detail in Chapter 22. Major points are reduction in the variability of bioavailability and potential increase in bioavailability. Possible formulations are drink suspensions made from lyophilized or spray-dried nanosuspensions (sachet) or from an effervescent tablet. Other possibilities are the production of pellets using the aqueous nanosuspension for pellet production, or production of tablets using the nanosuspension in the granulation process. It is also possible to spray aqueous nanosuspensions on the surface of nonpareilles. Hard gelatin capsules can be filled with freeze-dried or spray-dried nanosuspensions, soft gelatin capsules with drug nanoparticles dispersed in PEG-400 or PEG-600. A very straightforward approach would be the production of nanosuspensions using liquid PEG as external phase instead of water.

D. Parenteral Formulations

Nanosuspensions can be used to transform poorly soluble, noninjectable drugs into a formulation suitable for intravenous injection. This opens the perspective to utilize many drugs for therapy, which have a too low bioavailability after oral administration or parenteral administration as microparticles (e.g., IM or IP). In addition, conventional formulations with undesirable side effects due to problematic excipients can be replaced by a new well-tolerated nanosuspension formulation. One drug candidate is paclitaxel, being presently marketed in Taxol (Bristol Myers Squibb). Taxol contains Cremophor EL, which can cause anaphylactic reactions. Paclitaxel can be transformed to drug nanoparticles by pearl milling (8) or by high-pressure homogenization (9). Paclitaxel nanosuspensions were prepared by high-pressure homogenization at 1500 bar and 10 cycles. Figure 10 shows the size distribution determined directly after production. The nanosuspension was lyophilized and showed little difference in size distribution after reconstitution (9).

In addition, the production of nanosuspensions is an elegant tool to make newly developed, poorly soluble compounds accessible for pharmacological screening. Rapid dissolution in the blood after intravenous injection will create a sufficiently high availability even for extremely low-solubility compounds.

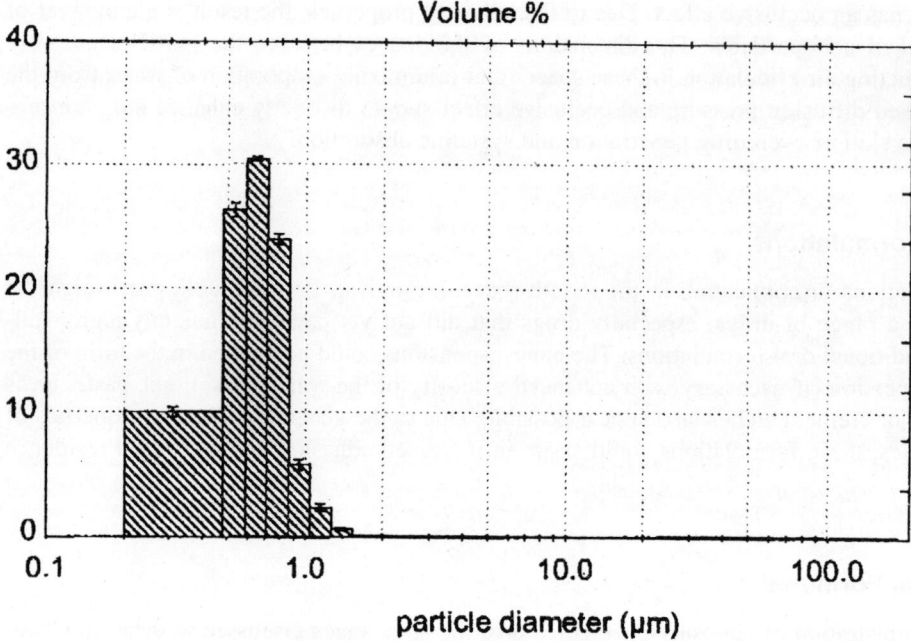

Figure 10 Particle size distribution of a paclitaxel nanosuspension. Laser diffractometry (LD) measurements on day of production. (Modified from Ref. 9.)

VI. PERSPECTIVES

The production of drug nanoparticles is an elegant approach to improve the in vivo performance of existing drugs and a simple, easy-to-perform method to formulate generally poorly soluble drugs. Nanosuspensions will be a very important formulation tool in the future because an increasing number of newly developed drugs are poorly soluble simultaneously in water and in organic media.

ACKNOWLEDGMENTS

We thank the Wissenschaftliche Verlagsgesellschaft for the permission to reproduce figures from R. H. Müller, G. E. Hildebrand, eds. *Pharmazeutische Technologie: Moderne Arzneiformen*, and we would like to thank the Controlled Release Society (CRS) for the permission to reproduce figures from the proceedings of the 22nd and 24th international symposia on controlled release of bioactive materials (6,9).

REFERENCES

1. R. H. Müller, G. E. Hildebrand, eds. Pharmazeutische Technologie: Moderne Arzneiformen. 2nd ed. Stuttgart: Wissenschaftliche Verlagsgesellschaft, 1997.
2. H. Sucker. Hydrosole, eine Alternative für die parenterale Anwendung von schwer wasserlöslichen Wirkstoffen. In: R. H. Müller, G. E. Hildebrand, eds. Pharmazeutische Technologie: Moderne Arzneiformen, 2nd ed. Stuttgart: Wissenschaftliche Verlagsgesellschaft, 1997, pp. 383–391.
3. P. Gassmann, M. List, A. Schweitzer, H. Sucker. Hydrosols: Alternatives for the parenteral application of poorly water soluble drugs. Eur. J. Pharm. Biopharm. 40: 64–72, 1994.
4. M. List, H. Sucker. Pat. No. GB 2200048, 1988.
5. P. Gassmann, H. Sucker. Pat. No. GB 2269536, 1994.
6. R. H. Müller, K. Peters, R. Becker, B. Kruss. Nanosuspensions for the i.v. administration of poorly soluble drugs; stability during sterilisation and long-term storage. Proc. Int. Symp. Control. Rel. Bioact. Mater. 22: 574–575, 1996.
7. S. Buchmann et al. Aqueous microsuspension, an alternative intravenous formulation for animal studies. Eur. J. Pharm. Biopharm. 42 (Suppl.): 10S, 1996.
8. E. Merisko-Liversidge et al. Formulation and antitumor activity evaluation of nanocrystalline suspensions of poorly soluble anticancer drugs. Pharm. Res. 13(2): 272–278, 1996.
9. B. H. L. Böhm, D. Behnke, R. H. Müller. Production of paclitaxel nanosuspensions by high pressure homogenisation. Proceed. 24th Int. Symp. Control. Rel. Bioact. Mater. 24: 927–928, 1997.
10. R. H. Müller. Nanosuspensionen —eine neue Formulierung für schwerlösliche Arzneistoffe. In: R. H. Müller, G. E. Hildebrand, eds. Pharmazeutische Technologie: Moderne Arzneiformen, 2nd ed. Stuttgart: Wissenschaftliche Verlagsgesellschaft, 1997, pp. 393–400.
11. G. Liversidge et al. Drug Nanocrystals for Improved Drug Delivery. Workshop "Particulate Drug Delivery Systems" on Int. Symp. Control. Rel. Bioact. Mater. 23, 1996.
12. R. H. Müller, R. Becker, et al., Pharmazeutische Nanosuspensionen zur Arzneistoffapplikation als Systeme mit erhöhter Sättigungslöslichkeit und Lösungsgeschwindigkeit, Int. Patent PCT/EP95/04401, 1996.
13. K. Peters. Nanosuspensionen—eine neue Formulierung für schwerlösliche Arzneistoffe. PhD thesis: Free University of Berlin, 1998.
14. M. Mosharraf, C. Nyström. The effect of particle size and shape on the surface specific dissolution rate of micronized practically insoluble drugs. Int. J. Pharm. 122: 35–47, 1995.
15. A. P. Simonelli, S. C. Mehta, W. I. Higuchi. Inhibition of sulfathiazole crystal growth by polyvinylpyrrolidone. J. Pharm. Sci. 56: 633, 1970.
16. H. Kala, U. Haack, et al. Zum kristallografischen Verhalten des Carbamazepins unter Pressdruck. Pharmazie 42(8): 524–527, 1987.
17. M. J. Grau. Physikalische Charakterisierung von Nanosuspensionen aus schwerlöslichen Arzeistoffen. PhD thesis: Free University of Berlin, in preparation.
18. W. Mehnert, A. zur Mühlen, A. Dingler, H. Weyhers, R. H. Müller. Solid Lipid Nanoparticles—ein neuartiger Wirkstoff-Carrier für Kosmetika und Pharmazeutika, 1. Mitteilung: Systemeigenschaften, Herstellung und Scaling-up. Pharm. Ind. 59, 5: 423–427, 1997.
19. W. Mehnert, A. zur Mühlen, A. Dingler, H. Weyhers, R. H. Müller. Solid Lipid Nanoparticles—ein neuartiger Wirkstoff-Carrier für Kosmetika und Pharmazeutika, 2. Mitteilung: Wirkstoff-Inkorporation, Freisetzung und Sterilisierbarkeit. Pharm. Ind. 59, 6: 511–514, 1997.
20. W. Mehnert, A. zur Mühlen, A. Dingler, H. Weyhers, R. H. Müller. Solid Lipid Nanoparticles—ein neuartiger Wirkstoff-Carrier für Kosmetika und Pharmazeutika, 3. Mitteilung: Langzeitstabilität, Gefrier- und Sprühtrocknung, Toxizität, Anwendung in Kosmetika und Pharmazeutika. Pharm. Ind. 59, 7: 614–619, 1997.
21. R. H. Müller, J. S. Lucks. Arzneistoffträger aus festen Lipidteilchen, Feste Lipidnanosphären (SLN). European Patent EP0605497B1, 1996.
22. R. H. Müller, S. Benita, and B. Bohm. Emulsions and Nanosuspensions for the Formulation of Poorly Soluble Drugs. Stuttgart. Med. Pharm, 1998.

18

Large-Scale Production of Solid Lipid Nanoparticles (SLN) and Nanosuspensions (DissoCubes)

R. H. Müller, A. Dingler, T. Schneppe, and S. Gohla
Free University of Berlin, Berlin, Germany

I. INTRODUCTION

A major obstacle for the introduction of particulate or colloidal drug carriers to the pharmaceutical market is the lack of a large-scale production method yielding a product of a quality that is acceptable by the regulatory authorities (e.g., Food and Drug Administration). This is no problem for traditional drug carriers like emulsions for parenteral administration. These emulsions for parenteral nutrition were introduced into therapy in the 1950s. Hence an accepted production method by high-pressure homogenization is available. The same technique was transferred to liposomes for large-scale production. For example, liposomes for the treatment of infant respiratory distress syndrome can relatively easily be prepared aseptically by high-pressure homogenization. The aseptic production makes a final sterilization redundant, thus preventing potential impairment of the physical stability of the liposomes. Large-scale production methods are also established for microparticles, e.g., spray drying or the solvent evaporation method (Parlodel LAR Decapeptyl, and Enantone). In contrast, there are still major problems to the establishment of large-scale production methods for solid nanoparticles, e.g., polymeric nanoparticles. It is considered to be one of the major obstacles preventing the successful introduction of the nanoparticles to the clinic and the pharmaceutical market. More than 30 years of intensive research has been invested in nanoparticle technology, the output in terms of products for the patient is rather low or practically nonexistent. To our knowledge, no product for chronic treatment based on nanoparticle technology is on the market. The company Nycomed did recently introduce a nanoparticulate product, but only for diagnostic purposes and not for chronic application (Abdomed).

Two major reasons for the lack of large-scale production methods for solid nanoparticles are as follows:

1. Basic technological problems (e.g., basic scale-up problem, toxicologically problematic residues from the production process), and
2. Regulatory aspects such as suitability of the production unit and production process to be qualified and validated.

For example, one approach to the production of polymeric nanoparticles is spraying of the polymer containing organic solvent via a nozzle into a supercritical fluid such as liquid carbon dioxide. Various methods are described using supercritical fluids, e.g., the aerosol solvent extraction system (ASES) (1). In principle, this spraying technique has the potential to be scaled up; however, by now no large production units seem to be available. Scaling up modifies the production conditions. In addition, a method is needed to collect the nanoparticles effectively from the supercritical fluid. The ASES system has been under development since the mid 1980s. Other production techniques based on supercritical fluids, such as the technique by York (2), are only able to produce about 100 g of solid polymeric nanoparticles in about 12 h (personal communication). This might possibly be sufficient for highly potent and very expensive drugs, but it is far from normal batch sizes required in pharmaceutical industry.

In addition, the production unit needs to be suitable for qualification according to regulatory requirements (e.g., PIC Draft Document 1/96). This needs to be considered when starting to design such a unit, e.g., the choice of materials used (e.g., quality of steel and inertness of materials used for fittings and tubes) and the product specification for the single parts of the unit (e.g., electropolished metal surfaces to reduce adhesion of bacteria). Furthermore, the system needs to be designed such that a proper qualification and validation is possible. For example, the unit needs to be suitable to undergo a cleaning validation. Surfaces in contact with the product being of a high adsorptivity should be avoided. Tubes and vessels must be designed to minimize areas and edges which are rather difficult for the access of the cleaning media. Preferentially cleaning in place (CIP) should be possible, as should sterilization in place (SIP).

As an alternative to nanoparticles made from polymers or natural macromolecules, the solid lipid nanoparticles (SLN) were developed a few years ago (3). SLN are particles consisting of a matrix made from solid lipids. In aqueous dispersion they are stabilized by surfactants or polymers; the aqueous dispersion can be transferred to a dry product by spray drying or lyophilization (4). They combine advantages of polymeric nanoparticles, emulsions, and liposomes. Similar to polymeric nanoparticles, they consist of a solid matrix protecting incorporated active substances against chemical degradation (5) and providing high flexibility to modify the release profiles (6). Similar to emulsions and liposomes, they are composed of well-tolerated, in vivo biodegradable lipids and can be produced on large industrial scale by high-pressure homogenization. In particular, the possibility of large-scale production provides a distinct advantage of the SLN over other solid nanoparticles. This chapter describes the production of SLN ranging from lab scale to medium and large industrial scale. It should be pointed out that the quantities required in industrial scale production differ very much depending on the nature of the product. For example, drug-loaded SLN (e.g., with corticoids) for incorporation into topical products such as cremes and lotions require quantities from 100 kg up to 1 ton and more. Highly potent and very expensive drugs, such as interferon-β and recombinant hormones such as follicle-stimulating hormone, require only a batch size of a few kilograms of aqueous nanoparticle dispersion (e.g., 10% or 20% solids content). This means that medium scale for one product is already large industrial scale for another product.

Incorporation of poorly soluble drugs into nanoparticles is a real problem if the drugs are simultaneously poorly soluble in aqueous media and in organic solvents. The poor solubility of drugs is no problem when producing microparticles because the drug particles can be finally dispersed in the solvent containing the polymer/macromolecule for particle formation. However, in general this is not possible for nanoparticles because of their small size. To be incorporated in, say, a 200-nm nanoparticle, the crystals of the poorly soluble drug need to be distinctly smaller, preferentially in the range of 5–10 nm. Such fine drug particles can only be achieved for a limited number of drugs, e.g., colloids for γ-scintigraphy and iron oxides for MRT (7). For most poorly soluble drugs this is not possible. An alternative is the production of nanoparticles consisting of pure drug without any matrix material. Such drug nanoparticles can be produced by a highly efficient milling process. Depending on the disintegration process, the obtained particles are called NanoCrystals or DissoCubes. NanoCrystals are produced by using pearl mills.

A potential problem might be erosion from the pearls (pearls made from glass or zircon oxide). Alternatively, the poorly soluble drugs can be milled by high-pressure homogenization. The high sheer forces and cavitation forces are able to disintegrate drug microparticles to drug nanoparticles. High-pressure homogenization has the advantage of being a continuous process (8). In addition, the homogenizers used for the production of DissoCubes are already established in the production lines for parenterals such as emulsions for parenteral nutrition (Lipofundin MCT, Intralipid). The homogenizers are accepted by the regulatory authorities. Of course, the cavitation forces lead to a limited erosion of metal from the homogenization valve. However, the contamination of the most prevalent metal in steel—iron—was found to be below 1 ppm, even after 20 homogenization cycles of a nanosuspension (9). For the production of nanosuspensions the same equipment can be used as for the production of SLN. To summarize, basically the same production equipment can be used for two different nanoparticulate delivery systems.

II. LABORATORY-SCALE PRODUCTION

Laboratory scale production of SLN and DissoCubes is performed using a piston-gap homogenizer (Micron LAB 40, APV Homogenizer GmbH, Lübeck, Germany). Minimum batch size is 20 mL, maximum size is 40 mL. Pressures applied range from 100 bar to a maximum of 1500 bar. The aqueous dispersion is pressed by a piston through a small homogenization gap that is approximately 25 μm (at a pressure of 500 bar). The process is discontinuous, i.e., the system needs to be dismantled and the dispersion poured back into the central cylinder for the next homogenization cycle. This is somewhat time consuming but the machine has the big advantage of an extremely low sample volume. This is of high interest for compounds that are expensive or of limited availability. Figure 1 shows the principle mode of operation and Fig. 2 a picture of the LAB 40 unit.

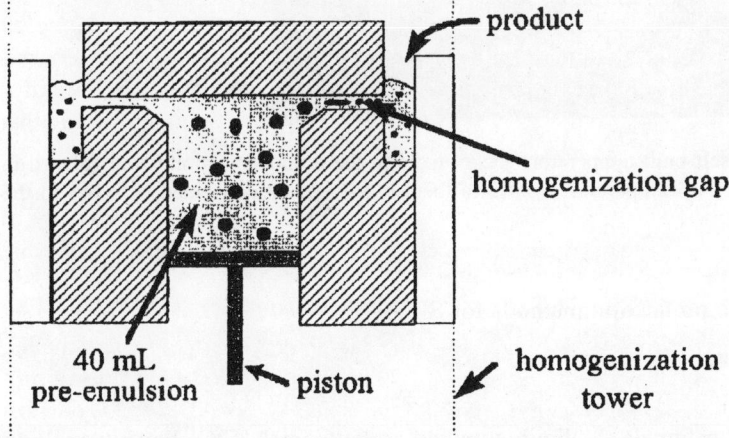

Figure 1 Production mode of discontinuous Micron LAB 40. The dispersion is pressed through a small gap (approximately 25 μm). For the next homogenization cycle the system must be dismantled and the central cylinder of the homogenization tower refilled.

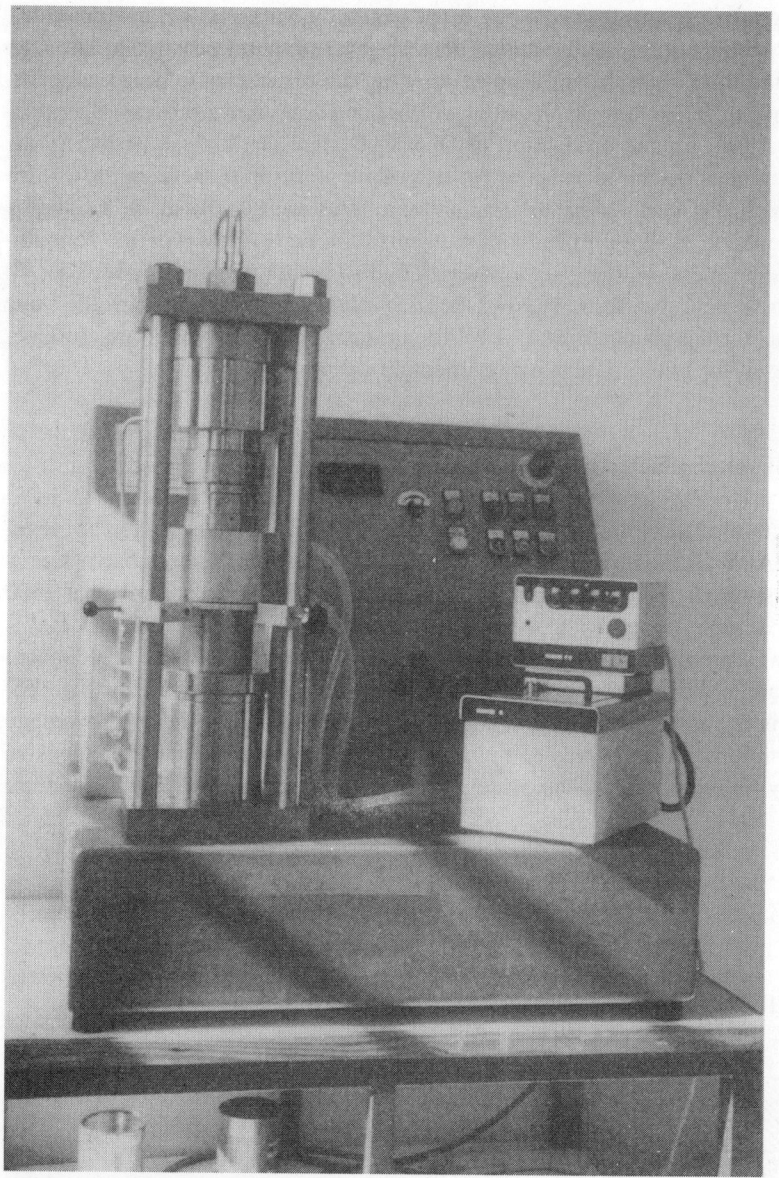

Figure 2 The LAB 40 with self-built temperature jacket fixed at the homogenization tower (placed in height of homogenization gap). For temperature control a thermostat/cryostat connected by tubes to the jacket is used.

There are basically two production methods for SLN:

Hot homogenization, and
Cold homogenization

For the hot homogenization technique the lipid is melted approximately 5°C above its melting point and the drug is dissolved or solubilized in the melted lipid. The drug-containing lipid melt is poured into a hot surfactant dissolution of identical temperature and dispersed by a high-speed stirrer to form a coarse preemulsion. The obtained preemulsion is then homogenized, typically at 500 bar for two to three homogenization cycles. The produced hot oil-in-water nanoemulsion is then cooled, the lipid recrystallizes and forms solid lipid nanoparticles. For the cold homogenization technique the drug-containing melt is solidified and milled by, for example, a mortar mill. The produced microparticles (50–100 μm) are suspended in a cold surfactant solution and this microparticulate suspension is then homogenized at room temperature or below. The cavitation and sheer forces are strong enough to break the solid lipid microparticles into solid lipid nanoparticles without melting of the lipid. The homogenization temperature needs to be sufficiently below the melting temperature of the lipid to avoid a lipid melting due to the heat generated by the homogenization process itself. Typically, the lipid suspension increases in temperature by about 20°C during one homogenization cycle. For multiple cycling it might be necessary to cool the suspension prior to the next homogenization cycle.

The production of nanosuspensions is comparable to the cold homogenization process for SLN. Generally it is beneficial to use drug particles as fine as possible, i.e., a jet-milled powder. The size distribution of a jet-milled powder is relatively broad, i.e., typically from about 0.1 μm to a maximum of about 25 μm (10). However, that means that most of the particles are below the size of the homogenization gap (approximately 25 μm at 500 bar). This avoids or minimizes the risk of blocking the homogenization gap. In general, suspensions can be processed with a solid content of 10%; sometimes 15% also is possible depending on the size of the starting material. The reduction in size per homogenization cycle depends on the hardness of the drug and the percentage of amorphous fraction of drug present. Soft drugs lead to a relatively fine product, e.g., paclitaxel yielding particles of about 200–300 nm (11). For other drugs such as RMKP 22 sizes between 500 and 700 nm have been reported (12), extremely hard drugs yield values of about 800–900 nm, e.g., RMMG (13).

The discontinuous Micron LAB 40 is highly suitable in case expensive drugs or compounds with limited availability are processed, but is very time consuming when performing a

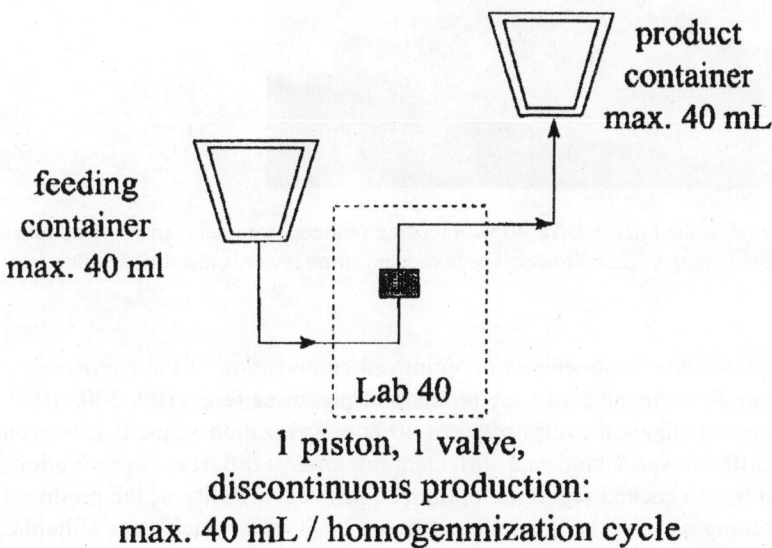

Figure 3 Schematic setup of continuous LAB 40. (Modified from Ref. 14.)

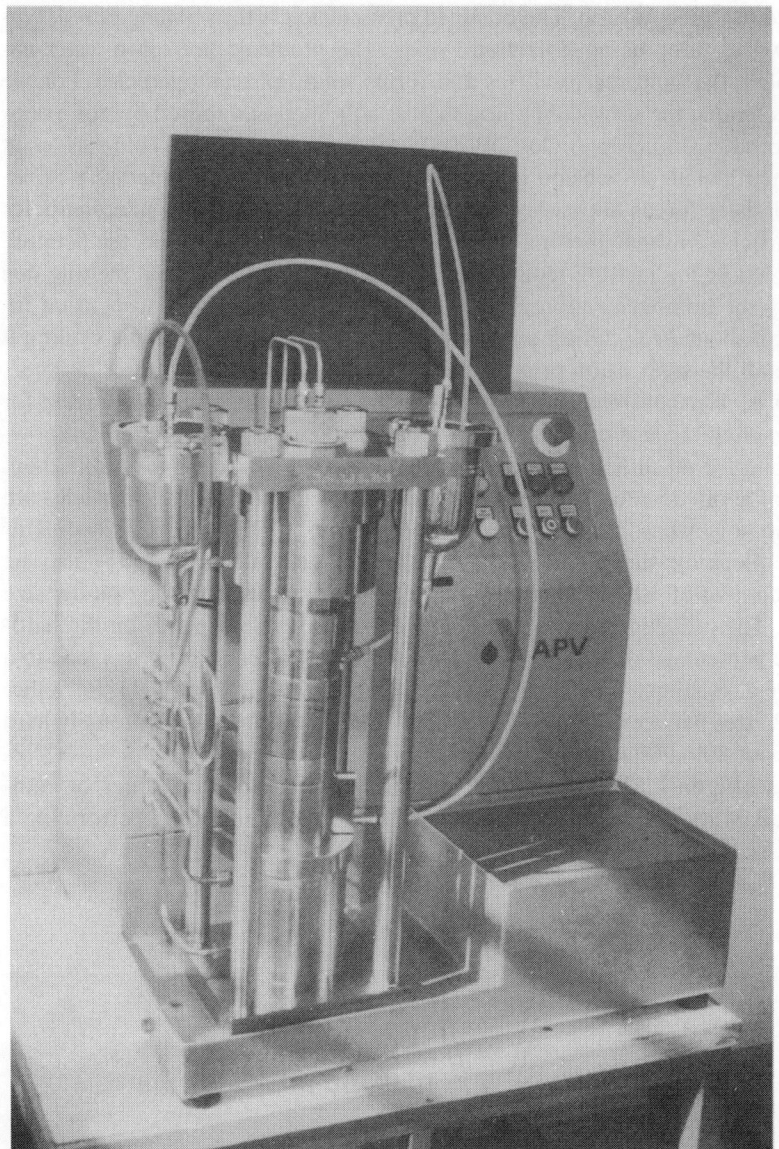

Figure 4 Continuous version of the Micron LAB 40 with feeding/production vessels (arrows) and tubes connecting the vessels and the homogenization tower. The homogenization tower is also fitted with a temperature control jacket.

screening for optimized production parameters and optimized composition of the nanosuspension formulation. For example, screening of four production pressures (e.g., 100, 500, 1000, and 1500 bar) up to 10 homogenization cycles requires 40 homogenization steps. It gets even more complicated when different surfactants and surfactant mixtures at different concentrations in a nanosuspension need to be checked regarding optimized physical stability of the produced nanosuspension. For screening purposes, a continuous Micron LAB 40 is much more suitable.

The continuous LAB 40 has a feeding vessel and a product vessel of a typical size of 0.5 L (Fig. 3). It is only necessary to switch two tubes before running the next homogenization cycle. Product samples for size analysis can be drawn directly from the vessels between the homogenization cycles. This speeds up the screening procedure enormously but requires a sample volume of at least 200 mL. This minimum volume of suspension cannot be accepted in the case of very expensive drugs, e.g., paclitaxel (normal price for 1 g is approximately 10.000,-$ US). On the other hand the continuous LAB 40 provides the possibility of producing lab scale batches of up to 0.5–1 L (to fit larger vessels to the systems). Producing 0.5 L of suspension by using the discontinuous LAB 40, i.e., by pooling 40-mL batches, is extremely tedious and time consuming, especially when, for example, five homogenization cycles is required. Half a liter of a suspension would be equivalent to about 60 times dismantling and mantling of the discontinuous LAB 40. Figure 4 shows a picture of the continuous LAB 40 machine.

III. GMP PRODUCTION OF 2-kg CLINICAL BATCHES

Depending on the nature and potency of the drug, the size of clinical batches might be between 2 kg and 10 kg aqueous nanoparticle dispersion. The solid content of the nanoparticle dispersions can vary from about 10% to 30% depending on the final formulation. For aqueous suspensions of nanoparticles a suspension with 10% solid content might be optimal. For some formulations as high a solid content as possible is preferred, i.e., 30% in case the nanoparticle dispersion is an intermediate product, e.g., in the production of pellets or for granulation to produce tablets. The production of 2-kg batches should be performed in a reasonably short time, especially when SLN are produced by the hot homogenization technique to minimize the temperature load. In addition, the homogenizer needs to be suitable for cleaning in place and for sterilization in place. This is not possible with the Micron LAB 40.

Therefore, a production unit was designed based on the Micron LAB 60. The Micron LAB 60 is a homogenizer for continuous production with a production capacity of 60 L/h. It consists of two pumps yielding a product flow with minimized fluctuations in homogenization pressure. The dispersion is subsequently passed through two homogenization valves: a first main homogenization valve, and a second valve that creates a certain reverse pressure and is also in charge of redispersing coalesced droplets or aggregates in the case of solid suspensions. As a general rule, the homogenization pressure of the second valve should be about one-tenth of the pressure used in the first valve. That means that using a pressure of 200 bar for the first valve would result in a pressure of 20 bar for the second valve. Intensive investigations have been performed modifying the pressure of the first valve and the second valve; the "10% rule" was found to be most efficient in most applications.

The Micron LAB 60 was modified according to the needs of a Good Manufacturing Practices (GMP) production. A feeding vessel and a product vessel were fitted to the basic homogenizer unit (Figs. 5 and 6). The two vessels are double-walled to allow a separate temperature control of the feed dispersion (preemulsion or microparticle suspension) and the resulting product. The product vessel is fixed above the feeding vessel, which allows refilling by gravity of the feeding vessel from the product vessel after each homogenization cycle to run the next cycle. The connecting tubes between vessels and homogenization tower, as well as between the two vessels, are all double-walled and allow separate temperature control. The homogenization tower itself can also be separately controlled, i.e., it is possible to perform a fine tuning of the production process by selecting optimum production temperatures in each part of the production unit. All surfaces in contact with the product are electropolished to minimize adhesion of bacteria. The homogenizer itself can be sterilized by streaming steam. CIP is possible by flushing through cleaning solutions, e.g., detergent solution, organic solvents, and mixtures of organic solvents with water. Fittings are available that are solvent-resistant. The vessels and the

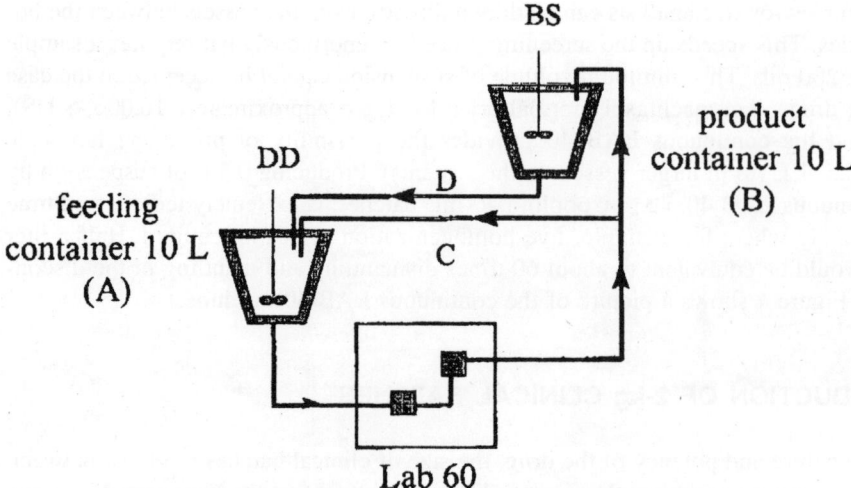

Figure 5 Scheme of the LAB 60 homogenizer for the production of 2- to 10-kg SLN batches in a continuous or discontinuous production mode, respectively. The feeding container (A) is equipped with a dissolver disk (DD) and the product container (B) with a blade stirrer (BS). In the continuous mode the dispersion is fed back after passing the tower directly to the feeding container via tube C. (Modified from Ref. 15.)

tubes can be dismantled, cleaned separately (e.g., in ultrasonic baths), and sterilized by heat or autoclaved. Assembling of the unit can be performed under laminar airflow. The modified Micron LAB 60 system was especially designed that it fits underneath a laminar airflow (LAF) unit fixed to the ceiling of the production facility (Fig. 6).

The preemulsion or presuspension is prepared in the feeding vessel using a dissolver disk. The product is kept in constant slow movement using a blade stirrer or a propeller stirrer. The dissolver disk and the stirrer are driven by two driving units with controllable stirring speed. The driving unit for the stirrer in the product container is placed horizontally to ensure that the total production unit is suitable to be positioned under a commercially available LAF unit. The temperatures in the different parts of the production unit are controlled by temperature control fluids, each fluid separately heated/cooled by a thermostat.

The production unit with the LAB 60 requires a batch size of approximately 2 L (approximately 2 kg). It is not possible to run such a low volume in the discontinuous production mode because of the relatively large dead volume of the machine (0.5 L). That means that when running the unit in the discontinuous mode about 25% of the suspension would remain in the machine without being homogenized prior to the next homogenization cycle. From this it is more sensible to run the unit in a continuous circulating mode, with the product fed back after having passed the homogenization tower directly to the feeding vessel. A double-walled tube goes directly from the homogenization tower to the feeding vessel (Fig. 5, tube C). It can be theoretically calculated as to how many minutes of circulation is required to guarantee that 99.9% of the droplets have at least passed the homogenization gap *once*. For 2 kg this is approximately 10 min. Figure 7 shows the mean diameters obtained when comparing the continuous mode of the LAB 60 to the discontinuous mode with the LAB 40 on lab scale. About

Solid Lipid Nanoparticles and Nanosuspensions

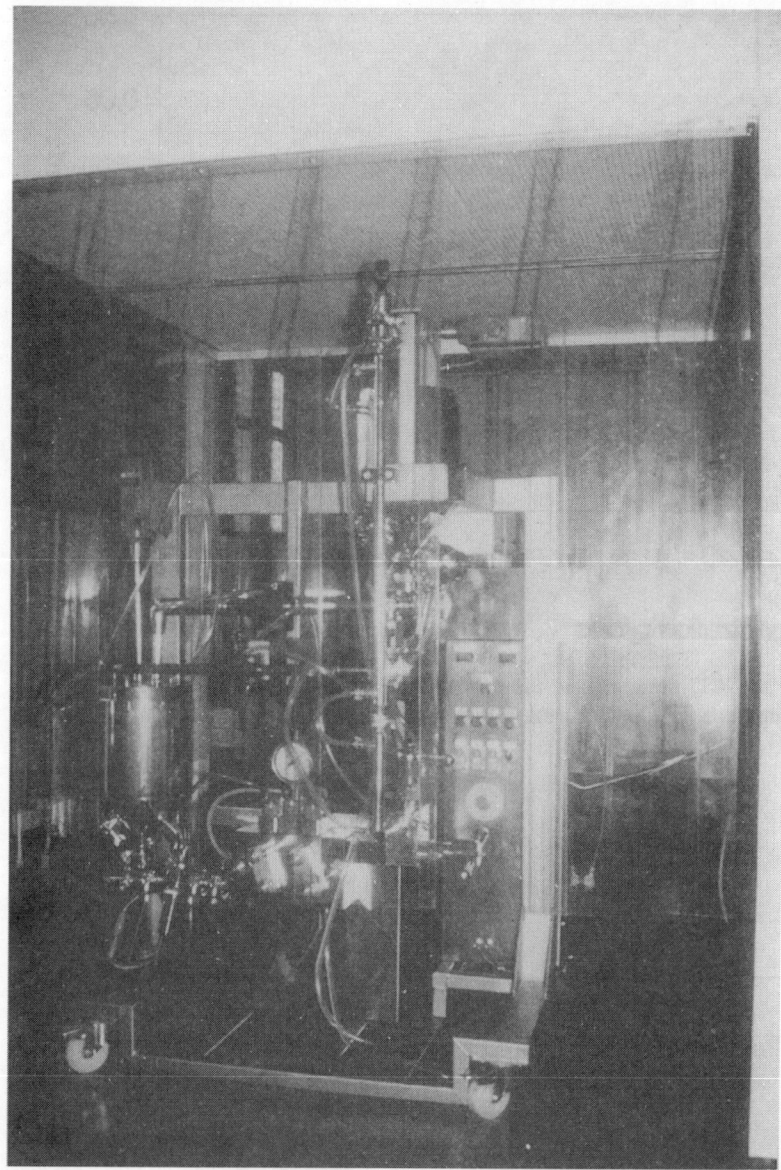

Figure 6 The LAB 60 for production under laminar airflow.

10 min circulation in the LAB 60 yields the same mean PCS diameter as three discontinuous homogenization cycles of the LAB 40.

IV. GMP PRODUCTION OF 10-kg BATCHES

The production of larger volumes cannot be performed in the continuous mode because the circulation times increase to an unacceptable level. The temperature load onto the product would be too high, leading possibly to chemical decomposition of drugs or excipients. For a 10-kg

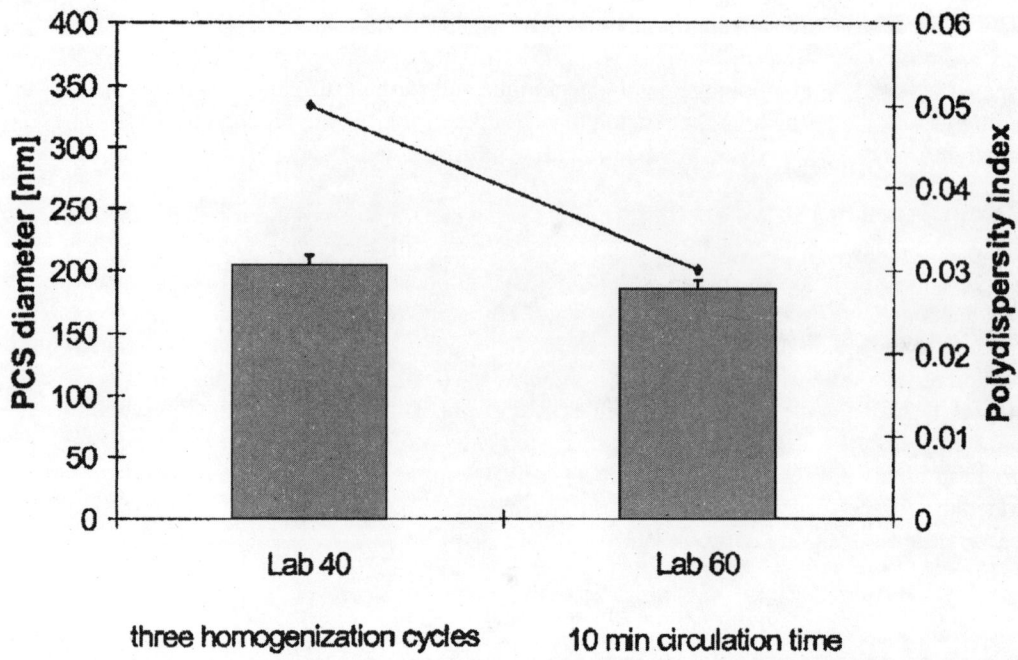

Figure 7 Comparison of the PCS diameter and the polydispersity index of a cetylpalmitate SLN dispersion produced in a discontinuous mode with the LAB 40 and in a continuous mode with the LAB 60.

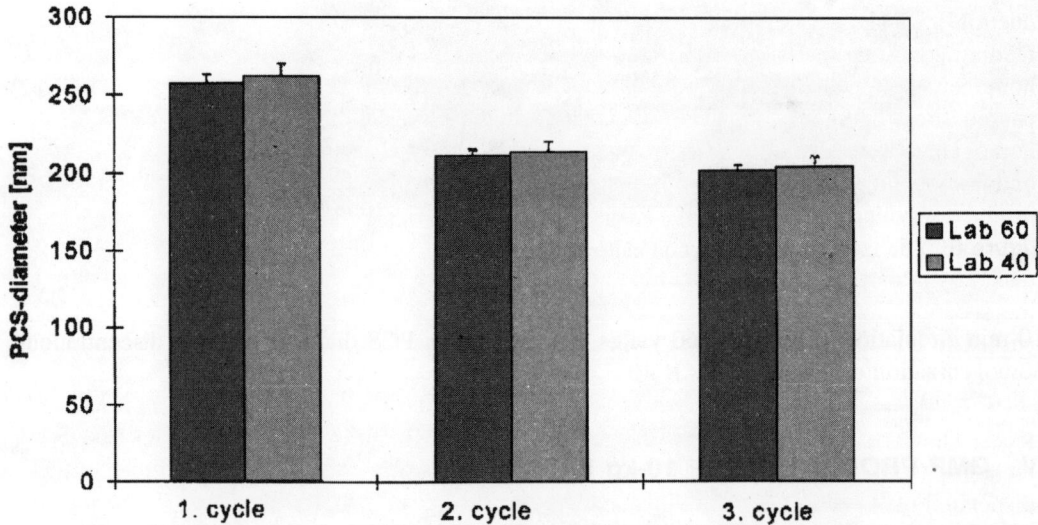

Figure 8 PCS diameter of [nm] of cetylpalmitate SLN dispersions produced with the LAB 40 and LAB 60 homogenizers and analyzed after one, two and three homogenization cycles.

batch a circulation time of approximately 1-1/2 h would be required. Therefore, such batch sizes are produced in the discontinuous mode. The predispersion (preemulsion for SLN, presuspension for SLN/cold homogenization technique and for nanosuspensions) is prepared in the feeding vessel, fed to the homogenization tower, and collected in the production vessel. The filling height in the feeding vessel is electronically controlled and the machine stops automatically when the minimum level has been reached. Then the product is fed back by gravity from the product vessel to the feeding vessel via tube D (Fig. 5) for passing the tower for the next homogenization cycle. In general, two or three homogenization cycles is sufficient for SLN produced by the hot homogenization technique. The number of cycles required for nanosuspensions depends on the hardness of the drug and the required fineness of the nanosuspension. The experiences with the homogenization of SLN show that one cycle with the LAB 60 is at least as efficient than one cycle with the discontinuous LAB 40. Especially the distribution is more uniform, that means the polydispersiy index is reduced. This is attributed to the second dispersion step when the dispersion passes this second homogenization valve. Loose aggregates formed after the passage of the first valve—which are due to still insufficient stabilization by surfactants—are effectively dispersed during the passage of the second valve. In general two cycles with the LAB 60 are approximately equivalent to three cycles with the discontinuous LAB 40 (Fig. 8).

V. PRODUCTION OF 50-kg BATCHES

Production of batches larger than 10 kg requires a priori the use of larger feeding and product containers. In addition, it is not possible to run a discontinuous production using a LAB 60 as it is being performed for 10-kg batches. One homogenization cycle would require approximately 1 h (homogenization capacity: 60 L/h). In the case of the hot homogenization technique for SLN this would require keeping the intermediate product for about 1 h before running the second cycle. The total production time for two cycles would be 2 h, i.e., a relatively high temperature load to the product. Therefore, two homogenizers are placed in series to run two homogenization cycles in a continuous process (Fig. 9). Identical to the 10-kg (10-L) production unit, the preemulsion (for SLN) and the presuspensions are prepared directly in the feeding container. From the 60-L feeding container the dispersion is fed to the APV LAB 60 homogenizer to undergo the first homogenization cycle. From the LAB 60 the product is passed directly into an APV Gaulin 5.5 homogenizer. The Gaulin 5.5 has three pistons and two homogenization valves; the maximum capacity is 160 L/H (approximately 160 kg). The second homogenizer needs to possess a higher capacity than the first one to ensure that all of the product provided by homogenizer 1 can be processed. It is possible to regulate the capacity of the Gaulin 5.5 up and down, i.e., it can be electronically adjusted exactly to the amount produced by homogenizer 1. Even if homogenizer 1 (LAB 60) produces slightly more than 60 L/h the second homogenizer can handle this amount. From the Gaulin 5.5 the final product is passed to a product container, cooled down in a controlled way, and filled into primary containers for transport.

Feeding and product containers are made from stainless steel with electropolished surfaces. They are double-walled for temperature control. The containers can be sterilized by autoclaving (121°C, 2 bar pressure). They can be pressurized up to 3 bar, which is favorable if the dispersion needs to be transported against gravity or if protective gassing needs to be used (e.g., nitrogen). Filling of the containers is performed through the top lid; dispersion leaves the container at bottom. The feeding container is again equipped with a dissolver disk, the product container with a blade stirrer or propeller stirrer.

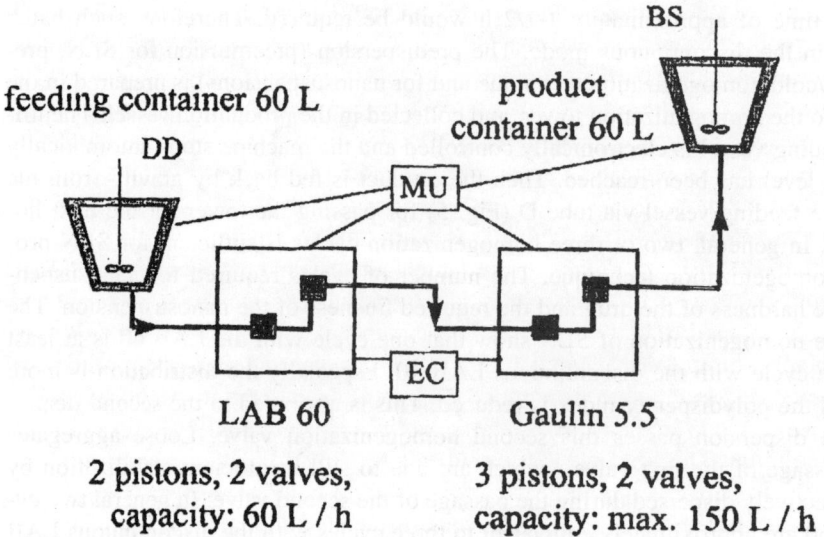

Figure 9 Production of 50-kg SLN dispersions by placing two homogenizers in series. DD, dissolver disk; BS, blade stirrer; EC, electronic control unit; MU, monitoring unit. (Modified from Ref. 16.)

The capacity of the second homogenizer is controlled by an especially designed electronic control unit (Fig. 9, EC). Production parameters such as temperatures at various points of the production unit and homogenization pressures are recorded by a special monitoring unit. The data are stored directly on disk and are therefore available for further computer processing. All parameters are recorded automatically, thus excluding human errors. The production unit is equipped with an automatic emergency stop in case the filling level in the feeding container falls below a critical level.

At the beginning of the production the design of the unit was slightly different. The Gaulin 5.5 was placed first, than the LAB 60 as second homogenizer (16). The present arrangement has the advantage that the product can be fed to the first homogenizer by gravity. The inlet of the homogenizer is below the outlet of the feeding container. This makes pressuring of the feeding container redundant.

VI. CONTINUOUS LARGE-SCALE PRODUCTION WITH 60–150 kg/h

For many applications 50-kg batches are fully sufficient. For many cosmetics as well as topical pharmaceutical products (creams, lotions), the particle dispersion is diluted by a factor of 10–20 during production of the final product. This leads to a batch size of 500–1000 kg of final product, a sufficient quantity for, say, highly priced cosmetics.

For the production of larger dispersion batches it is possible to further increase the capacity of the feeding and product containers, e.g., up to 500 kg. However, this is not sensible in case the dispersion contains temperature-sensitive active agents or excipients. A feeding container with 500 kg requires 8 h homogenization time (combination LAB 60 plus Gaulin 5.5) or, alternatively 3.5 h when combining two Gaulin 5.5. This is definitely no problem when temperature-resistant drugs are processed (e.g., in the production of nanosuspensions).

Alternatively, the excipients can be mixed by a continuous process prior to feeding the homogenizers. This production method is especially suited for preparing SLN by the hot homogenization technique. A factor determining the chemical stability of active agents incorporated in the lipid phase is very often the contact time between melted lipid and water phase. This can be minimized by continuous mixing of the melted lipid phase with the surfactant-containing water phase prior to homogenization. Mixing can be performed by static blenders. Figure 10 shows the arrangement.

In the continuous production mode the water is taken directly from the sterile water supply system. This water is sterile according to the United States Pharmacopeia (USP XXIII), meaning that the product has a priori an extremely low bacterial load. Dosing is performed via a gear pump and the water led directly to the static blender number 1 (SB 1). A second gear pump pumps a high concentrated surfactant solution to SB 1; water and surfactant solution are mixed to yield the final surfactant concentration of the outer phase in the dispersion. In a second static blender (SB 2) the lipid melt containing the active ingredient will be admixed to the aqueous surfactant solution. The lipid melt is stirred in a feeding container; transportation to the static blender is again performed by a gear pump. It should be noted that the sterile water in the supply system is stored at 80°C, and the aqueous surfactant solution has already reached the temperature required for the hot homogenization technique of SLN. Of course, tubes and static blenders are isolated or temperature-controlled, respectively. From the two homogenizers the product is fed to the product container. Filling to the packing containers is performed continuously.

Depending on the type of homogenizers used, the capacity of the production unit is 60 kg/h or 160 kg/h (combination of LAB 60 + Gaulin 5.5 or Gaulin 5.5 + Gaulin 5.5,

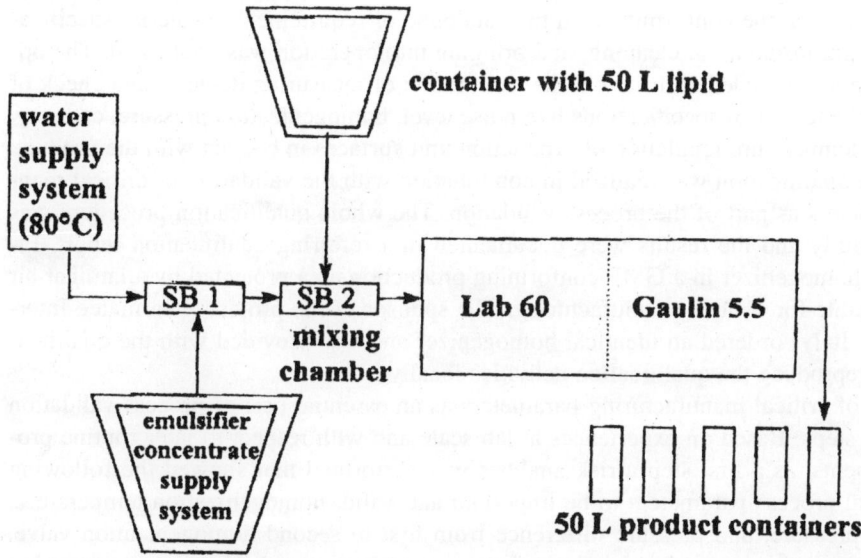

Figure 10 Arrangement of the production line to produce up to 300-kg SLN batches. Distilled water is mixed in the static blender 1 (SB1) with emulsifier concentrate. In a second static blender (SB2) surfactant containing water phase is mixed with the melted lipid for the preemulsion. (Modified from Ref. 14.)

respectively). For some active ingredients, not the contact with water but rather the temperature itself is the critical parameter for chemical stability. Such active agents cannot be dissolved in the lipid melt and kept for a few hours during the production. The solution is to dissolve the active ingredient in a liquid oil and admixing this liquid cold oil to the hot lipid blend in a separate static blender. Alternatively, the cold oil joins the lipid melt in static blender 2 (SB2). Blending of solid lipids with a liquid oil is basically no problem. It needs only to be ensured that the melting point depression is not too strongly pronounced. In some cases higher melting lipids such as carnauba wax can be easily blended with relatively large amounts of miglyol.

VII. QUALIFICATION OF THE PRODUCTION UNIT AND VALIDATION OF THE MANUFACTURING PROCESS

Prerequisites for manufacturing in accordance with current GMP standards are qualified production equipment and validated production processes. To allow an organized know-how transfer, to avoid redundent activities, and to ensure GMP compliance, a detailed strategy was invented in cooperation with the sponsor of the project.

The qualification of the homogenizer, used for 2-kg and 10-kg batches (LAB 60), was performed as a joint project together with the engineering company that built the homogenizer. The detailed activities were fixed in a qualification protocol. In the phase of design qualification a catalogue of requirements was elaborated to identify the necessary adaptations of the commercially available homogenizer to fulfill the project-specific GMP requirements, e.g., feasibility for CIP and SIP, adaptation of tubing and container design (e.g., double-walled for heating/cooling) to allow discontinuous or continuous production mode, and adequate material quality to minimize the risks of erosion and microbiological contamination. Furthermore, the measuring instrumentation for critical manufacturing parameters had to be calibratable. In the phase of installation qualification the conformity with the catalogue of requirements, material specifications, agreed design, installation, cleaning, and bringing into operation was confirmed. The operational qualification included security checks, calibration of measuring devices, and check of conformity with the technical specifications like noise level, homogenization pressure, capacity, and thermostatic temperature regulation of production unit surfaces in contact with the product. The performance qualification was realized in combination with the validation of critical manufacturing parameters as part of the process validation. The whole qualification procedure was finalized successfully and the results were documented in a referring qualification report. Finally a qualified homogenizer in a GMP conforming production area protected by a laminar air flow unit is available for contract manufacturing. The sponsor of the project (Pharmatec International, Milano, Italy) ordered an identical homogenizer and was provided with the qualification protocol to reproduce the qualification activities locally.

Validation of critical manufacturing parameters as an essential part of process validation was done in two steps. Based on experiences at lab scale and with respect to later routine production requirements, as a first step a risk analysis was performed that showed the following potentially critical process parameters to be important and valid: homogenization temperature, homogenization pressure, and pressure difference from first to second homogenization valve, and count of homogenization cycles in discontinuous production mode, i.e., homogenization time in continuous production mode. In the second step these parameters were screened, not to identify the worst cases but to detect proven acceptable ranges for reproducible and controlled manufacturing of product in conformity with the particle specification agreed with the sponsor. The most promising parameters and results from screening were verified by producing three consecutive placebo batches (active ingredient replaced by equal amount of lipid). After confirmation of their specification conformity, these batches were followed by a verum batch, conforming to specifications as well. The results of validation were fixed in the final version of manufacturing instruction that was provided to the sponsor. Based on this document the sponsor produced additional verum validation batches under full GMP conditions as a basis for further treatment (spray drying) and packaging for clinical trials.

VIII. PRODUCT QUALITY: LARGE-SCALE PRODUCTION LABORATORY SCALE

Formulation development for SLN and nanosuspensions takes place on the lab scale homogenizer LAB 40 (discontinuous or continuous version). The question is to what extent the production parameters on lab scale correlate to the production parameters on large scale, i.e., to what extent is an adaptation of the production parameters necessary. Intensive studies have been performed on the effect on production parameters when increasing the production scale, i.e., moving from 40–200 mL to 2 kg and up to 50 kg.

The correlation is demonstrated using the production of cetylpalmitate SLN by the hot homogenization technique. The cetylpalmitate SLN are produced on lab scale using 500 bar and three homogenization cycles at 80°C. This results in a mean PCS diameter of 220 nm and a polydispersity index of about 0.100 (PCS, photon correlation spectroscopy). The 2-kg batch was produced in the continuous mode on the LAB 60. Figure 11 shows the decrease in the mean diameter of the particles as a function of circulation time. Pressure and production temperature were kept unchanged. After 10 min of homogenization the same mean diameter produced on lab scale with three homogenization cycles could be reached (Fig. 7). This is below the theoretically calculated 30 min for the percentage of 99.9% of the droplets to have passed the homogenization gap three times. The polydispersity index as measure of the width of distribution is about 0.046, showing the more effective dispersion by the LAB 60 (narrower size

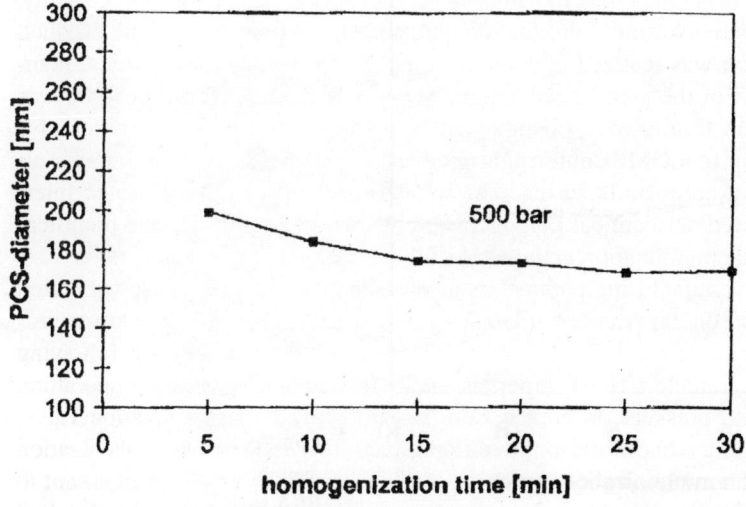

Figure 11 Mean diameter of a 2-kg SLN dispersion as a function of circulation time, cetylpalmitate SLN produced with the LAB 60 in the continuous mode. (Modified from Ref. 17.)

distribution). In summary, 2-kg batches could be produced without change of production pressure and temperature within 10 min.

A 10-kg batch was produced at identical pressure and temperature, but using the discontinuous mode, i.e., running three homogenization cycles (Fig. 12). Just three cycles with the LAB 60 is sufficient to reach a size of about 220 nm of the lab scale. Further increase of the cycle number confers no further size-reducing effect because the maximum dispersivity has been reached at the given production parameters. Applying more than three homogenization cycles can potentially increase the particle size due to aggregation (18). In summary, without changing homogenization pressure and temperature a 10-kg batch can be produced within 30 min.

The 50-kg production unit was tested for preparing 20-kg batches of SLN. The stirring rates of the dissolver disk in the feeding container and the propeller stirrer in the product container were optimized prior to running batches at identical pressure and production temperature as on lab scale. One pass of cetylpalmitate SLN through the two homogenizers yielded a particle dispersion with 238 nm mean diameter and a polydispersity index of 0.054. These values are again rather close to the data obtained on lab scale. The minor differences in mean diameter and polydispersity index do not impair te quality of the particle dispersion and its performance in the final product. Scaling up to larger production units creates differences in the heat transfer between product and surfaces/metal parts of the production unit, as well as in the cooling rate in the final product. Obviously, these heat transfer effects had little impact on the mean size and size distribution of the lipid particle dispersion. The passage of two homogenizers is again approximately equivalent to three homogenization cycles when using the lab scale unit. In summary, increasing the production scale from 40 g to 20 kg, i.e., by a factor of 500, could be performed without changing the production parameters of pressure and temperature.

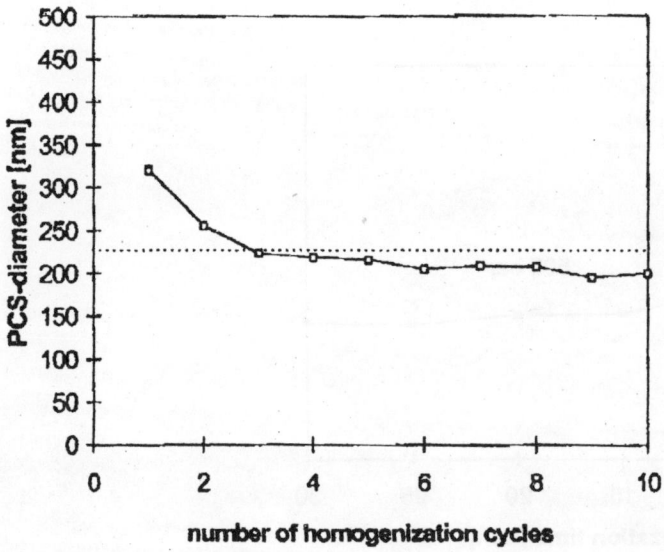

Figure 12 Mean diameter of a 10-kg SLN dispersion as a function of the number of homogenization cycles, produced with the LAB 60 in a discontinuous mode. (Modified from Ref. 17.)

IX. CONCLUSIONS AND PERSPECTIVES

The high-pressure homogenization technique provides relatively easy scaling up for the production of solid nanoparticles, i.e., SLN and nanoparticles from pure drug (nanosuspensions). The basic advantage of the equipment is that it is already used in the production of parenteral products on the market. Therefore, it is basically accepted by the regulatory authorities. Another advantage is that the equipment is already available in industry. It can be used, sometimes even without any modification (e.g., production of SLN by hot homogenization technique). Possible product contamination by metals from the production unit was found to be below the critical values. From this a major obstacle for the introduction of solid lipid nanoparticles into the clinic—the lack of large-scale production—could be removed by using high-pressure homogenization techniques.

Products based on SLN and DissoCubes technology are under development for both cosmetics and pharmaceuticals. The regulatory threshold for cosmetics is distinctly lower than for pharmaceutical products. Therefore, it is expected that the cosmetic formulations will be first on the market. There might be a similar development compared to the introduction of liposomes. Dior was the first company to introduce liposomes to the cosmetic market in 1986 (antiaging product "Capture"); a few years later, the pharmaceutical products followed. A similar development is expected for SLN and DissoCubes.

REFERENCES

1. Müller, B. W. Fischer, W. Method and apparatus for the manufacture of a product having a substance embedded in a carrier, US Patent No. 5043.280 (1991).
2. Hanna, M., York, P., Shekunov, B. Yu. Control of the polymeric forms of a drug. Substance by solution enhanced dispersion by supercritical fluids, Proc. 5th Meeting of Supercritical Fluids, Nice, France, March 1998.
3. Müller, R. H., Lucks, S. Arzneistoffträger aus festen Lipidteilchen-Feste Lipidnanosphären (SLN), European Patent No. 0605497 (1996).
4. Freitas, C. Feste Lipidnanopartikel (SLN): Mechanismen der physikalschen Destabilisierung und Stabilisierung, Dissertationsschrift Freie Universität Berlin, 1998.
5. Dingler, A., Lukowski, G, Pfegel, P., Müller, R. H., Gohla, S. Production and characterization of Lipopearls for cosmetics, Proc. Int. Symp. Control. Rel. Bioact. Mater., 24, 935–936, 1997.
6. zur Mühlen, A., Schwarz, C., Mehnert, W. Solid lipid nanoparticles (SLN) for controlled drug delivery-Drug release and release mechanism, Eur. J. Phar. Biopharm. 45, 149–155 (1998).
7. Weitschies, W. Kontrastmittel für die bildgebende medizinische Diagnostik. In: Müller, R. H, Hildebrand, G. E. (Eds.), Pharmazeutische Technologie: Moderne Arzneiformen, 2. Auflage, Wissenschaftliche Verlagsgesellschaft Stuttgart, 1998, pp. 259–292.
8. Müller, R. H., Becker, R., Kruss, B., Peters, K. US Patent 5.858.410 (1999).
9. Krause, K., Herstellung und Charakterisierung von Nanosuspensionen aus Arzneistoffen und Makromolekülen, PhD thesis, in preparation.
10. Müller, R. H., Peters, K., Becker, R., Kruss, B. Nanosuspensions for the i.v. Administration of Poorly Soluble Drugs: Stability During Sterilization and Long-Term Storage, Proc. Int. Symp. Control. Rel. Bioact. Mater., 22, 574–575, 1995.
11. Böhm, B. H. L., Behnke, D., Müller, R. H., Production of paclitaxel nanosuspensions by high pressure homogenization, Proc. Int. Symp. Control. Rel. Bioact. Mater 24, 927–928, 1997.
12. Peters, K., Müller, R. H., Nanosuspensions for the oral application of poorly soluble drugs, Eur. Symposium on Formulation of Poorly-Available Drugs for Oral Administration, APGI, Paris, 1996.
13. Grau, M. J., Müller, R. H., Increase of dissolution velocity and solubility of poorly soluble drugs by formulation as nanosuspension, Proc. 2nd World Meeting APGI/APV, Paris, 1998, 623–624.

14. Müller, R. H., Weyhers, H., zur Mühlen, A., Dingler, A., Mehnert, W., Solid Lipid Nanoparticles (SLN)—ein neuartiger Wirkstoff-Carrier für Kosmetika und Pharmazeutika, I. Systemeigenschaften, Herstellung und Scaling up, Pharm. Ind. 59(5), 423–427, 1997.
15. Hildebrand, G. E. Dingler, A., Runge, S. A., Müller, R. H., Medium scale production of solid lipid nanoparticles (SLN), Proceed. Intern. Symp. Control. Rel. Bioact. Mater., 25, 963–964, 1998.
16. Müller, R. H., Dingler, A., The next generation after the liposomes: Solid lipid nanoparticles (SLN/Lipopearls) as dermal carrier in cosmetics, Eur. Cosmet., 7/8, 19–26, 1998.
17. Dingler, A., Feste Lipid-Nanopartikel als kolloidale Wirkstoffträgersysteme zur dermalen Applikation, Dissertationsschrift Freie Universität Berlin, 1998.
18. Müller, R. H., Mehnert, W., Lucks, J. S., Schwarz, C., zur Mühlen, A., Weyhers, H., Freitas, C., Rühl, D., Solid Lipid Nanoparticles (SLN)—An Alternative Colloidal Carrier System for Controlled Drug Delivery, Eur. J. Pharm. Biopharm. 41(1), 62–69, 1995.

19
Solid Lipid Nanoparticles (SLN) as a Carrier System for the Controlled Release of Drugs

R. H. Müller, A. Lippacher, and S. Gohla

I. INTRODUCTION

A high potential for drug delivery has been attributed to particulate drug carriers, especially small particles such as microparticles and colloidal systems in the nanometer range. Looking at the types of colloidal/particulate drug carriers on the pharmaceutical market, one will find a number of systems being present in the majority of these products:

Emulsions
Liposomes
Micellar systems/mixed micelles
Microparticles.

The question arises, where are the solid nanoparticles? More than 30 years of intensive academic and industrial research did not lead to a product class. The dosage form based on solid polymeric nanoparticles is practically nonexistent on the market. Just recently, the company Nycomed launched a nanoparticulate product (Abdoscan); however, this is for diagnostic purposes and not for treatment. The registration criteria regarding toxicity are less strict for products which are administered only once compared to formulations for disease treatment, especially chronic treatment. Therefore, it is easier to realize a nanoparticulate product for diagnostic purposes.

The lack of nanoparticulate products seems to be surprising at first glance. Compared to emulsions and liposomes they have some distinct advantages. Advantages of solid particles are:

1. The solid matrix provides highest flexibility in controlling the release profile.
2. The slower degradation velocity in vivo (e.g., compared to liposomes) allows drug release for prolonged periods.
3. The solid matrix can (but need not) protect incorporated active ingredients/drugs against chemical degradation.

Drug release from emulsions is very fast. It takes place according to the partitioning coefficient and the phase ratios of oil and water phase. Typical release times are within milliseconds (1). Longer release times can be achieved with liposomes; however, release times are limited not only by liposome physical properties but also by metabolization in vivo. Compared to this solid polymeric particles provide a higher flexibility. In addition, release periods are longer because degradation times can be designed from days over weeks to months (2–5). Solid matrices are able to protect incorporated ingredients against chemical reactions with, say, water or oxygen. However, in the case of polymer-derived drug carriers, in some cases incorporated drugs may degrade within the carrier prior to their release (6).

Quite a few factors are problems in introducing solid polymeric nanoparticles to the market. Examples are:

Solvent residues from production
Sterilization problems
Cytotoxicity
Lack of suitable large-scale production methods
Cost effectiveness, affordable for health systems?

We will not discuss these points in detail but rather will highlight cytotoxicity and large-scale production. Polyester polymers such as poly(lactic acid) (PLA) and poly(lactic acid/glycolic acid) (PLA/GA) are accepted for parenteral administration by regulatory authorities (e.g., FDA, BfArM in Germany). They proved to be nontoxic and tolerated when used as implants or microparticles. However, the story is different when using them as nanoparticles or as particles with the size of a few micrometers. The particles can be internalized by macrophages, will be degraded intracellularily, and can show cytotoxicity (7).

The availability of a large-scale production method is the prerequisite for the introduction of a product to the market. In many cases the production methods for polymeric nanoparticles are only developed on lab scale. Large-scale methods are not available, or sometimes the equipment cannot be qualified or does not yield a product of a quality that is acceptable to the regulatory authorities. Of course, the production method needs to be low cost to make the nanoparticulate product competitive to traditional dosage forms. If the therapeutic benefit of a new nanoparticulate dosage form is limited, the public health systems could tend to go for the cheaper traditional product. A cost-intensive large-scale production method is no problem if the nanoparticulate product is the only way of treatment or if it is distinctly superior in therapy (e.g., more effective reducing treatment time, hospilization time of patients, and subsequently reducing the total treatment costs).

In summary, from our point of view major obstacles for the introduction of solid polymeric nanoparticles to the market are the status of excipients (e.g., polymers, toxicity, etc.) and lack of large-scale production methods yielding a product of acceptable quality.

The alternative is to replace the solid polymer by solid lipids, i.e., producing solid lipid nanoparticles (8,9). The solid lipid nanoparticles combine the advantages of traditional colloidal/particulate drug carriers but simultaneously avoiding some of their major disadvantages. The SLN can be produced on large industrial scale by high-pressure homogenization similar to emulsions but avoiding the problem of burst release due to the partitioning of the drug in emulsions. Similar to emulsions and liposomes, the SLN are composed of physiological compounds or toxicologically acceptable compounds (e.g., excipients of GRAS* status). Like polymeric nanoparticles, they possess a solid matrix which provides higher flexibility in controlling the drug release but avoids the problem of polymer particles, which implies a lack of large-scale production. This chapter focuses on the possibilities for modifying the drug release from SLN in a controlled way.

---

*Generally regarded as safe.

II. DEFINITION OF SLN

The SLN system can be easily explained. It is identical to an oil-in-water emulsion for parenteral nutrition (e.g., Intralipid, Lipofundin), but the liquid lipid (oil) of the emulsion has been replaced by a solid lipid, i.e., yielding solid lipid nanoparticles. SLN are particles made from solid lipids or lipid blends produced by high-pressure homogenization. The mean photon correlation spectroscopy (PCS) diameter is typically between approximately 80 nm and 1000 nm. Particles below 80 nm are more difficult to produce because very often they do not recrystallize (10). The same is valid for particles made from glycerides with short-chain fatty acids, e.g., Dynasan 112 (11). Of course, the Dynasan 112 SLN can be solidified applying some technological tricks. The SLN are dispersed in an aqueous outer phase and stabilized by surfactants, e.g. Tween-80, sodium dodecyl sulfate (SDS), lecithin. Alternatively, they can be produced surfactant-free using steric stabilizers (e.g., Poloxamer 188) or an outer phase of increased viscosity [e.g., ethylcellulose solution (12)]. SLN can also be produced in nonaqueous media, e.g., PEG-600 or oils like Miglyol 812. Production in PEG-600 gives a dispersion which can be directly filled into soft gelatin capsules.

The aqueous SLN dispersion can be incorporated in traditional dosage forms like tablets and pellets. For producing pellets, the water for the extrusion mass is replaced by aqueous SLN dispersion. The pellets disintegrate and release the SLN completely nonaggregated (13). SLN can be transformed to a dry product by spray drying or lyophilization.

III. HISTORICAL BACKGROUND

The lipid particle itself is not new. Lipid pellets have been known for many years. Oral products with lipid pellets filled into hard gelatin capsules are on the market (e.g., Mucosolvan, Thomae-Boehringer) (14). Lipid microparticles have been described by Speiser; they were produced by spray congealing (15). The next development step by Speiser was to reduce the size further and to produce lipid nanopellets for oral delivery (16,17). The lipid nanopellets were produced by dispersing a melted lipid into a surfactant solution by using high-speed stirrers or, alternatively, a sonication bath. Using low surfactant concentrations, the lipid nanopellets were a mixture of nanoparticles and microparticles, or contained at least a larger fraction of microparticles. Figure 1 shows a formulation described in the Speiser patent produced by stirring compared to SLN prepared with high-pressure homogenization. Liposheres are also described by Domb (18,19), who prepares them by a similar process to Speiser. Lipid nanoparticles made from solid lipids are also described by Gasco using a microemulsion technique (20–24). A hot microemulsion is prepared containing the lipid and the drug. This hot microemulsion is poured into a cold surfactant solution and the lipid nanoparticles precipitate. The preparation of the microemulsion requires organic solvents which can potentially cause a toxicological problem. Precipitation of the lipid particles in water leads to a dilution of the system; in general, the particle concentration is lower than the one obtained by using high-pressure homogenization. In contrast to these lipid particle systems, the SLN are produced by high-pressure homogenization (8,9). High-pressure homogenization can produce particle dispersions with a solid content of 20–30%. The drug-loaded lipid melt is dispersed in an aqueous surfactant solution to give a preemulsion. This preemulsion is passed through a high-pressure homogenizer to yield a hot oil-in-water emulsion which cools down. The lipid recrystallizes and forms solid lipid nanoparticles. Alternatively, the drug-loaded lipid can be homogenized in its solid state, which implies use of a high-pressure milling process and not a dispersion process as applied in emulsion

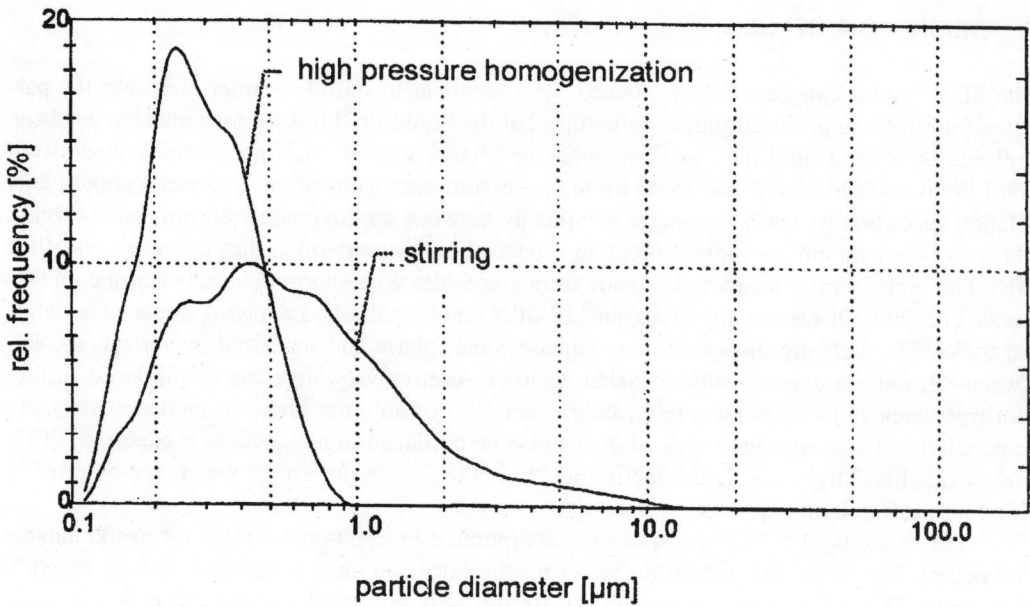

Figure 1 Volume size distribution of lipid particles produced by high-speed stirring and alternatively by high-pressure homogenization (composition of particles: 5% tristearin, 2% Tween-80, 4% Span-80, water up to 100%; size analysis by laser diffractometry). (Modified from Ref. 33.)

production. High-pressure homogenization leads generally to homogeneous products, that means one of the special features of SLN is the homogeneity in particle size distribution. Other research groups are also applying high-pressure homogenization for the lipid particle production (25–27).

IV. STATUS OF EXCIPIENTS

Depending on the route of administration, SLN must be differentiated in terms of the status of excipients (28). The three major routes are

1. External administration (e.g., topical)
2. Oral administration
3. Parenteral administration

For external administration the complete range of excipients used for cosmetics and pharmaceutical ointments/creams can be used. This provides a vast variety, especially with regard to the cosmetic excipients. There is no need to use any excipient which has not yet been accepted.

For oral administration of SLN all excipients can be employed that are frequently used in traditional oral dosage forms such as tablets, pellets, and capsules. Even surfactants with cell membrane–damaging potential, e.g., sodium dodecyl sulfate (SDS), can be used. SDS is contained in many oral products and accepted as an excipient by the regulatory authorities. In general, all GRAS substances and materials of approved GRAS status can be employed. In addition, SLN can be made from food lipids and using surfactants contained in food (e.g., surfactants from ice cream, such as e.g., sugar esters). Of course it needs to be considered that an excipient used in the food industry is not automatically accepted in pharmaceutical products; however, the required documentation process is relatively unproblematic.

The situation is different for parenteral administration. The basic point is that solid lipid nanoparticles are a novel system; solid lipids have not yet been administered parenterally before—in contrast to liquid lipids (o/w emulsions for intravenous administration, prolonged release oil-based injectables for intramuscular administration). However, the glycerides used for SLN production are composed of compounds (glycerol, fatty acids) which are also present in emulsions for parenteral nutrition. This means that, apart from drug delivery, the SLN are an additional nutritive, so to speak. The only difference to emulsions for parenteral nutrition is that the composition of the glycerides is different. The oils contain glycerides of mixed composition of medium- and long-chain triglycerides (MCTs, LCTs). The glycerides used for SLN production need to be solid, i.e., are composed of longer chain fatty acids. In addition, many lipids are monoacid glycerides, i.e., composed of just one fatty acid. Examples are Dynasan 114 with myristic acid, Dynasan 116 with palmitic acid, and Dynasan 118 with stearic acid. In some cases, the lipids used are mixtures of mono-, di-, and triglycerides. Some of them are more or less just one glyceride type or contain preferentially one glyceride, e.g., triglyceride of behenic acid in the commercial lipid Compritol [with smaller fractions of mono- (12–18%) and diglycerides]. In summary, for parenteral administration the toxicity needs to be investigated but because of the composition of compounds a good tolerability can be predicted.

V. BASIC PRODUCTION TECHNIQUES

There are two basic production techniques for SLN:

1. Hot homogenization
2. Cold homogenization

For hot homogenisation the lipid is melted to approximately 5°C above its melting point, the drug is dissolved or solubilized in the melted lipid, and the drug-containing lipid melt is dispersed in an aqueous surfactant solution of the same temperature. Dispersion is performed by a high-speed stirrer, e.g., a Silverson homogenizer or an Ultraturrax. The obtained preemulsion is then passed through a high-pressure homogenizer, e.g., a piston-gap homogenizer (Micron LAB 40, APV Homogeniser GmbH). The product of this process is a hot o/w emulsion. Cooling of the emulsion leads to the crystallization of the lipid and the formation of solid lipid nanoparticles.

The hot homogenization technique cannot be employed to incorporate hydrophilic active ingredients/drugs. Dispersing the lipid melt in the aqueous surfactant solution would lead to partitioning of drug to the water phase, which means that with hydrophilic drugs more than 90% would be lost to the water phase. To solve this problem the cold homogenization technique was developed. As with the hot homogenization technique, the drug is incorporated into a melted lipid. Then the lipid melt is cooled and after solidification ground by a mortar mill. The obtained lipid microparticles are dispersed in a cold surfactant solution at room temperature; the obtained lipid presuspension is then homogenized at room temperature or even at temperatures distinctly below room temperature (e.g., 0°C). The solid state of the matrix minimizes partitioning of the drug to the water phase. Even during storage of the aqueous SLN dispersion the entrapment efficiency remains unchanged (12). For details of the production method, especially large-scale production, the reader is referred to Chapter 18.

VI. DRUG RELEASE AND PARTICLE INTERNAL STRUCTURE

A major problem when developing lipid nanoparticles was the observed burst release. Surprisingly, the first lipid nanopellets behaved as an o/w emulsion. It seemed that the system is not feasible for a prolonged drug release. The breakthrough was in developing the first SLN, which showed a prolonged in vitro drug release up to 5–6 weeks (29,30). Of course, to develop controlled release SLN one needs to understand the drug release mechanism to allow a controlled development of formulations. Therefore, our group focused on investigating drug release profiles and the related drug release mechanisms.

At the very beginning of SLN development particles were produced using model drugs with different physicochemical properties, e.g., lipophilicity and hydrophilicity. Examples for lipophilic drugs studied were tetracaine base (31) and etomidate base (32), but also very hydrophilic drugs such as the x-ray contrast agent iotrolan produced by Schering AG in Berlin (33). For tetracaine and etomidate a burst release was observed. Study was done on the extent to which the burst release depends on particle size/surface area. It was found that the burst release diminished with increasing particle size and a prolonged release could be obtained when the particles were sufficiently large, i.e., lipid microparticles (Fig. 2) (11). From these data it was concluded that the drug was enriched in an outer shell of the particles. This lead to the core shell model of SLN with enriched drug in the outer shell (Fig. 3, upper left). The drug has a relatively short distance of diffusion and will be released in a burst. The formation of the shell is explained by the stepwise crystallization process of the drug–lipid mixture. After the hot homogenization step the produced o/w emulsion is cooled, the lipid precipitates first forming a more or less drug-free lipid core. The remaining liquid drug–lipid mixture will enrich continuously in drug content until the eutecticum is reached. Reaching the eutecticum leads to the simultaneous crystallization of lipid and drug, forming an outer shell surrounding the drug-free lipid core.

In addition, it must be considered that surfactant is present. This surfactant will interact with the outer shell and affect its structure. The existence of a shell can be proven by atomic force microscopy (AFM) measurements. With a special technique, noncontact imaging, the

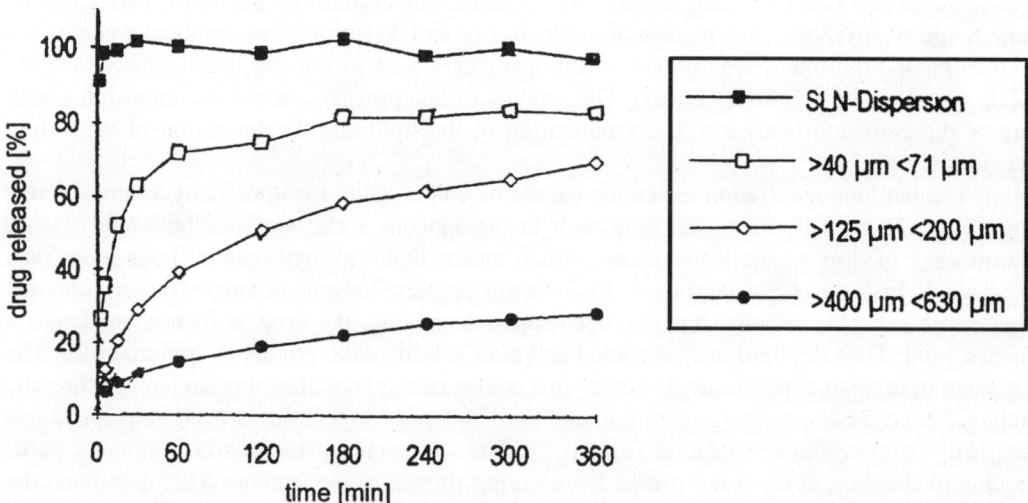

Figure 2 Release of etomidate from lipid nanoparticles (SLN) and lipid microparticles of increasing particle size. (Modified from Ref. 12.)

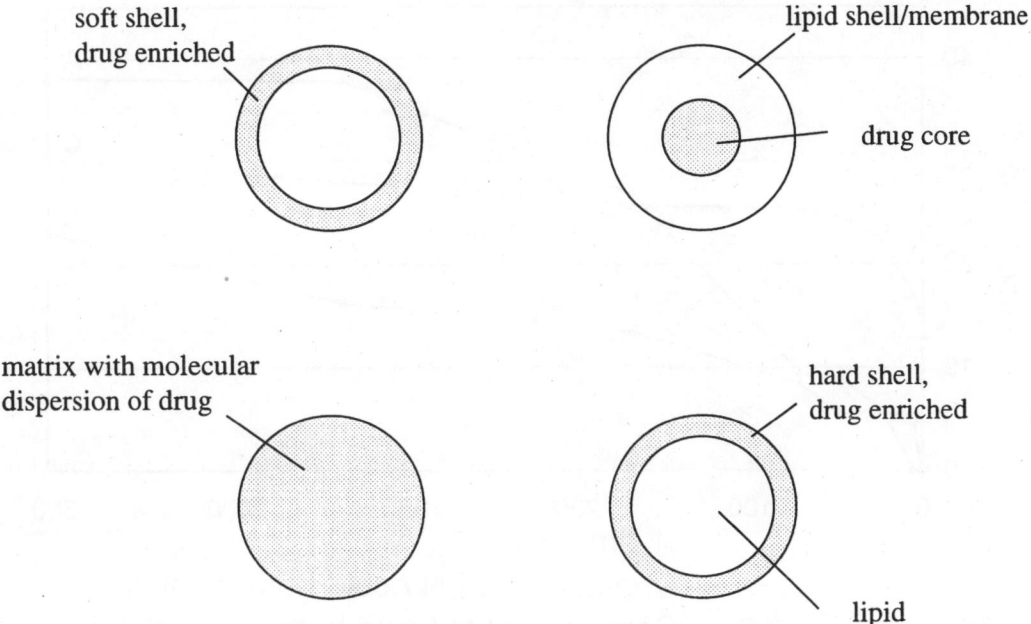

Figure 3 Proposed models for the internal structure of SLN: (1) Soft drug-containing shell surrounding a lipid core (upper left). (2) A drug core surrounded by a lipid shell being drug-free or of low drug content (upper right). (3) Homogeneous particle matrix with molecular dispersion of drug (lower left). (4) Drug-free lipid core surrounded by a hard shell composed of lipid–drug mixture (eutecticum) (lower right).

hardness of the particle is determined by pressing the cantilever of the AFM instrument into the particle. The force required to press the cantilever into the particle is a measure of the viscosity of the particle matrix. It can be shown that there is an outer shell of relatively low viscosity that is composed of lipid, drug, and partially incorporated surfactant (34). That means the model could be specified to be the so-called soft shell–hard core model.

In contrast, with the model drug prednisolone a prolonged release was observed over a period up to 6 weeks (29). The prolonged release can be explained by molecular distribution of the drug in the lipid matrix (= solid dispersion, Fig. 3 lower left). Figure 4 shows the release profiles obtained with prednisolone-loaded SLN of identical lipid composition but produced with different homogenization techniques (hot v. cold) and of SLN being produced under identical conditions (cold homogenization) but composed of different lipids (Compritol v. cholesterol). The very interesting feature is that the release profile changes with production parameters and also changes by using a different lipid. A slow release without distinct burst was obtained by applying the cold homogenization technique. This was attributed to the presence of a solid solution, i.e., prednisolone was distributed in a molecular dispersed form homogeneously in the solid lipid matrix. This is very likely because cooling the drug-containing lipid will lead to the formation of a solid dispersion. This solid dispersion was just milled by high-pressure homogenization, which means that no or limited melting occurred; the particles were just broken down and retained their structure of a solid dispersion. Of course, we are well aware of the fact that temperature peaks occur during the homogenization process. In addition, there will be a warming up of the dispersion by approximately 20°C. However, this does not lead to a melting if the difference between reached temperature and melting point of the lipid is

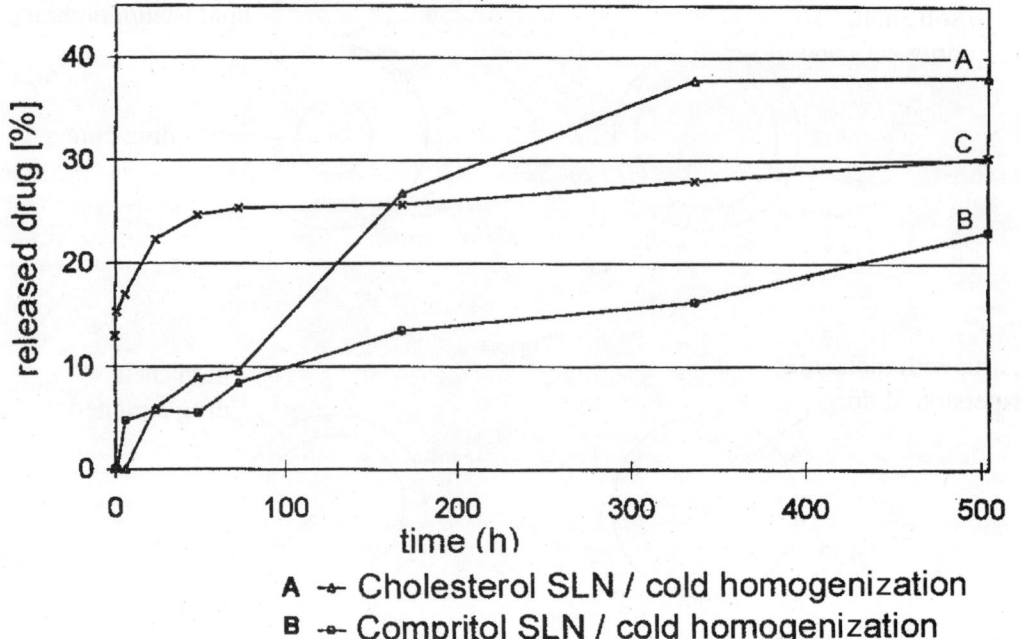

A ─▲─ Cholesterol SLN / cold homogenization
B ─■─ Compritol SLN / cold homogenization
C ─✕─ Compritol SLN / hot homogenization (40°C)

Figure 4 Drug release from SLN produced with identical lipid (Compritol) but different production methods (cold v. hot homogenization) and identical cold homogenization but different lipids (Compritol v. cholesterol). (Modified from Ref. 43.)

sufficiently high. Based on these results, the existence of a "solid dispersion model" for SLN was proposed (Fig. 3, lower left). Drug release is governed by diffusion of the drug in the solid matrix (solid phase diffusion).

Producing the prednisolone-loaded SLN by the hot homogenization technique led to a burst release followed by a prolonged release. The burst release was intensively investigated by changing the production parameters (temperature) and changing the composition of the SLN formulation (that means preferentially surfactant concentration) (29). It was found that the extent of burst release increased with increasing temperature and increasing surfactant concentration (Fig. 5). The explanation for this effect was very simple: With increasing temperature and increasing surfactant concentration, the solubility of the drug in the water phase increased. Applying the hot homogenization technique lead to an o/w emulsion. At high temperature the solubility of prednisolone in the outer aqueous phase was higher. Cooling down the emulsion lead to the precipitation of the drug-containing lipid core; simultaneously, the solubility of the prednisolone in the water phase decreased. Continuing decrease in temperature and prednisolone solubility in the water phase led to an drug enrichment in the outer shell of the SLN. The better the prednisolone solubility in the water phase, the higher was the enrichment in the outer shell of the SLN. That means that burst release consequently needed to be increased with increased production temperature and increased surfactant concentration. When replacing the cold homogenization technique with the hot homogenization technique, one moves away from the solid dispersion again to the core shell type of SLN. This presents the possibility for an optimal design of drug release profiles. If an initial dose is required, one can adjust the production parameters and/or the formulation composition (surfactant concentration) to obtain exactly the initial burst release required.

SLN as a Carrier System

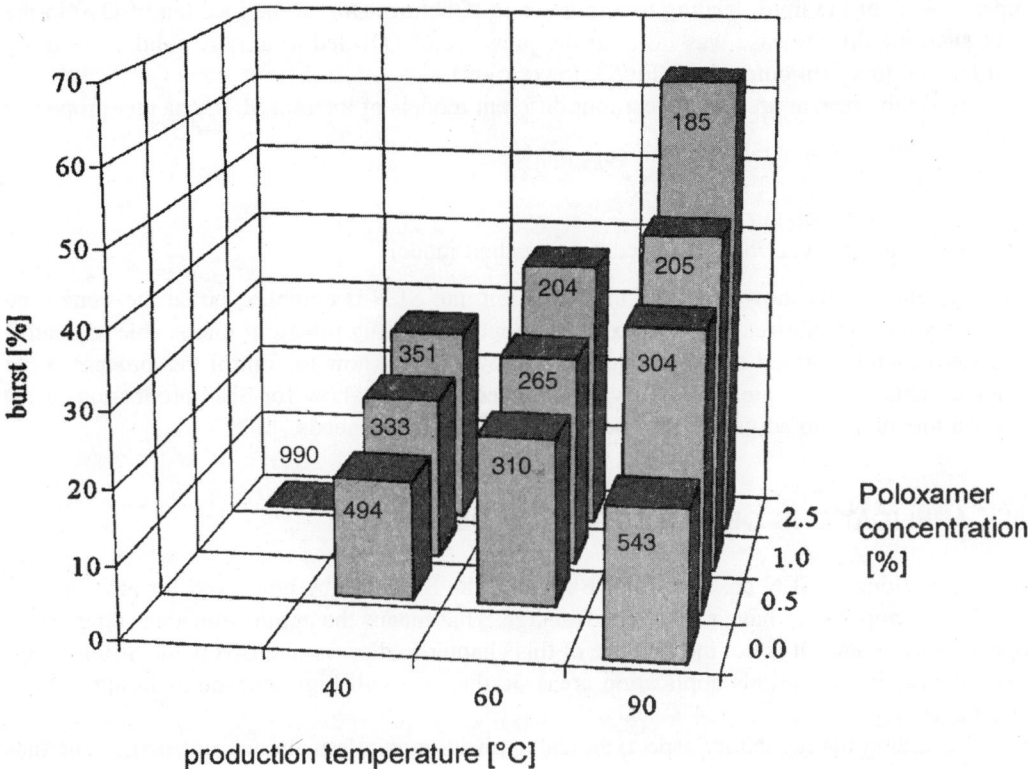

Figure 5 Extent of burst release as a function of production temperature and surfactant concentration. The particle sizes of the SLN are given in nanometers. (Modified from Ref. 30.)

Applying the hot homogenization technique and simultaneously using low surfactant concentration led to a minimal burst and a prolonged drug release. This cannot necessarily be explained by the prednisolone–lipid mixture crystallizing as a solid dispersion. Solubility of prednisolone in the lipid was very limited; maximum solubility obtained in the lipid melts was approximately 1%. The SLN were produced incorporating prednisolone at its maximum solubility in the heated lipid. From this it appears possible that during the cooling process instead of the lipid precipitating first, the drug precipitates first. It depends on where one is in a TX diagram. In the soft shell core model one moves down the isoplethe and reaches the solubility limit of the lipid first; then the lipid crystallizes and the remaining liquid enriches with drug. In this model one first reaches the solubility limit of the drug, the drug precipitates, the liquid mixture enriches with lipid until the euteticum precipitates as a mixture drug lipid. This eutecticum forms more or less a membrane through which the drug diffuses from the inner core (Fig. 3, upper right).

Recently it was discovered that there is additionally the hard shell core model of SLN. Within an industrial product development the SLN were loaded with Coenzym Q10. The Q10-loaded SLN were routinely investigated by contact AFM. It was assumed that a solid dispersion of Q10 in lipid would be present. Contact AFM revealed that there was an outer shell of increased rigidity; the core was distinctly less rigid. Q10 was released relatively fast. Obviously the Q10 had accumulated in the outer shell but promoted crystallization of the lipid. Possibly Q10 and the lipid had structural properties such that they fitted together very well to form a solid structure (like brick layers). It could be possible that the molecule Q10 fitted into the imperfections of the lipid, leading to a more solid structure. Due to the location of Q10 in the outer shell the drug release was fast, but the presence of Q10 led to a more solid state of the lipid leading to a firm outer shell (Fig. 3, lower right).

To summarize, at present there a four different models of internal SLN structure proposed:

1. Soft drug–containing shell core model
2. Drug core/lipid shell model
3. Solid dispersion model
4. Drug-free core/hard drug–containing shell model

The different models show that drug incorporation into SLN is complex, but at the same time the variety of models gives highest flexibility to modulate drug release if one is able to control the SLN structure formed during production. Knowledge of how to control this process is the major advantage of the companies having the adequate know-how for SLN production. It requires a fine tuning to adjust the release profile exactly to the needs.

VII. APPLICATIONS OF SLN FOR DRUG DELIVERY

The applications of SLN are manifold. Basically, the SLN can be employed for any purpose for which nanoparticles have a distinct advantage. That means the application areas range from topical to parenteral. It is not the purpose of this chapter to discuss intensively the different options of SLN in the various application areas. Rather, we will highlight the main application advantages.

Regarding the regulatory aspect, topical application is relatively unproblematic. The major advantages for topical products are the protective properties of SLN for chemically labile drugs against degradation and the occlusion effect due to film formation on the skin (35,36). Especially in the area of cosmetics there are many compounds such as retinol or vitamin C which cannot be incorporated because of the lack of chemical stability. Incorporation of retinol is only possible when applying certain protective measures during production (e.g., noble gasing) and using special packing materials (e.g., aluminum). This increases production costs, and it would be better to achieve the protection against degradation by the SLN and use a normal production process and a highly acceptable packing material (e.g., polyethylene elastic tube). It could be shown that incorporation of cosmetic ingredients into SLN can change their penetration profile (37,38). By choosing a controlled composition of the cream the release of the active ingredient/drug can be triggered. In addition, the occlusion effect of the SLN film formed onto the skin promotes penetration of active ingredients. In vitro occlusion tests showed a superior effect of solid lipid nanoparticles v. solid lipid microparticles and demonstrated the increase in occlusion by admixing SLN to traditional creams (35,36). Apart from the change in penetration, the occlusion can lead to an increased hydration and the smoothing of wrinkles.

Many investigations have been made to use nanoparticles for the prolonged release of drugs to the eye. The basic problem of ophthalmological formulation is the fast removal from the eye, which implies clearance of the applied drug through the nose. It could be shown for nanoparticles that an increased adhesiveness is available leading to higher drug levels at the desired site of action. However, the basic problem was that the nanoparticles are of limited toxicological acceptance, e.g., polyalkylcyanoacrylate nanoparticles which lead to the release of potentially cancerogenic formaldehyde. Other particles are too slowly biodegradable and therefore are not acceptable to the regulatory authorities. It was shown by Gasco that SLN have a prolonged retention time at the eye. This was confirmed by using radiolabeled formulations and γ-scintigraphy (Gasco, personal communication). The lipids of the SLN are easy to metabolize and open a new potential for ophthalmological drug delivery without impairing vision.

A very interesting application appears to be the pulmonary administration of SLN. SLN powders cannot be administered to the lung because the particle size is too small and they will be exhaled. A very simple approach is the aerosolization of aqueous SLN dispersions. The important point is that the SLN should not aggregate during the aerosolization process. Figure 6 shows the particle size distribution of SLN prior to and after aerosolization. The nebulizer employed was a Pari-boy (Paul Ritzau Pari-Werk GmbH, Starnberg, Germany). The aerosol droplets were collected by collision of the aerosol with a glass wall of a beaker. This basically demonstrates that SLN are suitable for lung delivery. After localization into the bronchial tube and in the alveoli, the drug can be released in a controlled way from the lipid particles. Afterward the lipid can be degraded by nonspecific enzymes or incorporated into macrophages. A special feature of SLN is that they are susceptible to nonspecific hydrolysis. This could be shown by degrading SLN produced from a wax, cetylpalmitate. In vivo the cetylpalmitate, despite being a nonphysiological wax, was much more quickly degraded than the glyceride mixture of behenic acid (Compritol) (39–42). A major field of administration is the gastrointestinal tract for SLN. Regarding the status of excipients, it is a very uncomplicated area. SLN can reduce the variability of absorption (erratic absorption). It is hoped to reduce the difference between fed/nonfed subjects. Undesired plasma peaks can be removed due to the prolonged release from SLN (45). Absorption might be improved because the SLN behave as other nanoparticles, i.e., they have adhesive properties and stick to the mucosa of the gastrointestinal wall. In addition, the fat of the SLN will be processed and absorbed like normal food fat. Therefore, it

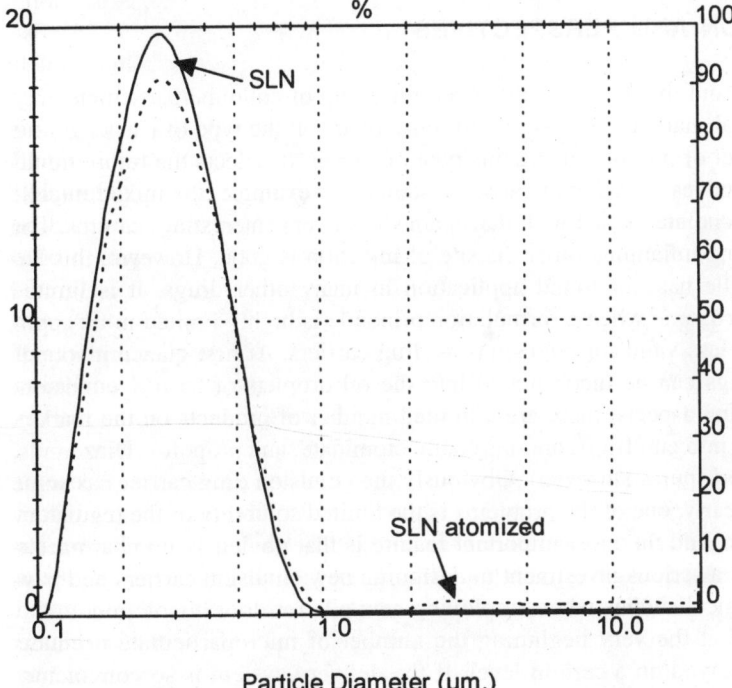

Figure 6 Volume size distribution of SLN before aerosolization and after aerosolization using a Pari-boy (laser diffractometry data).

appears possible that drugs will be absorbed like a "Trojan horse," i.e., they will be taken up simultaneously with the fat and lead to a sufficiently high bioavailability. An additional application is treatment of diseases directly located in the gastrointestinal tract, e.g., colitis ulcerosa.

Parenteral application is a very wide field for SLN. Subcutaneous injection of drug-loaded SLN can be employed for many interesting drugs, not only from the academic point of view but also from the commercial aspect, e.g., erythropoetin (EPO), interferon-β. Other routes are intraperitoneal and also intra-articular. Intraperitoneal application of drug-loaded SLN will prolong the release because of the application area. In addition, incorporation of the drug into SLN might reduce irritancy compared to injecting drug microparticles. Possible applications for intra-articular applications are treatment of arthritis. Arthritic inflammation in joints is caused by hyperactivation of macrophages releasing inflammation mediators. The basic concept is to give corticoids to the macrophages to reduce their hyperactivity. Corticoids are generally poorly soluble in water; incorporation in a lipophilic matrix is therefore possible. Macrophages can internalize the SLN. Release of corticoid will follow, leading to a reduction in hyperactivity and consequently inflammation of the joint. Another broad application area is intravenous injection. Critical excipients like Cremophor EL can be avoided by incorporating the drug into SLN stabilized with well-accepted and tolerated surfactants. An example is Taxol by Bristol-Myers Squibb. Since the surfactant Cremophor EL can lead to anaphylactic reactions, administration of the product can only be performed by applying medical precautions. Basic studies have been performed to incorporate paclitaxel into SLN. From SLN they can be released in a burst, i.e., infusion of SLN should be equivalent to infusion of Taxol. There should be no change in the pharmacokinetic profile, thus providing few only limited problems with regulatory authorities. One product might be exchanged by the new generation product.

VIII. MARKET SITUATION AND PERSPECTIVES

At the beginning we pointed out that there is only a certain group of colloidal/particulate drug carriers on the pharmaceutical market. One should not only focus on the type of carrier on the market but also on the number of products using this type of carrier. It reflects the future trends of the market and the perspectives of different carrier systems. For example, the mixed micelle of lecithin and sodium glycocholate loaded with diazepam shows very interesting features. The product performance regarding inflammation at the site of injection is good. However, this basic principle of mixed micelle has not found application in many other drugs. It is limited mainly to diazepam. It is worrisome when a formulation principle is highly limited in its application. The same is more or less valid for emulsions as drug carriers. At first glance it sounds intriguing that lipophilic drugs can be incorporated into the oil droplets of an o/w emulsion; however, despite this intriguing aspects, there are a limited number of products on the market. The main drugs incorporated into emulsions are diazepam, etomidate, and propofol (Diazemuls, Diazepam-Lipuro, Etomidate-Lipuro, Diprivan). Obviously the emulsion drug carrier has some problems in performance. Clearly, one of the problems is the limited solubility of the regulatory accepted oils for many drugs. And the most important feature is that obviously no pharmaceutical company wants to make a serious investment in designing new emulsion carriers and paying for the required toxicological studies when employing new oils for drug dissolution.

It is also amazing that at the very beginning the number of microparticulate products increased sharply and then stayed on a certain level. If the delivery system is so convincing, why do we not have an increasing number of products? It appears a bit strange that a delivery system—basically described as highly innovative and with potential—shows little or no increase in the number of products on the market.

The same is valid for liposomes. There was a lot of enthusiasm about liposomes at the very beginning; one hoped to solve each delivery problem by applying liposomes. Of course, when the expectations were too high the results were necessarily disappointing. One did not realize sufficiently the limitations to liposomes and nobody can expect that one delivery system will solve all problems. From our point of view, these overly high expectations were damaging to the basically good system liposome.

In summary, the present colloidal/particulate systems on the market are of limited success. Especially worrisome is that the number of products based on these technologies has not increased as expected or predicted. Obviously these technologies possess some major obstacles (ranging from technological problems to cost problems, i.e., the "cheap" liposome is not available).

Based on these considerations, there seems to be a need for an improved drug carrier system. SLN might be an alternative to the existing drug carrier systems providing more flexibility with regard to the area of applications and also the aspects for commercialization (43,44). The excipients are accepted (e.g., GRAS status), the production technique is simple and large-scale production is possible, the release profile can be modified in a controlled way, and it is a technology that has exclusivity, i.e., is patent-protected. The latter is a major point because companies investing in this new technology have to be sure that they can have a repayment of investments after market introduction.

We believe that the success of a delivery system has to be judged on the number of products reaching the pharmaceutical market. This is also valid for the delivery system SLN, which means that final judgment might be possible in about 5–8 years. However, the startup conditions are quite good because the other delivery systems are limited in their performance. This is clearly demonstrated by the relatively low number of drugs on the market in parenteral emulsions and as liposomal formulations. One has to consider the number of products in relation to the number of years spent in research. Liposomes are more than 30 years old; the number of products is limited. Emulsions for parenteral nutrition were introduced in the 1950s; the number of drug-loaded emulsions is also limited. Especially the polymeric nanoparticles, despite their high potential, have performed extremely below the expectations. After more than 30 years of research having just one diagnostic product is really disappointing. The excellent delivery system of polymeric nanoparticles has not deserved this limited success. Based on these frame conditions, the novel delivery system SLN is considered as having a good chance to perform much better.

REFERENCES

1. Washington, C., Drug release and interfacial structure in emulsions, in R. H. Miller, S. Benita, B. Böhm (Eds.), Emulsions and Nanosuspensions for the Formulation of Poorly Soluble Drugs, Medpharm, Stuttgart (1998) 101–117.
2. Wallis, K. H., Müller, R. H., Comparative measurements of nanoparticle degradation velocity using an accelerated hydrolysis test, Pharm Ind. 55(2) (1993) 168–170.
3. Grislain, L., Couvreur, P., Lenaerts, V., Roland, M., Deprez-Decampeneere, D., Speiser, P., Int. J. Pharm. 15, (1983) 335.
4. Kitchel, J. P., Wise, D. L., Poly(lactic/glycolic acid) biodegradable drug-polymer matrix systems, in K. J. Widder, R. Green (Eds.), Meth. Enzymol. 112 (1985) 436.
5. Müller, R. H., Colloidal Carriers for Controlled Drug Delivery and Targeting, Wissenschaftliche Verlagsgesellschaft, Stuttgart (1991).
6. Schwendeman, S. P., Costantino, H. R., Gupta, R. K., Langer, R., Progress and challenges for peptide, protein and vaccine delivery from implantable polymeric systems, in K. Park (Eds.), Controlled

Drug Delivery: Challenges and Strategies, American Chemical Society, Washington (1997), 229–267.
7. Smith, A., Hunneyball, I. M., Evaluation of of poly(lactic acid) as a biodegradable drug delivery system for parenteral administration, Int. J. Pharm. 30 (1986), 215–220.
8. Müller, R. H., Lucks, J. S., Arzneistoffträger aus festen Lipidteilchen, Solid Lipid Nanospheres (SLN), European Patent 0605497 (1996).
9. Müller, R. H., Mehnert, W., Lucks, J. S., Schwarz, C., zur Mühlen, A., Weyhers, H., Freitas, C., Rühl, D., Solid lipid nanoparticles (SLN)—an alternative colloidal carrier system for controlled drug delivery, Eur. J. Pharm. Biopharm. 41(1) (1995), 62–69.
10. Westesen, K., Bunjes, H., Do nanoparticles prepared from lipids solid at room temperature always possess a solid lipid matrix? Int. J. Pharm. 115 (1995), 129–131.
11. zur Mühlen, A., Schwarz, C., Mehnert, W., Solid Lipid Nanoparticles (SLN) for controlled drug delivery—drug release and release mechanism. Eur. J. Pharm. Biopharm. 45 (1998), 149–155.
12. Schwarz, C., Feste Lipidnanopartikel: Herstellung, Charakterisierung, Arzneistoffinkorporation und -freisetzung, Sterilisation und Lyophilisation, Ph. D. thesis, Free University of Berlin, 1995.
13. Pinto, J. F., Müller, R. H., Pellets as carriers of solid lipid nanoparticles (SLN) for oral administration of drugs, Die Pharmazie (in press).
14. Müller, R. H., Feste Lipidnanopartikel (SLN), in R. H. Müller, G. E. Hildebrand, Pharmazeutische Technologie: Moderne Arzneiformen, Wissenschaftliche Verlagsgesellschaft, Stuttgart (1997), 265–272.
15. Eldem, T., Speiser, P., Hincal, A., Optimization of spray-dried and congealed lipid micropellets and characterization of their surface morphology by scanning electron microscopy, Pharm. Res. 8 (1991), 47–54.
16. Speiser, P., Lipidnanopellets als Trägersystem für Arzneimittel zur peroralen Anwendung, Europäisches Patent EP0167825, 1990.
17. Haller-Dillier, F., Ultrafeine Lipidpellets als Trägersysteme für Arzneistoffe, Ph. D. thesis, ETH Zürich, 1982.
18. Domb, A., Liposheres for controlled delivery of substances, U.S. Patent 5,188,837 (1993).
19. Bergelson, L., Domb, A., The surface structure of lipid drug carriers—influence on carrier–cell interaction, in R. H. Müller, W. Mehnert (Eds.), Particle and Surface Characterization Methods, Medpharm, Stuttgart (1997).
20. Gasco, M. R., Method for producing solid lipid microspheres having a narrow size distribution, U.S. Patent 5,250,236 (1993).
21. Gasco, M. R., Morel, S., Carpignano, R., Optimization of the incorporation of deoxycorticosterone acetate in lipospheres, Eur. J. Pharm. Biopharm, 38, (1992) 7–10.
22. Morel, S., Ugazio, E., Cavalli, R., Gasco, M. R., Thymopentin in solid lipid nanoparticles, Int. J. Pharm. 132 (1996), 259–261.
23. Morel, S., Gasco, M. R., Cavalli, R., Incorporation in lipospheres of [D-Trp-6]LHRH, Int. J. Pharm 105 (1994), R1–R3.
24. Cavalli, R., Morel, S., Gasco, M. R., Chetoni, P., Saettone, M. F., Preparation and evaluation of colloidal lipospheres containing pilocarpine as ion pair, Int. J. Pharm. 117 (1995), 243–246.
25. Siekmann, B., Westesen, K., Sub-micron sized parenteral carrier systems based on solid lipids, Pharmaceut. Pharmacol. Lett. 1 (1992), 123–126.
26. Heiati, H., Tawashi, R., Phillips, N. C., Drug retention and stability of solid lipid nanoparticles containing azidothymidine palmitate after autoclaving, storage and lyophilization; J. Microencap. 15(2) (1998), 173–184.
27. Heiati, H., Phillips, N. C., Tawashi, R., Evidence for phospholipid bilayer formation in solid lipid nanoparticles formulated with phospholipid and triglyceride, Pharm. Res. 13(9) (1996), 1406–1410.
28. Müller, R. H., Weyhers, H., zur Mühlen, A., Dingler, A., Mehnert, W., Solid Lipid Nanoparticles—ein neuartiger Wirkstoff-Carrier für Kosmetika und Pharmazeutika, I. Systemeigenschaften, Herstellung und Scaling-up, Pharm. Ind. 59(5) (1997), 423–427.
29. zur Mühlen, A., Mehnert, W., Drug release and release mechanism of prednisolone loaded solid lipid nanoparticles, Die Pharmazie 53 (1998), 8.

30. zur Mühlen, A., Feste Lipid Nanopartikel mit prolongierter Wirkstoffliberation Herstellung, Langzeitstabilität, Charakterisierung, Freisetzungsverhalten und -mechanismen, Ph.D. thesis, Free University of Berlin, 1996.
31. Müller, R. H., Schwarz, C., zur Mühlen, A., Mehnert, W., Incorporation of lipophilic drugs and drug release profiles of solid lipid nanoparticles (SLN), Proc. Int. Symp. Control. Rel. Bioact. Mater., 21 (1994) 146–147.
32. Schwarz, C., Freitas, C., Mehnert, W., Müller, R. H., Sterilization and physical stability of drug-free and etomidate-loaded solid lipid nanoparticles, Proc. Int. Symp. Control. Rel. Bioact. Mater., 22 (1995) 766–767.
33. Weyhers, H., Feste Lipid Nanopartikel (SLN) für die gewebsspezifische Arzneistoffapplikation, Ph.D. thesis, Free University of Berlin, 1995.
34. zur Mühlen, A., zur Mühlen, E., Niehus, H., Mehnert, W., Atomic force microscopy studies of solid lipid nanoparticles, Pharm. Res. 13 (1996), 1411–1416.
35. Müller, R. H., Dingler, A., Feste Lipid-Nanopartikel als neuartige Carrier für Wirkstoffe, Pharmazeutische Zeitung, 49(143) (1998), 4237–4242.
36. Müller, R. H., Dingler, A., The next generation after the liposomes: solid lipid nanoparticles (SLN, Lipopearls) as dermal carrier in cosmetics, Eurocosmetics 7–8, (1998), 19–26.
37. Jenning, V., Schäfer-Korting, M., Gohla, S., Vitamin A loaded solid lipid nanoparticles for topical application: drug release properties, J. Contr. Rel. (submitted).
38. Jenning, V., Gysler, A., Gohla, S., Schäfer-Korting, M., Vitamin A loaded solid lipid nanoparticles for topical use: occlusive properties and penetration into porcine skin, J. Contr. Rel. (submitted).
39. Weyhers, H., Ehlers, S., Mehnert, W., Hahn, H., Müller, R. H., Solid lipid nanoparticles—determination of in vivo toxicity, Proc. 1st World Meeting APGI/APV Budapest (1995), 489–490.
40. Olbrich, C., Mehnert, W., Müller, R. H., Effect of surfactant and lipid composition on the in vitro degradation time of solid lipid nanoparticles (SLN), Proc. Int. Symp. Control. Rel. Bioact. Mater., 24 (1997) 921–922.
41. Olbrich, C., Mehnert, W., Müller, R. H., In vitro degradation properties of solid lipid nanoparticles SLN, Proc. 2nd World Meeting APGI/APV, Paris (1998), 577–578.
42. Olbrich, C., Mehnert, W., Müller, R. H., Development of an in vitro degradation assay for solid lipid nanoparticles, Proc. 2nd World Meeting APGI/APV, Paris (1998), 627–628.
43. Mehnert, W., zur Mühlen, A., Dingler, A., Weyhers, H., Müller, R. H., Solid Lipid Nanopartikcles (SLN)—ein neuartiger Wirkstoff-Carrier für Kosmetika und Pharmazeutika, II. Wirkstoff-Inkorporation, Freisetzung und Sterilisierbarkeit, Pharm. Ind. (1997) 511–514.
44. Müller, R. H., Dingler, A., Weyhers, H., zur Mühlen, A., Mehnert, W., Solid Lipid Nanoparticles (SLN)—ein neuartiger Wirkstoff-Carrier für Kosmetika und Pharmazeutika, III. Langzeitstabilität, Gefrier- und Sprühtrocknung, Anwendung in Kosmetika und Pharmazeutika, Pharm. Ind. (1997) 614–619.
45. Medac GmbH, Hamburg, SLN information leaflet, 1999.

20
Stability of Encapsulated Substances in Poly(Lactide-co-Glycolide) Delivery Systems

Steven P. Schwendeman, Anna Shenderova, Gaozhong Zhu, and Wenlei Jiang
The Ohio State University, Columbus, Ohio

I. INTRODUCTION

Controlled release of bioactive substances requires that the encapsulated material retain its biological activity or the activity of acceptable degradation products. Encapsulation of these molecules is commonly performed not only to retain and/or to slowly release them, but to provide a more stable environment for the encapsulated species. For example, encapsulation of enzymes within a support material containing fixed ionogenic groups (e.g., ion exchangers) can provide an optimal microenvironmental pH for stability by altering the partitioning of H^+ (1). However, in certain instances the microclimate within the matrix is more destabilizing than if the substance were not encapsulated at all. Such has been found for some substances encapsulated in poly(lactide-co-glycolide) (PLGA). For example, a commonly observed phenomenon of proteins encapsulated in PLGA is that during release the protein ceases to come out of the polymer (e.g., entrapment due to aggregation), or once released the protein is devoid of biological activity. An additional problem concerns destabilization of the substance during encapsulation. Since PLGA is a particularly important biodegradable polymer to deliver drugs for periods exceeding 1-3 months (2,3), the task of optimizing the encapsulated molecule in an apparently deleterious environment becomes a critical obstacle to overcome. Herein we will describe our approach to examining the stability of encapsulated substances in PLGA as well as our important findings on this topic to date.

The applied scientific disciplines relevant to the stability of substances encapsulated in PLGA consist of physical and chemical stability of the substance (under deleterious conditions existing in the encapsulated environment), controlled release, and microencapsulation. If one examines (a) the physical–chemical events affecting the encapsulated substance that take place between the times of microencapsulation and release from the polymer (4), and (b) the complexity of the background disciplines involved, it becomes clear that this open-ended problem requires substantial simplification if valuable mechanistic interpretations are to be made. To this end, we have developed several experimental methodologies that delineate individual factors of the problem. First, the physical–chemical events affecting the stability of the molecule can be separated into three subcategories: (a) microencapsulation, (b) drying and storage, and (c) release incubation. More success and information is available on the stability during part a than during part b and c. Our primary interest currently concerns part c, and we expect that this is the most difficult step in the time line to overcome from encapsulation to drug release. We have had success retaining the stability of several proteins during microencapsulation (i.e., >90% biological activity recoverable from the encapsulated protein after removal of the polymer) by exposing the lyophilized protein to the organic solvent, as opposed to an aqueous solution in which the protein is dissolved. This works presumably due to the lack of molecular motions in the solid state in the absence of significant water [as is known to be the reason for the exceptional thermostability of lyophilized enzymes in organic solvents (1)]. Others have successfully applied the Timasheff theory by incorporating sugars during exposure of the aqueous solution to organic solvents (immiscible with water) to increase the water activity around the protein molecule (5). We have thus far not encountered large difficulties with part b (although that is not to say we will not in the future).

II. MECHANISMS OF STABILIZATION OF CAMPTOTHECINS

A. Remarkable Stabilization of Camptothecins in PLGA Microspheres

Camptothecins (CPTs) are potent anticancer drugs that exhibit a poor chemical stability (6). In physiological solutions (pH = 7.4, T = 37°C), the potent lactone form of drug undergoes rapid chemical hydrolysis with formation of the carboxylate form. The half-time of the reaction is only 25 min. Chemical hydrolysis of CPT is reversible and pH-sensitive (7). Under acidic conditions (pH < 5) CPT exists in the lactone form; with an increase in pH lactone fraction of drug gradually decreases. Under basic conditions (pH > 8) CPT is completely converted to the carboxylate form. The analogue of CPT, 10-hydroxycamptothecin (10-HCPT), was encapsulated in PLGA microspheres to investigate their potential to slowly release the potent lactone form of drug (8). It was hypothesized that the microclimate in PLGA microspheres is acidic and therefore would stabilize the lactone. Microspheres were exposed to the release media of pH = 7.4 at 37°C and drug stability inside the particles was assessed at various time intervals of microsphere degradation. Remarkably, the hydrolysis of CPT did not occur inside microspheres. The drug was stabilized in the PLGA microenvironment for as long as 2 months (Fig. 1). Hence, the microclimate in PLGA microspheres is significantly different for the environment of external physiological media, which dramatically affects the chemical stability of encapsulated substances.

B. Potential Mechanisms of Camptothecin Stabilization

During erosion in aqueous media, the environment inside PLGA devices begins to develop at least two phases with different physicochemical properties: a gel-like polymer phase and aqueous pores. The presence of two phases was observed on a confocal micrograph of PLGA microsphere containing CPT after 1-month erosion in aqueous media (Fig. 2A). The polymer phase is hydrophobic with limited water, which can potentially promote the partitioning of lipophilic molecules. The aqueous phase contains dissolved drug and excipients as well as PLGA degradation products, which will affect aqueous media pH and ionic strength. The parameters determining the rate of chemical reaction in solution are the reaction rate constant and the activities of reagents participating in reactions. Hydrolysis of the polymer itself was found to be catalyzed by the presence of soluble acidic degradation products (9) and upon encapsulation of acidic drugs (10), consistent with fundamentals of chemical kinetics (11). However, the reaction rates and reactants' activities could be substantially different in PLGA matrix microclimate compared to solutions. In addition, the encapsulated drug could exist in the following forms: (a) dissolved in aqueous pores; (b) partitioned in the polymer phase; or (c) as precipitate

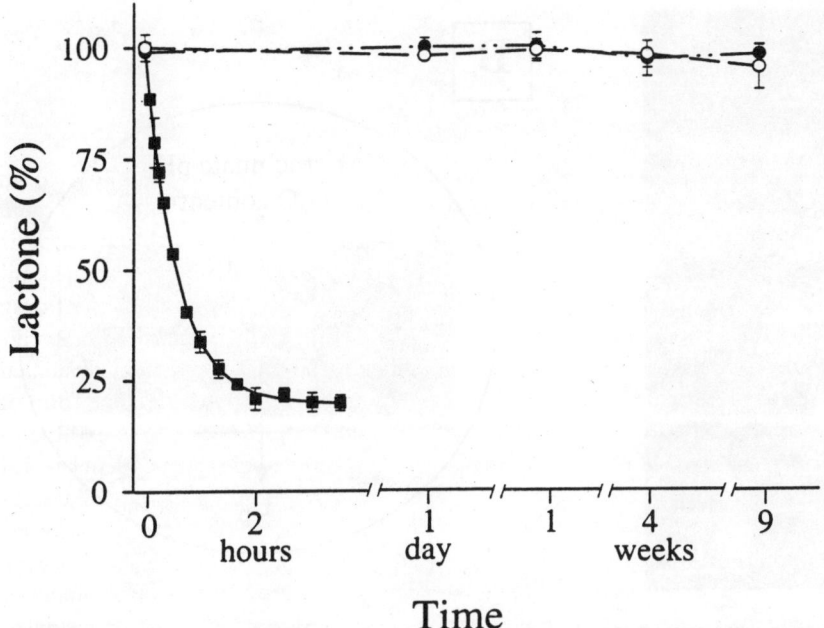

Figure 1 Stability of 10-HCPT remaining in the microspheres v. rapid hydrolysis in a simulated physiological environment. To find kinetic parameters of hydrolysis of the free drug in PBS pH = 7.4 at T = 37°C the equation $f = a + b \exp(-k_1 t)$ was fitted to the fraction of the intact lactone (f) v. time data (■). The fit yielded a $t_{1/2} = \ln(2)/k_1$ of 24 ± 2 min and a lactone fraction at equilibrium (a) of 19 ± 2% (n = 3, mean ± SEM). Drug stability inside the microspheres was examined by two methods: ○, 10-HCPT was captured in the release media (n = 2 ± SEM); ●, microspheres were dissolved in organic solvent (n = 2, mean ± SEM). Reproduced with permission (8).

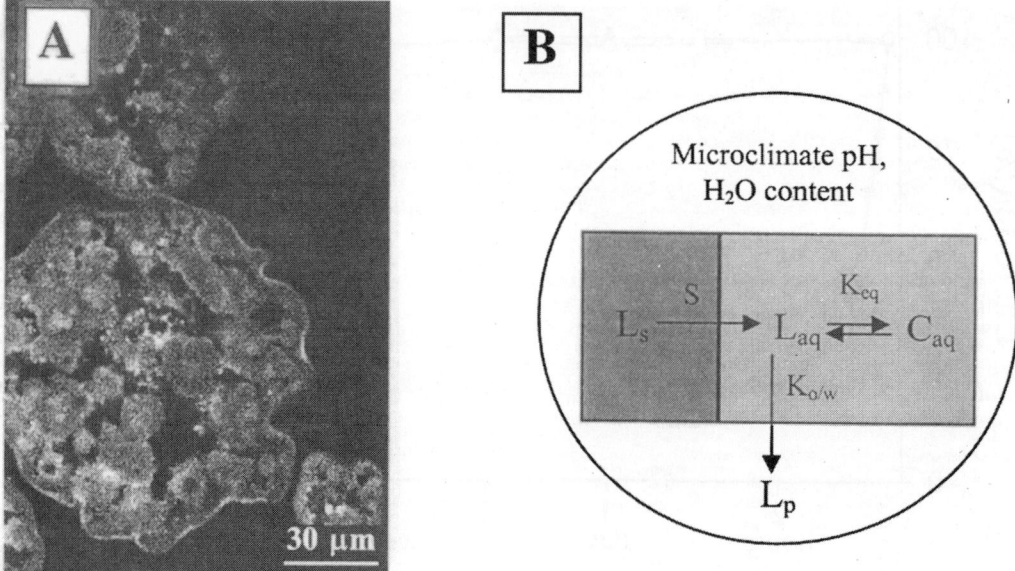

Figure 2 (A) Confocal microscopy image of medium cross-sections of PLGA microspheres containing the fluorescent drug 10-HCPT, after a month of degradation in PBS/0.02% Tween-80 (pH = 7.4) buffer at 37°C. (B). Schematic representation of drug distribution in PLGA microsphere microclimate. Drug exists in one or more of the following forms: as a lactone precipitate (L_s), dissolved in the microclimate (L_{aq} and C_{aq}), and as the lactone in the polymer (L_p). The faction of precipitated drug is determined by lactone solubility (S) and microsphere water content. The ratio between L_{aq} and C_{aq} is determined by interconversion equilibrium constant (K_{eq}) and the microclimate pH. Fraction of the CPT partitioning in the polymer is determined by the lactone partition coefficient ($K_{o/w}$).

in the matrix, if the drug loading is greater then the product of its solubility and water available for dissolution. The relative distribution of drug between these forms will influence its overall stability.

We have identified several possible sources that favor the CPT lactone in microspheres. The potential scheme of CPT distribution and stabilization in the microclimate is given in Fig. 2B. First, camptothecins exist in the lactone form at a pH <5, and a low microenvironmental pH in PLGA microspheres is expected during hydrolysis of the polymer ester bonds. Second, a preferential partitioning of the hydrophobic lactone into a polymer phase relative to the carboxylate could increase the lactone content in microspheres at equilibrium. Third, due to the relatively low aqueous solubility of the lactone and low water content in the microspheres, 10-HCPT could precipitate in the lactone form, which would also increase the overall lactone content recovered from the microspheres. Several experiments were performed to test each of these potential equilibrium sources of stabilization.

1. Acidic pH

The microenvironment of PLGA devices has a major effect on the stability and release of large macromolecules as well as small labile drugs. The presence of an acidic pH and accelerated degradation inside large specimens of PLGA is well known (4,9). However, the microclimate pH in PLGA microspheres remains controversial (12–15). The development of acidic microclimate likely depends on (a) the rate of formation of acidic monomers and oligomers, and the rate of their release from the microspheres; (b) neutralization of the microenvironmental acidity by encapsulated species or by buffering salts that have penetrated into the particles from the erosion media; and (c) the water uptake in the microspheres. Therefore, the microclimate pH depends on the raw materials used in microsphere preparation, buffering and osmotic capacities of the encapsulated substances, and microsphere properties such as porosity and size. All of these parameters are affected by the technique of microsphere preparation and therefore can vary between formulations. The microenvironmental pH of PLGA particles prepared by Pro-Lease technology was found to be neutral (pH = 6.4) by NMR nuclear magnetic resonance (12). In two different studies the microclimate pH was found to be acidic with a values of pH < 4.7 (15) and pH = 3.5 (13) by electron paramagnetic resonance (EPR) upon encapsulation of pH-sensitive spin probe. In both studies, microspheres were prepared by w/o/w emulsion–solvent evaporation technique. The encapsulation of a free base of antibiotic gentamicin and the use of basic buffer in the inner water phase (pH = 9, IS = 1.87 M) caused an increase in microenvironmental pH to 5.7 and 5.9, respectively (15). The microclimate pH was found to be as low as 1.5 in the center of microsphere and higher at the surface by imaging of pH-sensitive fluorescent probe with a confocal microscopy (14). The overall microenvironmental pH was reported to be influenced by the microsphere particle size.

Microspheres containing camptothecins were prepared by standard o/w emulsion solvent evaporation techniques form poly(lactide-co-glycolide) 50:50 polymer with inherent viscosity of 0.15 dL/g. The particle size was on the order of 50–200 μm. Two methods were used to assess the microclimate pH: (a) encapsulation of a pH-sensitive fluorescent probe, fluorescein, and mapping microclimate pH by confocal microscopy, and (b) direct measurement of proton activity with glass electrode after microsphere dissolution in mixed-solvent systems.

Mapping Microenvironment with a pH-Sensitive Fluorescent Probe. Fluorescein is a highly fluorescent compound frequently used to label macromolecules, track intracellular movement of proteins, and as a pH-sensitive probe (16). The intensity of fluorescein emission decreases with the decrease in pH (17). Calibration images of fluorescein solutions confirmed that virtually no signal is observed at a pH below 5. Therefore, if the microsphere microclimate were acidic we would expect to observe no emission from microsphere interior. The black and

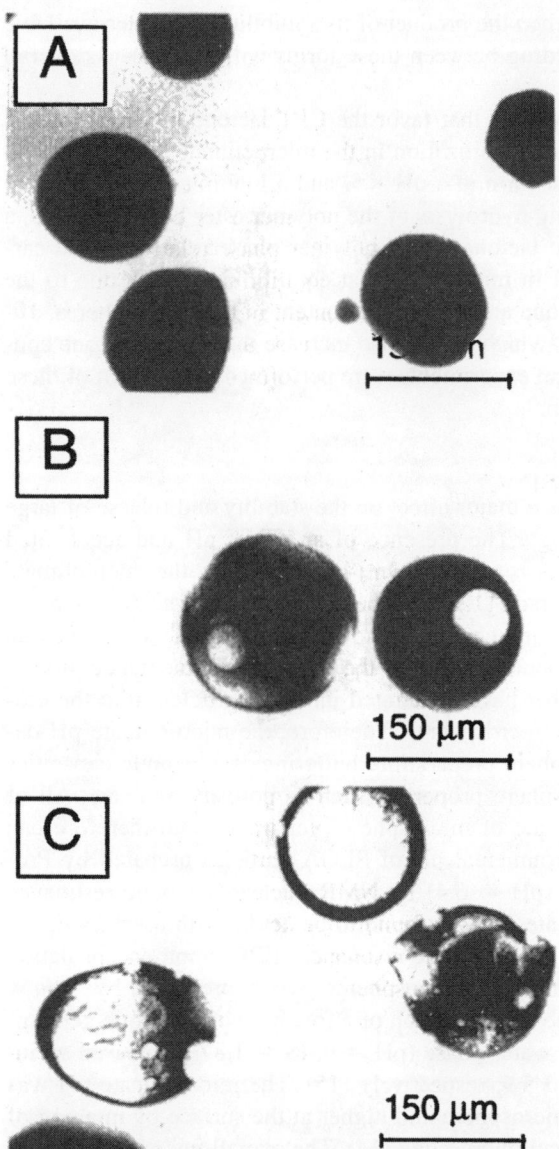

Figure 3 Confocal microscopy images of the microspheres containing the pH-sensitive fluorescent probe, fluorescein, and 0% (A), 1% (B), and 3% (C) of $Mg(OH)_2$ after 3 days of hydration in Hepes buffer containing 0.02% Tween-80 (pH = 7.4) and 0.1 mg/mL fluorescein at 37°C.

white images of PLGA microspheres after 3 days of hydration are shown in Fig. 3. No fluorescence from interior confirmed the presence of an acidic microclimate (Fig 3A). When black and white images were transformed into colors, a pH gradient approximately 5 μm in width was observed on the microsphere surface (18), although the potential artifact of poor focusing of the microscope in this region cannot be ruled out. In addition, the compressing of color image of microspheres with calibration images of probe solutions at different pH suggested that the microclimate pH was around 2 (18). However, it was impossible to determine the exact pH by the fluorescein mapping technique since the emission intensity depends both media pH and probe concentration.

Poorly soluble bases such as $Mg(OH)_2$ have been used successfully to increase the microclimate pH of poly(ortho-esters) and inhibit polymer degradation (19). We hypothesized that the coencapsulation of $Mg(OH)_2$ with fluorescein in PLGA microspheres would neutralize the microenvironmental pH and induce the emission of the dye from the microsphere interior. The images of microspheres containing 1% and 3% of base (w/w) are represented in Fig. 3B and C. As expected, the intensity from microsphere interior increased with the increase in base loading, demonstrating that $Mg(OH)_2$ can be used to increase microenvironmental pH of PLGA. However, *the neutralization occurred in a heterogeneous manner*. The microclimate was neutralized near the location of basic salt particles rather than homogeneously throughout the particle. Additional efforts are being made to provide total neutralization of the acidic pH and to assure the stability of acid-labile drugs.

Determination of H^+ Content in Dissolved Microspheres by pH Electrode. The second method to determine microclimate pH was to measure of hydronium ion concentration by a pH electrode after microsphere dissolution in an organic solvent–water mixture. Microspheres were eroded for various periods of time, removed from the erosion media, and dissolved in an acetonitrile (ACN)/H_2O 4:1 (v/v) mixture. The pH was measured immediately after particle dissolution by a glass pH electrode equilibrated with aqueous standards. The actual proton activity in organic–water mixture (pa^*_H) correlates with pH meter reading (pH) by $pa^*_H = pH + \delta$, where δ is a combined correction factor (20,21). The value of δ is a function of solvent composition, and $\delta = 0.95$ for an ACN/H_2O 4:1 (v/v) mixture (22). The pa^*_H is a relative measure of microsphere acidity. The pa^*_H changes with time were measured to observe relative changes in microclimate acidity upon polymer degradation and microsphere erosion. The neutralization effect of $Mg(OH)_2$ coencapsulation on pa^*_H of the microspheres was also determined. In addition, the actual microclimate pH was calculated from the ratio of proton content of the microspheres measured by pH electrode to water content of the particles determined gravimetrically.

If an acidic microclimate were present, then we would expect to detect a low pa^*_H reading upon microsphere dissolution. In contrast, if an acidic species were either absent or neutralized by buffering species from the erosion medium or encapsulated basic substances, then the pa^*_H should be neutral. Consistent with the acidic microclimate hypothesis, a low pa^*_H was detected, which increased upon coencapsulation of $Mg(OH)_2$ (Fig. 4). The pa^*_H of blank microspheres increased initially from 3.3 to 4.6 after 3 days of hydration, which is consistent with the known loss of oligomers and monomers upon hydration. As polymer degradation proceeded, the pa^*_H decreased substantially to as low as 2.8 after 4 weeks of microsphere incubation (Fig. 4A). Similar kinetics of an initial increase followed by a subsequent decrease in polymer molecular weight and glass transition temperature was observed for PLGA microspheres by Park (23). As base was added the pa^*_H increased gradually with the increase in $Mg(OH)_2$ loading (Fig. 4B). The neutralization of microclimate at 3% and 6% base loading was more complete and had longer duration than at 1% base loading. The pa^*_H of microspheres containing more than 3% of base remained unchanged for 2 weeks of microsphere incubation. This suggests that at a loading higher than 3%, the polymer degradation may be slowed down significantly, since the

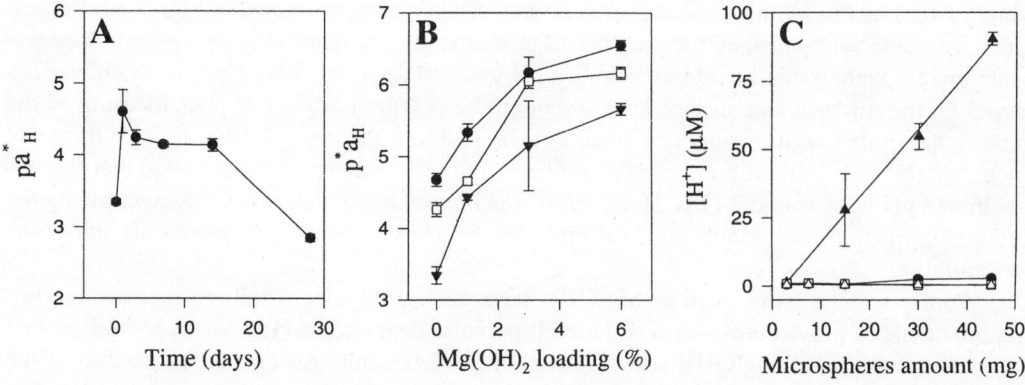

Figure 4 Determination of the H^+ content in microspheres by pH electrode after dissolution in an ACN/H_2O mixture. pa^*_H = pH(measured) − 0.95 for 80:20 v/v ACN/H_2O. (A) The pa^*_H of the blank microspheres (capped-end PLGA 0.15 dL/g IV) as a function of time of incubation in PBS containing 0.02% Tween-80 (pH = 7.4) at 37°C. (B) The pa^*_H from microspheres as a function of $Mg(OH)_2$ loading after 0 (▼), 3 (●), and 14 days (□) of degradation in Hepes containing 0.02% Tween-80 (pH = 7.4) at 37°C. (C) The effect of microsphere concentration in ACN/H_2O 80:20 (v/v) solutions on measured H^+ concentration. In the microspheres without $Mg(OH)_2$ (▲) and with 1% base (●), the $[H^+]$ increased linearly with microsphere concentration, with the slopes of 2.1×10^{-6} M/mg ($r^2 = 0.997$) and 5.6×10^{-8} M/mg ($r^2 = 0.967$), respectively. The $[H^+]$ was constant at $\sim 5 \times 10^{-7}$ M (independent of the microsphere concentration) for 3% (□) and 6% (Δ) $Mg(OH)_2$ loading. Reproduced with permission (8).

increase in microclimate pH leads to suppression of an acid-catalyzed hydrolysis of ester bonds. The decrease in rate of polymer degradation was observed previously for PLGA films containing $Mg(OH)_2$ (24). In addition, the base release occurs slowly due to its low aqueous solubility providing an extended duration of neutralization.

The actual microclimate pH was determined after microsphere hydration for 3 days. The dependency of hydronium ion concentration on the amount of microspheres dissolved in the ACN/H_2O mixture was measured (Fig. 4C). From the slope of the curve we determined that $\sim 2.1 \times 10^{-9}$ mol H^+ was liberated per mg of microspheres. The amount of water sorbed after 3 days of hydration was ~ 0.14 mg/mg of microspheres. The simple calculation gives the microclimate pH value of ~ 1.8. However, this calculation does not account for a potential change in degree of ionization of carboxylic moieties providing H^+ in the ACN/H_2O mixture compared to the microsphere microclimate. In the ACN/H_2O mixture all ionizable species (i.e., polymer chains and monomers) are dissolved, while in the microclimate polymer chains are hydrated with 14% of water sorbed. It is a known phenomenon from hydrogel drug delivery research that polymer end groups are capable of ionization upon hydration and the ionization does not require complete dissolution of the polymer chains. For PLGA devices the kinetics of water uptake was found to correlate closely with formation of new carboxylic groups upon polymer chain degradation (25). Hence, we postulated that ionizability of polymer end groups and monomers in the microenvironment is close to their ionizability in aqueous solution. On the other hand, the dissociation constant of carboxylic acids, K_a, decreases in aprotic solvents such as ACN compared to water (20). Hence, the K_a is expected to be greater in the microclimate compared to ACN/H_2O mixtures providing the microenviromental pH value even lower than the calculated 1.8. This value is consistent with pH measured by a glass electrode for large PLGA specimens (pH < 2) (4). It should be noted that the microclimate pH was calculated after 3 days of microsphere hydration at a maximum of measured pa*$_H$ (Fig. 4A). Therefore, the microclimate pH could decrease upon further polymer degradation, as was observed for the relative acidity measure (pa*$_H$). However, the increase in relative proton concentration could be compensated by an increased amount of sorbed water. Hence, the conclusions about the kinetics of microclimate pH change could not be made without further investigation.

2. Solid State Stabilization

The acidic microclimate of PLGA microspheres obviously plays an important role in CPT stabilization. However, the acidic pH only benefits the stability of CPT that is dissolved in the microclimate. When CPT stability in the microspheres is determined, the drug is extracted from the particles and the overall lactone-to-carboxylate ratio is measured (8). The total lactone content includes the contributions of lactone precipitated in the matrix, lactone dissolved in the aqueous pores, and lactone partitioning in the polymer (Fig. 2B). It was interesting to estimate what fraction of the drug is actually dissolved in the microclimate. The water uptake of the blank microspheres during the first 2 weeks of degradation was ~12–30% (weight water/weight polymer). The 10-HCPT loading is ~0.2% and the lactone solubility ~0.002 mg/mL. A simple calculation reveals that only ~0.01% of the encapsulated drug is dissolved, assuming that all of the microsphere water is available to dissolve the drug. Therefore, precipitation in the matrix could be a primary stabilization pathway for drugs with low aqueous solubility. Two experiments were designed to assess the impact of solid state precipitation on the overall stability of encapsulated CPTs.

In the first experiment, microenvironmental pH was neutralized by encapsulation of $Mg(OH)_2$ (6% w/w). We hypothesized that drug dissolved in the microclimate would convert to the carboxylate form according to the neutralized pH value, whereas drug precipitated in the matrix would remain in the lactone form. Drug will precipitate as the lactone rather than as the carboxylate, since the ionized carboxylate has much higher aqueous solubility. The loading of 10-HCPT was varied from 0.001% to 0.4%. At low drug loading we expected to observe higher carboxylate content of the microspheres, since 10-HCPT would be completely dissolved in the microclimate and the lactone-to-carboxylate ratio would reflect the neutralized pH value. In contrast, at a high drug loading the fraction of drug precipitated in the matrix increases, leading to higher overall lactone content. Therefore, a sharp increase in overall lactone content of the microspheres with the increase in drug loading was expected, which corresponds to a 10-HCPT transition from the solution to the solid state.

The expected trend was observed. In Fig. 5A the lactone fraction in microspheres is plotted as a function of drug loading remaining in the particles after 3 and 7 days of hydration. As drug content increased to greater than 0.01% (w/w), roughly 80% of 10-HCPT was recovered in the lactone form, whereas a sharp decrease in lactone content occurred at a loading of ~0.005–0.001%. For the microspheres with 6% encapsulated $Mg(OH)_2$ the water uptake during the first 2 weeks was ~120%. A rough calculation shows that 10-HCPT will be completely dissolved in the microsphere environment at a loading on the order of ~10^{-3}%, which is close to the curve minimum in Fig. 5A. Interestingly, this minimum is represented by different initial drug loading on different days, since the drug is released rapidly, and this drug loss was accounted by plotting lactone fraction v. the *actual drug content* in the polymer on the given day. Thus, the minimum will occur for each preparation throughout the release as the remaining 10-HCPT loading reaches the critical value of ~10^{-3}%. The plateau of lactone content at 80% in the microspheres at high drug loading can be explained by the precipitation of the carboxylate

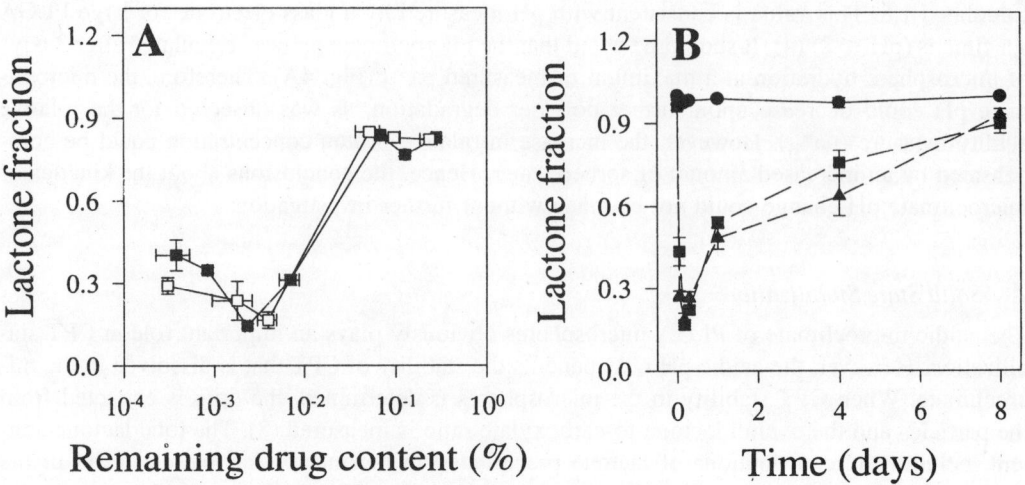

Figure 5 (A) The effect of 10-HCPT loading on its composition in PLGA microspheres containing 6% (w/w) Mg(OH)$_2$ after 3 (■) and 7 (□) days of hydration in Hepes buffer containing 0.02% Tween-80 (pH = 7.4) at 37°C. (B) The effect of camptothecin lipophilicity and solubility on its conversion in PLGA microspheres containing 20% (w/w) Mg(OH)$_2$ upon hydration in Hepes buffer containing 0.02% Tween-80 (pH = 7.4) at 37°C. Three camptothecins were studied: CMDC (●), 10-HCPT (▲), and TPT (■). Their corresponding lipid partition coefficients and solubility were approximately 400 M^{-1} and 0.0001 mg/mL, 75 M^{-1} and 0.02 mg/mL, 10 M^{-1} and 1 mg/mL, for CMDC, 10-HCPT, and TPT, respectively. Reproduced with permission (8).

with magnesium ion. This salt formation can be easily observed by the mixing of solutions of 10-HCPT carboxylate and MgCl$_2$.

In the second experiment, we encapsulated three CPTs with various aqueous solubilities in PLGA microspheres containing 20% Mg(OH)$_2$. The selected CPTs—topothecan (TPT), 10-HCPT, and 9-chloro-10,11-methylenedioxy-camptothecin (CMDC)—exhibit identical pH dependence of lactone to carboxylate equilibrium ratio (26), while the aqueous solubility of their lactones are ~2, 0.002, and 0.0001 mg/mL, respectively. With an increase in aqueous solubility of encapsulated CPT the greater fraction of total drug would be dissolved in the microclimate and converted into the carboxylate according to the neutralized pH value. Hence, we expected to see larger extent of conversion to carboxylate for more water-soluble drugs. The expected trend was observed. The response of the encapsulated agents on the neutralized environment is shown in Fig. 5B. The two more water-soluble agents, TPT and 10-HCPT, exhibited a fast conversion into the carboxylate form, whereas the least soluble, CMDC, remained in its lactone form even in very basic microspheres with 20% Mg(OH)$_2$. The results of these experiments emphasize that although a low microclimate pH must favor CPT stabilization, the contribution to stability from their low solubility can also be significant, allowing some analogues to remain in the lactone form even in the case of a neutralized microenvironment.

3. Preferential Partitioning in the Polymer

The preferential partitioning of the unionized lactone form of 10-HCPT in the polymer phase compared to the anionic carboxylate could also increase the lactone content of PLGA microspheres at equilibrium. The increase in equilibrium lactone fraction due to the partitioning of the lactone into lipid membranes was observed when camptothecins were equilibrated with red blood cells and encapsulated into liposomes (27,28). The structure of CPT was found to substantially affect drug partitioning into the lipid phase. The equilibrium binding constants for CMDC, 10-HCPT, and TPT with unilamellar vesicles composed of lipid dimyristoylphosphatidylcholine were found to be 400, 75, and 10 M^{-1}, respectively (29). The results of the kinetics of interconversion following the encapsulation of the three CPTs (Fig. 5B) also can be used to address the partitioning phenomena. The lactone of CPTs with higher lipid binding constant would partition into polymer matrix to a greater extent, leading to higher microsphere lactone content at equilibrium. If no partitioning of lactone in the polymer occurs, then all three drugs should exhibit the identical conversion kinetics in the microspheres. Virtually identical conversion kinetics was observed for the two more hydrophilic drugs, TPT and 10-HCPT (Fig. 5B), suggesting no significant interactions between PLGA and these CPTs with ~10-fold lipophilicity difference. The low aqueous solubility of CMDC explains its exceptional stability in this case, although the interactions between CMDC and PLGA cannot be ruled out. The CMDC stability is analogous to the improved stability of suspensions relative to solutions (30). Overall, we can conclude that no significant drug–polymer interaction occurs for more the hydrophilic CPTs (e.g., TPT and 10-HCPT) that has any substantial impact on the lactone equilibrium content. The partitioning of drug into the polymer phase as well as PLGA drug interactions could play a substantial role in stabilization of encapsulated drugs, although the partitioning was not observed for CPTs. Whether the drug will partition or interact with the polymer would largely depend on drugs' lipophilicity, charge, and molecular weight. Small and lipophilic molecules could partition in the polymer, while positively charged molecules could potentially interact with negatively charged PLGA carboxylic end groups. Additional definitive experiments should be carried on to address the polymer–drug interactions and partitioning phenomena for drugs with various physical–chemical characteristics.

III. MECHANISMS OF INSTABILITY OF BOVINE SERUM ALBUMIN

A. Kinetics of Release and Aggregation of Encapsulated Bovine Serum Albumin

Perhaps the most commonly encapsulated protein is bovine serum albumin (BSA). However, very few reported continuous release of BSA from the polymer and none have demonstrated release of the native protein. Some suggested that the incomplete release might be due to aggregation of encapsulated BSA or adsorption to the polymer (32). To investigate the nature of BSA instability in PLGA, we encapsulated solid BSA particles (<90 μm) into PLGA 50:50 (inherent viscosity = 0.63 dL/g) millicylinders (0.8 mm in diameter) by an acetone extrusion method as described previously (31). Then, we monitored both the release of BSA in PBS/0.02% Tween-80 (PBST, pH 7.4) and the formation of water-insoluble BSA extracted from the polymer at certain periods of incubation at 37°C. As seen in Fig. 6A, the continuous release of BSA from the millicylinders only lasted about 4 days and no significant amount of BSA was further released during the 28-day study. This incomplete release suggested that most of the encapsulated BSA formed insoluble aggregates, which was confirmed by the aggregation kinetics (Fig. 6B). As shown in the figure, the encapsulated BSA formed aggregates in a rapid rate during the first 2 weeks. After 28 days of incubation, almost all of the remaining BSA became water-insoluble aggregates.

B. Characterization of the Denatured State of Bovine Serum Albumin: Non-covalent Aggregation and Peptide Bond Hydrolysis

Since the formed BSA aggregates extracted from the polymer were totally soluble in a denaturing solvent (i.e., 6 M urea), this indicated that the interactions between the BSA molecules

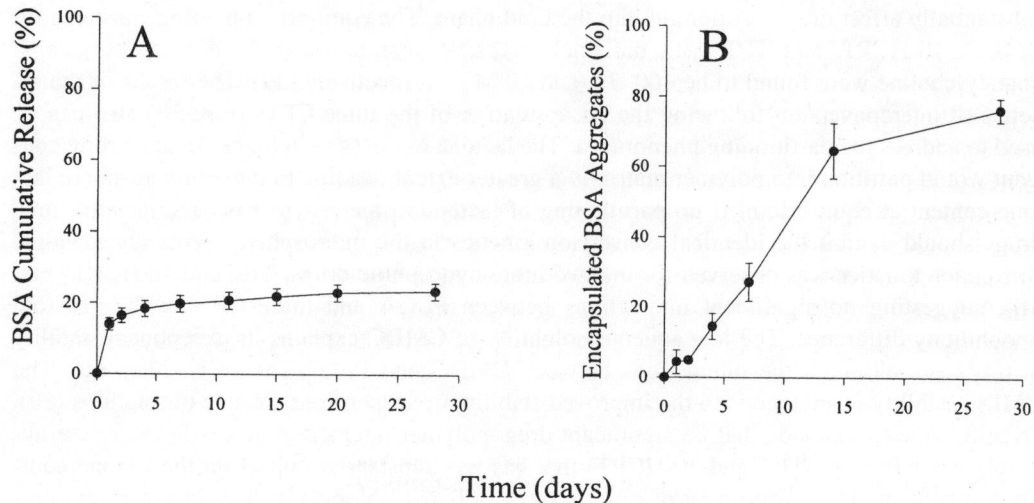

Figure 6 The BSA release (A) and aggregation (B) kinetics of 15% BSA/PLGA50:50 millicylinders in a phosphate buffer (pH 7.40) at 37°C (average ± SEM, n = 3). Reproduced with permission (31).

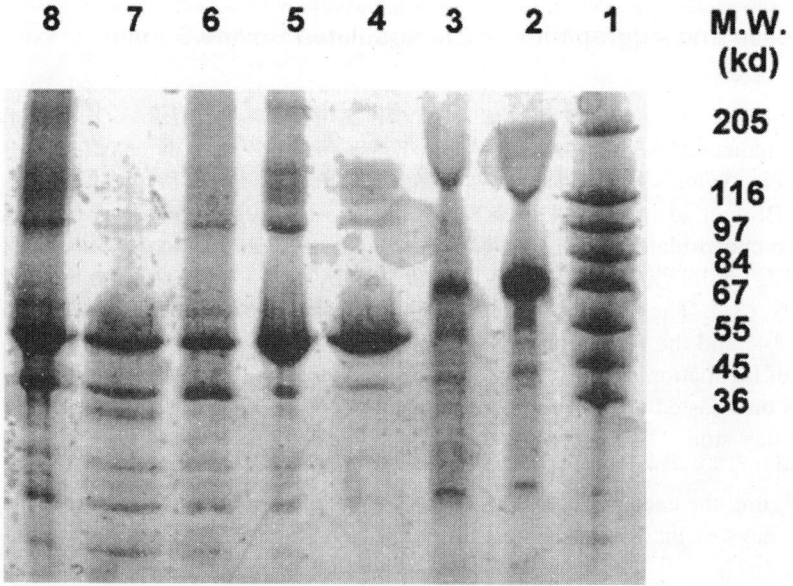

Figure 7 SDS-PAGE of BSA aggregates and degradation products from 15% BSA/PLGA (lanes 2, 5, and 7) and from the simulation (lanes 3, 6, and 8). Lane 1: High molecular weight markers; lanes 2 and 3: insoluble BSA treated with SDS and β-mercaptoethanol; lane 4: standard BSA treated with SDS buffer only; lanes 5 and 6: insoluble BSA treated with SDS only; lanes 7 and 8: soluble BSA treated with SDS only. Reproduced with permission (31).

in the aggregates were non-covalent bonded linkages. This was further confirmed by the fact that the aggregates were also completely soluble in 2.5% SDS buffer (pH 8) during the analysis of SDS-Polyacrylamide gel electrophoresis (PAGE). To obtain additional information about the instability of BSA, we examined the integrity of both the soluble BSA recovered from the polymer (28 days incubation) and insoluble aggregates by reducing and nonreducing SDS-PAGE. As seen in Fig. 7, for the soluble protein (lane 7), several peptide fragments (e.g., 55, 40, and 25 kDa) were observed, indicating that significant peptide bond hydrolysis occurred during incubation. For the insoluble protein (lane 2 and lane 5), beside some peptide fragments and small amount of dimeric and trimeric BSA, most of the BSA remained in the monomeric form. Therefore, based on these analyses, we conclude that two major instability pathways for the encapsulated BSA in PLGA during release are the formation of non-covalent water-insoluble aggregates and peptide bond hydrolysis.

C. Simulations of Stresses Responsible for Instability of Encapsulated Bovine Serum Albumin

In order to investigate the sources responsible for the BSA instability, we first hypothesized that the primary deleterious characteristics of the polymer microclimate at physiological temperature consists of one or more of the following: elevated moisture, an acidic pH, and the polymer surface (4). To test this hypothesis for the inactivation of BSA in PLGA, we simulated the microclimate conditions by exposing BSA at 37°C to various levels of moisture and pH, and the presence or absence of a polymer surface. If one or more of the chosen conditions adequately described the microclimate, we would expect to create a similar denatured state of BSA to that observed for encapsulated BSA and to find the instability occurring over similar time scales.

Following this methodology, the acidity of the polymer was simulated by exposing solid BSA, which had been lyophilized from pH 2, 3.1, 4.1, or 5.1 solutions, to a humid environment (86% RH and 37°C) for a week. Of the pH conditions tested, only the highly acidic preparation (pH 2) induced observable aggregation (43 ± 6% insoluble BSA, n = 3). Above this pH, no aggregation was observed. To further describe the aggregation and denatured state under the highly acidic condition, the kinetics of BSA aggregation was examined. As shown in Fig. 8, aggregation of BSA was nearly complete within 10 days.

Moisture had an effect on the rate of aggregation but did not affect the mechanism. When small amounts of water were added to the BSA powder lyophilized at pH 2, variable aggregation was observed. For water/protein ratios (w/w) of 0 and 0.2, no aggregates were observed after a week at 37°C; for a ratio of 0.8–1.0, aggregates were produced (~70% insoluble BSA), which were >94% soluble in 6 M urea (31). Since adsorption also may cause BSA unfolding and aggregation, BSA solutions at a pH range of 2–7 were incubated in the presence of PLGA microspheres (to provide a polymer surface) at 37°C for a week. Negligible losses in BSA concentration were recorded in each of these simulations, strongly suggesting a negligible effect of polymer adsorption on the stability of encapsulated BSA (31).

D. Matching Denatured States of Real and Simulated Instability of Bovine Serum Albumin: Implication of Acidic Microclimate as the Inactivating Source

The inactivation of BSA under real (polymer microclimate) and simulated (pH 2 and 86% RH) conditions is compared in Table 1. The aggregates generated in both conditions were com-

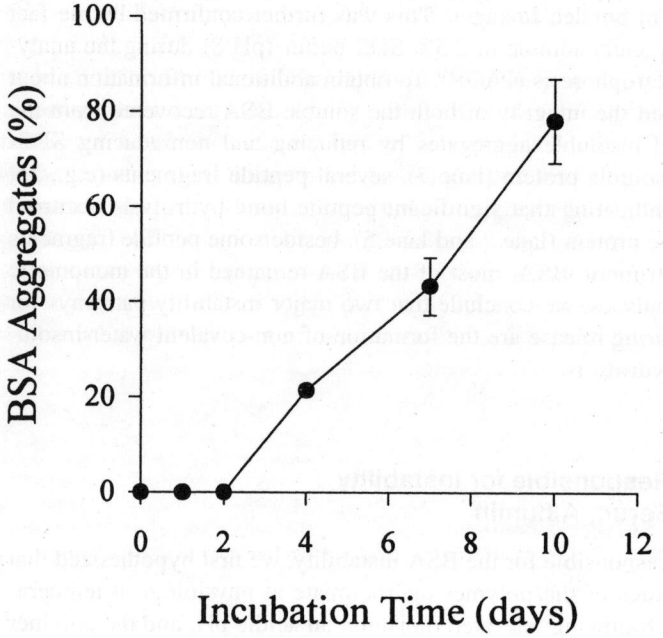

Figure 8 Aggregation kinetics of BSA at 37°C in the presence of 86% RH. BSA was lyophilized from pH 2 (simulated) solution. (Average ± SD, n = 2). Reproduced with permission (31).

Table 1 Irreversible Inactivation of BSA Under Simulated and Encapsulated Conditions at 37°C

	Encapsulated[a]	Simulated[b]
Time to 50% aggregation	12 days	7 days
Aggregates soluble in denaturing solvent[c]	>98%	>94%
Peptide fragmentation[d]	25, 40, and 55 kDa	25, 40, and 55 kDa

[a]15% BSA in PLGA millicylinders incubated in PBST at 37°C;
[b]lyophilized BSA at pH 2 incubated under 86% R.H. at 37°C;
[c]PBST containing 6 M urea and 1 mM EDTA;
[d]from SDS-PAGE of BSA samples treated with SDS and β-mercaptoethanol.
Source: Ref. 31

pletely soluble in the denaturing solvent (Table 1). Moreover, the soluble and insoluble fractions produced under both conditions exhibited nearly identical peptide bond fragmentation, as shown by SDS-PAGE (Fig. 7). Hence, incubation of solid protein (lyophilized at pH 2) in the presence of moisture produced a denatured state in BSA that was essentially identical to the denatured state when encapsulated in PLGA (Table 1). The type of aggregates (non-covalent), peptide bond fragments (e.g., 25, 40, 55 kDa), and time scale of aggregation (e.g., time to 50% aggregation) were equivalent. These results implicate that the moist and acidic polymer microclimate, not protein adsorption as previously suggested (32), is responsible for BSA instability in PLGA. We remark that the apparent discrepancy of protein adsorption can be clarified by the fact that the insoluble aggregates are also soluble in 2.5% SDS, the agent used to cause release of sequestered BSA in PLGA microspheres (32). Furthermore, during incubation in the release medium the polymer microenvironment should become extremely acidic, close to the simulated (near 2) and measured pH values in the polymer (4, 13–15, 18).

E. Developing a Hypothesis for the Mechanism of Instability of Encapsulated Bovine Serum Albumin

It is well established that an acidic microclimate develops in large PLGA specimens (4,9) due to the accumulation of acidic degradation products upon hydrolysis of the polyester. A highly acidic pH (<3) was also required for the formation of non-covalent aggregates of BSA in our simulations of the polymer microclimate. This indicates that the presence of 15% BSA does not significantly alter the acidic pH (e.g., by creating water channels in the polymer to allow buffer ions to diffuse in). Instead, the encapsulated BSA is rehydrated at a pH that causes the protein to unfold [BSA undergoes a conformational transition from the F to E isoform at pH 2.7 (33)], thus providing the driving force for non-covalent aggregation via hydrophobic interactions (33). Peptide bond hydrolysis is also particularly rapid under such acidic conditions or when labile peptide bonds [e.g., Asp-X linkage (34)] become exposed during unfolding. Hence, the mechanism of instability of BSA indicates that the microclimate pH is highly acidic (<3).

F. Stabilization of Bovine Serum Albumin by Neutralization of the Acidic Microclimate pH

The nature of the sources of BSA inactivation (i.e., acidic pH and intermediate moisture levels) and the mechanism of instability under these conditions (i.e., non-covalent aggregation by hydrophobic interactions and peptide bond hydrolysis) suggested a rational approach to stabilize encapsulated BSA. Since (a) aggregation of BSA did not occur in our simulations of the microclimate as the pH was raised above 3, and (b) peptide bond hydrolysis would be slow at higher pH, we tried an established method of increasing the microclimate pH in a biodegradable polymer akin to PLGA, the poly(ortho-esters). $Mg(OH)_2$ has been routinely incorporated into poly(ortho-esters) to extend the release time of drugs, since the stability of the ortho-ester bond is increased as the pH is raised to neutral levels (19). In addition, as described above, we used confocal microscopy of an encapsulated pH-sensitive fluorescent probe to verify that the microclimate pH in PLGA was effectively raised toward neutral pH as $Mg(OH)_2$ was incorporated (18).

Consequently, to test the ability of $Mg(OH)_2$ to inhibit the inactivation of BSA, we coencapsulated the base with BSA at 0.5% and 3% by weight. Then we compared the release and aggregation kinetics of these samples with those observed for the same preparation without any base. As predicted, as more $Mg(OH)_2$ was added, more BSA was released and less en-

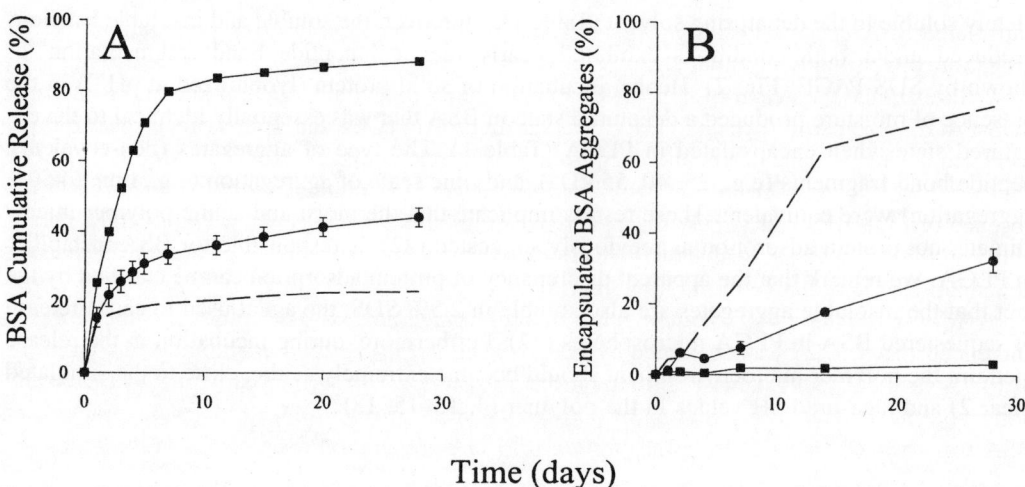

Figure 9 Stabilization effect of Mg(OH)$_2$ on encapsulated BSA release (A) and encapsulated BSA aggregation (B) kinetics during incubation of the polymer at 37°C in a phosphate buffer (pH 7.40) are shown. PLGA millicylinders were loaded with 15% BSA and 0% (———), 0.5% (●), and 3.0% (■) Mg(OH)$_2$ (Average ± SE, n = 3). Reproduced with permission (31).

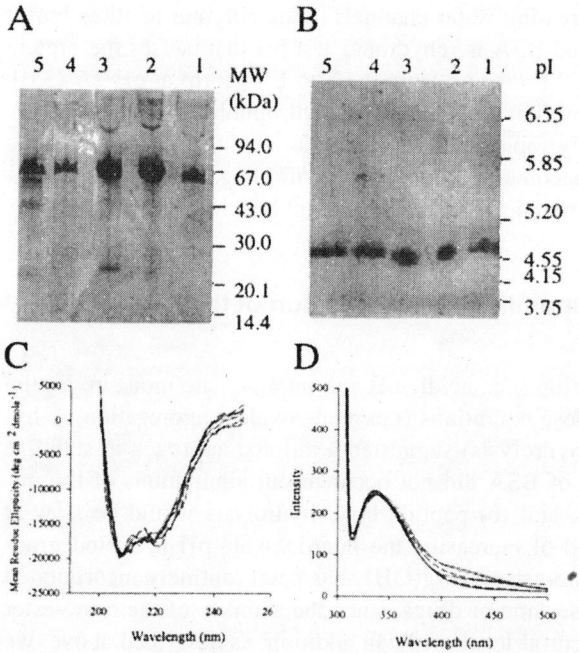

Figure 10 Structural analyses of BSA from incubated PLGA millicylinders by SDS-PAGE (A), IEF (B), CD spectra (C), and fluorescence emission spectra (D). In SDS-PAGE and IEF analyses, lanes 1–5 are standard BSA, released BSA on day 1, day 5–7, and day 21–28, and residual BSA on day 28, respectively. In CD and fluorescence emission spectra, released BSA samples were from day 1 (—), days 6–7 (———), days 16–20 (—-), and days 21–28 (●●●●), and residual BSA (-●-●). Reproduced with permission (31).

capsulated BSA became insoluble (Fig. 9A and B). For the 3% Mg(OH)$_2$ preparation, the aggregation was virtually eliminated.

To examine the extent of hydrolysis and any other potential structural alterations of BSA, SDS-PAGE, isoelectric focusing (IEF), circular dichroism (CD) and fluorescence spectroscopy were employed to characterize the encapsulated and released BSA from the Mg(OH)$_2$/PLGA devices (Fig. 10). As seen in Fig. 10A, the large degree of fragmentation that occurred in the absence of Mg(OH)$_2$ had largely disappeared. Some faint low molecular weight bands, particularly in the residual encapsulated BSA after 28 days, were noticeable, but these were present at a small fraction relative to the monomeric band.

To test for the most common route of protein degradation—deamidation—the released and encapsulated BSA was examined by IEF. As seen in Fig. 10B, no alteration of the protein's pI (4.7) was detected. Likewise, no alterations in secondary or tertiary structure of BSA were noticeable in the CD (Fig. 10C) and fluorescence spectra (Fig. 10D). Hence, the structure of BSA was retained (>90%) from the Mg(OH)$_2$/PLGA preparation for a period of 1 month.

IV. CONCLUSIONS

Our results indicate that the microclimate pH in PLGA 50:50 microspheres is acidic when prepared by standard solvent evaporation techniques. The microclimate can be neutralized by encapsulation of a poorly soluble base such as Mg(OH)$_2$, although this acid neutralization is not homogeneous. The neutralization effect appears to be limited by transport of the soluble fraction of the base throughout the polymer.

Careful examination of the denatured state of encapsulated BSA and simulations of the irreversible instability in the polymer have definitively implicated the acidic microclimate pH as the principal external stress responsible for BSA instability. BSA undergoes unfolding to an expanded form (E), which is most susceptible to non-covalent aggregation and hydrolysis. Data with the CPTs suggested that 3% Mg(OH)$_2$ should be useful to stabilize BSA from acid-induced instability. This is exactly what we observed. Finally, the very low pH that can develop inside this polymer is likely the most significant destabilizing stress of proteins during release from the polymer.

REFERENCES

1. Volkin, D. B. and Klibanov, A. M., Minimizing protein inactivation. In: Protein Function: A Practical Approach, T. E. Creighton, Ed. 1985, Oxford University Press: Oxford, pp. 1–24.
2. Johnson, O. F. L., Cleland, J. L., et. al., A month-long effect from a single injection of microencapsulated human growth hormone. Nature Med., 1996. 2(7): 795–799.
3. Ogawa, Y., Okada, H., Yamamoto, M., and Shimamoto, T., In vivo release profiles of leuprolide acetate from microcapsules prepared with polylactide acids or co-poly(lactic/glycolic acids) and in vivo degradation of these polymers. Chem. Pharm. Bull., 1988. 36: 2576–2581.
4. Schwendeman, S. P., Cardamone, M., Brandon, M. R., Klibanov, A., and Langer, R., Stability of proteins and their delivery from biodegradable polymer microspheres. In: Microparticulate Systems for the Delivery of Proteins and Vaccines, S. Cohen and H. Bernstein, Eds. 1996, Marcel Dekker: New York, pp. 1–49.
5. Cleland, J. L. and Jones, A. J. S., Stable formulations of rocombinant human growth hormone and interferon-γ for microencapsulation in biodegradable microspheres. Pharm. Res., 1996. 13(10): 1464–1475.

6. Potmesil, M. and. Pinedo., H., Camptothecins: New Anticancer Agents. 1995, Ann Arbor: CRC Press.
7. Fassberg, J. and Stella, V. J., A kinetic and mechanistic study of the hydrolysis of camptothecin and some analogues. J. Pharm. Sci, 1992. 81: 676–684.
8. Shenderova, A., Burke, T. G., and Schwendeman, S. P., Stabilization of 10-hydroxycamptothecin in poly(lactide-co-glycolide) microsphere delivery vehicles. Pharm. Res., 1997. 14:1406–1414.
9. Li, S. M., Garreau, H. and Vert, M., Structure-property relationships in the case of the degradation of massive aliphatic poly-(a-hydroxy acids) in aqueous media. J. Mater. Sci. Mater. Med., 1990. 1: 123–130.
10. Huffman, K. R. and Casey, D. J., J. Polym. Sci., 1985. 23: 1939–1945.
11. Connors, K. A., Chemical Kinetics. The Study of Reaction Rates in Solution. 1990, New York: VCH.
12. Burke, P., Determination of internal pH in PLGA microspheres using ^{31}P NMR spectroscopy. Proc. Int. Symp. Control. Rel. Bioact. Mater., 1996. 23: 237–238.
13. Mader, K., Bittner, B., Li, Y., Wohlauf, W. and Kissel, T., Monitoring microviscosity and microacidity of the albumin microenvironment inside degrading microparticles from poly(lactide-co-glycolide) (PLG) or ABA-triblock polymers containing hydrophobic poly(lactide-co-glycolide) A blocks and hydrophilic poly(ethyleneoxide) B blocks. Pharm. Res., 1998. 15(6): 787–793.
14. Fu, K., Pack, D. W., Laverdiere, A., Son, S., and Langer, R., Visualization of acidic environment within degrading poly(lactic-co-glycolic acid) (PLGA) microspheres. Pharm. Res., 2000. 17: 100–106.
15. Bunner, A., Mader, K. and Gopferich, A., pH and osmotic pressure inside biodegradable microspheres during erosion. Pharm. Res., 1999. 16: 847–853.
16. French, T., So, P. T. C., Weaver Jr., D. J., Coelho-Sampaio, T., Grattton, E., Voss Jr., E. W., and Carrero, J., Two-photon fluorescence lifetime imaging microcopy of macrophage-mediated antigen processing. J. Microsc., 1997. 185: 339–353.
17. Chen, S.-C., Nakamura, H., and Tamura, Z., Supplemental studies on relationships between structure and spectrum of fluorescein. Chem. Pharm. Bull., 1979. 27: 475–479.
18. Shenderova, A., Burke, T. G., and Schwendeman, S. P., The acidic microclimate in poly(lactide-co-glycolide) microspheres stabilizes camptothecins. Pharm. Res., 1998. 16: 241–248.
19. Heller, J., Development of poly(orto esters): a historical overview. Biomaterials, 1990. 11: 659–665.
20. Bates, R. G., Determination of pH. Theory and Practice. 1973, Wiley-Interscience: New York.
21. Bates, R. G., Paabo, M. and Robinson, R. A., Interpretation of pH measurements in alcohol–water solvents. J. Phys. Chem., 1963. 67: 1833–1838.
22. Douheret, G., Potentiels de jounction liquide et effet de milieu en solvants mixtes eau-solvant aprotique dipolaire. Bull. Soc. Chim. France, 1968. 8: 3122–3131.
23. Park, T. G., Degradation of poly(D,L-lactic acid) microspheres: effects of molecular weight. J. Controlled Release, 1994. 30: 161–173.
24. Zhang, Y., Zale, S., Alukonis, L. and Bernstein, H., Effects of metal salts on PLGA hydrolysis. Proc. Int. Symp. Control. Rel. Bioact. Mater., 1995. 22: 83–84.
25. Hutchinson, F. G. and Furr, B. J. A., Biodegradable polymer systems for the sustained release of polypeptides. J. Controlled Release, 1990. 13: 279–294.
26. Shenderova, A., Burke, T. G., and Schwendeman, S. P., Characterization of the microclimate in PLGA microspheres with a camptothecin probe. Pharm. Res., 1996. 9: S-254.
27. Mi, Z. and Burke, T. G., Differential interactions of camptothecin lactone and carboxylate forms with human blood components. Biochemistry, 1994. 33(34): 10325–36.
28. Burke, T. and Gao, X., Stabilization of topotecan in low pH liposomes compoused of distearoylphosphatidylcholine. J. Pharm. Sci., 1994. 83: 967–969.
29. Burke, T. G., Mishra, A. K., Wani, M. C., and Wall, M. E., Lipid bilayer partitioning and stability of camptothecin drugs. Biochemistry, 1993. 32: 5352–5364.
30. Carstensen, J. T., Drug Stability: Principles and Practices. 1995, Marcel Dekker: New York.
31. Zhu, G., Mallery, S. R., and Schwendeman, S. P., Stabilization of proteins encapsulated in injectable poly(lactide-co-glycolide). Nature Biotechnol. 2000. 18: 52–57.

32. Crotts, G., Sah, H., and Park, T. G., Adsorption determines in-vitro protein release rate from biodegradable microspheres: quantitative analysis of surface area during degradation. J. Controlled Release, 1997. 47: 101–111.
33. Peters, T. J., Serum Albumin. Adv. Protein Chem., 1985. 37: 161–245.
34. Manning, M. C., Patel, K. and Borchardt, R. T., Stability of protein pharmaceuticals. Pharm. Res., 1989. 6: 903–918.

21
Development of Polysaccharide Nanoparticles as Novel Drug Carrier Systems

C. Vauthier and P. Couvreur
Université de Paris XI
Chatenay Malabry, France

I. INTRODUCTION

Nanoparticles are submicronic structures (diameter below 1 μm) made with polymers. They are mainly developed as drug delivery systems as an alternative to liposome technology in order to overcome the problems related to the stability of these vesicles in biological fluids and during storage (1). Nanoparticles were first designed using albumin (2) and nonbiodegradable synthetic polymers such as polyacrylamide and poly(methyl methacrylate) (3,4). The risk of chronic toxicity due to the intracellular and/or tissue overloading of nondegradable polymers was soon considered as a major limitation for the systemic administration in man of polyacrylamide and poly(methyl methacrylate) nanoparticles. With the administration of protein-based material, the major concern was the possible antigenic response. As a consequence, the type of nanoparticle that received much attention was designed with synthetic biodegradable polymers including polyalkylcyanoacrylate, poly(lactic-co-glycolic acid), and polyanhydride (5–11). The therapeutic potential of these biodegradable colloidal systems was investigated for various applications (10–19). Despite the very interesting results reported in the literature, these systems may also be concerned with toxicological problems (20,21). In addition, they often present limitations for the administration of hydrophilic molecules such as peptides, proteins, and nucleic acids (oligonucleotides and genes) which are recognized to have great potential in therapeutics. These limitations are mainly because the polymers forming these nanoparticles are mostly hydrophobic, whereas proteins, peptides, and nucleic acids are hydrophilic. This leads to difficulties for the drug to be efficiently encapsulated and protected against enzymatic degradation (16,22–24). Therefore, the preparation of nanoparticles using more hydrophilic and naturally occurring materials has been explored (25–29).

As mentioned above, the first naturally occurring material used for the preparation of nanoparticles consisted of two proteins, albumin and gelatin (2,8,30,31). A good and extensive review of these systems already exists (32). Since it appeared, only a few papers were published on these nanoparticles (33–35).

More recently, polysaccharides have received much attention, and a few authors proposed the design of nanoparticles from naturally occurring polysaccharides for the administration of peptides, proteins, and nucleic acids (26,28,36). Some authors even designed a family of biomimetic particles presenting a core shell type of structure in which the core consisted of a chemically modified polysaccharide nanoparticle and the shell was formed by a lipid layer. These specific systems were named SupraMolecular BioVectors (SMBV) by their authors (25,27,37). This chapter will focus on the different polysaccharide nanoparticles that have been proposed in the literature including SMBV. Research in this area is very active and our knowledge of the biopharmaceutical potential of the different proposed systems is increasing. This chapter will present the way the different polysaccharide nanoparticles are produced and the state of present knowledge regarding their application as drug delivery systems. The different nanoparticles have been classified according to the polysaccharide used for their preparation.

II. ALGINATE NANOPARTICLES

Alginate is a naturally occurring polysaccharide composed of two types of uronic acids (Fig. 1a). The monomeric units consisting of guluronic (G) and manuronic acids (M) are arranged in three types of grouping: blocks of alternating mannuronic and guluronic residues (MGMG-MGM. . .) and blocks of guluronic acids (GGGGGGG. . .) and of mannuronic acids (MMM-MMM. . .) (38,39). Carboxylic groups from the uronic acid confer negative charges to alginate. The solubility of alginate in water depends on the associated cations. Sodium alginate is soluble in water, whereas calcium induces the formation of a gel. Alginate is widely used in the food industry as a thickening and gelling additive. It was also extensively proposed for the encapsulation of living cells showing good compatibility with living materials (39,40). The structure of the gel formed with calcium has been extensively studied (38,41). Calcium interacts

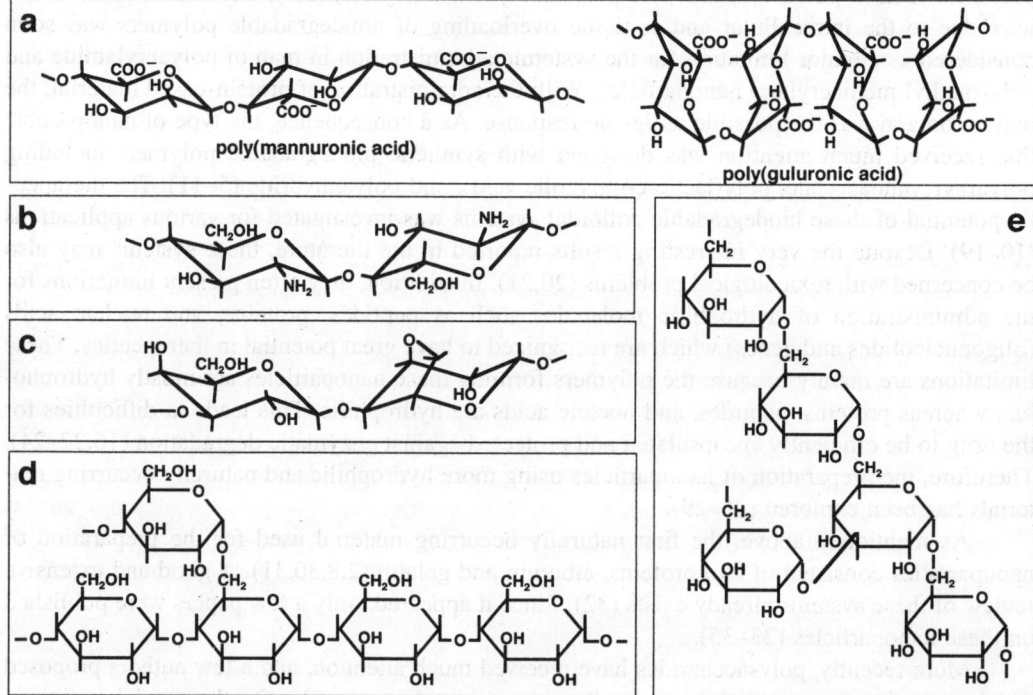

Figure 1 General structure of polysaccharides encountered in nanoparticle technology. (a) Polymannuronic and polyguluronic sequences of alginate; (b) chitosan; (c) agarose; (d) starch; and (e) dextran.

preferentially with homoguluronic sequences forming complexes that induce a parallel arrangement of the chains. This arrangement is caused by the entrapment of calcium within the interval created by guluronic residues of two distinct segments. The resulting structure was depicted as an "egg-box" model after spatial molecular arrangement arising from the interaction of calcium with alginate (Fig. 2a) (41). Gel forms even at low alginate concentrations (below 1%). Apart from the interaction with calcium, alginate may also form complexes with polycations such as polyethylenimine (PEI), chitosan, or basic peptides like polylysine and polyarginine (42,43). For example, complexes with polylysine occurred preferentially with the alternate guluronic-mannuronic acid sequences (43).

Alginate particles are usually produced by dropping sodium alginate solution into a calcium chloride solution (44,45). The instantaneous gelation of alginate caused by the calcium ions forms beads of alginate gel with a diameter depending on the size of the drop that fell within the calcium solution. The smallest particles produced according to such a process had a minimum size of 1 to 5 μm. These particles were obtained using a sophisticated device allowing the atomization of the sodium alginate within the calcium chloride solution (46). The major difficulty in further reducing the particle size by such methods is the fact that the particles always resulted from the gelation of sodium alginate drops poured into a calcium chloride solution.

The preparation of alginate particles of smaller size (diameter ± 300 nm) was directly achieved from a diluted aqueous sodium alginate solution in which gelation was induced by the addition of a low concentration of calcium. This lead to the formation of invisible clusters of calcium alginate gels which can be monitored by measuring the viscosity of the system (47,48). The clusters formed may also be observed by transmission electron microscopy after negative staining (Fig. 3). These clusters of small size are also named *pregels* and can be stabilized by

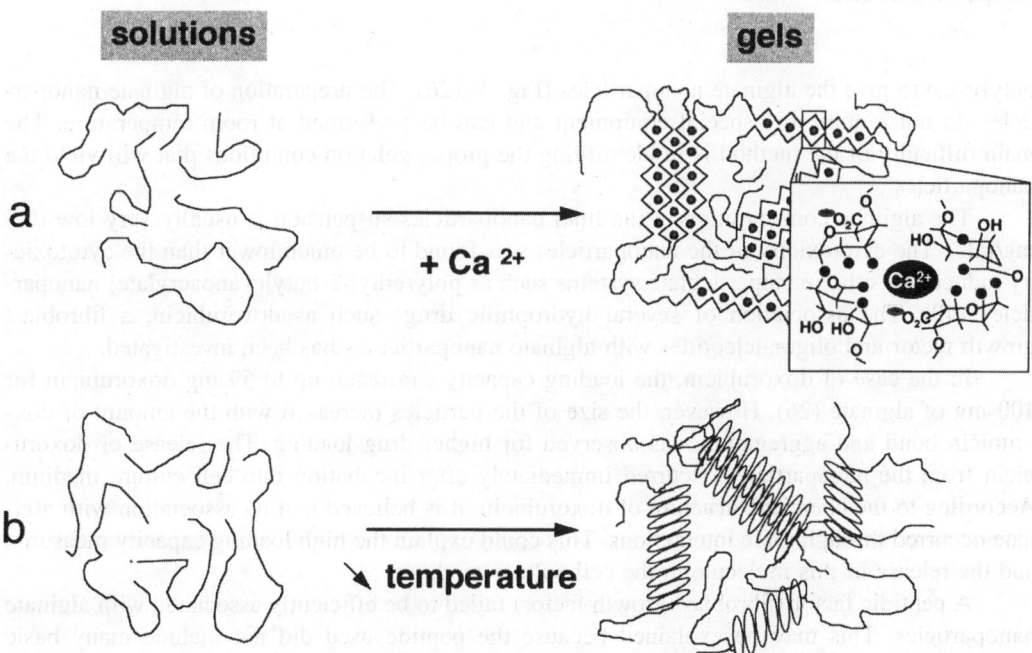

Figure 2 Structures of the gels obtained by ionic gelation of alginate induced by calcium (a) and by thermal gelation of agarose (b).

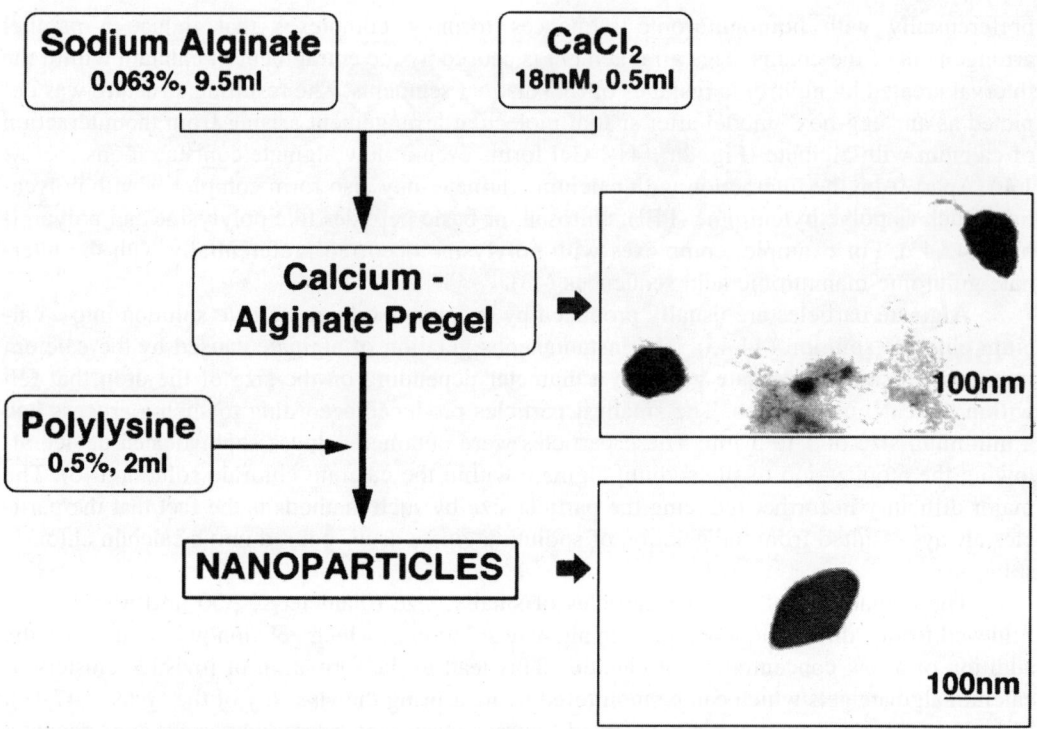

Figure 3 Scheme illustrating the formation of alginate nanoparticles. The transmission electron micrographs were performed by H. Alphandary (UMR 8612, Université de Paris XI) after negative staining with phosphotungstic acid.

polylysine to give the alginate nanoparticles (Fig. 3) (26). The preparation of alginate nanoparticles do not require any special equipment and can be performed at room temperature. The main difficulty of the method is in identifying the proper gelation conditions that will yield the nanoparticles.

The alginate concentration in the final nanoparticles suspension is usually very low (0.5 mg/mL). The cytotoxicity of the nanoparticles was found to be much lower than the cytotoxicity induced by other nanoparticulate systems such as poly(ethyl-2-butylcyanoacrylate) nanoparticles (49). The association of several hydrophilic drugs such as doxorubicin, a fibroblast growth factor and oligonucleotides with alginate nanoparticules has been investigated.

In the case of doxorubicin, the loading capacity can reach up to 59 mg doxorubicin for 100 mg of alginate (26). However, the size of the particles increased with the amount of doxorubicin bond and aggregation was observed for higher drug loading. The release of doxorubicin from the nanoparticles occurred immediately after incubation into cell culture medium. According to the chemical structure of doxorubicin, it is believed that its association with alginate occurred through ionic interactions. This could explain the high loading capacity measured and the release of this molecule in the cell culture medium.

A peptidic factor (fibroblast growth factor) failed to be efficiently associated with alginate nanoparticles. This may be explained because the peptide used did not include many basic amino acids within its composition. However, as in the case of polylysine, a basic peptide entering into the composition of the alginate nanoparticles, it can be expected that therapeutic peptides with a more basic structure could represent better candidates for an association with the alginate nanoparticles.

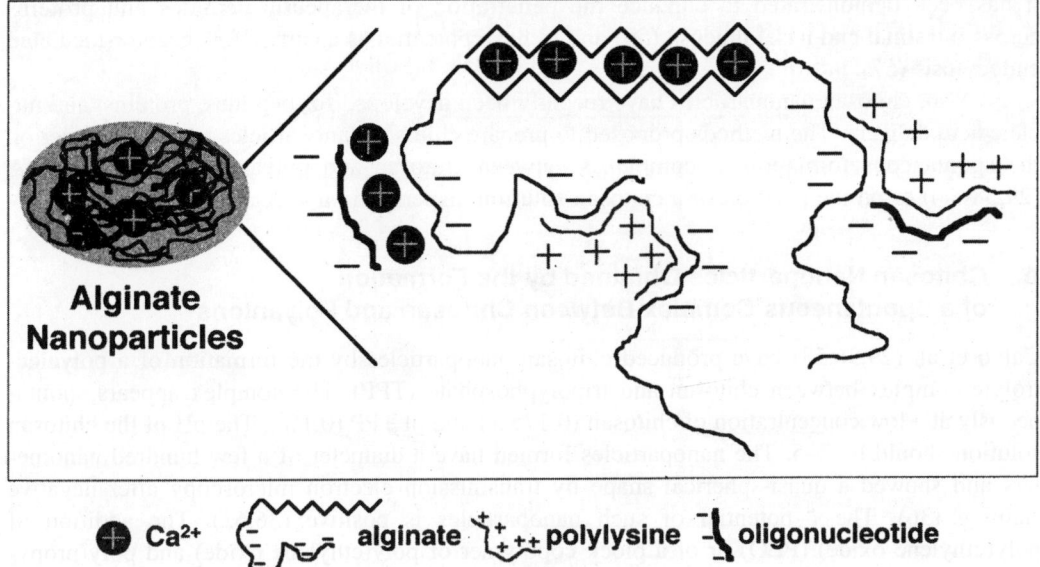

Figure 4 Hypothesis about the interactions responsible for the association of oligonucleotides with the alginate nanoparticles.

The association of antisense oligonucleotides has also been considered very recently (50–52). These molecules are polyanions and were used as complexes with polylysine in various experiments of cell transformation (53). Indeed, polylysine–oligonucleotide complexes are known to improve cell penetration of nucleic acid material. Oligonucleotides were found to associate with alginate nanoparticles by different ways. They can be added as a polylysine–oligonucleotide complex to the pregel or as a simple oligonucleotide solution either to the pregel or to the already formed nanoparticles. In all cases, efficient association requires a delay of a few days (51,52). The association of oligonucleotides with the alginate nanoparticles is believed to result from crossed interactions between the oligonucleotide and the polylysine on one side and between the polylysine and the alginate on the other side (Fig. 4). Other interactions between the oligonucleotide and the alginate that could be mediated by calcium ions may also be involved since the association occurred even in the absence of polylysine (Fig. 4). The size as well as the negative ζ potential of the nanoparticles were not affected by the oligonucleotide loading rate. Alginate nanoparticules were found to provide an effective protection of oligonucleotides from degradation in serum. After intravenous administration, they were observed to allow the targeting of oligonucleotides to the lungs, the liver, and the spleen (50–52).

III. CHITOSAN NANOPARTICLES

Chitosan is a naturally occurring biopolymer made up of $\beta(1,4)$-linked glucosamine units (Fig. 1b). It is produced by deacetylation of chitin extracted from shells of crabs, shrimps, and krills (54). The amino groups confer to the molecule a high charge density and are readily available for chemical reactions and salt formation with acids. Chitosan is soluble in various acids; it can also interact with polyanions to form complexes and gels (42–54). It has high biocompatibility and biodegradability. In vivo, it is degraded by lyzozyme (55). The development of pharmaceutical preparations with chitosan has been examined for different purposes (54). For example, it has been demonstrated to enhance the penetration of therapeutic peptides and proteins across intestinal and nasal mucosa (56) and to have potential as a carrier for receptor-mediated endocytosis (57).

Also, chitosan nanoparticles have recently been developed for peptides, proteins, and nucleic acid delivery. The methods proposed to prepare chitosan nanoparticles are based either on the spontaneous formation of complexes between chitosan and polyanions including DNA (29,58–60) or on the gelation of a chitosan solution dispersed in a water-in-oil emulsion (61).

A. Chitosan Nanoparticles Obtained by the Formation of a Spontaneous Complex Between Chitosan and Polyanions

Calvo et al. (29,36,58) have produced chitosan nanoparticles by the formation of a polyelectrolyte complex between chitosan and tripolyphosphate (TPP). The complex appears spontaneously at a low concentration of chitosan (0.175%) and of TPP (0.1%). The pH of the chitosan solution should be 3–5. The nanoparticles formed have a diameter of a few hundred nanometers and showed a quasi-spherical shape by transmission electron microscopy after negative staining (36). The ζ potential of such nanoparticles is positive (36,62). The addition of poly(ethylene oxide) (PEO) or of a block copolymer of poly(ethylene oxide) and poly(propylene oxide) (PEO-PPO) to the chitosan solution led to chitosan nanoparticles coated with POE (36,58). Varying the chitosan/PEO-PPO ratio, the ζ potential and the particle size can be conveniently modulated from +20 mV to +60 mV and from 200 nm to 1000 nm, respectively (36–58). Surface modification of the nanoparticles can also be achieved by the chemical coupling of methoxy-PEO (Me-PEO) using a carbodiimide (58). In this case, the ζ potential of the particles drop to a fixed value of +23 mV for Me-PEO concentrations higher than 1 mg/mL. The PEO-coated chitosan nanoparticles were less cytotoxic than the uncoated nanoparticles, indicating that PEO noticeably improved the biocompatibility of the particles.

This formulation was evaluated as a carrier for therapeutic peptides such as insulin (62), for vaccines and proteins (36), and as a delivery system for antisense oligonucleotides (58).

The encapsulation efficiency can reach 100% for the proteins and peptides which have a low pI such as bovine serum albumin (BSA) (pI 4.5–4.8) (36) and insulin (pI 5.5) (62). The highest entrapment efficiency was described when the chitosan solution had a pH of 5 and when the protein was dissolved in the TPP solution at pH 8 before its addition to the chitosan solution. In these conditions, the protein was negatively charged and its interaction with the amino groups of chitosan favored. Almost no association of the protein with the chitosan nanoparticles occurred when the protein was added to the completed nanoparticles. Proteins which have slightly higher pI can also be associated with chitosan nanoparticles, but their entrapment efficiency was lower (36). The entrapment efficiency is also lowered with PEO-PPO/chitosan nanoparticles. In this case, it is believed that PEO chains on the nanoparticle surface cause steric hindrance reducing protein–chitosan interactions. From data reported with insulin, it appears that both the size and the ζ potential of the chitosan nanoparticles were not dramatically influenced by the peptidic content of the nanoparticles (62).

The release kinetic profile of proteins from the chitosan nanoparticles showed no burst effect when studies were performed in trehalose solution at a concentration of 5%. In this medium, the release occurred slowly over several days. Tetanus toxoid was released under its active form for 18 days (36). In contrast, the release of insulin occurred rapidly as soon as the nanoparticles were transferred in a phosphate buffer at pH 7.4. The release was total indicating that the interactions which occurred between insulin and chitosan nanoparticles were reversible (62).

Oligonucleotides were also associated with chitosan nanoparticles formed with TPP. The entrapment efficiencies were quite high (over 95%) (58). The association was achieved by the addition of the oligonucleotide dissolved in the TPP solution. The particle size of the oligonucleotide-loaded chitosan nanoparticles ranged from 150 to 200 nm, whereas the positive ζ potential could be modulated as a function of TPP/oligonucleotide ratio. In vivo applications are under investigations.

Chitosan–DNA nanoparticles were developed on the model of PEI–DNA complex (63) to propose a novel nonviral gene delivery system made of biodegradable polymer to replace the nonbiodegradable PEI (59,60).

Chitosan–DNA nanoparticles were obtained by preparing complexes of chitosan with plasmid-DNA. The size of the particles formed was influenced by the positive to negative charge ratio (Table 1). The ζ potential of the particles appeared positive for positive to negative charge ratios higher than 1. In vitro assays of cell transformation performed with DNA-chitosan nanospheres appeared almost as efficient as those carried out with PEI–DNA complexes used as a reference (60). Other authors tested DNA–chitosan nanoparticles for their oral immunization potential using two different plamids encoding for luciferase, used as a model antigen and for a peanut allergen (59). A low immune response against the encoding antigens was reported after the oral administration of the DNA delivered with the aid of the chitosan nanoparticles. According to the authors, DNA administered under this formulation was protected against degradation and may be effective to generate an immune response against the encoding antigens administered (59).

B. Chitosan Nanoparticles Produced by an Emulsification-Based Method

Another way to produce chitosan nanoparticles is to induce the gelation of a chitosan solution dispersed in a water-in-oil emulsion. To achieve this preparation, two water-in-oil emulsions containing a high concentration of a nonionic surfactant (5%) are prepared (61) (Fig. 5). One emulsion contains a chitosan solution (concentration 2.5%) together with the molecule to be encapsulated; the second emulsion contains a concentrated solution of sodium hydroxide (3 M). The continuous phase of both emulsions is composed of paraffin oil in which the surfactant is dissolved. To induce the gelation of chitosan, the two emulsions are mixed together. A high-speed homogenizer is used to enhance the formation of very small aqueous globules and to promote collision between chitosan and sodium hydroxide containing globules responsible for their solidification. The particles formed can be isolated in water after successive washing steps with toluene and ethanol (Fig. 5). Chitosan nanoparticles with a diameter of 400 nm can be produced by this method. Compared to the previously described method, this technique presents the major disavantage to involve organic solvents during the isolation of the particles that are always difficult to remove from the particles and that may cause toxic problems.

Such particles were developed for gadolinium-neutron capture therapy, a cancer therapy which utilizes the nuclear neutron capture reaction of gadolinium by thermal neutron irradiation (61). A key success factor for this kind of therapy is to achieve the efficient delivery of gadolinium into the tumor tissue to be irradiated and to retain it in the tissue. Chitosan nanoparticles

Table 1 Chitosan-DNA Nanoparticle Size as Given by Different Positive to Negative Charge Ratio

+/− Charge ratio	Particle diameter (nm)
1.5 : 1	110
2.4 : 1	120
9.6 : 1	400

Source: Data from Ref. 60.

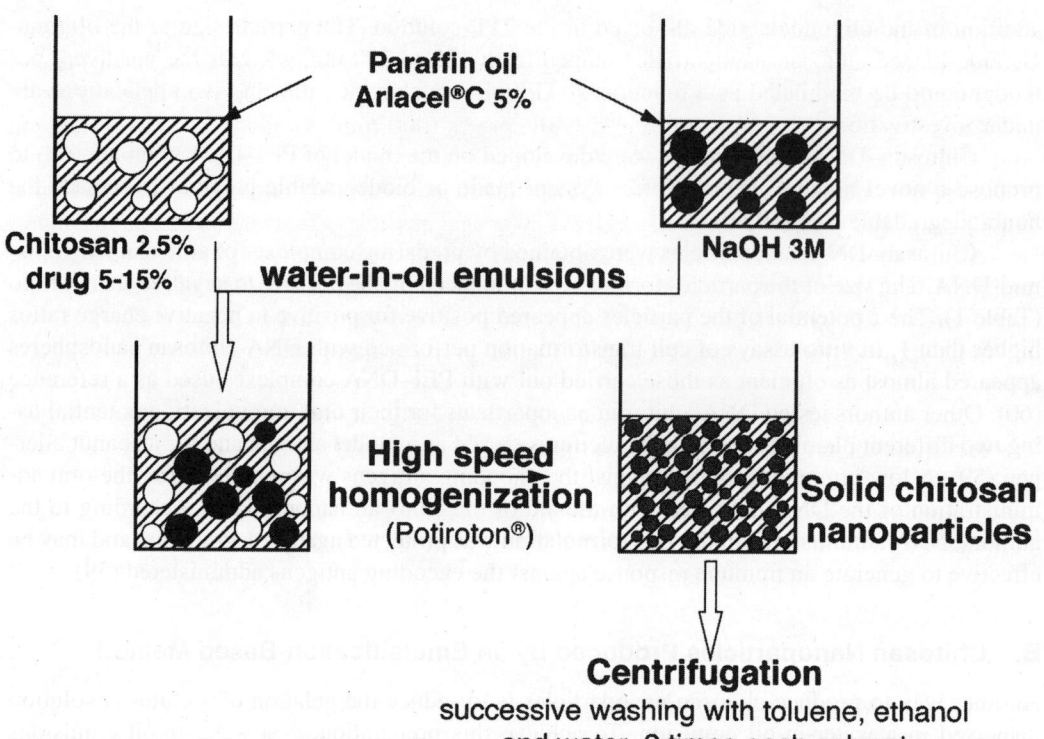

Figure 5 Preparation of chitosan nanoparticles by inducing the gelation of a chitosan solution dispersed in a water-in-oil emulsion. (Adapted from Ref. 60.)

containing up to 13% gadolinium could be prepared by dissolving gadopentetate into the chitosan solution used for the preparation of the nanoparticles. Results from in vivo experiments carried out on a solid tumor model bearing mice demonstrated that the gadolinium-loaded chitosan nanoparticles represented a very useful device for the intratumoral administration and retention of gadolinium into solid tumors. Therefore, these nanoparticles can be used to improve gadolinium-neutron capture therapy (61).

IV. AGAROSE NANOPARTICLES

Agarose nanoparticles were developed for the administration of therapeutic proteins and peptides (28,64,65). The purpose of the work was to design hydogel nanoparticles which may be administered by different parenteral routes: subcutaneous, intramuscular, or intravenous injection. Agarose (Fig. 1c) aqueous solution forms thermally reversible hydrogels while being cooled down below the gelling temperature (31–36°C). Thermic gelation results from the formation of helicoidal structures responsible for the appearance of a tridimensional network in which large amounts of water can be entrapped (Fig. 2b). The hydrogel, being hydrophilic, inert, and biocompatible, forms a suitable matrix for proteins and peptides which can be easily embedded in the gel during formation.

Agarose nanoparticles were produced using a technology termed the emulsion-converted-to-suspension in situ method and adapted from a method originally designed to make microparticles (66). This methodology requires the preparation of a water-in-oil emulsion in which agarose solution is dispersed in corn oil at 40°C (28). Peptides and proteins to be encapsulated in the particles are added to the agarose solution. The small size of the dispersed aqueous globules is achieved using an homogenizer at high speed (7000 rpm). Gelation of agarose is then induced by diluting the emulsion with cold corn oil (12°C) under agitation (7000 rpm) and the emulsion is placed at 5°C. The liquid globules of protein-containing agarose solution are then converted to protein-containing agarose hydrogel particles. To isolate the nanoparticles from the corn oil, the suspension is diluted with hexane prior to its filtration over a nylon membrane with such a porosity (0.1 μm) that it retains the nanoparticles. The nanoparticles are extensively washed with heptane to remove the oil before drying under vaccuum in a desiccator. An example of the complete procedure for the preparation of such nanoparticles is given in Fig. 6.

Some critical points should be carefully considered for the successful preparation of agarose nanoparticles. First, the emulsion must be prepared over the agarose gelling temperature and the size of the dispersed globules must be very small; otherwise, microparticles will form. Emulsion globules of agarose solution with a diameter of 1,000–2,000 nm lead to hydrogel nanoparticles with a mean diameter of 500 nm; more than 80% of the particles show a diameter below 1,000 nm. To reach such a size for the nanoparticles, only methods of agitation providing enough energy and producing high homogenization are suitable. Second, the gelation of agarose must occur rapidly. Therefore, the cooling procedure should provide fast drop of the temperature of the agarose solution globules. This is generally achieved by dilution of the emulsion with cold continuous phase. Indeed, the temperature of the emulsion will suddenly drop below the gelling point of agarose after the cold continuous phase has been added. Consequently, this induces quasi-instantaneous solidification of the globules. Hydrogel nanoparticles produced in this way tend not to aggregate because there is no time for the globules to remain in the intermediate stage between solution and hydrogel in which particles are generally sticky. Finally, the isolation of dry nanoparticles requires careful and progressive elimination of the oil to avoid aggregation phenomena.

The size of the nanoparticles formed is a function of the homogenization conditions and of the agarose concentration solution. In principle, the higher the homogenization speed and/or the longer the homogenization duration, the smaller the droplet size will be in the emulsion and consequently the smaller the agarose hydrogel particles should be. However, the authors mentioned that droplets of desirable size should be obtained within the first 30 s of homogenization because further homogenization increases the risk of aggregation and fusion of the droplets (28). To make nanoparticles, the viscosity of the solution should be low corresponding to low concentrations in agarose (1–3%). A high ratio between organic phase and aqueous phase should be used to reduce the possibility of aggregation of the agarose solution droplets followed by fusion to larger size.

Electron microscopy examination of agarose hydrogel nanoparticles shows single and almost spherical items (28). The dryed agarose nanoparticles obtained at the end of the preparation can be rehydrated in water. The amount of water taken up by the particles depends on the temperature. For example, the nanoparticles resulting from the preparation given in Fig. 6 were taking up to 76% of water at 25°C after 20 h soaking within distilled water. At 42°C, the amount of water in the nanoparticles increased to 84%. This is an important parameter to consider since the water content of a hydrogel greatly influences the diffusional migration process of the entrapped drug molecules and even facilitates diffusion of the drug out of the hydrogel matrix (67). The release of a model protein, ovalbumin, entrapped in the agarose hydrogel nanoparticles has been measured from dried particles soaked in PBS buffer (28). In these conditions, the release of the entrapped protein was controlled by a diffusion mechanism following

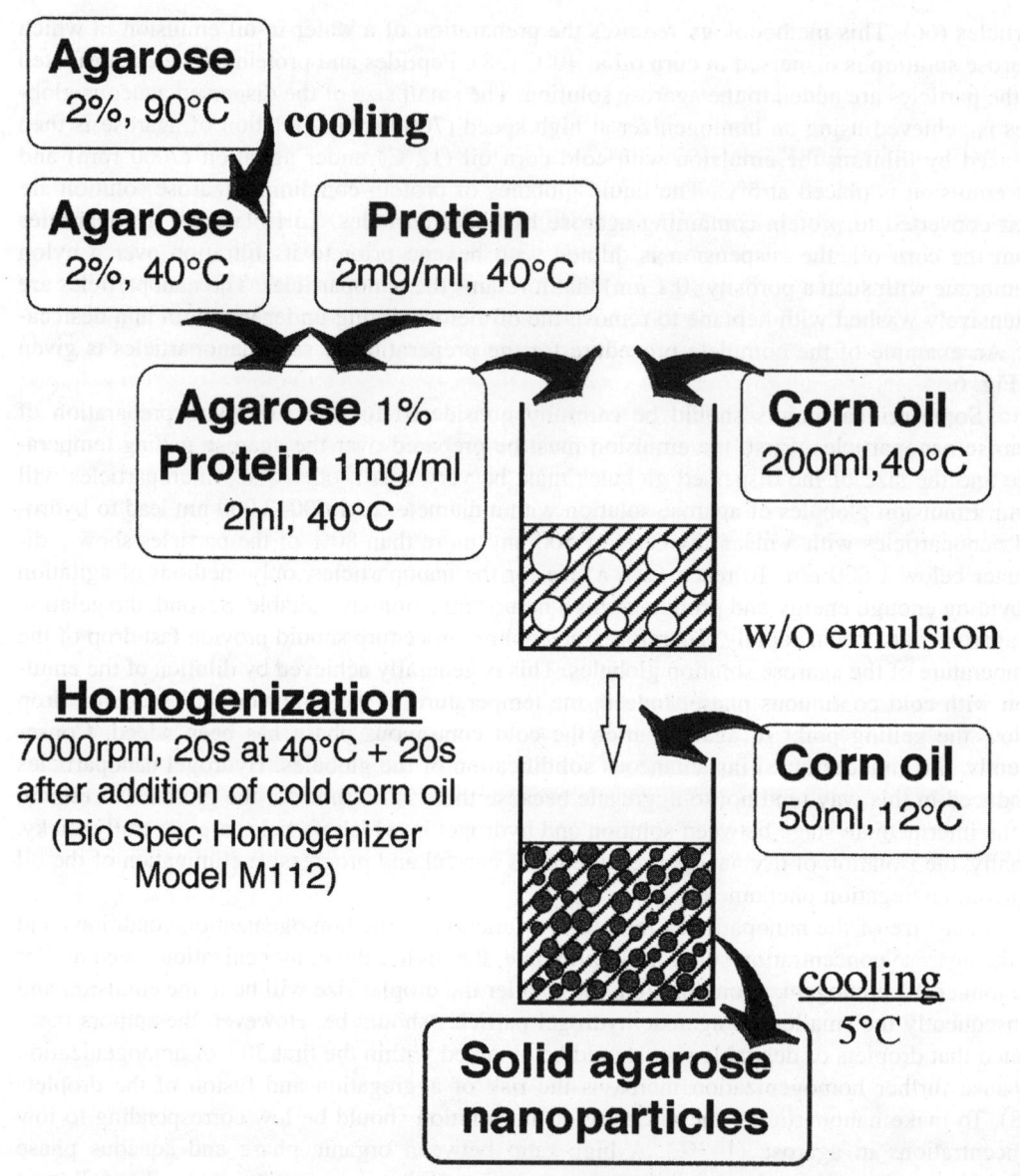

Figure 6 Preparation of agarose nanoparticles by the emulsion converted to suspension in situ method. (Adapted from Ref. 28.)

Fick's law of diffusion within the range of 0–90% of protein released at 37°C. The swelling of the nanoparticles did not control the release of protein (28).

V. SUPRAMOLECULAR BIOVECTORS

SupraMolecular BioVectors (SMBVs) consist of a family of biomimetic drug carrier systems made up as a complex sort of polysaccharide nanoparticles (25,37,68). They were imagined as analogous to low-density lipoproteins (LDLs), which are natural supramolecular structures carrying lipids within the bloodstream (25,68). LDLs present a lipid core containing cholesterol esters, surrounded by a layer of fatty acid plus an outer layer of lipids (Fig. 7a) (69). To create SMVBs on the LDL model, the lipid core of LDL was replaced by a polysaccharide nanoparticle conferring to the SMBV particles a hydrophilic core (Fig. 7b). Different SMBVs can be prepared by varying the polysaccharide forming the particle core and the lipids forming the outer membrane (37). These systems have been patented (25). Light Biovectors, a subclass of SMBVs, are composed of neutral, anionic, or cationic polysaccharidic core nanoparticles surrounded by phospholipids which organize in bilayers (37).

All SMBVs are prepared according to a general procedure in two steps, as illustrated in Fig. 8. Metabolizable polysaccharides such as dextran and starch (Fig. 1d and e), were used to make the SMBV core consisting of a polysaccharide nanoparticle. To achieve this goal, polysaccharides are crosslinked with bifunctional reagents to produce a gel. The gel is then functionalized with ligands conferring either negative or positive charges as the manner of an ion exchange resin. The drug loading of the polysaccharide particles may be achieved by the means of electrostatic interactions. The functionalized gel is divided into very small fragments under high pressure. By this way, particles as small as 30 nm in diameter can be produced. The particles are then dried under

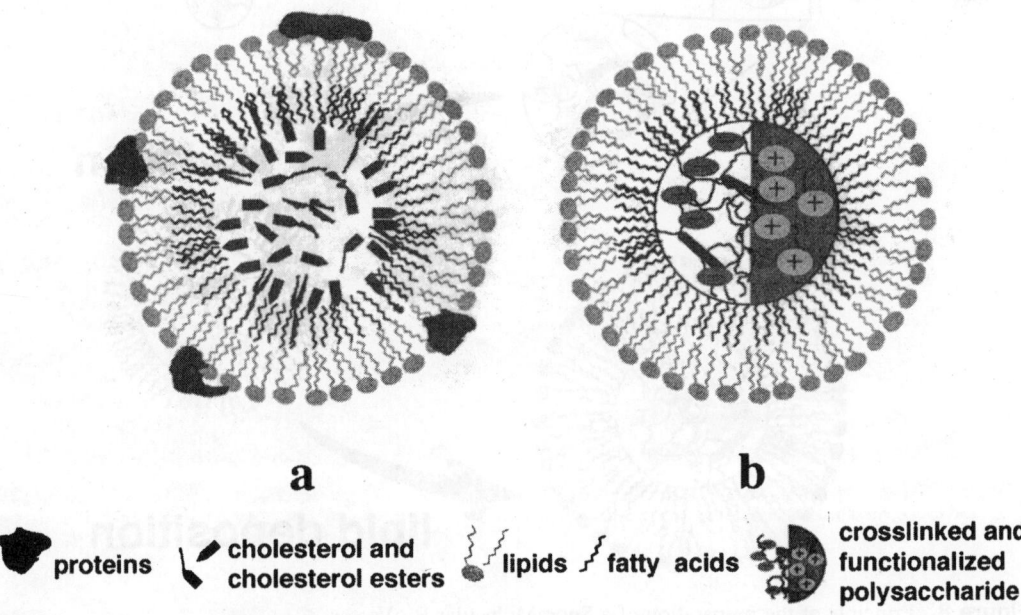

Figure 7 Schematic structure of (a) a low-density lipoprotein and of (b) the Supramolecular BioVector. (Adapted from Refs. 68 and 69.)

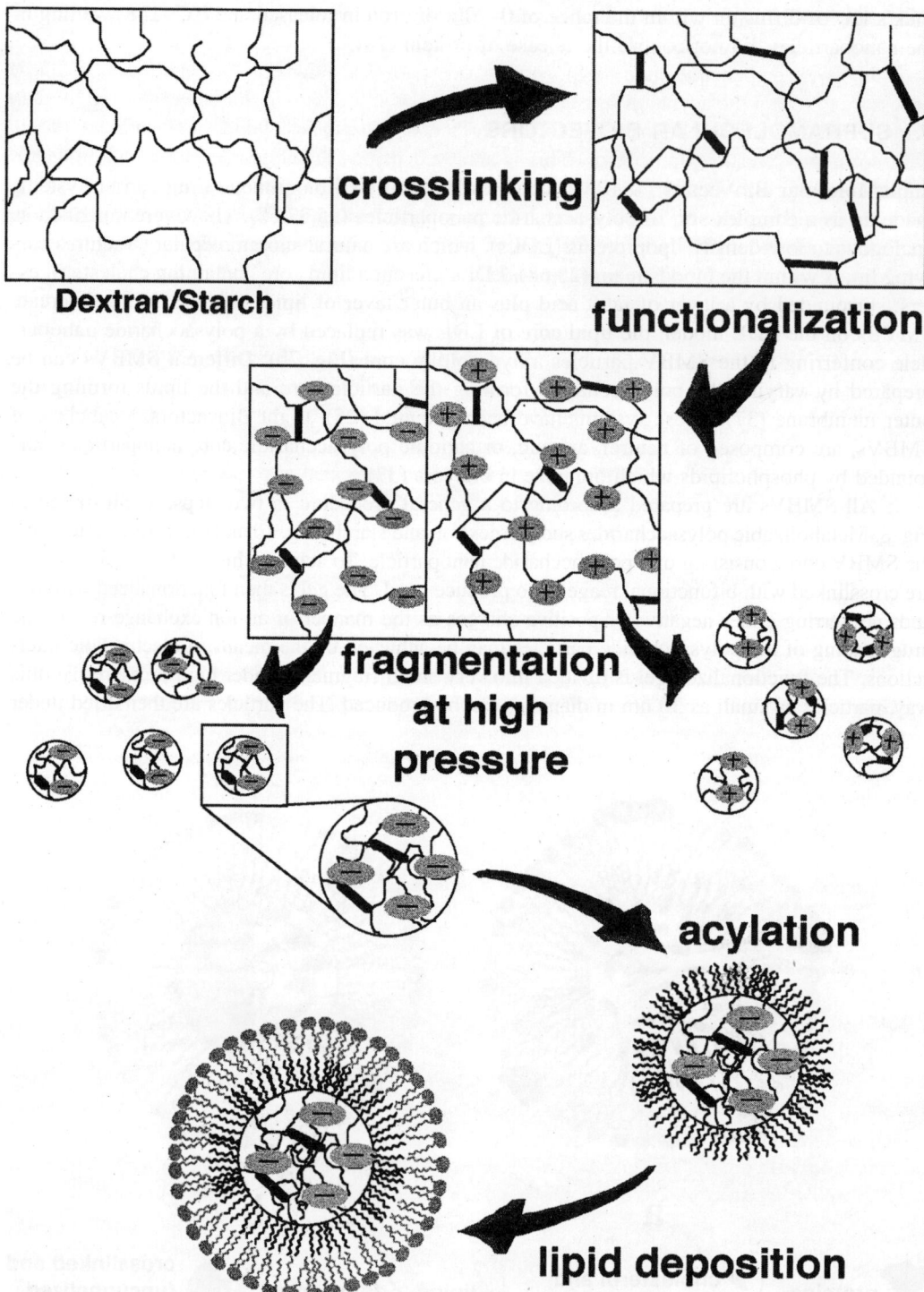

Figure 8 Principle of the preparation of a SupraMolecular BioVector.

mild conditions and dispersed in an organic solvent to achieve the attachment of fatty acid onto their surface. The acylation reaction is limited to the particle surface when the organic solvent does not swell or penetrate into the polysaccharide particles. For very small particles, it can be necessary to repeat the acylation several times before the entire particle surface is covered by fatty acids. Finally, lipids are deposited onto the surface of the polysaccharide nanoparticles coated with covalently attached fatty acids. This is achieved using techniques developed for liposome preparation. Sterilization of SMBVs can be performed by sterile filtration (27).

The drug loading of SMBVs may be achieved according to the ionic charge of the polysaccharidic core of the particles. SMBVs with an anionic core were designed for cationic drugs, whereas cationic cores were more adapted to anionic molecules.

The incorporation of cationic drugs in SMBVs has been considered by De Miguel et al. (27). Gentamicin, a polycation, doxorubicin, a monovalent cation, and interleukin-2 (IL-2), a hydrophobic and basic protein, were successfully associated with the anionic SMBVs. The acylated polysaccharide nanoparticles were loaded with the drug before the addition of the surrounded lipid layer that completed the formation of the SMBVs. The highest encapsulation efficiency was reported with the polycationic molecules. In the same way, the interaction stability of the polycationic molecule in biological media was improved and the release within the intracellular medium was better controlled compared to the monovalent cation. The association of IL-2 to the anionic SMBVs led to an improvement of its biological activity as measured on cell cultures in vitro.

SMBVs with a cationic core were specifically designed for the incorporation of nucleic acid materials (70). Oligonucleotides were incorporated into the acylated cationic polysaccharide core of the SMBVs prior to the formation of the outer lipid layer. Oligonucleotide loading capacity could reach 2.2% w/w with a loading efficiency of 90%. A minimal leakage of 10% of the total incorporated oligonucleotide was measured after 2 months. The SMBVs were found to confer a better protection against nuclease degradation attack than the single acylated cationic polysaccharide core. In vitro, SMBVs also improved the cellular uptake of the oligonucleotide. The internalization into cells was characterized according to an endosomal pathway. The amount of the oligonucleotide fraction that could be found within the cell cytoplasm could be up to 10 times higher than if the oligonucleotide was given in its free form (70). Finally, the specific and nontoxic action of an antisense oligonucleotide delivered to cells using an SMBV have been proven in vitro (71). This underscores the potential of SMBVs as carriers of oligonucleotides for in vivo applications.

The pharmacokinetics of SMBVs has been investigated as well. After intravenous administration, these drug carriers showed a half-life in the blood of 8 h. After 24 h they showed the same distribution pattern as liposomes. This indicated that the SMBVs were able to escape the immediate capture by the macrophages of the mononuclear phagocytes system (MPS) which is currently observed with many other drug carrier particulate systems (68). Specific cellular recognition of SMBVs was demonstrated in vitro with two models: SMBVs in which the apolipoprotein B was incorporated within the lipid outer membrane were internalized by fibroblasts (72), and SMBVs with chemically grafted monoclonal antibody directed against T lymphocytes were specifically targeted against the cells showing the corresponding surface antigen (73).

VI. CONCLUSION

Nanoparticles made up of polysaccharides show promise as carriers for the delivery of hydrophilic drugs. Such particles can be obtained under mild conditions according to various processes; some of these processes, being very easy, do not require any special equipment. In addition, the use of organic solvent or chemical crosslinking agents that may induce toxicological problems are generally not needed. Polysaccharide nanoparticles also present interesting features in terms of drug loading and releasing properties. After association with these nanoparticles, the biological activity measured for certain drugs was improved. Up to now little has been known about the in vivo behavior of polysaccharide nanoparticles as drug delivery systems. As suggested by the number of recent papers published on this subject, polysaccharide nanoparticles may be considered as a very active field of investigation for the development of new delivery systems specifically designed for the administration of peptides, proteins, antisense oligonucleotides, and even genes. However, much work is still required to evaluate their actual in vivo potential.

REFERENCES

1. Oppenheim R. C., 1981. Solid colloidal drug delivery systems: nanoparticles. Int J. Pharm., 8: 217–234.
2. Scheffel U., Rhodes B. A., Natarajan T. K. and Wagner H. N., 1972. Albumin microspheres for the study of the reticulo-endothelial system. J. Nucl. Med., 13: 498–503.
3. Birrenbach G. and Speiser P., 1976. Polymerized micelles and their use as adjuvant in immunology. J. Pharm. Sci., 65: 1763–1766.
4. Kreuter J. and Speiser P., 1976. New adjuvants on a polymethylmethacrylate base. Infect. Immunol., 13: 204–210.
5. Couvreur P., Kante B., Roland M. Guiot P., Baudhuin P. and Speiser P., 1979. Polycyanoacrylate nanoparticles as potential lysosomotropic carriers: preparation, morphological and sorptive properties. J. Pharm. Pharmacol., 31: 331–332.
6. Gurny R., 1981. Development of biodegradable and injectable latices for controlled release of potent drugs. Drug Dev. Ind. Pharm., 7: 1–25.
7. De Keyser J. L., Poupaert J. H. and Dumont P., 1991. Poly(diethyl methylidenemalonate) nanoparticles as potential drug carrier: preparation, distribution, and elimination after intravenous and peroral administration to mice. J. Pharm. Sci., 80: 67–70.
8. Vauthier-Holtzscherer C., Benabbou S., Spenlehauer G., Veillard M. and Couvreur P., 1991. Methodology for the preparation of ultradispersed polymer systems. STP Pharma Sci., 1: 109–116.
9. Allemann E., Leroux J. C., Gurny R. and Doelker E., 1993. In vitro extended-release properties of drug loaded poly(DL-lactic acid) nanoparticles produced by salting-out procedure. Pharm. Res., 10: 1732–1737.
10. Brannon-Peppas L., 1995. Recent advances on the use of biodegradable microparticles and nanoparticles in controlled drug delivery. Int. J. Pharm., 116: 1–9.
11. Mathiowitz E., Jacob J. S., Jong Y. S., Carino G. P., Chickering D. E., Chaturverdi P., Santos C. A., Vijayaraghavan K., Montgomery S., Basset M. and Morrel C., 1997. Biologically erodable microspheres as potential oral drug delivery systems. Nature, 386: 410–414.
12. Couvreur P. and Vauthier C., 1991. Polyalkylcyanoacrylate nanoparticles as drug carrier: present state and perspectives. J. Contr. Rel., 17: 187–198.
13. Couvreur P. and Vauthier C., 1994. Nanoparticles: therapeutic applications and prospects. In: Drug Absorption Enhancement: Concepts, Possibilities, Limitations and Trends. A. G. De Boer (Ed.), Harwood Academic, Chur, Switzerland, Chap. 15, pp. 457–486.
14. Couvreur P. and Puisieux F., 1993. Nano-and microparticles for the delivery of polypeptides and proteins. Adv. Drug Del. Rev., 10: 141–162.
15. Couvreur P., Dubernet C. and Puisieux F., 1995. Controlled drug delivery with nanoparticles: current possibilities and future trends. Eur. J. Pharm. Pharmacol., 41: 2–13.
16. Fattal E., Vauthier C., Aynié I., Nakada Y., Lambert G., Malvy C. and Couvreur P., 1998. Biodegradable polyalkylcyanoacrylate nanoparticles for the delivery of oligonucleotides. J. Control. Rel., 53: 137–143.

17. Brannon-Peppas L., and Vert M., 2000. Polylactic and polyglycolic acids as drug delivery carriers. This volume, pp. 99–130.
18. Labhasetwar V., Song C. and Levy J. R., 1997. Nanoparticle drug delivery system for restenosis. Adv. Drug Deliv. Rev., 24: 63–85.
19. Dubernet C., Fattal E. and Couvreur P., 1999. Nanoparticulate controlled release systems for cancer therapy. This volume.
20. Maassen S., Fattal E., Muller R. H. and Couvreur P., 1993. Cell cultures for the assessment of toxicity and uptake of polymeric particulate drug carriers. STP Pharma Sci., 3: 11–22.
21. Fernandez-Urrusuno R., Fattal E., Porquet D., Feger J. and Couvreur P., 1995. Evaluation of liver toxicological effects induced by polyalkylcyanoacrylate nanoparticles. Toxicol. Appl. Pharmacol., 130: 272–279.
22. Felgner P. L., 1990. Particulate systems and polymers for in vitro and in vivo delivery of polynucleotides. Adv. Drug Deliv. Rev. 5: 163–187.
23. Chavany C., Saisonbehmoaras T., LeDoan T., Puisieux F., Couvreur P. and Hélène C., 1992. Polyalkylcyanoacrylate nanoparticles as polymeric carriers for antisense oligonucleotides. Pharm. Res., 9: 441–449.
24. Emile C., Bazile D., Herman F., Hélène C. and Veillard M., 1996. Encapsulation of oligonucleotides in stealth Me.PEG-PLA$_{50}$ nanoparticles by complexation with structured oligopeptides. Drug Deliv., 3: 187–195.
25. Samain D., 1989. Les biovecteurs supramoléculaires: une nouvelle famille de transporteurs biomimétiques de médicaments. Biofutur, Décembre 1989: 64–66.
26. Rajaonarivony M., Vauthier C., Couarraze G., Puisieux F. and Couvreur P., 1993. Development of a new drug carrier made from alginate. J. Pharm. Sci., 82: 912–917.
27. De Miguel I., Ioualalen K., Bonnefous M., Peyrot M., Nguyen F., Cervilla M., Soulet N., Dirson R., Rieumajou V., Imbertie L., Solers C., Cazes S., Favre G. and Samain D., 1995. Synthesis and characterization of supramolecular biovector (SMBV) specifically designed for the entrapment of ionic molecules. Bioch. Biophys. Acta., 1237: 49–58.
28. Wang N. and Wu X. S., 1997. Preparation and characterization of agarose hydrogel nanoparticules for protein and peptide drug delivery. Pharm. Dev. Technol., 2: 135–142.
29. Calvo P., Remunan-Lopez C., Vila-Jato J. L. and Alonso M. J., 1997a. Novel hydrophilic chitosan-polyethylene oxide nanoparticles as protein carriers. J. Appl. Polym. Sci., 63: 125–132.
30. Marty J. J., Oppenheim R. C. and Speiser P., 1978, Nanoparticles—a new colloidal drug delivery system. Pharm. Acta Helv., 53: 17–23.
31. Keuter J., 1978. Nanoparticles and nanocapsules—new dosage forms in the nanometer range. Pharm. Acta Helv., 53: 33–39.
32. Oppenheim R. C., 1986. Nanoparticulate drug delivery systems based on gelatin and albumin. In: Polymeric Nanoparticules and Microspheres, P. Guiot and P. Couvreur (Eds.), CRC Press, Boca Raton, FL, pp. 1–25.
33. Leo E., Arletti R., Forni F. and Cameroni R., 1997. General and cardiac toxicity of doxorubicin-loaded gelatin nanoparticles. Il Farmaco, 52: 385–388.
34. Li J. K., Wang N. and Wu X. S., 1997. A novel biodegradable system based on gelatin nanoparticules and poly(lactic-co-glycolic acid) microspheres for protein and peptide drug delivery. J. Pharm. Sci., 86: 891–895.
35. Li J. K., Wang N. and Wu X. S., 1998. Gelatin nanoencapsulation of protein/peptide drugs using an emulsifier-free emulsion method. J. Microencapsul., 15: 163–172.
36. Calvo P., Remunan-Lopez C., Vila-Jato J. L. and Alonso M. J., 1997b, Chitosan and chitosan-ethylene oxide-propylene oxide block copolymer nanoparticles as novel carriers for proteins and vaccines. Pharm. Res., 14: 1431–1436.
37. Major M., Prieur E., Tocanne J. F., Betbeber D. and Sautereau A. M., 1997. Characterization and phase behavior of phospholipid bilayers adsorbed on spherical polysaccharidic nanoparticles. Biochim. Biophys. Acta., 1327: 32–40.
38. Gacesa P., 1988. Alginates. Carbohydr. Polym., 8: 161–182.
39. Guiseley K. B., 1989. Chemical and physical properties of algal polysaccharides used for cell immobilization. Enzyme Microb. Technol., 11: 706–716.

40. Sun A. M., Vacek I. and Tai I., 1994. Microencapsulation of living cells and tissues. In: Microcapsules and Nanoparticles in Medicine and Pharmacy, M. Donbrow (Ed.), CRC Press, Boca Raton, Fl, pp. 315–322.
41. Rees D. A. and Welsh E. J., 1977. Secondary and tertiary structure of polysaccharides in solutions and gels. Angew. Chem. Int. Ed. Engl., 16: 214–224.
42. Takahashi T., Takayama K., Machida Y. and Nagai T., 1990. Characteristics of polyion complexes of chitosan with sodium alginate and sodium polyacrylate. Int. J. Pharm., 61: 35–41.
43. Bystricky S., Malovikova A. and Sticzay T., 1991. Interaction of acidic polysaccharides with polylysine enantiomers. Conformation probe in solution. Carbohydr. Polym., 15: 299–308.
44. Wong H. and Chang T. M. S., 1991. The encapsulation of cells within alginate poly-L-lysine microcapsules prepared with the standard step drop technique: histological identified membrane imperfections and the associated graft rejection. Biomater. Art. Cells Immob. Biotech., 19: 675–686.
45. Arshady R., 1993. Microcapsules for food. J. Microencapsul., 10: 413–435.
46. Kwok K. K., Groves M. J. and Burgess D. J., 1991. Production of 5–15 μm diameter alginate-polylysine microcapsules by an air-atomization technique. Pharm. Res., 8: 341–344.
47. Mutin P. H., 1986. Etude de la gélification physique du poly(chlorure de vynyle). Ph.D. thesis, University of Strasbourg, France.
48. Vauthier C., Rajaonarivony M., Couarraze G., Couvreur P. and Puisieux F., 1994. Characterization of alginate pregel by rheological investigation. Eur. J. Pharm. Biopharm., 40: 218–222.
49. Nemati F., Dubernet F., Fessi H., Colin de Verdière A., Poupon M. F., Puisieux F. and Couvreur P., 1996. Reversion of multidrug resistance using nanoparticles in vitro: influence of the nature of the polymer. Int. J. Pharm., 138: 237–246.
50. Vauthier C., Aynié I., Couvreur P. and Fattal E., 1998. Pharmacokinetic and tissue disposition of oligonucleotides associated with alginate nanoparticles. Proc. Int. Symp. Control. Rel. Bioact. Mater., 25: 228–229.
51. Aynié I., Vauthier C., Fattal E., Foulquier M. and Couvreur P., 1998. Alginate nanoparticles as a novel carrier for antisens oligonucleotides. In: Future Strategies for Drug Delivery with Particulate Systems, J. E. Diederichs and R. H. Muller (Eds.), CRC Press, Boca Raton, FL, pp. 11–16.
52. Aynié I., Vauthier C. Fattal E., Puisieux F. and Couvreur P., 1998. Role of a small polylysine in a hydrogel nanoparticulate system for the antisense oligonucleotide strategy. Proc. 2nd World Meeting APGI/APV, Paris, May 25–28, pp. 583–584.
53. Rojanasakul Y., 1996. Antisens oligonucleotide therapeutics: drug delivery and targeting. Adv. Drug. Del. Rev., 18: 115–131.
54. Kas H. S., 1997. Chitosan: properties, preparations and application to microparticulate systems. J. Microencaps., 14: 689–711.
55. Nordtveit R. J., Vaarum K. M. and Smidsroed O., 1996. Degradation of partially N-acetylated chitosans with hen egg white and human lyzozyme. Carbohydr. Polym. 29:163–167
56. Illum L., Rarraj N. F. and Davis S. S., 1994. Chitosan as a novel nasal delivery system for peptide drugs. Pharm. Res., 11: 1186–1189.
57. Olsen R., Schwartzmiller D., Weppner W. and Winandy R., 1989, Biomedical applications of chitin and its derivatives. In: Chitin and Chitosan Sources: Chemistry, Biochemistry, Physical Properties and Applications, G. Skjak-Braek (Ed.), Elsevier, Amsterdam, pp. 813–829.
58. Calvo P., Boughaba A. S., Appel A., Fattal E., Alonso M. J. and Couvreur P., 1998. Oligonucleotide-chitosan nanoparticles as new gene tharapy vector. Proc. 2nd Worl Meeting APGI/APV, Paris, May 25–28, 1998, pp. 1111–1112.
59. Roy K., Mao H. Q., Lin K. Y., Lin J., Huang S. K. and Leong K. W., 1998. Oral immunization with DNA-chitosan nanospheres. Proc. Int. Symp. Control. Rel. Bioact. Mater., 25: 348–349.
60. Köping-Höggård M., Nilsson M., Edwards K. and Artursson P., 1998. Chitosan-DNA polyplex: a new efficient, biodegradable gene delivery system. Proc. Int. Symp. Control. Rel. Bioact. Mater., 25: 368–369.
61. Tokumitsu H., Ichikawa H., Fukumori Y., Hiratsuka J., Sakurai Y and Kobayashi T., 1998. Preparation of gadopentetate-loaded chitosan nanoparticle for gadolinium neutron capture therapy of cancer

using a novel emulsion droplet coalescence technique. Proc. 2nd Worl Meeting APGI/APV, Paris, May 25–28, 1998, pp 641–642.
62. Fernandez-Urrusuno R., Calvo P., Vila-Jato J. L. and Alonso M. J., 1998. Chitosan nanoparticles as carriers for mucosal administration of peptides. Proc. Int. Symp. Control. Rel. Bioact. Mater., 25: 520–521.
63. Boussif O., Lezoualc'h F., Zanta M. A., Mergny M. D., Scherman D., Demeneix B. and Behr J. P., 1995. A versatile vector for gene and oligonucleotide transfer into cells in culture and in vivo: polyethylenimine. Proc. Natl. Acad. Sci. USA, 92: 7297–7301.
64. Wang N., Wu X. S. and Mesiha M., 1995, A new method for the preparation of protein-loaded agarose nanoparticles. Pharm. Res., 12: S 257.
65. Wang N. and Wu X. S., 1996. Agarose nanospheres for protein drug delivery. Proc. Int. Symp. Control. Rel. Mater., 23: 829–230.
66. Burgess D. J. and Hickey A. J., 1994. Microsphere technology and application. In: Encyclopedia of Pharmaceutical Technology, J. Swarbrick and J. C. Boylan (Eds.), Vol. 10., Marcel Dekker, New York, pp. 1–29.
67. Peppas N. A. and Lustig S. R., 1986. Solute diffusion in hydrophilic network structures. In: Hydrogels in Medicine and Pharmacy, Vol. 1, Fundamental, N. A. Peppas (Ed.,), CRC Press, Boca Raton, FL, pp. 57–84.
68. Berton M., 1996. Application des biovecteurs supramoléculaires (BVSM) à la stratégie antisens: Incorporation et protection d'oligonucléotides, étude de leur devenir cellulaire et effet antisens. Ph.D. thesis 1996, Université de Paris XI, France.
69. Kostner G. M. and Lagger P., 1989. Chemical and physical properties of lipoproteins. In: Human Plasma Lipoproteins, J. C. Fruchart and J. Sherphed (Eds.), Walter de Gruyter, Berlin, pp. 23–54.
70. Berton M., Sixou S., Kravtzoff R., Dartigues C., Imbertie L., Allal C. and Favre G., 1997. Improved oligonucleotide uptake and stability by a new drug carrier, the SupraMolecular BioVector (SMVB). Biochim. Biophys. Acta, 1355: 7–19.
71. Allal C., Sixou S., Kravtzoff R., Soulet N., Soula G. and Favre G., 1998. SupraMolecular BioVectors (SMBV) improve antisens inhibition of erbB-2 expression. Br. J. Cancer, 77: 1448–1453.
72. Samain D., Favre G., Nguyen F., Peyrot M., Mercier P., Soulet N., Dirson R., Demiguel I. and Meniali J., 1992. Particulate vectors having selective tropism: method of preparation and pharmaceutical composition. French patent, PCT/FR 92/00506.
73. Courbon F., Picault P., Petereau C., Cigagna F., Al Saati T., Dirson R., Delson G. and Favre G., 1995. Targeting of cells with biovector drug delivery carriers by a monoclonal antibody. Proc. Am. Assoc. Cancer Res., 36: 1836.

22
An Overview of Controlled Release Systems

S. Venkatraman, N. Davar, A. Chester, and L. Kleiner
ALZA Corporation, Mountain View, California

I. INTRODUCTION

The term *drug delivery* covers a very broad range of techniques used to get therapeutic agents into the human body. The limitations of the most obvious and trusted drug delivery techniques, those of the ingested tablet and of the intravenous (IV)/subcutaneous/intramuscular (IM) injections, have been recognized for some time now. The former delivers drug into the blood only through the hepatic system, and hence the amount in the bloodstream may be much lower than the amount formulated into the tablet (i.e., it has low bioavailability); furthermore, liver damage is an unfortunate side effect of many soluble tableted drugs. The injection mode of delivery can be used to deliver any size of drug molecule and is versatile in this regard, but it suffers from the obvious disadvantage of being invasive and painful, and the less obvious disadvantage of shortness of duration (for drugs with short half-lives). To overcome some of these limitations, other modes of delivery of drugs into the body were investigated, beginning in the early 1970s. Transdermal (through the intact skin), transmucosal (through the intact mucosa of the mouth, intestine, rectum, vagina, or nose), transocular (through the eye), transalveolar (inhalation, through lung tissue), implantable (subcutaneous and deeper implants, delivery into surrounding tissue), and injectable (IM or subcutaneous) modes of delivery have all been explored extensively over the last 25 years, with varying degrees of commercial and therapeutic success. Of the above modes, the transdermal, transmucosal (specifically intestinal), transocular, injectables and the subcutaneous implant have found varying degrees of commercial acceptance. Of the rest, the inhalation route appears promising for a limited class of agents and at least three companies have products in advanced clinical trials. In the next 5 years, this route of administration is very likely to become acceptable to patients and hence commercially successful.

Currently, two other modes of injectable drug delivery are receiving increased attention. One focuses on the use of nanoparticles for delivering DNA or genes to cells for transfection. These particles have the unique ability to be taken up by targeted cells via various transcellular entry mechanisms. Another mode is needleless (and hence painless) injectables, which are being investigated by at least two companies. These approaches are in feasibility or early clinical trials.

The common theme underlying these delivery modes is increased therapeutic efficiency as well as increased patient compliance. The common key ingredient of all these technologies is polymeric material. In this chapter we focus on the demands made on the polymer material, which is often the component that controls drug delivery.

A. Drug Delivery Technologies

The main focus of this chapter will be four delivery modes: oral controlled release, transdermal, implantable, and particulate drug delivery. As mentioned above, all four modes have found commercial acceptance to varying degrees. The thrust of this chapter will be on the polymeric component and the requirements that each mode of delivery places on the polymer component. As can be imagined, the polymeric component must not only satisfy the design criteria for each mode of delivery, but also its toxicological and manufacturing requirements. Innovations in polymers drive improvements in these delivery technologies; therefore, each section will highlight the need for polymer improvements.

Regardless of the delivery mode, the polymer in each instance is required to perform a set of functions. To understand these functions, it is instructive to review the features and some of the shortcomings of the most popular forms of drug delivery, i.e., oral tablets and intravenous injections. In broad terms, these are summarized below as follows:

1. Tablets

1. All drugs enter the main circulation via the liver; a portion of the delivered drug is metabolized. In addition, for certain drugs, liver toxicity is an issue.
2. Drugs are typically absorbed in the stomach and in the small intestine (SI), where pH effects can influence extent of delivery.
3. For drugs with short half-lives, duration of action is limited to the maximum transit time through the stomach and SI, approximately 6 h.
4. The delivery profile typically has "peaks" and "valleys," i.e., fast onset followed by rapid decay. Constancy of drug levels in blood is rarely achieved.
5. There is a low level of patient compliance, i.e., patients forget to take the required dose at the correct time.

2. Intravenous Delivery

1. There is no metabolism by the liver.
2. Duration of action of a drug is determined solely by clearance rates for the drug; no control is possible (except for infusion control).
3. Macromolecules can be delivered.
4. The method is invasive and often painful, and therefore is not suitable for chronic indications.

Thus, alternative drug delivery modalities are needed to address the above shortcomings. The most important shortcomings are the duration of action and its control, by which is meant not only extended release of drug into the bloodstream, but also controlled release, i.e., achieving the desired plasma profile for the drug. In addition, the alternative modality must be acceptable to the patient (noninvasive) and must increase the level of patient compliance. There are also pharmacoeconomics and quality-of-life issues to be addressed.

Therefore, what the polymer is required to do, in these alternative drug delivery approaches, is to extend and control the release of the drug into the bloodstream via the various portals of entry (skin, oral mucosa, etc.). This is true of all modalities, except those where external fields are used to modulate drug delivery, such as iontophoresis (covered elsewhere in this book) and sonophoresis. The primary role of the polymer is diffusional control of active agents, and the secondary role is disintegration or dissolution control of the dosage form employed.

For reasons of editorial space, we will not be able to cover extensively the fields of buccal, rectal, or vaginal drug delivery, each of which is an active area of research. References to some of these concepts will be made in Section V.

B. Commercialized Technologies

As mentioned above, the transdermal delivery mode (commonly referred to as "patches") and controlled release orals are perhaps the most successful alternative delivery modes. Because of their similarity to bandages, transdermals found easy acceptance with patients. The duration of action of the first patch introduced (Transderm-Scop® developed by ALZA Corporation for Novartis Co. in 1981) was 72 h, easily surpassing the capability of existing tablets (Dramamine®) to provide continuous relief from sea or air sickness. The next type of transdermal introduced was for nitroglycerin delivery, and it also found immediate acceptance. Several companies introduced nitroglycerin transdermals, examples being Transderm-Nitro®, Nitro-Dur®. The duration of action was 24 h. With the introduction of Estraderm® by the then Ciba-Geigy Corporation, 3.5 days of delivery was achieved. Since then, we have seen the introduction of 7-day systems (Catapres TTS® for clonidine delivery, Climara® and FemPatch® for estradiol delivery). The transdermal market witnessed a surge in the early 1990s when the first nicotine patches were introduced for smoking cessation. Since then, the overall market has climbed to over $1 billion per annum for this mode of delivery.

Controlled release orals enjoy a large share of the drug delivery marketplace as well. Extended release dosage forms were introduced fairly early, but since these dosage forms do not strictly controlled drug delivery, they will not be discussed here (with the exception of dissolution-controlled delivery, Section II.A). The earliest from of controlled release oral dosage form was the osmotic tablet, developed by ALZA Corporation, for controlled delivery of phenylpropanolamine. This early product has been succeeded by several ethical pharmaceutical products, the most successful introduction being that of Procardia XL® by Pfizer: this product delivers a calcium channel blocker (CCB), nifedepine, in a controlled manner for 24 h using ALZA's proprietary osmotic tablet technology. To date, this technology is the most successful oral controlled release technology with about $2 billion of the total $6.2 billion in annual revenues for oral controlled release (CR) products. Other commercialized oral delivery technologies include R.P. Scherer's Zydis® (rapid-dissolve) and Elan Corporation's SODAS®, PRODAS®, and IPDAS® technologies. Of these, Zydis is not, strictly speaking, a controlled release technology, and it should be treated in the same manner as extended release branches of non-CR drug delivery technology. By our estimate, the CR share of the oral drug delivery market is about $3.5 billion—still much larger than the closest competing technology, transdermal delivery.

The other commercialized technology is implants. This delivery mode had about $1 billion in sales in 1996, largely from Norplant® (contraception), Atrisorb® and Atridox® from Atrix (dental implants for caries). Polymers play a large role in this technology as well, and we will explore this in detail in Section IV.

C. Technologies in Development

There are some CR technologies in various stages of development that have yet to see the marketplace. Noteworthy among these are controlled release via the alveoli (inhalation CR), controlled release via buccal tissue (buccal CR), and controlled release using microparticles or nanoparticles (particulate CR). The last named could have any of several modes of entry into the body. The most common mode of delivery for microparticles is as injectables (where the product Lupron Depot® is a commercial success), the nasal mucosa and the gastrointestinal (GI) tract being the other two routes. While discounting extended duration nasal sprays for congestion as being an extended rather than a controlled release system, it must be said that truly controlled release products in this category are still in the research or early clinical phase. Inhalation CR is now being pursued by three or four major companies, with Inhale Therapeutic Systems and Aradigm Corporation in the lead with products in phase II or phase III clinicals, and the Dura Corporation concentrating on delivery to the upper lung (local delivery). Whether the inhalation products being developed are strictly controlled release products is debatable; however, their potential for displacing injections as a route for administering important new therapeutic entities (proteins and peptides) is beyond any debate. In any event, the role of polymers in the delivery of inhalation products is clearly peripheral rather than central, and therefore these products will not be discussed. While polymers do play a central role in buccal controlled release products, products are still in pre-clinical or phase I, with the 3M Company finding it relatively difficult to market its proprietary buccal platforms (as of 1998, no partner deals have been announced for its CyDot® transmucosal delivery (TMD) technology). Theratech (now part of Watson Pharmaceuticals) is the other major player in this arena, and has announced a *peptide* development agreement with Eli Lilly for an undisclosed peptide. Therefore, in Section V, we will concentrate on particulate drug delivery, since polymers do play a central role in this technology, and products have either been commercialized or are likely to be commercialized soon.

D. Synthetic vs. Natural Polymers

Natural polymers can be defined for our purposes as polymers derived from natural sources, such as cellulose. In the broadest sense, sources of such polymers may include animals (bovine collagen, chitosan) and plants (cellulose); recently, polymers that are identical to or similar to those occurring in the human body have also received closer attention. Examples are poly(lactic acid), poly(glycolic acid), and hyaluronic acid. The naturally occurring type of polymer continues to be expensive and therefore is indicated for use only when stringent biocompatibility is required, such as in long-term implants. Animal-derived polymers have found limited use in drug delivery systems, although they have been used extensively in applications such as wound healing. Plant-derived polymers have been used extensively in drug delivery systems; hydroxy derivatives have in particular, being found to be benign for oral delivery. In general, synthetic polymers have found far wider application in drug delivery systems, for reasons that will be made clearer in the following sections.

E. Some General Toxicological Considerations

The potential adverse effects of polymers must be evaluated prior to testing a drug delivery system in humans. Potential adverse effects may result from contact with the polymer or from leachables such as residual monomers, reactive agents, or processing additives. The effects of polymers or extracts will be dependent on unique chemical characteristics and the amount (or dose) of polymer/extract administered. There should be an evaluation of whether the polymer is in direct or indirect contact with the drug-containing component of the system or with tissues of the patient. These evaluations will assist in the determination of the types of safety assessments that may be required during the various stages of the development process. To assist in the selection of materials, a review of the manufacturer's and published scientific literature should be conducted to gather clinical and nonclinical safety information. If necessary, in vivo and in vitro tests are used to evaluate the biocompatibility of the polymer and/or extract and of the drug delivery system, ensuring the safety of the system. In vitro studies should be conducted prior to initiating in vivo studies. Cytotoxicity tests are simple, rapid in vitro procedures that can provide predictive information on in vivo biocompatibility of polymeric materials (1). In vivo tests can then be conducted on the polymer and the drug delivery system.

II. ORAL DRUG DELIVERY SYSTEMS

Among all routes of administration, the oral route has been most popular and successful. This is, in part, because of the inherent simplicity of both the oral route and oral delivery systems. On the other hand, the oral route is constrained by short and variable GI transit time, first-pass metabolism, limited absorption in the lower part of the GI tract, and the size of the system.

A. Designs

Oral controlled delivery systems can be broadly divided into following categories, based on their mechanism of drug release:

1. Dissolution-controlled release
   a. Encapsulation dissolution control
   b. Matrix dissolution control
2. Diffusion-controlled release
   a. Reservoir devices
   b. Matrix devices
3. Ion exchange resins
4. Osmotic controlled release
5. Gastroretentive systems

1. Dissolution-controlled release

Dissolution-controlled release can be obtained by slowing the dissolution rate of a drug in the GI medium, incorporating the drug in an insoluble polymer, and coating drug particles or granules with polymeric materials of varying thickness. The rate-limiting step for dissolution of a drug is the diffusion across an aqueous boundary layer. The solubility of the drug provides the source of energy for drug release, which is countered by the stagnant-fluid diffusional boundary layer (2). The rate of dissolution (dm/dt) can be approximated by Eq. 1.

$$\frac{dm}{dt} = \frac{ADS}{h} \tag{1}$$

In Eq. 1, S is the aqueous solubility of the drug, A is the surface area of the dissolving particle or tablet, D is the diffusivity of the drug, and h is the thickness of the boundary layer.

Some examples of drugs with limited dissolution rate include digoxin, griseofulvin, salicylamide (3), and nifedipine (Adalat Retard tablet) (2). Unfortunately, this approach does not allow for a constant release rate because the surface area (A) changes with time. Also, the solubility (S) of the drugs, which are weak acids or bases, is affected by the variable pH of the GI tract.

Drug delivery using rate of dissolution as a controlled release mechanism can be achieved by *encapsulation* of a drug–polymer matrix with a relatively insoluble polymeric membrane. The coated beads can be compressed into tablets or capsulated, as was done with the Spansule® products (4). Since the time required for the membrane coat to dissolve is a function of membrane thickness, granules with varying thicknesses can be employed to achieve sustained release of the drug. Examples of drugs delivered in this manner include antispasmodic–sedative combinations (5), phenothiazines (6,7), and anticholinesterase agents (8).

One of the most common approaches used to achieve sustained release is to incorporate a drug in a hydrophobic matrix such as wax, polyethylene, polypropylene, and ethylcellulose; or a hydrophilic matrix such as hydroxypropylcellulose, hydroxypropylmethylcellulose, methylcellulose, and sodium carboxymethylcellulose. The rate of drug availability is controlled by the rate of penetration of the dissolution fluid into the matrix. It depends on the porosity of the compressed structure. In the case of a water-soluble drug in a hydrophobic matrix, the rate of drug availability.

2. Diffusion-Controlled Release

Diffusion of a drug molecule through a polymeric membrane forms the basis of these controlled drug delivery systems. Similar to the dissolution-controlled systems, the diffusion-controlled devices are manufactured either by encapsulating the drug particle in a polymeric membrane or by dispersing the drug in a polymeric matrix. Unlike the dissolution-controlled systems, the drug is made available as a result of partitioning through the polymer. In the case of a reservoir type diffusion-controlled device (9), the rate of drug released (dm/dt) can be calculated using Eq. 2.

$$\frac{dm}{dt} = ADK\frac{\Delta C}{\ell} \qquad (2)$$

In Eq. 2, A is the area, D is the diffusion coefficient, K is the partition coefficient of the drug between the drug core and the membrane, ℓ is the diffusional pathlength, and ΔC is the concentration difference across the membrane. In order to achieve a constant release rate, all of the terms on the right side of Eq. 2 must be held constant. It is very common for diffusion-controlled devices to exhibit a non-zero-order release rate due to an increase in diffusional resistance and a decrease in effective diffusion area as the release proceeds.

Another configuration of diffusion-controlled systems includes matrix devices, which are very common because of ease of fabrication. Diffusion control involves dispersion of drug in either a water-insoluble or a hydrophilic polymer (10–13). For instance, bupropion hydrochloride (Zyban®, Glaxo Wellcome) is formulated using carnuba wax and hydroxypropylmethylcellulose (13). The release rate is dependent on the rate of drug diffusion through the matrix but not on the rate of solid dissolution. Equation 3 describes the amount of drug released from the systems as derived by Higuchi (14):

$$Q = \left[\frac{D\epsilon}{\tau}(2C - \epsilon S)St\right]^{1/2} \qquad (3)$$

In Eq. 3, Q is the amount of drug released per unit surface area, D is the diffusion coefficient of the drug in the release media, ϵ is the porosity, τ is the tortuosity of the matrix, S is the solubility of the drug in the release media, and C is the concentration of the drug in the tablet.

3. Osmotically Controlled Release

In the early 1970s, Theeuwes et al. (15) developed an elementary osmotic pump (EOP) to achieve controlled drug delivery. The delivery of the drug from the system is controlled by solvent influx across a semipermeable membrane, which in turn carries the drug outside through a laser-drilled orifice. The osmotic and hydrostatic pressure differences on either side of the semipermeable membrane govern fluid transport into the system. Therefore, the rate of drug

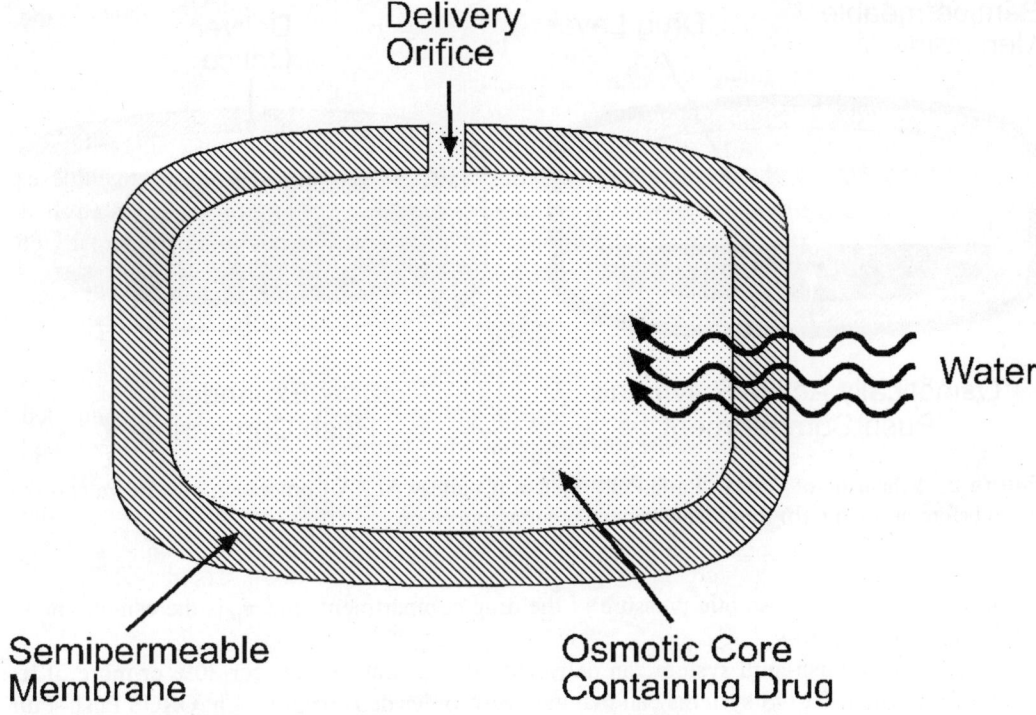

Figure 1 Schematic of elementary osmotic pump (EOP). (Courtesy ALZA Corporation.)

delivered from the system is dependent on the osmotic pressure of the formulation (π_s) as shown in Eq. (4). A schematic of an elementary pump is shown in Fig. 1 (16,17).

$$\frac{dm}{dt} = \frac{A}{h}k\pi_s S \qquad (4)$$

where A is the membrane area, k is the membrane permeability, and h is the membrane thickness.

More recently, ALZA Corporation has developed several other controlled release technology platforms based on the original concept of osmosis across a semipermeable membrane. OROS Push-Pull technology has proven to be very useful for delivering compounds of very high or very low solubility such as oxybutynin chloride and nifedipine (18), respectively. OROS Push-Pull technology is capable of zero-order drug delivery for 24 h. As shown in Fig. 2, the system is made of two compartments that are compressed into a bilayer core. The top layer contains the drug and the lower layer contains an osmotic polymeric driving agent. The bilayer tablet is coated with a semipermeable membrane that is drilled on the drug side to allow delivery of the drug formulation through an orifice. During operation, OROS systems imbibe water across the membrane. The push layer expands and drives the drug out of the system in the form of a solution or suspension through the orifice. The release rate of the drug from a push–pull system can be estimated by Eq. 5:

$$\frac{dm}{dt} = \frac{k}{h}\left[A_p(\pi_p - \pi_d) + A\pi_d\right]FC_0 \qquad (5)$$

Where F is the initial drug fraction in the drug compartment, C_0 is the solid concentration of the suspension dispensed from the system, A_p is the area of the push layer, A is the total area

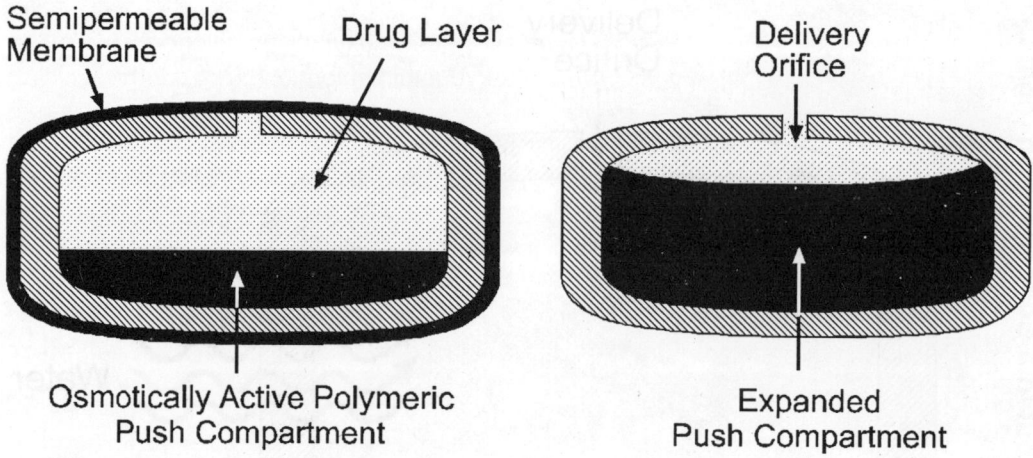

Figure 2 Schematic of OROS "Push–Pull" System (Courtesy ALZA Corporation.) (a) Represents the pump before operation. (b) Represents the pump during operation.

of the system, π_d is the osmotic pressure of the drug compartment, and π_p is the osmotic pressure of the push layer.

Typically, a push–pull system can deliver drug at a constant rate for 80% or more of its theoretical content. OROS systems can maintain zero-order delivery for 24 h. OROS Push–Pull technology has been applied to several commercial products, including oxybutynin chloride (Ditropan XL®), nifedipine (Procardia XL®), and isradipine (Dynacirc CR®). A typical release-rate profile for Ditropan XL® developed by Alza Corporation demonstrates a constant zero-order drug delivery (Fig. 3). The OROS technology has also been customized to suit the needs of a particular drug therapy. A classic example of such an application is OROS verapamil HCl (Covera HS®) for the treatment of hypertension and angina pectoris. The once-a-day system is programmed to provide a delayed onset of drug release after 4–5 h administration. The peak concentration (C_{max}) coincides with early morning hours (when the probability of a stroke is maximum), followed by a constant zero-order delivery.

4. Ion Exchange Resins

The idea of using ion exchange resins for controlled drug delivery was adapted from analytical and protein chemistry. Resins are water-insoluble materials containing anionic groups such as amino or quaternary ammonium groups, cationic groups such as carboxylic groups, or sulfonic groups in repeating positions on the resin chain. A drug–resin complex is formed by prolonged exposure of drug to the resin.

Theoretically, this controlled delivery approach is relatively immune to the conditions of the GI tract because an ionic environment is required to displace the drug from the resin. Biphetamine®, a capsule containing equal quantities of amphetamine and dextroamphetamine complexed to a sulfonic acid cation exchange resin, has been used as an antiobesity drug and for behavior control in children (20). Nicorette® is a widely used product based on ion exchange technology as an adjunct to smoking cessation programs. It contains nicotine absorbed to a carboxylic acid ion exchange resin (nicotine polacrilex) in a flavored chewing gum (21). Delsym® (dextromethorphan, Pennwalt), a 12-h cough medication taken as a liquid suspension, is another example of this type of dosage form (22). Further improvement of the ion exchange type of delivery system is illustrated by the development of the Pennkinetic® system (Fig. 4).

An Overview of Controlled Release Systems

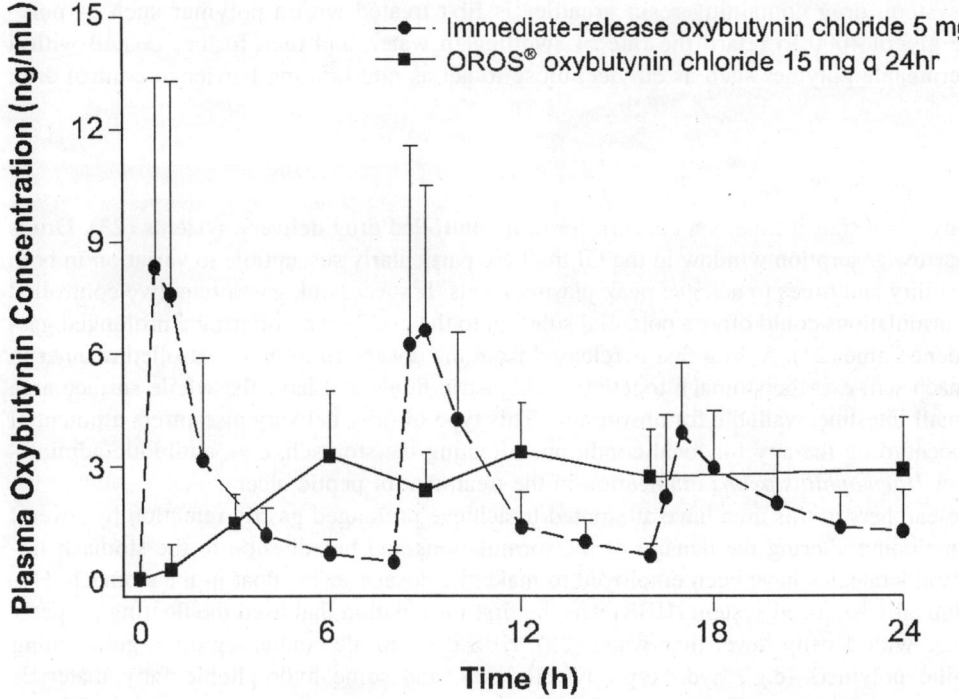

Figure 3 Comparison of mean plasma concentration of immediate release oxybutynin chloride (5 mg, administered every 8 h) with once-a-day OROS oxybutynin chloride (15 mg, administered once daily) after 1 day of administration.

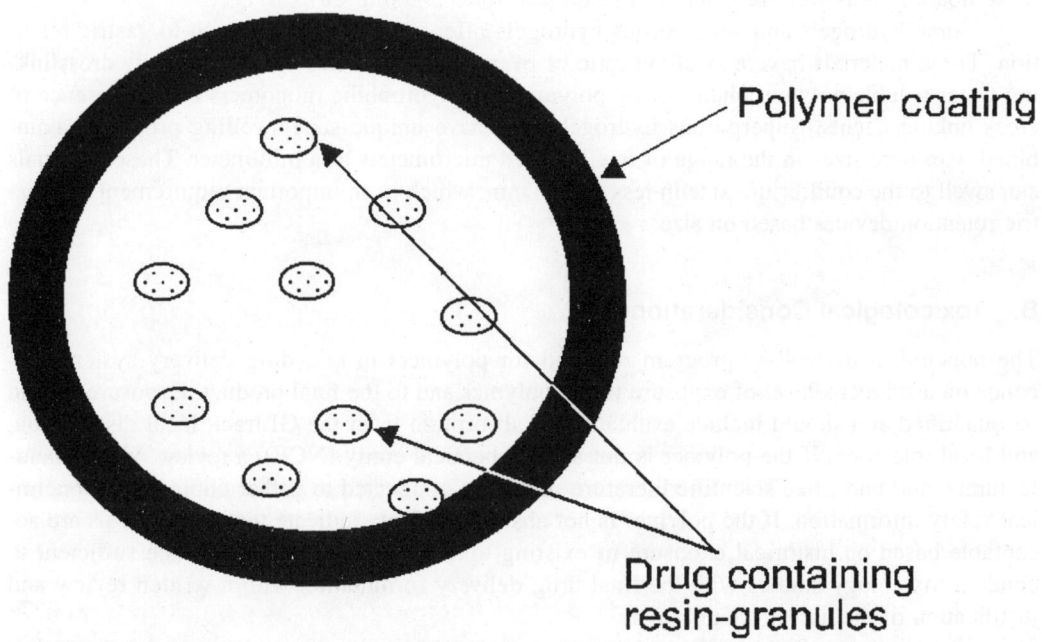

Figure 4 Polymer-coated drug-resin design.

In this system, drug containing resin granules is first treated with a polymer such as polyethylene glycol 4000 to retard the rate of swelling in water, and then further coated with a water-permeable polymer such as ethylcellulose to act as rate-limiting barrier to control drug release.

5. Gastroretentive Systems

Variability in GI transit time is a concern for oral controlled drug delivery systems (23). Drugs with a narrow absorption window in the GI tract are particularly susceptible to variation in both bioavailability and times to achieve peak plasma levels. If successful, gastroretentive controlled release formulations could offer a potential solution to the problem by offering a prolonged gastric residence time (24). A drug that is released from the dosage form in a controlled manner in the stomach will exit the stomach together with gastric fluids and have the whole surface area of the small intestine available for absorption. This type of drug delivery also offers a potential for enhanced drug therapy for local conditions affecting the stomach, e.g., antibiotic administration for *Haemophilus pylori* eradication in the treatment of peptic ulcer.

Researchers in this area have attempted to achieve prolonged gastric retention by several means, including altering the density of the formulations and bioadhesion to the stomach lining. Several strategies have been employed to make the dosage forms float in the stomach. Hydrodynamically balanced system (HBS) was the first formulation that used the floating property of a device with density lower than water (25). HBS is a capsule containing drug, gel-forming hydrophilic polymers (e.g., hydroxypropylcellulose), and some hydrophobic fatty materials (e.g., stearates) (26). In a different approach for gastric retention, ion exchange resin beads are loaded with bicarbonate, which, on contact with media containing hydrochloric acid, release carbon dioxide, causing the resin to float (27). Extension of the floating time is achieved by coating the bicarbonate-coated beads with a semipermeable membrane. Recently, a multiple-unit floating dosage form has been prepared from freeze-dried calcium alginate. In fed subjects, these floating units were retained in the stomach for 5.5–9.0 h (28).

Some hydrogels and superporous hydrogels offer a promising approach to gastric retention. These materials have a swelling ratio of over 1000 (23). They can be made by crosslinking water-soluble polymer chains or by polymerizing hydrophilic monomers in the presence of cross-linking agents. Superporous hydrogels (29) have unique superswelling properties combined with pore sizes in the range of few hundred micrometers to a millimeter. These materials can swell to the equilibrium size in less than 1 min, which is an important requirement for gastric retention devices based on size.

B. Toxicological Considerations

The nonclinical toxicology program required for polymers in oral drug delivery systems depends on a subject's level of exposure to the polymer and to the final product. Exposure should be quantified and should include evaluation of absorption from the GI tract, local distribution, and local tolerance. If the polymer is not a new chemical entity (NCE), a review of the manufacturers' and published scientific literature should be conducted to gather clinical and nonclinical safety information. If the polymer is not absorbed or data indicate that blood levels are acceptable based on historical exposure or existing toxicology data, then it may be sufficient to conduct toxicology studies with the final drug delivery formulation with a written review and justification of the use of the polymer.

If the polymer is an NCE, a series of in vitro and in vivo (animal) genotoxicity studies should be conducted. These mutagenicity and clastogenicity studies determine if the polymer harms the cell's DNA. If the assays reveal a genotoxic result in multiple assays, development of the polymer should be halted. If no genotoxic activity is present, the next step is to quantify exposure. Is the polymer absorbed from the GI tract? If the polymer is absorbed, a full toxicology program consisting of acute, chronic, reproduction, and carcinogenicity testing is likely to be required. If the polymer is not absorbed, studies up to 6 months long may be required with an evaluation of any proliferative changes. If proliferative changes occur, a carcinogenicity study might be indicated. Whether the polymer is absorbed or not, additional toxicology studies need to be conducted with the final formulation at multiple doses.

C. Functions of Polymers in Oral Controlled Release

For the most part, oral controlled release systems utilize principles such as diffusion, dissolution, and permeation for achieving a constant rate of drug delivery. Polymers are uniquely suited as materials of construction for oral delivery systems. They offer a wide range of properties such as diffusivity, permeability, and solubility that are important to achieving controlled delivery. They can be processed relatively easily into tablets and membranes by a variety of methods. Active ingredients and property modifiers can be incorporated either by physical or chemical means. In reservoir-type devices, polymers are ideal materials to form a membrane around the tablet or granule. These membranes are strong enough to maintain their integrity during normal handling and operation of these systems. Drugs can be dispersed or dissolved into polymers to manufacture matrix-type oral dosage forms. Ion exchange resins are types of polymers to which the drug substances are attached chemically. In general, polymers have little or no toxicity. Superporous hydrogel systems offer excellent ability to swell at a very fast rate, making them potential candidates for gastroretentive devices.

1. Polymer Properties That Affect the Release of Active Substances

A good understanding of polymer properties such as diffusion, solubility, and structural considerations is important in the selection of materials to be used as system components to regulate the fluxes of active ingredients. This section reviews some of these important properties affecting drug permeation.

The flux of a species migrating through a polymeric film is given by Eq. 6:

$$\text{Flux} = \frac{\text{area}}{\text{length}} \times (\text{permeability}) \times (\text{concentration difference}) \qquad (6)$$

Area is the surface through which a species is diffusing, and length is the film thickness. Permeability is given by the product of partition coefficient and diffusivity (30).

a. Diffusivity. Diffusivity is the component of permeability that accounts for the geometrical constraints encountered by the diffusing species in weaving across the polymeric film. Consequently, diffusivity increases as the free volume of the polymer increases relative to the dimensions of the diffusing species. Jacobs and Mason (31) have listed various factors that affect the diffusivity of a molecule in a polymeric medium as shown below:

Increases in factor	Effect on diffusivity
Interchain forces	−
Segmental mobility	+
Permeant molecular weight	−
Polymer crystallinity	−
Plasticizer	+
Copolymerization	+

Increases in factor	Effect on diffusivity
Temperature	+
Glass transition	−

b. Solubility Parameter. The active ingredient is either suspended or dissolved in a polymeric matrix in monolithic controlled release systems. Polymers are dissolved in a solvent and coated onto tablets and granules. In reservoir-type systems, for both monolithic and reservoir-type systems, the addition of a second component, such as a drug or solvent, to a polymer can change the strength of polymer intermolecular forces and therefore the physical properties of the polymer. The strength of the intermolecular forces of a polymer is measured by its cohesive energy density (CED). The solubility parameter of a polymer also describes intermolecular forces. The relationship between the solubility parameter, δ, and CED is shown in Eq. 7:

$$\delta = (CED)^{0.5} \tag{7}$$

The solubility parameters for many polymers are documented elsewhere (32). The choice of an ideal solvent to dissolve a polymer for any further processing can be made by comparing the solubility parameters of both polymer and solvent. For example, solvents and polymers with similar solubility parameters will most likely be compatible and soluble in each other. A polymer will precipitate from a solvent with a significantly different solubility parameter.

c. Structural Considerations. The structure of the polymer used in the drug delivery system is a very important parameter determining the mechanism of drug release. The diffusivity of a drug molecule dispersed in a hydrophobic polymer is dependent on the porous structure of the polymer (33,34). The solute diffuses through the solvent-filled pores. As the porosity increases, the release rate of the drug increases. For instance, in macroporous polymers, it is necessary to correct the diffusion coefficient for the porosity, tortuosity, and partition coefficient. For microporous polymers, additional steric hindrance and frictional resistance of the pores also need to be included. For nonporous polymeric networks, both solute molecule and structure of the polymeric network become important in determining the diffusion coefficient. The polymer structure–related factors affecting diffusivity include the degree of crystallinity, the size of the crystallites, the degree of swelling, the molecular weight between crosslinks, and the state of the polymer (whether glassy or rubbery) (35).

Many controlled release tablets and granules utilize hydrophilic polymers for retarding drug release. The mechanism of drug release is dependent on the swelling and dissolution process. An example of such a release mechanism could be demonstrated using tablets manufactured by dispersing drug in hydroxypropyl and hydroxymethylcellulose matrix. In this case, the early part of the release process is marked by swelling due to conversion of the polymer from a glassy to a rubbery state due to water penetration. Subsequently, when the water concentration at the polymer surface exceeds a critical concentration of macromolecular disentanglement, the true dissolution process occurs. Diffusivity through a swollen polymer is much higher than through nonswollen polymers and in fact approach diffusion coefficients in solution.

A detailed listing of polymers used in controlled release oral dosage forms is given in Table 1.

D. Fabrication Techniques

Oral controlled release forms most commonly involve either dispersing the drug into a polymeric matrix, or encapsulating the drug containing core or granules with a rate-controlling membrane. This section describes the most common unit operations involved in the manufacture of oral controlled release products.

Table 1 Polymers Used in Oral Controlled Release Technologies

Method of achieving controlled release	Polymer used	Examples of dosage forms
Matrix or Embedding		
(a) Hydrophillic Carriers	Methyl Cellulose Sodium Carboxymethylcellulose [38] Carboxymethylcellulose Hydroxypropylmethylcellulose [36,37] Hydroxylethylcellulose Methacrylate Hydrogels [39] Polyethylene Glycols Galactose Mannate Sodium Alginate Polyacrylic acid	Multilayer tablets with slow releasing cores Compression-coated tablets
(b) Hydrophobic Carriers		
(i) Soluble Carrier (digestible base)	Glycerides Waxes Fatty Alcohols Fatty Acids	
(ii) Insoluble Carrier (nondigestible base)	Polyethylene Polyvinyl chloride Polyvinyl acetate Waxes [40] Calcium Sulfate	Matrix tablets
Reservoir Type		
(a) Coating with insoluble membrane	Ethyl Cellulose [36, 37]	Granules, pellets, tablets
Osmotic Systems	Vapor permeable walls [41] - Tenite 808A polyethylene - Kynar 460 polyvinylidene fluoride Hydroxypropyl methyl cellulose Hydropropyl cellulose Sodium carboxymethyl cellulose Ethyl cellulose	Vapor permeable capsules Vapor permeable tablets Single and bilayer tablets
Ion-exchange Resins	Dowex® 50, 1, 2 [19] Amberlite® IR 120, 400, 4B [19] Amberlite® IRC 50 [19] With polystyrene-based polymeric backbone	Controlled release capsules Chewable tablets Chewable gums Liquid suspension
Gastric Retention Systems	Hydroxypropyl methylcellulose [24] Agar, Carrageenans, Alginic acid [24] Oils, porous calcium silicate [24] Superporous hydrogels [29] Ion-exchange resin beads coated with bicarbonate [27,29] Ethyl cellulose for coatings	Compressed tablets Gelatin Capsules

1. Wet Granulation

Drug is uniformly dispersed into a polymeric matrix using traditional high-shear granulation (HSG) or fluidized-bed granulation (FBG) techniques. In an HSG technique, an aqueous or a hydroalcoholic binder solution, such as 5% polyvinylpyrrolidone in water, is sprayed onto a polymeric powder bed, such as 85% hydroxypropylmethylcellulose containing the drug. The powder bed is subjected to a very high shear rate to obtain granules incorporating a uniform mixture of drug, binder, and the polymeric excipient. The wet granules could be dried either in a traditional tray dryer, fluidized-bed dryer, or microwave dryer. In an FBG technique, a powder bed consisting of drug, polymer, and other excipients is fluidized in an expansion chamber. The binder solution is sprayed through a nozzle from the top or bottom of the bed depending on the equipment design. The droplet size and bed humidity are the two most important process parameters, which control the granule size and other mechanical properties. The agglomerated mixture can be dried in the same equipment.

2. Spray Drying

Spray drying has been used to produce microencapsulated and matrix formulations of several drug substances including theophylline, acetaminophen, and sulfaethylthiazole. It involves three basic steps. First, a liquid feed is atomized into fine droplets. Second, these fine droplets are mixed with heated gas stream, allowing the liquid to evaporate and leave dried solids. Finally, the dried powder is separated from the gas stream and collected. The final product usually has the same size and shape as the atomized droplet.

3. Spray Congealing

This process consists of suspending the drug particles in a low-melting polymer or wax and pumping the resultant slurry through an atomizer into a spray dryer in which cold air is circulated. The slurry droplets congeal on coming in contact with the air and are collected in the same manner as the spray-dried product. The spray congealing process requires a much higher ratio of coating agent to active material than does spray drying because only the molten coating agent constitutes the liquid phase.

Encapsulation of drug-containing cores and granules in the manufacture of reservoir-type oral controlled released product can be accomplished by the following coating methods:

4. Pan Coating

Pan coaters are one of the earliest types of equipment to be used for encapsulating a drug-containing tablet core. Pan coating involves spraying an atomized coating solution through nozzles on a moving bed of tablets. The distribution of the coating is accomplished by movement of the tablets perpendicular to the application of the coating solution. Drying of the coating solution from the tablet bed is accomplished by directing heated airflow from the front to the back of the partially or fully perforated pan. The popular models include the Hi-Coater from Vector Corporation and the Glatt coater from Glatt Air Techniques Inc.

5. Air Suspension Coating

Granules and pellets are often coated in an air suspension process. Sometimes this technology is also used to apply release-controlling membranes around tablets. Fluidization of tablets or granules is achieved in a columnar chamber with upward flow of drying air. The airflow is controlled so that more air enters the center of the column, causing the tablets to rise in the center. The movement of the tablets is upward toward the center of the chamber. They then fall toward the chamber wall and move downward to reenter the air stream at the bottom of the chamber. Because tablets and granules hit against the chamber wall during coating, friable tablets are prone to chipping. The drying efficiency of the air suspension coaters is very good. Constant motion of the tablets and granules in the fluidized bed, along with efficient drying, prevents any twinning of tablets or particle agglomeration. Coating solution is applied continuously from a spray nozzle located either at the bottom of the chamber, as in the Wurster process, or atop the cascading tablet bed by nozzles located in the upper region of the chamber. Several models available on the market offer fully automated process capability. Coating uniformity is excellent.

6. Compression Coating

Rate-controlling polymer in the dry powder state can be compressed around the drug-containing core using a special tablet press. This process eliminates the use of any solvents from the manufacturing process. Most often the core tablets containing the drug are prepared prior to the compression coating step. During the compression coating operation, a lower layer of rate-controlling membrane is dosed at the bottom. The drug-containing core is guided to the center of the die followed by another layer of the polymer. Finally, the die contents are compressed under rolls to achieve a hard tablet encapsulated in a rate-controlling polymer. Geomatrix technology uses compression coating to lay a barrier coating of ethylcellulose on a hydrophilic core made of hydroxypropylmethylcellulose to achieve a near-zero-order release rate (36).

E. Future Research

Advances in the design of oral drug delivery systems can be realized by a better understanding of the biology of the GI tract and drug absorption process. So far polymers have contributed immensely to the development of technologies for delivering drug over extended periods. The present state of the art restricts the duration of delivery of oral CR forms to about 24 h. More research effort is needed to retain the dosage forms in the stomach to achieve prolonged as well as higher absorption from the upper GI tract. For instance, new polymers could be designed not only with an extremely rapid onset of swelling, but also with a higher extent of swelling, resulting in prolonged gastric retention. In addition, peptides and proteins are evolving as an important class of therapeutic agents in drug therapy, and absorption of these unstable substances from oral medications is challenging. Polymers could be designed to safely carry these moieties through the GI tract without presystemic clearance, resulting in substantially higher bioavailability.

III. TRANSDERMAL DRUG DELIVERY SYSTEMS

Transdermal systems are currently enjoying widespread consumer acceptance of both prescription and over-the-counter (OTC) products. To many users, the technology is an extension of the "bandage" concept, and therefore relatively noninvasive and easy to use. To a large extent, materials found acceptable for bandages were the starting points for transdermal delivery systems.

A. Designs

There are two predominant designs in transdermal systems: membrane-controlled systems and matrix systems. A brief discussion of the features of each, based mostly on a review article (42), is given below

1. Membrane-Controlled Systems

This type of design essentially consists of three major components: the drug reservoir (often a liquid-containing "form-fill-seal," or FFS, type), the rate-controlling membrane (RCM), and the adhesive. The drug permeates the membrane and the adhesive to reach the skin. Typically, the drug reservoir contains a solution of the drug and liquid excipients. One common excipient used is an enhancer, which also permeates the layers to the skin, where it exerts its enhancing effects by modulating the skin permeability in some fashion. (A variation of this design is the "multi-laminate" RCM design, whereby the drug reservoir is made of solid polymer, with drug dispersed/ dissolved in it; an example is Transderm-Scop.®) In the matrix-type design, the adhesive performs the roles of drug reservoir and adhesive, and to some extent, the role of the rate-controlling membrane as well. (See Fig. 5 for schematics of the two systems.)

The major material components of membrane-controlled systems are as follows:

1. The membrane
2. The adhesive
3. The backing, which is also the FFS material

2. Matrix Systems

In this design, the role of the drug reservoir is performed by the adhesive. The drug and excipients are formulated into the adhesive, typically into adhesive solution, and the solvent evaporated to yield the matrix film. The matrix-adhesive film is then laminated to a backing film. Thus, the major components in a matrix design are as follows:

1. The adhesive
2. The backing

The chief advantage of a matrix system is that the entire system can be made thin and elegant, as well as very comfortable to wear. In principle, it is much easier to make an extended wear system (>3 days) using a matrix design than using a membrane-controlled design, as the bulkiness of the FFS type of RCM systems is usually detrimental to comfortable wear. On the other hand, stability issues are more likely to occur in the case of matrix systems, as the drug

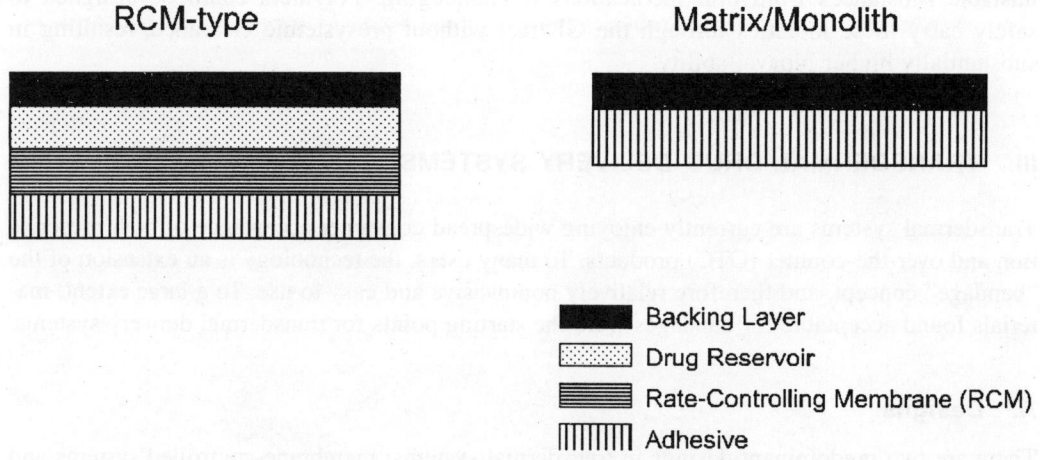

Figure 5 Schematic of membrane-controlled and matrix types of transdermal design.

and excipient may undergo phase changes (e.g., dissolved drug may crystallize or dispersed drug may agglomerate). Both of these causes of instability could adversely affect adhesive properties.

B. Toxicological Considerations

Polymers used in transdermal drug delivery systems may not penetrate the skin themselves, but there may be components of the polymer that migrate. The polymer and extracts should be biocompatible since they are in contact with components that do penetrate the skin. The tests listed in ISO/ANSI/AAMI Standard 10993, Biological Evaluation of Medical Devices are intended to provide testing strategies for medical devices. There are similar guidelines in the U.S. Pharmacopoeia 23 for plastics used as drug containers. These tests may also be used to test biocompatibility of polymers used in transdermal drug delivery systems. Extracts may also be tested for the potential to cause topical sensitization. Preparation of polymer extracts is defined by the guidelines, but the choice of conditions should come close to the conditions of manufacture of the drug delivery system. Extracts are evaluated in in vitro cytotoxicity tests and in in vivo irritation, intracutaneous injection, systemic injection, and implantation studies. A sample of the polymer may also be evaluated in these in vivo tests. The final transdermal drug delivery system must also be evaluated in standard nonclincal toxicology studies to evaluate the safety of the system. These studies should detect adverse effects of the system as well as any adverse effects of polymer extracts that are not detected in the previous tests. Study duration will depend on whether the active drug is an NCE and on its duration of use.

C. Delivery Profiles/Performance

The strength of the RCM-based design is constancy of drug delivery to the skin. In kinetic terms, the RCM design affords the possibility of zero-order release, i.e., the rate of drug delivery to the skin is constant with time. On the other hand, the matrix design can yield only a nonconstant rate of drug delivery to the skin. Typically, this rate decreases with time such that the amount delivered is proportional to the square root of time rather than to time. In either case, the likelihood of constancy of delivery of drug to the bloodstream is determined by the flux through skin relative to flux through the system alone. In limiting cases, the following is true:

> When drug flux through skin is very low (< approximately 10% of flux through device), the skin is termed rate controlling: in this instance, both types of designs can yield zero-order delivery to the bloodstream.
> When drug flux through skin is high (> approximately three times the rate through device), then only the RCM design can yield zero-order kinetics for drug delivery to the bloodstream.

When dealing with potent drugs or with drugs that have a narrow therapeutic window, the RCM design yields a greater margin of safety, but the level of safety is contingent on the level of control attained by the device as opposed to the skin. In addition, RCM systems also tend to demonstrate a lesser degree of patient-to-patient variability, for the same reasons outlined above. Matrix systems, on the other hand, are preferred for drugs that have very low skin flux, as they can achieve higher release rates. In addition, as mentioned above, matrix systems tend to be more appealing to the patient and may lead to greater acceptance.

Table 2 shows the commercial transdermal systems by type of design, and lists the materials used in each system.

Table 2 Family of Commercial Transdermal Systems

Product name	Innovator	Marketer	Active ingredient	Systems area(s)	Delivery rate(s)	Rated duration	Enhancer	Type
Alora®	TheraTech	P&G Pharm.*	17β-estradiol	18, 27, 36 cm²	0.05, 0.075, 0.1 mg/d	4 days	sorbitan monoleate	Adhesive matrix
Climara®	3M Pharm.	BerlexLabs	17β-estradiol	12.5 & 25 cm²	0.05 & 0.1 mg/d	7 days	fatty acid esters	Adhesive matrix
Deponit®	Lohman Pharma	Schwarz	Nitroglycerin	16 & 32 cm²	0.2 & 0.4 mg/h	12–14 hr	"a plasticizer" propylene glycol	Adhesive matrix
FemPatch®	Cygnus	ParkeDavis	17β-estradiol	30 cm²	0.025 mg/d	7 days	propylene glycol monolaurate	Adhesive matrix
Habitrol®	Novartis	Novartis	Nicotine	10, 20, 30 cm²	7, 14, 21 mg/d	24 hrs	none	Pad in adh. matrix
Minitran®	3M Pharm.	3M Pharm.	Nitroglycerin	20 cm²	0.6 mg/h	12–14 hr	fatty acid esters	Adhesive matrix
Nitrodur®	Key Pharm.	Key Pharm.	Nitroglycerin	10, 20, 30, 40 cm²	0.2,0.3,0.4,0.6,0.8 mg/h	12–14 hr	none	Adhesive matrix
Testoderm® with adhesive	Alza	Alza	Testosterone, USP	60 cm²	6 mg/d	24 hrs	none	Matrix, striped adh
Menorest®, Vivelle®	Noven	Ciba, RPR-Novo	17β-estradiol	11 & 29 cm²	4 Rates, 25–100 ug/d	3–4 days	oleic acid, propylene glycol	Adhesive matrix
Nicotrol®	Cygnus	McNeil	Nicotine	30 cm²	15 mg/16 h (1 day)	16 hr	none	Adhesive matrix
Androderm®	TheraTech	SmithKline Beecham	Testosterone, USP	37 & 44 cm²	2.5 & 5 mg/d	24 hrs	ethanol, glyceryl mono oleate, methyl laureate, glycerin	FFS***, peripheral adhesive
Prostep®	Elan	Elan	Nicotine	3.5 & 7 cm²	11 or 22 mg/d	24 hrs	none	Matrix, peripheral adhesive
Nitrodisc®	Searle	Searle	Nitroglycerin	8, 12, 16 cm²	0.2, 0.3, 0.4 mg/h	24 hrs	polyethylene glycol, isopropyl palmitate	Matrix, peripheral adhesive
Catapres TTS®	Alza	Boehringer Ingelheim	Clonidine	3.5, 7 & 10.5 cm²	0.1, 0.2, 0.3 mg/d	7 days	none	rate-control memb.
Duragesic®	Alza	Janssen	Fentanyl	10,20,30,40 cm²	25,50,75,100 ug/d	3 days	ethanol	rate-control memb.
Estraderm®	Alza	CibaGeneva SmithKline	17β-estradiol	10 & 20 cm²	0.05 & 0.1 mg/d	3 days	ethanol	rate-control memb.
Nicoderm®CQ	Alza	Beecham	Nicotine	7, 15 & 22 cm²	7, 14 & 21 mg/d	24 hrs	none	rate-control memb.
Transderm-Nitro®	Alza	CibaGeneva	Nitroglycerin	5,10,20, & 30 cm²	0., 0.2, 0.4 & 0.6 mg/h	12–14 hrs	none	rate-control memb.
Transderm Scop®	Alza	Novartis	Scopolamine	2.5 cm²	0.5 mg/3 d	3 days	none	rate-control memb.

*Proctor and Gamble Pharmaceutical; **RPR = Rhone-Poulenc Rohrer; ***FFS = Form-fill-seal.

An Overview of Controlled Release Systems

D. Polymer Requirements

For the sake of convenience, this discussion of materials used is divided in terms of the design type.

1. RCM-Based Systems

As mentioned above, the chief components of RCM a designs are the FFS material, the rate-controlling membrane itself, and the adhesive.

a. FFS materials. The requirements for the FFS material is that it should be as follows:

1. Thermoformable
2. Sealable to the membrane material
3. Occlusive (low moisture–vapor transmission rate; MVTR)
4. Impermeable to volatile excipients of the formulation
5. Nonabsorptive for the drug

Materials that meet these requirements include polyester (PET)/heat-seal layer laminates, or PET/metal/heat-seal layer laminates. Available trade names include Scotchpak® from 3M Company and Mediflex® from Bertek, Inc., in a range of thicknesses. These two vendors are also willing to custom-fabricate laminates. The PET layer confers the impermeability and low-MVTR attributes to the device backing, while the occlusivity is attained by the combination of material and thickness. Thermoformability is not a requirement when the drug formulation has high viscosity and can be contained relatively easily. However, when the drug formulation is predominantly liquid-like, the material must be capable of being formed (preferably by thermal means) into a cavity. An example of such material includes is polypropylene.

Examples of products that use the RCM design include Estraderm®, Transderm-Nitro®, and Testoderm TTS®; the first two are marketed by Novartis, while ALZA Corporation markets Testoderm TTS.

b. Membranes. The RCM is the critical component of the membrane design. It must satisfy the following criteria:

1. A diffusion coefficient for the drug under consideration that ranges from about 10^{-7} to 10^{-9}
2. Capable of being fabricated into a film of thickness from 1 to 5 mils
3. Low solubility for the drug and its excipients
4. Should be capable of being laminated to the FFS material on one side and the adhesive on the other
5. Should soften well above shipping temperatures
6. Modulus should be about 1000 to 1 MM Pa

Both homopolymer and copolymer films can be found that satisfy the above criteria. The 3M Company has developed the CoTran® series of membranes based on polyethylene and ethylene vinyl acetate (EVA, 9% vinyl acetate). The polyethylene films can be nonporous or microporous, whereas EVA is an extruded film. Also noteworthy are the Celgard® membranes from Hoechst-Celanese; these are also microporous films based on polyethylene and polypropylene. These are produced by a patented stretching process that introduces pores into the film. Celgard films are available with both hydrophobic and hydrophilic surfaces.

The copolymer EVA has long been the polymer of choice in this category. This is primarily because the vinyl acetate content can be varied to tune its permeability to meet the requirements of the drug under consideration. In general, the variables available for manipulation of the permeability of the material are the vinyl acetate content, thickness, crystallinity of the ethylene components, and domain structure of the fabricated film. The following table lists the various grades of EVA available and measured diffusion coefficients for selected drugs (43):

	9% EVA		18% EVA		40% EVA	
Percent EVA	K.I	$D \times 10^9$	K.I	$D \times 10^9$	K.I	$D \times 10^9$
19-nor-Progesterone	4.9	4	18	3	105	5
Testosterone	4.0	4			88	5
Estriol	0.0048	4	0.025	3		

K.I = normalized permeability coefficient, μg/cm.s.
D = coefficient of diffusion, cm^2/s.

Note that in the above examples, the diffusion coefficient remains unchanged for the different EVAs, whereas the permeability changes by factors of 10–25. This is explained by postulating that the diffusion coefficient is dependent on factors such as pore size, which in turn is determined by the amount of crystallinity in the material and how the crystallites are distributed (morphology). In this instance, as long as the average pore size is above a threshold value, the diffusion coefficient is unchanged in going from 9% to 40% EVA. The permeability, which is also dependent on the partition coefficient, is expected to change as the EVA content changes. This is borne out experimentally.

    c. *Adhesives.* In membrane-controlled systems, the adhesive must exhibit permeability for the drug and the enhancer that is defined by the delivery profile of the drug under consideration. At any time it is likely that the adhesive has measurable amounts of drug and enhancer dissolved in it to their solubility limits, as the typical process is one of partitioning followed by diffusion. If the solubility of either component is low, then the permeation process does not appreciably affect the adhesive. If it is substantial (>3% by weight), then the following effects may be anticipated: liquid excipients (including drug) will "plasticize" the adhesive to some degree; if the period of wear is long (>24 h), this could lead to unsightly residue and oozing on skin. The "oozing", in addition to being unsightly, also collects dirt and lint, and occasionally sticks to clothing. If the drug and excipients are solids, the adhesive may increase in cohesive strength and lose some of its adhesive characteristics, particularly tack. Thus, the optimum choice of adhesive for the RCM design depends on drug and excipient solubility.

    All of the commonly used adhesives are derived from the pressure-sensitive adhesive (PSA) industry. Used in such products as Post-It® notes, and also in automotive decals, office labels, and other applications, the same basic adhesives have been requalified for use in the transdermal field. Requalification typically involves animal and human toxicology testing, as well as incorporation of the material into a Drug Master File (DMF).

    Classes of PSAs available include:

1. Polyacrylate are copolymers of acrylates with vinyl acetate, alkyl acrylate, acrylic acid, or other functional monomers and are by far the most commonly used. Major suppliers include National Starch & Chemical Co., Morton-Thiokol, the Solutia division of Monsanto Chemical Co., and Adhesives Research. The 3M Company formulates its own acrylic adhesives for incorporation into 3M transdermal products (predominantly matrix-type constructions).
2. Silicones are also used in many transdermal systems, due primarily to their excellent adhesion characteristics and a perceived hypoallergenic nature. However, these are

made by two suppliers, Dow-Corning and NuSil Technology, and continue to be expensive.
3. Polyisobutylenes (PIBs), in mixtures with polybutene and tackifiers, are also heavily used. Suppliers, including Adhesives Research, Inc. ALZA Corporation, and Cygnus, Inc., have their own versions of PIB adhesives in some of their transdermal systems.
4. Natural rubber–and synthetic rubber–based adhesives are also available from National Starch Co. However, some of these suffer from complexity in their composition, while the natural rubber–based adhesives tend to be also somewhat more irritating than their counterparts.

2. Matrix Designs

The major components of this type of design are the backing material and the adhesive.

a. Backing Materials. The backing material must satisfy the following criteria:

1. Occlusive (low MVTR)
2. Impermeable to volatile excipients of the formulation
3. Nonabsorptive for the drug

Since the requirements are less stringent than those for FFS materials, a wider choice is available. Typically, polyesters, e.g., poly(ethylene terephthalate) (PET), polyolefins (HDPE or LDPE), multilayered films (Saranex from Dow Chemical), or elastomers can be used. In fact, it is claimed (44) that the elastomeric backings have more acceptable long-term wear. A sandwich of polyurethane/polyisobutylene/polyurethane has also been claimed (45). The commercial system, Fempatch®, utilizes an elastomeric backing layer. Patents for other elastomeric backings also exist (46).

b. Adhesives. Although the same classes of adhesives mentioned above are also used for the matrix systems, other additives have to be formulated into these adhesives. Therefore, the demands made of the adhesive in this design are far more exacting. The adhesive contains all of the drug and any excipients. The drug and excipient could be dissolved or dispersed, depending on the amount needed for the appropriate delivery profile. If the additives need to be dissolved and stay dissolved, then the choice of adhesive is determined solely by solubility characteristics. In the case of dispersed systems, the range of useful adhesives increases, but the effect on properties is different. Dissolved additives tend to decrease moduli and render the adhesive more susceptible to creep/cohesive failure. Dispersed additives tend to reinforce the adhesive, especially if the additive is a solid. Thus, adhesive selection for matrices is more complicated and entails compatibility studies, long-term stability studies of the adhesive, and optimization of the formulation, based on the nature of the additives.

E. Fabrication

For RCM designs, fabrication involves the incorporation of the drug formulation into an FFS construction. This process may involve forming, filling, and sealing, or just filling and sealing, depending on the state of the formulation (paste, viscous liquid, or liquid). Once the formulation is contained, the subsequent steps involve sealing the FFS material to the membrane and the lamination of membrane to adhesive. Sometimes the membrane is made part of the FFS material by a suitable lamination process prior to incorporation of drug formulation.

The major steps in the fabrication process for RCM systems are as follows:

1. Mixing of drug formulation
2. Form, fill, and seal

3. Lamination to adhesive
4. Die-cut, pouch, label, and package

The throughput is mostly dependent on the first of these processes. The FFS operation itself is dependent on formulation viscosity or dispensing speed. Metering pumps are often used for the dispensing process. Typical line speeds are about 30 ft/min.

For matrix designs, fabrication includes the following steps:

1. Mixing of drug formulation with adhesive solution
2. Casting mixture onto backing material or release liner
3. Evaporation of solvent
4. Laminating to backing material
5. Die-cut, pouch, label, and package

The throughput is determined mostly by the casting operation, which involves spreading the adhesive/drug formulation onto a moving web, and then evaporation of the volatile components. The line speed is determined by the nature of the solvent. Typical speeds are about 5–20 ft/min.

F. Issues and Opportunities

The factors limiting the advancement of transdermal technology are not related to polymers. The key factors are the ability to push small molecules through the skin faster and the problems associated with sensitization from certain drug classes. For example, the so-called lag time in transdermal administration (the time required for the drug to reach efficacious blood levels) is still of the order of 2–4 h for most drugs, and this may be unacceptable if immediate relief is desired. In another example, the flux requirements for a given drug are so high that very large patches are needed. In these cases, advancement will occur through the invention/discovery of new enhancers rather than new polymers, although new polymers may be needed to accommodate and deliver the new enhancers at an acceptable rate. Similarly, the issue of sensitization by certain drugs cannot be overcome by the use of new polymers. Coadministration of immune suppressants or modification of drug structure to an immunologically inert form may be required. Such advances will enable the transdermal administration of antihistamines, for example.

IV. IMPLANTABLE DRUG DELIVERY SYSTEMS

For the purposes of this chapter, implantable drug delivery systems are defined as long-term (greater than 30 days) implantable products that are resorbable or removable. The resorbable "implants" are really injectables incorporating lyophilized microspheres and will be discussed further in Section V. The removable version is typically a subcutaneous implant, requiring a minor outpatient procedure for both insertion and removal. The main commercialized product in this category is Norplant®, a contraceptive implant. A limited number of other companies have announced products in various stages of development, the leading candidate being the Duros technology from ALZA Corporation (currently in phase III trials). Medtronic Corporation has two products in the implantable area that allow drug delivery into the intrathecal space (where the spinal fluid circulates). One of these products delivers baclofen for spasticity and the other delivers anesthetics for pain control. Both products utilize Medtronic's SynchroMed® infusion pump, which can be electronically programmed to deliver any type of preset dose. However, this type of product falls outside the scope of this chapter, which will focus on removable implanted passive devices.

A. Designs

The Norplant® product was developed by the International Committee for Contraception Research (ICCR) of Population Council, Inc. It is marketed in the United States as a 5-year implant by Wyeth-Ayerst. The first-generation product consists of a set of five cylindrical pieces that are inserted subdermally using a simple procedure. This particular version of Norplant is a capsule system (labeled case I in Fig. 6) in that crystals of levonorgestrel (LN) are encapsulated by Silastic® polymer. Later designs being tested internationally by the ICCR include a Silastic matrix (case II in Fig. 6), in which micronized LN is dispersed and a covered rod (case III in Fig. 6), which is a membrane-coated matrix. The three designs are depicted schematically in Fig. 6. The three designs yield very different release profiles, partly due to the nature and amount of drug loading, and partly due to design features. The three release profiles (47) are shown schematically in Fig. 7.

As can be seen from the figures, the drug release rate in case I is constant after 450 days (~15 months), whereas case II (matrix) yields a rate that varies as the square root of time, and case III yields a nearly constant rate over time. Although in principle cases I and III (membrane-controlled systems) are expected to yield constant-rate (zero-order) profiles, case I yields an initial nonconstant rate because of the nature of the drug present in the capsules. Levonorgestrel is present as crystals in the capsule, and it has been noted that water permeates slowly into the capsule. At about ~450 days, the drug is virtually suspended in water, and the rate-determining step becomes the dissolution rate of levonorgestrel in water (48). Case II exhibits the classical matrix rate profile, whereas case III yields the classical membrane-controlled rate profile.

Research on optimizing the design in order to achieve constant rates over long periods, as well as to maximize drug loading (so that the size or number of rods can be reduced), continues, with contraception as the main focus.

Using a totally different approach, ALZA Corporation has developed the Duros® implant (see discussion elsewhere in this book) to deliver constant amounts of drug over periods

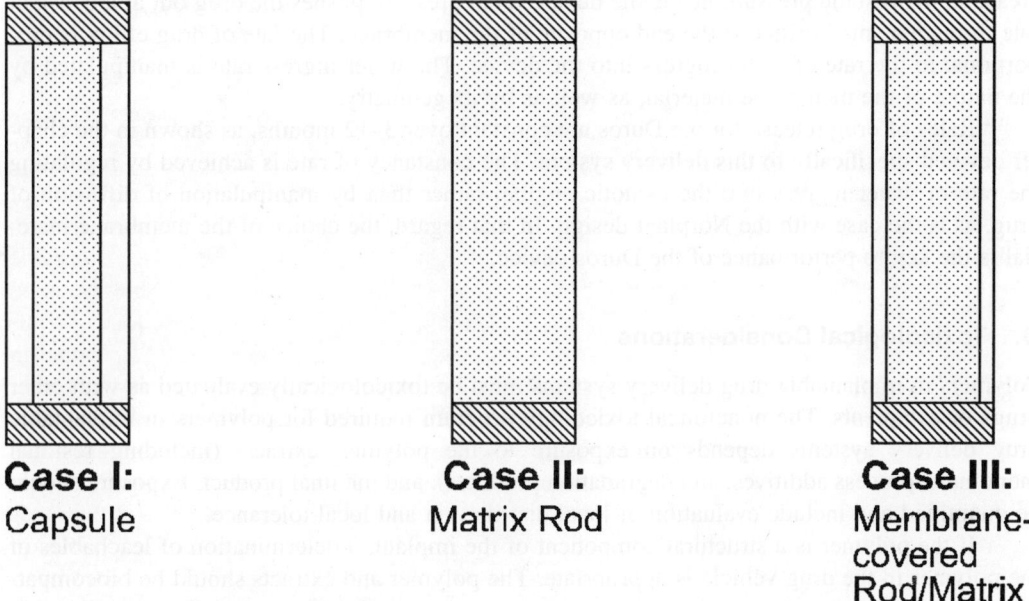

Case I: Capsule **Case II:** Matrix Rod **Case III:** Membrane-covered Rod/Matrix

Figure 6 Three types of long-term implant designs.

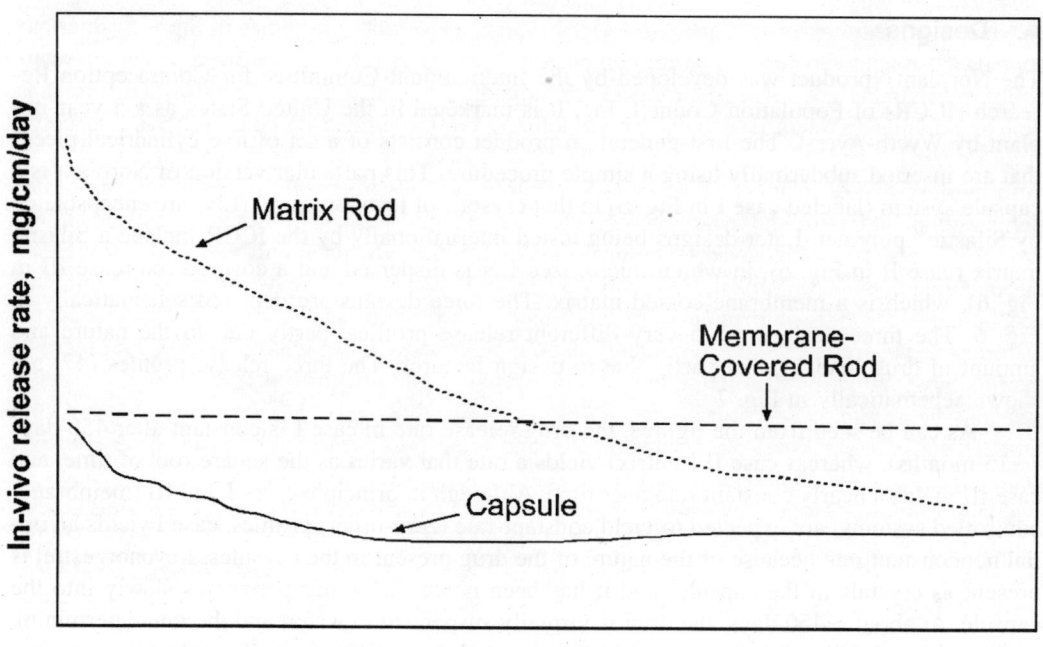

Figure 7 Drug release characteristics of three types of implants.

ranging from 3 to 12 months. The principle used in this design is essentially the same as the one used in the OROS system for oral controlled release. Basically, the osmotic engine draws in water at a constant rate through a semipermeable membrane, and this water causes an increase in hydrostatic pressure inside the device. That pressure pushes the drug out at a constant rate through a small orifice at the end opposite of the membrane. The rate of drug efflux is proportional to the rate of water ingress into the device. The water ingress rate is manipulated by the nature of the membrane material, as well as by its geometry.

Rates of drug release for the Duros are constant over 3–12 months, as shown in the chapter devoted specifically to this delivery system. The constancy of rate is achieved by regulating the rate of water ingress into the osmotic engine, rather than by manipulation of diffusion of drug, as is the case with the Norplant design. In that regard, the choice of the membrane material is the key to performance of the Duros device.

B. Toxicological Considerations

Polymers in implantable drug delivery systems must be toxicologically evaluated as with other drugs or excipients. The nonclinical toxicology program required for polymers in implantable drug delivery systems depends on exposure to the polymer, extracts (including residual monomers, process additives, and degradation products), and the final product. Exposure should be quantified and include evaluation of local distribution and local tolerance.

If the polymer is a structural component of the implant, a determination of leachables of the polymer in the drug vehicle is appropriate. The polymer and extracts should be biocompatible since they are in contact with components that are systemically released. The tests listed in ISO/ANSI/AAMI Standard 10993, Biological Evaluation of Medical Devices are intended to provide testing strategies for medical devices. There are similar guidelines in the U.S. Pharmacopoeia 23 for plastics used as drug containers. These tests may also be used to test biocompatibility. Extracts may also be tested for the potential to cause topical sensitization. Preparation of polymer extracts is defined by guidelines, but the choice of conditions should come close to the conditions of manufacture of the drug delivery system. Extracts are evaluated by in vitro cytotoxicity tests and in vivo irritation, intracutaneous injection, systemic injection, and implantation studies. A sample of the polymer may also be evaluated in these in vivo tests.

If the polymer is released systemically and not a new chemical entity (NCE), a review of the manufacturers' and published scientific literature should be a conducted to gather clinical and nonclinical safety information. If data indicate that blood levels are acceptable based on historical exposure or existing toxicology data, then conduct of toxicology studies that include the final drug delivery formulation with a written review and justification of the use of the polymer may be all that is necessary.

If the polymer is released systemically and is an NCE, a series of in vitro and in vivo genotoxicity studies should be conducted. These mutagenicity and clastogenicity studies will evaluate if the polymer and/or extract harms the cell's DNA. If the assays reveal a genotoxic result in multiple assays, development of the polymer should be halted. If no genotoxic activity is present, a full toxicology program consisting of acute, chronic, reproduction, and carcinogenicity testing will in all likelihood be required. Additional toxicology studies would necessarily be conducted with the final formulation.

C. Polymer Requirements

In the Norplant-type system, the membrane material has to satisfy the following criteria:

1. Should satisfy the long-term toxicological requirements, as outlined in Section IV.B.
2. Should not promote fibrotic tissue growth upon itself.
3. Should have the appropriate diffusion coefficient for small molecule drugs.
4. Should be capable of being fabricated into cylinders of varying sizes.
5. Should have low solubility for the drug in question.
6. Must be flexible enough so as not to be "felt" by the user. Typically, the modulus should be in the elastomer range of about 10^6 dynes/cm^2 or 100,000 Pa.

In actual use, the last of these requirements turns out to be inappropriate. While it is true that flexibility led to user acceptance, removal of the rods after use for prolonged periods in the body (~2 years or more) presented problems, as it became difficult to locate the rods. The ALZA design circumvents this problem by substituting a harder material for the body of the implant, at some cost to user acceptance. For the ALZA design, the two most important materials (outer container material and the rate-controlling membrane plug) must satisfy not only the toxicological and fibrotic growth requirement, but the container material must be rigid, and locatable either by feel or by other techniques, after prolonged use. This material must also have negligible solubility for the drug or the excipients, and negligible diffusion coefficient for the components of the drug formulation. The membrane plug material, on the other hand, must (in addition to the first two requirements above) have the following characteristics:

1. Possess a reproducible and well-defined permeability coefficient for water
2. Be moldable by standard polymer fabrication procedures
3. Retain its shape (under the constraints of the container material) without appreciable swelling in the presence of bodily fluids

In the next section, some of the materials and their characteristics will be explored.

D. Materials of Use

The earliest version of Norplant used six identical cylindrical rods (2.4 mm o.d., 1.57 mm i.d., 30 mm filled length) made of Silastic, a polydimethylsiloxane polymer made by Dow-Corning. The particular one used was Silastic medical-grade elastomer 382. This is a catalyst-cured siloxane elastomer, which for the implant application is also filled with silica. Essentially, thin-walled tubes were fabricated from this material, and sealed at the ends after having been filled with levonorgestrel crystals.

Later versions of Norplant include the rod and the covered rod. The rod is essentially a matrix of drug homogeneously dispersed inside the Silastic elastomer, whereas the covered rod comprises a core rod of PDMS and levonorgestrel, sealed inside thin-walled medical-grade Silastic tubing, using medical-grade Silastic adhesive. Practically all of this work derives from the early work of Folkman and Long (49), which evaluated the diffusion of small molecules through Silastic material. Repeated use of this material has ensured its continuance as an implant material, whereas others have not been subject to enough long-term studies to warrant use as a long-term implant material. In developmental work, however, poly (ϵ-capralactone) has been studied extensively in a development product called Copranor® (50). In the reported study, effective diffusion rates were obtained for levonorgestrel, testosterone, and progesterone. Biodegradable polymers such as esters of poly(lactic acid) and poly(glycolic acid), while acceptable as implant materials, generally exhibit too low a diffusion rate for most drugs of interest. The reason for this is that the PLA-PGA copolymers generally have too high a T_g, whereas both poly(ϵ-capralactone) and silicone elastomers have low, subambient T_g values.

In the Duros system, the outer container is constructed from a titanium alloy. The critical rate-controlling membrane is fabricated from a proprietary polyurethane developed specifically for ALZA Corporation. Early clinical data show little to no fibrotic growth around the implant body or its ends; more details are available elsewhere in this book.

E. Fabrication

The Norplant capsules are fabricated by first extruding tubes of Silastic, then filling with crystals of levonorgestrel, and then subsequently sealing the ends of the tube with silicone medical adhesive. Presumably, diffusion through the thin walls of the tube (approximately 15 mils) is the rate-controlling step, whereas diffusion through the ends (~150 mils) is much slower because of the higher pathlength.

The rods are fabricated by mixing about 25% by weight of steroid with a stannous octoate catalyst and Silastic 382, then pouring into a mold. Typical dimensions of rods are 2.4 mm diameter and 2 or 3 cm length.

Sterilization is carried out using ethylene oxide rather than radiation, since radiation further crosslinks the silicone and leads to a reduction in diffusion rates. Earlier studies had indicated that radiation affects the drug more than the polymer, but later studies have not borne this out. In any case, the preferred method of sterilization is by use of ethylene oxide.

Details of fabrication of the Duros device are given elsewhere in this book.

F. Issues and Opportunities

The use of biomaterials in human implants underwent a significant change in the early 1980s when the first of the silicone breast implant suits hit the courtrooms. Favorable and substantial awards to the plaintiffs resulted in bankruptcy for Dow-Corning. Subsequent lawsuits were directed at the parent companies of Dow-Corning, resulting in Dow Chemical making payments as well. All of this had very adverse consequences for the use of silicone materials

An Overview of Controlled Release Systems

in humans. Several companies, particularly the larger ones such as DuPont, Shell Chemical, and Exxon, made it corporate policy to not allow the use of any of their materials in inside-the-body applications.

In this context, the passage of the recent Biomaterials Access Assurance Act (H.R.872, Public Law 105-230, passed 8/98) is of great significance to biomaterial suppliers. The Act specifically exempts a supplier from liability for harm to a client caused by an implant, provided the supplier is not the implant manufacturer, and provided the supplier has supplied raw materials that meet contractual requirements and specifications. This should open the door for small and big firms to enter or reenter the biomaterials supplier market, but economics may drive the decision more than the perceived exemption from liability. Certainly, if the market is sizable for the polymer in question and/or if manufacturers of the implant are willing to pay a premium for implantable biomaterials, bigger firms will reenter the field. Otherwise the status quo will prevail, with smaller firms supplying materials to the industry. However, in all likelihood, the number of suppliers for any given biomaterial will increase, eventually driving prices down to manageable levels. The onus of testing and proving the safety of the implanted biomaterial will rest squarely on the implant manufacturer in each instance.

V. MICRO- AND NANOPARTICLE DELIVERY

Microparticles and nanoparticles incorporate drug in matrix or encapsulated form, delivered to the body via injection (IM, IV, or subcutaneous), via the oral cavity or via the nose. Control of delivery is typically achieved by one of the following mechanisms:

1. Diffusion through the coating of the capsules (for encapsulated particles)
2. Diffusion through the matrix of the particles
3. Erosion of the coating material
4. Erosion of the matrix material

For nasal and oral delivery, the particles are typically in the $20\text{-}\mu$ to $100\text{-}\mu m$ range, since smaller particles can be inhaled and may make their way to the lung for alveolar delivery. For injectable delivery, to achieve prolonged duration of effect, the particles tend to be in the 50- to $100\text{-}\mu m$ range. Nanoparticles are classified as having diameters below $1\ \mu m$ and tend to be used specifically for targeted drug delivery, usually via the injectable route.

The field of micro- and nanoparticles used in drug delivery is so broad an area of research that to list all of the applications and associated polymers is not practicable. It is convenient to subdivide this category as follows:

1. Bioadhesive microparticles
2. Injectable biodegradable depot formulations
3. Nanoparticles

The bioadhesive particles are typically formulated for mucosal delivery; this includes GI, buccal, nasal, and vaginal delivery. Injectable depot formulations invariably use biodegradable polymers, whereas nanoparticles may employ biodegradable and nonbiodegradable polymers. The rationale behind this subclassification is that for prolonged duration of delivery some bioadhesiveness is required of mucosal delivery vehicles, while depot formulations do not have this requirement. Nanoparticles are conceived to be used exclusively in injectable delivery and so are not required to bioadhere.

It is pertinent to make some general observations before proceeding to the specifics of each of these types of microparticulate delivery.

1. No product using bioadhesive particles has found commercial success to date. The products that offer prolonged action in mucosal delivery are nasal sprays, which do not employ bioadhesive microparticles. Therefore, we will survey the research on these particles to date and the materials employed in such formulations.
2. Depot formulations using biodegradable particles have been commercially successful, e.g., Lupron Depot®.
3. Nanoparticulate delivery is in early stages of research.
4. It is fair to say that, except for the case of biodegradable polymer matrices, formulations with microspheres tend not to have sustained or controlled release characteristics. Even in the case of microcpasules, the coating uniformity determines the degree of control over the release characteristics, even though in principle, membrane-coated particles can possess a controlled release profile. Furthermore, there is always a distribution of sizes in any of these preparations, and since surface-to-volume ratio also influences release kinetics, there is bound to be a distribution of rates achievable with any given preparation.

A. Mucosal Delivery: Bioadhesive Materials

In the field of mucosal delivery, the focus has been on two aspects of delivery:

1. Improving duration of action using mucoadhesive particles
2. Improving bioavailability of peptide drugs by enhanced delivery across the mucosa

For improving mucoadhesion, a variety of polymers have been tried with varying degrees of success. Perhaps the most mentioned polymer is a poly(acrylic acid) that is sold under the trade name Carbopol® by B.F. Goodrich. A variety of in vitro studies have claimed superior mucoadhesion for this polymer (51). In particular, the crosslinked poly(acrylic acid) known as polycarbophil has been claimed to have superior mucoadhesive properties. The crosslinking is usually carried out using divinyl glycol; crosslinked resins are available from B.F. Goodrich under the trade name Noveon®. This polymer has found successful use in three commercial products from Columbia Laboratories. These are not strictly microparticulate formulations but involve gels made of mucoadhesive polymer. They are discussed here as examples of commercialized mucoadhesive formulations:

Replens®—a vaginal moisturizer product utilizing polycarbophil in an aqueous gel formulation; duration of action is claimed to be several days

Advantage 24®—a vaginal contraceptive product, also utilizing a polycarbophil aqueous gel but containing a spermicide, nonoxynol 9 (3.5%); and

Crinone®—a vaginal delivery system for progesterone, utilizing a suspension of progesterone in an oil-in-water emulsion, with the polycarbophil swollen to a gel by the water phase. The advantage of this delivery system is that the drug is localized in the vagina, supplying progesterone to the uterus where it is needed. The indications for Crinone are for use in assisted reproductive technology (ART) as well as for menopausal women. Duration of action is claimed to be 24 to 72 h, with the polycarbophil assisting in adhesion to the vaginal wall, and delivering the progesterone locally, from where it travels to the uterus to exert its effect. It is not clear exactly how control of release is achieved in the case of Crinone; the formulation composition suggests that it could be a combination of dissolution control and diffusion control. The contraceptive gel does not require controlled release of nonoxynol 9, as it is a one-use application.

In oral gastrointestinal applications, the efficacy of adhesion in humans of microparticles made of poly(acrylic acid) and polycarbophil continues to be controversial. One study using γ-scintigraphic techniques (52) demonstrated that while gastric retention in rats may be enhanced by the use of these polymeric microparticles, no such effect was observed in humans. Previous studies in rats had observed bioadhesion for these polymer particles (53,54). Currently, it is acknowledged that the unique environment of the human GI tract and the composition of its mucin layer may preclude the extrapolation of rat studies to humans, and that no effective bioadhesive works in the human GI tract. Research into this problem continues, and there may be a need for newer types of polymers that exhibit enhanced adhesion.

Several studies in humans have claimed bioadhesive characteristics for hydroxypropylcellulose (55,56) in both nasal and buccal delivery. In the nasal application, duration of action (or of adhesion) is approximately 2–4 h after application of a powder spray, whereas in the buccal application, the best patches adhere only for 30 min to 1 h.

The 3M Company has used a different approach to buccal adhesion. They investigated blends of polyolefins—polyisobutylene (PIB), polyisoprene (PIP), and poly(acrylic acid) (PAA)—and optimized the adhesion based on both invitro (peel strength) and in vivo studies (duration of adhesion). The optimization was directed to development of a removable buccal patch or tablet, which 3M markets under the name of the CyDot® delivery system. From reports of in vivo studies (57), it appears that the adhesive mixture consists of Vistanex® L-100 PIB (8%), Vistanex LMMH PIB (32%), and Polycarbophil poly(acrylic acid) (60%). In dogs, the duration of adhesion appears to be about 12–24 h, while another study using melatonin (58) shows data for 10-h adhesion in human volunteers.

In summary, the following points can be made regarding bioadhesive materials for drug delivery:

1. To date, no effective mucoadhesive has been identified for prolonging GI retention time in humans.
2. Some human data exist for biadhesion of particles delivered intranasally.
3. A much bigger database attests to the viability of buccal adhesion using a variety of polymeric materials.

B. Injectable Depot Formulations/Materials and Performance

As mentioned above, all commercially successful depot formulations rely on the use of controlled biodegradation to prolong delivery of active agents. Duration of action ranges from a few weeks to several months. Two companies that are involved in the development of such formulations are TAP Pharmaceuticals and Alkermes. TAP has one line of depot products on the market, for delivery of leuprolide acetate, indicated for prostate cancer. Alkermes has announced preclinical and clinical studies for their products based on ProLease® technology. Both of these technologies utilize polylactide (PLA) or polyglycolide (PGA) in either homopolymer or copolymer form. (PLA is defined as the polylactic acid derived from polymerization of the lactide, and PGA is the polyglycolic acid derived from the glycolide.) Other biodegradable polymers that have been developed include the polyanhydrides (59), poly(ortho esters) (60), and the poly(ε-capralactones) mentioned in Section IV.D, all of which have found limited commercial success when compared to the PLA-PGA polymers. Consequently, the discussion in this chapter will focus on the PLA-PGA-based systems.

Polylactide is a stereoregular polymer that occurs in crystalline D or L forms, and is also available as the racemic DL-lactide. The DL form is mostly amorphous with a T_g of about 58°C. The glycolide is available mostly as a semicrystalline material with a T_g of 36°C and T_m of

230°C. The copolymers are amorphous with intermediate T_g values. Biodegradation of all of these polymers is thought to occur via simple hydrolytic cleavage of the ester bond, leading ultimately to the monomeric lactic or glycolic acids, which are metabolized via the Krebs cycle and excreted. Enzymes are speculated to be involved in the cleavage mechanism at later stages of degradation. The rate of degradation is dependent mostly on polymer composition, pH, surface area, and temperature. Therefore, these polymers do not show much variability in degradation rates from one body site to the next, a fact that accounts for their popularity in drug delivery applications.

The range of in vivo biodegradation times is from 2 months for a 50:50 copolymer to about 2 years for a poly(L-lactide). Both fabrication (manipulation of surface area) and polymer composition can be used to obtain a wide range of in vivo duration of action. The commercial product Lupron Depot®, sold by TAP pharmaceuticals, will serve to illustrate this versatility.

Lupron Depot is an injectable formulation of leuprolide acetate that is available in lyophilized microsphere form. It is available in 1-month, 3-month, and 4-month dosages, and is administered via intramuscular injection. Dosages cover the indications of endometriosis and the palliative treatment of prostate cancer. The duration of action (1 month vs. 3 months) is manipulated strictly via the polymer composition. The 1-month injectable formulation contains approximately 75% of poly(DL-lactide-co-glycolide) and 15% D-mannitol as plasticizer, whereas the 3-month formulation contains 75% of poly(DL-lactide) and 15% D-mannitol. Clearly, the copolymer degrades faster in vivo than the poly(DL-lactide), and this accounts for the 1-month and 3-month periods of action. Although not specifically mentioned, the drug is dispersed in the polymer matrix and fabricated into microspheres via any one of the following techniques:

1. Solvent evaporation of an organic phase in water emulsion (useful for water-insoluble drugs)
2. Coacervation processes whereby the polymer is precipitated from an organic phase by addition of an aqueous drug solution (useful for water-soluble drugs)
3. Wurster air suspension coating process involving solution of drug and polymer in an organic solvent (useful for water-insoluble drugs, with the possibility of microcapsule formation)

The other product category where these polymers have been successfully used is the long-acting contraceptive category. Here microcapsules of norethisterone have been fabricated using poly(DL-lactide-co-glycolide) as the membrane material (61). The resulting microcapsules are formulated as a suspension in a sterile saline solution and injected intramuscularly. Up to 3 months of duration of action has been reported in clinical studies (62). These two categories (delivery of low molecular weight peptides and of steroids) continue to attract a lot of attention in the depot formulation attempts. More recent research is focusing on bigger entities such as human growth hormone and interferon.

C. Issues and Opportunities

In the injectable depot field, the major issues areas follow:

1. The lack of suitable polymers besides the PLA-PGA type with clearly defined in vivo degradation rates
2. The capability of delivering a range of proteins and peptides of differing solubility characteristics

The two issues are related in that the second capability is influenced to a large extent by the lack of suitable polymers. The lack of suitable polymers is really a lack of commercialized polymers, since a variety of polymers have been synthesized and studied in laboratories. With the hysteria surrounding breast implants and the liability issues arising from it, most companies have been reluctant to undertake large-scale manufacturing of suitable polymers. Remarks attributed to the implant field are equally applicable here in terms of opportunities for biomaterial suppliers.

REFERENCES

1. Denizot, F. and Lang, R., 1986, Rapid colorimetric assay for cellular growth and survival. J Immunol Meth. 89, 211.
2. Theeuwes, F., Wong, P. S. L. and Yum, S. I. 1991, Drug delivery and therapeutic systems. In: Encyclopedia of Pharmaceutical Technology (J. Swarbrick and J. C. Boylan Eds.), Vol. 4, Mercel Dekker, New York.
3. Hui, H., Robinson, J. R. and Lee, V. H. 1987. In: Controlled Drug Delivery, Fundamentals and Applications, 2_{nd} ed. (J. R. Robinson and V. H. Lee, Eds.), Marcel Dekker, New York.
4. Benita, S. and Donbrow, M. 1982. Release kinetics of sparingly soluble drugs from ethylcellulose walled microcapsules. Theophylline microcapsules, J. Pharm. Pharmacol., 34, 547.
5. Steigmann, F., Kaminski, L. and Nasatir, S. 1959. Clinical-experimental evaluation of a prolonged acting antispasmodic-sedative, Am. J. Dig. Dis. 4, 534.
6. Mellinger, T. J. 1965. Serum concentration of thioridazine after different oral medication forms, Am. J. Psychiatry 121, 1119.
7. Hollister, L. E., 1965. Studies of prolonged action medication. II. Two phenothiazine tranquilizers (thoradizine and chlorpromazine) administered as coated tablets and prolonged action preparations, Curr. Pharmacol. Ther. 6, 486.
8. Magee, K. R. and Westerberg, M. R. 1959. Treatment of myasthenia gravis with prolonedaction mestinon, Neurology 9, 348.
9. Baker, R. W. and Lonsdale, H. K. 1973. Controlled release: mechanism and rates, Adv. Exp. Med. Biol. 47, 15.
10. Viega, F., Salsa, T. and Pina, M. E. 1998. Oral controlled release dosage forms. Part 2. Glassy polymers in hydrophillic matrices, Drug. Dev. Ind. Pharm. 24 (1), 1.
11. Viega, F., Salsa, T. and Pina, M. E. 1997. Oral controlled release dosage forms. I. Cellulose ether polymers in hydrophillic matrices, Drug. Dev. Ind. Pharm., 23(9) 929.
12. Khan, M. A. and Reddy, I. K. 1997. Controlled drug delivery development of solid oral dosage forms with acrylate polymers, STP Pharma Sci. 7(6), 483.
13. Physician's Desk Reference, 1999, 53_{rd} ed, Medical Economics, Oradell, NJ, p. 1277.
14. Higuchi, T. 1961. Rate of release of medicaments from ointment bases containing drugs in suspension, J. Pharm. Sci., 50, 847.
15. Theeuwes F. and Higuchi, T. U. S. patent 3,916,899.
16. Theeuwes F. 1983. Evolution and design of "rate controlled" osmotic forms, Curr. Med. Res. Opin., 8, Suppl.2, 20
17. Theeuwes, F. 1975. Elementary osmotic pump, J. Pharm. Sci., 64, 1987.
18. Swanson, D. R., Barclay, B., Wong, P. S. L. and Theeuwes, F. 1987. Nifedipine gastrointestinal therapeutic system, Am. J. Med., 83 (6B), 3.
19. Borodkin, S. 1991. Ion-exchange resin delivery systems. In: Polymers for Controlled Drug Delivery (P. J. Tarcha, Ed.), CRC Press, Boca Raton, FL, p. 215.
20. Deeb, G. and Becker, B. 1960. Absorption of sustained-release amphetamine preparations in the rat, Toxicol. Appl. Pharmacol., 2, 410.
21. Lichtneckert, S., Lundgren, C. and Ferno, O. 1975. Chewable smoking substitute composition, U.S. patent 3,901,248.

22. Amsel, L. P., Hinsvark, O. N. and Raghunathan, Y. 1980. Dissolution and blood level studies with a new sustained release system, Proc. Res. Sci. Dev. Conf., Washington, D.C., Proprietary Association, 94.
23. Deshpande, A. A., Rhodes, C. T., Shah, N. H. and Mallick, A. W. 1996. Controlled release drug delivery systems for prolonged gastric residence: an overview, Drug. Dev. Ind. Pharm., 22(6), 531.
24. Hwang, S., Park, H. and Park, K. 1998. Gastric retentive drug-delivery systems, Crit. Rev. Ther. Drug Carrier Syst. 15(3), 243.
25. Sheth, P. R. and Tossounian, J. 1978. Sustained release pharmaceutical capsules, U.S. patent, 4,126,672.
26. Sheth, P. R. and Tossounian, J. 1984. The hydrodynamically balanced systems (HBS), Novel drug delivery system for oral use, 10, 313.
27. Atyabi, F., Sharma, H. L., Mohammad, H. A. H. and Fell, J. T. 1996. In vivo evaluation of a novel gastric retention formulation based on ion-exchange resins, J. Control. Rel., 42, 105.
28. Whitehead, L., Fell, J. T., Collett, J. H., Sharma, H. L. and Smith, A. M. 1998. Floating dosage forms: an in vivo study demonstrating prolonged gastric retention., J. Control. Rel., 55, 3.
29. Park, K., Chen, J. and Park, H. Superporous hydrogel composites having fast swelling, high mechanical strength and superabsorbent properties, U.S. patent 5,750,585.
30. Berner, B. and Dinh, S. 1992. Fundamental concepts in controlled release. In: Treatise on Controlled Drug Delivery (A. Kydonieus, Ed.), Marcel Dekker, New York.
31. Jacobs, I. C. and Mason, N. S. 1993. Polymer delivery systems concepts. In: Polymeric Delivery Systems: Properties and Applications (M. A. El-Nokaly, D. M. Piatt, and B. A. Charpentier, Eds.), American Chemical Society, Washington, DC.
32. Burrell, H. 1975. Solubility Parameter Values Polymer Handbook (J. Brandrup, E. H. Immergut, and W. McDowell, Eds.), John Wiley, New York, IV-337.
33. Peppas, N. A. and Meadows, D. L. 1983. Macromolecular structure and solute diffusion in membrane: an overview of recent theories, J. Membrane Sci., 16, 361.
34. Peppas, N. A. and Lustig, S. R. 1986. Solute diffusion in hydrophilic network structures. In: Hydrogels in Medicine and Pharmacy, Vol. 1, Fundamentals (N. A. Peppas, Ed.), CRC Press, Boca Raton, FL.
35. Reinhart, C. T., Korsmeyer, R. W. and Peppas, N. A. 1981. Macromolecular network structure and its effects on drug and protein diffusion, Int. J. Pharm. Tech. Prod. Mfr., 2, 9.
36. Conte, U., Maggi, L., Colombo, P. and Manna, A. L. 1993. Multi-layered hydrophilic matrices as constant release devices (Geomatrix systems), J. Controlled Rel., 26, 39.
37. Conte, U. and Maggi, L. 1996. Modulation of the dissolution profiles from Geomatrix multi-layer matrix tablets containing drugs of different solubility, Biomaterials 17, 889.
38. Ritschel, W. A. 1973. Peroral solid dosage forms with prolonged action. In: Drug Design, Vol. 4 (E. J. Arien, Ed.), Academic Press, New York, Chapter 2.
39. Andrade, J. D. 1976. Hydrogels for Medical and Related Applications, ACS Symp. Series 31, American Chemical Society, Washington, DC.
40. John, P. M. and Becker, C. H. 1968. Surfactant effects of spray-congealed fomrulations of sulfaethylthiadazole-wax, J. Pharm. Sci., 57, 584.
41. Cussler, E. L., Herbig, S. M., Smith, K. L. and Van Eikeren, P. 1995. Osmotic devices having vapor permeable coatings, U.S. patent 95/03033.
42. Venkatraman, S. and Gale, R. M., 1998. Skin adhesives and skin adhesion 1. Transdermal drug delivery systems: a review. Biomaterials, 19, 1119.
43. Michaels, A. S., Wong, P. S. L., Prather, R. and Gale, R. M., 1975. A thermodynamic method of predicting the transport of steroids in polymer matrices. AIChE J., 21(6), 1073.
44. Cleary, G. W., 1993. In: Dermal and Transdermal Drug Delivery: New Insights and Perspectives (R. Gurny and A. Teubner, Eds.), Wiss Verl. Ges., Chapter 1.
45. Cleary, G. W., 1990. U.S. patent 4,906,463.
46. Venkatraman, S., and Scott, S. E, 1994. U.S. Patent 5,246,705.
47. Nash, H. A., Robertson, D. N., Moo-Young, A. J., Atkinson, L., 1978. Steroid release from Silastic capsules and rods. Contraception, 18(4), 367.

48. Robertson, D. N., 1984. In: Zatuchni, G. I., Goldsmith, A., Shelton, J. D. and Sciarra, J. J. (Eds.), Long-acting Contraceptive Delivery Systems, Harper and Row, New York, Chapter 11.
49. Folkman, J. and Long, D. M., 1964. The use of silicone rubber as a carrier for prolonged drug therapy. J. Surg. Res., 4, 139.
50. Pitt, C. G. and Schindler, A., 1984: Zatuchni, G. I., Goldsmith, A., Shelton, J. D. and Sciarra, J. J. (Eds.), Long-acting Contraceptive Delivery Systems, Harper and Row, New York, Chapter 5.
51. See, for example, the review by Pecosky, D. A. and Robinson, J. R., 1991. In: Polymers for Controlled Drug Delivery (P. J. Tarcha, Ed.), CRC Press, Boca Raton, FL, Chapter 6.
52. Harris, D., Fell, T. J., Sharma, H., Taylor, D. C. and Linch, J., 1989. Studies on potential bioadhesive systems for oral drug delivery. STP Pharmacol., 5, 582.
53. Longer, M. A., Ch'ng, H. S. and Robinson, J. R., 1985. Bioadhesive polymers as platforms for oral-controlled drug delivery. III. Oral delivery of chlorthiazide using a bioadhesive polymer. J. Pharm. Sci., 74, 406.
54. Beerman, B. and Groschinsky-Grind, M., 1987. Enhancement of the gastrointestinal absorption of hydrochlorothiazide by propantheline. Eur. J. Pharmacol., 13, 385.
55. Discussion on nasal delivery by Nagai, J. and Machida, Y., 1990. In: Bioadhesive Drug Delivery Systems, V. Lenoerts and R. Gurny, (Eds.), CRC Press, Boca Raton, FL, Chapter 9.
56. Discussion on buccal delivery by Merkle, H. P., Anders, R and Wernerskirchen, A., 1990, ibid., Chapter 6.
57. Scherrer, R. A., Scholtz, M. T., McQuinn, R. C., Barkhaus, J. K. and Marecki, N. M., 1992. A transmucosal drug delivery system based on polyisobutylene and polyacrylic acid. Presentation at AAPS annual meeting, November 1992.
58. Benes, L., Brun, J., Claustrat, B., Degrande, G., Ducloux, N., Geoffriau, M., Horriere, F., Karsenty, H. and Lagain, D., 1993. Plasma melatonin (M) and sulfatoxymelatonin (aMT6s) kinetics after transmucosal administration to humans. Proc. Int. Symp. the Pineal Gland, Paris, France, March 1993.
59. Chasin, M., Domb, A., Ron, E., Mathiowitz, E., Leong, K., Laurencin, C., Brem, H., Grossman, S. and Langer, R., 1990. In: Biodegradable Polymers as Drug Delivery Systems, M. Chasin, and R. Langer, (Eds.), Marcel Dekker, New York, Chapter 2.
60. Heller, J., Sparer, R. V. and Zentner, G. M., 1990, ibid., Chapter 4.
61. Beck, L. R., Flowers, C. E. (Jr.)., Pope, V. Z., Tice, T. R., Dunn, R. L. and Gilley, R. M., 1984. Zatuchni, G. I., Goldsmith, A., Shelton, J. D. and Sciarra, J. J. (Eds.), Long-acting Contraceptive Delivery Systems, Harper and Row, New York, Chapter 39.
62. Beck, L. R., Flowers, C. E., Jr., Pope, V. Z., and Tice, T. R., 1983. Clinical evaluation of an improved microcapsule contraceptive system. Am. J. Obstet. Gynecol., 147, 815.

23
Research and Development Aspects of Oral Controlled-Release Dosage Forms

Yihong Qiu
Abbott Laboratories, North Chicago, Illinois

Guohua Zhang
Andrx Corportation, Florida

I. INTRODUCTION

Controlled release may be defined as a technique or approach by which active chemicals are made available to a specified target at a rate and duration designed to accomplish an intended effect. More specifically, an oral controlled release drug delivery system is, in principle, a device or dosage form that controls drug release into the absorption site in the gastrointestinal (GI) tract. It controls the drug absorption rate to achieve the desired plasma profiles defined by the steady-state pharmacology (1). A typical controlled release system is designed to provide constant or nearly constant drug levels in plasma with reduced fluctuation via slow release of drug over an extended period of time. Controlled release systems are sometimes called extended release or sustained release systems. In practical terms, an oral controlled release should allow a reduction in dosing frequency as compared to that drug presented as a conventional dosage form (2).

Over the last two decades, controlled technology has received increasing attention from the pharmaceutical industry and academia. As new technologies emerge, they not only open up a wide range of new therapeutic opportunities, but also offer the benefits of product differentiation, market expansion, and patent extension. By 1998 over 70 chemical entities had been formulated into more than 90 oral controlled release products that were approved for marketing by the U.S. Food and Drug Administration (FDA) (3).

Controlled release technology may provide increased clinical value as well as extended product life. The advantages of an ideal controlled release dosage form over an immediate release product include improved patient compliance due to a reduced dosing frequency, a decreased incidence and/or intensity of the side effects, a greater selectivity of pharmacological activity, and a more constant or prolonged therapeutic effect, as well as an increase of cost effectiveness. A typical example is diltiazem hydrochloride, a calcium antagonist for the treatment of hypertension. To enhance drug therapy and competitiveness, this compound was formulated into three generations of dosage forms, including immediate release tablets (Cardizem) approved from 1982 to 1986, twice-daily controlled release capsules (Cardizem SR) approved in 1989, and once-daily controlled release capsules (Cardizem CD) approved from 1991 to 1992.

With the growing need for optimization of therapy, controlled release technologies providing programmable delivery rates other than immediate input have increasingly become more important, especially for drugs for chronic use or with a narrow therapeutic index. Thus, understanding and utilizing the fundamentals of controlled release technologies is essential to the successful formulation research and development of a controlled release product.

II. CONTROLLED RELEASE SYSTEMS FOR ORAL ADMINISTRATION

The basic concepts of controlled release have been reviewed thoroughly in the literature (1,4–6). Various physical and chemical approaches have been applied to produce a well-characterized dosage form that controls drug input into the body within the specifications of the desired release profile. In this section, commonly used methods based on application of physical and polymer chemistry to oral drug delivery systems will be briefly discussed with emphasis on polymeric systems.

A. Common Oral Polymeric Controlled Release Systems

The thrust of oral controlled release efforts has been focused mostly on the dosage forms with well-defined controlled release profiles. Almost all of the oral solid controlled release products on today's market are based on the designs of matrix, membrane-controlled, and osmotic systems (see Table 1). The application of polymeric systems to the oral controlled release dosage form designs and release-controlling mechanisms of these systems have been extensively investigated (1,7). The mechanisms of these controlled release dosage forms generally involve drug diffusion through a viscous gel layer, tortuous channels, or a barrier; drug dissolution via system erosion; and drug solution or suspension forced out of the device by osmotic pressure.

1. Matrix Systems

Both hydrophilic and hydrophobic polymeric matrix systems are widely used to provide controlled delivery of drug substances because of their versatility, effectiveness, and low cost. These types of systems are also suitable for in-house development since they are usually manufactured using conventional equipment and processing. In a matrix system, a drug is incorpo-

Table 1 Common Oral Controlled Release Polymeric Systems Feasible for Commercial Development

Matrix systems	Reservoir systems	Osmotic systems
Hydrophilic matrix	Coated beads or tablets	Elementary osmotic pump
• Swellable	Microencapsulation	Push-Pull system
• Swellable and erodible		Push-Layer system
Hydrophobic matrix		Push-Stick system
• Homogeneous (nonporous)		
• Heterogeneous (porous)		
1. Inert (monolithic)		
2. Erodible		
3. Degradable		

rated into the polymer matrix by either particle or molecular dispersion. The former is simply a suspension of drug particles homogeneously distributed in the polymer matrix, whereas the latter is a matrix with drug molecules dissolved in the polymer. Drug release occurs by diffusion and/or erosion of the matrix system.

In a hydrophilic matrix, there are two competing mechanisms involved in the drug release: Fickian diffusional release and relaxational release. Diffusion is not the only pathway by which a drug is released from the matrix; the erosion of the matrix following polymer relaxation also contributes to the overall release. The relative contribution of each component to the total release is primarily dependent on the properties of a given drug. For instance, the release of a sparingly soluble drug from hydrophilic matrices involves the simultaneous absorption of water and desorption of drug via a swelling-controlled diffusion mechanism. As water penetrates into a glassy polymeric matrix, the polymer swells and its glass transition temperature is lowered. At the same time, the dissolved drug diffuses through this swollen rubbery region into the external releasing medium. This type of diffusion and swelling generally does not follow a Fickian diffusion mechanism. A simple semiempirical equation was introduced to describe drug release behavior from hydrophilic matrix systems (8,9):

$$Q = kt^n \quad (1)$$

where Q is the fraction of drug released in time t, k is the rate constant incorporating characteristics of the macromolecular network system and the drug, and n is the diffusional exponent. It has been shown that the value of n is indicative of the drug release mechanism (10–14). For $n = 0.5$, drug release follows a Fickian diffusion mechanism that is driven by a chemical potential gradient. For $n = 1$, drug release occurs via the relaxational transport that is associated with stresses and phase transition in hydrated polymers. For $1 > n > 0.5$, non-Fickian diffusion behavior is often observed as a result of contributions from diffusion and polymer erosion (10).

In order to describe relaxational transport, Peppas and Sahlin derived the following equation by introducing a second term into Eq. 1 (12):

$$Q = k_1 t^n + k_2 t^{2n} \quad (2)$$

where k_1 and k_2 are constants reflecting the relative contributions of Fickian and relaxation mechanisms. In the case where surface area is fixed, the value of n should be 0.5. Thus, Eq. 2 becomes:

$$Q = k_1 t^{0.5} + k_2 t \quad (3)$$

where the first and second terms represents drug release due to diffusion and polymer erosion, respectively. This equation was later successfully applied to describe drug release from the hydrophilic matrices (14,15).

In a hydrophobic inert matrix system, the drug is dispersed throughout a matrix that involves essentially negligible movement of the device surface. For a homogeneous monolithic matrix system, the release behavior can be described by the Higuchi equation subject to the matrix boundary conditions (16):

$$M_t = [DC_s(2A - C_o)t]^{1/2} \quad (4)$$

where M_t is the drug released per unit area at time t, A is the drug loading per unit volume, C_s is the solubility, and D is the diffusion coefficient in the matrix phase. Equation 4 was derived based on the assumptions that (a) a pseudo–steady state exists, (b) the drug particles are small compared to the average distance of diffusion, (c) diffusion coefficient is constant, (d) perfect sink conditions exist in the external media, (e) only the diffusion process occurs, (f) the drug concentration in the matrix is greater than the drug solubility in the polymer, and (g) no interaction between drug and matrix takes place. In the case of $A \gg C_s$, Eq. 4 reduces to:

$$M_t = [2DAC_s t]^{1/2} \tag{5}$$

Thus, the amount of drug released is proportional to the square root of time, A, D, and C_s.

Drug release from a porous monolithic matrix system involves the simultaneous penetration of surrounding liquid, dissolution of drug, and leaching out of the drug through interstitial channels or pores. The volume and length of the openings in the matrix must be accounted for in the diffusion equation, leading to a second form of the Higuchi equation (17):

$$M_t = \left[\epsilon C_s (2A - \epsilon C_s) \frac{D_a}{\tau} t \right]^{1/2} \tag{6}$$

where ϵ and τ are the porosity and tortuosity of the matrix, respectively, and D_a is the drug diffusion coefficient in the aqueous phase. Similarly, Eq. 7 can be derived based on pseudo-steady-state approximation ($A \gg C_s$):

$$M_t = \left(2D_a AC_s \frac{\epsilon}{\tau} t \right)^{1/2} \tag{7}$$

The porosity, ϵ, in Eqs. 6 and 7, is the fraction of matrix that exists as pores or channels into which the surrounding liquid can penetrate. It is the total porosity of the matrix after the drug has been extracted. The total porosity consists of the initial porosity, ϵ_a, due to air, or void space in the matrix before the leaching process begins, and the porosity created by extracting the drug, ϵ_d, and the water-soluble excipients, ϵ_{ex} (18, 18a):

$$\epsilon = \epsilon_a + \epsilon_d + \epsilon_{ex} = \epsilon_a + \frac{A}{\rho} + \frac{A_{ex}}{\rho_{ex}} \tag{8}$$

where ρ is the drug density, and ρ_{ex} and A_{ex} are the density and the concentration of water-soluble excipient, respectively. In a case where no water-soluble excipient is used in the formulation and initial porosity, ϵ_a, is smaller than the porosity, ϵ_d, Eq. 8 becomes:

$$\epsilon \cong \epsilon_d = \frac{A}{\rho} \tag{9}$$

Hence, the Eqs. 6 and 7 yield:

$$M_t = A \left[\left(2 - \frac{C_s}{\rho} \right) \frac{D_a C_s}{\tau \rho} t \right]^{1/2} \tag{10}$$

$$M_t = A \left(\frac{2 D_a C_s}{\tau \rho} t \right)^{1/2} \tag{11}$$

In contrast to the homogeneous monolithic matrix system, the release from a porous monolith is expected to be directly proportional to the drug concentration in the matrix, A.

It should be noted that the Higuchi equation was originally derived for planar diffusion into a perfect sink. More recently, a simple exponential relation was introduced by Ritger and Peppas to describe the general release behavior from hydrophobic matrices in the form of slabs, spheres, and cylinders (19):

$$Q = \frac{M_t}{M_\infty} = kt^n \tag{12}$$

where Q is the fractional release, k is a constant, and n is the diffusional exponent. In the case of pure Fickian release, the exponent n has a limiting values of 0.50 for smooth slabs, 0.45 for smooth spheres, and 0.43–0.50 for smooth cylinders depending on the aspect ratio.

2. Reservoir Polymeric Systems

In developing reservoir polymeric systems, commonly used methods include microencapsulation of drug particles, coating of tablets or multiparticulates, and press coating of tablets. A polymeric membrane offers a predetermined resistance to drug diffusion from the reservoir to the sink. The driving force of such systems is the concentration gradient of active molecules between reservoir and sink. The resistance provided by the membrane is a function of film thickness and characteristic of both the film and the migrating species in a given environment. The mechanisms of drug release from the film-coated dosage forms may be categorized into (a) transport of the drug through a network of capillaries filled with dissolution media; (b) transport of the drug through the homogeneous film barrier by diffusion; (c) transport of the drug through a hydrated swollen film; and (d) transport of the drug through flaws, cracks, and imperfections within the coating matrix (20–22).

Based on Fick's first law of diffusion, the release rate of a drug from a reservoir polymeric system at steady state is given by:

$$\frac{dM_t}{dt} = \frac{DSK}{L} \Delta C \qquad (13)$$

where M_t is the total amount of drug released at time t, D is the diffusion coefficient of the drug, S is the effective membrane or barrier surface area for drug diffusion, L is the diffusional pathlength (such as thickness of the film), K is the partition coefficient of drug between the barrier and aqueous phases, and ΔC is the concentration gradient. In a case where D, S, K, L, and ΔC are constant in Eq. 13, the amount of drug released as a function of time can be obtained by integration:

$$M_t = \left(\frac{DSK\,\Delta C}{L}\right) t = kt \qquad (14)$$

where k is the release rate constant. The apparent zero-order release from this type of system is often desired for a controlled release dosage form in many situations.

3. Osmotic Pump Systems

In an osmotic pump system, a tablet core is encased by a semipermeable membrane with an orifice. When the system is exposed to body fluids, water will penetrate through the semipermeable membrane into the tablet core containing osmotic excipients and the active drug. There are two types of osmotic pump systems that have been described: a one-chamber elementary osmotic pump (EOP) and a two-chamber system (e.g., push-pull). In both systems, drug release via the orifice of the dosage form is controlled by an osmotic pressure formed in the device. The rate of water penetration into the system in terms of volume can be expressed as:

$$\frac{dV}{dt} = \frac{Ak}{l}(\Delta\pi - \Delta P) \qquad (15)$$

where dV/dt is the rate of water flow, k is the hydraulic permeability, A is the membrane area, l is the thickness, $\Delta\pi$ is the osmotic pressure difference, and ΔP is the hydrostatic pressure difference. Since the system is usually rigid, the volume of the device is constant during operation, the amount of drug released at time t can be expressed by:

$$\frac{dM}{dt} = \frac{dV}{dt}[S] \tag{16}$$

where [S] is the drug solubility. When the hydrostatic pressure difference is negligible, Eq. 16 becomes:

$$\frac{dM}{dt} = \frac{kA}{l}\Delta\pi[S] \tag{17}$$

In summary, the osmotic delivery systems can be more readily programmed to obtain various desired release profiles, such as zero-order and pulsatile release. For most drug molecules, the release rate is independent of the drug properties and release environment. However, the manufacturing of this type of system often requires specialized equipment and processes.

4. Other Systems

Other controlled release systems include ion exchange systems, such as, Biphetamine capsules containing amphetamine and dextroamphetamine, manufactured by Penwalt (23). Ion exchange systems generally utilize resins composed of water-insoluble crosslinked polymers. These polymers contain salt-forming functional groups in repeating positions on the polymer chain. The drug is bound to the resin and released by exchanging with appropriately charged ions in contact with the ion exchange groups.

B. Materials Used for Controlling Drug Release

Materials used for controlling drug release from oral tablets and capsules include polymers from natural products, chemically modified natural products, and synthetic products. Some of the common materials that have regulatory clearance are discussed briefly in this section based on their applications in different types of controlled release systems. The list is not intended to be comprehensive but rather serves as a starting point for interested readers.

1. Materials Used for Matrix Systems

The materials most widely used in preparing matrix systems include both hydrophilic and hydrophobic polymers. Commonly available hydrophilic polymers include hydroxypropylmethylcellulose (HPMC), hydroxypropylcellulose (HPC), hydroxyethylcellulose (HEC), xantham gum, sodium alginate, poly(ethylene oxide), and crosslinked homopolymers and copolymers of acrylic acid. They are usually supplied in micronized forms because small particle size is critical to the rapid formation of gelatinous layer on the tablet surface.

Hydroxypropylmethylcellulose is a nonionic water-soluble cellulose ether made by Dow Chemical under the brand name Methocel. Methocel is available in four different chemistries (E, F, J, and K series) based on varying degrees of hydroxypropyl and methyl substitution. The specially produced Methocel of ultrafine particle size for controlled release formulations include K100LV, K4M, K15M, K100M, E4M, and E10M. When dissolved at a concentration of 2% in water, the viscosity ranges from 100 to 100,000 cps. Similar grades of HPMC (Metolose SR) are also available from ShinEtsu of Japan.

Both HPC and HEC are also nonionic water-soluble cellulose ethers made by the Aqualon division of Hercules Inc. under the brand names Klucel and Natrosol, respectively. For controlled release applications, they are available in high- and low-viscosity grades, such as Klucel HXF, EXF, and Natrosol 250HX.

Xanthan gum is a water-soluble polysaccharide gum produced by the Kelco division of Monsanto Co. under the brand name of Keltrol. It is composed of D-glucosyl, D-mannosyl, and D-glucosyluronic acid residues and differing proportions of O-acetyl and pyruvic acid acetal. The primary structure consists of a cellulose backbone with trisaccharide side chains.

Sodium alginate is a water-soluble gelling polysaccharide also made by Kelco under the brand name Keltone. Keltone HVCR and LVCR are forms that are used in controlled release products.

Poly(ethylene oxide) polymer is a nonionic water-soluble resins made by Union Carbide under the brand name of Polyox. Its common structure is $-(OCH_2CH_2)_n-OH$. For controlled release applications it is available in a variety of viscosity grades. Examples include Polyox WSR N-12K, WSR N-60K, WSR-301, WSR-coagulant, WSR-303, WSR-308 with molecular weights ranging from 100,000 to 8 million.

Crosslinked homopolymers and copolymers of acrylic acid are water-swellable, but insoluble, resins made by the B. F. Goodrich Company under the brand name Carbopol. Carbopol 971P NF, 974P, and 934P NF are specifically designed for preparing hydrogel controlled release systems.

Hydrophobic and monolithic polymer matrix systems usually use waxes and water-insoluble polymers in their formulation. Many waxes are long carbon chain wax esters, glycerides, and fatty acids. Natural and synthetic waxes of differing melting points have been used as controlled release matrix materials. Examples include carnauba wax, beeswax, candelilla wax, microcrystalline wax, ozokerite wax, paraffin waxes, and low molecular weight polyethylene, to name a few. Insoluble polymers used in preparing controlled release matrices include fine powders of ammoniomethacrylate copolymers (Eudragit RL100, PO, RS100, PO) by Rohm America, Inc., ethylcellulose (Ethocel FP7, FP10, FP100) by Dow Chemical Co., cellulose acetate (CA-398-10), cellulose acetate butyrate (CAB-381-20), cellulose acetate propionate (CAP-482-20) by Eastman Chemical Co., and latex dispersion of methacrylic ester copolymers (Eudragit NE30D).

2. Materials Used for Reservoir Systems

The most common materials to form a drug release barrier surrounding a core tablet, drug particles, beads, or pellets for diffusion-controlled reservoir systems include water-insoluble acrylic copolymers and ethylcellulose. These film-coating polymers have historically been used in an organic solution. In recent years, they have been mostly applied as aqueous dispersions that form films by a process of coalescence of submicrometer polymer particles. Ammoniomethacrylate copolymers (Eudragit RL 30D, RS 30D) are water-permeable and swellable film formers based on neutral methacrylic esters with a small proportion of trimethylammonioethyl methacrylate chloride. Methacrylic ester copolymers (Eudragit, NE30D) is a neutral ester without any functional groups. They are supplied by Rohm America as 30% aqueous dispersions without the need of plasticizers unless improved film flexibility is desired. Ethylcellulose for film coating is available as an aqueous polymeric dispersion containing plasticizers under the brand name of Surelease (Colorcon) and as pseudolatex dispersion, Aquacoat ECD (FMC), which requires addition of plasticizers to facilitate film formation during coating.

Enteric polymers may also be incorporated into the coating film to modify release rate, such as cellulose acetate phthalate (CAP), hydroxypropylmethylcellulose phthalate (HPMCP), methacrylic acid and methacrylic esters (Eudragit L and S). Enteric polymers are pH-dependent polymers. At high pH (e.g., >5.5), the polymer dissolves. At low pH, the polymer is impermeable and insoluble.

3. Polymers Used for Osmotic Pump Systems

Cellulose acetate comprising a certain percentage of acetyl content can be used together with other pH-dependent and pH-independent soluble cellulose derivatives to form a semipermeable film. Other polymers including polyurethane, ethylcellulose, poly(ethylene oxide) polymers, PVC, and PVA may be used in the osmotic pump systems.

C. Development Technologies

Most oral controlled release systems are in the forms of tablets and capsules. Development technologies for these dosage forms include tableting, spheronization (or pelletization), and film coating of single unit or multiparticulates.

1. Tableting Process

Controlled release tablet dosage forms are usually manufactured using conventional processes of granulation, blending, compression, and coating where necessary. Each unit operation of the development technologies has been extensively addressed (24). In manufacturing matrix formulations, precompression may have to be considered to ensure product quality because high concentrations of polymers are often used in these systems.

2. Spheronization/Pelletization Process

Controlled release pellets, beads, or spheres may offer certain advantages over single unit dosage forms in that they minimize the risk of unexpected drug release (e.g., dose dumping) which may occur when a single-unit device is defective (25). In addition, multiparticulate dosage forms can be designed to provide customized release profiles by combining beads with different release rates or to deliver incompatible drugs in the same dosage unit (26).

The basic methods for pellet or bead production include (a) microencapsulation, (b) spray congealing, (c) formation of particles from a plastic mass, and (d) agglomeration. Most microencapsulation techniques are based on processes by which coatings of natural or synthetic polymers are applied to solid or liquid agents via coacervation or polymerization (27,28). The spray-congealing process consists of embedding the active drug in an excipient, such as wax or plastic. Formation of particles from a plastic mass is achieved using a machine known as a marumerizer or a spheronizer (29,30). The spheronization process in the marumerizer involves partial shaping of pellets followed by utilization of friction and surface forces to form spheres. Powdered raw materials are converted into a plastic mass using water or solvents in conjunction with binding agents. This mass is extruded under pressure through a perforated screen or die. The cylindrical, spaghetti-like extrudates are then broken down by spinning in the marumerizer until the length is equal to the diameter. The process continues until they are rolled into spheres by centrifugal and frictional forces. To produce solid spheres, the extrudate must break into short segments and short cylinders must be sufficiently plastic to be rounded by spheronization. The materials that break into short cylinders without sufficient plastic properties do not yield a spherical product (31). Microcrystalline cellulose is found to exhibit the elasticity required for extrusion and spheronization. Thus, it is an excipient most commonly used for pelletization/spheronization (32).

Agglomeration is one of the oldest processes for manufacturing spherical particles. It is based on the layering technology derived from sugar coating in a coating pan. Traditionally, these spheronization processes involving surface forces can be divided into two stages: nucleation (seed growth) and sphere growth (bead preparation). With the layering technique, the active drug or other ingredients in the form of either a dry powder or solution/dispersion are agglomerated to form seeds. There are commercially available nonpareil seed or seeds containing active drugs. This process can be performed in a coating pan, a rotary granulator, or a fluidized bed.

3. Coating Technologies

In the pharmaceutical industry, significant advances have been achieved in polymer coating of solid dosage forms over the last two decades. Polymer coating involves deposition of a uniform membrane of polymer onto the surface of the substrates, such as tablets, spheres, or pellets, and drug particles. Coating techniques that are used in developing controlled release reservoir or osmotic systems include (a) film coating, (b) layering coating, and (c) compressed coating. The properties of the resulting functional coating are influenced by coating formulations as well as processing variables.

The film coating process is performed in a coating pan, a fluidized bed or a rotary granulator. Ethylcellulose, methacrylic ester copolymers, methacryl ester copolymers, cellulose acetate, and enteric polymers are widely used either alone or in combination with water-soluble polymers for the preparation of controlled release films. Since the integrity of the film and the absence of flaws or cracks are important factors in controlling the drug release from such preparation, it is imperative that the film formulation be optimized. Plasticizers are often added to such films to increase the film flexibility and minimize the incidence of flaws. Other factors affecting film coating and drug release include formulation (e.g., pigment, plasticizer, solvent) and process variables (e.g., equipment, batch scale, airflow, spray rate, temperature.).

The layering coating process is often performed in a sugar coating pan or a fluidized bed. This type of coating process is noncontinuous. For example, in coating beads, the seeds may first be coated with one layer of active drug, then coated with one layer of polymer followed by another active drug layer. The process is repeated until multiple layers are completed to meet the predetermined requirement. In some cases, the active drug may be dissolved or dispersed with the coating materials. Factors affecting coating quality and performance of the final product are similar to those discussed in the film coating process.

The compression coating process is performed using a tablet press to make a compress coat surrounding a tablet core (tablet-in-tablet). The compress coat may function as a barrier to drug release or as part of formulation to provide biphasic release. The process involves initial compression of the core formulation to produce a relatively soft tablet followed by transferring to a larger die for final compression of the compress coat layer. This process can be used to develop a controlled release product with unique release profiles or to formulate two incompatible drugs by incorporating one in the core and the other one in the compress coat layer.

III. IN VITRO AND IN VIVO CONSIDERATIONS

A. Feasibility Assessment of Chemical Entity for Controlled Release Delivery

The first step in developing a controlled release product for a compound should be feasibility assessment. In today's competitive market conditions, pharmaceutical companies are being forced to develop increasingly aggressive strategies to enable them to prosper. Differentiation of existing and future products by developing once- or twice-daily controlled release dosage forms is one of the key components of such strategies. However, the feasibility of extended oral delivery of a compound is often dictated by its physicochemical, biopharmaceutical, and therapeutic properties, as well as physiological constraints. It should be emphasized that it is not difficult to extend or control the in vitro drug release for almost any compound by using nonproprietary matrix or reservoir systems. However, achieving desired in vivo effects may be difficult or impossible due to physicochemical and biopharmaceutical limitations of a particular compound. To help better understand the suitability of a particular drug for controlled release delivery, some of the important factors and their impact on the development of a controlled release product are summarized in Table 2.

Drug solubility is one of the most important factors that needs to be considered in controlled release design. In general, the dissolution of a compound with low solubility (e.g.,

Table 2 Factors Affecting the Feasibility in Developing Oral Controlled Release Systems

a. **Solubility/Dose**
Absorption of poorly soluble drugs is often naturally extended due to the slow dissolution rate of the drug particles. However, the dissolution kinetics of these particles is typically nonlinear and varies with surface properties, particle size, and size distribution. In addition, the absorption of such drugs may be incomplete and variable if the in vivo release is extended past the ileocecal junction ($>7-8$ h) where the amount of fluid available for dissolution is progressively limited and the rate of absorption is decreased. Furthermore, poorly soluble drugs combined with a prohibitively high dose can further limit the suitability for developing a controlled release system.

b. **Stability**
Drugs must be stable to pH, enzymes, and flora throughout the entire intended delivery regions of the GI tract. For example, a drug that will be degraded by the colonic bacterial population is not a suitable candidate for once- or twice-daily dosing that requires an in vivo absorption of at least 12 h.

c. **Lipophilicity/Permeability**
Absorption of hydrophilic drugs with poor permeability may be limited by membrane permeation, which is known to vary with the surface area and enzymatic activities in different regions of the GI tract. Changing the release rate of such drugs may have little effect on the shape of plasma profiles and may even result in decreased absorption.

d. **Elimination $t_{1/2}$**
The need for controlled release systems is primarily a result of short half-life (2–6 h). However, other variables (e.g., minimum effective concentration, volume of distribution, and dose) are also important in determining the feasibility of extended delivery. Developing a twice-daily (or once-daily) system may be possible for one particular molecule but may not be feasible for another drug having similar half-life.

e. **Therapeutic Window**
One of the important characteristics of oral controlled drug delivery is the ability to maintain plasma levels within therapeutic range with reduced fluctuation. For drugs with relatively short half-lives, the lower the minimum effective concentration (MEC) is, the more likely it is to achieve prolonged drug exposure above MEC with controlled release systems. However, this will result in greater fluctuation in steady-state plasma levels, which is often undesirable for narrow therapeutic index drugs.

f. **First-Pass Metabolism**
For drugs with saturable first-pass metabolism (hepatic or gut), bioavailability will be decreased due to slow systemic input from the controlled release systems, thus limiting the chance of success of a controlled release system.

g. **PK/PD Relationship**
In many cases, the relationship between drug concentration (C) and the pharmacological effect (E) is described by a sigmoidal E_{max} model. For a particular drug, a relatively shallow E-C profile indicates that only very modest attenuation in E is expected even for large degrees of change in C. In such cases, there is no pharmacodynamic rationale to develop controlled release systems. In addition, for those pharmacodynamic properties that are concentration-dependent and require only short exposure time, an intermittent bolus regimen is preferred over the slow presentation of the drug.

<0.01 mg/mL) is inherently sustained in the GI tract. Therefore, it may not be necessary to develop a controlled release dosage form for such compound unless release kinetics need to be changed or absorption enhancers are required. It is also important to realize that drug solubility often limits the choice of release mechanism to be used in the controlled release dosage form. For instance, for a drug having reasonable solubility, both diffusion and erosion mechanisms of matrix systems may be utilized. For drugs with low solubility, the erosion system or osmotic pump is better suited to ensure complete drug release. Dosage strength is another factor affecting the suitability of controlled release development. In general, a single dose of 1.0 g for an immediate-release (IR) dosage form is considered maximum for a controlled release dosage form.

Drug molecules must cross biological membranes upon their release from a controlled release delivery system to produce a therapeutic effect. Thus, the partition coefficient of the drug becomes important in determining the potential of penetration across the membrane barriers. Drugs of a relatively high partition coefficient often have low aqueous solubility, which may affect the design of the delivery system. On the other hand, large molecules with low partition coefficient (e.g., peptides) often show low membrane permeability due to their poor lipophilicity or slow and site-specific penetration because of the mechanism of active transport.

Orally administered drugs may be subject to acid or base hydrolysis and to other chemical or enzymatic degradation. Stability of the drugs in the GI tract can affect the bioavailability and design of the delivery system. For example, drugs that are unstable in the stomach require delayed onset of drug release until the dosage form enters the small intestine. This may result in shortened GI residence time for extended absorption. On the other hand, drugs that are unstable in the lower GI tract would require complete drug delivery in the upper GI tract (i.e., a gastric retention device).

The residence time of drug dosage forms in the GI tract is a very important biological parameter for assessing the suitability of controlled release delivery. In general, the transit time of most dosage forms in the upper GI tract is 6–8 h, which becomes a limitation for a drug requiring absorption beyond this time frame after dosing (32a). In some cases, absorption from the lower colon may allow continued drug delivery for up to a total of 24 h. Hence, it is very important to define the absorption regions of a specific drug candidate in the GI tract before further development proceeds. If drug release is not completed by the time the dosage form passes the absorption region, bioavailability will be significantly decreased. In this regard, scintigraphic techniques have made valuable contributions to screening of drug candidates for once- or twice-daily oral formulations (35). Techniques typically used in assessing regional absorption potential of a compound include in vitro permeability and site-specific delivery in animal and human subjects. For instance, regional differences in absorption are determined by administering drug solution via indwelling access ports to the jejunum, ileum, and colon in dogs. In humans, this can be achieved by using a noninvasive delivery device, such as an InteliSite® capsule developed by Scintipharma, Inc. This radiolabeled capsule, loaded with a drug solution or powder formulation, can be externally activated to release the drug when it reaches the desired location in the GI tract as determined via gamma scintigraphy. To quantify colonic absorption for extended delivery potential, intubation study has also been used via bolus and/or continuous colonic delivery of a drug solution in transverse colon in healthy volunteers. These types of studies provide useful information for feasibility assessment, release rate design, as well as reducing development time and risk.

To maintain therapeutic blood levels of a drug over an extended period of time, the rate at which drug enters the systemic circulation must approximately equal the rate of elimination. Since the elimination rate is determined by the half-life ($t_{1/2}$), drugs with very short half-lives and high volumes of distribution undergo rapid clearance, which can make extended delivery

very difficult. Compounds with relatively long half-lives often exhibit intrinsically extended plasma levels. In general, an ideal candidate compound for controlled release delivery typically has a half-life of 2–8 h. The therapeutic window of a candidate drug is also a critical factor in suitability consideration. For drugs with a very narrow therapeutic index, patients may be exposed to a potentially harmful dose should the controlled release dosage form fail.

B. In Vitro Evaluation

Although the state of science is such that in vivo testing is essential in the development and evaluation of dosage forms, assessment of the in vitro characteristics and quality of the product is also necessary. For solid controlled release dosage forms, drug release characterization is the most important among various in vitro tests because the in vivo absorption is determined by the release kinetics of the dosage forms. A validated in vitro dissolution test can serve the purposes of (a) providing necessary quality and process control, (b) determining stability of the relevant release characteristics of the product, and (c) facilitating certain regulatory determinations and judgments concerning minor formulation changes, change in site of manufacture, etc. However, the dissolution rate of a specific dosage form is essentially an arbitrary parameter that may vary with the dissolution methodology, such as type of apparatus, medium, agitation, etc. Unless it is demonstrated that the in vitro release behavior reflects the in vivo performance in humans, the data can be of no relevant value in predicting or judging the clinical effectiveness of a drug product. Therefore, development of a dissolution testing method for controlled release formulations should have in vivo considerations (34). For the in vitro test to be predictive, it should be discriminative and correlated with the in vivo performance. For the in vitro test to be reliable, the in vitro specifications must be relevant to bioavailability variables and to the critical manufacturing variables that might be expected during normal manufacturing procedures.

Many issues and challenges related to dissolution testing of controlled release dosage forms have been addressed by regulatory authorities (35–37) and in a recent review by Khan (38). After a prototype formulation with acceptable ranges of process and composition variables has been identified, test variables should be studied, which include variations in pH, effect of surfactants, agitation, ionic strength etc. The key elements during the dissolution evaluation include (a) reproducibility of the method; (b) maintenance of sink conditions; (c) dissolution profile with a narrow limit on 1-h specification to assure lack of dose dumping; and (d) at least 75% of drug released at the last sampling interval to assure complete release.

Commonly used USP dissolution methods are recommended for determination of drug release from oral controlled release dosage forms as follows. Table 3 lists the test conditions commonly used in in vitro dissolution testing for controlled release dosage forms.

1. *USP Apparatus I (basket method):* preferred for capsules and dosage forms that tend to float or disintegrate slowly
2. *USP Apparatus II (Paddle method):* preferred for tablets
3. *USP Apparatus III (Bio-Dis dissolution method, or modified disintegration):* useful for bead-type dosage forms
4. *USP Apparatus IV (Flow-through cell method):* for insoluble drugs

It should be pointed out that none of the existing in vitro methods can perfectly mimic the in vivo situation given the nature of the GI tract and factors that affect its activity, and various mechanisms employed to achieve controlled release. In vivo drug absorption from dosage forms is known to be dependent on many factors other than dissolution, such as transit time, permeability, solubility, luminal contents, metabolism, and chemical stability in the GI tract. Nevertheless, dissolution is an essential and critical step, particularly for controlled release drug prod-

Table 3 Conditions Recommended for Dissolution Testing of Controlled Release Dosage Forms

Media	1. Buffers over the full range of physiological pH (1–1.5, 4–4.5, 6–6.5, 7–7.5 for topographical plot);
	2. Simulated gastric/intestinal fluids, i.e., 1 h acid plus pH 7.4 buffer from 1 h on;
	3. Solutions of gradient pH: 1.2, 2.1, 5.5, 6.5, 6.7, 7.4;
	4. Water
	5. In some cases, surfactant may be used in dissolution media.
Volume of media	Sufficient to maintain "sink" conditions: the entire dose should dissolve in <33% of the dissolution media
Mixing	Different agitation rates including the standard conditions. Apparatus I and II may be more useful at higher rpm (e.g., paddle at 100 rpm).
Sampling schedule	1. At a minimum, three time points (1–2 h, t_{50} and t_{80}).
	2. Early sampling times for assurance against premature release: 1,2,4 h and every 2 h thereafter, until 80% of the drug is released
No. units to be tested	12
Temperature	37 ± 0.5°C

ucts, even though it is only one of the processes involved in drug absorption. Therefore, the ability to predict in vivo absorption characteristics from dissolution data of a controlled release dosage form has become one of the current emphases in the development of controlled release products. Development of an in vitro/in vivo correlation (IVIVC) for this purpose has been extensively discussed and explored over the last decade (2,39–43). The existence of workshops, research, and publications led to the issuance of a guidance on this topic by the FDA in 1997 (2). The guidance presented a comprehensive perspective on the methods of developing and validating an IVIVC and its applications in setting dissolution specifications and using an in vitro test as a surrogate for an in vivo bioequivalence study in certain regulatory submissions. Interested readers are advised to refer to Chapter 25 devoted to this topic.

C. In Vivo Performance Evaluation

The successful design and development of a controlled release delivery system is ultimately determined by the ability of the product to modulate the magnitude and duration of the drug action. In most cases, it is evaluated by the reduction of the dosing frequency and/or fluctuation in plasma levels based on the assumption that the magnitude of response elicited by the drug is closely related to changes in plasma concentrations. This is normally achieved by conducting in vivo studies following prototype formulations with acceptable in vitro characteristics have been identified.

1. Animal Models

As product development progresses, in vivo studies are frequently conducted in animal models to obtain basic information about the in vivo absorption characteristics of the formulation design. These studies are typically carried out in a species that can accommodate a human scale dosage form. Selection of an animal model for oral drug absorption study of controlled release dosage forms is a difficult task due to the differences in the anatomy and physiology of the GI tracts between available species and humans. It also depends on different physicochemical and biological properties of the tested compound. Over the years, dogs have been used extensively as a model for oral drug absorption because of the similar gastric anatomy and physiology and the similar general upper GI motility patterns between dogs and humans (e.g., similar gastric emptying, similar pattern and periodicity of motility cycle, similar motility response to feeding, and similar profiles of bile secretion) (44). Some of the GI physiological parameters of the dog and of human are given in Table 4 (45,46). For controlled release dosage forms, the potential differences include higher total bile salt concentration, less bacterial metabolism, higher agitation intensity, and, most importantly, shorter GI transit time in dogs (44,47). As a result, decreases in the extent of absorption from controlled release dosage forms of certain compounds (e.g., SR acetaminophen and valproic acid formulations) have been observed (44). Thus, data obtained in animal models should be interpreted with caution. For dosage forms designed to release drug over a period beyond the GI transit time in dogs or for compounds not well absorbed in the colon, incomplete availability from controlled release dosage forms would be expected in dogs. To increase the intestinal residence time of the dosage forms, use of dogs pretreated with anticholinergic drugs, such as propantheline bromide, has been reported (48,49). Other models, such as pigs and stomach-emptying-controlled rabbits, have also been used with limited success (50–52). An alternative approach is to use the dog as a model for preliminary evaluation of release control in vivo by the designed dosage forms only within the time frame of transit through the absorption site in dogs, e.g., 4–5 h for drugs with low solubility and 9–12 h for soluble and permeable drugs (53,54). Different rates of in vivo absorption should result from formulations with different in vitro release rates if the in vitro test method is discriminative and the tested formulations are truly different. Unlike immediate release formulations, the extent of absorption should not be a major concern in the screening of controlled release formulations in dogs. The reduced bioavailability from the slower releasing formulations may be considered as a result of truncated absorption.

2. Studies in Humans

The in vivo studies in humans required to evaluate controlled release dosage forms have been categorized into four cases depending on the types of drug products (39). For a controlled release oral dosage form of a marketed immediate-release drug for which extensive pharmacokinetic/pharmacodynamic (PK/PD) data exist, a minimum of three studies are required. The first study is a single dose, randomized, crossover study under fasting conditions. The second is a single-dose, randomized, crossover study under fasting and nonfasting conditions with potential for maximum perturbation. If significant differences in bioavailability are found, it would be necessary to carry out additional studies to define the cause of the food effect and the effect of time

Table 4 Comparison of Dog and Human Gastrointestinal Physiology

Parameter	Human (70 kg)	Dog (10 kg)
Gastric acid secretion (mEq/h)	2.2 (female)	0.1
	3.7 (male)	
Intestinal pH (fed), beginning	5.4	6.2
Intestinal pH (fed), end	7.5	7.5
Periodicity of phase III MMC activity (min) (mean ± SE)	113.11 ± 11	106 ± 8
Cutoff size for emptying of multiple units (mm)	11–13	2–7
Stomach transit time (min)	78	96
Small intestine transit time (min) (mean ± SD)	180 ± 60	111 ± 17
Whole-gut transit time (min)	2350	770

MMC, migrating myoelectric (motor) complex.

on the food–drug effect. The third, definitive study should be a multiple-dose, steady-state, randomized, crossover study under fasting or nonfasting conditions. The in vivo bioequivalence studies for a generic version of an approved controlled release product are outlined in the FDA Guidance (37). First, the test product should be compared with the reference in a single-dose, randomized, two-period, two-sequence, crossover study under fasting conditions. The limited food effects study should follow a single-dose, three-treatment, three-period, six-sequence, crossover design, comparing equal doses of the test product administered under fasting conditions with those of the test and reference products given after a standard breakfast. The final study should be a multiple-dose, steady-state, two-treatment, two-period, two-sequence, crossover study under fasting conditions comparing the test and reference formulations. For safety reasons, this study may also be performed in the nonfasting state. In developing a controlled release dosage form of a new chemical entity for New Drug Application (NDA) submission, besides a clinical study, linearity of dose, food effects, and absorption characteristics must be characterized.

3. In Vivo Metrics

In bioequivalence studies, extent of absorption is usually evaluated by the area under the curve (AUC), which may be determined by linear trapezoidal summation or its combination with logarithmic trapezoidal summation. Parameters for assessing rate of absorption often include C_{max} and t_{max} obtained directly from the data without interpolation. However, C_{max} depends on both the rate and extent of absorption and is quite insensitive to changes in rate (55). t_{max} is unreliable because it only has discrete values depending on the sampling time and its frequency distribution is not normal. For controlled release products, use of t_{max} is further discouraged because formulations having the same or similar t_{max} values can have different release rates depending on the shape of plasma profiles. Other alternative measures of rate of absorption, such as C_{max}/AUC and C_{max}/AUC_{max}, have been proposed for immediate-release dosage forms under single dosing conditions and found to have advantages and limitations that depend on the kinetics of the drug and formulations (56).

In the statistical comparison of different products, the currently accepted criteria for equivalence require that the mean pharmacokinetic parameters (e.g., AUC and C_{max}) of the test product should be within 80–125% of the reference dosage form using a 90% confidence interval and the upper and lower bounds must be within the 90% confidence interval. Since many biological data are known to correspond more closely to a log-normal distribution than to a normal distribution, AUC and C_{max} are skewed and their variances tend to increase with the means. The usual assumptions of normality and variance homogeneity underlying the ANOVA may not be met. Therefore, a log transformation is often made on the derived pharmacokinetic parameters to make the variances independent of the mean and to make the frequency distribution more symmetrical. Using log transformation, the general linear statistical model applied in the analysis of data allows inferences about the difference between two means on the log scale, which can then be transformed to inferences about the ratio of two averages on the original scale (57).

The definitive in vivo studies of controlled release dosage forms are usually carried out in humans at steady state as required by the FDA (37,55). Reasons put forward for this include the following: (a) Controlled release products are often intended for chronic use. (b) Smaller intersubject variability has been found in steady-state studies that may permit the use of fewer subjects. (c) Steady-state results in higher plasma concentrations which need only be measured over a dosing interval. In assessing the steady-state performance of a controlled release dosage form, degree of fluctuation (DOF), or peak trough fluctuation ratio (PTC), is usually employed in addition to AUC and C_{max}:

$$DOF = \frac{C_{max} - C_{min}}{\overline{C}} \tag{17}$$

where $\overline{C} = \dfrac{AUC_{0-\tau}}{\tau}$ and τ is the dosing interval. It is a measure of maximum deviation during a dosing interval and an indirect measure of absorption rate. Reppas et al. (55) recently compared the performances of various in vivo metrics using simulated as well as actual data and found that most of the metrics, including C_{max}/AUC and C_{max}/AUC_{max}, do not provide reliable information about changes in the rate of absorption from controlled release dosage forms at steady state. Although DOF is a most sensitive measure, it is also the most imprecisely measured. Another potentially important parameter to consider is C_{min}. Based on our experiences, the FDA may also require evaluation of C_{min} at steady state for certain types of drugs. For example, a controlled release product may be required to meet the bioequivalence criteria of C_{min} similar to those set for C_{max} and AUC.

Other measures that have been proposed for assessing the in vivo performances of controlled release products involve assessment of duration of drug plasma levels or absorption profiles. For instance, retard quotients were used for screening and comparing controlled release formulations (58):

$$R_\Delta = \frac{HVD_{CR}}{HVD_{IR}} \tag{18}$$

where HVD (half-value duration) is defined as the time span for which the plasma concentration exceeds $1/2\ C_{max}$. R_Δ is independent of dose and quantifies the factor by which the HVD is prolonged for controlled release product relative to the IR product. However, it doesn't provide information regarding the duration within the therapeutic range. When the minimum effective of concentration of a given drug is not known, the trough level of an IR dosage regimen at steady state may be used instead. In 1983, Vallner et al. proposed controlled-release effectiveness (CRE) for comparing controlled release with IR dosage forms (59):

$$CRE = \frac{AUC_{\Delta C}^{CR}}{AUC_{\Delta C}^{IR}} \tag{19}$$

where $AUC_{\Delta C}^{CR}$ is the area within C_{max} and C_{min} limits over the dosing interval. This method is based on the assumption that a controlled release product should yield plasma levels that lie within the minimum and maximum levels produced by sequential doses of the IR product. Treatment equivalence can be demonstrated by the ratio near unity. Another parameter used to measure in vivo behavior of a controlled release dosage form is therapeutic occupancy time, defined as the length of time that a controlled release product produces drug levels within the therapeutic range at steady state. For a particular product and dosing frequency, it is dependent on dose and bioavailability, as well as other factors (e.g., variability in clearance). Therefore, a low occupancy time cannot necessarily be construed as indicative of poor product performance. It may represent only an inappropriate dosing regimen (58).

Direct examination of the entire in vivo time course of absorption is very important in the design and evaluation of a controlled release product. The cumulative amount or fraction absorbed in vivo estimated by deconvolution can provide useful information about in vivo release and absorption kinetics, intersubject variability in absorption, and correlation with in vitro release.

Finally, it should be noted that a known potential risk associated with controlled release dosage forms is dose dumping. Dose dumping is defined as the release of more than the usual fraction of drug or the release at a greater rate than the customary amount of drug per dosing interval such that potentially adverse plasma levels may be reached (58). It may be caused by a product's faulty manufacture or by its susceptibility to the influence of food or other variables in the GI tract. For drugs of which the therapeutic range is unknown, the relationship between relatively high drug levels and adverse effects cannot be accurately assessed. An evaluation of dose dumping may be based on a relative comparison with a reference product, i.e., the profile for the controlled release product should generally remain within the successively increasing peak and trough levels of the IR product over the interval t of the test controlled release product. In addition, the determination of dose dumping may also be based on deviation from a theoretically desirable rate of release and absorption (58).

4. In Vivo Variables

Due to drug release over an extended or the entire region of the GI tract, controlled release dosage forms are subject to a much wider range of physiological variables. Hence, higher variability in absorption is usually expected. The critical in vivo variables that affect the absorption from a controlled release dosage form include GI motility, gastric emptying, intestinal residence, blood flow, luminal contents, pH, GI mucus, gut flora, and first-pass metabolism, to name a few. One parameter that plays a key role in determining in vivo performance is the susceptibility of the controlled release device to physiological constraints created by transit through the GI tract. In view of the differences in the local environment and absorption capacity of the three sections of the GI tract, the duration of residence times of a controlled release product in each section can greatly affect its performance. Even if a product can be designed to release drug independently of the local environment, its performance may still be determined by the orocaecal transit time if the drug is not well absorbed in the colon. Therefore, the study of transit properties of dosage forms in the GI tract has received increased attention in the research and development of controlled release products in recent years. Scintigraphy techniques are used to monitor the integrity and fate of the dosage form in the GI tract and allow correlation between the location of the system and the resulting in vivo profile (33).

The residence time of any dosage form in the GI tract can be highly variable and unpredictably dependent on inter- and intrasubject variation, food effect, and type of dosage form. A basic review of GI motility and its relationship with the dosage form transit is helpful in designing a controlled release dosage form and understanding its in vivo behavior.

   (a) **Gastric Emptying.** In general, the variable residence times of a dosage form is a result of highly variable gastric emptying. Overnight and during daytime intervals between food, the stomach and small intestine exhibit a striking cycle of motility. Approximately every 90 min there is a brief (2–10 min) burst of intense muscle contraction that begins in the stomach and passes progressively along the small intestine to the distal ileum. This interdigestive cycle is designated as phase I (quiescence, basal), phase II (irregular activity, preburst), and phase III (intense burst of contractile activity). The passage of phase III from the stomach down the small bowel is known as the migrating myoelectric (motor) complex (MMC, or housekeeper effect) (60). The emptying of dosage forms is influenced by multiple chemical factors and physical size. It is also influenced by whether it is taken on an empty stomach (interdigestive state), or with or soon after a meal (digestive state). The emptying of solid dosage forms ranges from 5 min to over 5 h, depending on the size of the dosage form, the time of administration, and the time of the next housekeeper wave. Since the interval between two housekeeper contractions is highly variable from one individual to another, this further contributes to differences between subjects. It has been well documented that gastric emptying varies with different types of dosage forms. Examples of gastric residence times of single-unit tablets and multiparticulates are given in Tables 5–8 (61–65). It has been generally accepted that liquid emptying follows a monoexponential process and digestible solids empty in a linear fashion with time. The variable time to empty a single tablet is dependent on time of onset of MMC. The gastric emptying of a single-unit nondisintegrating dosage form is a simple all-or-none process, while the emptying of multiunit formulations is more complex (63). Gastric processing of multiunit formulations has been studied using beads of defined size. Following a heavy meal, test beads were emptied

Table 5 Gastrointestinal Transit Parameters of Hydrophilic Matrix Tablets Under Fasting Conditions (700 mg, 40% HPMC, oval with 19 mm length)

Subject	Gastric emptying (min)	Small intestine transit (min)	Colon arrival (min)
1	8	187	195
2	8	135	143
3	102	131	233
4	38	160	198
5	8	222	230
6	23	210	233
mean	**33**	**173**	**205**

Source: S. S. Davis et al. Int. J. Pharm., 94:235–238 (1993).

Table 6 Gastrointestinal Transit Times for Felodipine CR Hydrophilic Matrix

Section	Gastric emptying (h)		Small intestine transit (h)		Colon arrival (h)	
	Fasting	Fed	Fasting	Fed	Fasting	Fed
Mean	0.6	3.2	4.7	5.1	5.3	8.3
Range	0.1–1.1	1.9–4.8	3.9–5.9	2.2–7.7	4.0–7.0	6.0–11.0
p	<0.001		>0.05		<0.01	

Source: B. Abrahamsson et al. Pharm. Res. 10:709–714 (1993).

Table 7 Gastric Emptying Parameters of Multiparticulate Pellets (1.18–1.4 mm)

Subject		$t_{50\%}$ Emptied (min)		$t_{100\%}$ Emptied (min)	
Fasted	Fed	Fasted	Fed	Fasted	Fed
1	7	11	183	16	196
2	8	88	179	184	315
3	9	24	183	41	255
4	10	8	118	18	165
5	11	154	176	215	230
6	12	136	246	187	380
Mean		70	181	110	257
SE		27	17	38	32
P		0.005		0.015	

Source: K. H. Yuen et al. Int. J. Pharm., 97:61–77 (1993).

Table 8 Representative Data for Gastric Residence Times (GRT) of Various Sized Dosage Forms in the Fasted and Fed States in Humans

Dose size (mm)	State	GRT (min)
1	Fasted	60–150
3	Fasted	15–420
14	Fasted	15–210
1	Fed	101 (±53)
3.2	Fed	152 (±40)
9	Fed	105 to >600
14	Fed	180 to >780

Source: J. B. Dressman et al. Pharm. Res., 15: 11–22 (1998).

more slowly than in a lightly fed state. The timing of bead administration relative to eating has no influence on the emptying rate (63). Beads dosed before, during, and after a meal were shown to have similar half-lives of emptying. Furthermore, beads dosed predispersed with food emptied at the same rate as those taken in a capsule. The distribution of the beads in the stomach depends on their surface characteristics. In general, the beads were emptied as a series of small boluses. It has also been reported that some volunteers were consistently rapid emptiers, whereas some were consistently slow emptiers (63).

When food is ingested, the interdigestive cycle is inhibited. It is replaced by a prolonged period of irregular, mild to moderate activity (>1 h). It delays the onset of the MMC that is necessary for emptying of large, indigestible spheres or tablets. Davis et al. showed that 0.8- to 1.1-mm beads and an 8-mm tablet exited from the stomach in a wide time range when taken 1 h after a fatty meal (61). It was suggested that items approximately 7 mm in size may exit during the digestive state, while larger items definitely require phase III motor activity. During the digestive state, larger dosage forms are retained in the stomach until the meal is essentially emptied. Furthermore, the stomach can discriminate between particles of less than 2 mm in diameter and digestible food. Coupe et al. showed that in the fed state, beads in the size range 0.8–1.1 mm diameter reside in the base of the stomach away from antral flow. Emptying only occurs when the stomach becomes nearly empty and the contractions both increase in force and originate further up the stomach. However, beads can resist these contractions and are then emptied later with phase II and III contractions of the MMC (63).

In summary, the stomach represents a complex system that differentiates between differences in density, size, and meal composition. The emptying process of dosage forms cannot be described by one mechanism. Many processes are probably involved that may vary both within and between subjects. The in vivo data of controlled release dosage forms should not be interpreted solely based on a mean curve when the individual data are clearly different. The individual curves may describe several different patterns of gastric emptying. Once the mean curve was plotted, such features may no longer be apparent.

(b) Small Intestinal Transit. According to Davis et al., transit times through the small intestine generally varied between 1 and 6 h. Liquids, small solids (beads, small tablets), and larger capsule-sized units moved essentially at the same rates and the transit is unaffected by food status (61). An example of small intestinal transit (SIT) of a multiparticulate dosage form is given in Table 9 (64). Some evidence suggests that terminal ileum can store residue between meals and that the eating of a subsequent meal stimulates the emptying of ileal contents into the colon. The presence of dietary residues in the ileum, especially fat and carbohydrate, can stimulate mechanisms by which gastric emptying and transit through the upper small intes-

Table 9 Numerical Values of Cecum Arrival and Small Intestinal Transit Time of Multiparticulate Pellets (1.18–1.4 mm)

Subject		$t_{50\%}$ arrival (min)		Small intestine transit time (min)	
Fasted	Fed	Fasted	Fed	Fasted	Fed
1	7	239	318	228	135
2	8	390	413	302	234
3	9	342	388	318	205
4	10	244	412	236	294
5	11	279	454	125	278
6	12	425	503	289	257
Mean		320	415	250	234
SE		32	25	29	24
P		0.042		0.681	

Source: K. H. Yuen et al. Int. J. Pharm., 97:61–77 (1993).

tine is slowed. In a more recent study concerning dosing in relation to the timing of food intake, Digenis et al. found that although SIT is relatively independent of food and dosage form, it was actually shortened significantly if the dose is given 30 min before food intake. This can have adverse impact on the in vivo performance of the dosage forms (66).

(c) Colonic Transit. In the stomach and small intestine, food residue and endogenous secretions are exposed to an essentially sterile environment through which their transit can be measured by hours. On entering the large intestine, dosage forms encounter a rich bacterial flora and transit through the large intestine can be as long as several days. It was reported that overall mean transit time is 36 h with a range of 1 to 72 h and that the transit of liquids and small solids is equal (67). Thus, absorption from colon may be incomplete and erratic depending on the dose and physicochemical properties of a particular drug. In general, absorption of an insoluble drug with high dose or a drug with limited permeability is unfavorable in this region because of the limited volume of fluid available for dissolution and the significantly reduced surface area.

5. Relationship Between Pharmacokinetics and Pharmacodynamics

The basic goal in the development of controlled release dosage forms is to achieve optimal drug treatment through rate and time programmed drug delivery (68). However, the major emphasis in the design of controlled release products is, in many cases, placed on reducing the dosing frequency or fluctuation of plasma concentrations (pharmacokinetics) associated with IR formulations, rather than on the improved pharmacological effect profile (pharmacodynamics). As a result, it is not uncommon to see new drug delivery systems looking for a suitable drug candidate (68). This can be attributed to the often overly simplified linear PK/PD relationship, as well as to the fact that the PK consequences of controlled drug delivery are generally well understood and easy to monitor. In reality, the relationship between systemic drug concentration (C) and intensity of effect (E) is often nonlinear as described by a sigmoidal E_{max} model (69). Thus, different fluctuations in pharmacological response (ΔE) may result from the same or similar concentration changes (ΔC) depending on different concentration ranges (69). In addition, the slow and constant mode of drug input provided by controlled release dosage forms may have varying therapeutic impacts depending on different drugs and PK/PD relationships. Furthermore, the time course of drug effects can be quite different from the time course of drug concentrations. A short elimination half-life will not necessarily imply short duration of action (68). Therefore, the design of release characteristics from a controlled release product should be based on the desired optimal drug concentration time profile defined by the quantitative information of the PK/PD relationship, i.e., information on the kinetics of drug effects and its potential dependence on the rate and time of drug input.

The importance of using integrated PK/PD and clinical research strategies in the design of an optimal drug delivery regimen has been emphasized with examples by Breimer (68). More recently, a thorough review was published by Hoffman on the therapeutic and safety implications of the complex relationship between drug input and pharmacodynamics (69). For instance, the shape factor (n) which determines the slope of the E-C curve based on an E_{max} model can have significant impact on the design of a controlled release system. A relatively shallow E-C profile (small n) may suggest a lack of pharmacodynamic rationale to develop a controlled release product because E is relatively insensitive to even a large change in concentration. When the concentration range required to elicit drug response is very small (large n), such as for levodopa, the E-C profile represents an all-or-none phenomenon. Thus, as long as the drug concentrations remain above MEC, the drug effect is essentially independent of the fluctuation in plasma levels. The impact of input rate on the efficacy and safety ratio is best illustrated by the classical example of nifedipine. Comparative studies of slow vs. rapid input have led to the realization and confirmation that the rate of increase of nifedipine concentration, rather than absolute concentration, is the determining factor for the observed haemodynamic effects, i.e., gradual decrease in blood pressure was observed without side effect (increase in heart rate) occurring with the slow regimen, while the opposite was observed with the rapid regimen (68). It is known that the non-steady-state E-C curves of certain drugs may exhibit clockwise or counterclockwise hysteresis due to desensitization or equilibrium delay and formation of an active metabolite. In the former case, either pulsatile or constant rate input may be designed depending on the desired pharmacological responses of the drugs (e.g., gonadotropin-releasing hormone) (69). On the other hand, a slow input rate may minimize the counterclockwise hysteresis and thus require lower C_{max} to achieve the desired response. Methylphenidate is another example whereby rate of delivery can have a significant impact on the efficacy of the drug. To overcome the acute tolerance acquired from administering the commercial sustained release product (Ritalin SR), a new controlled release dosage form with constantly ascending release rate was designed and clinically proven to be effective with less adverse effects (70).

IV. PRODUCT AND PROCESS DEVELOPMENT

A. System Design Considerations

Each drug possesses inherent properties that require considerations specific to that drug and its dosage forms. A defined therapeutic rationale, the drug's biological properties, and physicochemical characteristics must be integrated for rational development of controlled release formulations (71). The basic therapeutic rationale of a controlled release product is that it must offer one or more advantages in efficacy, safety, and patient compliance. The required drug input rate and pharmacokinetic properties of the drug determine the design of the controlled release products. The physicochemical characterization is similar to that required for IR product. However, it becomes more critical because properties of a drug not only affect the absorption but also influence the design of the delivery system. For example, for a drug with low solubility, an erodible matrix system may be more effective than a diffusion system where the release driving force is concentration gradient. On the other hand, a diffusion-controlled system would be more appropriate for soluble drugs. A drug with pH-dependent solubility may have low solubility in

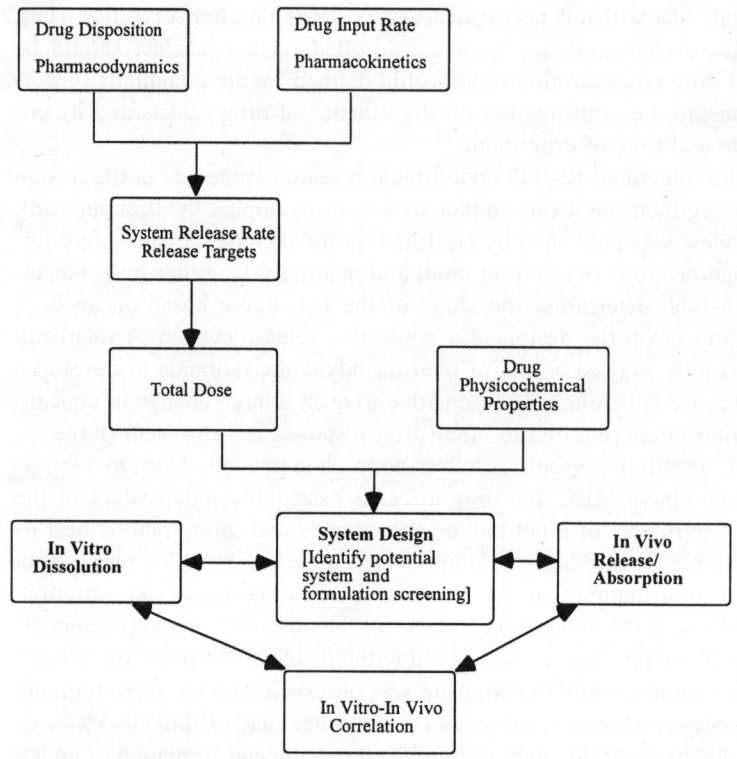

Figure 1 Stages in the design of a controlled release dosage form.

the specific sites of absorption. In this case, a pH-independent release system or a system that may be retained in the area preceding absorption may be desirable.

1. Therapeutic Demand

In principle, the design of a controlled release dosage form should be based on the clinical needs and typically involves several stages as described in Fig. 1 (71). In some cases, a demand can arise to satisfy specific clinical requirements, such as delivery of the drug during a particular chronological cycle. It was reported that many patients with myocardial infarction exhibit a clinical incidence of this syndrome that shows a circadian distribution with high frequency in the morning hours between 4:00 a.m. and 9:00 a.m. (72–74). Hence, a once-daily controlled release system that provides a higher blood level during this time period is desired. In most other cases, however, the desired drug input into the body is zero order in order to obtain a constant plasma level within therapeutic windows.

In many cases, the most important goal in successful design of a controlled release system is to maintain plasma concentrations above the MEC during a dosing interval. Critical factors determining the duration above MEC include intrinsic clearance ($t_{1/2}$ and V_d), levels of MEC, kinetics of drug input, extent of absorption, window of absorption, GI physiology, and residence time of the dosage form at the site of absorption. Rational design that takes into account these factors should result in fewer development iterations, reduced number of failed formulations, and accelerated product development. Two of these factors that are extrinsic to a particular drug and can be altered during the system design process are extent of absorption and kinetics of input (linear vs. nonlinear). The key to a successful formulation design is to achieve the optimal rate of absorption with a minimal decrease in the extent of absorption.

2. Drug Properties

The physicochemical characteristics of the drug, in particular its aqueous solubility, should first be considered in the selection of an appropriate delivery mechanism. Recommended polymer delivery systems based on drug aqueous solubility are summarized in Table 10. Other drug properties affecting system design include drug stability in the system and at the site of absorption, pH dependency of the solubility, particle size, and specific surface area. These will be addressed in a later section of this chapter.

In practice, either of the two single-unit systems (matrix and reservoir) should be able to provide linear or near-linear controlled release for most compounds. However, if a multiparticulate dosage form is desired, release kinetics will vary depending on the selected systems. The drug release profile from a multiparticulate hydrophobic matrix (e.g., wax matrix) generally exhibits a high degree of curvature. This results from the decreasing surface area with time. In theory, coated multiparticles can be used if constant rate of drug release is desired to reduce fluctuations and to provide extra duration of plasma concentrations over MEC. But in reality the feasibility of using a reservoir system is limited by the properties of the compound. Based on steady-state diffusion, the time (T) required to release the entire dose (M_t) from a multiunit spherical reservoir system can be estimated with the following rearranged equation:

$$T = \frac{M_t L}{SDPC_s} \tag{20}$$

where L is the apparent diffusion thickness including coating and unstirred layer, S is the total surface area of the particles, D is diffusion coefficient in water, P is the partition coefficient, and C_s is the solubility. For a multiparticulate system (e.g., beads), the total surface area, S, is:

$$S = NA = \frac{4V}{3r} \tag{21}$$

where N is the number of beads in a dosage form with a total volume of V, A is the surface area of a single bead with the radius of r. For a given drug, M_t, L, D, P, C_s, and V can be assumed to be constant. The time (T) required to release the entire dose (M_t) from a multiunit spherical

Table 10 Recommendations to Polymer Delivery System

Polymer delivery system	Drug release mechanism	Drugs not recommended
Matrix systems		
Hydrophilic:		
Swellable/erodible	Diffusion and erosion	Very soluble
Erodible	Erosion	Freely soluble
Hydrophobic:		
Monolithic	Diffusion	Practically insoluble
Multiparticulate	Diffusion	Freely soluble
Erodible/Degradable	Erosion/enzymatic Degradation of polymer	—
Reservoir systems	Diffusion	Practically insoluble
Osmotic pumps		
Elementary	Osmotic pressure	Practically insoluble
Two-chamber	Osmotic pressure	—

reservoir system should be directly proportional to the bead size (radius) as described by the following equation:

$$T = kr \tag{22}$$

$$\frac{T_1}{T_2} = \frac{r_1}{r_2} \tag{23}$$

where k is a constant. In designing a multiparticulate reservoir system (coated beads) for a slightly soluble drug (see Tables 11 and 12), the time to release the entire dose from coated beads with a radius of 250 μm is 36.5 h according to Eq. 20 because of the limited solubility/dose ratio. This may result in incomplete release within the desired 24-h dosing interval. Based on Eqs. 22 and 23, the time to release the entire dose of the same drug can be adjusted by changing the particle size. For example, T can be reduced to 29.2 h and 21.9 h, respectively, if particle sizes (r) of 200 μm and 150 μm are used with coating thickness unchanged. Thus, the potential incomplete absorption from the coated beads of 250 μm can be overcome by using smaller particles or by reducing the coating thickness. It should be noted that perfect coating on uniform spheres is assumed in this example. In reality, drug release time may be shortened because of nonideal coating and size distribution.

3. Impact of Release Kinetics and Extent of Absorption

Incomplete absorption from controlled release dosage forms, although not uncommon, is undesirable because it can result in a controlled release product that is non-bioequivalent to the IR counterpart, and it may also lead to shortened duration above MEC. The potential causes for reduced bioavailability of controlled release dosage forms may include (a) increased extraction due to saturable first-pass metabolism, (b) decreased absorption in the lower GI tract (due to less fluid, lower surface area, and bacterial metabolism), (c) incomplete release from the dosage form, and (d) extending drug release beyond the "window" of absorption. The relationships among the designed drug release kinetics, absorption characteristics, and duration above MEC at steady state are shown in Fig. 2 using the relevant parameters in Table 12. In generating the graphs, three different release or absorption characteristics are considered and a 1:1 IVIVC is assumed. The results clearly indicate that zero-order or near-zero-order release (release II) not

Table 11 Relevant Parameters of a Given Compound for Estimation of Release Duration from a Multiparticulate Controlled Release System

Mt (mg)	500
Cs (μg/mL)	1
h (μm)	25
A (cm^2)	159
D (cm/s)	1×10^{-7}
K	1
Density (g/cm^3)	0.9

Table 12 Properties of a Hypothetical Drug

Design objective	Once-daily controlled release dosage form
Physicochemical properties	Solubility = 1 mg/mL (pH-independent); stable and permeable
Biopharmaceutical properties	$t_{1/2}$ = 8 h; V/F = 200 L; F = 80%
Therapeutic properties	Dose = 500 mg; MEC = 0.5 μg/mL

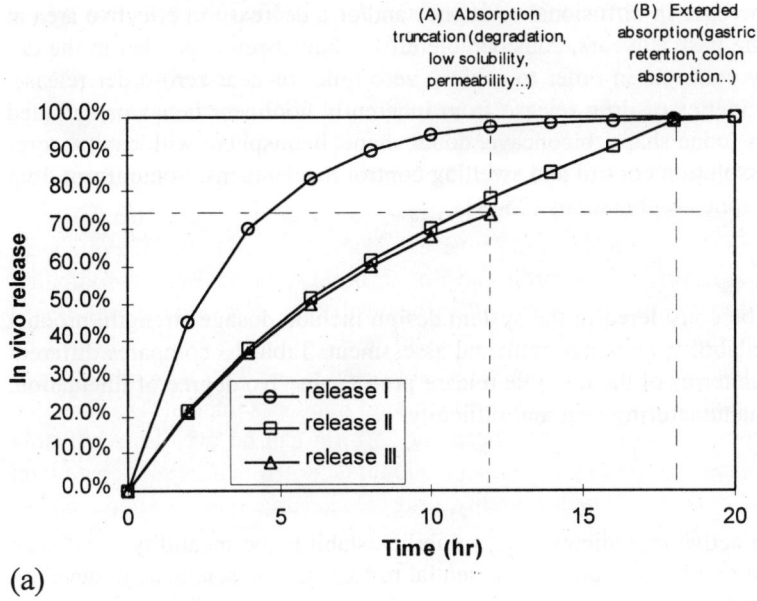

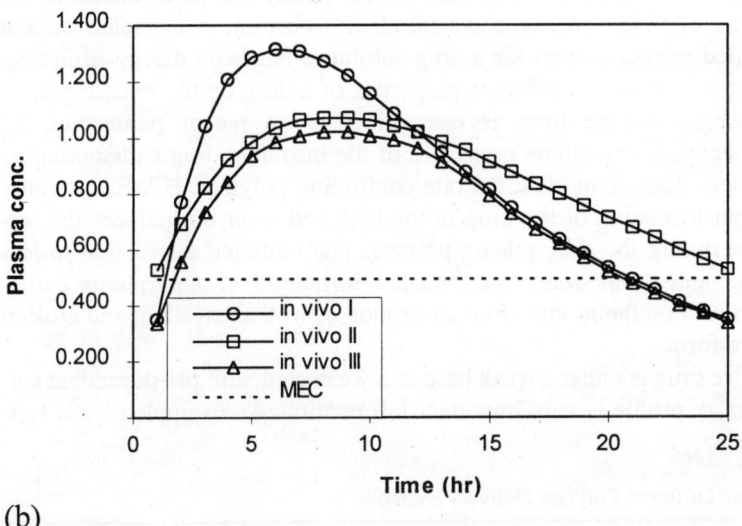

Figure 2 Relationship between absorption "window" and designed release rate for a hypothetical drug.

only reduces the peak-to-trough ratio of the in vivo plasma concentration but also provides longer duration above MEC when compared with the non-zero-order release (release I) over an absorption duration of 18 h. However, if the in vivo absorption is only limited to 12 h due to truncation and the designed release rate remains unchanged (release III), then a significantly decreased AUC and shortened duration above MEC would be expected. Hence, customized design of an optimal release rate with minimum loss of bioavailability via the intelligent matching of the rate of drug release to the site(s) of drug absorption for a specific drug is not only critical but also challenging in the formulation development of controlled release products.

In many diffusion-controlled matrix systems, drug release behavior is inherently nonlinear in nature, with a continuously diminishing release rate. This is a result of decreasing release rate with time due to an increase in diffusional resistance and/or a decrease in effective area at the diffusion front. Over the past 30 years, considerable efforts have been expended in the development of new delivery concepts in order to achieve zero-order or near-zero-order release. Examples of altering the kinetics of drug release from inherently nonlinear behavior included the use of geometry factors (cone shape, biconcave, donut shape, hemisphere with cavity, core-in-cup, etc.), erosion or dissolution control and swelling control mechanisms, nonuniform drug loading, and matrix–membrane combinations (75–83).

4. Other Factors

Other factors that need to be considered in the system design include dosage strength, product manufacturability, cost, scalability, and environmental assessment. Table 13 compares different polymer delivery systems in terms of the possible release profiles, in vivo degree of fluctuation, duration of above MEC, manufacturing cost and difficulty.

B. Preformulation

Preformulation data for the active ingredients (e.g., solubility, stability, permeability, solid-state properties, and compatibility with excipients) are essential to formulation scientists in developing stable, safe, and effective dosage forms. This type of information can provide a rational basis for the formulation approaches, maximize the chances of success in developing an acceptable product, and ultimately provide a basis for optimizing the quality and performance of the product. The importance of a complete physicochemical characterization in the selection and rational design of a controlled release system for a drug substance has been discussed in Sec. III. A and IV. A. The potential impact of solid-state properties of a drug on the release performance of a controlled release dosage form is exemplified by a recent publication by Katzhendler et al. (84). In studying crystalline properties of the insoluble drug carbamazepine in a hydrophilic matrix system, they found that the rate-controlling polymer, HPMC, not only inhibits the polymorphic transformation of the drug in the hydrated layer but induces the formation of amorphous phase during the drug release process. The inhibited conversion to less soluble dihydrate from the anhydrous form and induced formation of amorphous carbamazepine can have direct impact on the in vivo drug absorption as well as swelling and erosion characteristics of the dosage form.

In most cases, the active drug is either a weak base or a weak acid with pH-dependent solubility. Thus, the pH–solubility profile is very important information. An example of this type

Table 13 Comparison Among Different Polymer Delivery Systems

Polymer delivery system	Release kinetics	In vivo degree of fluctuation	Duration above MEC	Manufacturing cost and difficulty
Matrix systems				
Hydrophilic	Varies[a]	Low–high	Long—short	Low
Hydrophobic	Varies[b]	Low–high	Long—short	Low—medium
Monolithic	Non-zero-order	Higher	Shorter	Medium
Reservoir systems	Near-zero-order	Lower	Longer	Medium—high
Osmotic pumps	Zero-order	Lower	Longer	High

[a]Dependent on solubility and dose.
[b]Mostly non-zero-order, depending on whether the device is erodible and whether it is a single unit or multiparticulate.

of compound is etodolac, a nonsteroidal anti-inflammatory drug indicated for the management of the signs and symptoms of osteoarthritis and rheumatoid arthritis. It is very slightly soluble below pH 3. The solubility increases gradually with pH up to 5 followed by a 30-fold increase at pH 7. To minimize the dependency of its solubility on pH, a release rate–modifying agent (e.g., dibasic sodium phosphate) was incorporated into the controlled release tablet formulation, Lodine XL, to enhance drug release in the acidic environment (85). However, the effectiveness of this approach often depends on the properties of the drug and the release-modifying agent, as well as the ratio of drug to release-modifying excipient. For example, in a diffusion-controlled matrix system, a small inorganic molecule (e.g., dicalcium phosphate) that is soluble at low pH can leach out of the viscous gel layer fairly rapidly, resulting in limited change of the pH in the gel over the extended duration of drug release. Thus, it is important to design a system that retains the release-modifying agent in a delivery device.

The stability of drug in the solid state is essential information in formulation development. It was reported that bupropion hydrochloride, an antidepressant, undergoes extensive degradation in an alkaline environment. To develop an acceptable controlled release solid dosage form, weak acids or salts of strong acids are used as stabilizers in the formulation, such as citric acid, tartaric acid, ascorbic acid, L-cystine hydrochloride, and glycine hydrochloride. These stabilizers serve to provide an acidic environment surrounding the active drug that prevents its decomposition (86).

C. Formulation and Process Development

In this section, controlled release tablets and capsules of verapamil hydrochloride (soluble) and nifedipine (insoluble) are used to illustrate the formulation and process development aspects of oral controlled release delivery systems

1. Verapamil Hydrochloride Controlled Release Systems

Verapamil, a calcium channel blocker, is indicated for the management of essential hypertension. Verapamil hydrochloride is a water-soluble compound. It is well absorbed (>90%) with the elimination half-life ranging from 2.8 to 7.4 h. These basic properties indicate that all three release mechanisms, i.e., diffusion, erosion, and osmotic pressure, may be applied to the design of controlled release dosage forms of this compound. Presently there are three types of once-daily oral controlled release products available commercially: matrix tablets (Isoptin SR), a reservoir system (Verelan capsules), and an osmotic pump (Covera-HS tablets).

(a) **Matrix Tablets.** Several U.S. patents have been issued for controlled release matrix systems of verapamil. It was reported that Isoptin SR tablets were designed based on alginates, a pH-dependent gelling polymer (87). Since sodium alginate is insoluble in water at pH below 3, drug release from the matrix tablets is pH-dependent as shown in Fig. 3.

At low pH (e.g., pH 1.2), sodium alginate at the tablet surface converts to insoluble alginic acid and loses its ability to swell and to form a viscous gel layer that is critical in controlling drug release. In the dissolution vessels, it was found that stress cracks were created on the tablet surface, allowing undesirable drug diffusion via water filled cracks. To overcome this problem, Howard and Timmins of Squibb invented a new controlled release matrix system of verapamil by incorporating pH-independent polymer in the alginate-based formulation (88). In an acidic environment (e.g., stomach), the pH-independent polymer (e.g., HPMC) hydrates to form a gel layer at the surface of the tablet. Drug dissolves in the gel layer and slowly diffuses into the surrounding aqueous environment. As the pH increases with passage of the tablets from the stomach to the intestinal tract, the alginate in the tablets starts to swell and form a hydrogel

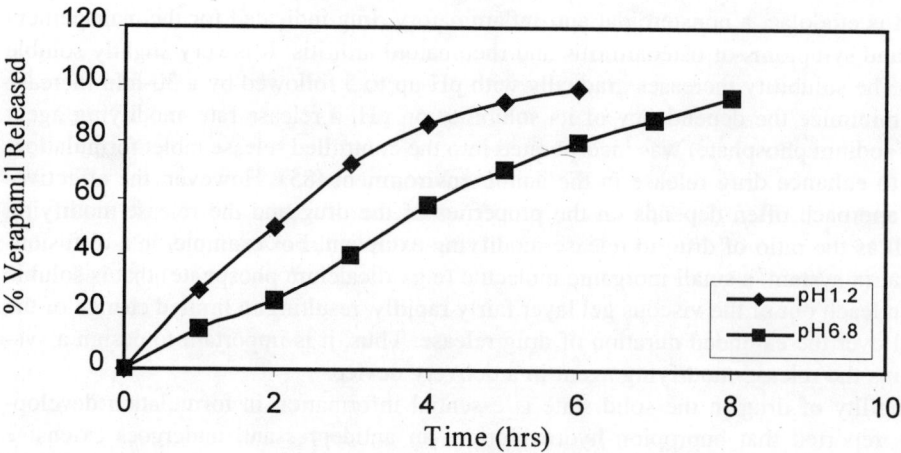

Figure 3 Effect of pH of dissolution medium on verapamil release from alginate-based tablets.

contributing to the overall barrier to drug diffusion and matrix erosion. Drug release from this system is independent of pH. In some cases, a zero-order release profile for up to 80% of the dose can be obtained with such a system.

One of the potential shortcomings of this type of design is that at a high pH, the drug release rate may decrease with time due to the reduction of surface area by system erosion. To design a more rugged pH-independent zero-order controlled release system, Zhang and Pinnamaraju of Duramed Pharmaceuticals recently invented a matrix system consisting of three different types of polymers: (a) an alginate component, such as sodium alginate; (b) an enteric polymer, such as methacrylic acid copolymer; and (c) a pH-independent polymer, such as HPMC (89). It was demonstrated that drug release from this system is pH-independent. At higher pH, the decreasing release rate due to the change in surface area is compensated for by dissolution of the enteric polymer in the matrix, thus maintaining a constant dissolution rate. The results of zero-order release from both types of system designs are shown in Fig. 4. A zero-order release profile can be obtained for up to nearly 100% of drug release with the three-polymer system design.

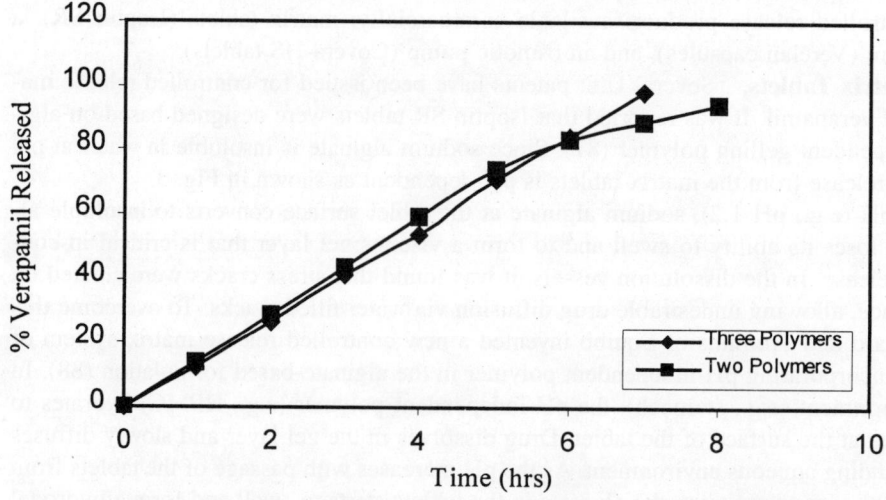

Figure 4 Comparison of drug release from a three-polymer matrix and a two-polymer matrix.

(b) **Reservoir System.** Drug release from a reservoir delivery system is predominantly controlled by diffusion. In this type of system, water permeates the coated dosage form through a membrane followed by dissolution of the drug and diffusion through a network of capillaries filled with aqueous medium or a homogeneous film barrier. In general, drug release from a reservoir delivery system is less pH-dependent. A controlled release capsule of verapamil hydrochloride, Verelan, developed by Elan Corporation, contains a mixture of rapid and slow-release coated beads (90). The manufacturing processes for coated beads include (a) preparation of core beads and (b) film coating of the beads as follows:

(a) Formulation and preparation of core beads:

Sugar/starch seeds (0.4–0.5 mm)	9 kg
Verapamil hydrochloride	30 kg
Malic acid	10 kg
Talc	2.4 kg
Hydroxypropylmethylcellulose suspension in methanol/methylene chloride (60:40)	5%

Preparation of core beads was performed in a standard coating pan using the layering coating technology discussed previously. The spherical seeds were first thoroughly dampened with sufficient polymer suspension followed by dusting of a portion of the powder blend of the active drug until no more adhesions occurred. The coated seeds were allowed to dry after each application of polymer suspension. This step was repeated until all of the powder blend was applied. The last step involves the drying of the coated beads to an acceptable level of moisture content.

(b) Formulation and preparation of membrane coating:

5% Hydroxypropylmethylcellulose suspension in methanol/methylene chloride (60:40)	2 parts
5% Ethylcellulose in methanol/methylene chloride (60:40)	8 parts
Talc	5 parts

The membrane coating process was performed in a standard coating pan by spraying the coating suspension onto the core beads.

The final commercial capsules contain 20% of the core beads and 80% of the membrane-coated beads. The dissolution profile in Fig. 5 indicates that the drug release from this system is pH-independent.

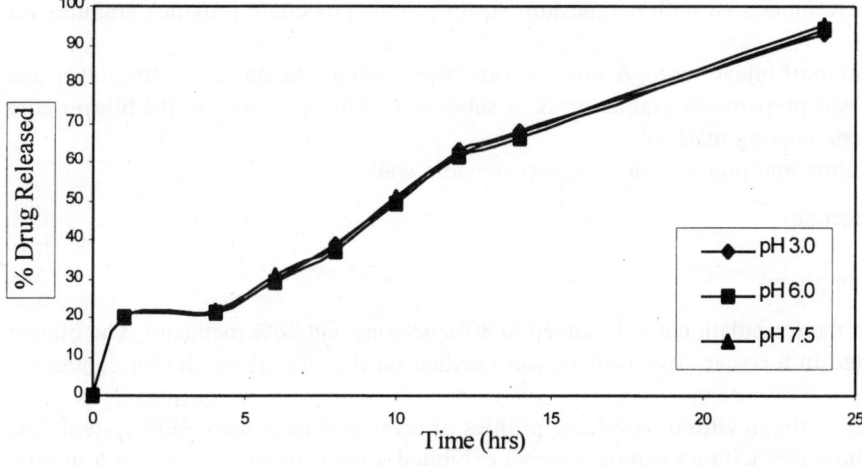

Figure 5 Dissolution profiles of verapamil capsules in different pH media.

(c) Osmotic Pump. In general, high blood pressure for many patients with myocardial infarction often occurs during morning hours from 4:00 a.m. to 9:00 a.m. Ideally, a formulation of verapamil may be designed to be administered at bedtime and to initiate the drug release 4–5 h after ingestion. Covera-HS tablet developed by Alza and marketed by G. D. Searle is a two-chamber OROS Push-Pull osmotic system that consists of an active drug core and an osmotic push compartment. The device is designed to provide delayed initial drug release by an extra coating layer between the tablet core and outer semipermeable membrane. As water in the GI tract enters the tablet, this subcoating is solubilized and released. As tablet hydration continues, the osmotic layer expands and pushes against the active drug layer, releasing the drug through precision laser-drilled orifices in the outer membrane at a constant rate. This controlled rate of drug delivery in the GI tract is independent of posture, pH, GI motility, and fed or fasting conditions. The biologically inert components of the delivery system remain intact during transit through the GI tract and are eliminated in the feces as an insoluble shell.

A controlled release osmotic device containing verapamil intended for dosing at bedtime for releasing verapamil to coincide with an early-morning rise of blood pressure associated with hypertension and angina is prepared by the following steps (91–93):

(a) Formulation and preparation of active drug layer:

Verapamil hydrochloride	600 g
Poly(ethylene oxide)	305 g
Sodium chloride	40 g
Polyvinylpyrrolidone	50 g
Magnesium stearate	5 g

All ingredients except magnesium stearate were granulated with anhydrous ethyl alcohol. The dried granules were lubricated with magnesium stearate. This procedure provides granules for the active drug layer.

(b) Formulation and preparation of osmotic layer:

Poly(ethylene oxide)	735 g
Sodium chloride	200 g
Hydroxypropylmethylcellulose (Methocel E5)	50 g
Ferric oxide	10 g
Magnesium stearate	5 g

All ingredients except magnesium stearate were granulated with anhydrous ethyl alcohol. The dried granules were lubricated with magnesium stearate. This procedure provides granules for the osmotic layer.

(c) Preparation of bilayer core: A bilayer core tablet comprising an active drug layer and an osmotic layer was prepared in a tablet press. A subcoat may be applied on to the bilayer core tablets using enteric coating material.

(d) Formulation and preparation of semipermeable wall:

Cellulose acetate	55%
Hydroxypropylcellulose	40%
Polyethylene glycol	5%

All ingredients in the formulation are dissolved in 80% acetone and 20% methanol. The bilayer tablets were coated in a coater. Two orifices were drilled on the side of the device containing the active drug.

Figure 6 shows the in vitro drug release profiles of verapamil from the OROS system. The dosage form without and with an enteric subcoat exhibited a lag time of 1.5 and 3.0 h in drug release, respectively, followed by zero-order controlled release of verapamil.

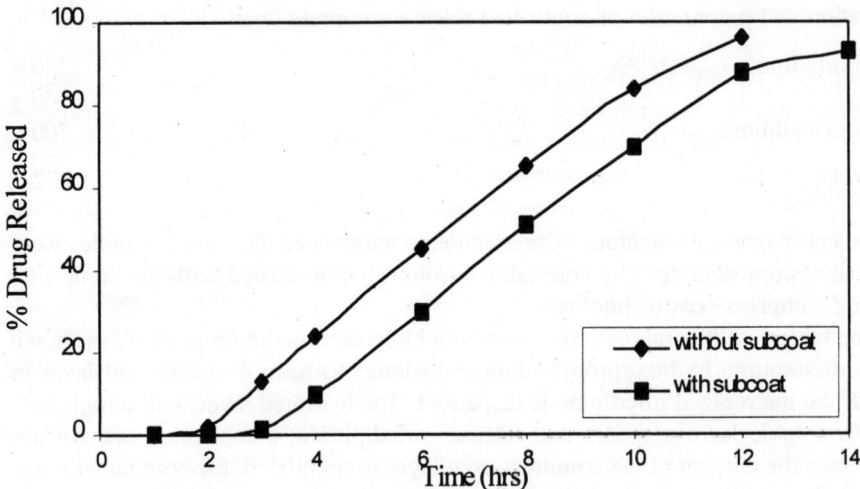

Figure 6 Dissolution profiles of verapamil from osmotic pump system with and without enteric subcoat.

2. *Nifedipine Controlled Release Systems*

Nifedipine is another antihypertension drug in the class of the calcium channel blockers. It is practically insoluble in water with an elimination half-life of approximately 2 h. Oral absorption of nifedipine is known to be proportional to the dose. Due to its poor aqueous solubility, the drug is usually micronized to increase the specific surface area for enhanced drug absorption. Based on the properties of nifedipine, a controlled release dosage form can be designed utilizing erosion-and osmotic pressure–controlled mechanisms. In fact, there are two types of once-daily commercial oral controlled release delivery systems: matrix tablets (Adalat CC tablets) and an osmotic pump (Procardia XL tablets).

(a) **Osmotic Pump System.** The controlled release osmotic pump system for nifedipine consists of an osmotically active drug core tablet surrounded by a semipermeable membrane. The core itself is divided into two layers: (a) an active drug layer and (b) an osmotic push layer. The compositions and principles for developing the controlled release osmotic system for nifedipine are similar to those for verapamil (Covera HS). The tablet was designed to release drug at a constant rate over 24 h.

(b) **Matrix Tablets—Compress-Coated System.** A controlled release matrix system of nifedipine for dosing at bedtime was developed to release nifedipine to coincide with the early-morning rise in blood pressure associated with hypertension and angina. This was achieved using a design that slowly delivers one portion of the drug from the compress coat followed by rapid release of the remaining dose from the tablet core (94):

(a) Formulation and preparation of IR core tablets:

Micronized nifedipine	50 g
Lactose	388 g
Corn starch	150 g
Microcrystalline cellulose	50 g
Magnesium stearate	2 g

All ingredients except microcrystalline cellulose and magnesium stearate were granulated with water. The dried granules were blended with microcrystalline cellulose and magnesium stearate followed by compression into the core tablets. An optional enteric coating may be applied to the core tablets.

(b) Formulation and preparation of controlled release compress coat:

Micronized nifedipine	250 g
Lactose	400 g
Hydroxypropylcellulose	700 g
Citric acid	320 g
Magnesium stearate	27 g

All ingredients except magnesium stearate were granulated with water. The dried granules were lubricated with magnesium stearate. The core tablets from (a) were coated with the compress-coat granules using compress-coat technology.

The resulting tablets with compress coats exhibit a biphasic dissolution profiles, as shown in Fig. 7. During dissolution, hydroxypropylcellulose hydrates to form a viscous gel layer in which a portion of the micronized nifedipine is dispensed. The hydrated layer with a high concentration of water-soluble lactose erodes and releases nifedipine at a controlled rate for approximately 8 h. Once the erosion of the compress-coat layer is completed, the core tablet is exposed to the dissolution medium, resulting in an immediate release of the remaining dose.

V. POSTAPPROVAL CHANGES

Following the successful launch of a new product, it is not uncommon for development scientists to make continuous efforts to improve its quality or to reduce its manufacturing cost. The modifications typically involve changes in the formulation components or composition, the site of manufacturing, scale-up or scale-down of the manufacturing process and/or equipment. The issues involved in these changes of controlled release products are different and usually more complex than their IR counterparts. Thus, the FDA issued a separate guidance on the scale-up and postapproval changes (SUPAC) for modified-release solid dosage forms in September 1997 (95). Based on fundamental pharmaceutical principles and the scientific database, acceptable ranges of these changes are defined and categorized into three different levels depending on their likelihood of having significant impact on the product quality and performance. Additional in-process

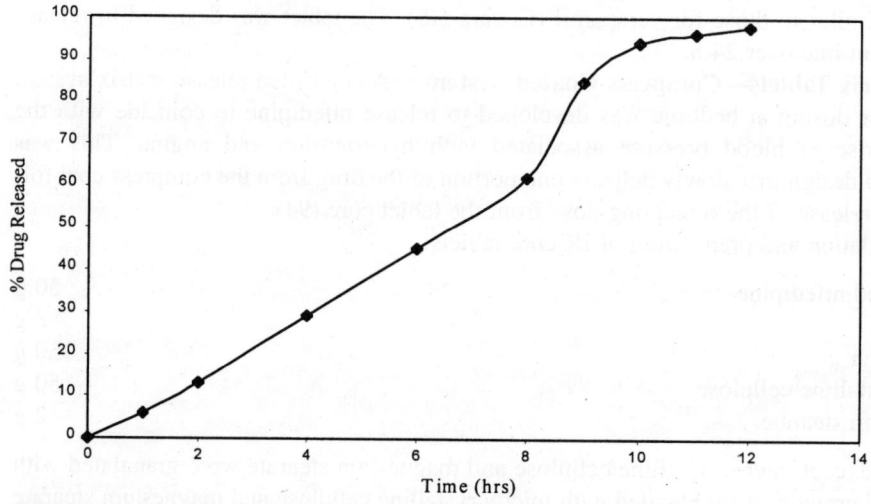

Figure 7 Dissolution profile of nifedipine from compress-coated tablets.

and finished product control parameters are also specified for use in supporting these changes. Formulation and process changes discussed in this section are mostly based on SUPAC Guidance for modified-release solid oral dosage forms published by the Center for Drug Evaluation Research, Food and Drug Administration.

A. Formulation Changes

For modified-release solid dosage forms, consideration should be given as to whether the excipient is critical or not critical to drug release.

1. Nonrelease-Controlling Excipient

Three levels of changes for nonrelease-controlling excipients are defined as follows:

1. Level 1 changes are those that are unlikely to have any detectable impact on formulation quality and performance.
2. Level 2 changes are those that could have a significant impact on formulation quality and performance.
3. Level 3 changes are those that are likely to have a detectable impact on formulation quality and performance.

Table 14 summarizes the changes, test documentation, and filing documentation required for nonrelease-controlling excipient changes.

Table 14 Nonrelease-Controlling Excipient Changes

Factor	Level 1	Level 2	Level 3
Filler	±5%	±10%	Beyond level 2 changes
Disintegrant:			
Starch	±3%	±3%	
Other	±1%	±1%	
Binder	±0.5%	±1%	
Lubricant:			
Ca or Mg stearate	±0.25%	±0.25%	
Other	±1%	±1%	
Glidant:			
Talc	±1%	±1%	
Other	±0.1%	±0.1%	
Film coat	±1%	±2%	
Test documentation			
Chemistry	Annual report on stability (one lot)	Supplement with 3 months AST	Supplement with 3 months AST[a]
Dissolution	None beyond approved specifications	Multiple dissolution profiles	Multiple dissolution profiles
Bioequivalence	None	None	Single-dose bioequivalence study[b]
Filing documentation	Annual report	Prior approval supplement and annual report	Prior approval supplement and annual report

[a]AST, accelerated stability testing.
[b]Waived in the presence of an established *in vitro/in vivo* correlation.

2. Release-Controlling Excipient

The changes for the release-controlling excipient are categorized into three levels similar to the nonrelease-controlling excipients:

1. Level 1 changes are those that are unlikely to have any detectable impact on formulation quality and performance.
2. Level 2 changes are those that could have a significant impact on formulation quality and performance. Test documentation for a level 2 change would vary depending on whether the product could be considered to have a narrow therapeutic range.
3. Level 3 changes are those that are likely to have any detectable impact on formulation quality and performance affecting all therapeutic ranges of the drug.

Table 15 summarizes the changes, test documentation, and filing documentation required for release-controlling excipient changes. Changes exceeding the ranges defined in each level may be allowed if considered to be within normal batch-to-batch variation and contained within an approved original application.

B. Process Changes

If a manufacturing process that is not identical to the original manufacturing process used in the approved application is to be used, appropriate validation studies should be conducted to demonstrate that the new process is similar to the original process. For oral controlled release dosage forms, consideration should be given to whether or not the change in manufacturing process is critical to drug release. Three levels of process changes are defined as follows:

Table 15 Release-Controlling Excipient Changes

Factor	Level 1	Level 2	Level 3
Total release–controlling excipients	Less than 5%	Less than 10	Beyond level 2 changes.
Test documentation			
Chemistry	Annual report on stability (first lot)	Non-NTD[a]: Supplement with 3 months AST (first lot) NTD: Supplement with 3 months AST (three lots)	Supplement with 3 months AST (three lots)
Dissolution	None beyond approved specifications	Multiple dissolution profiles and similarity testing for two dissolution profiles	Multiple dissolution profiles
Bioequivalence	None	Non-NTD[a] None NTD: Single-dose bioequivalence study[b]	Single-dose bioequivalence study[b]
Filing documentation	Annual report	Prior approval supplement and annual report	Prior approval supplement and annual report

[a]NTD, narrow therapeutic range drugs.
[b]Waived in the presence of an established *in vitro/in vivo* correlation.

Table 16 Process Changes

Factor	Level 1	Level 2	Level 3
Test documentation			
Chemistry	None beyond approved specifications	Supplement with 3 months AST	Supplement with 3 months AST[a]
Dissolution	None beyond approved specifications	Multiple dissolution profiles	Multiple dissolution profiles
Bioequivalence	None	None	Single-dose bioequivalence study[b]
Filing documentation	Annual report	Prior approval supplement and annual report	Prior approval supplement and annual report

[a]AST, accelerated stability testing.
[b]Waived in the presence of an established *in vitro/in vivo* correlation.

1. Level 1 changes: This category includes process changes involving adjustment of equipment operating conditions such as mixing times and operating speeds within original approved application ranges affecting the nonrelease-controlling and/or release-controlling excipient(s).
2. Level 2 changes: This category includes process changes involving adjustment of equipment operating conditions such as mixing times and operating speeds outside of original approved application ranges.
3. Level 3 changes: This category includes change in the type of process used in the manufacture of the product, such as a change from wet granulation to direct compression of dry powder.

Table 16 summarizes test documentation and filing documentation required for process changes.

VI. CONCLUSIONS

This chapter summarizes the research and development aspects of oral controlled release dosage forms with focus on drug release mechanisms of three major delivery systems: (a) matrix systems, (b) reservoir polymeric systems, and (c) osmotic pump systems. Selecting a delivery system to develop a controlled release dosage form is mainly based on considerations of the therapeutic demand, pharmacokinetic and pharmacodynamic parameters, and physicochemical properties of the chemical entity. Using verapamil hydrochloride and nifedipine as examples, it is demonstrated that different controlled release technologies and release mechanisms can be applied to the design of various dosage forms for a given drug in order to meet the therapeutic requirement.

ACKNOWLEDGMENT

We are grateful to Dr. W. Porter and Mr. P. Pinnamaraju for their critical reading and comments of the manuscript.

REFERENCES

1. Berner, B. and Dinh, S., Fundamental concepts in controlled release, 1992. In: Kydonieus, A. (Ed.), Treatise on Controlled Drug Delivery: Fundamentals, Optimization, Applications, Marcel Dekker, New York, pp. 1–35.
2. Guidance for Industry: Extended Release Oral Dosage Forms: Development, Evaluation, and Application of In Vitro/In Vivo Correlations. FDA, September 1997.
3. Approved Drug Products with Therapeutic Equivalence Evaluations, 18th Ed., U.S. Department of Health and Human Services, 1998.
4. Robinson, J. R., 1976. Controlled-release pharmaceutical systems. In: F. W. Long, W. P. O'Neill and R. D. Stewart (Eds.), Chemical Marketing and Economics Reprints, p. 212.
5. Robinson, J. R. and Lee, V. H. L. (Eds.), 1987. Controlled Drug Delivery: Fundamentals and Applications, 2nd ed.
6. Kydonieus, A., 1980. Fundamental concepts of controlled release. In: A. F. Kydonieus (Ed.), Controlled Release Technologies: Methods, Theory, and Applications, Vol. 1, p. 7.
7. Korsmeyer, R. W., Gurny, R., Doelker, E., Buri, P. and Peppas, N. A. 1983. Mechanisms of solute release from porous hydrophilic polymers. Int. J. Pharm., 15: 25–35.
8. Peppas, N. A., 1985. Analysis of Fickian and non-Fickian drug release from polymers, Pharm. Acta Helv., 60: 110–111.
9. Ford, J. L., Mitchell, K., Rowe, P., Armstrong, D. J., Elliott, P. N. C., Rostron, C. and Hogan J. E., 1991. Mathematical modeling of drug release from hydroxypropyl-methylcellulose matrices: effect of temperature. Int. J. Pharm., 71: 95–104.
10. Ford, J. L., Rubinstein, M. H., McCaul, F., Hogan, J. E. and Edgar, P. J., 1987. Importance of drug type, tablet shape and added diluents on drug release kinetics from hydroxypropylmethylcellulose matrix tablets. Int. J. Pharm., 40: 223–234.
11. Baveja, S. K. and Ranga Rao, K. V., 1986. Sustained release tablet formulation of centperazine. Int. J. Pharm., 31: 169–174.
12. Peppas, N. A. and Sahlin, J. J., 1989. A simple equation for the description of solute release. III. Coupling of diffusion and relaxation. Int. J. Pharm., 57: 169–172.
13. Ranga Rao, K. V., Padmalatha D. K. and Buri, P. 1990. Influence of molecular size and water solubility of the solute on its release from swelling and erosion controlled polymeric matrices. J. Controlled Release, 12: 133–141.
14. Harland, R. S., Gazzaniga, A., Sangalli, M. E., Colombo, P. and Peppas, N. A., 1988. Drug/polymer matrix swelling and dissolution. Pharm. Res. 5: 488–494.
15. Catellani, P., Vaona, G., Plazzi, P. and Colombo, P. 1988. Compressed matrices: formulation and drug release kinetics. Acta Pharm. Technol. 34: 38–41.
16. Higuchi, T. 1961. Rate of release of medicaments from ointment bases containing drugs in suspension. J. Pharm. Sci., 50: 847.
17. Higuchi, T. 1963. Mechanism of sustained release medication, theoretical analysis of rate of release of solid drugs dispersed in solid matrices. J. Pharm. Sci., 52: 1145.
18. Martin, A., Swarbrick, J. and Cammarata, A. 1983, Physical Pharmacy, chap. 15. Crank, J. 1975. The Mathematics of Diffusion, 2nd ed.
18a. Crank, J. 1986. Diffusion in Heterogeneous Media. In: Crank, J. (Ed.) The Mathematics of Diffusion, 2nd edition, Claren Don Press, Oxford, pp-266-285.
19. Ritger P. L. and Peppas N. A. 1987, A simple equation for description of solute release I. Fickian and non-Fickian release from non-swellable devices in the form of slabs, spheres, cylinders or discs, J. Controlled Release 5: 23–26.
20. Donbrow, M. and Friedman, M., 1975. Enhancement of permeability of ethyl cellulose films for drug penetration. J. Pharm. Pharmacol., 27: 633.
21. Donbrow, M. and Samuelov, Y. 1980. Zero order drug delivery from double-layered porous films: release rate profiles from ethyl cellulose, hydroxypropyl cellulose and polyethylene glycol mixtures. J. Pharm. Pharmacol., 32: 463.
22. Rowe, R. C. 1986. The effect of the molecular weight of ethyl cellulose on the drug release properties of mixed films of ethyl cellulose and hydroxypropyl methylcellulose. Int. J. Pharm., 29: 37–41.

23. Grass IV, G. M. and Robinson, J. R. 1990. Sustained- and controlled release drug delivery systems, In: G. S. Banker and C. T. Rhodes (Eds.), Modern Pharmaceutics, pp. 657–658.
24. Lieberman, H. A., Lachman, L. and Schwartz, J. B. (Eds.) 1990. Pharmaceutical Dosage Forms: Tablets, Vols. 1–3. Marcel Dekker, New York.
25. Gamlen, D. J. 1985. Pellet manufacture for controlled release. Mfg. Chem., 56(6): 55–63.
26. Gajdos, B. 1984. Drug Made Ger. 27: 30.
27. Madan, P. L. and Shanbhag, S. R. 1978. Cellulose acetate phthalate microcapsules: method of preparation. J. Pharm. Pharmacol., 30: 65.
28. Moldauer, H. and Kala, H. 1974. Pharmacie, 29: 521.
29. Reynolds, A. D. 1970. Mfg. Chem. Aerosol News, 41(6): 40.
30. Woodruff, C. W. and Nuessle, N. O. 1972. Effect of processing variables on particles obtained by extrusion-spheronization processing. J. Pharm. Sci., 61: 787
31. Conine, J. W. and Hadley, H. R. 1970. Preparation of small solid pharmaceutical spheres. Drug Cosmet. Ind., 106: 38.
32a. O'Conner and Schwartz, J.B., 1989. Extrusion and spheronizing technology. In: Ghebre-Sellassie, I. (Ed.) 1989. Pharmaceutical Pelletization Technology. Marcel Dekker, Inc. New York, pp-187-216.
32b. Bauer, K.H., Lehmann, K., Osterwald, H.P. and Rothgang, G., 1998. Environmental conditons in the digestive tract and their influence on the dosage form. In: Coated Pharmaceutical Dosage Forms, Fundamentals, Manufacturing Techniques, Biopharmaceutical Aspects, Test Methods and Raw Materials. Medpharm GmbH Scientific Publishers, Birkenwaldstr, Stuttgart. pp.-126-130.
33. Digenis, G. A., Sandefer, E. P., Page, R. C. and Doll, W. J. 1998. Gamma scintigraphy: an evolving technology in pharmaceutical formulation development, Parts 1 and 2. PSTT, 1: 100–165.
34. Skelly, J. P., et al. 1993. Report on workshop: scaleup of oral extended-release dosage forms. Pharm. Res., 10(12): 1800–1805.
35. Cohen, J., Hubert, B. B., Leeson, L. J., Rhodes, C. T., Robinson, J. R., Roseman, T. J. and Shefter, E. 1990. The development of USP dissolution and drug release standards. Pharm. Res., 7: 983–987.
36. Pharmacopeial Forum, 1993. In vitro and in vivo evaluation of dosage forms. 19: 5366–5379.
37. FDA Guidance for Industry: Oral extended (controlled) release dosage forms: in vivo bioequivalence and in vitro dissolution testing, 1997.
38. Khan, M. Z. I., 1996. Dissolution testing for sustained or controlled release oral dosage forms and correlation with in vivo data: challenges and opportunities. 140: 131–143.
39. Skelly, J. P., et al., 1987. Report of the workshop on controlled release dosage forms: issues and controversies. Pharm. Res., 4: 75–78.
40. Pharmacopeial Forum Stimuli Article, 1988. In vitro–in vivo correlation for extended release oral dosage forms. 4160–4161.
41. Skelly, J. P. and Shiu, G. F., 1993. In vitro/in vivo correlations in biopharmaceutics: scientific and regulatory implications. Eur. J. Drug Metab. Pharmacokin., 18: 121–129.
42. Siewert, W. 1993. Perspectives of in vitro dissolution tests in establishing in vitro/in vivo correlations. Eur. J. Drug Metab. Pharmacokin., 18: 7–18.
43. Skelly, J. P. et al. 1990. In vitro and in vivo testing and correlation for oral controlled/modified-release dosage forms, Pharm. Res., 7(9): 975–982.
44. Dressman, J. B. and Yamada, K. 1991. Animal models for oral drug absorption. In: Welling, P. G., Tse, F. L. and Dighe, S. (Eds.), Pharmaceutical Bioequivalence, Marcel Dekker, New York. pp. 235–266.
45. Davis, S. S., Wilding, E. A. and Wilding, I. R., 1993. Gastrointestinal transit of a matrix tablet formulation: comparison of canine and human data. Int. J. Pharm., 94: 235–238.
46. Davis, B. and Morris, T. 1993. Physiological parameters in laboratory animals and humans. Pharm. Res., 10: 1093–1098.
47. Akimoto, M., Furuya, A. Maki, T., Yamada, K., Suwa, T. and Ogata, H. 1993. Evaluation of sustained release granules of chlorphenesin carbamate in dogs and humans. 100: 133–142.
48. Yamakita, H., Maejima, T. and Osawa, T. 1995. Preparation of controlled release tablets of TA-5707F with wax matrix type and their in vivo evaluation in beagle dogs. Biol. Pharm. Bull., 18: 984–989.

49. Yamakita, H., Maejima, T. and Osawa, T. 1995. In vitro/in vivo evaluation of two series of TA-5707F controlled release matrix tablets prepared with hydroxypropyl methyl cellulose derivatives with entero-soluble or gel formation properties. Biol. Pharm. Bull., 18: 1409–1416.
50. Hussain, M., Abramowitz, W., Watrous, B. J., Szpunar, G. J. and Ayres, J. W. 1990. Gastrointestinal transit of nondisintegrating, nonerodible oral dosage forms in pigs. Pharm. Res., 7: 1163–1166.
51. Hildebrand, H., McDonald, F. M. and Windt-Hanke, F., 1991. Characterization of oral sustained release preparations of iloprost in a pig model by plasma level monitoring. Prostaglandins, 41: 473–486.
52. Kostewicz, E., Sansom, L., Fishlock, R., Morella, A. and Kuchel, T. 1996. Examination of two sustained release nifedipine preparations in humans and in pigs. Eur. J. Pharm. Sci., 4: 351–357.
53. Qiu, Y., Cheskin, H., Briskin, J. and Engh, K., 1997. Sustained-release hydrophilic matrix tablets of Zileuton: formulation and in vitro/in vivo studies. J. Controlled Release, 45: 249–256.
54. Qiu, Y., Flood, K., Marsh, K., Carroll, S., Trivedi, J., Arneric, S. P. and Krill, S. L. 1997. Design of sustained-release matrix systems for a highly water-soluble compound, ABT-089. Int. J. Pharm., 157: 43–52.
55. Roppas, C., Lacey, L. F., Keene, O. N., Macheras, P. and Bye, A. 1995. Evaluation of different matrices as indirect measures of rate of drug absorption from extended release dosage forms at steady-state. Pharm. Res., 12: 103–107.
56. Bois, F. Y., Tozer, T. N., Hauck, W. W., Chen, M., Patnaik, R. and Williams, R. 1994. Bioequivalence: performance of several measures of rate of absorption. Pharm. Res., 11: 966–974.
57. Metzler, C. M. 1991. Statistical criteria. In: Welling, P. G., Tse, F. L. and Dighe, S. (Eds.), Pharmaceutical Bioequivalence, Marcel Dekker, New York. pp. 35–66.
58. Dighe, S. V. and Adams, W. P. 1991. Bioavailability and bioequivalence of oral controlled-release products: a regulatory perspective. In: Welling, P. G., Tse, F. L. and Dighe, S. (Eds.), Pharmaceutical Bioequivalence, Marcel Dekker, New York, pp. 35–66.
59. Vallner, J. J. et al. 1983. A proposed general protocol for testing bioequivalence of controlled-release drug products. Int. J. Pharm. 16: 47–55.
60. Bass, P. 1993. Gastric emptying; differences among liquid, fiber, polymer and solid dosage forms of medications. In: Current Status on Targeted Drug Delivery to the Gastrointestinal Tract. Capsulegel Library, pp. 11–18.
61. Davis, S. S. et al. 1986. Transit of pharmaceutical dosage forms through the small intestine. Gut, 27: 886–892.
62. Abrahamsson, B. et al. 1993. Absorption, gastrointestinal transit, and tablet erosion of felodipine extended-release (ER) tablets. Pharm. Res., 10(5): 709–713.
63. Coupe, A. J. et al. 1993. Do pellet formulations empty from the stomach with food? Int. J. Pharm., 92: 167–175.
64. Yuen, K. H. et al. 1993. Gastrointestinal transit and absorption of theophylline from a multiparticulate controlled-release formulation. Int. J. Pharm., 97: 61–77.
65. Dressman, J. B., Amidon, G. L., Reppas, C. and Shah, V. P. 1998. Dissolution testing as a prognostic tool for oral drug absorption: immediate release dosage forms. Pharm. Res., 15: 11–22.
66. Digenis, G. A., Sandefer, E. P., Parr, A. F., Beihn, R., McClain, C., Scheinthal, B. M., Ghebre-Sellassie, I., Nesbitt, R. U. and Randinitis, E. 1990. Gastrointestinal behavior of orally administered radiolabeled erythromycin pellets in man as determined by gamma scintigraphy. J. Clin. Pharmacol., 30: 621–631.
67. Phillips, S. F. 1993. Gastrointestinal physiology and its relevance to targeted drug delivery. In: Current Status on Targeted Drug Delivery to the Gastrointestinal Tract. Capsulegel Library, pp. 11–18.
68. Breimer, D. D. 1996. An integrated pharmacokinetic and pharmacodynamic approach to controlled drug delivery. J. Drug Target., 3: 411–415.
69. Hoffman, A. 1998. Pharmacodynamic aspects of sustained release preparations. Adv. Drug Deliv. Rev., 33: 185–199.
70. Gupta, S. K., Guinta, D. R., Christopher, C. A. and Samuel, S. 1998. Dosage form and method for administering drug. PCT. WO 98/14168.
71. Tabusso, G. 1992. Regulatory aspects of development pharmaceutics (1). The Regul. Affairs J., 11: 909–912.

72. Andreotti, F., Davies, G. J., Hackett, D. R., Khan, M. I., De Bart, A. C. W., Aber, V. R., Maseri, A. and Kluft, C. 1988. Major circadian fluctuations in fibrinolytic factors and possible relevance to time of onset of myocardial infarction, sudden cardiac death and stroke. Am. J. Cardiol., 62: 635–637.
73. Ridker, P. M., Manson, J. E., Buring, J. E., Muller, J. E. and Hennekens, C. H. 1990. Circadian variation of acute myocardial infarction and the effect of low-dose aspirin in a randomized trial of physicians. Circulation, 82: 897–902.
74. Straka, R.J., Benson, S.R., 1996. Chronopharmacologic considerations when treating the patient with hypertension: a review. J. Clin. Pharmacol. 36:771-782.
75. Hildgen P. and McMullen, J. N. 1995. A new gradient matrix: formulation and characterization. J. Controlled Release, 34: 263–271.
76. Danckwerts M. P. 1994. Development of a zero-order release oral compressed tablet with potential for commercial tabletting production. Int. J. Pharm., 112: 34–45.
77. Kim C. 1995. Compressed donut-shaped tablets with zero-order release kinetics. Pharm. Res. 12: 1045–1048.
78. Benkorah A. Y. and McMullen J.-N. 1994. Biconcave coated, centrally perforated tablets for oral controlled drug delivery, J. Controlled Release, 32: 155–160.
79. Conte U., Maggi L., Colombo P. and Manna A. L. 1993. Multi-layered hydrophilic matrices as constant release devices (Geomatrix Systems). J. Controlled Release, 26: 39–47.
80. Scott D. C. and Hollenbeck R. G. 1991. Design and manufacture of a zero-order sustained-release pellet dosage form through nonuniform drug distribution in a diffusional matrix. Pharm. Res., 8: 156–161.
81. Brooke D. and Washkuhn R. J. 1977. Zero-order drug delivery system: theory and preliminary testing. J. Pharm. Sci., 66: 159–162.
82. Lipper R. A. and Higuchi W. I. 1977. Analysis of theoretical behavior of a proposed zero-order drug delivery system. J. Pharm. Sci., 66: 163–164.
83. Qiu, Y., Chidambaram and Flood, K. 1998. Design and evaluation of layered diffusional matrices for zero-order sustained-release. J. Controlled Release, 51: 123–130.
84. Katzhendler, I., Azoury, R. and Friedman, M. 1998. Crystalline properties of carbamazepine in sustained release hydrophilic matrix tablets based on hydroxypropyl methylcellulose. J. Controlled Release, 54: 69–85.
85. Michelucci, J. J., Sherman, D. M. and DeNeale, R. J. 1990. Sustained release etodolac. US patent 4,966,768.
86. Ruff, M. D., Kalidindi, S. R. and Sutton, Jr., J. E., 1994. Pharmaceutical composition containing bupropion hydrochloride and a stabilizer. US Patent 5,358,970.
87. Baiz, E. and Einig, H. 1992. Alginate-based verapamil-containing depot drug form. US Patent 5,132,295.
88. Howard, J. R. and Timmins, P. 1988. Controlled release formulation. US Patent 4,792,452.
89. Zhang, G. and Pinnamaraju, P. 1997. Sustained release formulation containing three different types of polymers. US patent 5,695,781.
90. Panoz, D. E. and Geoghegan, E. J., 1989. Controlled absorption pharmaceutical composition. US patent 4,863,742.
91. Jao, F., Wong, P. S., Huynh, H. T., McChesney, K. and Wat, P. K., 1992. Verapamil therapy. US patent 5,160,744.
92. Jao, F., Wong, P. S., Huynh, H. T., McChesney, K. and Wat, P. K., 1993. Verapamil therapy. US patent 5,190,765.
93. Jao, F., Wong, P. S., Huynh, H. T., McChesney, K. and Wat, P. K., 1993. Verapamil therapy. US patent 5,252,338.
94. Ohm, A. and Luchtenberg, H., 1990. Press coated DHP tablets. US patent 4,892,741.
95. Food and Drug Administration, Guidance for Industry: Modified Release Solid Oral Dosage Forms: Scale-up and Postapproval Changes: Chemistry, Manufacturing and Controls, In Vitro Dissolution Testing and In Vivo Bioequivalence Documentation. September 1997.

24
A Gastrointestinal Retentive Microparticulate System to Improve Oral Drug Delivery

Y. Kawashima, H. Takeuchi, and H. Yamamoto
Gifu Pharmaceutical University, Gifu, Japan

I. INTRODUCTION

A number of oral controlled release systems have been developed to improve the delivery of drugs to the systemic circulation. Although such systems can control precisely and predictably the drug release rate for extended periods of time, even over a number of days, they do not always perform satisfactorily if they pass through the drug absorption site, e.g., the small intestine, before the release of loaded drug is complete. Thus, attention must be given to prolonging the residence time of the system to achieve complete drug release in the gastrointestinal (GI) tract (stomach or small intestine) as well as to modulating the drug release rate as predicted by the system in order to obtain an ideal oral controlled release system. Several approaches to extend the gastric residence time have been developed including an intragastric floating system; a high-density system; a mucoadhesive system; a magnetic system; unfoldable, extendible, or swellable systems; and a superporous hydrogel system (1). An important issue in the development of these systems is how to avoid interunit and intersubject variations in GI residence time. Another problem is how to improve the absorption of a poorly absorbed drug by using such systems.

In this chapter, we will focus on microparticulate systems, such as microspheres, nanospheres, and liposomes, used for multiparticulate forms. Such multiparticulate (or multiple-unit) dosage forms can disperse as individual units in the stomach so that they can pass randomly through the pylorus and thus become widely distributed in the GI tract. For this reason, they have a longer reproducible gastric residence time than single-unit systems. We describe one such promising system, multiple-unit hollow microspheres (microballoons) developed by our group (2) as a floating controlled drug delivery system in the stomach, and we will also refer to other systems that have appeared in the literature.

A submicronized particulate system (colloidal drug carrier), when administered orally, may be able to penetrate into the deep mucous layer and prolong the residence time at the mucin–epithelial cell surface. It is likely that they are able to maintain the concentration of drug released there and reduce its exposure to enzymatic digestion. This helps improve the absorption of poorly absorbed drugs, such as peptides. This can be achieved by providing them with a mucoadhesive function to improve their retention at the mucus layer of the GI tract. Recently, mucoadhesive colloidal drug carriers, such as surface-modified liposomes and DL-lactide/glycolide copolymer nanospheres with a mucoadhesive polymer, have been successfully developed by us to improve and extend the biological action of peptides absorbed from the GI tract (3). We describe how to prepare such surface-modified (coated) microparticulate systems with polymer and how to evaluate the mucoadhesive properties of these systems in vitro and in vivo. This is done by referring to case studies involving the improved oral delivery of peptides, e.g., calcitonin and insulin, by using such systems.

II. INTRAGASTRIC FLOATING MICROPARTICULATE SYSTEMS (MICROBALLOONS)

Floating systems having a specific density lower than that of gastric fluids can remain buoyant in the stomach contents, thereby prolonging the gastric residence time. A hydrodynamically balanced system (HBS) was the first to be developed as a floating system with single-unit formulations (4). A disadvantage of this system is the high variability in the gastric emptying time, due to the all-or-nothing emptying process. To overcome this problem, multiple-unit floating systems have been developed.

One successful system involves multiple-unit hollow microspheres prepared by the emulsion solvent diffusion process that we developed (2). Such microspheres are termed "microballoons" due to their characteristic internal hollow structure and excellent floatability in vitro. To prepare this device, the drug and enteric acrylic polymer soluble at pH >7.0 (Eudragit S) are dissolved in an ethanol–dichloromethane mixture (1:1 v/v) at room temperature. The drug solution is then poured into the aqueous polyvinyl alcohol (PVA) solution (<1%) that is thermostatically controlled at 40°C under agitation. The finely dispersed droplets of the polymer solution of drug solidify in the aqueous phase due to diffusion of the solvent. Evaporation of dichloromethane from the solidified droplets leaves the cavity in the microspheres filled with water. During the drying procedure, the cavity inside each microsphere becomes filled with air, generating the microballoon.

A cross-section of such a microballoon is shown in Fig. 1. The characteristic internal structure of the microballoon, a spherical cavity enclosed within a rigid shell constructed of drug and polymer, is clearly apparent.

The drug (e.g., riboflavin) release rate from the shell of the microballoon can be controlled by varying the polymer concentration and by coformulating a water-soluble polymer, such as hydroxypropylmethylcellulose (HPMC), as shown in Fig. 2 and Table 1. In acidic medium, very little release of drug occurs at a Eudragit S content >90%, due to solubility limitations of the polymer; and almost 90% of the microballoons float on the surface of the test solution because they are filled with air. The floatability of the microballoons is also modified by the amount of coformulated HPMC in the shell. The drug release rate is pH-dependent, as expected, since the polymer is an enteric polymer, being soluble above pH 7. Therefore, the subunits that lose buoyancy should subsequently pass through the stomach and release significant amounts of drug in the upper gut, i.e., the absorption site.

An in vivo oral absorption study with microballoons (Eudragit S100/HPMC = 9:1) containing riboflavin has been conducted in fasted and fed human subjects. As a control, nonfloating sustained released microspheres were administered under the same conditions. The pharmacokinetic parameters obtained from the urinary excretion data are summarized in Table 1. The excretion half-life of the dose administered in the form of microballoons was longer than that of the nonfloating microspheres, irrespective of the feeding conditions, indicating a longer gastric transit time for the microballoons. Concomitant food ingestion increased the gastric residence time of the microballoons because the meal most likely induces closing of the pylorus and promotes buoyancy in the stomach (5).

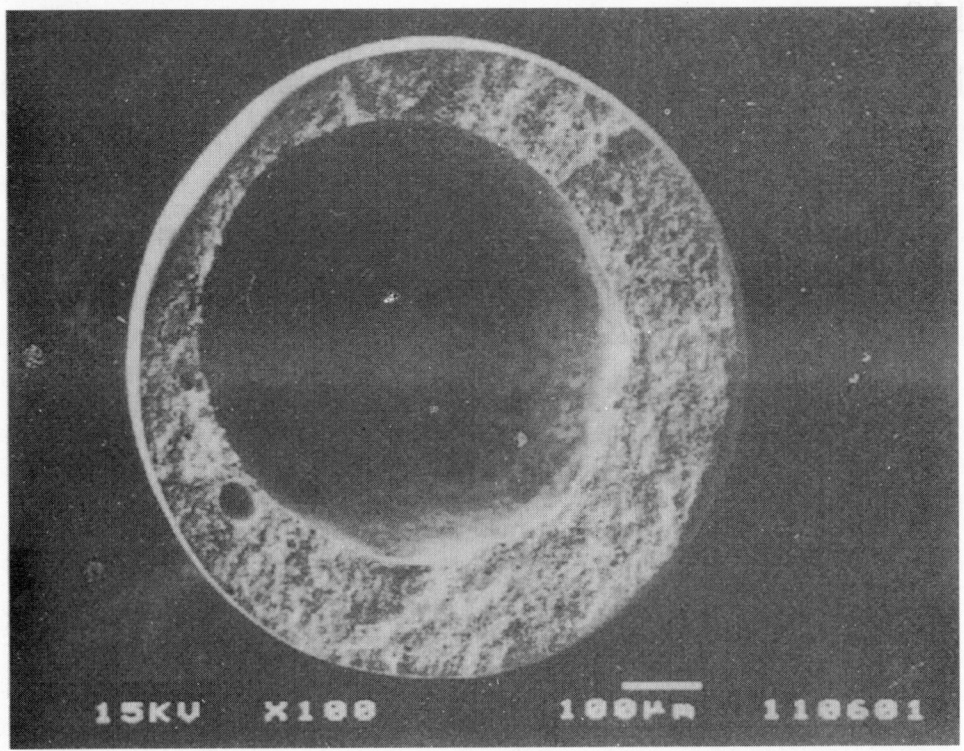

Figure 1 Scanning electron microphotograph of a cross-section of microballoon.

The intragastric behavior of ^{99m}Tc-labeled nonfloating microspheres (control) and microballoons after their oral administration to fasted and fed humans has been investigated by γ-scintigraphy as shown in Fig. 3. In the fed state, the microballoons disperse in the upper part of the stomach and are retained for over 3 h compared with the nonfloating microspheres, which gradually descend to the lower part of the stomach within 90 min. In the fasted state, the microballoons float for only 60 min, after which they are emptied rapidly by peristaltic contractions. The nonfloating microspheres are emptied more rapidly, within less than 60 min. It has been found that the pharmacokinetic parameters, e.g., excretion half-life and excretion %, correlate well with the gastric retention time determined by γ-scintigraphy in Fig. 3 and shown in Fig. 4.

These microballoons can be used with a wide variety of drugs as novel drug delivery systems. Although hydrophilic drugs can be used in such systems, hydrophobic drugs are generally preferable. The drug entrapment efficiency in the microballoons is determined by the solubility of the drug in water and its partition coefficient between water and dichloromethane.

Other floating devices have been described in the literature, including a carbon dioxide–generating system and an air-entrapping system. In the former, the carbon dioxide–generating material is coformulated in the preparation formulation, forming an effervescent layer or matrix inside a swellable polymer particulate device. The carbon dioxide produced by interaction of the carbon dioxide–generating material with the gastric medium imparts buoyancy to the device (6). While the system floats over a period of 5 h, the drug is released in a sustained manner from the system. In addition to our air-entrapping, i.e., microballoon, system, another smart system, termed an air compartment multiple-unit system, has been described by Iannuccelli et

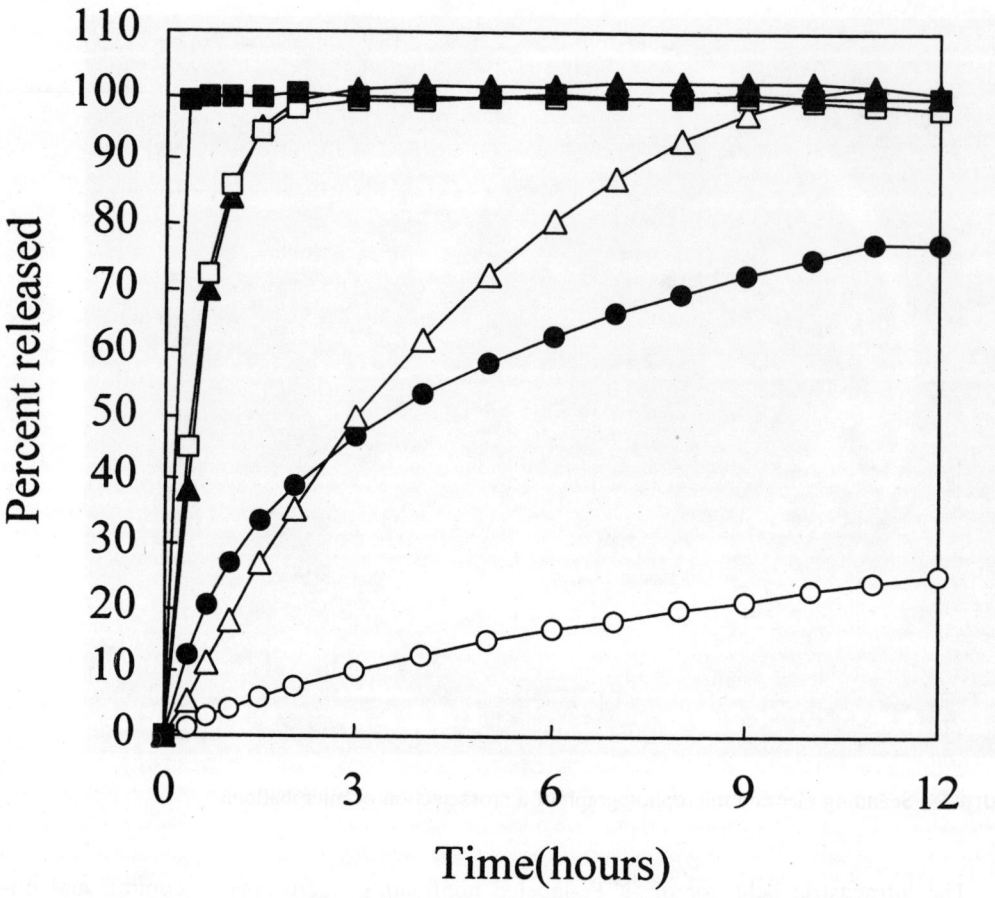

Figure 2 Release profiles of riboflavin from microballoons. ○, pH 1.2 (S100/HPMC = 9:1); ●, pH 1.2 (S100/HPMC = 7:3); △, pH 6.8 (S100/HPMC = 9:1); ▲, pH 6.8 (S100/HPMC = 7:3); □, pH 7.2 (S100/HPMC = 9:1); ■, pH 7.2 (S100/HPMC = 7:3).

Table 1 Physicochemical Properties and Pharmacokinetic Parameters of Microballoons and Nonfloating Microspheres

Ratio of polymer (S100/HPMC)	Buoyancy (%)	% Released			$t_{1/2}$		Excretion (%)	
			pH1.2	pH6.8	pH1.2	pH6.8	pH1.2	pH6.8
Microballoons (9:1)	93.6 (12h)	20min	1.3	5.3	5.63[a]	4.67[b]	27.1[a]	25.0[b]
		12h	25.0	100.1	(n=3)	(n=3)	(n=3)	(n=3)
Microballoons (7:3)	38.0 (12h)	20min	12.7	38.4	3.85[a]		40.4[a]	
		12h	77.1	100.6	(n=1)		(n=1)	
Nonfloating microspheres	9.2 (4h)	20min	0.6	3.3	4.35[a]	4.50[b]	20.7[a]	19.3[b]
		12h	22.2	100.3	(n=3)	(n=3)	(n=3)	(n=3)

[a]Fed state.
[b]Fasted state.
Excretion (%) = excretion (0–22 h, mg) × 10^4/dose (mg)/content (%)

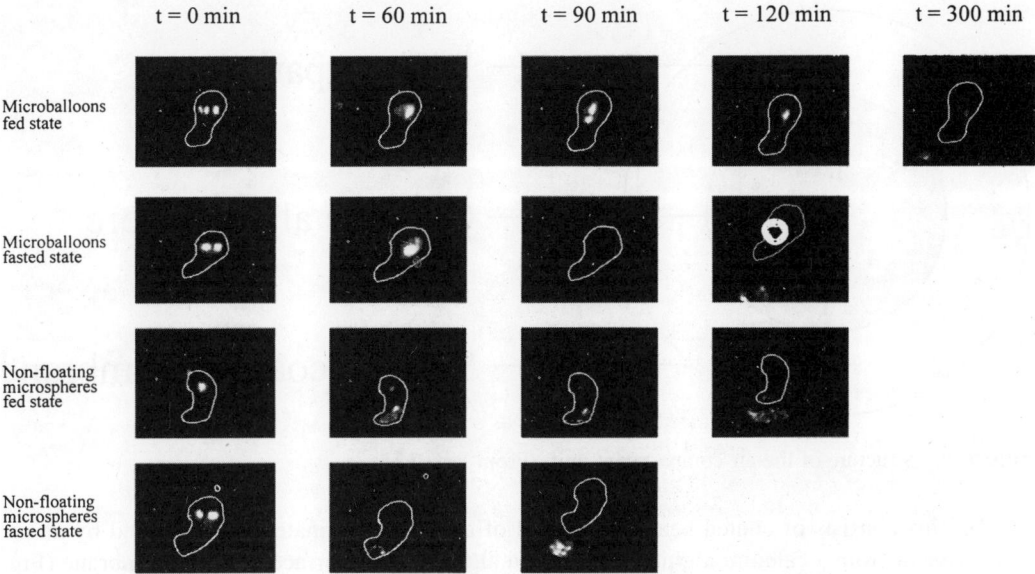

Figure 3 Scintigraphic images of in vivo behavior of microballoons and nonfloating microspheres.

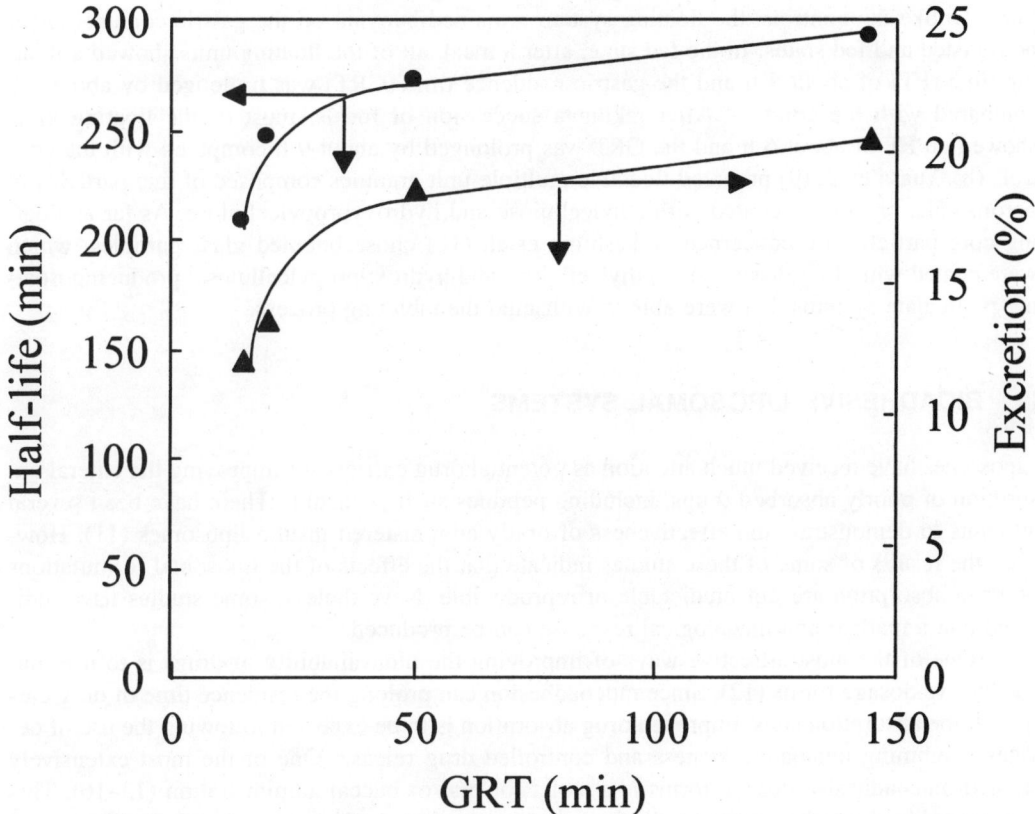

Figure 4 Effect of gastric retention time (GRT) on the half-life of excretion and cumulative urinary excretion (t = 22 h), ●: half-life (min), ▲: excretion (%).

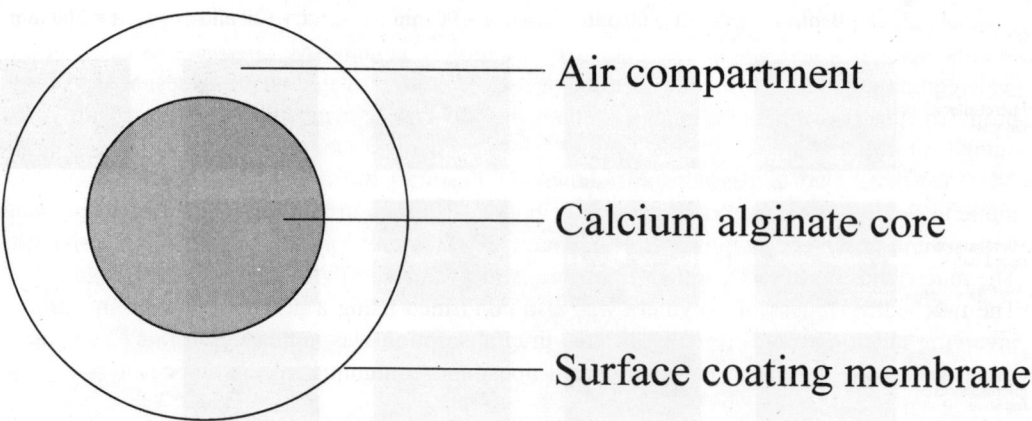

Figure 5 Structure of the air compartment unit. (From Ref. 7.)

al. (7). This consists of coated beads composed of a calcium alginate core separated by an air compartment from a calcium alginate or calcium alginate/PVA surface-coating membrane (Fig. 5). This system is able to float immediately when coming into contact with artificial gastric juice and remains floating for a long period in vivo. The intragastric behavior of this system loaded with barium sulfate was investigated by x-raying humans under different feeding conditions. Unlike the controls, the floating system remained buoyant on the gastric contents under both fasted and fed states. In the fed state, after a meal, all of the floating units showed a floating time (FT) of about 5 h and the gastric residence time (GRT) was prolonged by about 2 h compared with the controls. After taking a succession of meals, most of the floating units showed an FT of about 6 h and the GRT was prolonged by about 9 h compared with the controls (8). Yuasa et al. (9) prepared floatable multiple-unit granules composed of fine particles of porous calcium silicate coated with ethylcellulose and hydroxypropylcellulose. As far as floating core particles are concerned, Takashima et al. (10) chose bubbled glass particles, which were coated with drug dissolved in ethylcellulose and hydroxypropylcellulose, producing floating particulate systems that were able to withstand the tableting process.

III. BIOADHESIVE LIPOSOMAL SYSTEMS

Liposomes have received much attention as potential drug carriers for improving the enteral absorption of poorly absorbed drugs, including peptides such as insulin. There have been several attempts to demonstrate the effectiveness of orally administered insulin liposomes (11). However, the results of some of these studies indicate that the effects of the liposomal formulations on drug absorption are not predictable or reproducible. Nevertheless, some studies have indicated that a marked pharmacological response can be produced.

One of the most attractive ways of improving the bioavailability of drugs is to use mucoadhesive dosage forms (12). Since mucoadhesion can prolong the residence time of drug carriers at the absorption sites, improved drug absorption is to be expected following the use of devices combining mucoadhesiveness and controlled drug release. One of the most extensively studied mucoadhesive dosage forms is a tablet for oral or buccal administration (13–16). This is prepared by formulating mucoadhesive polymers such as hydroxypropylmethylcellulose and Carbopol (CP), which is a high molecular weight poly(acrylic acid) copolymer, loosely crosslinked with divinyl glycol.

A multiunit bioadhesive system has also been reported to have been prepared by coating microspheres of polyhydroxyethylmethacrylate with mucoadhesive polymers using laboratory scale equipment (17,18). Recently, Pimienta et al. (19) investigated the bioadhesion of hydroxypropyl methacrylate nanoparticles or isohexylcyanoacrylate nanocapsules coated with poloxamers and poloxamine on rat ileal segments in vitro using a labeled compound.

We have tried to develop mucoadhesive liposomes by using the polymer coating technique to facilitate the enteral absorption of poorly absorbed drugs. The liposomes were coated with several polymers including chitosan and CP, which are expected to be mucoadhesive (20). The mucoadhesion of the resultant liposomes was evaluated in vitro using isolated rat intestine. The mucoadhesiveness of polymers was also confirmed using a newly developed in vitro test involving mucin particles. Finally, in vivo drug absorption was monitored in rats following intragastric administration of polymer-coated liposomes containing insulin and calcitonin.

A. Polymer-Coated Liposomes

Polymer coating of liposomes is an attractive method for modifying the surface properties of liposomes. Sunamoto et al. (21) have demonstrated an improvement in the chemical and physical stability of polymer-coated liposomes prepared with polysaccharide derivatives such as mannan or amylopectin. So far, several substances, such as poloxamer (22), polysorbate-80 (23), carboxymethyl chitin (24), carboxymethyl chitosan (25), and dextran derivatives (26), have been reported to be suitable for such liposomal systems.

In order to design a mucoadhesive liposomal system, we examined the feasibility of coating liposomes with some mucoadhesive polymers such as chitosan (3,27). Negatively charged liposomes were prepared with L-α-dipalmitoylphosphatidylcholine (DPPC) and dicetyl phosphate (DCP) by a thin-film hydration method. A phosphate buffer (1mL, pH 7.4) was used in the hydration process. The polymers used for liposome coating were chitosan (CS), PVA having a long alkyl chain (PVA-R), and poly(acrylic acid) bearing a number of cholesterol moieties (PAA-Chol), prepared using poly(acrylic acid) (28). The properties of these polymers are summarized in Table 2. PVA-R and PAA-Chol dissolved in a phosphate buffer (pH7.4) and CS dissolved in an acetate buffer (pH 4.4) were used to coat the liposomes. In coating with CP, positively charged liposomes with sterile amine (SA) were prepared. Polymer coating was carried

Table 2 Properties of Polymers Used for Liposome Coating

Polymer	Structure	Note
Chitosan		Degree of deacetylation = 85% Molecular weight = approx. 150,000
PVA-R	$C_{16}H_{33}-S-[CH_2-CH(OH)]_n-H$	Degree of polymerization = 480
PAA-Chol	$H-[CH_2-CH(COOH)]_n-[CH_2-CH(CO-O-Chol)]_m-H$	Molecular weight of PAA = 250,000

out by mixing the resultant liposomal suspensions with the same amount of polymer solution, followed by incubation.

The formation of a polymer layer on the surface of the liposomes was confirmed by comparing the ζ potential of the liposomes before and after coating (27). The values of the ζ potential of the polymer-coated liposomes were found to be affected by increasing the concentration of polymer solution used in coating (Fig. 6). The change in the ζ potential of PAA-Chol-coated liposomes was largely due to the electric charge of the polymers attached to the surface of the liposomes. Formation of an ion complex of CS with DCP on the surface of the liposomes during the coating process could explain the decrease in the ζ potential of the CS-coated liposomes. In the case of the noncharged polymer, PVA-R, formation of a polymer layer on the surface of the liposomes could move the shear plane to the solution side, which could then be responsible for the change in ζ potential. These results confirmed the existence of a fixed polymer layer on the surface of the liposome particles. On changing the pH of the dispersing medium of the liposomes from acidic to neutral, the ζ potential of the CP-coated liposomes shifted from zero to higher negative values, supporting the formation of a polymer layer on the surface of the positively charged liposomes (29).

B. Mucoadhesive Tests for Particulate Systems

Various methods have been proposed to measure the mucoadhesive properties of polymers and devices composed of polymers (16,30). One possible way is to use a labeled compound to estimate the mucoadhesiveness of particulate systems including liposomes (19). We tried to develop a simpler in vitro method to evaluate the mucoadhesiveness of polymer-coated liposomes and have called this the particle counting method (27).

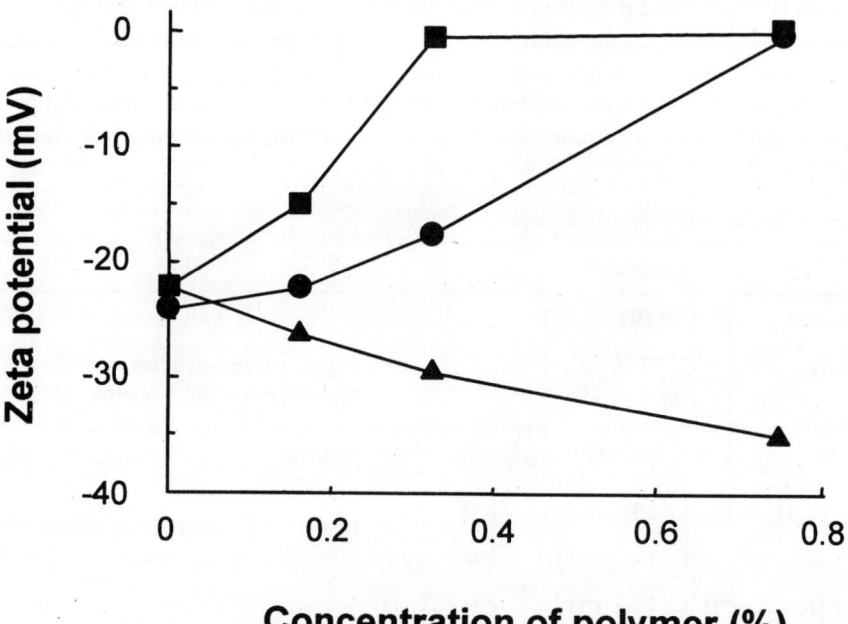

Figure 6 The ζ potential of liposomes coated with various polymers at pH 7.4. ●, Chitosan, ■, PVA-R; ▲, PAA-Chol. Lipid composition: DPPC/DCP = 8:2. (From Ref. 27.)

In the particle counting method, a length of intestine (15 cm) isolated from Wistar rats was filled with liposomal suspensions diluted 100-fold with appropriate buffer after a washing of the inside of the intestinal preparation with saline. The length of intestine was sealed and incubated in saline at 37°C for more than 15 min. By measuring the number of liposomal particles in a Coulter counter, both before and after incubation, the mucoadhesive percentage could be calculated from the following equation.

$$\text{Adhesive \%} = (N_o - N_s)/N_o \times 100$$

where N_o and N_s are the number of liposomes, before and after incubation, respectively.

As shown in Fig. 7, CS-coated liposomes showed the highest adhesive percentage among the three different polymer-coated liposomes tested. The mucoadhesive function was thought to be due to the polymer layer attached to the surface of the liposomes because noncoated liposomes had an adhesive percentage of zero. Interpenetration between the polymeric and mucous networks is considered to be responsible for this adhesion. The adhesive percentage of CS-coated liposomes depended on the CS concentration used for coating (Fig. 8). Combining the results shown in Figs. 6 and 8 allows us to conclude that a more effective coating leads to a higher adhesive percentage.

The mucoadhesive properties of positively and negatively charged liposomes were compared using the particle counting method (Fig. 9) (29). Positively charged liposome had a higher adhesive percentage to a mucin layer than negatively charged ones, and this was attributed to the negatively charged surface of the mucin layer of the intestine. However, the

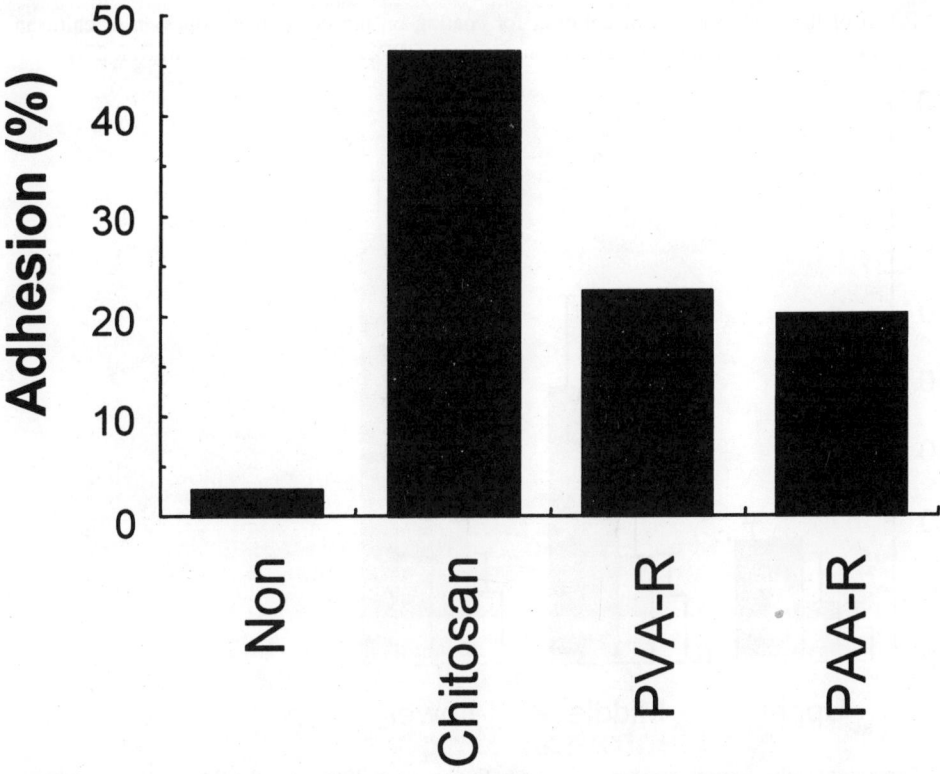

Figure 7 Percentage adhesion of liposomes coated with various polymers to rat intestinal tube. (From Ref. 27.)

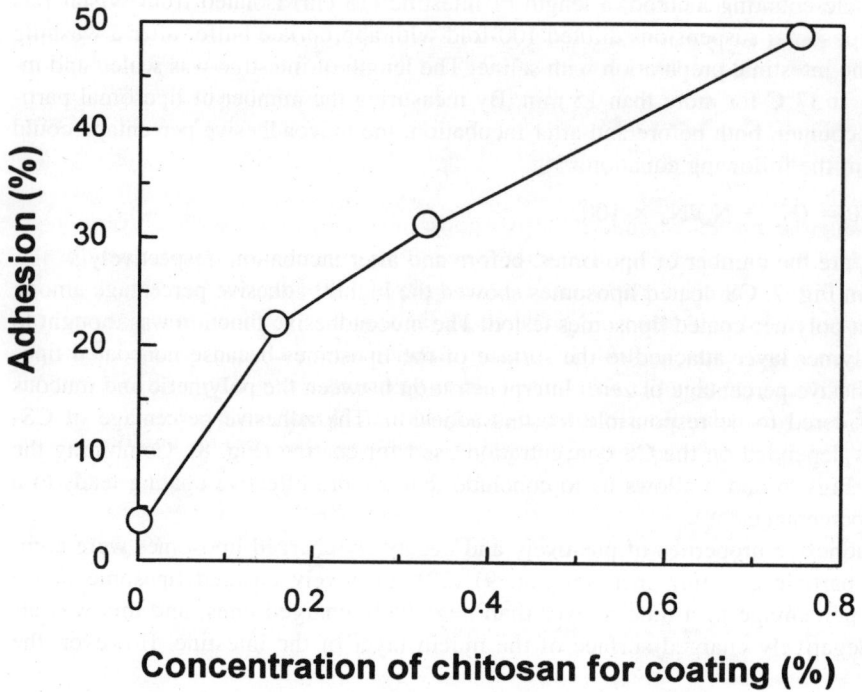

Figure 8 Effect of the concentration of chitosan for coating on the percentage adhesion of chitosan-coated liposomes to the rat intestinal tube. Lipid composition: DPPC/DCP = 8:2. (From Ref. 27.)

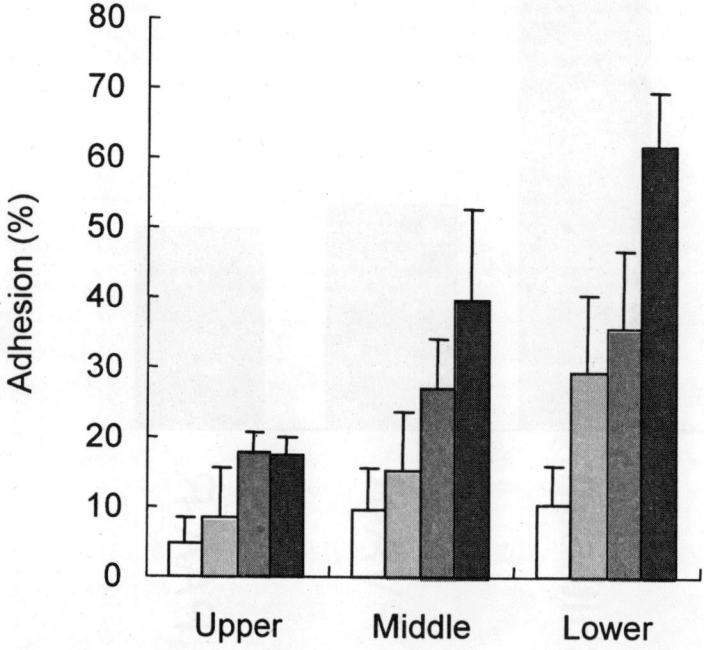

Figure 9 Percentage adhesion of liposomes coated with various polymers to the three different sections of rat intestinal tube (n = 4). Lipid compositions: DPPC/DCP = 8:2, DPPC/SA = 40:1. Medium: saline (pH 6.1). (From Ref. 30.) ☐, Negatively charged MLVs; ☐, positively charged MLVs; ■, carbopol-coated MLVs; ■, chitosan-coated MLVs.

CP-coated, and thus negatively charged, liposomes, as well as positively charged CS-coated liposomes, showed a higher adhesive percentage than positively charged noncoated liposomes. This result suggests again that a physical interaction between the polymer and mucous layer is an important factor in facilitating the mucoadhesion of polymer-coated liposomes.

C. Improved Enteral Absorption of Peptide Drugs

The most important role played by mucoadhesive liposomes is to improve the absorption of poorly absorbed drugs, such as peptides. The effectiveness of polymer-coated liposomes for the oral administration of peptide drugs has been evaluated in rats (3).

Insulin-encapsulating liposomes were prepared by the thin-film method with 1 mg/mL insulin solution, prepared by mixing 0.01 N HCl insulin solution with the same volume of acetate buffer (pH 4.4). Coating of the polymer was carried out as described above. The insulin liposomal suspensions (24 IU/rat) were administered intragastrically to male Wistar rats previously fasted for 24 h and the plasma glucose levels were measured using a commercially available kit (glucose CII

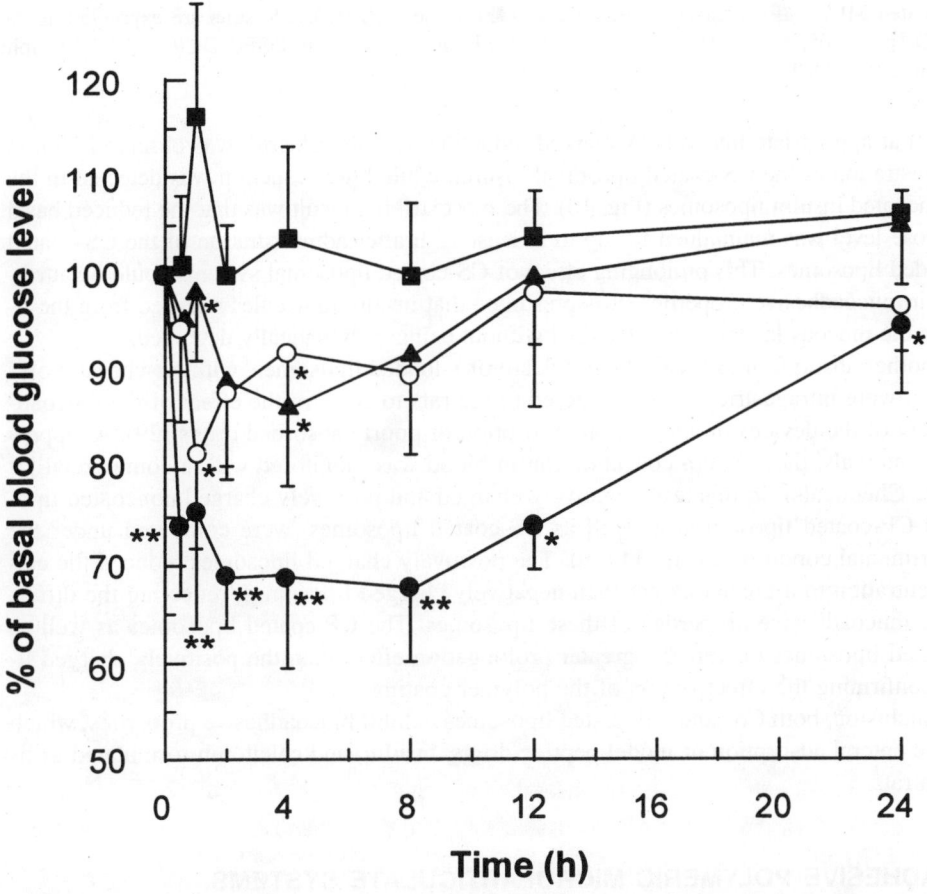

Figure 10 Change in basal blood glucose (%) after oral administration of an insulin solution or insulin-encapsulated liposomes. ○, Noncoated liposome; ●, CS-coated liposome; ■, control; ▲, insulin solution. The dose of insulin for oral administration was 24 IU/rat. Symbols represent mean ± SD of six experiments for oral administration of insulin solution. Statistically significant compared with control: $p < 0.01$, **; $p < 0.05$, *.

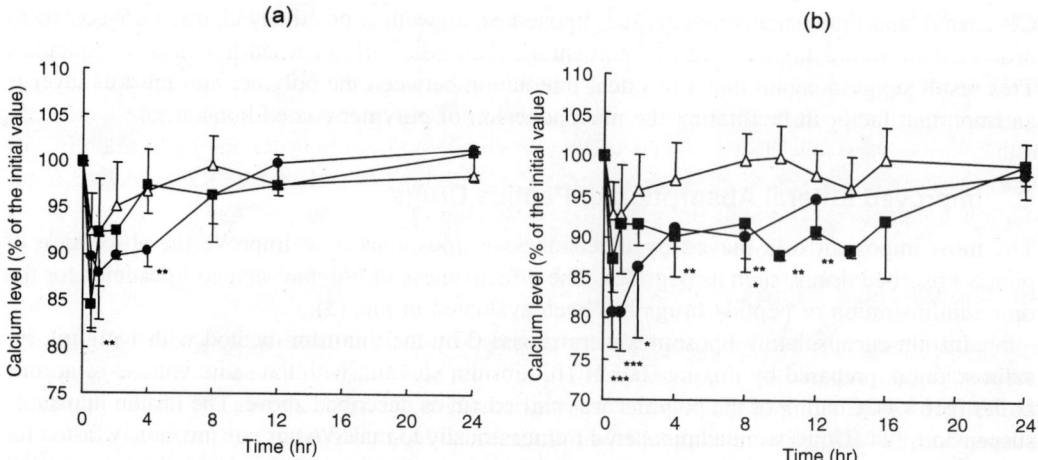

Figure 11 Profiles of plasma Ca level (a) after oral administration of calcitonin solution (△), negatively charged MLVs (■), positively charged MLVs (●); (b) after oral administration of calcitonin solution (△), carbopol-coated MLVs (■), chitosan-coated MLVs (●). Dose: 500 IU/kg. Results are expressed as the mean ± SD *$p < 0.05$, **$p < 0.01$, ***$p < 0.001$. (a) Lipid composition; DSPC/DCP = 8:2. (b) Lipid composition; DPPC/DCP = 8:2 or DPPC/SA = 40:1.

test WAKO) at appropriate intervals. A marked reduction in blood glucose was observed 30 min after administration of the CS-coated liposomal insulin, while little reduction was detected in the case of noncoated insulin liposomes (Fig. 10). The most striking result was that the reduced basal blood glucose level was maintained for up to at least 12 h after administration of the CS-coated insulin-loaded liposomes. This prolonging effect of CS-coated liposomal systems could be attributed to their mucoadhesive properties. It is presumed that insulin molecules released from the liposomes in the mucous layer can be absorbed without being enzymatically degraded.

In another absorption test, calcitonin (elcatonin)–loaded liposomes, with or without polymer coating, were intragastrically administered to the rats to confirm the effect of the mucoadhesive ability of the devices on the enteral absorption of poorly absorbed drugs (29). At appropriate time intervals, the calcium concentration in blood was monitored with a commercial kit (Wako Pure Chemicals). In this test, negatively charged and positively charged noncoated liposomes and CP-coated liposomes, as well as CS-coated liposomes, were compared under the same experimental conditions. (Fig. 11a, b). The positively charged liposomes reduced the calcium concentration to a greater extent than negatively charged liposomes, reflecting the difference in the mucoadhesive properties of these liposomes. The CP-coated liposomes as well as the CS-coated liposomes exhibited a greater prolongation effect than the positively charged liposomes, confirming the effectiveness of the polymer coating.

In conclusion, both CS- and CP-coated liposomes exhibit mucoadhesive properties, which improve the enteral adsorption of model peptide drugs, insulin, and calcitonin formulated as liposomes in rats.

IV. BIOADHESIVE POLYMERIC MICROPARTICULATE SYSTEMS

The polymeric microparticulate systems, consisting of nano- and microspheres, have been studied extensively as oral drug delivery systems to control drug release and improve drug bioavailability. Polymeric drug delivery systems are physically and physiologically more stable than liposomes or emulsions. Orally administered microparticulate systems are captured by gut-associated lymphoid tissue (GALT), and then adhere to the intestinal mucosa or are eliminated in the feces. Several papers have reported that solid nanoparticles are taken up directly into the systemic circulation through the gut wall. However, the percentage of microparticles taken up in this way is very low (1–2%). However, an alternative way to improve the bioavailability of poorly absorbed drugs is to use bioadhesive systems, which can extend the GI transition time to allow completion of the absorption of the released drug.

A. Bioadhesive Microspheres

Longer et al. were the first to show that a delayed GI transit induced by bioadhesive polymer can lead to an increased oral bioavailability of a drug (31,32). They demonstrated that albumin microspheres admixed with 30% polycarbophil particles successfully adhered to the stomach mucosa and increased the bioavailability of chlorothiazide, a drug whose absorption window is limited to the proximal parts of the GI tract. The distribution of microspheres in the rat small intestine, in the presence and absence of polycarbophil, after oral administration is shown in Fig. 12. In polycarbophil dosage forms, nearly 90% of the albumin beads remain in the stomach after 6 h, with few beads being seen beyond the stomach. It was evident that polycarbophil binds to the gastric mucin–epithelial cell surface. However, the majority of microspheres, in the absence of polycarbophil, moved at least halfway down the small intestine, with some moving even further. The relative bioavailability from such a polycarbophil–albumin dosage form is

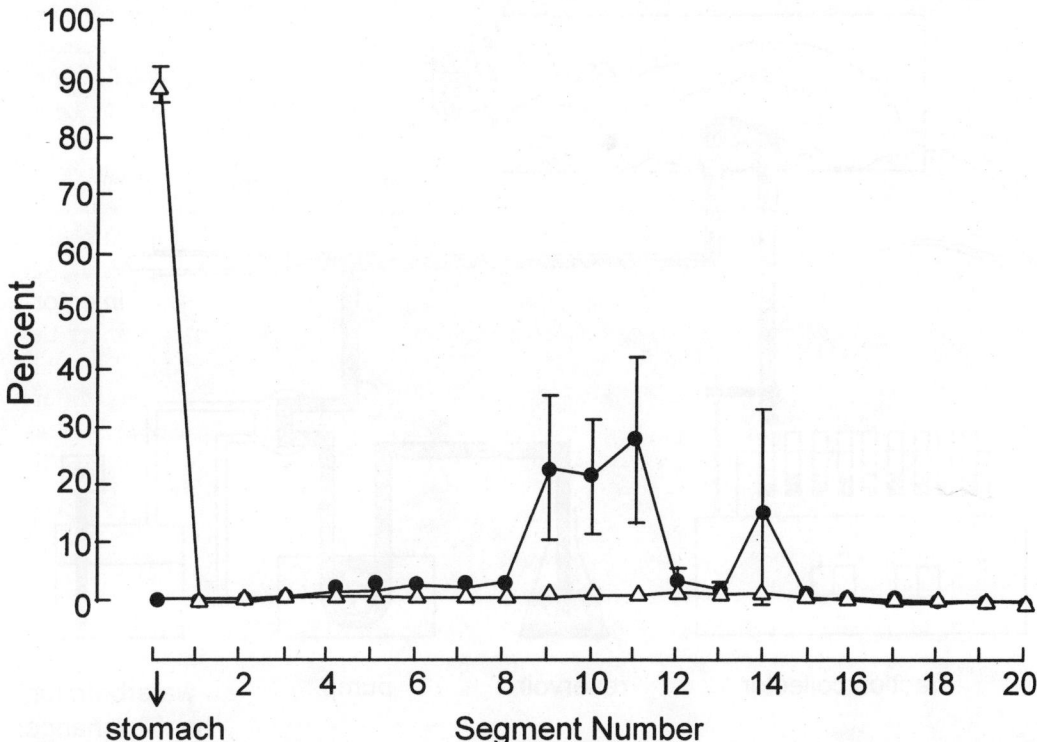

Figure 12 Distribution of albumin beads in the rat small intestine after 6 h. ●, Albumin beads; △, bioadhesive polycarbophil–albumin bead dosage form. (From Ref. 33.)

1.95 times greater than that from albumin microspheres. These data indicate that the bioadhesion system is useful for improving the bioavailability of poorly absorbed drugs by delaying the gastric emptying time. However, in this case, the polycarbophil particles and albumin microspheres form a simple physical mixture. It is thought that particles could not be properly incorporated into polymer gel in such an environment and coating particles with mucoadhesive polymers would be preferable.

Junginger et al. evaluated the mean residence time of poly(2-hydroxyethyl methacrylate) microspheres coated with polycarbophil, Carbomer, and Eudragit RL100 after injection into a gut segment perfused in situ (Fig. 13) (16,17,33). Fifty microspheres were injected and the loop was perfused at a constant flow of 1.0 mL/min. Fractions of the perfusate were collected at intervals of 5 min and the particles in each fraction were counted. The rank order of mucoadhesiveness was polycarbophil > Eudragit RL > Carbomer. However, even in the case of microspheres coated with polycarbophil, the bioadhesive effect was only apparent for about 2 h. Thereafter, the microspheres adhering to the mucosal tissue became detached. It was believed that either turnover of the mucus occurred or these polymers exhibited poor mucoadhesive properties.

Akiyama et al. prepared three types of microspheres (177–500 μm in diameter), i.e., (a) PGEF microspheres prepared by spraying and chilling a melted mixture of tetraglycerol pen-

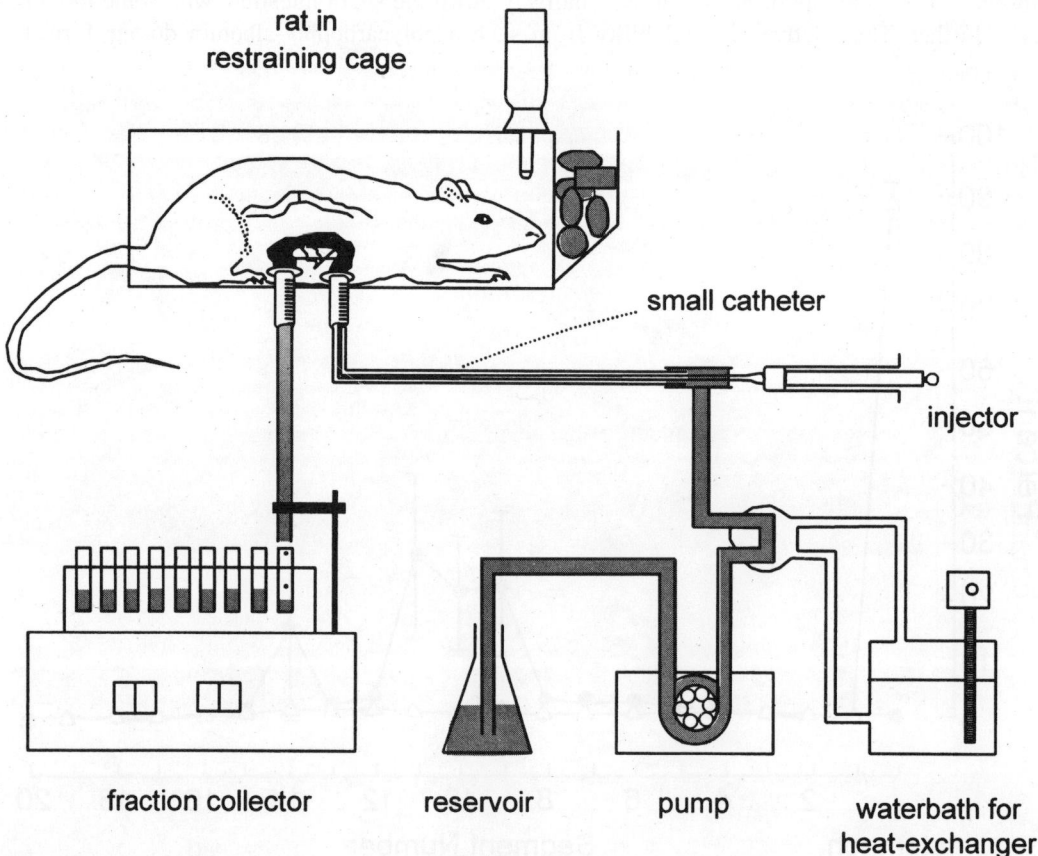

Figure 13 Experimental setup to investigate the intestinal transit of microspheres in a chronically isolated loop in the rat. (From Ref. 35.)

tastearate (TGPS) and tetraglycerol monostearate (TGMS); (b) PGEF microspheres coated with Carbopol 934P prepared using a centrifugal fluidizer; and (c) CPD microspheres prepared by spraying and chilling the CP dispersion with a mixture of TGPS and TGMS (34). In a series of in vitro studies of mucoadhesiveness, 100 microspheres were placed on stomach and small intestine that had been removed from rats. After 20 min, the stomach and small intestine were tilted at 45° and rinsed with JP No. 1 fluid and saline for 5 min, respectively. Over 90% of the CPD microspheres remained on each tissue. However, less than 10% of PGEF microspheres or CPC microspheres remained on the stomach. Furthermore, no microspheres could be found on the small intestine. This pattern was also observed in a series of in vivo studies (Fig. 14). In general, mucoadhesive dosage forms are prepared by coating microspheres with mucoadhesive polymer, as in the case of CPC microspheres. Carbopol forms a gel layer around the microspheres in acidic solution and the gel layer soon detaches itself from the surface due to a lack of affinity for PGEF. In the case of CPD microspheres, CP was buried in the microspheres and, therefore, the swollen CP particles were strongly associated with the microspheres. Consequently, CPD microspheres adhered tightly to the mucosal surfaces (Fig. 15). These data suggest that a comparison of the interaction between polymer and mucin and between polymer and core particles is necessary in order to design suitable particles.

B. Mucoadhesive Lactide/glycolide Copolymer Nanospheres to Improve Peptide Delivery

We have developed mucoadhesive lactide/glycolide copolymer (PLGA) nanospheres coated with chitosan by using the emulsion solvent diffusion method in water (WSD) or oil (OSD) (35–37). In the WSD method, PLGA dissolved in the acetone/methanol mixture was poured into aqueous chitosan and PVA solution. The emulsion droplets were submicronized due to the rapid diffusion of the organic solvent in the aqueous solution (Marangoni effect). The emulsion

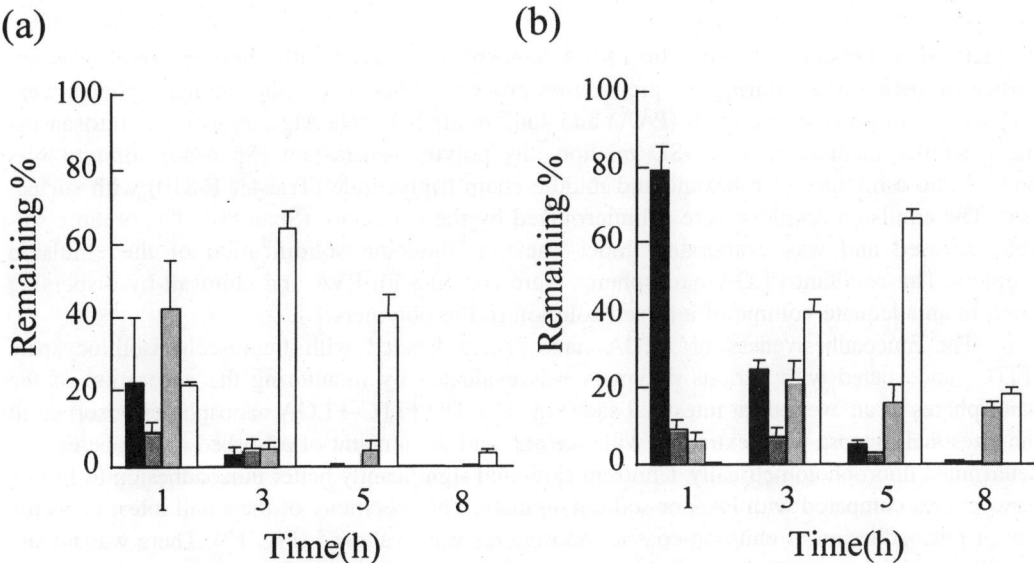

Figure 14 Distribution of (a) PGEF microspheres and (b) CPD microspheres in the stomach and upper, middle, and lower segment of the small intestine in rats. ■, Stomach; ☐, upper segment; ☐, middle segment; ☐, lower segment. Data are shown as mean ± SEM (n = 3). (From Ref. 37.)

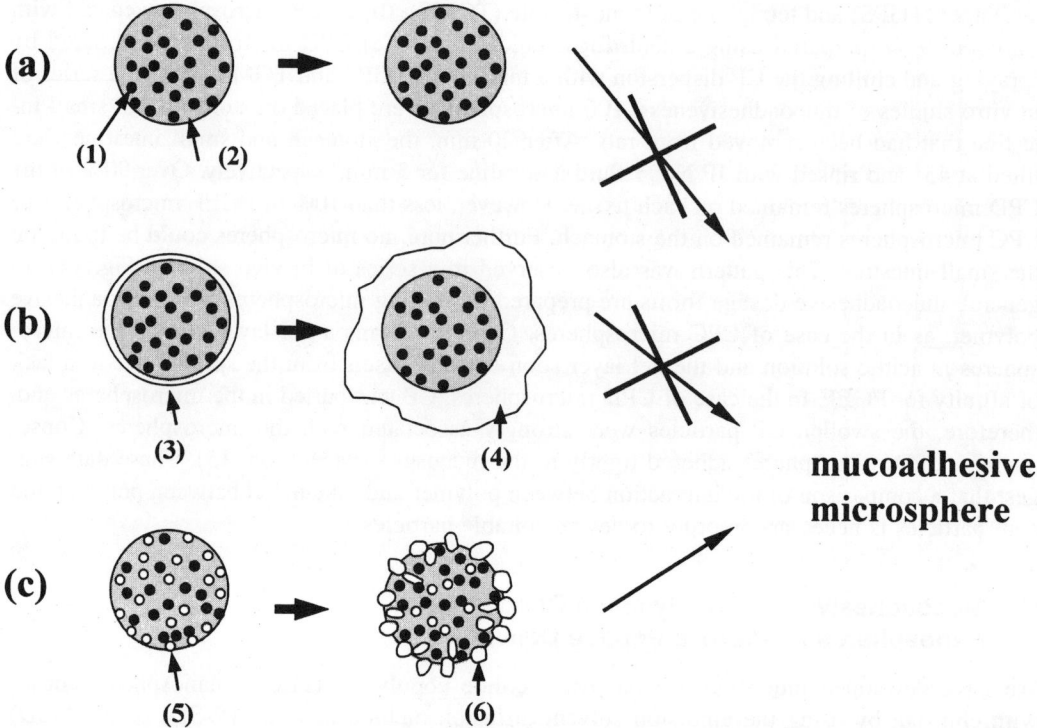

Figure 15 Schematic description of the mucoadhesion process with microspheres. (a) PGEF microsphere; (b) CPC microsphere; (c) CPD microsphere; (1) drug; (2) PGEF; (3) coated CP layer; (4) swollen CP layer; (5) dispersed CP; (6) swollen CP. (From Ref. 37.)

droplets were transformed into solid PLGA nanospheres coated with chitosan which was adsorbed on their surface during the preparation process. Other mucoadhesive nanospheres were prepared from poly(acrylic acid) (PAA) and sodium alginate (Na Alg), as well as chitosan using a similar method. In the OSD method, the polymer–surfactant (Span-80) solution was poured into a mixture of n-hexane and middle-chain triglyceride (Triester F-810) with surfactant. The emulsion droplets were submicronized by the surfactant (Span-80). The organic solvent diffused and was evaporated under vacuum, inducing solidification of the emulsion droplets. The resultant PLGA nanospheres were coated with PVA and chitosan by dispersing them in an adequate volume of a mixed solution of the polymers.

The mucoadhesiveness of PLGA nanospheres labeled with fluorescein isothiocyanate (FITC) and coated with various polymers was evaluated by monitoring the adsorption of the nanospheres to an everted rat intestinal sac (Fig. 16). The FITC–PLGA nanospheres adsorbed to the intestinal mucosa were extracted with acetone and the amount of adsorbed nanospheres was determined fluorophotometrically. Chitosan exhibited significantly better mucoadhesion to PLGA nanospheres compared with PAA or sodium alginate. The specificity of the small intestine as the site of mucoadhesion of chitosan-coated nanospheres was evaluated (Fig. 17). There was no site specificity of the mucoadhesion of chitosan-modified nanospheres as far as the gut sac was concerned, although there was a trend in reduced mucoadhesion in the order duodenum > jejunum > ileum. This behavior should help improve the intestinal absorption of a drug released from nanospheres due to the prolonged residence of the nanospheres in the small intestine.

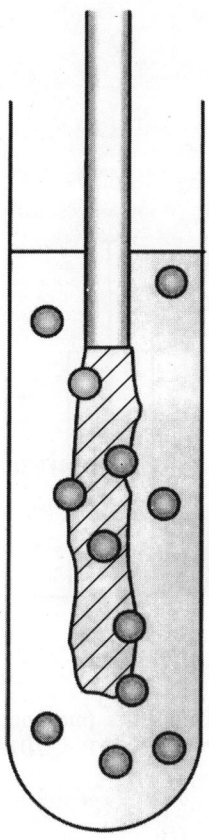

Figure 16 Evaluation of mucoadhesive properties of PLGA nanospheres in vitro with an everted rat intestinal sac. ◯, Nanospheres; ▨ , everted intestine.

Chitosan-coated nanospheres loaded with elcatonin were prepared by the OSD method. Coating the nanospheres with chitosan did not alter the content of drug, its recovery, or its release pattern. Elcatonin solution or PLGA nanosphere suspensions loaded with elcatonin corresponding to 125, 250, and 500 IU/kg were intragastrically administered via a sonde to male Wistar rats. The blood calcium levels fell temporarily by about 80–85% over 1 h after intragastric administration of elcatonin solution (125–500 IU/kg), as shown in Fig. 18. The noncoated nanospheres exhibited almost the same blood calcium time profile as the solution of 250 IU/kg or less. By increasing the dose administered, the noncoated nanospheres were able to maintain the reduced Ca level up to 10 h. A further prolonged reduction in blood Ca after administration of the chitosan-coated nanospheres was seen up to 12 h at doses of 125 IU/kg or 250 IU/kg. Increasing the dose further, e.g., 500 IU/kg, dramatically reduced the blood calcium and the action was prolonged up to 48 h following the administration of chitosan-coated nanospheres. Generally, peptides are assumed to be poorly absorbed through the gut wall due to their instability in the digestive tract due to the action of digestive enzymes and poor mucosal permeability. However, the extent of drug absorption attributed to their mucoadhesiveness as shown in Figs. 17 and 18 could be significantly improved by increasing the residence time and time of intimate contact between nanospheres and the wall of the small intestine.

The effect of feeding on the mucoadhesiveness of nanosphere encapsulating elcatonin, with or without a chitosan coating, was investigated by administering them intragastrically to

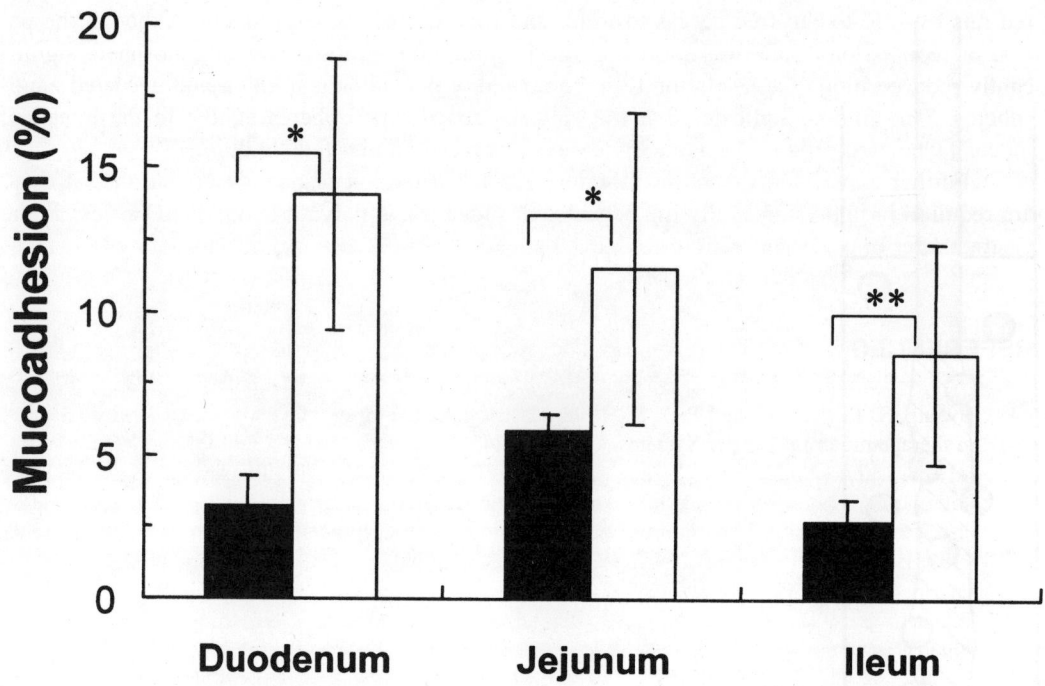

Figure 17 Effect of the intestinal site of the rat intestine on the mucoadhesive properties (medium; saline). ■, Noncoated nanospheres; □, chitosan-coated nanospheres. Mean ± SD. *P < 0.05, **P < 0.01.

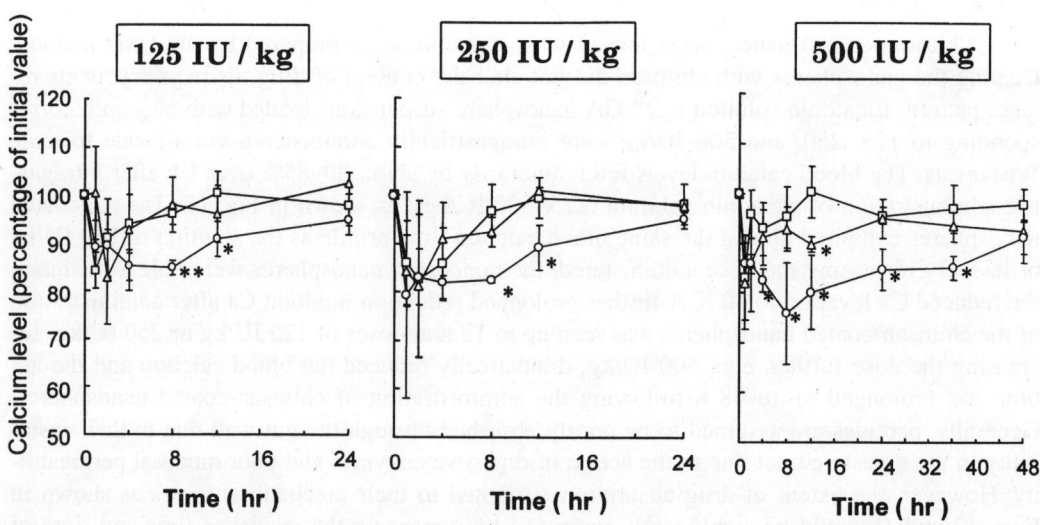

Figure 18 Profiles of calcium levels (percentage of the initial value) after intragastric administration to the fasted rats (n = 3). Mean ± SD. *P < 0.05, **p < 0.01. □, Elcatonin solution; △, noncoated nanospheres; ○, chitosan-coated nanospheres.

fed rats (39). Rats had free access to water and food during the experiment. Although the period of reduced blood Ca was shorter in the fed state, the chitosan-coated nanosphere significantly reduced blood Ca levels for 12 h, compared with elcatonin solution and uncoated nanospheres. This finding indicates that the chitosan-coated nanospheres adhere to the intestinal mucus layers and produce sustained release of drug even under fed conditions.

Further experiments, such as monitoring the distribution of nanospheres in the GI tract, are required to understand fully the behavior of bioadhesive polymeric colloidal carriers in the GI tract after oral administration.

REFERENCES

1. Hwang, S. J., Park, H. and Park K., 1998, Gastric retentive drug delivery systems, critical reviews in therapeutic drug. Carrier Systems, 15: 243–284.
2. (a) Kawashima, Y., Niwa, T., Takeuchi, H., Hino, T., and Itoh, Y., 1991, Preparation of multiple unit hollow microspheres (microballoons) with acrylic resin containing tranilast and their drug release characteristics (in vitro) and floating behavior (in vitro). J. Control. Release, 16: 279–290. (b) Ibid., 1992, Hollow microspheres for use as a floating controlled drug delivery system in the stomach. J. Pharm. Sci., 81: 135–140.
3. Takeuchi, H., Yamamoto, H., Niwa, T., Hino, T. and Kawashima, Y., 1996, Enteral absorption of insulin in rats from mucoadhesive chitosan-coated liposomes. Pharm. Research, 13: 896–901.
4. Sheth, P. R. and Tossounian, J. L., 1978, Sustained release pharmaceutical capsules. U.S. patent 4,126,672.
5. Sato, Y., Kawashima, Y., Takeuchi, H., Yamamoto, H., Fujibayashi, Y., Preparation of multiple unit hollow microspheres (microballoons) as a floating controlled drug delivery system in the stomach and in vivo evaluation. Proceedings of 119th Meet Pharmaceutical Society of Japan 4:30.
6. Ichikawa, M., Watanabe, S. and Miyake, Y., 1991, A new multiple-unit oral floating dosage system. I: Preparation and in vitro evaluation of floating and sustained-release characteristics. J. Pharm. Sci., 80: 1062–1066.
7. Iannuccelli, V., Coppi, G., Bernabei, M. T. and Cameroui, R., 1998, Air compartment multiple-unit system for prolonged gastric residence. I: Formulation study. Int. J. Pharm., 174: 47–54.
8. Iannuccelli, V., Coppi, G., Sansone, R. and Ferolla, G., 1998, Air compartment multiple-unit system for prolonged gastric residence. Part. In vivo evaluation. Int. J. Pharm., 174: 55–62.
9. Yuasa, H., Takashima, Y. and Kanaya, Y., 1996, Studies on the development of intragastric floating and sustained release preparation. I: Application of calcium silicate as a floating carrier. Chem. Pharm. Bull., 44: 1361–1366.
10. Takashima, Y., Yuasa, H. and Kanaya, Y., 1998, Studies on production of higher functional pharmaceutical preparations by using various additives. III: Application of hollow glass beads for intragastric floating granules. Chem. Pharm. Bull., 46: 1173–1176.
11. Patel, H. and Ryman, B. E., 1981, Systemic and oral administration of liposomes. In: C. G. Knight (Ed.), Liposomes: From Physical Structure to Therapeutic Applications, Elsevier, Amsterdam, pp. 409–441.
12. Guputa, P. K., Leung, S-H. S. and Robinson, J. R., 1990, Bioadhesives/mucoadhesives in drug delivery to the gastrointestinal tract. In: V. Lenaerts and R. Gurny (Eds.), Bioadhesive Drug Delivery Systems, CRC Press, Boca Raton, FL, pp. 65–92.
13. Ishida, M., Nambu, N. and Nagai, T., 1982, Mucosal dosage form of lidocaine for toothache using hydroxypropyl cellulose and carbopol. Chem. Pharm. Bull., 30: 980–984.
14. Satoh, K., Takayama, K., Machida, Y., Suzuki, Y., Nakagaki, M. and Nagai, T., 1989, Factors affecting the bioadhesive property of tablets consisting of hydroxypropyl cellulose and carboxyvinyl polymer. Chem. Pharm. Bull., 37: 1366–1368.
15. Chen, W.-G. and Hwang, G. C.-C., 1992, Adhesive and in vitro release characteristics of propranolol bioadhesive disc system. Int. J. Pharm., 82: 61–66.

16. Peppas, N. A. and Mikos, A. G., 1989, Experimental methods for determination of bioadhesive bond strength of polymers with mucus. STP Pharm., 5: 187–191.
17. Lehr, C.-M., Bouwstra, J. A., Tukker, J. J. and Junginger, H. E., 1990, Intestinal transit of bioadhesive microspheres in an in situ loop in the rat: a comparative study with copolymers and blends based on poly acrylic (acid). J. Control. Release, 13: 51–62.
18. Lehr, C-M., Bouwstra, J. A., Kok, W., De Boer, A. G., Tukker, J. J., Verhoef, J. C., Breimer, D. D. and Junginger, H. E., 1992, Effects of the mucoadhesive polymer polycarbophil on the intestinal absorption of a peptide drug in the rat. J. Pharm. Pharmacol., 44: 402–407.
19. Pimienta, C., Chouinard, F., Labib, A., and Lenaerts, V., 1992, Effect of various poloxamer coatings on in vitro adhesion of isohexylcyanoacrylate nanospheres to rat ileal segments under liquid flow. Int. J. Pharm., 80: 1–8.
20. Lehr, C.-M., Bouwstra, J. A., Schacht, E. H., and Junginger, H. E., 1992, In vitro evaluation of mucoadhesive properties of chitosan and some other natural polymers. Int. J. Pharm., 78: 43–48.
21. (a) Sunamoto, J., Iwamoto, K., Takada, M., Yuzuriha T. and Katayama K., 1983, Improved drug delivery to target specific organs using liposomes as coated with polysacchrides. Polym. Sci. Technol., 23: 157–168; (b) Sunamoto, J., Iwamoto, K., Takada, M., Yuzurihat, and Katayama K., 1984, Polymer coated liposomes for drug delivery to target specific organs. In: Recent Advances in Drug Delivery Systems, J. M. Anderson and S. W. Kim (Eds.), pp. 153–162.
22. Jamshaid, M., Farr, S. J., Kearney, P. and Kellaway, I. W., 1988, Poloxamer sorption on liposomes: comparison with polystyrene latex and influence on solute efflux. Int. J. Pharm., 48: 125–131.
23. Kronberg, B., Dahlman, A., Carlfors, J., Karlsson, J. and Artursson, P., 1990, Preparation and evaluation of sterically stabilized liposomes: colloidal stability, serum stability, macrophage uptake, and toxicity. J. Pharm. Sci., 79: 667–671.
24. Dong, C. and Rogers, J. A., 1991, Polymer-coated liposomes: stability and release of ASA from carboxymethyl chitin–coated liposomes. J. Contl. Rel., 17: 217–224.
25. Alamelu, S. and Rao K. P., 1991, Studies on the carboxymethyl chitosan–containing liposomes for their stability and controlled release of dapson. J. Microencaps., 8: 505–515.
26. Elferink, M. G. L., de Wit, J. G., Veld, G. In't, Reichert A., Driessen, A. J. M., Ringsdorf, H. and Konings W. N., 1992, The stability and functional properties of proteoliposomes mixed with dextran derivatives bearing hydrophobic anchor groups. Biochim. Biophys. Acta, 1106: 23–30.
27. Takeuchi, H., Yamamoto, H., Niwa, T., Hino, T. and Kawashima, Y., 1994, Mucoadhesion of polymer-coated liposomes to rat intestine in vitro. Chem. Pharm. Bull., 42: 1954–1956.
28. Arnold, S. C., Ferritto, M. S., Lenz, R. W. and Tirrell, D. A., 1986, pH dependent modification of phospholipid vesicle membranes by poly(carboxylic acid)s bearing pendant cholesteryl esters. Polym. Prepr., 27: 42–43.
29. Takeuchi, H., Matsui, Y., Yamamoto, H. and Kawashima, Y., 1999, Mucoadhesive liposomes coated with chitosan or carbopol for oral administration of peptide drugs. Proc. 26th Int. Symp. on Controlled Release of Bioactive Materials, 988-989.
30. Smart, J. D., 1991, An in vitro assessment of some mucosaadhesive dosage forms. Int. J. Pharm., 73: 69–74.
31. Ch'ng, H. S., Park, H., Kelly, P. and Robinson, J. R., 1985, Bioadhesive polymers as platforms for oral controlled drug delivery. II: Synthesis and evaluation of some swelling, water-insoluble bioadhesive polymers. J. Pharm. Sci., 74: 399–405.
32. Longer, M. A., Ch'ng, H. S. and Robinson, J. R., 1985, Bioadhesive polymers as platforms for oral controlled drug delivery. III: Oral delivery of chlorothiazide using a bioadhesive polymer. J. Pharm. Sci., 74: 406–411.
33. Poelma, F. G. J. and Tukker, J. J., 1987, Evaluation of a chronically isolated intestinal loop in the rat for the study of drug absorption kinetics. J. Pharm. Sci., 76: 433–436.
34. Akiyama, Y., Nagahara, N., Kashihara T., Hirai, S., and Toguchi, H, 1995, In vitro and in vivo evaluation of mucoadhesive microspheres prepared for the gastrointestinal tract using polyglycerol esters of fatty acids and a poly(acrylic acid) derivative. Pharm. Res., 12: 397–405.
35. Niwa, T, Takeuchi, H., Hino, T. Kunou, N. and Kawashima Y., 1993, Preparations of biodegradable nanospheres of water soluble and insoluble drugs with DL-lactide/glycolide copolymer by a novel

spontaneous emulsification solvent diffusion method, and the drug release behavior. J. Control. Release, 25: 89–98.
36. Kawashima, Y., Yamamoto, H., Takeuchi, H., Hino, T. and Niwa. T., 1998, Properties of a peptide containing DL-lactide/glycolide copolymer nanospheres prepared by novel emulsion solvent diffusion methods. Eur. J. Pharm. Biopharm., 45: 41–48.
37. Kawashima, Y., Yamamoto, H., Takeuchi, H. and Kuno, Y., 1998, Mucoadhesive DL-lactide/glycolide copolymer nanospheres coated with chitosan to improve oral delivery of elcatonin. Pharm. Develop. Technol., in press.

25
In Vitro–In Vivo Correlations in the Development of Solid Oral Controlled Release Dosage Forms

Yihong Qiu
Abbott Laboratories, North Chicago, Illinois

Emil E. Samara
Chiron Corporation, Emeryville, California

Guoliang Cao
Abbott Laboratories, Abbott Park, Illinois

I. INTRODUCTION

The therapeutic efficacy of a drug is determined by the in vivo performance of the pharmaceutical dosage form, which is in turn dependent on the quality and characteristics of the product. With a controlled release product a patient is typically exposed to specific plasma levels over an extended period of time (e.g., 12 or 24 h). There should be specific in vitro methods to assure the consistent in vivo performance from each batch of the same product. Among various in vitro procedures used to control the product quality, the drug release test is the single most useful method for this purpose, particularly when differences in the release rate can be correlated quantitatively with the in vivo differences in product performance, i.e., in vitro–in vivo correlation (IVIVC). Over the last 10 years, there has been an increasing confidence in using in vitro dissolution as an indication of the in vivo bioavailability characteristics for the drug product based on IVIVC (1). As a result, an increasing number of IVIVC studies have been included in New Drug Application (NDA) submissions; particularly with controlled release dosage forms, and a guidance for industry on IVIVC was established by the FDA (1).

IVIVC has been defined by the U.S. Pharmacopeia (USP) and The Food and Drug Administration (FDA), respectively, as follows (1,2):

> *USP:* The establishment of a relationship between a biological property, or a parameter derived from a biological property produced by a dosage form, and a physicochemical characteristic of the same dosage form.
>
> *FDA:* A predictive mathematical model describing the relationship between an in vitro property (usually the extent or rate of drug release) and a relevant in vivo response (e.g., plasma concentration or amount of drug absorbed).

The goal of an IVIVC study is to define a relationship between two parameters. According to the FDA Guidance, the parameters to be correlated are normally specified as in vitro release rate and in vivo absorption rate (1). It should be noted that this relationship may be expanded to critical formulation parameters and "in vivo" input rate. The relationship is generally described as a linear function with or without time scaling. However, nonlinear models can also be suggested (3,4).

The usefulness of IVIVC has been recognized since the early 1960s. Exploring the preliminary in vitro–in vivo association or correlation is very useful in guiding formulation and process development in the early stages of product development. A validated IVIVC can facilitate scale-up, pre- and postapproval changes (1). The establishment of meaningful dissolution specifications and use of dissolution as a surrogate for bioequivalency testing is another advantage of a validated IVIVC since IVIVC provides a biological meaning to the specification limits and to the controls carried out with the in vitro dissolution test (1). In general, compared to immediate-release (IR) products, an IVIVC is more readily defined for controlled release dosage forms where drug release is rate limiting in the absorption process. It is believed that the availability of a well-defined, predictive IVIVC of high quality can result in a significant positive impact on product quality and reduced regulatory burden. Hence, the FDA has recommended investigation of the possibility of an IVIVC in the development of controlled release dosage forms (1).

II. CATEGORIES OF CORRELATIONS

Evaluation of in vitro–in vivo correlations by different levels was first proposed for controlled release dosage forms in the USP's Information chapter 1088 (5) and was later adopted globally. Presently, IVIVC is categorized by the FDA into levels A, B, C, and Multiple C depending on the ability of the correlation to predict the complete plasma profile of a dosage form (1).

Level A: A predictive mathematical model for the relationship between the entire in vitro release time course and the entire in vivo response time course, e.g., the time course of plasma drug concentration or amount of drug absorbed.

Level B: A predictive mathematical model for the relationship between summary parameters that characterize the in vitro and in vivo time courses, e.g., models that relate the mean in vitro dissolution time to the mean in vivo dissolution time, or to mean residence time in vivo.

Level C: A predictive mathematical model for the relationship between the amount dissolved in vitro at a particular time (e.g., Q_{60}) or the time required for dissolution of a fixed amount (e.g., $T_{50\%}$) and a summary parameter that characterizes the in vivo time course (e.g., C_{max} or AUC).

Multiple level C: Predictive mathematical models for the relationships between the amount dissolved at several time points of the product and one or several pharmacokinetic parameters of interest.

Level A is the most informative and useful correlation in that it represents a point-to-point relationship between in vitro release and in vivo release/absorption from the dosage form. It can be used to predict the entire in vivo time course from the in vitro data; thus, it is highly recommended for controlled release dosage forms. Multiple level C is also useful as it provides the in vitro release profile of a dosage form with biological meaning. Level C can be useful in early stages of product development, although it does not reflect the complete shape of the plasma concentration time curve. Level B utilizes the principles of statistical moment analysis. However, it is least useful for regulatory applications because there can be a number of different in vitro or in vivo profiles that will produce similar mean time values.

III. MATHEMATICAL METHODS USED IN DIFFERENT LEVELS OF CORRELATIONS

A. Convolution and Deconvolution

Convolution and deconvolution methods are essential tools for establishing level A IVIVC. Convolution is a model-independent method used in linear system analysis. Based on the superposition principle in a linear time–invariant system, a response, C(t), to an arbitrary input, f(t), of the system can be obtained using the following convolution integral (6):

$$C(t) = f(t)*C_\delta(t) = \int_0^\infty C_\delta(t-\tau)f(\tau)d\tau \qquad (1)$$

where $C_\delta(t)$ is the unit impulse response that defines the characteristic of the system. It is the response of the system to an instantaneous unit input, usually attainable from IV bolus or oral solution. By the same principle, f(t) can be obtained by deconvolution, the inverse operation of convolution. The representative systems used in pharmaceutical applications are given in Table 1. The definition of a system is flexible and is determined by the nature of the time functions involved (7). Depending on different $C_\delta(t)$ and input responses used to define a system, f(t) obtained by deconvolution in IVIVC may represent the dissolution process, absorption process, or the combined processes of the two. In exploring IVIVC, level A correlation is usually estimated by a two-stage procedure, i.e., deconvolution followed by correlating the fraction dissolved in vitro with the fraction dissolved or absorbed in vivo, or convolution followed by comparison of the observed with predicted plasma profiles. According to Eq. 1, the in vitro drug release and the in vivo input (release/absorption) estimated by deconvolution of the unit impulse response with the observed plasma data either are directly superimposable or can be made to be superimposable by the use of a scaling factor should an IVIVC exist. Similarly, the plasma concentration profile observed following oral administration should be in good agreement with that obtained by convolution of the unit impulse response with in vitro release data should there be a level A IVIVC.

1. General Solution

The exact solution of convolution or deconvolution can be obtained by operation of Laplace transform if each functional form is defined:

$$L\{C(t)\} = L\{(C_\delta * f)(t)\} = L\{C_\delta(t)\}L\{f(t)\} \qquad (2)$$

$$f(t) = L^{-1}\{\bar{f}(s)\} = L^{-1}\left\{\frac{\bar{c}(s)}{\bar{c}_\delta(s)}\right\} \qquad (3)$$

Table 1 Illustration of System Defintions for Oral Administration

Case	Unit Impulse Response $C_\delta(t)$	Input Response $C(t)$	Input Function $f(t)$
I	Plasma levels from iv bolus	Plasma levels from oral solution	Absorption in GI
II	Plasma levels from iv bolus	Plasma levels from oral solid dosage form	Dissolution and absorption in GI
III	Plasma levels from oral solution	Plasma levels from oral solid dosage form	Dissolution in GI

where L and L^{-1} denote Laplace transform and inverse Laplace transform, respectively. Deconvolution methods include explicit (numerical point–area and midpoint methods, least-squares curve fitting using polyexponential, polynomial, spline functions,) and implicit methods (prescribed function or deconvolution via convolution) (8–20).

Since the disposition of most drugs can be described by polyexponentials,

$$C_\delta(t) = \sum_{i=1}^{n} A_i e^{-\alpha_i t} \tag{4}$$

in vivo input function f(t) can be obtained using Eq. 3. For example, in the case of single-exponential disposition (n = 1), $C_\delta(t) = A_1 e^{-\alpha_1 t}$, and hence, f(t), the input rate, is given by (20):

$$f(t) = \frac{C'(t) + \alpha_1 C(t)}{A_1} \tag{5}$$

The amount of drug absorbed from time 0 to t, Xa(t), is then obtained by integration:

$$X_a(t) = \int_0^t f(t)dt = \frac{C(t) + \alpha_1 \int_0^t C(t)dt}{A_1} \tag{6}$$

In cases where C(t) or f(t) cannot be fitted to an explicit functional form, numerical methods are used to deal with raw data. In actual applications, computer programs, e.g., PCDCON or ADAPT II, are available for calculations.

2. Model-Dependent Deconvolution Methods

Two commonly used deconvolution methods for estimating the apparent in vivo drug absorption profiles following oral administration of a dosage form are Wagner–Nelson and Loo–Riegelman methods (21). Those are model-dependent approaches based on mass balance. The Wagner–Nelson equation is derived from a one-compartment model and the mass balance, $X_a = X_t + X_e$, where X_a, X_t, and X_e are amounts of drug absorbed, in the "body," and eliminated at time t, respectively. By derivation, the amount of drug absorbed up to time T, $(X_a)_T$, is given by:

$$(X_a)_T = VC_T + kV\int_0^T C_t\, dt$$

where V is the volume of central compartment, C_T is concentration of drug in the central compartment at time T and k is the first-order elimination rate constant. In the study of IVIVC, this is often expressed in terms of fraction (F) of the dose (D) absorbed for comparison with fraction released in vitro:

$$F_a(T) = \frac{(X_a)_T}{(X_a)_\infty} = \frac{C + k\int_0^T C_t\, dt}{k\int_0^\infty C_t\, dt} \tag{7}$$

where $F_a(T)$ or FD is the fraction of bioavailable drug absorbed at time T. It should be noted that Eq. 7 is identical to Eq. 6. Therefore, the Wagner–Nelson method represents a special case of deconvolution. When intravenous data are not available, the apparent in vivo fractional absorption profile can be obtained by using terminal phase elimination rate constant, k, and partial areas

In Vitro/In Vivo Correlation

under the plasma concentration curve in Eq. 7. However, it should be pointed out that (a) k value should be derived from the true elimination phase, which may be difficult for drugs with prolonged absorption and/or long half-life; and (b) only apparent absorption is estimated using this method.

The approximate equation used in absorption analysis for the two-compartment model was first published by Loo and Riegelman in 1968 (22). Wagner published an exact Loo–Riegelman method for a multicompartment model in 1983 (23). This is a general equation for absorption analysis of one- to three-compartment models. It requires IV data for the calculation of absorption profiles. For biexponential disposition, mass balance leads to $(X_a)_T = X_c + X_p + X_e$, where X_c and X_p are amounts of drug in the central and peripheral compartments at time T, respectively. By derivation (23), $(X_a)_T$ can be determined:

$$\frac{(X_a)_T}{V_c} = C_T + k_{12}e^{-k_{21}T}\int_0^{T_T} C_t\, e^{-k_{21}t}\, dt + k_{10}\int_0^{T_T} C_t\, dt \tag{8}$$

where k_{12}, k_{21}, and k_{10} are the microconstants that define the rates of transport between compartments. On the basis of mass balance, $(X_a)_T = X_c + X_{p1} + X_{p2} + X_e$, a similar equation can be derived for triexponential disposition. The corresponding exact Loo–Riegelman equation is given as:

$$\frac{(X_a)_T}{V_c} = C_T + k_{12}e^{-k_{21}T}\int_0^{T_T} C_t\, e^{-k_{21}t}\, dt + k_{13}e^{-k_{31}T}\int_0^{T_T} C_t\, e^{-k_{31}t}\, dt + k_{10}\int_0^{T_T} C_t\, dt \tag{9}$$

It can be shown that the Loo–Riegelman method is also a special case of deconvolution where in vivo disposition is described by two or three exponentials (20). The theoretical and practical aspects of absorption analysis using model-dependent approaches have been thoroughly summarized by Wagner (21).

3. Convolution Approach

A deconvolution-based IVIVC model is typically established using a two-stage approach, i.e., deconvolution calculation to estimate the time course of in vivo absorption and/or release followed by comparison with in vitro fraction released. An alternative modeling approach based on convolution can be utilized to directly predict the time course of plasma concentrations using Eq. 1 in a single step. Based on the assumption of equal or similar release rates between in vitro and in vivo, the input rate, f(t), is modeled as a function of the in vitro release data with or without time scaling to predict the in vivo plasma profiles by convolution with the dose-normalized plasma data from an IV or IR reference dose. The IVIVC is assessed and validated by statistically comparing the predicted with the observed plasma levels. This convolution-based modeling focuses on the ability to predict measured quantities rather than on indirectly estimated "in vivo" fraction absorbed and/or released. Thus, the results are more readily evaluated in terms of the effect of in vitro release on in vivo performances, e.g., AUC, C_{max}, and duration above minimum effective concentrations.

It should be noted that this single-stage approach is based on the assumption of a linear, time-invariant relationship between input (drug release) and plasma concentrations, and multiple formulations with different release rates are normally used in establishing an IVIVC. If a significant fraction of the dose of slow-release formulations is released beyond the site(s) of drug absorption (truncated absorption), overestimation of plasma concentrations can occur because Eq. 1 predicts the same dose-normalized AUC as the reference dose used to estimate $C_\delta(t)$ (24). To address the potential discrepancies between in vitro and in vivo release/absorption, Gillespie recently proposed an extended convolution-based IVIVC model using a function relating cumulative amounts released or release rate in vitro (x_{vitro}) to that in vivo, (x_{vivo}), $x_{vivo} = f(x_{vitro})$. Thus, plasma concentrations of multiple extended release (ER) formulations can be more accurately predicted by substituting f(t) with x_{vivo} in Eq. 1 should there be an IVIVC. Selection of a specific functional form of x_{vivo} can be based on a mechanistically understanding of the in vitro–in vivo relationship or semiempirically based on the goodness of model fitting. Certain plausible relationships include linear, nonlinear, or time-variant functions; and linear or nonlinear time scaling for taking into account the effects of lag time, truncated absorption, or saturable presystemic metabolism (24).

For controlled release systems, the apparent absorption in vivo is limited by the drug release from the dosage form of which the kinetics is determined by the system design. In most cases, the release kinetics can be described by one of the following models: zero-order, first-order, square root of time, or Peppas's exponent models (25). Therefore, the parametric function, C(t), describing the plasma concentrations of an ER dosage form can be defined via convolution of $C_\delta(t)$ with the input, $f(t)$, prescribed from the in vitro model according to Eq. 1. For instance, the functional form of C(t) can first be obtained by convolution of a prescribed function of input (e.g., first-order) with a known unit impulse response. The unknown parameters remaining in C(t) equation are those from the prescribed input function, $f(t)$, which can then be solved by fitting the C(t) equation to the observed plasma concentrations. The resulting $f(t)$ is compared with the observed in vitro data to evaluate IVIVC. This approach is also known as deconvolution through convolution.

In predicting C(t) by convolution, data from an IV or oral solution are desirable because they provide an estimate of $C_\delta(t)$ independent of the ER data. However, such a reference dose is not always available, particularly for compounds having low aqueous solubility. Nevertheless, estimation of C(t) by convolution for evaluation of IVIVC is still possible using only data from ER formulations (24). In such cases, the prescribed parametric functional forms of both $C_\delta(t)$ and $f(t)$ can be mechanistically or empirically selected and substituted into Eq. 1. The parameters of $C_\delta(t)$ are then estimated by fitting the overall convolution model to the plasma concentrations of ER formulations. Predictive performance of the IVIVC is evaluated by comparing the predicted and observed results. It should be pointed out that the ability of the model to predict changes of in vivo plasma concentrations with varying release rates should be validated by separately or simultaneously fitting the date from multiple formulations. In addition, by doing so a $C_\delta(t)$ function can be reliably defined. Thus, one of the most critical requirements of this approach is to use at least two ER formulations with different release rates in the assessment of IVIVC (24).

B. Mean Time Parameters

Level B correlation is based on correlating mean time parameters that characterize the in vitro and in vivo time courses, e.g., the in vitro or in vivo mean dissolution time (MDT), or in vivo mean residence time (MRT). Mean time parameters have been commonly utilized in pharmacokinetic studies and used to describe in vitro release. They are useful in studying specific models as well as less differentiated, more general system models. Many important concepts, definitions, and computations on this subject have been thoroughly discussed by Veng-Pedersen (26) and Podczeck (27).

1. In Vivo Parameters

By definition, MRT is the average total time the drug molecule spends in the introduced kinetic space. It depends on the site of input and the site of elimination. When the elimination of the molecule follows first-order kinetics, its MRT can be expressed by (26):

$$MRT = \frac{\int_0^{T_f} tCt\, dt}{\int_0^{\infty} Ct\, dt} = \frac{AUMC}{AUC} \qquad (10)$$

where AUMC is area under the moment curve. Estimates for MRT can be calculated by fitting $C(t)$ to polyexponential equation followed by integration or by using trapezoidal rules. For noninstantaneous input into a kinetic space, such as oral absorption, the MRT estimated from extravascular data includes a contribution of the mean transit time for input, known as mean absorption time (MAT, or mean arrival time, or mean input time) (26). The MAT of drug molecules represents the average time taken to arrive in that space, and it can be estimated as:

$$MAT = \frac{\int_0^{T_f} tf_{in}(t)dt}{\int_0^{\infty} f_{in}(t)dt} = \frac{AUMC}{AUC} \qquad (11)$$

where $f_{in}(t)$ denotes an arbitrary rate of input into the kinetic space. For oral delivery, the MAT can be determined according to the equation:

$$MAT = MRT_{po} - MRT_{iv} \qquad (12)$$

The term MAT thus obtained represents the mean transit time involved in apparent absorption process in the GI tract. When the formulation contains solid drug, the MAT includes in vivo dissolution as well as absorption. If data of the same drug given in solution state are available, the in vivo MDT can be estimated by:

$$MDT_{solid} = MAT_{solid} - MAT_{soln} = MRT_{solid} - MRT_{soln} \qquad (13)$$

2. In Vitro Parameters

The measured amount of drug substance in cumulative release profile can be considered as a probability that describes the time of residence of the drug substance in the dosage form. Therefore, a dissolution profile may be regarded as the distribution function of the residence times of each drug molecule in the formulation (27). By definition, the MDT is the arithmetic mean value of any dissolution profile. If the amount of the drug remaining in the formulation is plotted as a function of time, the arithmetic mean value of the residence profile is the MRT of the drug molecules in the dosage form.

The techniques that are used to calculate MDT or MRT can be divided into model-independent (pragmatic plane geometry and prospective area) and model-dependent methods (e.g., polyexponential, Weibull, and overlapping parabolic integration) (27). In general, model-independent approaches are used when release kinetics are unknown. These methods are based on area calculations from the amount released at various times. The following simple method is often used to determine the MDT and MRT using trapezoidal rules (127):

$$MDT = \frac{\int_0^{\infty} [M_{max} - M(t)]dt}{M_{max}} = \frac{ABC}{M_{max}} \qquad (14)$$

$$MRT = \frac{\int_0^\infty tA(t)dt}{\int_0^\infty A(t)dt} \qquad (15)$$

where ABC is the area between the drug dissolution curve and its asymptote, A(t) is the amount of drug remaining in the dosage form at time t, and M(t) and M_{max} are the amount of drug released at time t and the maximal amount released, respectively. The model-dependent methods are based on the derived parameters of functions that describe the release profiles. It should be noted that one important source of errors in calculations comes from the often incomplete release. The calculation of the moments in such case is based on the maximum drug release. For systems that have a complete drug release, the size of errors depends on the number of data points and the curve shape (27).

C. Summary Parameters

The extent and rate of drug release from a dosage form are often characterized by one or more of the single measurements (e.g., Q_{60}, $T_{50\%}$, or $T_{85\%}$), particularly when there are not enough data points available to define the time functions of the profiles or there is simply no suitable model that describes the dissolution curves. These parameters are most often obtained either directly from the dissolution measurements or by interpolation. Although they do not adequately characterize the whole dissolution process, they are utilized in quality control in vitro and are also commonly used in level C correlation studies. The in vivo parameters used to correlate with the in vitro parameters are bioavailability parameters reflecting the rate and extent of absorption (e.g., AUC, T_{max}, and C_{max}).

IV. DEVELOPMENT AND EVALUATION OF A CORRELATION

A. Study Design and Correlation Development

The formulation development work and the dissolution method development start hand by hand. Once a candidate formulation with adequate in vitro controlled release properties is identified, a study must be conducted to evaluate the in vivo performance of the formulation along with one or more of its variants. The additional formulations need to be designed to produce different in vivo release rates, ideally one with slower and one with faster release properties (1,28,29). The in vitro work of the correlation typically involves the development of a dissolution methodology that discriminates between the different formulation variants. Although it is generally acceptable to use any in vitro dissolution method, more standardized methods are usually adopted. Such methods include USP Apparatus I (basket) and II (paddle) in a buffered aqueous dissolution media with or without the use of surfactants such as SLS. Using the accumulated knowledge regarding the effect of the dissolution pH, agitation speed, and surfactant, the dissolution methodology could be finely tuned to allow differentiation between the different tested formulations.

The in vivo part involves comparison of the absorption characteristics of the tested formulation along with a reference standard in human subjects generally under fasting conditions. Although a crossover study design is ideal, data from parallel study design or data utilizing multiple studies could suffice. In the latter situation a standardized reference formulation must be included with each study. To better characterize the disposition kinetics of the drug, a reference such as IV administration, oral solution, or IR formulation is routinely used. This will allow for a better accuracy in the deconvolution calculations.

The percent absorbed–time profile of each controlled release formulation is estimated for each subject using an appropriate deconvolution methodology and data from the reference standard. The first element in the correlation development is visual inspection of the average in vitro dissolution rate and average in vivo absorption rate for each tested formulation. The second step involves fitting the data to an adequate correlation model. Either the two-stage approach or the single-stage approach can be utilized. In the two-stage approach, the in vivo percent absorbed is calculated by means of deconvolution and then correlated with the percent dissolved in vitro using a simple linear model with intercept (a) and slope (b):

$$\% \text{ absorbed}_{in\ vivo} = a + b^* \% \text{ dissolved}_{in\ vitro} \tag{16}$$

A slope closer to 1 indicates a 1:1 correlation and a negative intercept implies that the in vivo process lags behind the in vitro dissolution. A positive intercept has no clear physiological meaning. It can be a result of relatively high variability or curvature at the early time points.

Alternatively, in the single-stage approach the plasma concentrations are directly estimated from the in vitro dissolution data. A polyexponential unit impulse response with lag time could be used in the model as follows:

$$C_\delta(t) = \sum_{i=1}^{nex} A_i * e^{-\alpha_{(i)}(t - t_{lag})} \tag{17}$$

where "nex" is number of exponential terms in the model, t_{lag} is the absorption lag time, and $C(t)$ is the plasma concentration at time t. The input rate is modeled as a linear function of the in vitro cumulative amount dissolved.

To appropriately demonstrate a complete level A IVIVC for a controlled release product, the FDA Guidance indicated that it is necessary to have a single correlation fit, with the same time scale if used, for all tested formulations (1). As suggested by Cao (30) and others (35), the use of nonlinear mixed effect modeling in fitting the data (see next section) allows the use of individual in vivo data rather than the mean. This approach also allows for valid statistical comparison to whether the correlation lines are similar for all tested formulations.

As with any modeling program, criteria to evaluate the goodness of fit or the appropriateness of the IVIVC model should be adopted. The FDA Guidance suggested evaluating the goodness of fit by measuring the prediction error, i.e., differences between observed and predicted values. The FDA further suggested measurement of the internal prediction error using data from the same study used to develop the IVIVC. The internal prediction could be adopted for cases where the IVIVC was derived using three or more formulations with different release rates and provided the drug is not considered a narrow therapeutic index drug. The internal prediction error evaluates how well the model describes the data used to develop the IVIVC. The external prediction error approach involves the use of an external dataset that was not used in the development of the IVIVC, such as formulation with different release rate, formulations with minor manufacturing process changes, or formulation from a different manufacturing batch. A prediction error of 10% or lower generally signifies a well-established model for the IVIVC.

B. Statistical Assessment of a Correlation

Much of the research in the pharmaceutical field is based on longitudinal designs that involve repeated measurements of a variable of interest in each subject. A common example is a crossover design in many phase I clinical trials. Such designs can be very powerful, both statistically and clinically, because they enable one to compare measurements within individual subjects over time or under different conditions. Most standard statistical techniques, such as the paired t test and the simple linear regression, assume that each of the response variables in a dataset is independent of each other. Unfortunately, this assumption can be violated if the repeated observations are taken within subjects because the repeated measurements within each subject tend to be correlated with one another. If one takes two observations at random from the same subject, they are likely to be more similar in value than two random observations from two different subjects. If a standard statistical analysis that assumes independence among all observations is performed on data from repeated measurements, the results can be misleading. Fortunately, valid approaches do exist for the analysis of this type of data. In this section, we discuss a method in which the dependence of repeated observations is accounted by random effects in the framework of mixed-effects modeling.

In developing an IVIVC, the response observation can be plasma concentrations or the amount of drug absorbed in vivo. The latter is directly obtained from the observed plasma concentration–time curve by deconvolution. There are advantages and disadvantages for either type of response variable. When plasma concentration is used as a response variable, the link between the in vitro dissolution profile with the in vivo plasma concentration profile has clear clinical relevance because many pharmacokinetic parameters such as C_{max}, T_{max}, and AUC are directly derived from the plasma concentration–time profile. However, it is difficult to determine IVIVC and the unit impulse response function at the same time. Using the amount of drug absorbed as a response variable in establishing the IVIVC is intuitively straightforward because the in vitro and in vivo parameters are directly compared. The impulse response function needs to be defined first.

The general models for using the plasma concentration, C(t), and amount absorbed in vivo, X(t), as response variables can be written as follows, respectively:

$$C_{ij}(t) = \int_0^t C_\delta(t - \tau; \alpha_i) f[\tau, d(\tau; \beta_j); \gamma_{ij}] d\tau \tag{18}$$

and

$$X_{ij}(t) = g[t, D(t; \beta_j); \gamma_{ij}] \tag{19}$$

where $C_{ij}(t)$ is the plasma concentration at time t for the ith subject taking drug formulation j; the function $C_\delta(t)$ and associated parameter vector α_i describes the response of the ith subject to an instantaneous unit input, usually obtained from IV bolus or oral solution; the function f and associated parameter vector γ_{ij} describes the rate of in vivo absorption of the jth formulation by the ith subject, which depends on the rate of in vitro dissolution of the jth formulation represented by the function d and associated parameter vector β_j; $X_{ij}(t)$ is the amount of drug absorbed in vivo from time 0 to t for the ith subject taking formulation j; the function g and associated parameter vector γ_{ij} describes the relationship between in vitro amount dissolved $D(t; \beta_j)$ and in vivo amount drug absorbed $X_{ij}(t)$. Furthermore, $D(t; \beta_j)$ in Eq. 19 can be written as $\int_0^t d(\tau; \beta_j) d\tau$. Because variability among dosage units is typically much smaller than intersubject variability, $D(t; \beta_j)$ or $d(t; \beta_j)$ is the "average" in vitro dissolution at time t for formulation j. The functions f and g are dependent on formulation j since the parameter γ_{ij} is formulation-specific. That is, different formulations may have different IVIVCs.

The observed plasma concentration y_{ijk} or the estimated amount of drug absorbed z_{ijk} at time t_k from the ith subject and jth formulation can be given below:

$$y_{ijk} = C_{ij}(t_k) + \epsilon_{ijk} \tag{20}$$

or

$$z_{ijk} = X_{ij}(t_k) + \psi_{ijk} \tag{21}$$

where ϵ_{ijk} and ψ_{ijk} are error terms with a mean of zero. In the mixed-effects modeling framework, α_i and γ_{ij} are specified as random effects with mean zero, and β_j are fixed effects. Random effects α_i and γ_{ij} are independent of each other and independent of error terms ϵ_{ijk} or ψ_{ijk}. The dependence of repeated measurements from the same subject is accounted for by random effects α_i and γ_{ij}. Furthermore, all random effects are assumed to be normally distributed.

Statistical analyses and inference of such mixed effects models have been worked by Beal and Sheiner (31), Vonesh and Carter (32), Wolfinger (33), Davidian and Giltinan (34), Cao and Locke (30), and Mauger and Chinchilli (35). Software is available to make statistical inference under such a model framework. For example, the NONMEM package, introduced by Beal and Sheiner (31), can be used for the mixed-effects model. The SAS procedure MIXED (36) can be performed on the linear mixed-effects models.

To assess the validity of a level A correlation, the superiority of the reduced model wherein all tested controlled release formulations are fitted to a single correlation should be established over the full model wherein each formulation is fitted to a different correlation line. The following reduced model is compared to the full model described by Eq. 18 or 19:

$$C_{ij}(t) = \int_0^t C_\delta(t - \tau; \alpha_i) f[\tau, d(\tau; \beta); \gamma_i]) d\tau \tag{22}$$

or

$$X_{ij}(t) = g[t, D(t; \beta); \gamma_i] \tag{23}$$

In such a model, the plasma concentration or amount of drug absorbed for the jth formulation depends on j only through the in vitro dissolution function d or D and associated parameter vector β_j. Such models can be termed formulation-independent because the parameter γ_i is not formulation-specific. That is, it is possible to predict the plasma concentration or amount of drug absorbed based solely on its in vitro dissolution data. By comparing the fits of full and reduced models, it is possible to evaluate whether or not it is reasonable to use in vitro dissolution as a surrogate for in vivo bioavailability studies. If both models fit well, the IVIVC is considered validated. Hence, it would seem reasonable to conclude that in vitro dissolution is a suitable predictor of in vivo bioavailability. If the full model fits well but the reduced model does not, the IVIVC becomes formulation-dependent and therefore is invalid. If neither model fits well, it could be because the assumptions about the error structures were incorrect, the choice of functions (C_δ, d, f, or g) was incorrectly specified, or the current dataset is of insufficient quality to validate an IVIVC because it is too noisy or too sparse. It may be that the models fit well only for a subset of the formulation. In this case, the IVIVC is validated only for those formulations.

In evaluating an IVIVC, goodness of fit can be assessed graphically on a subject-by-subject basis by overlaying the observed data on the fitted plasma concentration profile. To assess goodness of fit across subjects, it is more useful to plot predicted vs. observed values. Systematic deviations from the unity line typically indicate misspecification of the model. Testing whether both full and reduced models give the same fit can be done using the change of -2 ln (likelihood function) from full model to reduced model. The change has approximate χ^2 distribution. The degree of freedom is the difference of the number of parameters for fixed effects in both models. If the full model is statistically different from the reduced model at significance level 0.05, the IVIVC is deemed invalid. Otherwise, the IVIVC is considered the same for all formulations.

C. Case Study

In order to develop a level A IVIVC, three controlled release tablet formulations (A, B, and C) of a proprietary compound were designed to have differing release rates by varying the concentration of the rate-controlling polymer in the formulation.

The absorption characteristics of the three formulations were tested in a single-dose, nonfasting, open-label, complete crossover study. An IV infusion was used as a reference formulation (D). Sixteen healthy adult subjects received all four treatments, one at a time, at weekly intervals. Each oral dose was given with approximately 180 mL of water under nonfasting conditions. Serial blood samples were collected prior to dosing and until 72 h after dosing in each period.

The release rates from the controlled release tablets were tested using a discriminative in vitro method that was developed following extensive experiments with the testing variables. The in vitro drug release was obtained from 12 tablets of each formulation using USP apparatus 2 (Paddle) in 500 mL of 0.1 N HCl for the first 45 min, followed by 900 mL of pH 5.5, 0.05 M potassium phosphate buffer containing 75 mM sodium dodecyl sulfate. The dissolution medium was thermostated at 37.0 ± 0.5°C and stirred with 100 rpm. Samples were collected at 1, 3, 5, 9, 12, 18, and 24 h.

In developing an IVIVC for this product, both the two-stage approach and the single-stage approach were utilized. For the two-stage approach, the percent absorbed was calculated from the plasma concentration data using the Wagner–Nelson method. The individual in vivo data were correlated to the average in vitro dissolution data using a linear model and the nonlinear mixed-effect approach. Data from the three formulations were fitted using the NONMEM (37) software either to a single regression line (same intercept and slope for all three formulations; reduced model) or to a full model in which data from each formulation were fitted to separate regression lines. Under the null hypothesis that the in vivo–in vitro relationship is the same for all three formulations, the difference in the minimum objective function values of the full and reduced models has an approximate χ^2 distribution with 4 degrees of freedom. A reduction of more than 9.5 in the minimum value of the objective function (MVOF) when the additional four parameters are included in the model is considered to be statistically significant at the 0.05 level.

For the single-stage approach, the average plasma concentration data of the drug were predicted from the in vitro dissolution data using ADAPT II (35,38). The mean plasma concentrations for each of the three regimens were used as the input function and the mean plasma concentrations obtained after the IV administration were used to determine the unit impulse response. A one-compartment model was used to describe the dispositional kinetics. The ADAPT II code also allowed a time scaling factor (t_{scale}) for the input function such that the cumulative amount dissolved at time t would correspond to the cumulative amount absorbed in vivo at time $t*t_{scale}$. The lag time was estimated to be approximately 0 and therefore was not included as a parameter in the final analysis.

To evaluate the goodness of IVIVC, the mean absolute prediction error (PE_{abs}) and the root mean square prediction error (PE_{rms}) were calculated. PE_{abs} is calculated as the mean absolute difference between predicted and observed mean percent absorbed at several time points of percent dissolved in vitro. PE_{rms} is calculated as the square root of the mean square difference between predicted and observed mean percent absorbed at the same time points of percent dissolved in vitro.

The IVIVC was also validated externally using data from a second study in which a different clinical batch of the drug product was administered to 24 healthy young male subjects. The established IVIVC model from the NONMEM analysis was used to predict the in vivo absorption rate of the tested formulation from its in vitro dissolution rate.

The mean fraction absorbed from each of the three ER formulations was found to be highly linearly correlated ($r^2 = 0.90$) with the in vitro dissolution results (Fig. 1), suggesting a level A IVIVC for all three formulations. Furthermore, the slopes and the intercepts of the regression lines were similar for the three formulations. The NONMEM analysis indicated that the three regression lines were not statistically significantly ($p = 0.284$) different at the 0.05 level and that a single regression line with a slope approximately equal to unity (0.90) and an intercept of 8.73 adequately fits the combined data from the three controlled release tablet formulations.

Using the monoexponential model, the in vitro dissolution data are predictive of the in vivo plasma concentration levels for all three ER dosage forms. The r^2 values for predicted and observed mean concentrations were 0.947, 0.967, 0.868, and 0.997 for the four regimens (Fig. 2), respectively. As shown in Table 2 and Fig. 3, both the internal validation (prediction

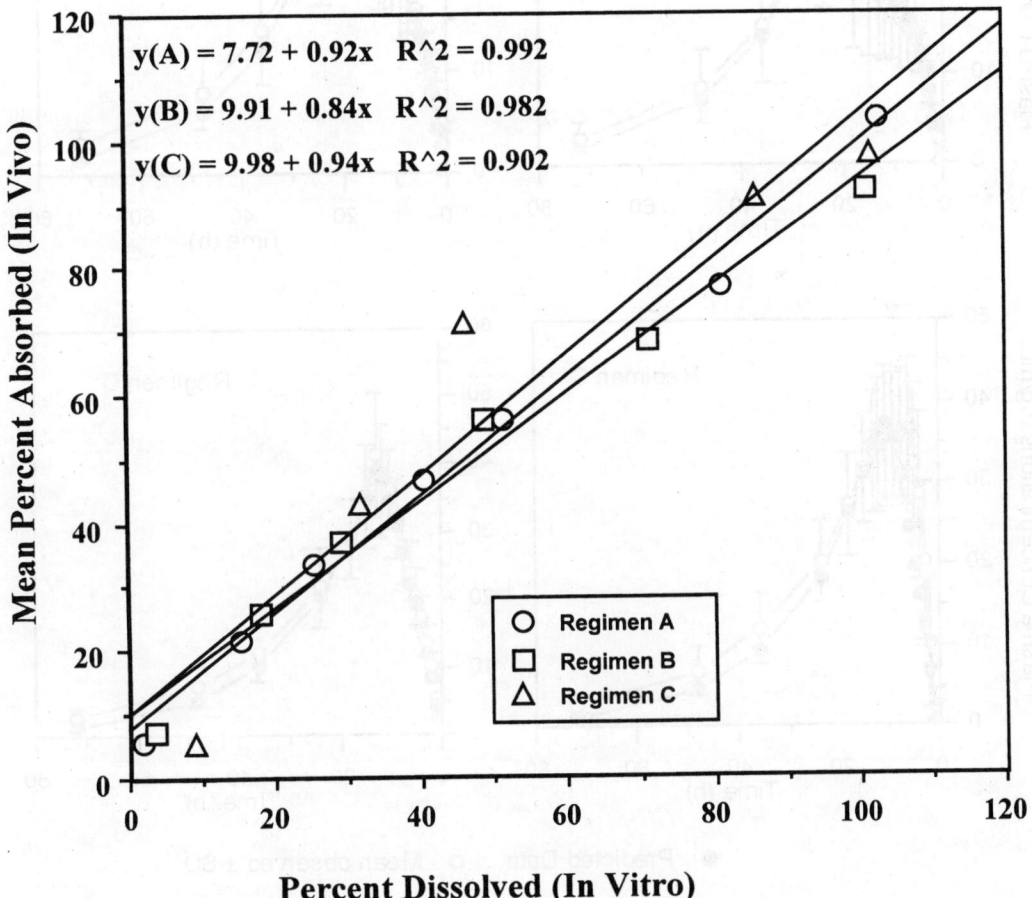

Figure 1 In vivo-in vitro correlation between mean percent absorbed and mean percent released from three different CR tablet formulations.

Table 2 Goodness of Fit of the NONMEM IVIVC Model

Regimen	N	r^2	PE_{abs}^*	PE_{rms}^*
A	7	0.9913	2.54	2.88
B	7	0.9826	3.50	4.21
C	7	0.9182	7.09	9.55
Combined	21	0.9652	4.38	6.25

*PE_{abs} and PE_{rms} are the mean absolute prediction error and the root mean square prediction error.

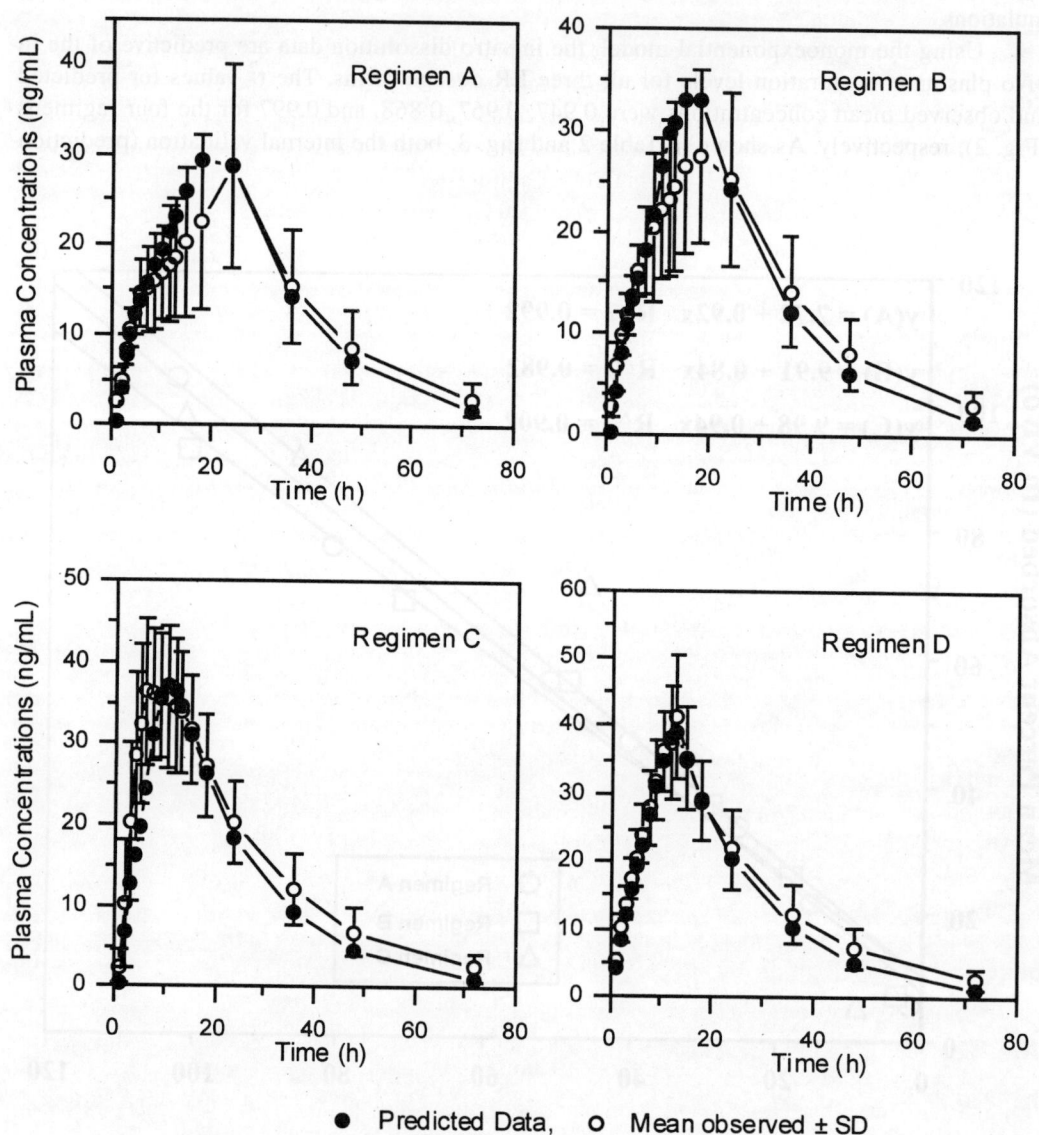

● Predicted Data, ○ Mean observed ± SD

Figure 2 Predicted vs. observed mean plasma concentrations obtained after oral administration of three different CR tablet formulations and an IV infusion.

In Vitro/In Vivo Correlation

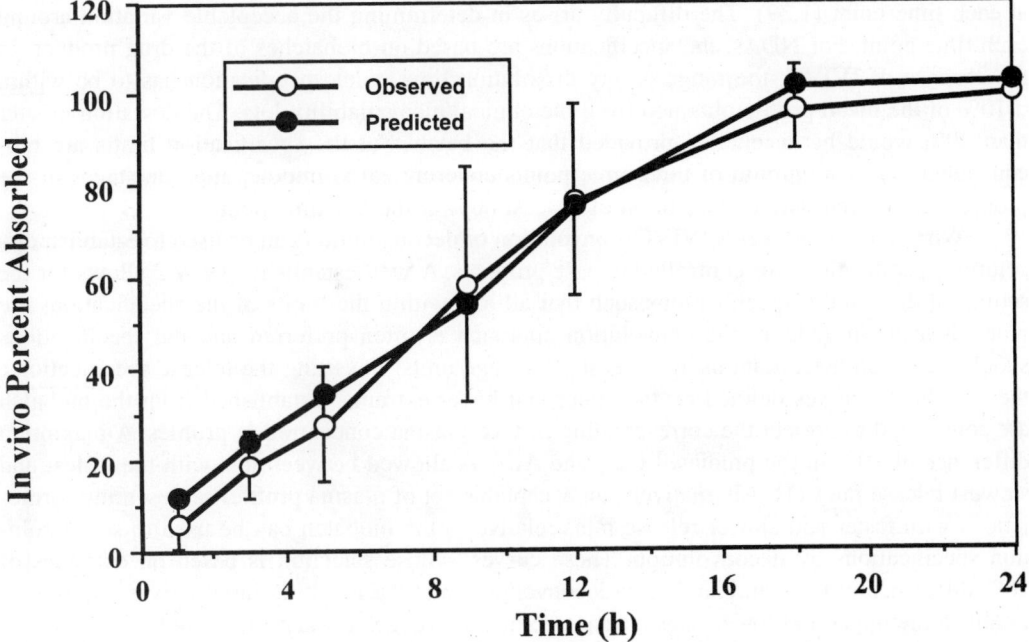

Figure 3 Observed vs. predicted in vivo drug absorption from a different batch of the to-be-marked formulation based on IVIVC model

error of less than 10%) and the external validation confirmed the suitability of the IVIVC developed for the tested controlled release formulations.

In conclusion, a level A IVIVC model was developed using both the single-stage and the two-step approaches. The mixed-effect model that accounts for inter- and intrasubject variabilities as well as the dependence of the observations from the same subject was successfully applied to the evaluation and validation of IVIVC.

V. APPLICATIONS AND LIMITATIONS

An important aspect of the development of IVIVC is to identify an in vitro test that can serve as an indicator of how well the formulation will perform in vivo. The main utility of such a predictive in vitro dissolution method is to serve as a surrogate marker for human bioequivalence studies so that the cost and time for product development can be significantly reduced. According to the FDA Guidance on IVIVC for ER solid dosage forms (1), a validated IVIVC can be used for setting meaningful dissolution specifications as well as for waiving bioequivalence requirements for approving and maintaining a product on the market.

A. Setting Dissolution Specifications

In vitro dissolution specifications are established to ensure batch-to-batch consistency and to differentiate between acceptable and unacceptable drug products, thus minimizing the possibility of releasing lots that might not have the desired in vivo performance. In general, dissolution behaviors of the clinical, pivotal bioavailability batches are used to define the amount released at each time point (1,39). The difficulty arises in determining the acceptable variation around each time point. For NDAs, the specifications are based on biobatches of the drug product. In the absence of IVIVC, the range at any dissolution time point specification has to be within ±10% of the mean profile obtained from the clinical/bioavailability lots. The deviation greater than 20% would be acceptable provided that the batches at the specification limits are bioequivalent (1). A minimum of three time points covering early, middle, and late stages of the profile are required with a dissolution of at least 80% at the last time point.

When there is a level A IVIVC, convolution or deconvolution can be used to establish dissolution specifications for controlled release products. A well-established IVIVC allows for the setting of dissolution specifications such that all lots within the limits of the specifications are bioequivalent. In general, the convolution approach is often preferred and the specifications should be set on mean data using at least 12 dosage units. In setting the release specifications, the dissolution curves defined by the upper and lower extremes established from the biobatch are convoluted to project the corresponding in vivo plasma concentration profiles. A maximum difference of 20% in the predicted C_{max} and AUC is allowed between lots with the fastest and slowest release rates (1). Alternatively, an acceptable set of plasma profiles representing formulations with faster and slower release rates relative to the biobatch can be used to set dissolution specifications by deconvolution. These curves, whose selection is based on extremes of 20% difference in C_{max} and AUC, are deconvoluted, and the resulting input curves are used to establish the upper and lower dissolution specification ranges at each time point.

In the case of level C and multiple level C IVIVC, the specification ranges should be set at the correlation time point such that there is a maximum of 20% difference in the predicted AUC or C_{max} (1). If the correlation involves more than one parameter, the one resulting in tighter limits should be used. In addition, drug release at the last time point should be at least 80%.

B. Supporting Waiver of In Vivo Bioequivalence Study

In addition to quality control tests, comparative dissolution tests have been used to waive bioequivalence studies required for multiple strength after approval of a bioequivalence study performed on single strength (40). A dissolution test based on a validated IVIVC can be used for obtaining a waiver for demonstrating in vivo bioavailability often required for scale-up, preapproval, and postapproval changes (1). According to the FDA Guidance on IVIVC, categories of biowaivers are based on therapeutic index of the drug, the extent of the validation performed on the developed IVIVC, and dissolution characteristics of the formulation (1). For instance, for nonnarrow therapeutic index drugs, IVIVC developed with two formulations can be used for biowaiver in level III manufacturing site changes and level III nonrelease-controlling excipient changes defined in SUPAC (Scale-up and Postapproval Changes) Guidance for Modified Release Solid Dosage Forms (40). If an IVIVC is developed using three formulations, or two formulations with external validation, biowaiver may include (a) level III process changes, (b) complete removal or replacement of nonrelease-controlling excipient without affecting release mechanism, (c) level III changes in the release-controlling excipients, and (d) change of strength (lower than the highest strength). The criteria for granting the biowaivers are that (a) the difference in predicted means of C_{max} and AUC is no more than 20% from that of the reference product and (b) dissolution meets specifications.

C. Limitations and Considerations

Limitations to the IVIVC methodology reside in the pharmacokinetic and physicochemical properties of the drug substance, the formulation design, as well as the methodology used to evaluate, predict, and validate the IVIVC.

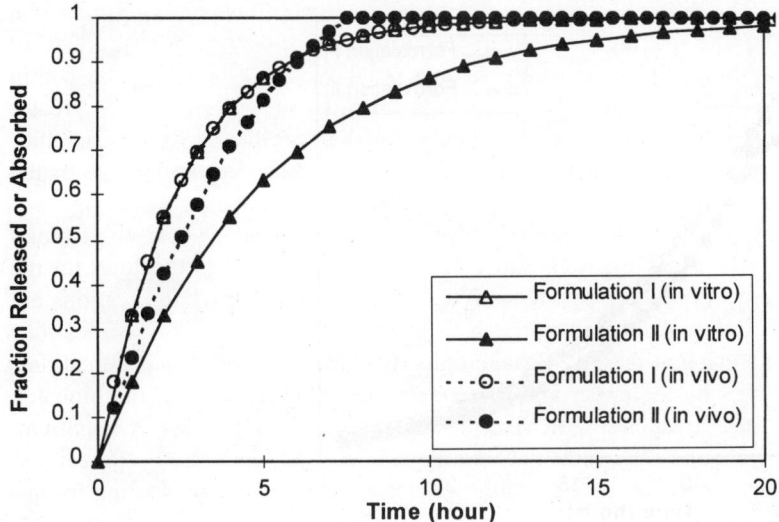

Figure 4 In vivo release vs. in vivo absorption profiles obtained by Wagner-Nelson method based on simulated data.

For any drug to be a good candidate for IVIVC development, it has to have linear dispositional pharmacokinetics. The lack of saturable absorption, lack of absorption windows, and lack of rate-dependent absorption or rate-dependent presystemic metabolism are important factors to consider when validating an IVIVC (41,42). In addition, IVIVC should not be developed using plasma concentrations of racemate when there is stereoselective dissolution or absorption between the two enantiomers. More importantly, the dissolution process should be the rate-limiting step in the absorption process. In most cases, IVIVC models are being established using the average in vivo response, thereby ignoring the inter- and intrasubject variability. For drugs that have a high intersubject variability this could result in difficulties in developing and establishing meaningful IVIVC.

The state of science is such that IVIVC is only valid for one particular type of dosage form containing certain rate-controlling excipients with the same release mechanism. Even with the same drug released from the same type of solid dosage form, such as tablet, different mechanisms (e.g., diffusion vs. osmosis) would require development of separate IVIVC. The absorption parameters calculated using the most widely used Wagner–Nelson method reflects only the rate and not the extent of absorption. Problems can arise from a correlation established using formulations that have different systemic bioavailability. For example, decreased or truncated absorption in the lower GI tract may occur with slow-releasing formulations due to there being less liquid for dissolution, lower surface area, bacterial metabolism, or short residence time. As a result, the IVIVC will be apparently formulation-dependent. This is illustrated using a simulated example. Two formulations (I and II) were originally designed to release a drug over approximately 8 and 14 h (Fig. 4). Following oral administration, reduced absorption from formulation II was observed because the "window" of absorption is 8 h (Fig. 5). The apparent in vivo absorption profiles of the two formulations obtained by the Wagner–Nelson method are also shown in Fig. 4. A comparison between the in vitro release and in vivo absorption indicates a good 1:1 relationship for formulation I and a significant deviation from the relationship for formulation II as a result of overestimation of the in vivo absorption. Therefore, in developing IVIVC, reduced AUC needs to be accounted for, e.g., by using a time-dependent function: $X_{in\ vivo} = g(t)X_{in\ vitro}$ where $g(t)$ is a step function for truncated or site-dependent absorption.

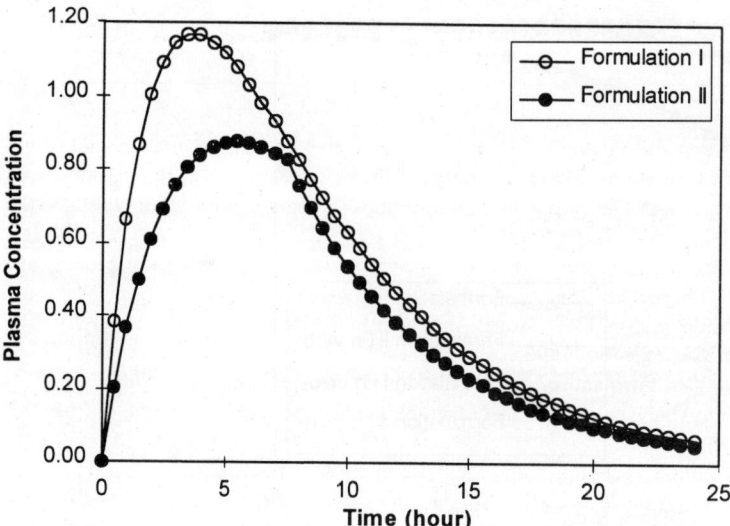

Figure 5 Simulated plasma concemntration profiles of two CR formulations with different release rates.

Finally, similar to bioavailability studies, the in vivo study used for development of the IVIVC is conducted in healthy volunteers under a semiartificial, well-controlled environment. Implementing this IVIVC model under circumstances that might affect the performance of the dosage form should be done cautiously. Factors such as the food effect, disease state, age, and drug–drug interactions might affect GI motility and/or GI transit time, and therefore might invalidate the IVIVC model.

VI. CONCLUSIONS

In the last few years the concept of in vitro–in vivo correlation has literally evolved from theory to practice. During the development of a controlled release product, where IVIVC is more readily defined, it is expected that an attempt will be made to develop an IVIVC. The methodology is not yet fully optimized and there is a need for further research of appropriate statistical methodology that could be used to evaluate the predictability and the validity of the IVIVC model, taking into consideration the inter- and intrasubject variability. IVIVC if properly developed is a cost-effective procedure that ultimately could reduce the time and cost of drug development. During the early stages of drug development, it provides guidance for optimizing drug delivery from the formulations. At later stages the dissolution test, as a reliable indicator of the in vivo performance, would reduce the number of required bioavailability studies. In addition, the correlation is being used to set meaningful dissolution specifications that take into account clinical consequences and therefore could facilitate regulatory approvals of scale-up and postapproval changes.

ACKNOWLEDGMENTS

The authors express their sincere thanks to Dr. William R. Gillespie for providing the ADAPT code, Dr. Patrick Marroum of the FDA for his valuable comments, and Ms. Paulette Johnson of Abbott Laboratories for her critical reading of the manuscript.

REFERENCES

1. Guidance for Industry: Extended Release Oral Dosage Forms: Development, Evaluation, and Application of In Vitro/In Vivo Correlations. FDA, September, 1997.
2. Tabusso, G. Regulatory Aspects of Development Pharmaceutics (2), Regulatory Affairs J. (12): 909-912, (1992).
3. Dunne, A., O'Hara, T. and Devane, J. Level A In vivo-In vitro Correlation: Nonlinear Models and Statistical Methodology. J. Pharm. Sci., 86: 1245-1249, 1997.
4. Polli, J. E., Crison, J. R. and Amidon, G. L. Novel Approach to the Analysis of in vitro-in vivo Relationships. J. Pharm. Sci., 85: 753-760, 1996.
5. Pharmacopeial forum. 1993. In vitro and in vivo evaluation of dosage forms. 19: 5366-5379.
6. Cutler, D. J. Linear System Analysis in Pharmacokinetics, J. Pharmacokin. Biopharm. 6: 265-282, (1978).
7. Moller, H., 1989. Deconvolution Techniques and their use in Biopharmaceutics. In: J. G. Hardy, S. S. Davis and C. G. Wilson (Editors), Drug Delivery to the Gastrointestinal Tract, Ellis Horwood Ltd., Chichester, pp 179-194.
8. Cutler, D. J. Numerical Deconvolution by least squares: Use of Prescribed Input Functions., J. Pharmacokin. Biopharm. 6: 227-241, (1978).
9. Langenbucher, F. Numerical Convolution/Deconvolution as a Tool for Correlating In vitro with In vivo Drug Bioavailability. Pharm. Ins. 4:1166-1172 (1982).
10. Gillespie, W. R. and Veng-Pedwesen, P. A Ployexponential Deconvolution Method. Evaluation of the "Gastrointestinal Bioavailability" and Mean In vitro Dissolution Time of Some Ibuprofen Dosage Forms. J. Pharmacokin. Biopharm. 13: 289-307, (1985).
11. Vajda, S. Godfrey, K. R. and Valko, P. Numerical Deconvolution Using System Identification Methods. J. Pharmacokin. Biopharm. 16: 85-107, (1988).
12. Cutler, D. J. Numerical Deconvolution by least squares: Use of Polynormils to Represent the Input Funciton., J. Pharmacokin. Biopharm. 6: 243-263, (1978).
13. Verotta, D. Two Constrained Deconvolution Methods Using Spline Functions. J. Pharmacokin. Biopharm. 21: 609-636, (1993).
14. Vaubhan, D. P. and Dennis, M. Mathematica Basis of the Point Area Deconvolution Method for Determining In vivo Input Fuctions. J. Pharm. Sci. 67: 663-665, (1978).
15. Veng-Pedersen, P. Model Independent Method of Analyzing Input in Linear Pharmacokinetic Systems Having Polyexponential Impulse Response. 1: Theoretical Analysis. J. Pharm. Sci. 69: 298-304, (1980).
16. Veng-Pedersen, P. Model Independent Method of Analyzing Input in Linear Pharmacokinetic Systems Having Polyexponential Impulse Response. 2: Numerical Evaluation. J. Pharm. Sci. 69: 305-312, (1980).
17. Veng-Pedersen, P. Novel Deconvolution Method for Linear Pharmacokinetic Systems with Polyexponential Impulse Response. 1: Theoretical Analysis. J. Pharm. Sci. 69: 312-318, (1980).
18. Veng-Pedersen, P. Novel Approach to Bioavailability Testing: Statistical method for Comparing Drug Input Calculated by a Least Squares Deconvolution Technique. J. Pharm. Sci. 69: 319-324, (1980).
19. Madden, F. N., Godfrey, K. R., Chappell, M. J., Hovorka, R and Bates, R. A. A Comparison of Six Deconvolution Techniques. J. Pharmacokin. Biopharm. 24: 283-299 (1996).
20. Veng-Pedersen, P. Personal Communications.
21. Wagner, J. G. Absorption Analysis and Bioavailability, in: Pharmacokinetics for the Pharmaceutical Scientist. Technomic Pub. Co. Inc., Lancaster, PA. 1993, pp. 159-206.
22. Loo, J. and Riegelman, S. New Mehtod for Calculating the Intrinsic Absorption Rate of Drugs. J. Pharm. Sci. 57: 918-928 (1968).
23. Wagner, J. G. Pharmacokinetic absorption plots from oral data alone or oral/intravenous data and an exact Loo-Riegelman equation. J. Pharm. Sci. 72: 838-842, (1983).

24. Gillespie, W. R. In vivo Modeling Strategies for IVIVC for Modified Release Dosage Forms. AAPS/CRS/FDA Workshop on Scientific Foundation and Applications for the Biopharmaceutics Classification System and In vitro-In vivo Correlations. Arlington, VA. April, 1997.
25. Ritger, P. L. and Pepas, N. A. A simple equation for description of solute release I. Fickian and non-Fickian release from non-swellable devices in the form of slabs, spheres, cylindres or disck, J. Controlled Release 5: 23-26, (1987).
26. Veng-Pedersen, P. Mean Time Parameters in Pharmacokinetics. Definition, Computation and Clincial Implications (Part I). Clin. Pharmacokin. 17: 345-366. (1989).
27. Podczeck, F. Comparison of In vitro Dissolution Profiles by Calculating Mean Dissolution Time (MDT) or Mean Residence Time (MRT). Int. J. Pharm. 97: 93-100. (1993).
28. Mojaverian, P. et al., 1997. In vivo-in vitro correlation of four extended release formulations of pseudophdrine sulfatre. J Pharm. Biomed Analysis 15: 439-445.
29. Mojaverian, P. et al., 1992. correlation of in vitro release rate and in vivo absorption characteristics of four chlorpheniramine maleate extended release formaulations. Pharm. Res. 9:450-456.
30. Cao, G. L. and Locke, C. (1997) Assessing whether controlled release products with differing in vitro dissolution rates have the same in vivo-in vitro relationship, In: In vitro-In vivo correlations. D. Young, J. Devane and J. Butler (Editors), Plenum Press, New York. p. 173-180.
31. Beal, B. L. and Sheiner, L. B. (1992) NONMEM User's Guide, NONMEM Project Group. USCF, CA.
32. Vonesh, E. F. and Carter, R. L. (1987). Efficient inference for random coefficient growth curve models with unbalanced data. Biometrics 43, 617-628.
33. Wolfinger, R. (1992). A tutorial on mixed models. SAS institute Inc.
34. Davidian, M. and Giltinan, D. (1995). Mixed effects models for repeated measurement data, Chapman and Hall.
35. Mauger, M. T. and Chinchilli, V. M. (1997) In vitro-In vivo Relationships for Oral Extended-Release Drug Products, Journal of Biopharmaceutical Statistics, 7(4) 565-578.
36. SAS Institue (1990). SAS Precedure Guide, Version 6, 3th ed.
37. Dunne, A., O'hara, T. and Devane, J., (1997) Level A in vivo-in vitro correlation: nonlinear models and statistical methodology. J. Pharm. Sci. 86: 1245-1249.
39. Guidance for Industry: Dissolution Testing of Immediate Release Solid Oral Dosage Forms. FDA, August, 1997.
40. Guidance for Industry: SUPAC-MR: Modified Release Solid Oral Dosage Forms; Scale-up and Postapproval Changes: Chemistry, Manufacturing, and Controls, In vitro Dissolution Testing, and In vivo Bioequivalence Documentation. FDA, Septmeber, 1997.
41. M. Siewert Perspective of in vitro dissolution test in establishing in vivo/in vitro correlations. Eur J Drug Metab Pharmacokinet 18(1); 7-18; 1993.
42. JM Cadot and E Beyssac, In vitro/in vivo correlations: Scientific implications and standardisation. Eur J Drug Metab Pharmacokinet 18(1); 113-120; 1993.
43. Skelly, J. P. and Shiu, G. F., 1993. In vitro/in vivo correlations in biopharmaceutics: scientific and regulatory implications. Eur. J. Drug Metab. Pharmacokin., 18: 121–129.
44. Siewert, W. 1993. Perspectives of in vitro dissolution tests in establishing in vitro/in vivo correlations. Eur. J. Drug Metab. Pharmacokin., 18: 7–18.
45. Skelly, J. P. et al. 1990. In Vitro and In Vivo Testing and Correlation for Oral Controlled/Modified-Release Dosage Forms, Pharm. Res. 7(9): 975–982.
46. Dressman, J. B. and Yamada, K. 1991. Animal models for oral drug absorption. In: Welling, P. G., Tse, F. L. and Dighe, S.. (Editors) Pharmaceutical Bioequivalence,., Marcel Dekker, Inc. New York. pp. 235–266.
47. *Davis, S. S. Wilding, E. A. and Wilding, I. R., 1993. Gastrointestinal Transit of a Matrix Tablet Formulation: Comparison of Canine and Human Data, Int. J. Pharm. 94: 235–238.
48. Davis, B. and Morris, T. 1993. Physiological Parameters in Laboratory Animals and Humans, Pharm. Res. 10: 1093–1098.
49. Akimoto, M., Furuya, A. Maki, T., Yamada, K., Suwa, T. and Ogata, H. 1993. Evaluation of sustained release granules of chlorphenesin carbamate in dogs and humans. 100: 133–142.

50. Yamakita, H., Maejima, T. and Osawa, T. 1995. Preparation of controlled release tablets of TA-5707F with wax matrix type and their in vivo evaluation in beagle dogs. Biol. Pharm. Bull. 18: 984–989.
51. Yamakita, H., Maejima, T. and Osawa, T. 1995. In vitro/in vivo evaluation of two series of TA-5707F controlled release matrix tablets prepared with hydroxypropyl methyl cellulose derivatives with entero-soluble or gel formation properties. Biol. Pharm. Bull. 18: 1409–1416.
52. Hussain, M., Abramowitz, W., Watrous, B. J., Szpunar, G. J. and Ayres, J. W. 1990. Gastrointestinal transit of nondisintingrating, nonerodible oral dosage forms in pigs. Pharm. Res. 7: 1163–1166.
53. Hildebrand, H., McDonald, F. M. and Windt-Hanke, F., 1991. Characterization of oral sustained release preparations of iloprost in a pig model by plasma level monitoring. Prostaglandins. 41: 473–486.
54. Kostewicz, E., Sansom, L., Fishlock, R., Morella, A. and Kuchel, T. 1996. Examination of two sustained release nifedipine preparations in humans and in pigs. Euro. J. Pharm. Sci. 4: 351–357.
55. Qiu, Y. Cheskin, H., Briskin, J and Engh, K., 1997. Sustained-Release Hydrophilic Matrix Tablets of Zileuton: Formulation and In Vitro/In Vivo Studies. J. Controlled Release 45: 249–256.
56. Qiu, Y. Flood, K., Marsh, K, Carroll, S, Trivedi, J., Arneric, S. P. and Krill, S. L. 1997. Design of Sustained-Release Matrix Systems for a Highly Water-Soluble Compound, ABT-089. Int. J. Pharm. 157: 43–52.
57. Roppas, C., Lacey, L. F., Keene, O. N., Macheras, P. and Bye, A. 1995. Evaluation of different matrics as indirect measures of rate of drug absorption from extended release dosage forms at steady-state. Pharm. Res. 12: 103–107.
58. Bois, F. Y., Tozer, T. N., Hauck, W. W., Chen, M., Patnaik, R. and Williams, R. 1994. Bioequivalence: performance of several measures of rate of absorption. Pharm. Res. 11: 966–974.
59. Metzler, C. M. 1991. Statistical Criteria. In: Welling, P. G., Tse, F. L. and Dighe, S.. (Editors) Pharmaceutical Bioequivalence, Marcel Dekker, Inc. New York. pp. 35–66.
60. Dighe, S. V. and Adams, W. P. 1991. Bioavailability and bioequivalence of oral controlled-release products: a regulatory perspective. In: Welling, P. G., Tse, F. L. and Dighe, S.. (Editors) Pharmaceutical Bioequivalence,., Marcel Dekker, Inc. New York. pp. 35–66.
61. Vallner, J. J. et al. 1983. A Proposed General protocol for Testing Bioequivalence of Controlled-release Drug Products, Int. J. Pharm. 16: 47–55.
62. Bass, P. 1993. Gastric emptying; differences among liquid, fiber, polymer and solid dosage forms of medications. IN: Current Status on Targeted Drug Delivery t the Gastrointestinal Tract. Capsulegel Library. pp. 11–18
63. Davis, S. S. et al. 1986. Transit of Pharmaceutical dosage forms through the small Intestine, Gut 27: 886–892.
64. Abrahamsson, B. et al. 1993. Absorption, Gastrointestinal Transit, and Tablet Erosion of Felodipine Extended-Release (ER) Tablets, Pharm. Res. 10(5): 709–713.
65. Coupe, A. J. et al. 1993. Do Pellet Formulations Empty from the Stomach with Food? Int. J. Pharm. 92: 167–175.
66. Yuen, K. H. et al. 1993. Gastrointestinal Transit and Absorption of Theophylline from a Multiparticulate Controlled-Release Formulation, Int. J. Pharm. 97: 61–77.
67. Dressman, J. B., Amidon, G. L., Reppas, C. and Shah, V. P. 1998. Dissolution testing as a prognostic tool for oral drug absorption: Immediate release dosage forms. Pharm. Res. 15: 11–22.
68. Digenis, G. A., Sandefer, E. P., Parr, A. F., Beihn, R., McClain, C., Scheinthal, B. M., Ghebre-Sellassie, I., Nesbitt, R. U. and Randinitis, E. 1990. Gastrointestinal behavior of orally administered radiolabeled erythromycin pellets in man as determined by gamma scintigraphy. J. Clin. Pharmacol. 30: 621–631.
69. Phillips, S. F. 1993. Gastrointestinal physiology and its relevance to targeted drug delivery. IN: Current Status on Targeted Drug Delivery t the Gastrointestinal Tract. Capsulegel Library. pp. 11–18.
70. Breimer, D. D. 1996. An integrated pharmacokinetic and pharmacodynamic approach to controlled drug delivery. J. Drug Targetting. 3: 411–415.

71. Hoffman, A. 1998. Pharmacodynamic aspects of sustained release preparations. Adv. Drug Delivery Rev. 33: 185–199.
72. Gupta, S. K., Guinta, D. R., Christopher, C. A. and Samuel, S. 1998. Dosage form and method for administering drug. PCT. WO 98/14168.
73. Tabusso, G. 1992. Regulatory Aspects of Development Pharmaceutics (1), The Regulatory Affairs J. (11): 909–912.
74. Andreotti, F., Davies, G. J., Hackett, D. R., Khan, M. I., De Bart, A. C. W., Aber, V. R., Maseri, A. and Kluft, C. 1988. Major Circadian Fluctuations in Fibrinolytic Factors and Possible Relevance to Time of Onset of Myocardial Infarction, Sudden Cardiac Death and Stroke. Amer. J. Cardiol., 62: 635–637.
75. Straka, R. J., Benson, S. R., 1996. Chronopharmacologic considerations when treating the patient with hypertension: a review. J. Clin. Pharmacol. 36: 771–782.
76. Ridker, P. M., Manson, J. E., Buring, J. E., Muller, J. E. and Hennekens, C. H. 1990. Circadian Variation of Acute Myocardial Infarction and the Effect of Low-Dose Aspirin in a Randomized Trial of Physicians. Circulation, 82: 897–902.
77. Hildgen P. and McMullen, J. N. 1995. A new gradient matrix: formulation and characterization, J. Controlled Release 34: 263–271.
78. Danckwerts M. P. 1994. Development of a zero-order release oral compressed tablet with potential for commercial tabletting production, Int. J. Pharm. 112: 34–45.
79. Kim C. 1995. Compressed Donut-shaped tablets with zero-order release kinetics, Pharm. Res. 12: 1045–1048.
80. Benkorah A. Y. and McMullen J-N. 1994. Biconcave coated, centrally perforated tablets for oral controlled drug delivery, J. Controlled Release 32: 155–160.
81. Conte U., Maggi L., Colombo P. and Manna A. L. 1993. Multi-layered hydrophilic matrices as constant release devices (GeomatrixTM Systems), J. Controlled Release 26: 39–47.
82. Scott D. C. and Hollenbeck R. G. 1991. Design and manufacture of a zero-order sustained-release pellet dosage form through nonuniform drug distribution in a diffusional matrix, Pharm. Res. 8: 156–161.
83. Brooke D. and Washkuhn R. J. 1977. Zero-order drug delivery system: Theory and Preliminary testing, J. Pharm. Sci. 66: 159–162.
84. Lipper R. A. and Higuchi W. I. 1977. Analysis of theoretical behavior of a proposed zero-order drug delivery system, J. Pharm. Sci. 66: 163–164.
85. Qiu, Y., Chidambaram and Flood, K. 1998. Design and evaluation of layered diffusional matrices for zero-order sustained-release. J. Controlled Release. 51: 123–130.
86. Katzhendler, I., Azoury, R. and Friedman, M. 1998. Crystalline properties of carbamazepine in sustained release hydrophilic matrix tablets based on hydroxypropyl methylcellulose. J. Controlled Release. 54: 69–85.
87. Michelucci, J. J., Sherman, D. M. and DeNeale, R. J. 1990. Sustained Release Etodolac, US Patent 4,966,768.
88. Ruff, M. D., Kalidindi, S. R. and Sutton, Jr., J. E., 1994. Pharmaceutical Composition Containing Bupropion Hydrochloride and a Stabilizer, US Patent 5,358,970.
89. Baiz, E. and Einig, H. 1992. Alginate-Based Verapamil-Containing Depot Drug Form, US Patent 5,132,295.
90. Howard, J. R. and Timmins, P. 1988. Controlled Release Formulation, US Patent 4,792,452.
91. Zhang, G. and Pinnamaraju, P. 1997. Sustained Release Formulation Containing Three Different Types of Polymers, US Patent 5,695,781.
92. Panoz, D. E. and Geoghegan, E. J., 1989. Controlled Absorption Pharmaceutical Composition, US Patent 4,863,742.
93. Jao, F., Wong, P. S., Huynh, H. T., McChesney, K. and Wat, P. K., 1992. Verapamil Therapy, US Patent 5,160,744.
94. Jao, F., Wong, P. S., Huynh, H. T., McChesney, K. and Wat, P. K., 1993. Verapamil Therapy, US Patent 5,190,765.

95. Jao, F., Wong, P. S., Huynh, H. T., McChesney, K. and Wat, P. K., 1993. Verapamil Therapy, US Patent 5,252,338.
96. Ohm, A. and Luchtenberg, H., 1990. Press Coated DHP Tablets, US Patent 4,892,741.
97. Guidance for Industry: Modified Release Solid Oral Dosage Forms: Scale-up and Postapproval Changes: Chemistry, Manufacturing and Controls, In Vitro Dissolution Testing and In Vivo Bioequivalence Documentation. FDA, September, 1997.

26
Gamma Scintigraphy in the Analysis of the Behavior of Controlled Release Systems

C. G. Wilson
Strathclyde Institute for Biomedical Sciences, Glasgow, Scotland

N. Washington
AstraZeneca, Loughborough, Leicester, England

To support the introduction of novel, controlled release dosage forms, regulatory bodies have increasingly accepted imaging technologies to validate proof of the concept over the past 10 years. Of all the modalities available, i.e., x-rays, nuclear medicine (gamma scintigraphy and positron emission tomography), magnetic resonance imaging, and ultrasound, gamma scintigraphy has become preeminent as a tool in the assessment of oral, pulmonary, and ophthalmic dosage forms. Many of the early applications in the study of controlled release dosage forms rode on the developments in diagnostic radiopharmaceuticals, which have steadily improved in terms of specificity, safety, and diversity. Advances in technology have allowed faster acquisition, and new computing techniques have allowed better characterization, of the pharmacokinetics of the radiopharmaceuticals incorporated in the formulation. Parallel to this, applications of scintigraphy in the study of drug formulations generated a new expertise quite separate from the diagnostic arena. Now radiology and nuclear medicine are utilizing this knowledge to obtain better imaging agents and in many respects the two paths criss-cross to the mutual benefit of both camps.

In view of the importance of gamma scintigraphy for the assessment of formulation deposition, the research groups active in this area are frequently asked to contribute reviews of the subject. In this chapter, we have drawn from our experience utilizing the use of the gamma camera to study oral drug delivery. In particular, we have tried to highlight issues that must be considered when contemplating scintigraphic studies of controlled release formulations. Examples have largely been drawn from our own studies, but one should not ignore the important contribution of the commercial groups in the United States and in Europe; in particular, the reader is referred to studies conducted by the Lexington- and the Nottingham-based groups who have published excellent reviews of the subject area.

In functional terms, progress in controlled release technology has branched into three main directions: *deposition* control, *temporal* control, and *barrier* control. The terms are not absolute descriptors as temporal control affects deposition control, especially in the gut, and increasing the residence time and concentration of a ligand at the target site allows more flux. Deposition control refers to the coverage of tissue achieved by the device, and *dispersion* and *accumulation* are the parameters measured. Temporal control refers to devices that delay release of the active component, usually after administration by the oral route allowing exposure further down the gut. This generally results in less dispersion when compared to devices that release in stomach. Barrier control refers to the construction of devices in which excipients or films modulate the release of the drug. This is especially important for drugs exhibiting a short half-life and hence having a short dosing interval. Prolonging the release rate not only reduces dosing frequency but allows smoothing of the peaks and drops in the plasma level, which can reduce side effects and avoid subtherapeutic levels.

Temporal control has become especially relevant for devices used to release drug in prophylaxis. It has long been the aim of the pharmaceutical industry to achieve delayed absorption of a drug to treat nocturnal and early-morning exacerbation of disease, e.g., asthma, rheumatoid disease, and cardiovascular disease. This attempt at controlling the transit of oral formulations requires a thorough understanding of the interaction of physiological and pharmaceutical processes.

I. GAMMA SCINTIGRAPHY

In medical diagnosis, gamma scintigraphy offers a noninvasive method for the measurement of organ function, perfusion, and receptor binding, but unlike x-rays it gives little anatomical information. The principle of conventional gamma scintigraphy measurements involves the administration of a suitably labeled formulation containing a small amount of a γ-emitting substance (Table 1). The gamma or scintillation camera detects gamma photons in a large crystal detector optically coupled to a bank of photomultipliers mounted behind the crystal. The crystal, usually composed of thallium-doped sodium iodide, is extremely fragile and has

Table 1 Selected Nuclides Used in Assessment of Controlled Release Products

Technetium 99m Half-life 6 h. Most widely used radionuclide, half-life 6 h and principle emission at 140 keV. Low radiation dose. Used in oral, parenteral, pulmonary, and especially ophthalmic dosing, where dosimetry to the lens is a concern. Generator produced as [^{99m}Tc]sodium pertechnetate and therefore routinely available as a sterile material.

Indium 111 Half-life 2.8 days. Emissions at 173 and 247 keV. Often used with technetium to label a second component of the formulation. Camera can be tuned in to register counts upper energy 247 keV although overlap into technetium channel is significant and must be accounted for. Relatively long half-life useful for labeling dosage forms and testing release in vitro prior to administration

Iodine 123 Half-life is 13 h, energy 160 keV. Generally the successor to iodine 131, which is associated with higher dosimetry. Incorporation of iodine into a diversity of formulations is generally more facile than technetium 99m.

Samarium 153 Half-life 47 h, energy 103 keV. Produced using stable isotope-labeled formulation (samarium 152) by neutron activation, usually of the oxide Sm_2O_3. Energy is suboptimal for the gamma camera but long half-life allows the user to decay out Na-24 and K-42 produced during activation

Erbium 171 Half-life 7.5 h, energy 296–308 keV. Produced from enriched Er-170 again as the oxide Er_2O_3. Short half-life and expense somewhat restrictive.

Krypton 81m Half-life 13 s, energy 191 keV. A gas with a rapid decay especially useful for examining relative deposition in lung studies

Carbon 11 Half-life 20 min, energy 511 keV. A positron emitter, like oxygen 15, nitrogen 13, and fluorine 18, the detection of positron emissions utilizes a special double-headed design to detect the simultaneous emission of rays produced during the annhilation of the positron. Generally used for functional imaging studies.

to be protected from rapid temperature transients and physical shocks. Collimation, using various designs of lead plates or cones, focuses the γ-ray photons on the crystal and the distribution is recorded as a matrix of 256 × 256, 128 × 128, or 64 × 64 pixels. The reader is referred to Refs. 1 and 2 for a more complete description of the instrumentation. Recently, a solid-state camera was introduced that is claimed to be lighter and more robust.

Dual-headed cameras, which allow simultaneous acquisition of anterior and posterior images, have become more common. Tomographic images produced by single photon emission computed tomography (SPECT) allow the construction of three-dimensional volume or surface-calculated structures. The routine is performed using a dedicated system or a rotating camera. The fastest acquisition is typically 20 min, so that dynamic processes in the upper gut are difficult to follow; however, it has been used to study topical delivery in the terminal ileum and colon (3). Figure 1 illustrates the use of tomographic imaging to monitor the appearance of activity released from a Pulsincap device toward the end of the small intestine; the tomographic images showed better delineation of the iliocecal junction.

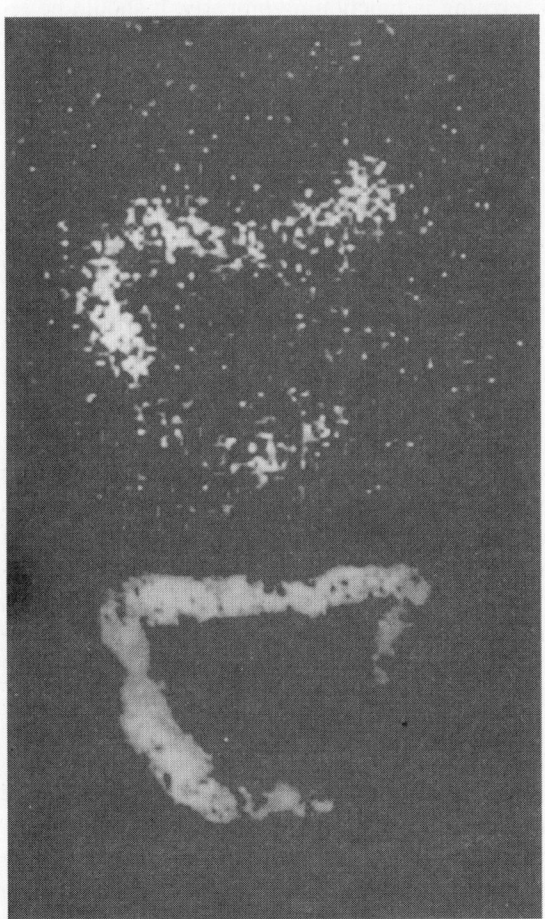

Figure 1 Comparison of a planar and three-dimensional SPECT image of the release of contents from a Pulsincap device toward the end of the small intestine. Note that the tomographic images showed better delineation of the iliocecal junction.

II. LABELING FORMULATIONS

The ingenuity of the radiopharmacist is generally highly taxed by the pharmaceutical scientist since the parameters to be studied are so varied. The list of available radionuclides is briefly covered in Table 1, and a variety of radiopharmaceuticals can be prepared on site using commercially available kits.

The drug entity generally cannot be directly labeled and a range of strategies are employed as follows:

1. The formulation matrix is radiolabeled with a tracer that remains associated with the matrix only and is not released. This gives position data. Generally, this is seen as a single spot of activity and there are no anatomical data. If the formulation is given orally, it is wise to give a ^{99m}Tc-DTPA-tagged drink at some point in the imaging schedule to give the relative positions and shape of the stomach and colon.
2. A radiopharmaceutical is admixed with drug and excipients during manufacture. The release of the tracer has to be tested rigorously in vitro to ensure that it is similar to that of the drug. This will give information about release rates, spreading, and position, e.g., confirming that an enteric coating is functioning properly. It should be remembered, however, that the drug will be absorbed whereas the radiotracer will not, and care should be taken when interpreting these data. For example, in pharmacoscintigraphic studies, if the drug dissolves rapidly after release and is absorbed, the subsequent distribution of the radiolabel is of no interest.

A. Solute Phase Markers

Sodium pertechnetate is available on demand from a generator in most nuclear medicine departments since it is used diagnostically in more than 90% of the clinical evaluation of organ function. Pertechnetate is absorbed through the gastrointestinal (GI) tract and accumulates in the thyroid and stomach since the radius and charge on the pertechnetate ion is similar to that of iodide. To avoid the resultant increase in dosimetry, ^{99m}Tc-pertechnetate is usually formulated as a chelate. Ring molecules of varying polarity can be formed with molecules containing electron-donating atoms such as nitrogen, oxygen, or sulfur. Space between multiple electron donor atoms is required to allow several bonds to form with the technetium that is located in the center of the complex. The stability of the complex increases with an increasing number of bonds. Alteration in chemistry produces an associated change in physicochemical characteristics of the chelate. This is exploited in the clinic to facilitate regional targeting to brain, heart, skeleton, hepatobiliary system, and lungs to assess function and pathological changes. Applications of technetium chelates in formulation studies were originally reviewed by Hardy and Wilson (4), and more general clinical applications by Hjelsteun (5). For more complex formulations, especially emulsions, radioiodination of a fat component is an obvious approach. The use of technetium 99m to label oil phases has also been reviewed by Wilson and colleagues (6).

Other directly labeled, solute radiopharmaceuticals used in studies of controlled release preparations include indium 111–labeled albumin, In-111 alginates (7, 8), and indium 111–labeled hyaluronic acid (9). In all cases, the total amount of radioligand administered is very small—usually less than 1 μg—and the effect on the formulation is low. Adverse reactions to radiopharmaceuticals are also comparatively uncommon. Samson (10) quotes an incident rate of one to six reactions per 100,000 injections; however, some formulations used clinically are associated with a greater incidence of adverse event reports. A 1 in 800 rate is quoted for the bone-seeking radiopharmaceutical methylene diphosphonate and 1 in 400 for the lung visualization agent macroaggregated albumin (10).

B. Colloids and Fine Suspensions

A number of colloidal preparations are used in lymphoscintigraphy including technetium 99m–labeled sulfur colloid, tin colloid, and the smaller antimony colloids. Recent developments in the design of nanocolloids for lymph node imaging have utilized amphiphilic block copolymers, which spontaneously form colloidal particles with a diameter of 20–100 nm (11) and polyethylene plycol (PEG)–coated liposomal formulations, which have prolonged circulation times (12). The potential for entrapment of imaging agents into liposomes was suggested a decade ago by various groups who speculated that formulation of liposomes with targeting moieties might be useful for both identifying and treating cancer (13).

C. Particulate Markers

Amberlite resins bind technetium 99m and indium 111 tenaciously and are widely used to radiolabel formulations for scintigraphic studies. For tablet formulations, the labeled resins are usually admixed with the granulate and compressed. Pellet formulations that are packed into hard gelatin capsules usually have the Amberlite resin, matched for particle size, added to the pellets within the capsule. Yuen and colleagues describe a technique for the preparation of a pellet formulation prepared by spheronization of a mix of Amberlite CG 400 ion exchange resin mixed with microcrystalline cellulose and lactose. The spheronized material was then labeled with the technetium 99m immediately before administration to the volunteers (14).

Another useful particulate is activated charcoal, which we have utilized to follow the behavior of radiolabeled perfluorodecalin suspensions and carbomer 940 preparations in humans (15,16). Sterilized activated charcoal can be labeled by direct addition of ^{99m}Tc-DTPA followed by freeze drying. The resulting powder binds the radiopharmaceutical avidly.

The most important group of particulates utilized in scintigraphic studies of controlled release formulations are the lanthanide earths, particularly samarium and erbium which are used as oxides and the radioisotope generated in situ by neutron activation. Although all of the naturally occurring isotopes are activated to some extent, the isotopes ^{170}Er and ^{152}Sm have the highest neutron capture cross-sections. Neutron activation overcomes some of the problems associated with handling high amounts of radioisotopes during the production of the radiolabeled formulation. It also allows the use of pilot scale production machinery without the risk of contamination, since only the parent nonradioactive material is handled. The final formulation is activated in a cyclotron. Daughter radionuclides of lower atomic weight elements (carbon, hydrogen, oxygen, and nitrogen) are not formed during the irradiation process, although the generation of short-lived isotopes of potassium and sodium may be a problem. Irradiation may also result in structural changes of the formulation causing an alteration in physical properties, so it is important to carefully examine the effects of the neutron activation process (17,18).

III. DEPOSITION AND DISPERSION OF FORMULATIONS

Following Fickian principles, dispersion of the dose will determine the rate and extent of drug entry into the body. In addition, deposition control provides a measure of selectivity through regional targeting. This is well illustrated in pulmonary delivery with β_2 agonists where the

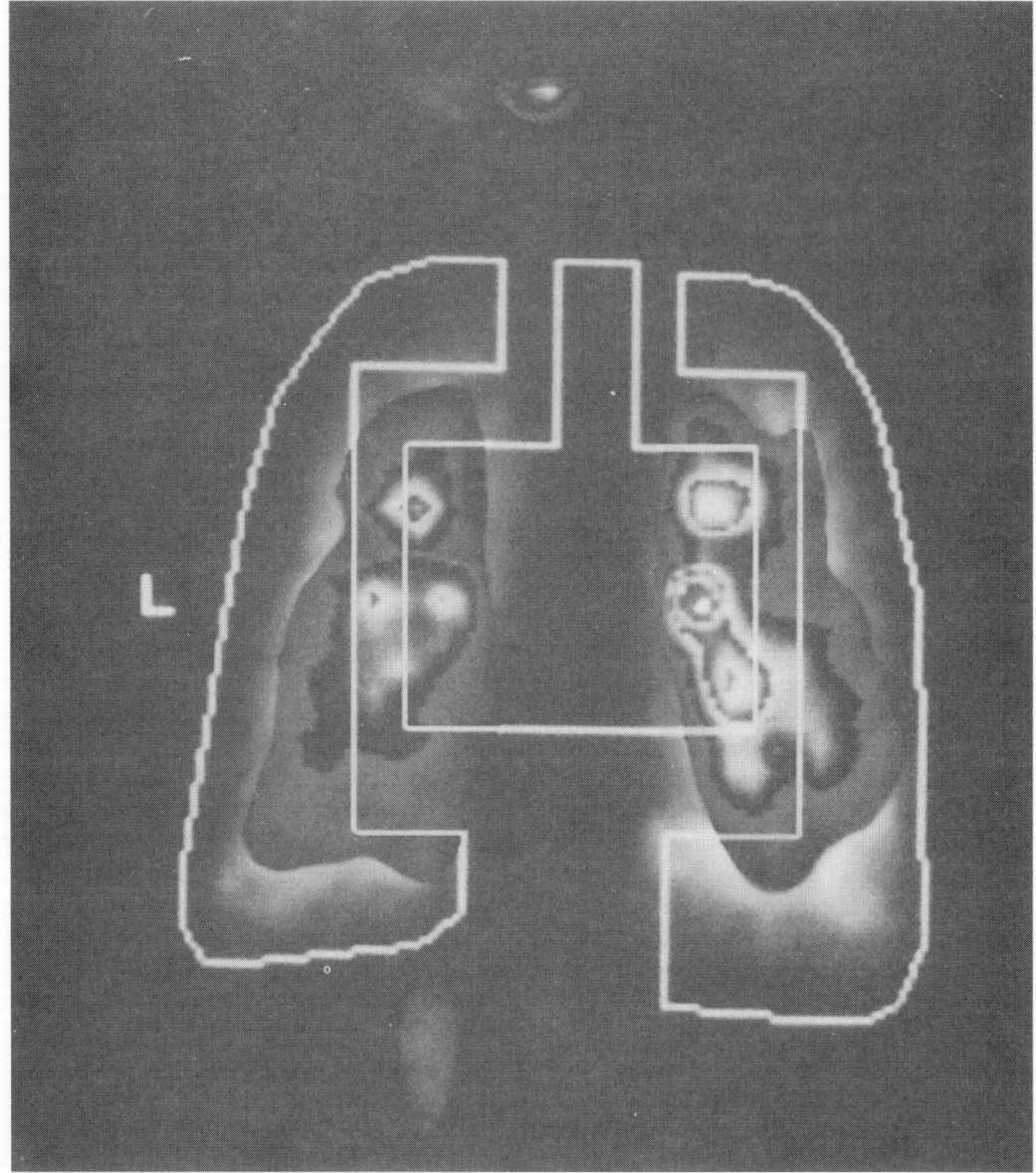

Figure 2 Overlay of Tc-99m HMPAO image on a krypton 81 m scan. The two acquisitions are taken sequentially as the generator-produced Kr-81m decays with a half-life of 13 s.

objective is to achieve targeted delivery to the smaller airways and minimize the proportion of drug that is swallowed. Gamma scintigraphy, using a radioactive gas such as krypton 81m to outline the lung margins, may be applied to measure the proportion of the dose delivered to central (bronchi) and to peripheral (alveolar) areas of the lung as shown in Fig. 2.

Scintigraphy has demonstrated that ion exchange resins can be used successfully to coat the stomach, which may be of value either for local delivery of drug to the gastric mucosa or for drugs that have a proximal window of absorption (19). Dividing the stomach images into three regions, each of approximately the same pixel area, assessed the distribution of the ion exchange resin. It was found to be evenly distributed within these regions and the gastric residence of about 15% of the total dose administered was greater than 6 h. Interestingly, a meal administered 4 h after dosing did not dislodge the resin attached to the mucosa (20).

Concerning oral dosing, the intake of food markedly alters the rate of presentation to the small intestine. This is particularly true for controlled or sustained release preparations. The pH, density, volume, and calorific effects on gastric emptying are fairly well appreciated physiological parameters that will affect the environment and transit of dosage forms. Alteration of the absorption profile by food of a once-a-day formulation will have greater consequences than alteration of a single dose of a three-times-daily formulation. For example, and ibuprofen matrix tablet (500 mg) given with a large breakfast and succeeding meals may not empty from the stomach until evening (21).

In these studies it is useful to utilize double labeling. For example, indium 111 is used to follow the behavior of the dosage form and technetium 99 is used to label the food. This enables the time of gastric emptying to be accurately assessed and provides some degree of anatomical definition of the stomach and colon. The two labels can also be used simultaneously to monitor the transit of different formulations administered at the same time, e.g., tablets and multiparticulates administered in a hard gelatin capsule.

A. Resolving Site of Release and Transit Parameters for Point Sources

Most protocols used to follow the intestinal transit of controlled release dosage forms involve periodic imaging of a batch of subjects. If scintigraphy is combined with plasma sampling, the interval between dosing can become extended and the best estimate of the time of gastric emptying has to be estimated as the midpoint of sequential views. Podczek and co-workers recently commented that because many laboratories follow strict protocols, parametric analysis is wrongly applied and statistical tests that define the general trend should be substituted. For example, a Wilcoxon test might be used to describe differences in gastric emptying times for two types of tablets distinguised by size or density. The authors calculate that imaging intervals no longer than 3 min should be chosen to allow accurate comparison of the gastric emptying of solid objects (22). Since anterior and posterior views take between 30 s and 1 min each to acquire, this would entail virtually continuous imaging of one subject at a time to ensure proper measurement. Although this might be impractical, in an analysis of previous data generated by the London-based group, the authors concluded that significant differences in gastric emptying of tablets cannot be detected using an acquisition interval or 15 min or more.

Resolving the anatomical location of a point source in the gut is problematic, and investigators be to be cautious in defining the regions of interest in the absence of suitable landmarks. Recently, we studied the behavior of small soft-gelatin capsules that showed erratic emptying after a high carbohydrate meal. The carbohydrate mass was formed in a partially hydrated mass that showed up on the magnetic resonance image as a spherical mass. The capsule taken after the meal remained above the food bolus and became located in the gastric rugae of the inner curvature. This unusual behavior was revealed when a ^{99m}Tc-labeled drink was taken and the position of the formulation was located as shown in Fig. 3.

The transverse colon is quite mobile and movements of gas in this region cause mark shifts in the orientation of the gut between images. This problem is illustrated in Fig. 4. In order to resolve whether the tablet was in the ascending colon or the transverse colon, images were taken with the subject standing sideways on the collimator. Similar techniques were used to confirm plug and body separation of a Pulsincap unit, since the separation of point sources was not evident in anterior and posterior images in some instances. This emphasizes the need

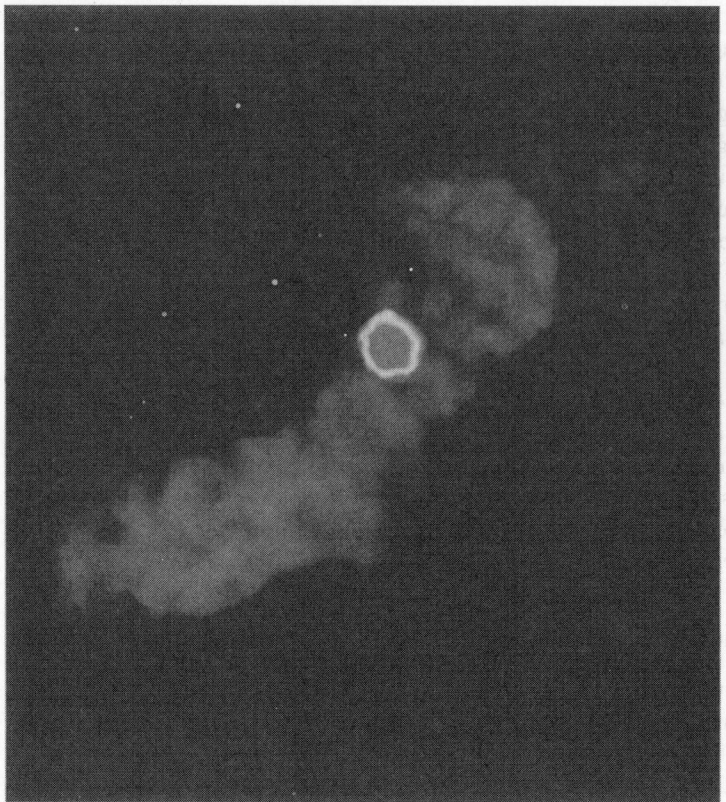

Figure 3 Shows sticking of a radiolabeled soft-gelatin capsule size #4 given with a high carbohydrate meal (filled baguette). The capsule has a low density and becomes lodged in the inner curvature.

for vigilance during a study, since the opportunity to take an extra acquisition may be lost and with it the ability to define the precise moment and location of release.

B. Locating Absorption Sites for Drugs

For sustained drug delivery to be successful, it is a necessary requirement that the drug is absorbed in adequate amounts from the colon. Ibuprofen, quinine, and oxprenolol are examples of drug that are well absorbed from the colon, whereas buflomedil, atenolol, and frusemide are not. For drugs that are poorly absorbed from the colon, the time for absorption would be no more than 7–8 h, i.e., the combined times for gastric emptying and small intestinal transit. Obviously, this would vary depending on food intake and whether or not drug was released from the dosage form whereas it was in the stomach. Several approaches have been made to study sites of absorption within the gut. Lennernas and colleagues have explored the use of a patented intestinal isolating system (Loc-I-Gut). It has been demonstrated that it is possible to determine the effective permeability for carrier-mediated transported compounds and hepatic extraction using this procedure (23). One of the most important restrictions of intubation is that some subjects find the procedure uncomfortable or stressing.

Other approaches to deliver drugs to specific sections of the gut are swallowable but large devices that can be triggered to release drug at the required site. In the early 1980s, Bieck and

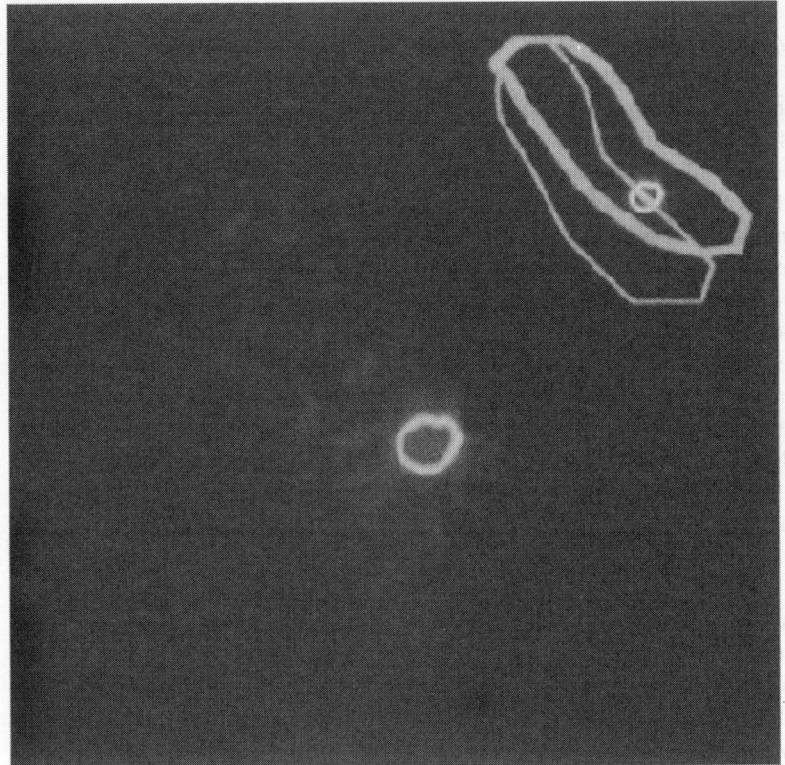

Figure 4 Resolving the position of a sustained release capsule. By taking images from the side, the location of the tablet in the transverse colon was resolved. Note how the anterior view fails to resolve the position of the main mass of the tablet.

colleagues used a small device, the high frequency (HF) capsule, containing the drug as a solution in a small latex balloon (24). Release of drug at the required part of the GI tract was accomplished externally by a radiofrequency pulse that energized a relay within the device. In order to ascertain the position in the GI tract, the subjects were fluoroscoped at regular intervals. The dosimetry associated with this radiologic procedure is relatively high and scintigraphic detection of location of the unit offers an obvious benefit. Gardner and colleagues have utilized an alternative device, i.e., the Intellisite capsule, which can be filled with powders, suspensions, or liquids. The system consists of a unit whose delivery ports are exposed by twisting of a section of the cap under the command of an externally applied radiofrequency pulse of around 120 W (25). Transit through the GI tract is followed using scintigraphy and the device actuated once it has reached the correct site.

C. Potential Sites for Adhesion or Lodging

Adhesion of dosage form was first detected in the 1970 when reports of "pill erosion" were made by gastroenterologists. In the last 20 years scintigraphy has been widely used to study this potential hazard. A recent review highlighted old studies in which four patients died from haemorrhages caused by sustained release potassium chloride tablets (26), and there are currently concerns with regard to the bisphosphonate analogues used in the treatment of osteoporosis in women after menopause (27). Scintigraphy has clearly established that some dosage forms, e.g., buoyant capsules, have greater potential to adhere to the esophagus than others do (28). A study of esophageal transit of capsule vs. tablet formulations show that the elderly have significant problems clearing buoyant formulations. The ability to swallow a hard gelatin capsule containing enteric-coated beads was examined in two cohorts of elderly subjects, mean age 66 years (both studies). The capsules were administered with 50 mL of water, which represents the average volume taken with a tablet in this group (Dansereau, personal communication). Mean transit times in the second study (n = 25 volunteers) were 3.3 s for the tablet and 23.8 s for the capsule (29). This compares with results obtained in the primary study (n = 23) with mean transit times ($\pm$ SD) of 4.3 $\pm$ 3 for the tablet and 20.9 $\pm$ 35.6 s for capsule (28).

Large units can lodge at anatomical junctions within the GI tract (personal observation), especially at the ileocaecal junction and the hepatic and splenic flexures. The overall transit through the entire GI tract is thus delayed to greater than 48 h in some cases; this represents an extremely unusual behavior which is not mimicked by most conventional and controlled release formulations. With this restriction in mind, triggered or passive pulse released systems provide a convenient method of studying windows of absorption in the gut for candidate therapeutic agents. Care must be taken to ensure full mass balance studies account for all release drug.

The complex salt of sucrose sulfate and aluminum hydroxide (Sucralfate, Carafate) is known to adhere to damaged gut epithelium by interacting with the protein exuded by the wound to form an adherent gel. Hardy and colleagues compared the gastric retention of sucralfate gel and suspension in healthy subjects and commented on the tendency of the gel to adhere to the walls of the esophagus (30). The study aroused much interest, although the extent of retention was never tacitly stated. A recent study conducted by our group confirms the superiority of retention of the gel in the esophagus; however, the extent of coating was extremely modest. Doses of three formulations, labeled with 2 MBq technetium added directly as pertechnetate, were administered to healthy volunteers. The retention after swallowing was 2.15% (gel), 0.99% (carafate), and 0.88% (vehicle control) between 30 s and 10 min (26). Bioadhesive polymer gels that undergo thermogelation have been recently investigated by our group as a method of delivering to the esophagus. A system based on poly(oxyethylene-b-oxypropylene-b-oxyethylene)-g-poly(acrylic acid) incorporating ^{99m}Tc-DTPA into the aqueous phase of the polymer was examined in a group of volunteer subjects. Good retention was seen up to half hour after dosing, which was superior to the Gastrogel association to the esophagus. Approximately 15% of the dose was associated with the esophagus after 30 min, which suggests use of these types of vehicles as delivery platforms in the treatment of esophageal inflammation and reflux disease.

D. Following Complex Pharmacokinetics

Fischer and colleagues are utilized gamma scintigraphy to unravel a complex absorption profile for isosorbide 5-mononitrate (IS-5-N) in which three distinct steps could be identified. The preparation consisted of 30% immediate dose; the remaining 70% was trapped in the core, surrounded by a controlled release membrane. The interior sustained release dose and the exterior immediate release dose were monitored using gamma scintigraphy following labeling of the formulation with In -111-labeled DTPA. During the first hour the immediate release dose and a fraction of the controlled release dose were absorbed whereas the pellets were still in the stomach. The second phase showed a near constant absorption for up to 6 h. After this, about 40% of the pellets were located in the colon and the rate of absorption was observed to decrease (31).

E. Temporal Control and Colonic Delivery

It has been appreciated for some time that disorders of the large intestine, such as inflammatory bowel disease and Crohn's disease, might be treated more effectively by local delivery of the appropriate therapeutic agent. Such a delivery system should deliver the payload of drug preferentially to the affected area and would be especially useful if it allowed exposure of tissue not accessible by rectal administration. The reservoir function of the ascending colon, with long contact times, permits extended delivery of drug, albeit at a lower flux than in the small intestine due to reduced surface area. The utilization of delayed delivery to help manage the plasma concentration–time profile while the patient is asleep offers significant advantages. A circadian rhythm is evident in many diseases, notably asthma and cardiovascular disease (32). A drug delivery system capable of bolus-releasing the drug to provide peak concentrations at the appropriate time would be a significant medical advance.

Based on known and robust physiological parameters, there are two mechanisms that can form the basis for the design of a colon-targeted formulation:

1. The relatively constant small intestinal transit time of 3–4 h.
2. The pH change observed on leaving the stomach and entering the small intestine. A much smaller pH change occurs moving from terminal ileum to cecum dependent on diet.

The Pulsincap delivery system developed by Rashid and colleagues is a time delayed pulsatile delivery system which in our studies has been configured to target drug release to the terminal small intestine and ascending colon (33). The device comprises an impermeable capsule body containing the drug formulation, sealed at the neck edge with a hydrogel polymer plug. On ingestion, the capsule becomes exposed to gastric fluids and the water-soluble gelatin cap dissolves allowing the hydrogel plug to hydrate. At a predetermined and controlled time point after ingestion, the swollen plug is ejected from the capsule body, thereby enabling the drug formulation to be released, with the time of plug ejection being controlled by the length of the hydrogel plug and its position relative to the neck of the capsule body. The dosage form is represented schematically in Fig. 5.

In studies of the permeability characteristics of the colon, the Pulsincap device provides a versatile tool that can be adapted to provide varying degrees of delay within the boundaries of 3–10 h. Addition of a gastric resistant layer allows exploration of the proximal and transverse colon with minimal interference. Originally, it was anticipated that the proximal and descending colon could be explored by administering units with 5-h and 15-h release characteristics. In practice, two problems were encountered that prevented this approach. The first problem was that the 15-h devices were too large (about the size of a 00 capsule) and several fasted volunteers showed delays in gastric emptying longer than 6 h. The second problem proved more interesting and provided an interesting suggestion as to how exposure of the proximal colon to drugs delivered by controlled delivery systems could be increased (e.g., topically acting agents or those fermented by bacteria). We anticipated that transit through the gut to reach the distal small intestine would take around 15 h, based on normal behavior following dosing in the morning. In order to run the arms in parallel, we dosed the 15-h device at 2200 h the night before the trial, anticipating that at 1300 h the next day, units would be distributed in the ascending colon (5 h devices) and proximal colon (15-h devices) to begin the permeability experiments. Quinine dihydrochloride was selected as the transcellular probe, ^{51}Cr-EDTA as the paracellular marker and ^{111}In-labeled resin as the position marker. The following morning it was found that the devices dosed the night before were located either in the proximal colon or in the sigmoid colon. This indicated that following dosing at night the colon becomes quiescent and

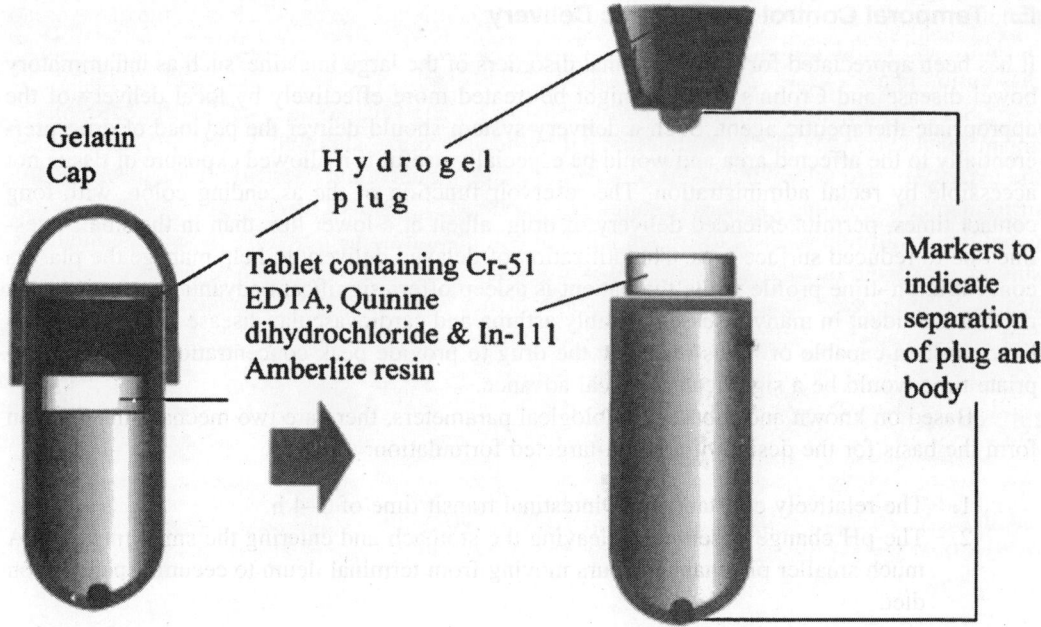

Figure 5 Gelatin caps.

that units located in the proximal large bowel on retiring do not move forward (34). Subsequent experiments showed that on waking, material travels very rapidly in the first 30 min after rising, irrespective of food cues, and that both disperse and monolithic devices show this effect.

Another factor influenced by temporal control is the availability of water. This is critical when considering the release of drug from devices where water cannot be transferred to the dissolving mass of material, e.g., when an object is encased by a water-impermeable layer and water in the lumen has to flow into the interior of the device. In the case of the Pulsincap, loss of the plug leaves an area of 3–4 mm to be bridged by luminal fluid after the mid–ascending colon, and the environment has insufficient fluid to ensure dispersion. Pharmacological manipulation by pretreatment with lactulose markedly increases the available fluid, resulting in a faster and more extensive absorption of the quinine dihydrochloride (35). The difference in fluidity between right- and left-sided regions of the colon also causes the steady-state distribution of contents to shift in favor of the ascending (right) colon; this difference is also seen in active left-sided ulcerative colitis, which has implications for drug delivery with controlled release formulations designed for topical delivery (36).

F. Barrier Control

The use of gamma scintigraphy to follow the performance of enteric coating and the performance of matrix systems has been fairly extensive, although the results in terms of selective release have been mixed. Early in vivo studies of the effectiveness of enteric coating employed x-ray techniques (37,38), although gamma scintigraphy is now the technique of choice in these studies. For example, Ashford and co-workers examined tablet cores protected with Eudragit S. In vivo disintegration was extremely variable with regard to both time (5.0–15 h) and position (39). Similar variability is often found with matrix tablets: sustained release tablets containing morphine labeled with indium 111 indicated that morphine is absorbed throughout the GI tract, although the release of the drug from matrix tablets is incomplete or too slow in the distal small intestine and in the colon, resulting in reduced bioavailability of tablets and a very prolonged dissolution phase (40).

Specific targeting to the large intestine using bacterial metabolism as the triggering mechanism for release (41) has been investigated by many groups, although reservations concerning the toxicity of azo polymers has generally caused pharmaceutical scientists to focus on the use of fermentable polymers including starch and pectin (42). Munjeri and colleagues recently evaluated the absorption of drug from radiolabeled amidated low-methoxyl pectin beads containing sulfamethoxazole or indomethacin (43). Rapid transit out of the stomach and bunching of the beads at the ileocasecal junction was observed. Once into the colon, fermentation of the polymer started and drug was released.

IV. CONCLUSIONS

Scintigraphy is currently one of the most powerful techniques that the pharmaceutical scientist has in the interpretation of the in vivo behavior of formulations. In the past there were few direct methods of assessing the behavior of drug formulations within the body. Information was gleaned from in vitro dissolution tests and plasma–concentration time curves for the drug and the true behavior and relationship within the body of the two could only be guessed. Radiological contrast studies produce good definition of anatomical structure but are not well suited to measurements of transit and dispersion of pharmaceutical formulations because the radiation burden of multiple x-rays and/or repeated studies would be prohibitively high. Gamma scintigraphy avoids artifacts produced by intubation studies, including stimulation of acid secretion and mechanical stimulation of the gut wall. When combined with techniques including magnetic resonance imaging, the power of the resolution and quantification offered by each modality provides the pharmaceutical research worker the ability to precisely quantify deposition kinetics. These tools will be critical for future developments in implant technology and the next generation of controlled release products.

REFERENCES

1. Perkins, A. C., 1996. Nuclear Medicine Science and Safety. London: John Libby.
2. Perkins, A. C., 1999. Instrumentation, imaging, data analysis and display. In: Nuclear Medicine in Pharmaceutical Research, A. C. Perkins and M. Frier, Eds. Taylor & Francis: London.
3. Perkins, A. C., Mann, C., and Wilson, C. G., 1995. Three dimensional visualisation of the large bowel: a potential tool for assessing targeted drug delivery and colonic pathology. Eur. J. Nucl. Med., 22: 1035–1038.
4. Hardy, J. G., and C. G. Wilson, 1981. Radionuclide imaging in pharmaceutical, physiological and pharmacological research. Clin. Phys. Physiol. Meas., 2: 71–121.
5. Hjelsteun, O. K., 1995. Tc-99m chelators in nuclear medicine—a review. Analyst, 120: 863–866.
6. Wilson, C. G., McJury, M., O'Mahony, B., Frier, M., and Perkins, A. C., 1997. Imaging of oily formulations in the gastrointestinal tract. Adv. Drug Deliv. Rev., 25: 91–101.
7. May, H. A., Wilson, C. G., and Hardy, J. G. 1984. Monitoring radiolabelled antacid preparations in the stomach. Int. J. Pharm., 19: 169–179.
8. Washington, N., Washington, C., Wilson, C. G., and Davis, S. S. 1986. The effect of inclusion of aluminum hydroxide in alginate containing raft-forming antacids. Int. J. Pharm., 28: 139–143.
9. Durani, A. M., Farr, S. J., and Kellaway, I. W. 1995. Influence of molecular weight and formulation pH on the precorneal clearance rate of hyaluronic acid in the rabbit eye. Int. J. Pharm., 118: 243–250.

10. Sampson, S., 1992. Adverse reactions and drug interactions with radiopharmaceuticals. Drug Safety, 8: 280–294.
11. Trubetskoy, V. S., 1999. Polymeric miceslles as drug carriers of diagnostic agents. Adv. Drug. Deliv. Rev., 37: 81–88.
12. Phillips, W. T., 1999. Delivery of gamma-imaging agents by liposomes. Adv. Drug Deliv. Rev, 37: 13–32.
13. Ogiharaumeda, A., Sasaki, T., and Nishigori, H. 1992. Development of a liposome encapsulated radionuclide with preferential tumor accumulation—the choice of radionuclide and chelating ligand. Nucl. Med. Biol., 19: 753–757.
14. Yuen, K. H., Deshmuhk, A. A., Newton, J. M., Short, M., and Melchor, R., 1993. Gastrointestinal transit and absorption of theophylline from multiparticulate controlled release formulation. Int. J. Pharm., 97: 61–77.
15. Wilson, C. G., Zhu, Y. P., Frier, M., Gilchrist, P., Perkins, A. C., and Rao, L. S. 1998 Ocular contact time of a carbomer gel (Geltears,) in humans. Br. J. Ophthalmol., 82: 1131–1134.
16. Zhu, Y. P., Wilson, C. G., Meadows, D., Olejnik, O., Frier, M., Washington, N., and Musson, R. (1999). Dry powder dosing in liquid vehicles: ocular tolerance and scintigraphic evaluation of a perfluorocarbon suspension. Int. J. Pharm. 191: 79–85.
17. Watts, P. J., Atkin, B. P., Wilson, C. G., Davis, M. C., and Melia, C. D. 1991. Radiolabelling of polymer microspheres for scintigraphic investigations by neutron activation. 1. Incorporation of samarium oxide and its effects on the properties of Eudragit R S: sulphasalazine microspheres. Int. J. Pharm., 76: 55–59.
18. Watts, P. J., Atkin, B. P., Wilson, C. G., Davies, M. C., and Melia, C. D. 1993. Radiolabelling of polymer microspheres for scintigraphic investigations by neutron activation. 2. Effects of irradiation on the properties of Eudragit RS: sulphasalazine microspheres. Int. J. Pharm., 98: 63–73.
19. Washington, N., Wilson, C. G., Greaves, J. L., Norman, S., Peach, J., and Pugh, K. 1989. A gamma scintigraphic study of gastric coating by Expidet, tablet and liquid formulations. Int. J. Pharm., 57: 17–22.
20. Thairs, S., Ruck, S., Feely, L., Steele, R. J. C., and Washington, N. 1998. Effect of dose size, food and surface coating on the gastric residence and distribution of ionic resins. Int. J. Pharm. 176: 47–53.
21. Wilson, C. G., Washington, N., Greaves, J. L., Kamali, F., Rees, J. A., Sempik, A. K., and Lampard, J. F. 1989. Bimodal release of drug in a sustained release ibuprofen formulation: a scintigraphic and pharmacokinetic open study in healthy volunteers under different conditions of food intake. Int. J Pharm., 50: 155–161.
22. Podczeck, F., Course, N. J., and Newton, J. M. 1999. Determination of the gastric emptying of solid dosage forms using gamma scintigraphy: a problem of image timing and mathematical analysis. Eur. J. Nucl. Med., 26: 373–378.
23. Lennernas, H., 1997. Human jejunal effective permeability and its correlation with preclinical drug absorption models. J. Pharm. Pharmacol., 49: 627–638.
24. Bieck, P. J., 1989. Drug absorption from the colon. In: Drug Delivery to the Gastrointestinal Tract, J. G. Hardy, S. S. Davis, and C. G. Wilson, Eds. Ellis Horwood, Chichester, pp. 147–159.
25. Gardner, G., Casper, R. Leith, F., and Wilding, I. 1997. Regional drug absorption from the gastrontestinal tract. Pharm. Tech., 9: 46–53.
26. Dansereau, R. J., R. N. Dansereau, and J. W. McRorie, 1999. Scintigraphic study of oesophageal transit and retention. In: Nuclear Medicine in Pharmaceutical Research, A. C. Perkins and M. Frier, Eds. Taylor & Francis, London. pp. 57–69.
27. de Groen, P. C., Lubbe, D. F, Hirsch, L. J., Daifotis, A., Stephenson, W., Freedholm, D., Pryor-Tillotson, S., Seleznick, M. J., Pinkas, H., and Wang, K. K. 1996., Esophagitis associated with the use of alendronate. N. Engl. J. Med., 335: 1016–1021.
28. Perkins, A. C., Wilson, C. G., Blackshaw, P. E., Vincent, R. M., Dansereau, R. J., Juhlin, K. D., Bekker, P. J., and Spiller, R. C., 1994. Impaired oesophageal transit of capsule versus tablet formulation in the elderly. Gut, 35: 1363–1367.
29. Perkins, A. C., Perkins, A. C. Wilson, C. G. Vincent, R. M. Frier, M. Blackshaw, P. E. Dansereau, R. J. Juhlin, K. D. Bekker, P. J., and Spiller, R. C. 1999. Oesophageal transit of cellulose film coated

tablet and gelatin capsule formulations for administration of risedronate to the elderly. Int. J. Pharm. 186: 169–175.
30. Hardy, J. G., Hooper, G., Ravelli, G-P., Steed, K. P., and Wilding, I. R. 1993. A comparison of the gastric retention of a sucralfate gel and a sucralfate suspension. Eur. J. Pharm. Biopharm. 39: 70–74.
31. Fischer, W., Boertz, A., Davis, S. S., Khoshla, R., Cawello, W., Sandrock, K., and Cordes, G., 1987. Investigation on the gastrointestinal transit and in vivo drug release of isosorbide-5-nitrate pellets. Pharm. Res., 1987. 4: 480–485.
32. Lemmer, B., 1991. Circadian rhythms and drug delivery. J. Contr. Rel., 16: 63–74.
33. Rashid, A., 1990. Dispensing device, U. K. patent 2230441A.
34. Hebden, J. M., Gilchrist, P. J., Blackshaw, E., Frier, M. E., Perkins, A. C, Wilson, C. G., and Spiller, R. C., 1999. Night-time quiescence and morning activation in teh human colon: effect on transit of dispersed versus large single unit formulations. Eur. J. Gastro. Hepatol. 11: 1379–1385.
35. Hebden, J. M., Gilchrist, P. J., Perkins, A. C., Wilson, C. G., and Spiller, R. C. 1999., Stool water content and colonic drug absorption: contrasting effects of lactulose and codiene. Pharm. Res. 16:(8) 1254–1259.
36. Hebden, J. M., Perkins, A. C., Frier, M., Wilson, C. G., and Spiller, R. C. 1999. Limited exposure of the healthy distal colon to orally dosed formulation is further exaggerated in active left-sided ulcerative colitis. Aliment. Pharmacol. Ther., 1999 submitted.
37. Dew, M. J., Hughes, P. J., Lee, M. G., Evans, B. K., and Rhodes, J. 1982. An oral preparation to release drugs in the human colon. Br. J. Clin. Pharm., 14: 405–408.
38. Dew, M. J., Ryder, R. E. J., Evans, N., Evans, B. K., and Rhodes, J. 1983 Colonic release of 5-aminosalicylic acid from an oral preparation in active ulcerative colitis. Br. J. Clin. Pharm., 16: 185–187.
39. Ashford, M., Fell, J. T., Attwood, D., Sharma, H., and Woodhead, P. J. 1993. An in vivo investigation into the suitability of pH dependent polymers for colonic targeting. Int. J. Pharmaceut. 95: 193–199.
40. Olsson, B., Wagner, Z. G., Mansson, P., and Ragnarsson, G. 1995. A gamma scintigraphic study of the absorption of morphine from controlled-release tablets. Int. J. Pharm., 119: 223–229.
41. Saffran, M., Kumar, G. S., Neckers, D. C., Pena, J., Jones, R. H., and Field, J. B. S. 1990. Biodegradable azopolymer coating for oral delivery of peptide drugs. Biochem. Soc. Trans., 18: 752.
42. Ashford, M., and Fell, J. T. 1994. Targeting drugs to the colon: delivery systems for oral administration. J. Drug Target., 2: 241–258.
43. Munjeri, O., Collett, J. H., Fell, J. T., Sharma H. L., and Smith, A. M. 1998. In vivo behavior of hydrogel beads based on amidated pectins. Drug Deliv., 5: 239–241.

27
Electrically Assisted Transdermal Delivery of Drugs

Ajay K. Banga
Mercer University, Atlanta, Georgia

I. INTRODUCTION

Several drugs, such as clonidine, estradiol, fentanyl, nicotine, nitroglycerin, scopolamine, and testosterone, are available as skin patches for transdermal delivery. These patches do not use any enhancement mechanisms and are considered to be "passive" patches. Sufficient delivery to achieve therapeutic dose without any enhancement is feasible for these drugs since they are relatively potent and have desirable physicochemical properties (small lipophilic molecules) to penetrate the skin. The scope of drug delivery via skin is limited to only a few drugs by passive delivery. However, the range of drugs that can be delivered via skin can be expanded by various physical and chemical enhancement methods. The latter involves the use of chemical penetration enhancers while the former can involve the use of ultrasonography (phonophoresis) or electricity. This chapter will discuss the electrically assisted transdermal delivery of drugs. The description "electrically assisted" is being used to refer to delivery by iontophoresis, electroosmosis, and electroporation. The topics of iontophoresis and electroporation are separately discussed in this book in more details as separate chapters. This brief chapter is written to provide a general overview of the field.

II. ELECTROTRANSPORT MECHANISMS

A. Iontophoresis

Iontophoresis is the use of electric current to drive charged drug molecules into the skin by placing them under an electrode of like charge. A positively charged drug would thus be placed under the anode or positive electrode and the resulting electric repulsion would provide the driving force to push the drug into the skin. The current used is small, typically 0.5 mA/cm^2 or less, and increasing body of literature seems to suggest that this amount of current does not cause any irreversible damage to the skin. The drug is delivered in proportion to the applied current, providing an opportunity to program delivery as needed. Our understanding of iontophoresis has advanced over the years from when the author first reviewed the field (1) to when he compiled research to date in a recent text (2). Iontophoresis is already used in clinical medicine in physical therapy clinics over the last several decades for topical or localized delivery of drugs into skin, such as delivery of lidocaine and epinephrine for local analgesia.

Devices available on the market for delivery of local anesthetics and corticosteroids include Phoresor II (Iomed, UT), Empi Dupel (Empi, Inc., St. Paul, MN), Life-Tech Iontophor (Houston, TX), and Henley Intl. Dynaphor (Houston, TX). In addition, devices for iontophoresis of pilocarpine for diagnosis of cystic fibrosis are on the market, and these include CF Indicator (Scandipharm, Birmingham, AL) and the system based on Webster sweat inducer with Pilogel discs and Macroduct collector (Wescor, Utah, USA). These topical applications of iontophoresis have not been discussed in this chapter. Instead, the focus of this chapter is the use of iontophoresis (and electroporation) for systemic delivery of drugs into the general circulation. Several companies are actively trying to commercialize miniaturized iontophoretic patch systems and are close to the market. A partial list includes Alza Corporation (USA), Becton Dickinson (USA), Fournier (France), Hisamitsu (Japan), and Cygnus (USA). Alza currently has a E-TRANS fentanyl product under development with Janssen Pharmaceutica. Currently in phase III clinical trials, the product is an on-demand delivery system intended to allow a patient to manage acute pain by self-titrating the level of fentanyl administered according to his or her need. Other companies doing iontophoresis research on their own or for larger pharmaceutical companies include Pharma Peptides (France), Sanofi Recherche (France), Dermion/Iomed (USA), and Novartis (Europe/USA). Much of the activity in the area is proprietary and will unfold over the next few years (2). Iontophoresis patches for systemic delivery are expected to be commercially available in the near future (3). This has been made possible partly due to the revolution in microelectronics, which has allowed the development of prototype iontophoretic patches not much larger than the traditional passive patches, with miniaturized circuitary and button cells.

B. Electro-osmosis

If a charged porous membrane is subjected to a voltage difference, a bulk fluid or volume flow, called electro-osmosis, occurs without concentration gradients, suggesting that this flow is not diffusion (4). This bulk fluid flow by electro-osmosis is a significant factor in iontophoresis and was found to be of the order of microliters per hour per square centimeter of hairless mouse skin (5). Since skin is a permselective membrane with negative charge at physiological pH (6), the electro-osmotic flow occurs from anode to cathode, thus enhancing the flux of positively charged (cationic) drugs and making it possible to deliver neutral drugs by iontophoresis. Electro-osmotic flow can also hinder drug flux in a situation where a negatively charged drug (anion) or a neutral drug is being delivered under the cathode. If the skin reverses its charge such as at a pH below its isoelectric point (somewhere between pH 3 and 4), the direction of electro-osmotic flow will also reverse. Some positively charged peptides may actually associate with the skin to reduce or neutralize its negative charge. In these cases, the cation permselectivity of the skin may be lost, resulting in a reversal of electro-osmotic flow to the cathode-to-anode direction. This was seen for the iontophoretic delivery of nafarelin across human skin in vitro (7). The same phenomenon was also observed for another luteinizing hormone–releasing hormone (LHRH) analogue, leuprolide (8), and more recently, with positively charged polypeptides (9). The classical Nernst–Planck equation to describe iontophoresis must be modified to include electro-osmosis component, as discussed elsewhere in this chapter. The origin of electro-osmotic flow lies in the realm of nonequilibrium or irreversible thermodynamics. Intuitively, one may visualize electro-osmotic flow as occurring because immobile charges in membrane require the flow of mobile counterions to maintain electroneutrality in the membrane.

Electro-osmosis is also the underlying mechanism for the phenomenon of reverse iontophoresis, which is the back iontophoretic extraction (by electro-osmotic flow) of a molecule from the body rather than forward iontophoretic delivery of drugs into the body. This technique can have important applications in medical diagnostics as it can allow noninvasive sampling of biological fluids. Reverse iontophoresis can thus be used as a noninvasive technique to perform clinical chemistry without blood sampling. This approach has been used for iontophoretic extraction of glucose from subcutaneous tissue in an attempt to develop an alternative for the commonly used invasive and inconvenient "fingerstick" technique. In a study in human subjects, iontophoresis at 0.25 mA/cm^2 for 60 min was applied to the ventral forearm surface to show that iontophoretic sampling of glucose is feasible (10). Based on the principles of reverse iontophoresis, a glucose-monitoring device (GlucoWatch) is under development by Cygnus (Redwood City, CA). Glucose is extracted from the body due to electro-osmosis induced by reverse iontophoresis. Using a electrochemical reaction linked with a sensor and a control module, blood glucose levels can be continuously monitored and displayed at the push of a button. The system can sound an alarm in the event of hypo- or hyperglycemia. The factors affecting electro-osmotic flow during reverse iontophoresis have been investigated. Since electro-osmotic flow normally takes place from anode to cathode, extraction at the cathode will be most efficient and is preferred. The electro-osmotic flow can be increased to increase extraction efficiency at either anode or cathode by the use of some excipients such as divalent ions or EDTA in the electrode formulations, respectively. The mechanism is believed to be modification of the net negative charge of the skin (11,12). If reverse iontophoresis is to be successfully commercialized, a sensitive analytical detection method for the target material will be required since the amount extracted is likely to be very low. Though the approach can sample several materials at the same time, the need to have separate detection methods for each will pose a challenge. For the measurement of glucose, calibration procedures for day-to-day use are required. Also, the collection formulation will need to be optimized to improve the efficiency of extraction and the "on-board" sensor will need to be perfected (13).

C. Electroporation

Electroporation involves the application of a high-voltage pulse for a very short duration to permeabilize the skin, unlike iontophoresis which uses a continuous low current to push drug into the skin. Electroporation has been used for DNA transfection in recombinant technology for a long time but its application to skin is relatively new. The technique of electroporation is normally used on the unilamellar phospholipid bilayers of cell membranes. However, it has been demonstrated that electroporation of skin is feasible, even though the stratum corneum contains multilamellar, intercellular lipid bilayers with few phospholipids (14). The approximately 100 multilamellar bilayers of the stratum corneum need about 100 V pulses for electroporation, or about 1 V per bilayer (15). The stratum corneum does not contain any living cells, but it can still be permeabilized by an electric pulse because electroporation is a physical process based on electrostatic interactions and thermal fluctuations within fluid membranes and no active transport processes are involved. The exact mechanism for electroporation is not clear although changes in the behavior of membranes seen following electroporation are consistent with the theory of pore formation (16). These new aqueous pathways are created on a time scale of microseconds or less and allow the entry of drug molecules by diffusion and local electrophoresis and/or electro-osmosis. The pathways then close over a time period that may vary from milliseconds to hours (17). In a recent study, methylene blue dye was delivered across full-thickness porcine skin by pulses (1 ms; up to 240 V) applied for 30 min. The dye was observed to be delivered into skin and the transport by pulsing was more than an order of magnitude greater than that seen following iontophoresis. The dye penetration was increased with increasing applied voltage (18).

The use of electroporation alone or in combination with iontophoresis can apparently deliver much larger molecules through skin than are feasible with iontophoresis alone. This can expand the scope of transdermal delivery to larger molecules such as therapeutic proteins and oligonucleotides. It may also be feasible to use electroporation as an alternative nonviral approach for gene therapy (19). Recently, the delivery of a protein or the delivery and expression of a plasmid carrying the reporter gene has been demonstrated in murine melanoma. This was achieved by a direct injection of the protein or plasmid in the tumor, followed by application of pulses with surface electrodes in contact with the skin (20). The delivery of particles into skin may also be feasible by "electroincorporation," a technique in which a drug encapsulated in vesicles or particles is delivered into the skin by applying a pulse that causes a breakdown of the stratum corneum (21,22). The technique involves placing particles on the skin and then pulsing with electrodes placed directly on top of the particles. This creates an electric field that breaks down the stratum corneum by a yet unknown mechanism and a slight pressure is applied to drive particles into skin. The particles apparently do not have to be charged for delivery. Particles of 0.2, 4.0, and 45.0 μm were shown to be embedded in hairless mouse skin when pulsed with three exponential decay pulses of amplitude 120 V and pulse length 1.2 ms (21). If "electroincorporation" can be commercialized to successfully deliver particulates in skin, then no molecular size limitations would exist in terms of what can be delivered through the skin. The commercial development of electroporation for transdermal delivery of drugs is in very early stages. Unlike iontophoresis, the miniaturization of technology to develop wearable patches is currently not feasible for electroporation due to the need for a capacitor. However, Genetronics (San Diego, CA) has developed palm-size generator that can deliver pulses to a medication patch attached to the skin (23). Patent activity by several universities or companies, such as the Masachusetts Institute of Technology, Genetronics, and others, illustrates the developing interest in this area (2).

D. Pathways of Delivery

During iontophoresis, the greatest concentration of ionized species is expected to move into some regions of the skin where the skin is damaged, or along the sweat glands and hair follicles, as the diffusional resistance of the skin to permeation is lowest in these regions. Thus, a preexisting pore or transappendageal pathway is generally assumed for iontophoretic delivery (24). In contrast, electroporation is considered to involve the creation of new aqueous pathways or pores during the application of an electric pulse. However, it has been suggested that even low-voltage iontophoresis may electroporate the epithelial layers of the skin appendages, which in turn allows transport from appendages to epidermal cells. At low voltages (<30 V), the drop in resistance of skin may be attributed to electroporation of appendageal ducts. At higher voltages (>30 V), electroporation of the skin itself leads to a further drop in resistance (25,26).

E. Theoretical Basis of Electrotransport

For iontophoresis, the flux (J_i) of an ionic species, i, is defined by a modified Nernst–Planck equation:

$$J_i = -D_i \, dC_i/dx - z_i m F C_i \, dE/dx \pm C_i J_v$$

The first term takes into account any passive contribution to flux by Fick's first law of diffusion, where D_i is diffusivity and C_i concentration. The second term is the equation for electrophoresis or the contribution of direct electrical repulsion during iontophoresis, where z_i is the valence of the ionic species, m the mobility, F Faraday's constant, and E the electrostatic potential. The last term of this equation corrects for electro-osmotic flow, with J_v being the velocity of convective flow, i.e., volume flow per unit time per unit area.

For electroporation, the steady-state, time-average, one-dimensional solute flux across the stratum corneum has been expressed (27) as:

$$<J> = 1/T \int_0^T J \, dt \approx K_1 <U^*> C_1$$

where J is the solute flux normal to the skin surface, T the time period of any oscillatory process, K_1 the skin/donor–solution equilibrium partition coefficient, U^* the mean solute velocity component normal to the skin surface (with $<U^*>$ its time average), and C_1 the time-independent solute concentration in the donor compartment.

F. pH Control Mechanisms

The electrochemistry at the electrode–solution interface where electronic current is converted to ionic current is controlled by the electrode material used. As oxidation occurs at the anode and reduction at the cathode, the following reactions take place:

$$H_2O \rightarrow 2H^+ + 1/2\, O_2 + 2e^- \text{ (at anode)}$$

$$2H_2O + 2e^- \rightarrow H_2 + 2OH^- \text{ (at cathode)}$$

The production of hydrogen and hydroxyl ions leads to a pH drop in the solution containing the anode and a rise in the pH at the solution containing the cathode. A better choice of electrode material with respect to pH changes is silver for anode and chloridized silver for cathode. Silver/silver chloride or so-called reversible electrodes prevent pH drifts as they are consumed by the active electrochemistry, thus avoiding the use of water in the electrochemistry:

$$Ag + Cl^- \rightarrow AgCl + e^- \text{ (at anode)}$$

$$AgCl + e^- \rightarrow Ag + Cl^- \text{ (at cathode)}$$

The amount of chloride added to the buffer should be just enough to drive the electrochemistry, as any excess will provide avoidable competition to the drug for transport. The ideal case would be where the drug itself exists as a hydrohalide salt (e.g., lidocaine hydrochloride) in which case the drug itself provides the ion for electrochemistry, resulting in high current efficiency (28). Other alternative methods to control pH drifts are also feasible. Ion exchange resins have been used for pH control under iontophoresis electrodes. The drug ions may be attached to an ion exchange resin; as the drug leaves the resin, the vacated site is filled by the ions of electrolysis products, so that relatively constant pH can be maintained. Alternatively, the drug need not be attached to the resin, and a more generalized mechanism may be involved (2).

III. SKIN SOURCE AND STUDY MODELS

The European Centre for the Validation of Alternative Methods has recommended that there be a concerted effort toward using human skin as the primary in vitro model for skin permeability studies. In case of difficulty in acquiring human skin, pig skin and hairless-guinea-pig skin may be acceptable alternatives (29). Since the supply of fresh and viable human skin is limited, animal skin will continue to be used. However, human skin should be used where possible. Animal skins are typically more permeable than human skin and thus will overestimate drug delivery. The permeability coefficients of morphine, fentanyl, and sufentanil across full-thickness hairless-mouse skin were found to be one order of magnitude higher than those for human epidermis (30). An exception is shed snake skin, which may be as much as 10 times less permeable than cadaver skin (31). Also, skin from animal species such as hairless rat often has a higher proteolytic activity than human skin. Pig skin is generally considered a close model for human skin, partly because the hair follicle density of pig and human skin (about 11 hair follicles/cm^2) is similar. Using a series of compounds, it has been shown that the skin of miniature swine has the closest permeability characteristics to that of human skin (32). In vitro studies with human skin have also been shown to correlate well with in vivo studies in pigs (33). In contrast, the hair follicle density is much higher for rat (289/cm^2), mouse (658/cm^2), or even hairless mouse (75/cm^2). Thus, even the use of hairless animals does not provide a good model since despite the fact that hair shafts are lacking, rudimentary follicles are still present (34). In recent years, a cultured or living-skin equivalent of human origin has also become available. This artificial skin closely resembles human skin as it has a epidermis and dermis, the former with a well-differentiated stratum corneum. However, it lacks appendages such as hair follicles and sweat glands and obviously lacks the vasculature as well. Also, the cost and commercial availability of the skin can be a drawback, and more thorough evaluation of its potential usefulness is not available. A potential alternative to in vitro studies is the use of the isolated perfused porcine skin flap (IPPSF) model, which was developed as a novel alternative animal model for dermatology and cutaneous toxicology (35) and has since been used in several transdermal delivery and/or iontophoresic investigations (36,37). While most in vitro models can only investigate the first step, the IPPSF model can go a step further to investigate the movement into the vasculature as well since a porcine flap with intact vasculature is maintained in a chamber in this model. All of these studies are then followed by in vivo studies in animals and humans. The skin is a complex biological tissue and thus permeability measurements across skin tend to have a high variation. Furthermore, the application of electric current can change skin permeability, thus making delivery more unpredictable in some cases. In order to avoid these problems, various synthetic membranes have been tried in iontophoresis research. However, these membranes may not be predictive of what to expect with skin precisely because skin is a complex biological tissue and these membranes are not. Nevertheless, they could be useful for preliminary studies. These membranes could also be useful for in vitro release studies that may be required to assure batch-to-batch uniformity of product.

IV. ADVERSE EFFECTS OF ELECTRICAL EXPOSURE

Clinical precedent for safely applying electrical pulses of hundreds of volts to the skin exists with the use of techniques such as transcutaneous electrical nerve stimulation (TENS) (14). TENS is commonly used to treat chronic conditions such as lower back pain, arthritis, and pain caused by a variety of neurologic disorders (38). Nevertheless, electroporation of skin or tissue is a relatively new area, and there is much to be learned about its safety. Electroporation of anesthetized hairless rats has been reported to result in direct stimulation of motor nerves, with each pulse resulting in a kicking of the hind legs of the rat (39). Toxicological effects of electroporation pulses have been evaluated ex vivo on pig skin using histological scores and by scaling the degree of erythema, edema, and the presence of petechiae. The changes following electroporation pulses were comparable to those seen with iontophoresis alone. Also, at both the gross and light microscopic level, electroporation did not result in any skin changes not previously seen with iontophoresis alone (40). A recent study has provided the first in vivo demonstration of the safety of the high-voltage pulses for transdermal delivery, using chromametry, transepidermal water loss, laser Doppler flowmetry, and corneometery techniques for noninvasive sensing of skin biophysical parameters. The changes in skin biophysical parameters for hairless rats following high-voltage pulse exposure were similar to those observed with skin penetration enhancers or iontophoresis (41).

V. FACTORS AFFECTING ELECTRICALLY ASSISTED DRUG DELIVERY

A. Factors Affecting Iontophoresis

If the transport pathways across the skin are current-dependent, then an increase in current density is expected to increase the amount of drug that will be delivered (24). Ideally, a linear dependence of the flux on the total current density applied at steady state is expected. Several published reports support this expected result. The delivery of various inorganic ions through various types of excised skin has been shown to be have a linear relationship with the current density (42). Similarly, a linear relationship was found between current density and steady-state flux of apomorphine through human skin in an in vitro study (43). Since the current is easily controlled by electronics, this technology provides a convenient means to control the rate of delivery of drugs (44). However, the current density and current intensity cannot be indefinitely increased as it will irritate and/or damage the skin, and also produce unpleasant electrical sensation. In general, 0.5 mA/cm^2 is often stated to be the maximum current density that should be used on humans. Iontophoresis is usually carried out by a continuous direct current, though the use of pulsed direct current has been promoted, in which direct current is interrupted in a periodic manner. A pulse waveform supposedly allows the skin to depolarize and return to its initial state before the onset of the next pulse. This is because the stratum corneum acts as a capacitance and this polarization may reduce the magnitude of a current applied as a constant current. It has also been suggested that pulse current will be less irritating to the skin, so that patients can tolerate higher levels of current if pulse direct current at high frequency is used. Also, it is hoped that higher drug fluxes could be achieved with pulsed current as compared to equivalent direct current. While several studies do show a higher delivery with pulsed current, several other do not, and any advantages of using pulsed direct current remain controversial (2).

The charge, size, structure, and lipophilicity of the drug will influence its potential to be a candidate for iontophoresis. Ideal candidates for iontophoresis should be water-soluble, potent drugs that exist in their salt form with high charge density (45,46). Structure–transport relationships are hard to predict due to a multitude of factors involved in iontophoretic delivery (47). The size of the solute molecule is a major factor determining the feasibility of iontophoretic delivery and the amount transported. The upper size limit for iontophoretic delivery is not known. However, in vitro electrotransport of cytochrome c, a 12,400-D protein, across human epidermis has been demonstrated ("Electrotransport: A technology whose time has come," 1993 brochure from Alza Corp., USA). Formulation factors such as the drug concentration, pH, ionic strength, and viscosity of the formulation will also affect the iontophoretic delivery of the drug. An increase in the drug concentration in the formulation will typically result in higher iontophoretic delivery, as seen with apomorphine (43). At some point, the flux may become independent of concentration due to the drug concentration reaching maximum solubility, or it could be because the boundary layer gets saturated with the drug while the bulk donor solution is still not saturated (48). Extraneous ions from the buffer system used to avoid pH changes will often compete with the drug for carrying the current and introduce a need for a carefully designed iontophoretic patch for maximum delivery efficiency. Extraneous ions can also be introduced at the electrodes, such as the generation of hydronium and hydroxide ions when platinum electrodes are used. The ionic strength of the buffer should be a compromise to achieve just adequate buffer capacity to avoid pH drifts but not be too high to minimize the competition for current. Maintaining the desired pH is critical since it can determine whether or not the drug is charged or can affect the ratio of the charged and uncharged species (49). In the case of polypeptides, the type of charge is also controlled by the formulation pH relative to the isoelectric point of the polypeptide. Lastly, biological factors should also be considered. For small ions, iontophoretic delivery may not be affected by the type of skin used. However, most drug molecules have complex structures that may interact with the skin in various ways. Thus, their iontophoretic delivery profile will have to be evaluated on a case-by-case basis. Statistical techniques such as response surface methodology can be used to minimize the number of experiments required to optimize the transdermal iontophoretic delivery of a drug under different operational conditions (50).

B. Factors Affecting Electroporation

Factors affecting electroporation include selection of the pulse voltage, pulse duration, number of pulses, and spacing between pulses. An optimum combination of these factors to maximize delivery without significant damage to the skin is not known and perhaps needs to be determined for each drug on a case-by-case basis. There is a significant voltage drop that occurs as a function of distance, and resistance of the solution and skin. Thus, applied voltages need to be significantly higher than the voltage intended to be delivered to the skin, for both in vitro (51) and in vivo studies (52). A typical applied voltage used is 100–300 V (53), though voltages as high as 1000 V have been used during in vitro transdermal studies. The electric field represents the voltage that is applied across the electrode gap (cm). For instance, if a pair of electrodes is put across a 5-mm tumor and a voltage of 500 V is applied, then the strength of the electric field is 500 V/0.5 cm = 1000 V/cm, or 1 kV/cm (54). Several studies have begun to evaluate the relative importance of these factors in drug delivery, but any general conclusions may be premature. It has been suggested that a large number of high-voltage/short-duration pulses may permeabilize the skin efficiently but may be less efficient than a small number of low-voltage/long-duration pulses to obtain an electrophoretic movement of drug (53). However, a long-duration pulse may be associated with increased skin irritation. In a study on the transport of metoprolol, a linear correlation was observed between pulse voltage (24–450 V; pulse time 620 ms) and cumulative metoprolol transported after 4 h. A linear correlation was also observed with pulse time (80–710 ms) at 100 V (55). For studies with calcein, the transport increased almost linearly with transdermal voltage above a threshold of about 80 V and then leveled off at higher voltages (>250 V) or shorter spacing (<10 s) between pulses (56). The current flowing through the skin during the first pulse is different from subsequent pulses because the resistance of the skin drops. Unpublished data from our laboratory with several drugs or model compounds such as buprenorphine, calcitonin, colchicine, dextran sulfate, and propranolol suggest that optimum delivery protocols may need to be developed for individual drugs. The electrodes used for pulsing in transdermal studies have mostly been Ag-AgCl. The material should be capable of accommodating a high instantaneous charge density and should not form harmful electrochemical products. Homogeneously mixed Ag-AgCl electrodes may be best since Ag wires electrochemically plated with AgCl may be susceptible to the detachment of the outer layer of coating during pulsing. While wire electrodes have been used for in vitro studies, more elaborate designs are required for in vivo studies. The effect of competitive ions and electrode polarity may be less significant in electroporation if passive permeation of the drug through electropermeabilized skin represents significant percentage of flux. Delivery of fentanyl following electroporation of hairless rats was not affected significantly by a 10-fold change in the buffer concentration or by reversal of electrode polarity (53).

VI. EXAMPLES OF ELECTRICALLY ASSISTED DRUG DELIVERY

Examples of electrically assisted drug delivery are too numerous to list here but can be found in a recent text (2). Some of the more recent studies are listed here, with more details on a few examples. Current dependent delivery of apomorphine in 10 patients with Parkinson's disease was recently demonstrated at acceptable levels of skin irritation (57). Some other drugs recently investigated include acyclovir (58), azidothymidine (59), hydrocortisone (60), ketorolac (61), and nicotine (62). A few examples are discussed in greater detail in the following sections.

A. Delivery of Fentanyl

Fentanyl is a synthetic opioid widely used as an analgesic and as a narcotic analgesic supplement. It undergoes extensive first-pass metabolism and is thus only available for parenteral and transdermal routes. The transdermal form currently marketed is approved for the management of chronic pain, especially cancer pain (63). Transdermal fentanyl patch has a slow onset of action and a long duration, so that efforts are under way to develop a patch with a faster onset and shorter duration of action for the control of postoperative pain. Titration of dose to individual patients is desirable and may be accomplished by iontophoretic delivery (64,65). It has been shown that clinically significant doses of fentanyl citrate can be administered to humans. Analgesic doses of fentanyl were administered by iontophoresis for delivery periods of 2 h. Mean times to detectable plasma concentration were 33 and 19 min for 1 and 2 mA deliveries, with corresponding maximum concentrations being 0.76 and 1.59 ng/mL after 122 and 119 min, respectively (66). A wearable iontophoretic patch for delivery of fentanyl is currently under commercial development, as discussed elsewhere in this chapter. The use of electroporation may further decrease the lag time of delivery of fentanyl. A recent in vivo study used fentanyl as the drug to demonstrate that skin electroporation can deliver therapeutic quantities of a drug, with an onset of action as fast as subcutaneous injection. Fentanyl was delivered to hairless rats using different pulse protocols: 15 pulses of 100 V–500 ms, or 15 pulses of 250 V–200 ms, or 60 pulses of 500 V–1.3 ms. The pulses were spaced 15 s apart. Significant voltage drop occurs across the electrodes, and skin resistance was observed to drop by three orders of magnitude during a pulse. The actual voltage achieved across the skin was only 30–45 V, with a current density of 0.04–0.3 mA/cm^2. Within a few minutes after pulsing, high-fentanyl plasma levels were reached and reached a peak half an hour after treatment. The effectiveness of delivery was also demonstrated by pharmacodynamic measurements. The pulses were applied by pinching a fold of the abdominal skin of rat into a clip. A slight erythema was observed following pulsing, with no visible skin damage (52).

B. Delivery of Peptides

Peptide drugs have short half-lives and would benefit from a continuous input (similar to an intravenous infusion) into a body, which can be made possible by iontophoretic delivery. Furthermore, the modulation of delivery by controlling current would be of benefit for pulsatile delivery, where desired. Also, the skin is relatively low in proteolytic activity, as compared to other mucosal routes, thereby reducing degradation at the site of administration. Peptides with a high isoelectric point such as vasopressin (pI $\sim$ 10.9) or salmon calcitonin (pI $\sim$ 10.4) are perhaps the ideal candidates for iontophoretic delivery. This is because they will have a positive charge with high charge density at physiological or lower pH values. Since these will be delivered under anode, electro-osmotic flow that flows from anode to cathode will assist delivery in addition to direct electrostatic repulsion. In contrast, for peptides with very low pI (<3) delivered from a pH 7.4 buffer, the electro-osmotic flow may hinder their transport. Iontophoretic delivery of peptides with a pI between 4 and 7.3 is faced with severe challenges. The pH of the stratum corneum can range from 4 to 6, with a lowest pH of 3.5–4.5 at some small distance below the surface of the stratum corneum. The pH of the hydrated tissue just under the basement membrane is about 7.3. Thus, a peptide with a pI of, say, 5 will be delivered into the skin up to some distance before it encounters a pH equal to its pI. At this point, the peptide will become uncharged and the iontophoretic force will no longer apply. As it diffuses a little further due to concentration gradient (or electro-osmotic flow), it will reverse its charge and may be pulled back toward the delivery electrode until it is again uncharged. Thus, the peptide will concentrate at some depth below the skin to form a depot or drug reservoir, and may even precipitate in the skin (44). It would then be obvious that this limitation applies to insulin (isoelectric point 5.3) as well. In the case of insulin, there are other barriers to delivery as well. For instance, insulin normally exists as a hexamer, which makes its effective molecular weight about 36,000 rather than the expected 6000. Nevertheless, insulin is being extensively investigated for the feasibility to deliver it iontophoretically (2). The iontophoretic delivery of LHRH across epidermis separated from human cadaver skin has been shown to be significantly enhanced following a single electroporation pulse. The pulse was an exponentially decaying type with an initial amplitude of 1000 V and a time constant of 5 ± 1 ms. At a current of 0.5 mA/cm^2, the flux was 0.27 ± 0.08 without the pulse and increased to 1.62 ± 0.05 μg/h/cm^2 with the pulse (67). The usefulness of electroporation to enhance the iontophoretic flux of LHRH has been verified using the IPPSF model. It was found that the application of a single pulse (500 V, 5 ms) immediately prior to 30 min of iontophoresis increased the LHRH concentration in the IPPSF perfusate by nearly twofold, whereas application of a pulse every 10 min resulted in a threefold increase (40). Repeated short-term iontophoresis has been shown to be a safe and effective technique for transdermal delivery of desmopressin acetate (68). Iontophoretic delivery of some other peptides such as calcitonin (69), δ sleep-inducing peptide (70), growth hormone–releasing peptide (71), and LHRH (72) has been recently investigated.

C. Delivery of Oligonucleotides

Conventional delivery routes such as oral are not suitable for oligonucleotides due to their large size, high negative charge, biological instability toward intra- and extracellular nucleases, rapid in vivo plasma elimination kinetics, poor cellular uptake, and ineffective delivery to target site. Transdermal delivery enhanced by iontophoresis and/or electroporation offers one possibility for the delivery of antisense oligonucleotides. Iontophoretic in vitro delivery of oligonucleotides across excised full-thickness hairless-mouse skin has been investigated. The flux was found to decrease with increasing size, with the 10-mer being transported at a rate about sixfold faster than the 30-mer and two-fold faster than the 20-mer. A steady-state lag time of about 30–60 min was observed before the oligonucleotides appeared in the receptor chamber following the start of current, using a current density of 0.3 mA/cm^2 (73). In another study, a small six-base-sequence oligonucleotide, TAG-6 (MW 1927), was delivered across hairless-mouse skin in an in vitro study. Cathodal iontophoretic delivery for 12 h using either the 5′-FITC or ^{35}S-labeled oligonucleotide resulted in a substantial flux, with steady-state levels of 273 ± 65 or 285 ± 71 ng/cm^2-h, respectively, suggesting that FITC labeling does not alter TAG-6 transport (74). In a recent study, the in vitro permeation of 16 biologically relevant phosphorothiolate oligonucleotides across hairless-mouse skin was studied. The transport in general decreased with increasing size, though molecular structure was also observed to important (75).

Electroporation technique has been successfully used to transport 15-mer (4.8 kDa) and 24-mer (7.0 kDa) antisense oligonucleotides through human skin in vitro with fluxes of 6.4

pM/cm^2-h and 11.5 pmol/cm^2-h, respectively. Transport was found to increase significantly with transdermal voltages greater than about 70 V, but it formed a plateau soon afterward. Transport also increased as the pulse length increased from 1.1 to 2.2 ms (76). In another study, the 15-mer phosphodiesters were delivered to hairless-rat skin by electroporation. It was shown that the 3'-protected phosphodiesters were better for topical delivery to the skin, due to good stability against skin nucleases as compared to phosphorothiolate oligonucleotides (77).

D. Electrochemotherapy

Electrochemotherapy is a new mode of cancer treatment that utilizes a combination of electroporation and chemotherapeutic agents (54). The rationale for this approach is that many cancer drugs are very poorly permeable to the tumor cells and pulsing the tumor site will increase the uptake of the drug from the systemic circulation into which the drug has previously been injected or even from a intratumoral injection. In a study with six patients, electrochemotherapy was used for delivery of bleomycin to a total of 18 nodules. Eight 99-μs pulses of 1.3 kV/cm were administered to the tumors 5–15 min after intravenous administration of bleomycin to the patients, using electrodes placed on both sides of the protruding tumors. Five of the six patients responded positively to the treatment, with partial to complete regression. Some nodules were left untreated as positive controls (78). In order to avoid systemic drug delivery for localized therapy, bleomycin can potentially be injected directly into the tumors for electrochemotherapy. Studies in mice have shown that intratumoral injection of bleomycin in combination with electric pulses is effective, and human studies are currently ongoing (79). A more recent study treated 30 tumor nodules for four patients with malignant melanoma, squamous cell carcinoma, and basal cell carcinoma, using cisplatin with appropriate controls. After 4 weeks, all tumors treated with electrochemotherapy showed a complete response. For these tumors, intratumoral administration of cisplatin was followed by delivery of electric pulses to the tumor nodules. When electric pulses alone were used with no cisplatin, there was no effect on tumor growth. When treatment was done with cisplatin alone, fewer than half of the nodules showed response. These promising results were supplemented by the observation that electrochemotherapy is easy to perform and can be carried out on an outpatient basis (80). The electrode geometry and distribution for better coverage of tumors with sufficiently high electric field for improved effectiveness of electrochemotherapy has been investigated (81).

REFERENCES

1. Banga, A. K. and Chien, Y. W., 1988. Iontophoretic delivery of drugs: fundamentals, developments and biomedical applications, J. Control. Release, 7: 1–24.
2. Banga, A. K., *Electrically Assisted Transdermal and Topical Drug Delivery,* Taylor & Francis, London, 1998.
3. Green, P., 1996. Iontophoretic delivery of peptide drugs, J. Control. Release, 41: 33–48.
4. Pikal, M. J., 1992. The role of electroosmotic flow in transdermal iontophoresis, Adv. Drug Del. Rev., 9: 201–237.
5. Pikal, M. J. and Shah, S., 1990. Transport mechanisms in iontophoresis. II. Electroosmotic flow and transference number measurements for hairless mouse skin, Pharm. Res., 7: 213–221.
6. Burnette, R. R. and Ongpipattanakul, B., 1987. Characterization of the permselective properties of excised human skin during iontophoresis, J. Pharm. Sci., 76: 765–773.
7. Bayon, A. M. R. and Guy, R. H., 1996. Iontophoresis of nafarelin across human skin in vitro, Pharm. Res., 13: 798–800.

8. Hoogstraate, A. J., Srinivasan, V., Sims, S. M. and Higuchi, W. I., 1994., Iontophoretic enhancement of peptides: behaviour of leuprolide versus model permeants, J. Control. Release, 31: 41–47.
9. Hirvonen, J. and Guy, R. H. 1998., Transdermal iontophoresis: modulation of electroosmosis by polypeptides, J. Control. Release, 50: 283–289.
10. Rao, G., Guy, R. H., Glikfeld, P., Lacourse, W. R., Leung, L., Tamada, J., Potts, R. O. and Azimi, N., 1995. Reverse iontophoresis: noninvasive glucose monitoring in vivo in humans, Pharm. Res., 12: 1869–1873.
11. Santi, P. and Guy, R. H., 1996. Reverse iontophoresis: parameters determining electroosmotic flow. I. pH and ionic strength, J. Control. Release, 38: 159–165.
12. Santi, P. and Guy, R. H. 1996., Reverse iontophoresis-Parameters determining electroosmotic flow. II. Electrode chamber formulation, J. Control. Release, 42: 29–36.
13. Merino, V., Kalia, Y. N. and Guy, R. H., 1997. Transdermal therapy and diagnosis by iontophoresis, Trends. Biotech., 15: 288–290.
14. Prausnitz, M. R., Bose, V. G., Langer, R. and Weaver, J. C., 1993. Electroporation of mammalian skin: a mechanism to enhance transdermal drug delivery, Proc. Natl. Acad. Sci., 90: 10504–10508.
15. Weaver, J. C. and Chizmadzhev, Y. in C. Polte and E. Postow (Eds.), *Biological Effects of Electromagnetic Fields,* CRC Press, Boca Raton, FL, 1996, p. 247.
16. Tomov, T. C. 1995. Quantitative dependence of electroporation on the pulse parameters, Bioelectrochem. Bioenerg., 37: 101–107.
17. Prausnitz, M. R. 1997. Reversible skin permeabilization for transdermal delivery of macromolecules, Crit. Rev. Ther. Drug Carr. Syst., 14: 455–483.
18. Johnson, P. G., Gallo, S. A., Hui, S. W. and Oseroff, A. R., 1998. A pulsed electric field enhances cutaneous delivery of methylene blue in excised full-thickness porcine skin, J. Invest. Dermatol., 111: 457–463.
19. Banga, A. K. and Prausnitz, M. R., 1998. Assessing the potential of skin electroporation for the delivery of protein- and gene-based drugs, Trends Biotechnol., 16: 408–412.
20. Rols, M. P., Delteil, C., Golzio, M., Dumond, P., Cros, S. and Teissie, J., 1998. In vivo electrically mediated protein and gene transfer in murine melanoma, Natl. Biotechnol., 16: 168–171.
21. Hofmann, G. A., Rustrum, W. V. and Suder, K. S., 1995. Electro-incorporation of microcarriers as a method for the transdermal delivery of large molecules, Bioelectrochem. Bioenerg., 38: 209–222.
22. Zhang, L., Li, L. N., An, Z. L., Hoffman, R. M. and Hofmann, G. A., 1997. In vivo transdermal delivery of large molecules by pressure- mediated electroincorporation and electroporation: a novel method for drug and gene delivery, Bioelectrochem. Bioenerg., 42: 283–292.
23. Shaw, K., 1997. The new transdermal technologies, Pharmacy Times., July: 38–41.
24. Cullander, C., 1992. What are the pathways of iontophoretic current flow through mammalian skin? Adv. Drug Del. Rev., 9: 119–135.
25. Hui, S. W. 1998. Low voltage electroporation of the skin, or is it iontophoresis? Biophys. J., 74: 679–680.
26. Chizmadzhev, Y. A., Indenbom, A. V., Kuzmin, P. I., Galichenko, S. V., Weaver, J. C. and Potts, R. O., 1998. Electrical properties of skin at moderate voltages: contribution of appendageal macropores, Biophys. J., 74: 843–856.
27. Edwards, D. A., Prausnitz, M. R., Langer, R. and Weaver, J. C., 1995. Analysis of enhanced transdermal transport by skin electroporation, J. Control. Release, 34: 211–221.
28. Sage, B. H., in J. Swarbrick and J. C. Boylan (Eds.), *Encyclopedia of pharmaceutical Technology,* Marcel Dekker, New York, 1993, p. 217.
29. Howes, D., Guy, R., Hadgraft, J., Heylings, J., Hoeck, U., Kemper, F., Maibach, H., Marty, J. P., Merk, H., Parra, J., Rekkas, D., Rondelli, I., Schaefer, H., Tauber, U. and Verbiese, N., 1996. Methods for assessing percutaneous absorption. The report and recommendations of ECVAM workshop 13, ATLA. Altern. Lab. Anim., 24: 81–106.
30. Roy, S. D., Hou, S. Y. E., Witham, S. L. and Flynn, G. L. 1994., Transdermal delivery of narcotic analgesics: comparative metabolism and permeability of human cadaver skin and hairless mouse skin, J. Pharm. Sci., 83: 1723–1728.

31. Lu, M. F., Lee, D. and Rao, G. S., 1992. Percutaneous absorption enhancement of leuprolide, Pharm. Res., 9: 1575–1579.
32. Bartek, M. J., LaBudde, J. A. and Maibach, H. I., 1972. Skin permeability in vivo: comparison in rat, rabbit, pig and man, J. Invest. Dermatol., 58: 114–123.
33. Slough, C. L., Spinelli, M. J. and Kasting, G. B., 1988. Transdermal delivery of etidronate (EHDP) in the pig via iontophoresis, J. Membr. Sci., 35: 161–165.
34. Monteiro-Riviere, N. A., Inman, A. O. and Riviere, J. E., 1994. Identification of the pathway of iontophoretic drug delivery: light and ultrastructural studies using mercuric chloride in pigs, Pharm. Res., 11(2): 251–256.
35. Riviere, J. E., Bowman, K. F., Monteiro-Riviere, N. A., Dix, L. P. and Carver, M. P., 1986. The isolated perfused porcine skin flap (IPPSF): I. A novel in vitro model for percutaneous absorption and cutaneous toxicology studies, Fund. Appl. Toxicol., 7: 444–453.
36. Heit, M. C., Monteiroriviere, N. A., Jayes, F. L. and Riviere, J. E., 1994. Transdermal iontophoretic delivery of luteinizing hormone releasing hormone (LHRH): effect of repeated administration, Pharm. Res., 11: 1000–1003.
37. Riviere, J. E., Brooks, J. D., Williams, P. L., McGown, E. and Francoeur, M. L., 1996. Cutaneous metabolism of isosorbide dinitrate after transdermal administration in isolated perfused porcine skin, Int. J. Pharm., 127: 213–217.
38. Prausnitz, M. R., 1996. The effects of electric current applied to skin: a review for transdermal drug delivery, Adv. Drug Deliv. Rev., 18: 395–425.
39. Prausnitz, M. R., Seddick, D. S., Kon, A. A., Bose, V. G., Frankenburg, S., Klaus, S. N., Langer, R. and Weaver, J. C., 1993. Methods for in vivo tissue electroporation using surface electrodes, Drug Delivery., 1: 125–131.
40. Riviere, J. E., Monteiroriviere, N. A., Rogers, R. A., Bommannan, D., Tamada, J. A. and Potts, R. O., 1995. Pulsatile transdermal delivery of LHRH using electroporation: drug delivery and skin toxicology, J. Control. Release., 36: 229–233.
41. Vanbever, R., Fouchard, D., Jadoul, A., DeMorre, N., Preat, V. and Marty, J. P., 1998. In vivo noninvasive evaluation of hairless rat skin after high-voltage pulse exposure, Skin Pharmacol. Appl. Skin Phys., 11: 23–34.
42. Phipps, J. B., Padmanabhan, R. V. and Lattin, G. A., 1989. Iontophoretic delivery of model inorganic and drug ions, J. Pharm. Sci., 78: 365–369.
43. vanderGeest, R., Danhof, M. and Bodde, H. E., 1997. Iontophoretic delivery of apomorphine I: in vitro optimization and validation, Pharm. Res., 14: 1798–1803.
44. Sage, B. H., Bock, C. R., Denuzzio, J. D. and Hoke, R. A., in V. H. L. Lee, M. Hashida and Y. Mizushima (Eds.), *Trends and Future Perspectives in Peptide and Protein Drug Delivery*, Harwood Academic, Chur, Switzerland, 1995, p. 111.
45. Gangarosa, L. P., Park, N. H., Fong, B. C., Scott, D. F. and Hill, J. M., 1978. Conductivity of drugs used for iontophoresis, J. Pharm. Sci., 67: 1439–1443.
46. Lattin, G. A., Padmanabhan, R. V. and Phipps, J. B., 1991. Electronic control of iontophoretic drug delivery, Ann. N. Y. Acad. Sci., 618: 450–464.
47. Yoshida, N. H. and Roberts, M. S. 1992. Structure–transport relationships in transdermal iontophoresis, Adv. Drug Del. Rev., 9: 239–264.
48. Sanderson, J. E., Riel, S. D. and Dixon, R., 1989. Iontophoretic delivery of nonpeptide drugs: Formulation optimization for maximum skin permeability, J. Pharm. Sci., 78: 361–364.
49. Cullander, C. and Guy, R. H., 1992. (D) Routes of delivery: case studies (6) Transdermal delivery of peptides and proteins, Adv. Drug Del. Rev., 8: 291–329.
50. Huang, Y. Y., Wu, S. M. and Wang, C. Y., 1996. Response surface method: a novel strategy to optimize iontophoretic transdermal delivery of thyrotropin-releasing hormone, Pharm. Res., 13: 547–552.
51. Prausnitz, M. R., Pliquett, U., Langer, R. and Weaver, J. C., 1994. Rapid temporal control of transdermal drug delivery by electroporation, Pharm. Res., 11: 1834–1837.
52. Vanbever, R., Langers, G., Montmayeur, S. and Preat, V., 1998. Transdermal delivery of fentanyl: rapid onset of analgesia using skin electroporation, J. Control. Release, 50: 225–235.

53. Vanbever, R., LeBoulenge, E. and Preat, V., 1996. Transdermal delivery of fentanyl by electroporation. 1. Influence of electrical factors, Pharm. Res., 13: 559–565.
54. Dev, S. B. and Hofmann, G. A., 1994. Electrochemotherapy-a novel method of cancer treatment, Cancer Treatment Rev., 20: 105–115.
55. Vanbever, R., Lecouturier, N. and Preat, V., 1994. Transdermal delivery of metoprolol by electroporation, Pharm. Res., 11: 1657–1662.
56. Pliquett, U. and Weaver, J. C., 1996. Transport of a charged molecule across the human epidermis due to electroporation, J. Control. Release, 38: 1–10.
57. vanderGeest, R., vanLaar, T., GubbensStibbe, J. M., Bodde, H. E. and Danhof, M., 1997. Iontophoretic delivery of apomorphine II: an in vivo study in patients with Parkinson's disease, Pharm. Res., 14: 1804–1810.
58. Volpato, N. M., Nicoli, S., Laureri, C., Colombo, P. and Santi, P., 1998. In vitro acyclovir distribution in human skin layers after transdermal iontophoresis, J. Control. Release, 50: 291–296.
59. Oh, S. Y., Jeong, S. Y., Park, T. G. and Lee, J. H., 1998. Enhanced transdermal delivery of AZT (zidovudine) using iontophoresis and penetration enhancer, J. Control. Release., 51: 161–168.
60. Chang, S. and Banga, A. K., 1998. Transdermal iontophoretic delivery of hydrocortisone from cyclodextrin solutions, J. Pharm. Pharmacol., 50: 635–640.
61. Park, K., Verotta, D., Gupta, S. K. and Sheiner, L. B., 1998. Passive versus electrotransport-facilitated transdermal absorption of ketorolac, Clin. Pharmacol. Ther., 63: 303–315.
62. Conaghey, O. M., Corish, J. and Corrigan, O. I., 1998. Iontophoretically assisted in vitro membrane transport of nicotine from a hydrogel containing ion exchange resins, Int. J. Pharm., 170: 225–237.
63. Southam, M. A., 1995. Transdermal fentanyl therapy: system design, pharmacokinetics and efficacy, Anti-Cancer Drug., 6: 29–34.
64. Thysman, S. and Preat, V., 1993. In vivo iontophoresis of fentanyl and sufentanil in rats: pharmacokinetics and acute antinociceptive effects, Anesth. Analg., 77: 61–66.
65. Thysman, S., Tasset, C. and Preat, V., 1994. Transdermal iontophoresis of fentanyl: delivery and mechanistic analysis, Int. J. Pharm., 101: 105–113.
66. Ashburn, M. A., Streisand, J., Zhang, J., Love, G., Rowin, M., Niu, S., Kievit, J. K., Kroep, J. R. and Mertens, M. J., 1995. The iontophoresis of fentanyl citrate in humans, Anesthesiology., 82: 1146–1153.
67. Bommannan, D. B., Tamada, J., Leung, L. and Potts, R. O., 1994. Effect of electroporation on transdermal iontophoretic delivery of luteinizing hormone releasing hormone (LHRH) in vitro, Pharm. Res., 11: 1809–1814.
68. Nakakura, M., Kato, Y. and Ito, K., 1998. Safe and efficient transdermal delivery of desmopressin acetate by iontophoresis in rats, Biol. Pharm. Bull., 21: 268–271.
69. Santi, P., Colombo, P., Bettini, R., Catellani, P. L., Minutello, A. and Volpato, N. M., 1997. Drug reservoir composition and transport of salmon calcitonin in transdermal iontophoresis, Pharm. Res., 14: 63–66.
70. Chiang, C. H., Shao, C. H. and Chen, J. L., 1998. Effects of pH, electric current, and enzyme inhibitors on iontophoresis of delta sleep–inducing peptide, Drug Dev. Ind. Pharm., 24: 431–438.
71. Ellens, H., Lai, Z. P., Marcello, J., Davis, C. B., Cheng, H. Y., Oh, C. K. and Okabe, K., 1997. Transdermal iontophoretic delivery of [H-3]GHRP in rats, Int. J. Pharm., 159: 1–11.
72. Bhatia, K. S. and Singh, J., 1998. Synergistic effect of iontophoresis and a series of fatty acids on LHRH permeability through porcine skin, J. Pharm. Sci., 87: 462–469.
73. Oldenburg, K. R., Vo, K. T., Smith, G. A. and Selick, H. E., 1995. Iontophoretic delivery of oligonucleotides across full thickness hairless mouse skin, J. Pharm. Sci., 84: 915–921.
74. Brand, R. M. and Iversen, P. L., 1996. Iontophoretic delivery of a telomeric oligonucleotide, Pharm. Res., 13: 851–854.
75. Brand, R. M., Wahl, A. and Iversen, P. L., 1998. Effects of size and sequence on the iontophoretic delivery of oligonucleotides, J. Pharm. Sci., 87: 49–52.
76. Zewert, T. E., Pliquett, U. F., Langer, R. and Weaver, J. C., 1995. Transdermal transport of DNA antisense oligonucleotides by electroporation, Biochem. Biophys. Res. Commun., 212: 286–292.
77. Regnier, V., Tahiri, A., Andre, N., Lamaitre, M., Preat, V. and Doan, T. L., 1997. Delivery of 3′-protected phosphodiester oligodeoxynucleotides to the skin, Pharm. Res., 14: S–640.

78. Heller, R., Jaroszeski, M. J., Glass, L. F., Messina, J. L., Rapaport, D. P., DeConti, R. C., Fenske, N. A., Gilbert, R. A., Mir, L. M. and Reintgen, D. S., 1996. Phase I/II trial for the treatment of cutaneous and subcutaneous tumors using electrochemotherapy, Cancer., 77: 964–971.
79. Heller, R., Jaroszeski, M., Perrott, R., Messina, J. and Gilbert, R., 1997. Effective treatment of B16 melanoma by direct delivery of bleomycin using electrochemotherapy, Melanoma Res., 7: 10–18.
80. Sersa, G., Stabuc, B., Cemazar, M., Jancar, B., Miklavcic, D. and Rudolf, Z., 1998. Electrochemotherapy with cisplatin: Potentiation of local cisplatin antitumour effectiveness by application of electric pulses in cancer patients, Eur. J. Cancer., 34: 1213–1218.
81. Miklavcic, D., Beravs, K., Semrov, D., Cemazar, M., Demsar, F. and Sersa, G., 1998. The importance of electric field distribution for effective in vivo electroporation of tissues, Biophys. J., 74: 2152–2158.

28
A Novel Method Based on Artificial Neural Networks for Optimizing Transdermal Drug Delivery Systems

Kozo Takayama and Tsuneji Nagai
Hoshi University, Shinagawa-ku, Tokyo, Japan

I. INTRODUCTION

A transdermal therapeutic system requires drugs to penetrate the stratum corneum into the systemic circulation in sufficient concentrations for the desired therapeutic effect. To achieve this, an absorption enhancer is usually needed. Many studies have discussed percutaneous absorption enhancers and mechanisms of their enhancing activity (1–3). We have found that cyclic monoterpenes such as d-limonene and l-menthol remarkably enhance the skin's permeability of several kinds of drugs (4–7). Recently, we synthesized O-alkylmenthol and O-acylmenthol derivatives, and investigated their ability to enhance percutaneous absorption of ketoprofen from alcoholic hydrogels in rats in vivo (8). The skin irritancy of these compounds was also evaluated based on histopathological findings (8). Among these compounds, O-ethylmenthol (MET, Fig. 1) was the most promising compound, with the greatest promoting action and relatively low skin irritancy (8,9).

For an efficacious transdermal formulation, sufficient amounts of enhancer are required to obtain favorable drug absorption. At the same time, the amount of enhancer should be kept as low as possible to avoid skin irritation. A response surface method (RSM) has often been used to solve this problem (10–13). However, prediction of pharmaceutical responses based on a second-order polynomial equation, which is commonly used in RSM, is often limited to a low level, resulting in the poor estimation of optimal formulations. In order to overcome this drawback, we developed a novel optimization technique in which an artificial neural network (ANN) was incorporated (14,15). ANNs are learning systems based on a computational techniques that can simulate the neurological processing ability of the human brain (16). ANNs have been successfully applied to solving various problems in pharmaceutical research such as product development (14,15,17), estimating diffusion coefficients (18), predicting the mechanism of drug action (19), and predicting pharmacokinetic parameters (20–23).

The aim of this study is to describe the basic concept of the multiobjective optimization technique incorporating ANNs. The usefulness and reliability of this ANN approach were demonstrated by the optimization for ketoprofen hydrogel ointment (15).

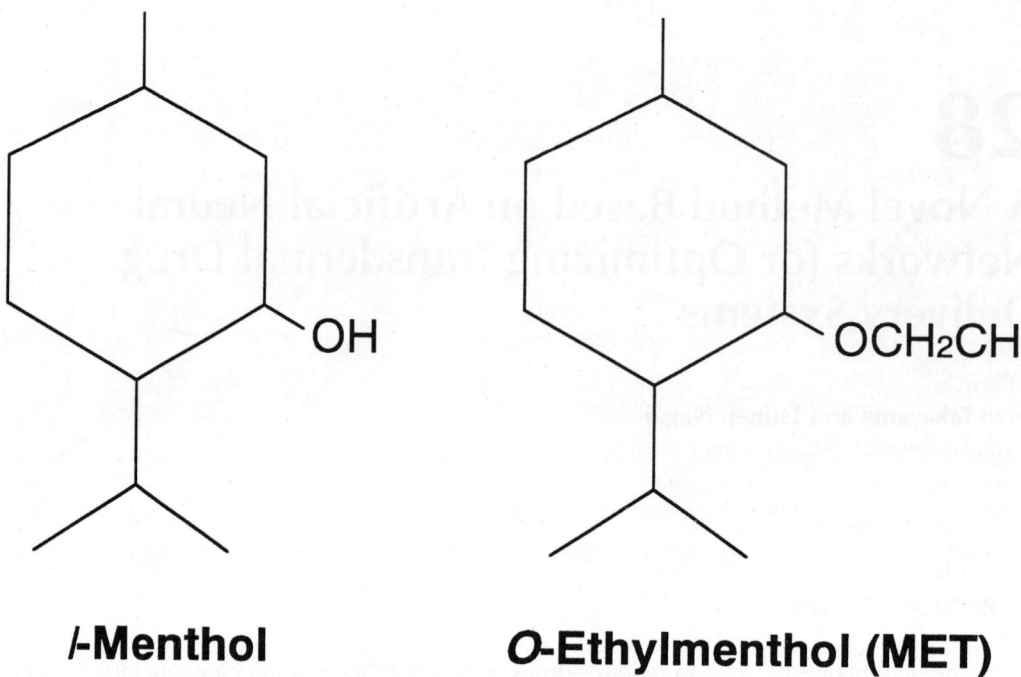

Figure 1 Chemical structures of menthol and O-ethylmenthol (MET).

II. ARTIFICIAL NEURAL NETWORK STRUCTURE

Theoretical details of a hierarchical ANN have been given elsewhere. Briefly, the general structure of an ANN has one input layer, one or more hidden layers, and one output layer (Fig. 2a). Each layer has some units corresponding to neurons. The units in neighboring layers are fully interconnected with links corresponding to synapses. The strengths of connections between two units are called "weights." In each hidden layer and output layer the processing unit sums its input from the previous layer and then applies the sigmoidal function to compute its output to the following layer according to the following equations:

$$y_q = \Sigma\, w_{pq} x_p \tag{1}$$

$$f(y_q) = 1/[1 + \exp(-\alpha y_q)] \tag{2}$$

where w_{pq} is the weight of the connection between unit q in the current layer and unit p in the previous layer, and x_p is the output value from the previous layer; $f(y_q)$ is conducted to the following layer as an output value; and α is a parameter relating to the shape of the sigmoidal function. Nonlinearity of the sigmoidal function is strengthened with an increase in α. ANN learns an approximate nonlinear relationship by a procedure called "training," which involves varying weight values. Training means a search process for the optimized set of weight values that can minimize the squared error sum between the estimation and experimental data of units in the output layer. A back-propagation method with the steepest descent algorithm has been widely applied for training ANNs (24). Training is very long iterative process, and ANNs often get stuck in local minima. Certain empirical techniques have been reported to improve the convergence of ANNs in the global minima (25,26). Another essential approach is to use an extended Kalman filter algorithm for ANN training (27–29). We can greatly reduce the number of

A Method Based on Artificial Neural Networks

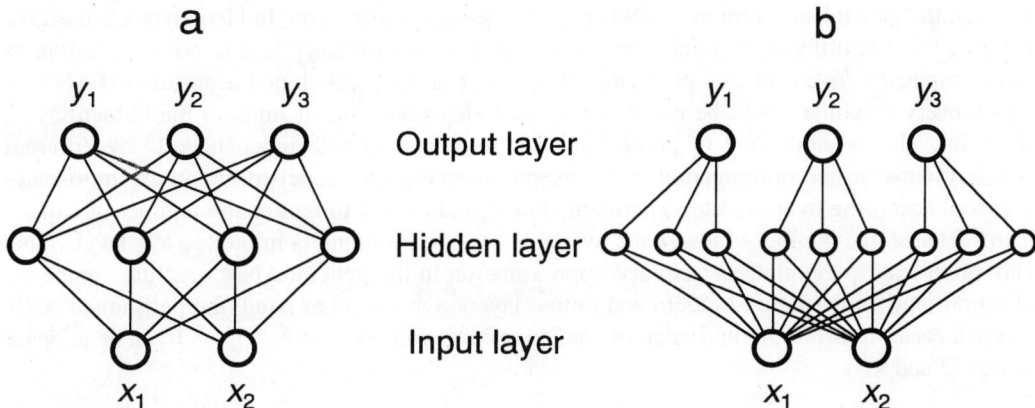

Figure 2 Typical structures of a hierarchical artificial neural network (ANN). (a) General ANN composed of two input units, four hidden units, and three output units. (b) Partitioned structure of ANN composed of two input units, three hidden units, and three output units. Every response (output unit) in the partitioned ANN can be estimated by the independent set of units in the hidden layer, although the same units in the hidden layer are used in common for the prediction of different responses in the case of general ANN.

iterative trainings by using the extended Kalman filter algorithm, and we can also avoid, to a certain extent, an ANN getting stuck in a local minimum (27). Although multiple layers can be set between the input layer and the output layer, many ANNs consist of one hidden layer (26). One layer is usually sufficient to provide adequate prediction even if continuous variables are adopted as the units in the output layer (30–32).

To enable reasonable prediction of each response variable by an ANN, Carpenter et al. (33) introduced an equation relating to the number of units in the input layer, the hidden layer, and the output layer:

$$N_{hidden} = (N_{sample}/\gamma - N_{output})/N_{input} + N_{output} + 1) \quad (3)$$

where N_{hidden} is the number of hidden units, N_{input} is the number of input units, N_{output} is the number of output units, and N_{sample} is the number of training data pairs. The constant γ is the parameter relating to the degree of overdetermination.

Equation 3 can be rewritten as:

$$N_{sample} = \gamma\{N_{hidden}(N_{input} + 1) + N_{output}(N_{hidden} + 1)\} \quad (4)$$

The unknown parameters associated with ANNs are the weights of the network. Overdetermined ($\gamma > 1$), exactly determined ($\gamma = 1$), and underdetermined ($\gamma < 1$) approximations have more, an equal number, or fewer training data pairs than the number of unknown parameters associated with the approximation. For example, $\gamma = 1.5$ would give a 50% overdetermined approximation. With an underdetermined approximation ($\gamma < 1$), each output data point is fitted perfectly by iterative training, but the approximation may vary widely between the output data points, i.e., the overtraining problem. Thus, the selection of $\gamma > 1$ is usually recommended to enable reasonable prediction of each response variable adopted as the unit in the output layer. However, it may be possible to reduce the γ value; i.e., $\gamma \cong 1$, when statistical experimental designs are employed to prepare the model formulations because the independency among the factors is highly ensured by use of such designs (10).

In the general structure of ANN (Fig. 2a), the same units in the hidden layer are used for the prediction of different response variables. This may occasionally lead to poor estimation of some responses. To avoid this problem, Fujikawa et al. (34) developed a partitioned ANN in which every response could be estimated by an independent set of units in the hidden layers (Fig. 2b). This is equivalent to predicting each response variable independently by different ANN systems. In the optimization study for pharmaceuticals, model formulations are usually prepared according to statistical experimental designs in order to reduce the number of experiments. Hence, the number of data pairs available for ANN training is limited to low levels. This may often lead to the underdetermined approximation in the general ANN structure composed of plural units in the input, hidden, and output layers. On the other hand, the partitioned ANN is much easier to avoid the underdetermined approximation because $N_{output} = 1$ can be adopted in Eqs. 3 and 4.

III. SINGLE-OBJECTIVE OPTIMIZATION

In general, the optimization problems of pharmaceutical formulations can be viewed in terms of minimization (or maximization) of the objective function, $F(\mathbf{X})$, under the following inequality and/or equality constraints:

$$G_i(\mathbf{X}) \geq 0 \qquad i = 1, 2, 3, \ldots \qquad (5)$$

$$H_j(\mathbf{X}) = 0 \qquad j = 1, 2, 3, \ldots \qquad (6)$$

where $G_i(\mathbf{X})$ is the inequality constraint and $H_j(\mathbf{X})$ is the equality constraint. In the case of a fully trained ANN, $F(\mathbf{X})$ corresponds to the predicted value of response variable adopted as the unit in the output layer and $\mathbf{X}$ is a set of causal factors used as the units in the input layer. As it is difficult to solve the constrained optimization problem described above without mathematical modifications, the constrained optimization problem is transformed to one that is unconstrained by adding a penalty function as follows:

$$\begin{aligned} T(\mathbf{X}, r) &= F(\mathbf{X}) + r^{-1} \Sigma [\phi_i G_i(\mathbf{X})]^2 + r^{-1} \Sigma [H_j(\mathbf{X})]^2 \\ &\text{when } G_i(\mathbf{X}) < 0, \phi_i = 1; \text{ when } G_i(\mathbf{X}) \geq 0, \phi_i = 0 \end{aligned} \qquad (7)$$

where $T(\mathbf{X}, r)$ is the transformed unconstrained objective function, r is a perturbation parameter ($r > 0$) of $T(\mathbf{X}, r)$, and ϕ_i is a step function by which the objective function, $F(\mathbf{X})$, is penalized. The second and third terms in Eq. 7 act as penalty functions because these values increase abruptly when the values of $G_i(\mathbf{X})$ are negative or the $H_j(\mathbf{X})$ values deviate from zero. The meaning of the perturbation parameter, r, and the means of obtaining a global optimum solution are described fully in a previous paper (35). The optimum solution is obtained as the point, $\mathbf{X}$ (r), which gives the minimum value of $T(\mathbf{X}, r)$ when the value of r is sufficiently close to zero.

IV. MULTIOBJECTIVE OPTIMIZATION

When the optimization problem includes several objectives, response variables should be incorporated into a single function in order to consider all of the responses simultaneously. Derringer and Suich (36) introduced general transformations based on the concept of desirability associated with a given response function. This transformation, a desirability function method, requires minimal and maximal acceptable values for every response. The individual response can be normalized to the desirability functions, $d_{1, 2, 3, \ldots, n}$, which have values inside the interval [0, 1] by using the distance between minimal and maximal acceptable values. The normalized functions are then combined into a multiobjective function, D_{total}, by means of the geometrical mean of predicted values of each function:

$$D_{total} = (d_1 \times d_2 \times d_3 \times \cdots \times d_n)^{1/n} \tag{8}$$

The desirability function method has widely been applied to the development of pharmaceutical products (37–39) and the method has been useful for solving practical optimization problems. However, one of the basic shortcomings of this approach is subjectivity in the selection of the minimal and maximal acceptable values for each response. Namely, improper values of minima and/or maxima may lead to inaccurate solutions for the optimum formulation. In order to avoid the problem of subjectivity in application of the desirability function method, we can employ another approach based on the generalized distance between the predicted value of each response and the optimum one that was obtained individually (12,40):

$$S(\mathbf{X}) = (\Sigma[\{FD_k(\mathbf{X}) - FO_k(\mathbf{X})\}/SD_k]^2)^{1/2} \tag{9}$$

where $S(\mathbf{X})$ is the distance function generalized by the standard deviation, SD_k, of the observed values for each response variable, $FD_k(\mathbf{X})$ is the optimum value of each response variable optimized individually over the experimental region, and $FO_k(\mathbf{X})$ is the estimated value of all the responses given in the same set of causal factors, $\mathbf{X}$. Substituting $F(\mathbf{X})$ in Eq. 7 with $S(\mathbf{X})$ in Eq. 9, the transformed function, $T(\mathbf{X}, r)$, in the case of multiobjectives can be given as follows:

$$T(\mathbf{X}, r) = (\Sigma [\{FD_k(\mathbf{X}) - FO_k(\mathbf{X})\}/SD_k]^2)^{1/2} + r^{-1} \Sigma\{\phi_i G_i(\mathbf{X})\}^2 \\ + r^{-1} \Sigma\{H_j(\mathbf{X})\}^2 \tag{10}$$

when $G_i(\mathbf{X}) < 0$, $\phi_i = 1$; when $G_i(\mathbf{X}) \geq 0$, $\phi_i = 0$

The simultaneous optimum solution is estimated as the point, $\mathbf{X}(r)$, which gives minimum value of $T(\mathbf{X}, r)$ when the value of r is sufficiently close to zero.

V. PROMOTING ACTIVITY OF MET

A promoting activity of MET on the percutaneous absorption of ketoprofen from the hydrogels was investigated in rats in vitro and in vivo (8,9). Results were compared with those of menthol. The hydrogels were prepared as follows: Ketoprofen was dissolved in ethanol containing MET or menthol. Separately, carboxyvinyl polymer and triethanolamine were dissolved in distilled water. Both compounds were then mixed well and the resulting hydrogel was stored at room temperature for 24 h under airtight conditions prior to use. The amounts of ketoprofen, carboxyvinyl polymer, triethanolamine, and ethanol were fixed at 0.30 g, 0.15 g, 0.20 g, and 4.00 g, respectively. The total amount of each hydrogel was adjusted to 10.0 g by the addition of water. For the in vitro skin permeation study, the excised abdominal skin was used as a permeation membrane. A vertical diffusion cell having an available diffusion area of 1.77 cm^2 was employed. The receiver side was filled with phosphate buffer solution (pH 7.2) and the donor side was filled with test hydrogel under occlusive conditions. The concentration of ketoprofen in the receiver solution permeated through the membrane was analyzed using an high-performance liquid chromatography. For the percutaneous absorption study in vivo, the hydrogel was applied on the shaved abdominal skin (2.01 cm^2) under occlusive conditions. The concentration of ketoprofen in blood samples was analyzed as in the in vitro permeation study.

Figure 3 shows the permeation profiles of ketoprofen in hydrogels containing MET or menthol through rat skin in vitro. When a small quantity of MET (0.25–0.5%) was added to the

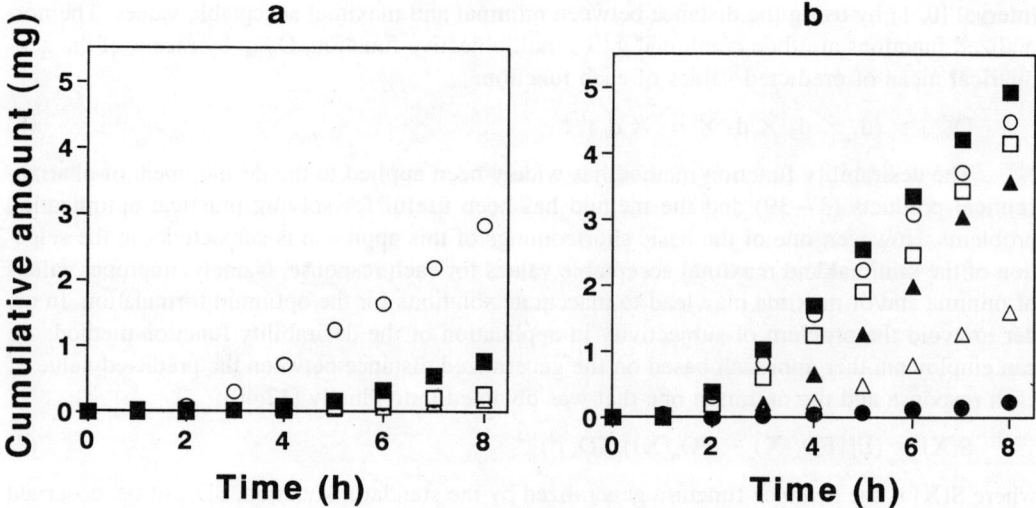

Figure 3 Effect of menthol (a) or MET (b) on the permeation of ketoprofen from hydrogels in rat skin. Each point is the mean of three determinations. Concentrations of enhancer: (●) 0%, (△) 0.125%, (▲) 0.25%, (□) 0.5%, (■) 1%, (○) 2%.

hydrogels, the permeation of ketoprofen increased remarkably, compared with the control (the hydrogel not containing MET or menthol), while further increases in the amounts of MET (1–2%) only resulted in limited increases in permeation. Only small changes in permeation were observed when small amounts of menthol were used (<1%), and at least 2% menthol was required to obtain a promoting efficiency comparable with 0.25% MET. To elucidate how MET promotes permeation, the profiles of ketoprofen permeation through the skin, shown in Fig. 3, were analyzed based on the following diffusion model (2):

$$Q_t = AK'C_0 [D't - (1/6) - (2/\pi^2) \Sigma\{(-1)^n \cdot \exp(-D'n^2\pi^2 t)/n^2\}] \qquad (11)$$

$$D' = D/L^2 \qquad (12)$$

$$K' = KL \qquad (13)$$

where D is the diffusion constant, L is the thickness of the membrane, K is the partition coefficient of the penetrant between the membrane and the donor phase, Q_t is the cumulative amount of penetrant in the receptor fluid at time t, A is the area of application, and C_0 is the concentration of the donor phase. The diffusion parameter, D', and the partition parameter, K', were simultaneously estimated by a curve fitting technique. Results are given in Table 1. An impressive elevation in the D' value of ketoprofen resulted from increasing MET concentrations (0.5–1%) in the hydrogels. The K' value was remarkably enhanced when a small amount of MET (0.125%) was added to the hydrogels, while no further enhancement of the K' value was observed at higher concentrations of MET (0.25–2%). These results suggest that the partitioning of ketoprofen from the hydrogel to the skin is improved by the addition of a small amount of MET, whereas the diffusivity of the drug is enhanced at higher concentrations of MET (0.5–1%). With lower concentrations of menthol (0.125–0.5%), the effect on permeation was negligible, compared with MET. More pronounced permeation, comparable with 0.25–0.5% MET, was only observed at higher concentrations of menthol (2%).

In order to evaluate the percutaneous absorption in vivo in rats, the rate of penetration (R_p) of ketoprofen was estimated based on the assumption that the rate of penetration of

Table 1 Effect of Enhancer Concentrations on the Diffusion Parameters (D′) and Partition Parameters (K′) of Ketoprofen in Hydrogels Containing 40% Ethanol

Enhancer	Conc. (%)	$D' \times 10^2$ (h^{-1})	$K' \times 10$ (cm)
Menthol	0.125	3.44 ± 0.40	0.335 ± 0.195
	0.25	3.78 ± 0.71	0.374 ± 0.065
	0.5	3.45 ± 0.48	0.476 ± 0.175
	1	2.69 ± 0.18	1.31 ± 0.08
	2	4.89 ± 1.19	2.51 ± 0.82
MET	0.125	3.75 ± 0.54	1.86 ± 0.87
	0.25	3.77 ± 0.71	2.54 ± 0.83
	0.5	5.79 ± 0.81	2.61 ± 0.10
	1	8.66 ± 0.12	1.83 ± 0.43
	2	8.04 ± 0.98	1.82 ± 0.43
Control (without enhancer)		3.41 ± 0.55	0.440 ± 0.120

Note: Each value represents the mean ± SD of three determinations.

ketoprofen absorbed from the hydrogel is constant after a lag time according to the following equation (12):

$$C = R_p [1 + (\beta - k_{10}) \times \exp\{-\alpha(t - t_L)\}/(\alpha - \beta) + (k_{10} - \alpha) \\ \times \exp\{-\beta(t - t_L)\}/(\alpha - \beta)]/(V_d k_{10}) \quad (14)$$

where C is the plasma concentration, R_p is the rate of penetration, t is time, t_L is lag time, V_d is the distribution volume of the central compartment, k_{10} is the elimination rate constant from the central compartment, and α and β are the hybrid first-order rate constants. The mean values of V_d, k_{10}, α, and β, estimated previously (12), were used in this study to determine R_p and t_L values. Results are summarized in Table 2. When the hydrogel containing menthol was applied, the R_p values gradually increased as a function of the amount of menthol. However, prominent increases in the R_p values were observed in hydrogels containing a small amount of MET (0.25–0.5%). At least 2% menthol was required to obtain the same results. Furthermore, t_L values were greatly reduced as the R_p values increased. Results observed in the in vivo experiments broadly correlated with the results from the in vitro study.

Table 2 Pharmacokinetic Parameters of Percutaneous Absorption of Ketoprofen in Hydrogels Containing 40% Ethanol in Rats In Vivo

Enhancer	Conc. (%)	R_p (mg/h)	t_L (h)
Menthol	0.125	0.0137 ± 0.0035	1.06 ± 0.00
	0.25	0.0164 ± 0.0034	1.06 ± 0.00
	0.5	0.0240 ± 0.0021	1.06 ± 0.01
	1	0.0580 ± 0.0056	1.04 ± 0.01
	2	0.753 ± 0.021	0.0618 ± 0.0101
MET	0.125	0.0314 ± 0.0097	1.04 ± 0.00
	0.25	0.315 ± 0.098	1.01 ± 0.02
	0.5	0.873 ± 0.255	0.0678 ± 0.0054
	1	0.942 ± 0.135	0.0575 ± 0.0051
	2	1.45 ± 0.03	0.0452 ± 0.0076
Control (without enhancer)		0.00781 ± 0.00164	1.08 ± 0.01

Note: Each value represents the mean ± SD of three determinations.

VI. OPTIMIZATION BASED ON ANN

Optimization based on the partitioned ANN was applied to the design of ketoprofen hydrogels containing MET as an absorption enhancer. The amounts of ethanol (X_1) and MET (X_2) in the hydrogels were selected as causal factors. A central composite spherical design with four center point replications was used for preparing the model formulations (Table 3). Pharmacokinetic parameters, the apparent penetration rate (R_p) and the lag time (t_L), of ketoprofen percutaneously absorbed from model formulations were determined in rats as prime response variables. The skin damage evoked by each formulation was microscopically judged and graded as the total irritation score (TIS) for skin safety factors (12). These response variables are summarized in Table 4.

A set of causal factors and response variables was used as tutorial data for the partitioned ANN (12,34). According to Eq. 3, $N_{hidden} = 2$ was employed as the number of units in the hidden layer. Degree of overdetermination in this partitioned ANN structure ($N_{sample} = 12$, $N_{input} = 2$, $N_{hidden} = 2$, $N_{output} = 1$) was estimated to be 33%. The extended Kalman filter algorithm

Table 3 Experimental Design and Model Formulas of Ketoprofen Hydrogels Containing Various Amounts of Ethanol (X_1) and MET (X_2)

Formulation	X_1	Ethanol (%)	X_2	MET (%)
1	$\sqrt{2}$	50.0	0	1.50
2	$-\sqrt{2}$	20.0	0	1.50
3	0	35.0	$\sqrt{2}$	3.00
4	0	35.0	$-\sqrt{2}$	0
5	1	45.6	1	2.56
6	1	45.6	−1	0.44
7	−1	24.4	1	2.56
8	−1	24.4	−1	0.44
9	0	35.0	0	1.50
10	0	35.0	0	1.50
11	0	35.0	0	1.50
12	0	35.0	0	1.50

Table 4 Experimental Values of Response Variables

Formulation	R_p (mg/h)	t_L (h)	TIS
1	1.45	0.900	17
2	0.468	0.626	4
3	1.84	0.190	16
4	0.00499	1.08	0
5	1.36	0.854	16
6	0.422	0.931	14
7	1.56	0.235	11
8	0.273	0.956	1
9	0.918	0.904	12
10	1.06	0.954	13
11	1.37	0.913	17
12	1.08	0.929	17

A Method Based on Artificial Neural Networks

was applied for training ANN (27). Figures 4 and 5 show the three-dimensional diagrams of each response variable as a function of X_1 (amount of ethanol) and X_2 (amount of MET). Nonlinear relationships between the causal factors and the response variables were well represented with response surface predicted by ANN (Fig. 4). On the other hand, the second-order polynomial equation exhibited relatively plain surfaces for all responses (Fig. 5). Furthermore, polynomial equation analysis predicted negative values in the boundary region of the experimental limits and were outside of physical reality (Fig. 5). Generally, the quantitative relationships

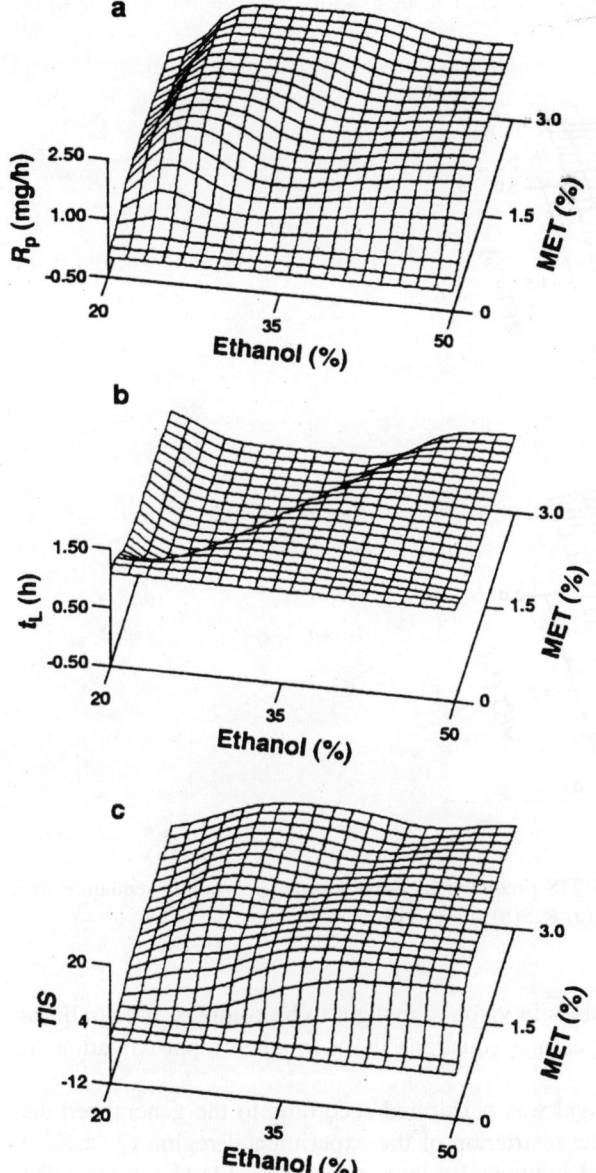

Figure 4 Response surfaces of R_p, t_L and TIS predicted by ANN as a function of the amounts of ethanol and MET. (a) R_p; (b) t_L; (c) TIS.

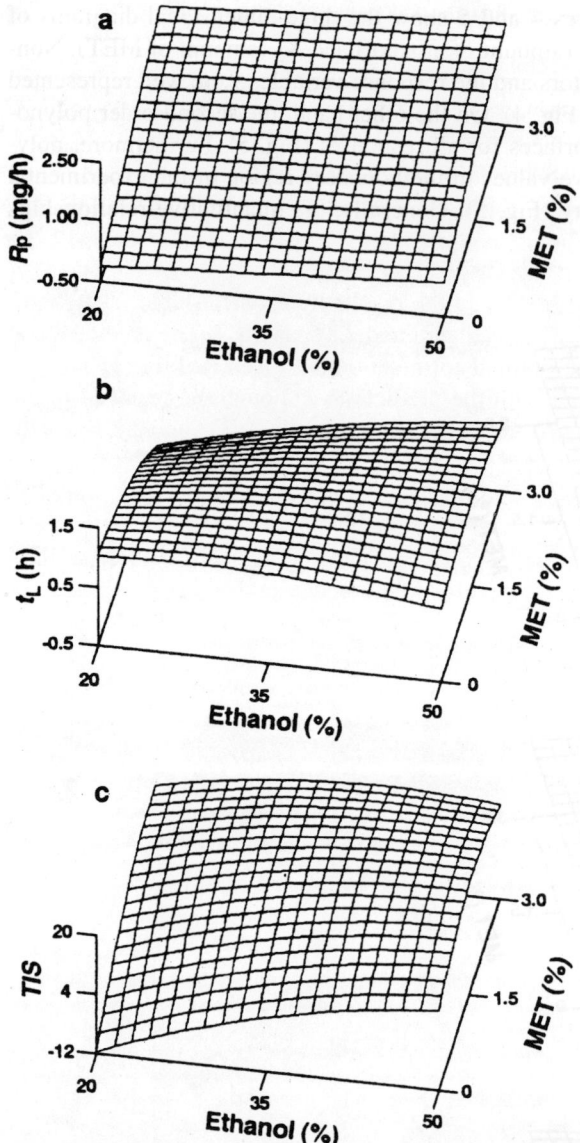

Figure 5 Response surfaces of R_p, t_L, and TIS predicted by second-order polynomial equation as a function of the amounts of ethanol and MET. (a) R_p; (b) t_L; (c) TIS.

between causal factors and response variables in vivo are thought to be complex and nonlinear. ANN seems to be more useful than polynomial equations in cases where approximations of such relationships are required.

Optimization of a ketoprofen hydrogel was performed according to the generalized distance function defined in Eq. 10 under the restriction of the experimental region ($2 \geq X_1^2 + X_2^2$; in coded form). The optimal values of individual response variables, $FD_k(\mathbf{X})$, were calculated before simultaneous optimization was carried out, i.e., the individual maximum R_p, the minimum t_L and the minimum TIS values, respectively. ANN training and the estimation of

Table 5 Predicted and Experimental Response Variables for the Optimal Formula

Response	Predicted	Experimental[a]
R_p (mg/h)	1.45	1.21 ± 0.19
t_L (h)	0.264	0.713 ± 0.106
TIS	9.42	10.8 ± 1.0

[a] The mean ± SD of four determinations.

simultaneous optima were repeated several times and the results were fairly stable. The simultaneous optimal solution was estimated at 23% as ethanol and 2.2% as MET. The predicted and the experimental response variables for the optimal formulation are given in Table 5. The observed results of R_p and TIS coincided well with the predictions although the result of t_L did not. The difference between the predicted and the experimental t_L value was about 30 min. In order to predict t_L more precisely, other experiments such as an in vitro permeation study are required. However, R_p and TIS, which are very significant for effectiveness and safety, were satisfactorily predicted.

In conclusion, the multiobjective simultaneous optimization technique incorporating ANNs is useful for optimizing pharmaceutical formulas when predictions of pharmaceutical responses based on the second-order polynomial equations are limited to low levels.

ACKNOWLEDGMENT

This work was supported by the Ministry of Education, Science, Sports, and Culture, Japan. The authors are grateful to Professor Hiroshi Ichikawa, Department of Information Science, Hoshi University, for his support and valuable advice in ANN, and Dr. Kimio Higashiyama, Department of Organic Chemistry, Hoshi University, for his help in synthesizing MET.

REFERENCES

1. Barry, B. W., 1987. Mode of action of penetration enhancers in human skin. J. Contr. Rel., 6: 85–97.
2. Okamoto, H., Hashida, M. and Sezaki, H., 1988. Structure–activity relationship of 1-alkyl- or 1-alkenylazacycloalkanone derivatives as percutaneous penetration enhancers. J. Pharm. Sci., 77: 418–424.
3. Kadir, R. and Barry, B. W., 1991. α-Bisabolol, a possible safe penetration enhancer for dermal and transdermal therapeutics. Int. J. Pharm., 70: 87–94.
4. Okabe, H., Takayama, K., Ogura, A. and Nagai, T., 1989. Effect of limonene and related compounds on the percutaneous absorption of indomethacin. Drug Design Deliv., 4: 313–321.
5. Obata, Y., Takayama, K., Okabe, H. and Nagai, T., 1990. Effect of cyclic monoterpenes on percutaneous absorption in the case of a water-soluble drug (diclofenac sodium). Drug Design Deliv., 6: 319–328.
6. Takayama, K., Kikuchi, K., Obata, Y., Okabe, H., Machida, Y. and Nagai, T., 1991. Terpenes as percutaneous absorption promoters. STP Pharma Sci., 1: 83–88.
7. Ohara, N., Takayama, K., Machida, Y. and Nagai, T., 1994. Combined effect of d-limonene and temperature on the skin permeation of ketoprofen. Int. J. Pharm., 105: 31–38.
8. Negishi, J., Takayama, K., Higashiyama, K., Chida, K., Isowa, K. and Nagai, T., 1995. Promoting effect of O-alkylmenthol and O-acylmenthol derivatives on the percutaneous absorption of ketoprofen in rats. STP Pharma Sci., 5: 156–161.

9. Nakamura, Y., Takayama, K., Higashiyama, K., Suzuki, T. and Nagai, T., 1996. Promoting effect of O-ethylmenthol on the percutaneous absorption of ketoprofen. Int. J. Pharm., 145: 29–36.
10. Box, G. E. P., Hunter, W. G. and Hunter, J. S., 1978. Statistics for Experimenters, Wiley, New York.
11. Fonner, Jr., D. E., Buck, J. R. and Banker, G. S., 1970. Mathematical optimization techniques in drug product and process analysis. J. Pharm. Sci., 59: 1587–1596.
12. Takayama, K. and Nagai, T., 1991. Simultaneous optimization for several characteristics concerning percutaneous absorption and skin damage of ketoprofen hydrogels containing d-limonene. Int. J. Pharm., 74: 115–126.
13. Levison, K. K., Takayama, K., Isowa, K., Okabe, K. and Nagai, T., 1994. Formulation optimization of indomethacin gels containing a combination of three kinds of cyclic monoterpenes as percutaneous absorption enhancers. J. Pharm. Sci., 83: 1367–1372.
14. Takahara, J., Takayama, K. and Nagai, T., 1997. Multi-objective simultaneous optimization based on artificial neural network in sustained release formulations, J. Contr. Rel., 49: 11–20.
15. Takahara, J., Takayama K., Isowa, K. and Nagai, T., 1997. Multi-objective simultaneous optimization based on artificial neural network in a ketoprofen hydrogel formula containing O-ethylmenthol as a percutaneous absorption enhancer. Int. J. Pharm., 158: 203–210.
16. Aoyama, T., Suzuki, Y. and Ichikawa, H., 1989. Neural networks applied to pharmaceutical problems. I. Method and application to decision making. Chem. Pharm. Bull., 37: 2558–2560.
17. Hussain, A. S., Yu, X. and Johnson, R. D., 1991. Application of neural computing in pharmaceutical product development. Pharm. Res., 8: 1248–1252.
18. Jha, B. K., Tambe, S. S. and Kulkarni, B. D., 1995. Estimating diffusion coefficients of a micellar system using an artificial neural network. J. Coll. I. Sci., 170: 392–398.
19. Weinstein, J. N., Kohn, K. W., Grever, M. R., Viswanadhan, V. N., Rubinstein, L. V., Monks, A. P., Scudiero, D. A., Welch, L., Koutsoukos, A. D., Chiausa, A. J. and Paull, K. D., 1992. Neural computing in cancer drug development: predicting mechanism of action. Sciences, 258: 447–451.
20. Hussain, A. S., Johnson, R. D., Vachharajani, N. and Ritschel, W. A., 1993. Feasibility of developing a neural network for prediction of human pharmacokinetic parameters from animal data. Pharm. Res., 10: 466–469.
21. Brier, E., Zurada, J. M. and Aronoff, G. R., 1995. Neural network predicted peak and trough gentamicin concentrations. Pharm. Res., 12: 406–412.
22. Gobburu, J. V. S. and Shelver, W. H., 1995. Quantitative structure–pharmacokinetic relationship (QSPR) of beta blockers derived using neural networks. J. Pharm. Sci., 84: 862–865.
23. Smith, B. P. and Brier, M. E., 1996. Statistical approach to neural network model building for gentamicin peak predictions. J. Pharm. Sci., 85: 65–69.
24. McClelland, J. L. and Rumelhart D. E., 1988. Explorations in Parallel Distributed Processing. MIT Press, Cambridge, MA.
25. Achanta, A. S., Kowalski, J. G. and Rhodes C. T., 1995. Artificial neural networks: Implications for pharmaceutical sciences. Drug Dev. Ind. Pharm., 21: 119–155.
26. Erb, R. J., 1993. Introduction to backpropagation neural network computation. Pharm. Res., 10: 165–170.
27. Murase, H., Koyama, S., Honami, N. and Kuwabara, T., 1991. Kalman filter neuron training. Bull. Univ. Osaka Pref., Ser. B., 43: 91–101.
28. Blank, T. B. and Brown, S. D., 1994. Adaptive, global, extended Kalman filters for training feedforward neural networks. J. Chemom., 8: 391–407.
29. Simutis, R., Havlik, I., Dors, M. and Luebbert, A., 1993. Training of artificial networks extended by linear dynamic subsystems. Process Control Qual., 4: 211–220.
30. Lippman, R. P., 1987. An introduction to computing with neural nets. IEEE ASSP Mag., April: 4–22.
31. Bounds, D. G. and Lloyd, P. J., 1988. A multilayer perceptron network for the diagnosis of low back pain. In: Proceedings of Second IEEE International Conference on Neural Networks, San Diego, CA, July 24–27, pp. II-481–II-489.
32. Cybenko, G., 1989. Approximations by superpositions of a sigmoidal function. Math. Control Signals Syst., 2: 303–314.

33. Carpenter, W. C. and Hoffman, M. E., 1995. Understanding neural network approximations and polynomial approximations helps neural network performance. AI Expert., March: 31–33.
34. Fujikawa, M., Takayama, K. and Nagai T., 1998. Application of partitioned artificial neural networks to optimize pharmaceutical formulations. In: Abstract of Conference on Challenges for Drug Delivery and Pharmaceutical Technology, Tokyo, June 9–11, p. 133.
35. Takayama, K. and Nagai, T., 1989. Novel computer optimization methodology for pharmaceutical formulations investigated by using sustained-release granules of indomethacin. Chem. Pharm. Bull., 37: 160–167.
36. Derringer, G. and Suich, R., 1980. Simultaneous optimization of several response variables. J. Quality Tech., 12: 214–219.
37. McLeod, A. D., Lam, F. C., Gupta, P. K. and Hung, C. T., 1988. Optimized synthesis of polyglutaraldehyde nanoparticles using central composite design. J. Pharm. Sci., 77: 704–710.
38. Müller, B. G., Leuenberger, H. and Kissel, T., 1996. Albumin nanospheres as carriers for passive drug targeting: an optimized manufacturing technique. Pharm. Res., 13: 32–37.
39. Wang, Y. M., Sato, H., Adachi, I. and Horikoshi, I., 1996. Optimization of the formulation design of chitosan microspheres containing cisplatin. J. Pharm. Sci., 85: 1204–1210.
40. Khuri, A. I. and Conlon, M., 1981. Simultaneous optimization of multiple responses predicted by polynomial regression functions. Technometrics, 23: 363–375.

29
Transdermal Drug Delivery by Skin Electroporation

Tani Chen, Robert Langer, and James C. Weaver
Massachusetts Institute of Technology Cambridge, Massachusetts

I. INTRODUCTION

Transdermal drug delivery has several noteworthy advantages over other drug delivery techniques, including avoidance of the metabolic "first-pass" effect (as in oral delivery techniques), the avoidance of pain (by not using needles), and, in some versions, the ability to control drug delivery rates (1–3). However, transporting drugs through the skin by passive diffusion is a slow process (3), and many techniques have been developed to "enhance" or increase molecular transport. Some of these enhancement techniques include chemical enhancers (2,4), sonophoresis (5–7), iontophoresis (8,9), and high-voltage pulsing (believed to cause skin electroporation) (10,11).

In high-voltage pulsing, a series of short (typically about 1 ms), high-voltage (typically about 100 V across the skin) pulses are applied to the stratum corneum, causing significant molecular transport to occur (10). A distinction should be made between the electrical conditions applied to the skin (a series of short, high-voltage pulses), and the skin electroporation hypothesis, where the high-voltage pulses cause "pores" or aqueous pathways to form in the lipid bilayer membranes composing the stratum corneum, through which ions (measured as electrical resistance) and molecular transport across the stratum corneum of the skin can occur (10,11). However, many refer to the overall process as skin electroporation.

To date, the application of high-voltage pulsing for transdermal drug delivery purposes has been tested primarily in in vitro systems using cadaver and animal skin (10,12,13), and a few in vivo studies using hairless mice, hairless rats, and pigs (10,14–16). Trials involving humans have not been performed yet, as the electrical conditions used for molecular transport have not been fully optimized, but related studies of electrochemotherapy using transdermal pulses show no damage (17).

II. SKIN ELECTROPORATION

The application of a series of high-voltage pulses to sheets of lipid bilayer membranes causes a a phenomenon known as electroporation to occur, where a rearrangement of the lipids within the membrane takes place, resulting in a transient aqueous pathway (termed a "pore") to form in the membrane. Molecular transport has been shown to occur through these pores (18–20). Applying high-voltage pulsing to cells cause the same phenomenon to occur, which can be used advantageously to transport many compounds, including DNA, into the cells without killing them (18,19). Since then, researchers have also applied high-voltage pulsing to larger structures, such as frog epithelium (21), and directly to human skin, for the purposes of transdermal drug delivery.

The first experiments in skin electroporation research used exponentially decaying high-voltage pulses, with an applied voltage of 1000 V and a time constant of about 1 ms (10). Pulses were applied at the rate of one pulse every 5 s for 1 h (about 720 pulses total). Although this protocol was originally chosen somewhat arbitrarily, many other studies since then have also used this same protocol (13,22–29) to facilitate comparisons between different experiments and different equipment. Thus this protocol has come to be regarded as a "standard" electroporation protocol for some research purposes.

In these first experiments, it was found that the molecular flux of several small molecular weight compounds (approximately 600 Da) increased dramatically during 1 h of pulsing, compared to background fluxes. Although a four order-of-magnitude increase in molecular transport over passive control levels was quoted (10), this was incorrect since the background fluorescence actually measured during the passive control was below the detection limit of the spectrofluorimeter. Thus, the amount of "enhancement" compared to the passive control was not specifically determined. After pulsing, the molecular flux through the skin appeared to drop back to background levels, over the course of 3 h (10). The electrical resistance of the skin was also found to decrease during high-voltage pulsing, with some recovery of the skin's resistance after pulsing (10,30).

Many electrical conditions have been studied in an effort to determine which factors control transport. Molecular transport generally increases with the transdermal voltage and the duration of each pulse (31). The shape of the applied pulse does not appear to be as important in determining molecular transport (32). Other factors that may be important in molecular transport include the overall amount of charge transported (31).

Fluorescent molecules with low molecular weights (typically less than 1000 Da) have successfully been transported across the skin during high-voltage pulsing, including lucifer yellow (457 Da, −2 charge) (10,28), cascade blue (596 Da, −3 charge) (28), sulforhodamine (607 Da, −1 charge) (13,24,28,33,34), and calcein (623 Da, −4 charge) (10,13,24,28,33,34). These four molecules were all negatively charged and had similar molecular weights (28). Another tracer molecule that has been used is methylene blue (374 Da, +1 charge) (35).

Larger, biologically relevant molecules have also been successfully transported across the skin (36), including luteinizing hormone–releasing hormone (LHRH, 1182 Da) (37,38), cyclosporin A (39), heparin (5–30 kDa) (22,26,27), and several oligonucleotides (4.8–7.0 kDa) (23). All of these molecules were successfully transported across human skin in detectable and biologically relevant amounts, although using differing electrical protocols. Even larger molecules such as fluorescent latex particles have been tried, although their transport across the skin is questionable at best (29,40–42).

Skin electroporation has also been combined with other transdermal drug delivery techniques, including iontophoresis (37), ultrasound, (43), and various pathway-enlarging molecules (26,27,44,45). In many cases, skin electroporation combines synergistically with these other techniques for an additional one order-of-magnitude enhancement in molecular transport.

III. THEORY

Theories of skin electroporation are based on cell and membrane electroporation, accounting for the more complicated geometry of the skin, including the corneocytes and the parallel sheets of lipid bilayers (11,46–48). Molecular transport has been predicted to occur through the corneocytes of the stratum corneum, unlike in iontophoresis (constant DC current, resulting in transdermal voltages of less than 5 V) where transport occurs primarily through the hair follicles and sweat ducts. Electroporation of the stratum corneum has been predicted to occur at transdermal voltages more than 30 V (49), consistent with experimental findings that electroporation occurs at voltages more than 50 V (28).

The molecular transport pathways are believed to be concentrated in regions of the skin known as localized transport regions, or LTRs (11,47,50), which for some transported fluorescent molecules appear as small, brightly fluorescent regions after pulsing (13,23,33,34,40). The LTRs form spontaneously and almost randomly on the surface of the skin, and in particular, did not appear near hair follicles or sweat ducts (13,33). The LTRs were typically about 100 μm in diameter. The surface density of LTRs increased with the transdermal voltage (33,34).

The appearance of the LTRs on the surface of the skin can differ greatly, depending on the molecular species being transported. In some cases, the LTRs appear as small regions of intense fluorescence (13,23); however, in other cases, the LTRs may appear as "rings" (13,33,34), dark spots (51), or may be missing altogether (51). The observed LTR structures are believed to involve interactions (staining) of the transported molecules with the electrically induced structural changes in the skin. Moreover, the regions of fluorescence have previously been shown to also be the regions where molecular transport takes place (33).

IV. FLOW-THROUGH SYSTEMS

Skin electroporation is a highly dynamic process, and it quickly became evident in early studies that more rapid measurements of the molecular flux across the skin would be necessary to quantify and understand molecular transport (24,52). This led to the development of "flow-through" systems, where the contents of the receptor compartment were continuously pumped through a spectrofluorimeter for real-time detection (24,28,52,53). Although the first generation of flow-through systems had time resolutions of several minutes, limiting pulsing frequencies to 1 pulse/min (24,52), later flow-through systems improved the time resolution to 14 s, thus allowing studies of pulsing rates of the "standard" 1 pulse/5 s (Fig. 1b) (28,53).

Since a spectrofluorimeter is used as the real-time detector, this technique is limited to fluorescent compounds, such as sulforhodamine, lucifer yellow, cascade blue, and calcein (24). Despite the close similarities in the molecular weights and physical characteristics of the compounds used in these experiments, very different molecular transport properties emerged. In some cases, steady-state molecular fluxes were achieved in less than 1 h with repeated pulsing of the skin. However, in other cases, steady-state fluxes were not achieved, even after more than 7 h of repeated pulsing; either the molecular flux continued to rise during pulsing (24), or the molecular flux peaked and then decreased with additional pulsing (28). The cause of these differences is still not understood.

V. TRANSDERMAL VOLTAGE MEASUREMENTS

The actual voltage that forms across the skin has been the most relevant quantity in understanding aqueous pathway creation and molecular transport. While this fact has been known since the earliest skin electroporation studies (10), it has often been omitted in favor of the applied voltage, which is much easier to measure (12,32,34,41,42,54–61) but complicates the interpretation. Typically, the transdermal voltage exponentially decays, directly following the applied voltage waveform; thus, only the "peak" transdermal voltage usually needs to be reported.

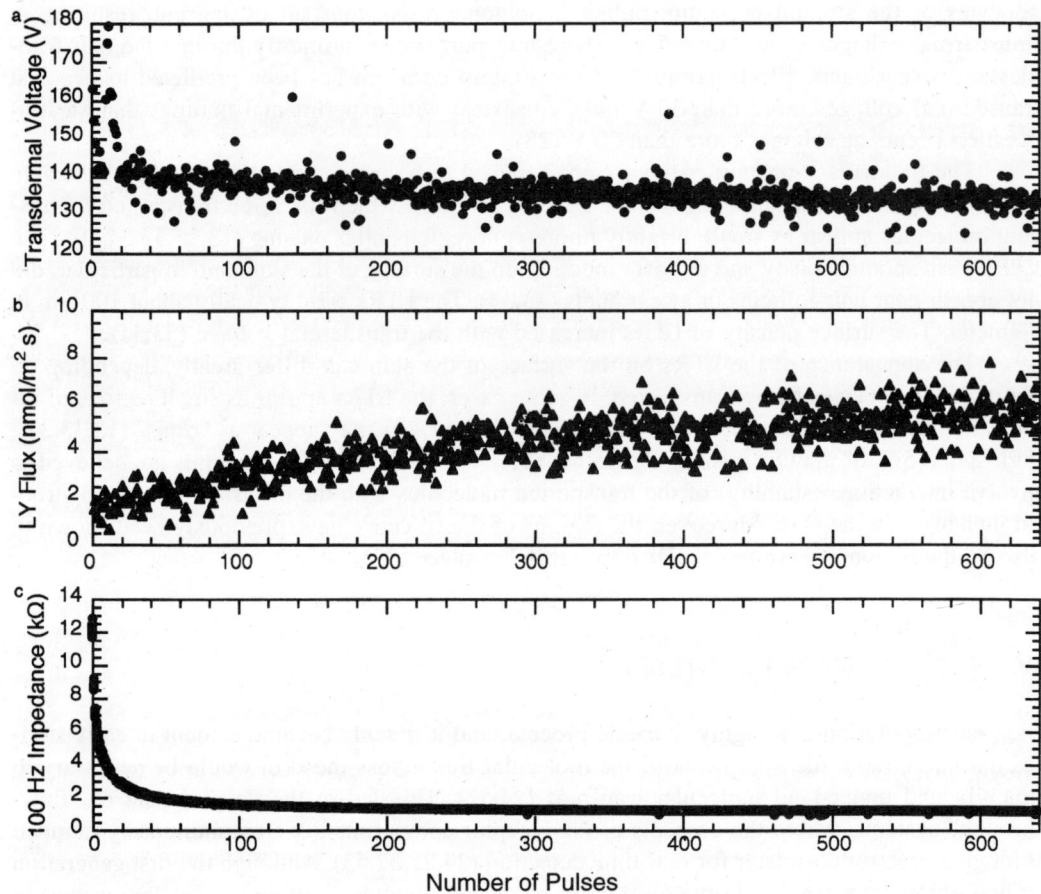

Figure 1 Simultaneous plot of the many changing parameters during skin electroporation. (a) The transdermal voltage drops very quickly with the first few pulses, then continues to decrease with additional pulsing. (b) The molecular flux (lucifer yellow shown here) reaches steady state with repeated pulsing. (c) The 100-Hz impedance of the skin decreases with continued pulsing, as new aqueous pathways through the skin are created. Measurement of all of these parameters is critical to understanding how molecular transport through the skin occurs during high-voltage pulsing.

The driving force for molecular transport across the skin is dependent on the transdermal voltage, not the applied (electrode) voltage. The transdermal voltage is a function of the applied voltage; however, it is also a function of many other parameters, such as the geometry of the system in use, the electrolyte–electrode interface, the resistivity of the saline, and the condition of the skin itself (11). With many different experimental chambers in use (10, 12–14,28,33,35,52,53), it is therefore often not possible to meaningfully compare the applied voltages.

The transdermal voltage does not remain constant with repeated pulsing but often decreases as new aqueous pathways are created across the skin, lowering the electrical resistance of the skin. However, this decrease in voltage is not always consistent and therefore should be measured for each pulse throughout the entire experiment (Fig. 1a). Decreases of 10 V to over 50 V during repeated pulsing have been observed; thus, using average values for the transdermal voltage (10,13,22,23,26,29,31,40) instead of instantaneous measurements can also result in misleading data (24,28,30). A single averaged transdermal voltage value often does not sufficiently describe the actual transdermal voltages experienced by the skin throughout an experiment.

VI. INTERPULSE SKIN IMPEDANCE AND SKIN RESISTANCE

The DC resistance of the skin gives a measure of the recovery of the barrier properties of the skin, as DC resistance is simply a measure of the resistance to the flow of ions across the skin. However, the DC resistance itself should never be directly measured. Measuring the DC resistance typically involves applying a potential drop across the skin to cause the flow of ions to occur, which is essentially iontophoresis of the skin. Many commercial ohmmeters apply voltages of 2–5 V during resistance measurements, which can cause currents of 1 mA/cm^2, more than enough to cause iontophoresis (51,53). In many skin electroporation experiments, the condition of the skin was checked using a DC ohmmeter (10,22,23,31,40). However, if the DC measuring voltage was applied briefly, the perturbation could still be negligible.

The impedance of the skin at a low frequency can be used as a surrogate for the resistance of the skin. The impedance of the skin should be measured by placing a bipolar, sinusoidal voltage across the skin. At higher frequencies, the capacitance of the skin does not have enough time to charge fully, which can lead to modified impedance measurements, but at lower frequencies (i.e., less than 100 Hz), the impedance of the skin is close to its DC resistance (62,63).

Before pulsing, the impedance of the skin is typically about 40 kΩ cm^2 at 100 Hz (10,62) (corresponding to $R_{skin} \sim$ 50 kΩ cm^2). However, during the first pulse, the impedance of the skin typically drops to about 100 Ω cm^2. After the pulse, there are two time constants for recovery (30). The skin usually recovers to about 1 kΩ cm^2 in less than 1 s, then recovers more slowly afterward, up to 70–80% of the original prepulse value, on a time scale of minutes (30).

However, with subsequent pulsing, the impedance of the skin continues to drop (Fig. 1c), and the skin does not recover its impedance quite as readily. After (more than 10 pulses), the impedance of the skin does not recover significantly and only reaches 5–10% of its prepulse impedance. Furthermore, this recovery is somewhat variable (30,51).

VII. ANIMAL MODELS

The most commonly used models of human skin are hairless rat skin and hairless mouse skin. Despite their names, they are covered with very fine hair, giving the appearance of hairlessness. In fact, both hairless mice and hairless rats are significantly more hairy than humans (13). Despite these differences, many molecules have been transported with varying electrical protocols, across hairless (rat or hairless) mouse skin, both in vitro or in vivo, such as metroprolol (12,54), fentanyl (16,32,55), alnitidan (56), domperidone (57), and several oligonucleotides (58–60). Pig skin has also been used as a model for human skin, although its hair is typically stiffer than human hair (15,35).

The presence of hair follicles is a large problem with these animal models. The LTRs responsible for molecular transport do not form near hair follicles or sweat ducts (13,33); thus, the formation of LTRs would be expected to be significantly different. Fluorescence microscopy studies directly examining LTR formation have confirmed that LTRs do not readily form in hairless-rat skin (13), which could potentially affect the molecular transport results.

Studies using shed snake skin, which lacks hair follicles and sweat ducts, have shown similar molecular transport characteristics and LTR formation as in human skin during high-voltage pulsing (13). Snake skin is a good model of human skin, due to a layer of the skin known as the "mesos" layer, which is analagous to human stratum corneum. It is composed of corneocytes and sheets of lipid bilayer membranes, similar to human skin (64,65). Thus, these experiments have shown that most of the molecular transport during skin electroporation occurs through the LTRs, and not through the hair follicles or sweat ducts, as in iontophoresis (13).

Thus, molecular transport through human skin during skin electroporation can be modeled with shed snake skin, but it should not be modeled with hairless rat or hairless mouse skin.

VIII. CONCLUSIONS

The application of a series of short, high-voltage pulses to the skin causes significant molecular transport across the skin, a phenomenon known as skin electroporation. However, both the molecular flux and the transdermal voltage change rapidly with repeated pulsing. Many studies have shown that skin electroporation is a dynamic process, requiring careful measurements with sufficiently high time resolution. It is vital that these parameters be measured in real time if any analysis of the mechanism of molecular transport can be made, or if any control of the skin electroporation process is to be achieved for drug delivery or extraction purposes.

REFERENCES

1. Bronaugh, R. L. and Maibach, H. I. (Eds.), 1989. Percutaneous Absorption. Mechanisms, Methodology, Drug Delivery. Marcel Dekker, New York.
2. Hadgraft, J. and Guy, R. H. (Editors), 1989. Transdermal Drug Delivery: Developmental Issues and Research Initiatives. Marcel Dekker, New York.
3. Schaefer, H., and Redelmeier, T. E. (Eds.), 1996. Skin Barrier: Principles of Percutaneous Absorption. Karger, Basel.
4. Chattaraj, S. C. and Walker, R. B., 1995. Penetration enhancer classification. In: E. W. Smith and H. I. Maibach (Eds.), Perucutaneous Penetration Enhancers. CRC Press, Boca Raton, FL.
5. Bommannan, D., Menon, G. K., Okuyama, H., Elias, P. M. and Guy, R. H., 1992. Sonophoresis. II. Examination of the mechanisms of ultrasound-enhanced transdermal drug delivery. Pharm. Res., 9: 1043–1047.
6. Bommannan, D., Okuyama, H., Stauffer, P. and Guy, R. H., 1992. Sonophoresis. I. The use of ultrasound to enhance transdermal drug delivery. Pharm. Res., 9: 559–564.
7. Mitragotri, S., Edwards, D. A., Blankenstein, D., and Langer, R., 1995. A mechanistic study of ultrasonically-enhanced transdermal drug delivery. J. Pharm. Sci., 84: 697–706.
8. Burnette, R. R., 1989. Iontophoresis. In: J. Hadgraft and R. H. Guy (Eds.), Transdermal Drug Delivery: Developmental Issues and Research Initiatives. Marcel Dekker, New York.
9. Guy, R. H., 1996. Current status and future prospects of transdermal drug delivery. Pharm. Res., 13: 1765–1769.
10. Prausnitz, M. R., Bose, V. G., Langer, R. and Weaver, J. C., 1993. Electroporation of mammalian skin: a mechanism to enhance transdermal drug delivery. Proc. Natl. Acad. Sci. USA, 90: 10504–10508.
11. Weaver, J. C., Vaughan, T. E. and Chizmadzhev, Y. A. (1999). Theory of electrical creation of aqueous pathways across skin transport barriers. Adv. Drug Deliv. Rev., 35: 21–39.
12. Vanbever, R., Lecouturier, N. and Préat, V. 1994. Transdermal delivery of metoprolol by electroporation. Pharm. Res., 11: 1657–1662.
13. Chen, T., Langer, R. and Weaver, J. C., 1998. Skin electroporation causes molecular transport across the stratum corneum through localized transport regions. J. Invest. Dermatol. Symp. Proc., 3: 159–165.

14. Prausnitz, M. R., Seddick, D. S., Kon, A. A., Bose, V. G., Frankenburg, S., Klaus, S. N., Langer, R. and Weaver, J. C., 1993. Methods for in vivo tissue electroporation using surface electrodes. Drug Deliv., 1: 125–131.
15. Riviere, J. E., Monteiro-Riviere, N. A., Rogers, R. A., Bommannan, D., Tamada, J. A. and Potts, R. O., 1995. Pulsatile transdermal delivery of LHRH using electroporation: drug delivery and skin toxicology. J. Control. Rel., 36: 229–233.
16. Vanbever, R., Langers, G., Montmayeur, S. and Préat, V., 1998. Transdermal Delivery of Fentanyl: Rapid Onset of Analgesia Using Skin Electroporation. J. Control. Rel., 50: 225–235.
17. Mir, L. M., Belehradek, M., Domenge, C., Orlowski, S., Poddevin, B., Belehradek, J., Schwaab, G., Luboinski, B. and Paoletti, C., 1991. Electrochemotherapy, a Novel Antitumor Treatment: First Clinical Trial. C. R. Acad. Sci. Paris Serle. III, 313: 613–618.
18. Neumann, E., Sowers, A. E. and Jordan, C. A. (Editors), 1989. Electroporation and Electrofusion in Cell Biology. Plenum Press, New York.
19. Chang, D. C., Chassy, B. M., Saunders, J. A. and Sowers, A. E. (Editors), 1992. Guide to Electroporation and Electrofusion. Academic Press, New York.
20. Weaver, J. C. and Chizmadzhev, Y. A., 1996. Electroporation. In: C. Polk and E. Postow (Editors), CRC Handbook of Biological Effects of Electromagnetic Fields, 2nd Edition. CRC Press, Boca Raton, FL.
21. Powell, K. T., Morgenthaler, A. W. and Weaver, J. C., 1989. Tissue Electroporation: Observation of Reversible Electrical Breakdown in Vaible Frog Skin. Biophys. J., 56: 1163–1171.
22. Prausnitz, M. R., Edelman, E. R., Gimm, J. A., Langer, R. and Weaver, J. C., 1995. Transdermal Delivery of Heparin by Skin Electroporation. Bio/Technology, 13: 1205–1209.
23. Zewert, T. E., Pliquett, U. F., Langer, R. and Weaver, J. C., 1995. Transdermal Transport of DNA Antisense Oligonucleotides by Electroporation. Biochem. Biophys. Res. Com., 212: 286–292.
24. Pliquett, U. and Weaver, J. C., 1996. Electroporation of Human Skin: Simultaneous Measurement of Changes in the Transport of Two Fluorescent Molecules and in the Passive Electrical Properties. Bioelectrochem. Bioenerg., 39: 1–12.
25. Pliquett, U. and Weaver, J. C., 1996. Transport of a Charged Molecule across the Human Epidermis due to Electroporation. J. Control. Rel., 38: 1–10.
26. Weaver, J. C., Vanbever, R., Vaughan, T. E. and Prausnitz, M. R., 1997. Heparin Alters Transdermal Transport Associated with Electroporation. Biochem. Biophys. Res. Com., 234: 637–640.
27. Vanbever, R., Prausnitz, M. R. and Préat, V., 1997. Macromolecules as Novel Transdermal Transport Enhancers for Skin Electroporation. Pharm. Res., 14: 638–644.
28. Chen, T., Segall, E. M., Langer, R. and Weaver, J. C., 1998. Skin Electroporation: Rapid Measurements of the Transdermal Voltage and Flux of Four Fluorescent Molecules Show a Transition to Large Fluxes Near 50 V. J. Pharm. Sci., 87: 1368–1374.
29. Chen, T., Langer, R. and Weaver, J. C., 1999. Charged Microbeads are Not Transported Across the Human Stratum Corneum in Vitro by Short High-Voltage Pulses." Bioelectrochem. Bioenerg, 48: 181–192.
30. Pliquett, U., Langer, R. and Weaver, J. C., 1995. Changes in the Passive Electrical Properties of Human Stratum Corneum due to Electroporation. Biochim. Biophys. Acta, 1239: 111–121.
31. Prausnitz, M. R., Lee, C. S., Liu, C. H., Pang, J. C., Singh, T.-P., Langer, R. and Weaver, J. C., 1996. Transdermal Transport Efficiency during Skin Electroporation and Iontophoresis. J. Control. Release, 38: 205–217.
32. Vanbever, R., Le Boulengé, E. and Préat, V., 1996. Transdermal Delivery of Fentanyl by Electroporation. I. Influence of Electrical Factors. Pharm. Res., 13: 559–565, 1996.
33. Pliquett, U., Zewert, T. E., Chen, T., Langer, R. and Weaver, J. C., 1996. Imaging of Fluorescent Molecule and Small Ion Transport through Human Stratum Corneum during High Voltage Pulsing: Localized Transport Regions are Involved. Biophys. Chem., 58: 185–204.
34. Vanbever, R., Pliquett, U. F., Préat, V. and Weaver, J. C., submitted. Transdermal Transport and Changes in Skin Electrical Properties due to Short and Long High-Voltage Pulses.
35. Gallo, S. A., Oseroff, A. R., Johnson, P. G. and Hui, S. W., 1997. Characterization of Electric-Pulse-Induced Permeabilization of Porcine Skin Using Surface Electrodes. Biophys. J., 72: 2805–2811.
36. Banga, A. and Prausnitz, M. R., 1998. Delivery of Protein and Gene-based Drugs by Skin Electroporation. Trends Biotech., 16: 408–412.

37. Bommannan, D., Tamada, J., Leung, L. and Potts, R. O., 1994. Effect of Electroporation on Transdermal Iontophoretic Delivery of Luteinizing Hormone Releasing Hormone (LHRH) in Vitro. Pharm. Res., 11: 1809–1814.
38. Riviere, J. E., Monteiro-Riviere, N. A., Rogers, R. A., Bommannan, D., Tamada, J. A. and Potts, R. O., 1995. Pulsatile Transdermal Delivery of LHRH Using Electroporation: Drug Delivery and Skin Toxicology. J. Control. Rel., 36: 229–233.
39. Wang, S., Kara, M. and Krishnan, R. R., 1998. Transdermal Delivery of Cyclosporin-A Using Electroporation. J. Control. Rel., 50: 61–70.
40. Prausnitz, M. R., Gimm, J. A., Guy, R. H., Langer, R., Weaver, J. C. and Cullander, C., 1996. Imaging of Transport Pathways across Human Stratum Corneum during High-Voltage and Low-Voltage Electrical Exposures. J. Pharm. Sci., 85: 1363–1370.
41. Hofmann, G. A., Rustrum, W. V. and Suder, K. S., 1995. Electro-incorporation of Microcarriers as a Method for the Transdermal Delivery of Large Molecules. Bioelectrochem. Bioenerg., 38: 209–222.
42. Zhang, L., Li, L., An, L., Hoffman, R. M. and Hofmann, G. A., 1997. In vivo Transdermal Delivery of Large Molecules by Pressure-Mediated Electroincorporation and Electroporation: A Novel Method for Drug and Gene Therapy. Bioelectrochem. Bioenerg., 42: 283–292.
43. Kost, J., Pliquett, U., Mitragotri, S., Yamamoto, A., Langer, R. and Weaver, J., 1996. Synergistic Effect of Electric Field and Ultrasound on Transdermal Transport. Pharm. Res., 13: 633–638.
44. Weaver, J. C., Zewert, T. E., Pliquett, U. F., Vanbever, R., Gowrishankar, T. R., Herndon, T. O., Martin, G. T., Vaughan, T. E., Ilic, L., Handwerker, J., Chen, T., Allen, D., Langer, R. and Monteiro-Riviere, N., submitted. Pathway-enlarging Molecules for Skin Electroporation: The Possibility of Macromolecule Delivery with Minimal Side Effects.
45. Zewert, T. E., Pliquett, U. F., Vanbever, R., Langer, R. and Weaver, J. C., submitted. Creation of Transdermal Pathways for Macromolecule Transport by Skin Electroporation and a Low Toxicity, Pathway-enlarging Molecule.
46. Chizmadzhev, Y. A., Zarnytsin, V. G., Weaver, J. C. and Potts, R. O., 1995. Mechanism of Electroinduced Ionic Species Transport through a Multilamellar Lipid Bilayer System. Biophys. J., 68: 749–765.
47. Weaver, J. C., Vaughan, T. E. and Chizmadzhev, Y. A., 1998. Theory of Skin Electroporation: Implications of Straight-Through Aqueous Pathway Segments that Connect Adjacent Corneocytes. J. Invest. Deramatol. Symp. Proc., 3: 143–147.
48. Chizmadzhev, Y. A., Kuzmin, P. I., Weaver, J. C. and Potts, R. O., 1998. Skin Appendageal Macropores as Possible Pathways for Electric Current. J. Invest. Dermatol. Symp. Proc., 3: 148–152.
49. Chizmadzhev, Y. A., Indenbom, A. V., Kuzmin, P. I., Galichenko, S. V., Weaver, J. C. and Potts, R. O., 1998. Electrical Properties of Skin at Moderate Voltages: Contribution of Appendageal Macropores. Biophys. J., 74: 843–856.
50. Vaughan, T. E., Chizmadzhev, Y. A. and Weaver, J. C., in press. Theoretical Issues in Understanding Local Transport Regions in Electroporated Stratum Corneum. In: Electricity and Magnetism in Biology and Medicine. Plenum Press, New York.
51. Chen, T. The Pathways and Mechanisms for Skin Electroporation, 1998. Massachusetts Institute of Technology, Sc. D. Thesis. Cambridge, MA.
52. Pliquett, U., Prausnitz, M. R., Chizmadzhev, Y. A. and Weaver, J. C. Measurement of Rapid Release Kinetics for Drug Delivery. Pharm. Res., 12: 549–555 (Errata in Pharm. Res., 12: 1244, 1995).
53. Chen, T., Langer, R. and Weaver, J. C., in press. An in Vitro System for Measuring the Transdermal Voltage and Molecular Flux across the Skin in Real Time. In: M. J. Jaroszeski, R. Gilbert and R. Heller (Editors), Electrically Mediated Delivery of Molecules to Cells: Electrochemotherapy, Electrogenetherapy, and Transdermal Delivery by Electroporation. Humana Press, Totowa, NJ.
54. Vanbever, R., and Préat, V., 1995. "Factors Affecting Transdermal Delivery of Metoprolol by Electroporation." Bioelectrochem. Bioenerg., 38: 223–228.
55. Vanbever, R., De Morre, N. and Préat, V. Transdermal Delivery of Fentanyl by Electroporation. II. Mechanisms Involved in Drug Transport." Pharm. Res., 13: 1359–1365.

56. Jadoul, A., Lecouturier, N., Mesens, J., Caers, W. and Préat, V., in press. Electrically Enhanced Transdermal Delivery of Alnitidan. J. Control. Rel.
57. Jadoul, A. and Préat, V., 1997. Electrically-Enhanced Transdermal Delivery of Domperidone. Int. J. Pharm., 154: 229–234.
58. Regnier, V., Le Doan, T. and Préat, V., 1998. Topical Delivery of Phosphorothioate Oligonucleotides to the Skin by Electroporation. J. Drug Target., 5: 275–289.
59. Regnier, V. and Préat, V., in press. Localisation of a FITC-labelled Phosphorothioate Oligodeoxynucleotide in the Skin after Topical Delivery by Iontophoresis or Electroporation. Pharm. Res.
60. Regnier, V. and Préat, V., in press. Mechanisms of a Phosphorothioate Oligonucleotide Delivery by Skin Electroporation. Int. J. Pharm.
61. Vanbever, R. and Préat, V., in press. Transdermal drug delivery by skin electroporation in the Rat. In: M. J. Jaroszeski, R. Gilbert and R. Heller (Editors), Electrically Mediated Delivery of Molecules to Cells: Electrochemotherapy, Electrogenetherapy, and Transdermal Delivery by Electroporation. Humana Press, Totowa, NJ.
62. Gowrishankar, T. R. Personal communication.
63. Pliquett, U. and Prausnitz, M. R. (in press). Electrical impedance spectroscopy for rapid and non-invasive analysis of skin electroporation. In: M. J. Jaroszeski, R. Gilbert, and R. Heller (Eds.), Electrically Mediated Delivery of Molecules to Cells: Electrochemotherapy, Electrogenetherapy, and Transdermal Delivery by Electroporation. Humana Press, Totowa, NJ.
64. Itoh, T., Magavi, R., Casady, R. L., Nishihata, T., and Rytting, J. H., 1990. A method to predict the percutaneous permeability of various compounds: shed snake skin as a model membrane. Pharm. Res., 7: 1302–1306.
65. Itoh, T., Xia, J., Magavi, R., Nishihata, T., and Rytting, J. H., 1990. Use of shed snake skin as a model membrane for in vitro percutaneous studies: comparison with human skin. Pharm. Res., 7: 1042–1047.

30
Enhancement of Transdermal Transport Using Ultrasound in Combination with Other Enhancers

Samir Mitragotri
University of California, Santa Barbara, Santa Barbara, California

Robert Langer
Massachusetts Institute of Technology, Cambridge, Massachusetts

Joseph Kost
Massachusetts Institute of Technology, Cambridge, Massachusetts
and Ben-Gurion University, Beer-Sheva, Israel

I. INTRODUCTION

Transdermal drug delivery offers several advantages over traditional drug delivery systems, such as oral delivery and injection including elimination of first-pass metabolism, increased patient compliance, and possible sustained release of drugs (1). However, transdermal transport of molecules is slow due to the low permeability of the stratum corneum, the uppermost layer of the skin. Therefore, it is difficult to deliver drugs across the skin at a therapeutically relevant rate. This, in fact, is the main reason why only a handful of low molecular weight drugs are administered by this route today. A possible solution to this problem is to increase the permeability of the skin using physicochemical driving forces, referred to as penetration enhancers, e.g., ultrasound, chemical enhancers, and electrical fields. Chemical enhancers are compounds that, when applied to the skin surface along with the drug, are believed to penetrate the skin and modify the transport pathways through it, thereby inducing higher drug transport (2). Electrical fields can also enhance drug transport through the skin in two ways. First, they can enhance the transport of a charged molecule across the skin by electrophoresis, a phenomenon referred to as *iontophoresis* (3). Second, application of short pulses of high-voltage electrical fields can also enhance transdermal transport through the formation of short-lived pores (4). This phenomenon is referred to as *electroporation*. Ultrasound may enhance transdermal transport through affecting skin structure or through inducing convection across the skin (5,6). This phenomenon is referred to as *sonophoresis*. Numerous literature reports have shown that application of ultrasound enhances transdermal transport of a variety of drugs in vitro, in vivo as well as in a clinical setting (5–53). The enhancement of transdermal transport induced by ultrasound varies from a few percents to several orders of magnitude depending on the condition. Ultrasound has also been shown to synergistically enhance transdermal transport along with other penetration enhancers, including chemicals (24) and electroporation (28). In this chapter we present a review of sonophoresis with an emphasis on its synergistic effects with various enhancers. We first give a brief review of the principles and mechanisms of sonophoresis and its effect on transdermal transport. We then discuss the synergistic effects of ultrasound with two enhancers: chemicals and electroporation. Mechanisms of such synergistic effects are also discussed.

II. SONOPHORESIS

Depending on the ultrasound frequency used, sonophoresis can be categorized into three regions: low-frequency (frequency <1 MHz), therapeutic frequency (frequency 1–3 MHz), and high-frequency (frequency >3 MHz). A brief summary of sonophoretic enhancement in each frequency region is discussed below.

A. Low-Frequency Sonophoresis

Tachibana et al. reported that application of low-frequency ultrasound (48 kHz) enhances transdermal transport of lidocaine (51) and insulin (49) across hairless-rat skin in vivo. They also showed that application of ultrasound under similar conditions enhances transdermal transport of insulin in rabbits (50). Mitragotri et al. have shown that application of ultrasound at even lower frequencies (20 kHz) enhances transdermal transport of various low molecular weight drugs, including corticosterone and salicylic acid (37), as well as high molecular weight proteins, such as insulin, across human skin in vitro (6). Transdermal transport induced by low-frequency ultrasound is much more significant than that induced by therapeutic or high-frequency ultrasound. For example, application of therapeutic ultrasound has no effect on transdermal permeation of lidocaine; however, low-frequency ultrasound has been shown to significantly enhance lidocaine transport across hairless-rat skin in vivo. Quantitatively, Mitragotri et al. found that the enhancement induced by low-frequency ultrasound is up to 1000-fold higher than that induced by therapeutic ultrasound (37). Low-frequency ultrasound has also been found to enhance transdermal transport drugs that do not permeate skin passively, e.g., high-molecular weight proteins (6).

B. Therapeutic Frequency Sonophoresis

Therapeutic frequency is the most commonly used frequency region for sonophoresis. Numerous clinical and nonclinical reports have been published concerning sonophoresis. Fellinger and Schmidt (16) reported successful treatment of polyarthritis of the hand's digital joints using hydrocortisone ointment with sonophoresis. Newman et al. (54) and Coodley (55) showed improved results of hydrocortisone injection combined with ultrasound "massage" compared to simple hydrocortisone injection for a bursitis treatment. Sonophoresis has also been tested for its ability to aid penetration in a variety of drug–ultrasound combinations, mainly for localized conditions. The major medications used include the anti-inflammatory agents, e.g., cortisol, dexamethasone, salicylates, and local anesthetics. Griffin et al. (20) treated 102 patients diagnosed with elbow epicondylitis, bicipital tendonitis, shoulder osteoarthritis, shoulder bursitis, and knee osteoarthritis with hydrocortisone and ultrasound. A significant beneficial effect of ultrasound in the treatment was observed. Moll presented similar effects for lidocaine delivery (56). McElnay et al. evaluated the influence of ultrasound on the percutaneous absorption of lignocaine from a cream base (31). Mean data indicated that there was a slightly faster onset time for local anesthesia when ultrasound was administered when compared with control values (no ultrasound). However, the differences were not statistically significant. Benson et al. reported on the influence of ultrasound on the percutaneous absorption of lignocaine and prilocaine from Emla cream (7). They demonstrated that ultrasound is also capable of enhancing the percutaneous absorption of methyl and ethyl nicotinate (10). McEnlay et al. also evaluated the skin penetration enhancement effect of sonophoresis on methyl nicotinate in healthy volunteers and found that ultrasound treatment applied prior to methyl nicotinate led to enhanced percutaneous absorption of the drug (33). Similar experiments were performed by Hofman and Moll (57) who studied the percutaneous absorption of benzyl nicotinate. Kleinkort and Wood (25) showed a significant effect of ultrasound cortisol delivery in human volunteers. On the other hand, Williams showed that ultrasound at intensities of 0.25 W/cm^2 at 1.1 MHz ultrasound had no detectable effect on the rate of penetration of anesthetic preparations through a human being. Levy et al. showed that 3–5 min of ultrasound exposure (1 MHz, 1.5 W/cm^2) increased transdermal permeation of mannitol and physostigmine across hairless-rat skin in vivo by up to 15-fold (58). They also reported that the lag time typically associated with transdermal drug delivery was nearly completely eliminated after exposure to ultrasound. Therapeutic ultrasound has been attempted to enhance transdermal transport of more than 15 drugs, although the degree of enhancement varies from drug to drug. An explanation for this variation has been provided by Mitragotri et al. based on their conclusion that ultrasound disorganizes the stratum corneum lipid bilayers (35). Although several attempts have been made to enhance transdermal drug transport using therapeutic ultrasound, a typical enhancement induced by therapeutic ultrasound is about 10-fold or smaller. This enhancement may be sufficient for local delivery of certain drugs such as hydrocortisone, but in most cases it is not sufficient for the systemic delivery of many drugs. Accordingly, despite significant attention dedicated to sonophoresis, there have been no commercially available sonophoresis systems for systemic drug delivery.

C. High-Frequency Sonophoresis

Bommanan et al. (11,12) hypothesized that since the absorption coefficient of the skin varies directly with the ultrasound frequency, high-frequency ultrasound energy would concentrate more in the epidermis, thus leading to higher enhancements. In order to assess this hypothesis, they studied the effect of high-frequency ultrasound (2–15 MHz) on the permeability of salicylic acid (dissolved in a gel) through hairless guinea pig skin in vivo. They found that a 20-min application of ultrasound (0.2 W/cm^2) at a frequency of 2 MHz did not significantly enhance amount of salicylic acid penetrating the skin. However, 10 MHz ultrasound under otherwise like conditions resulted in about a 4-fold increase and 16 MHz ultrasound resulted in about a 2.5-fold increase in transdermal salicylic acid transport. They also found that transdermally delivered salicylic acid appears much sooner in the urine if driven by sonophoresis than by passive permeation. These researchers also found that an electron-dense tracer, such as lanthanum, was driven deep into the dermis by a 5-min application of high-frequency ultrasound in hairless mouse in vivo.

III. MECHANISM OF SONOPHORESIS

Various mechanisms of sonophoresis have been considered. A brief description of the mechanisms of sonophoresis in each frequency region is discussed below. First, we provide a brief description of various ultrasound-related phenomena that may play an important role in sonophoresis.

A. Thermal Effects

Absorption of ultrasound increases temperature of the medium (59). Materials that possess higher ultrasound absorption coefficients, such as bones, experience severe thermal effects compared to muscle tissues, which have a lower absorption coefficient. The absorption coefficient of a medium increases proportionally with the ultrasound frequency. The increase in the temperature of a medium upon ultrasound exposure at a given frequency varies proportionally with the ultrasound intensity and exposure time (59).

B. Acoustic Streaming

Acoustic streaming is the development of time-independent large fluid velocities in a medium under the influence of an ultrasound wave (59). The primary cause of acoustic streaming is ultrasound reflections and other distortions that occur during wave propagation. Oscillations of cavitation bubbles may also contribute to acoustic streaming. The shear stresses developed by streaming velocities may affect the neighboring structures.

C. Cavitational Effects

Cavitation is the formation of gaseous cavities in a medium upon ultrasound exposure. The primary cause of cavitation is ultrasound-induced pressure variations in the medium. Cavitation involves either rapid growth and collapse of a bubble (transient cavitation) or slow oscillatory motion of a bubble in an ultrasound field (stable cavitation) (59). Cavitation affects tissues in several ways. Specifically, collapse of cavitation bubbles releases a shock wave, which can cause structural alterations in its surroundings. Biological tissues contain numerous air pockets trapped in the fibrous structures which act as nuclei for cavitation upon ultrasound exposure. Accordingly, a significant cavitation activity is known to occur in biological tissues upon ultrasound exposure. The cavitational effects vary inversely with ultrasound frequency and directly with ultrasound intensity. Below we discuss the roles of these phenomena in sonophoresis.

1. Mechanism of Low-Frequency Sonophoresis

Tachibana et al. (49) hypothesized that application of low-frequency ultrasound generates acoustic streaming in the hair follicles and sweat ducts of the skin, thus leading to enhanced transdermal transport. Mitragotri et al. hypothesized that transdermal transport during low-frequency sonophoresis occurs across the keratinocytes rather than hair follicles (37). They provided the following hypothesis for the high efficacy of low-frequency sonophoresis. Cavitation induced by low-frequency ultrasound may cause disordering of the stratum corneum lipids. In addition, oscillations of cavitation bubbles may result in significant water penetration into the disordered lipid regions. This may cause the formation of aqueous channels through the intercellular lipids of the stratum corneum through which permeants may transport. Transdermal transport through aqueous channels across the disordered lipid regions may enhance transdermal transport compared to passive transport because (a) the diffusion coefficients of permeants through saline, which is likely to primarily occupy the channels generated by ultrasound, are up to 1000-fold higher than those through the ordered lipid bilayers, and (b) the transport pathlength of these aqueous channels may be much shorter (by a factor up to 25) than that through the tortuous intercellular lipids in the case of passive transport. This hypothesis also explains why low-frequency ultrasound can induce transdermal transport of drugs, which exhibit very low passive transport. Drugs possessing low passive permeabilities are either (a) hydrophilic, which makes their partitioning into the stratum corneum bilayers difficult, or (b) large in molecular size (e.g., proteins), which reduces their diffusion coefficients in the stratum corneum. Low-frequency ultrasound may overcome both of these limitations by providing aqueous transport channels across the skin. Since these channels are filled with saline, hydrophilic drugs can easily partition into the stratum corneum. In addition, diffusion of drugs through water is much faster than that through ordered lipid bilayer regions, thus allowing drugs to transport across the skin at a faster rate. Therefore, hydrophilic drugs or proteins may permeate skin with relative ease in the presence of low-frequency ultrasound.

2. Mechanism of Therapeutic Sonophoresis

Simmonin et al. (47) hypothesized that cavitation occurs in the follicles of the skin upon ultrasound exposure and enhances transdermal permeation by convective velocities through follicles. However, no evidence was presented to support this hypothesis. Mortimer et al. performed sonophoresis of oxygen across frog skin in vitro (41,42). They found that the sonophoretic enhancement of transdermal oxygen transport depends on ultrasound intensity rather than on pressure amplitude. They hypothesized that cavitation cannot be responsible for sonophoresis. They proposed that ultrasound enhances transport due to acoustic streaming in the solution around the skin. Levy et al. (58) suggested that sonophoretic transport across polymeric membranes is induced by cavitation and not by thermal effects. Mitragotri et al. (35) suggested that ultrasound exposure in the therapeutic range causes cavitation in the keratinocytes of the stratum corneum. Oscillations of the ultrasound-induced cavitation bubbles near the keratinocyte–lipid bilayer interfaces may, in turn, cause oscillations in the lipid bilayers, thereby causing structural disorder of the stratum corneum lipids. Shock waves generated by the collapse of cavitation bubbles at the interfaces may also contribute to the structure-disordering effect. Since diffusion of permeants through a disordered bilayer phase can be significantly higher than that through a normal bilayer, transdermal transport in the presence of ultrasound is expected to be higher than passive transport.

3. Mechanism of High-Frequency Sonophoresis

Bommanan et al. (11) performed sonophoresis of lanthanum tracers across hairless-mice skin at an ultrasound frequency of 16 MHz in order to understand the transport pathways during high-frequency sonophoresis. They observed the skin under the electron microscope after sonophoresis and found that 5 min of sonophoresis results in penetration of lanthanum tracers to dermal levels of the skin. They further reported that the tracer was patchily distributed within the intercellular lipid bilayers of the stratum corneum. They provided the following hypothesis for the mechanism of high-frequency sonophoresis: The micronuclei (air pockets) present in the stratum corneum oscillate in response to oscillating pressure fields of ultrasound and eventually collapse. The oscillations of these bubbles result in enhanced skin permeation. They also hypothesized that the patchy distribution of the lanthanum tracer revealed in the micrographs corresponds to the location of oscillating air pockets in the stratum corneum. In a later report, Menon et al. presented additional microscopic studies of the hairless-mice skin after undergoing sonophoresis of lanthanum tracer (34). They reported the presence of long confluent channels in the intercellular lipids filled with lanthanum tracers in the hairless-rat skin exposed to ultrasound. They presented the following hypothesis for the mechanism of sonophoresis: application of ultrasound opens and expands gas-filled cavities in the stratum corneum much like pumping air through a collapsed rubber tubing. Enhanced transport of drugs may then occur through these confluent channels across the stratum corneum.

IV. SYNERGISTIC EFFECT OF ULTRASOUND WITH CHEMICAL ENHANCERS

Chemical enhancers have been found to increase transdermal drug transport via several different mechanisms, including increased solubility of the drug in the donor formulation, increased partitioning into the stratum corneum, fluidization of the lipid bilayers, and disruption of the intracellular proteins (2). Detailed reviews of the effects of chemical enhancers on transdermal transport may be found in Ref. 2. Below we present a summary of the synergistic effect of ultrasound with chemical enhancers.

Johnson et al. (24) performed a study of the synergistic effect of therapeutic ultrasound (1 MHz, 2 W/cm^2) with a series of chemical enhancer formulations, including (a) PEG-200 dilaurate (PEG), (b) isopropyl myristate (IM), (c) glycerol trioleate (GT), (d) ethanol/pH 7.4 phosphate-buffered saline (PBS) in a 1:1 ratio (50% EtOH), (e) 50% EtOH saturated with linoleic acid (LA/EtOH), and (f) phosphate-buffered PBS, using corticosterone as a primary model drug. Additional drugs, including dexamethasone, estradiol, lidocaine, and testosterone, were used to test the generality of the conclusions. A combination of LA/EtOH and ultrasound was found to be the most effective of these enhancers. One way to estimate the total enhancement of transdermal transport induced by a combination of chemical enhancers and ultrasound is to calculate the flux from a saturated solution in that enhancer in the presence of ultrasound. This is presented in Table 1 for corticosterone enhancement from various enhancers. The table shows corticosterone solubility in each enhancer used in their study C^{sat}, permeability in the absence of ultrasound $P^{passive}$, flux from the saturated solution in the absence of ultrasound J^{sat}, permeability in the presence of ultrasound P^{US}, and the flux from the saturated solution in the presence of ultrasound J^{sat-US}. Table 1 shows that the use of LA/EtOH and therapeutic ultrasound yields a flux greater than or equal to $15{,}600 \times 10^{-5}$ mg/cm^2/h, which is more than two orders of magnitude greater than that from 50% EtOH with ultrasound, 90×10^{-5} mg/cm^2/h. Thus the combination of LA/EtOH with ultrasound increases the corticosterone flux from the saturated solutions by up

Table 1 Corticosterone Transdermal Transport Properties with Chemical Enhancers and Ultrasound

Enhancer	Solubility C^{sat} (mg/mL)	Steady-state permeability $P^{passive}$ (cm/h × 10^5) ± SEM	Saturated flux J^{sat} 5 $P \times C^{sat}$ (mg/cm^2/h × 10^5)	Permeability with ultrasound P_{us} (cm/h × 10^5) ± SEM	Sonophoretic saturated flux $J^{sat-US} = P_{us} \times C^{sat}$ (mg/cm^2/h × 10^5)
PBS	0.12	10 ± 11%	1.2	50 ± 23%	6.0
PEG-200 dilaurate	0.94	2.4 ± 17%	2.2	4.5 ± 14%	4.8
Isopropyl myristate	0.77	7.0 ± 22%	5.4	25 ± 19%	19.4
Glycerol trioleate	0.14	7.1 ± 17%	1.0	9.3 ± 21%	1.3
50% Ethanol 50% PBS	9.2	5.2 ± 12%	48	9.8 ± 11%	91.2
Linoleic acid in 50:50 Ethanol PBS	12.4	87 ± 14%	1080	≥1260 ± 20%	≥15,552

to 13,000-fold (LA/EtOH), relative to the passive flux from PBS. Possible mechanisms for the synergistic effect of ultrasound and therapeutic ultrasound are discussed below.

Ultrasound may drive linoleic acid into the skin over time. This would increase the linoleic acid levels in the stratum corneum, which would likely result in increased bilayer fluidity relative to the passive case. However, the rates of uptake of radiolabeled linoleic acid were nearly identical over 24 h (24), indicating that linoleic acid is not being driven into the skin at a significantly greater rate by ultrasound than as compared to the passive case.

Ultrasound may be aiding the dispersion of linoleic acid in the stratum corneum lipids. Previous studies have shown that fatty acids, such as oleic acid, form segregated phases within the stratum corneum. Under passive conditions, linoleic acid may also tend to diffuse into the stratum corneum and collect in pools. The cavitation produced by ultrasound may induce mixing and facilitate the dispersion of linoleic acid and the stratum corneum lipids. The increased entropy of the resulting mixed system would make it a more favorable molecular arrangement that would remain stable even after ultrasound is turned off.

Mitragotri et al. (60) have also performed an evaluation of the synergistic effect of low-frequency ultrasound (20 kHz) with surfactants including sodium lauryl sulfate (SLS) and a model permeant mannitol. Application of SLS alone, as well as of ultrasound alone, increased skin permeability. Application of SLS alone for 90 min induced about threefold increase in mannitol permeability, while application of ultrasound alone for 90 min induced about eightfold enhancement. However, when combined, application of ultrasound from 1% SLS solution induced about 200-fold increase in skin permeability to mannitol. We considered various possible mechanisms of this synergistic effect, including (a) SLS enhances ultrasound-induced cavitation, (b) ultrasound drives more SLS into the skin, and (c) ultrasound may enhance dispersion of SLS and the stratum corneum lipids. The latter two mechanisms were found to be dominant.

V. SYNERGISTIC EFFECT OF ULTRASOUND WITH ELECTROPORATION

Electroporation has been shown to enhance transdermal transport of a variety of drugs. Typical voltages used in electroporation range from 100 V to 1000 V. Application of short pulses of high voltage is believed to induce formation of short-lived pores in the skin, through which enhanced transdermal transport may occur (4,61). Kost et al. (28) performed an evaluation of the synergistic effect of therapeutic ultrasound (1 MHz, 2 W/cm^2) with electroporation. Application of ultrasound increased the steady-state transport flux during electroporation of two model molecules, calcein and sulforhodamine. This enhancement was twofold in the case of calcein and threefold in the case of sulforhodamine. Application of ultrasound also reduced transdermal calcein transport lag time, defined as the time required to reach the steady state, from a typical value of 15 min in the presence of electric field alone to about 9 min in the presence of ultrasound and electric field. In this respect, it is important to note that application of ultrasound at the same level alone does not enhance transdermal calcein or sulforhodamine flux. Application of ultrasound also reduced the threshold voltage for electroporation. In the absence of ultrasound this threshold was about 53 ± 3 V, and in the presence of ultrasound it is about 46 ± 3 V, indicating that application of ultrasound reduces slightly the threshold electroporation voltage. In addition, electroporating voltage required to achieve a given transdermal flux was found to be smaller in the presence of ultrasound. The authors performed a mechanistic analysis of the synergistic effect of ultrasound and electroporation.

The authors hypothesized that the synergistic effect of ultrasound and electroporation may also be related to cavitation induced by ultrasound exposure. To test this hypothesis they simultaneously exposed the skin to electric pulses (100 V across the skin, 1-ms exponential pulse applied every minute) and ultrasound (3 MHz, 1.5 W/cm^2). It is known that the cavitational effects vary inversely with ultrasound frequency. Exposure to ultrasound at 3 MHz (intensity = 1.5 W/cm^2) did not affect transdermal transport by electroporation, based on which the authors suggested that cavitation may play a major role in the synergistic effect of ultrasound and electroporation.

Cavitation may play a twofold role in enhancing the effect of electrical field on transdermal transport. First, oscillations of cavitation bubbles induce partial structural disordering of the skin's lipid bilayers. Since the electrical resistance of the disordered bilayers is likely to be smaller than that of the normal lipid bilayers, the applied voltage may concentrate preferentially across the normal bilayers. This may increase the transdermal transport of calcein and sulforhodamine. Second, the oscillations of cavitation bubbles may also induce convection across the skin. In order to assess the role of convection in the synergistic effect of ultrasound and electroporation, the authors measured transdermal calcein and sulforhodamine transport sequentially in the presence of electric fields alone, ultrasound and electric fields together, ultrasound alone, and in the absence of ultrasound and electroporation. The authors hypothesized that if electrophoresis plays an important role in calcein and sulforhodamine transport, the transdermal flux is likely to decrease rapidly after electric fields is turned off while ultrasound is kept on. On the other hand, if cavitation-induced convection plays an important role, transdermal flux would rapidly decrease after turning ultrasound off while keeping electric fields on. Indeed, calcein flux decreases rapidly after turning electric field off and achieved a value comparable to the background. When ultrasound was turned off, calcein flux decreased only by a small amount (compared to the reduction after turning electric) and thereafter it remained nearly at the background level. This suggests that calcein transport is mainly driven by electrical forces. On the other hand, convection appears to play an important role in transdermal sulforhodamine transport in the presence of ultrasound and electroporation since the sulforhodamine flux did not decrease rapidly electric fields were turned off but decreased instantaneously after ultrasound was turned off.

VI. CONCLUSION

Application of ultrasound enhances transdermal transport of drugs. Cavitation has been suggested to play a dominant role in sonophoresis. Ultrasound may enhance transdermal transport through affecting skin structure as well as through inducing active transport. Various other means of transport enhancement including chemicals, iontophoresis, and electroporation may enhance transport synergistically with ultrasound. Application of ultrasound enhances transdermal transport synergistically with various chemicals. Ultrasound also exhibited a synergistic effect with electroporation. Specifically, ultrasound reduced the threshold voltage for electroporation as well as increased transdermal transport at a given electroporating voltage. The enhancement of transdermal transport induced by the combination of ultrasound and electroporation was higher than that induced by the sum of the enhancement induced by each enhancer alone. Further studies should focus on detailed investigations of these synergistic effects.

REFERENCES

1. Bronaugh, R. L., and Maibach, H. I. 1989. Percutaneous Absorption, Marcel Dekker, New York, pp. pp 1–12.

2. Walters, K. A., and Hadgraft, J. 1993. Pharmaceutical Skin Penetration Enhancement, Marcel Dekker, New York.
3. Burnette, R. R. In: Transdermal Drug Delivery: Developmental Issues and Research Initiatives (Hadgraft, J., and Guy, R. H., eds), Marcel Dekker, New York, 1989, pp. 247–291.
4. Prausnitz, M. R., Bose, V., Langer, R., and Weaver, J. C. 1993. Proc. Natl. Acad. Sci. USA, 90, pp. 10504–10508.
5. Kost, J., and Langer, R. 1993. In: Topical Drug Bioavailability, Bioequivalence, and Penetration (Shah V. P., and Maibach, H. I., eds.), Plenum Press, New York, pp. 91–103.
6. Mitragotri, S., Blankschtein, D., and Langer, R. (1995). Science, 269, pp. 850–853.
7. Benson, H. A. E., McElnay, J. C., and Harland, R. 1988. Int. J. Pharm., 44, pp. 65–69.
8. Antich, T. J. 1982. J. Orth. Sports Phys. Ther., 4, pp. 99–102.
9. Benson, H. A. E., McElnay, J. C., and R., H. 1989. Phys. Ther., 69, pp. 113–118.
10. Benson, H. A. E., McElnay, J. C., and J., H. 1991. Pharm. Res., 9, pp. 1279–1283.
11. Bommannan, D., Menon, G. K., Okuyama, H., Elias, P. M., and Guy, R. H. 1992. Pharm. Res., 9, pp. 1043–1047.
12. Bommannan, D., Okuyama, H., Stauffer, P., and Guy, R. H. 1992. Pharm. Res., 9, pp. 559–564.
13. Cameroy, B. M., 1966. Am. J. Orthoped., 8, pp. 47.
14. Ciccone, C. D., Leggin, B. Q., and Callamaro, J. J. 1991. Phys. Ther., 71, pp. 666–678.
15. Davick, J. P., Martin, R. K., and Albright, J. P. 1988. Phys. Ther., 68, pp. 1672–1675.
16. Fellinger, K., and Schmidt, J. 1954. Maudrich Vienna, Austria, pp. 549–552.
17. Fogler, S., and Lund, K. 1993. J. Acous. Soc. Am., 53, pp. 59–64.
18. Griffin, J. E., and Touchstone, J., Am. J. Phys. Med., 44, pp. 20–25 (1965).
19. Griffin, J. E. 1966. J. Am. Phys. Ther. Assoc., 46, pp. 18–26.
20. Griffin, J. E., Echternach, J. L., Proce, R. E., and Touchstone, J., C. 1967. Phys. Ther., 47, pp. 600–601.
21. Griffin, J. E., and Touchstone, J. C. 1968. Phys. Ther., 48, pp. 1136–1344.
22. Griffin, J., E., and Touchstone, J. C., Am. J. Phys. Med., 51 (1972), pp. 62–78.
23. Howkins, S. S. 1969. Ultrasonics, 8, pp. 129–130.
24. Johnson, M. E., Mitragotri, S., Patel, A,., Blankschtein, D., and Langer, R. 1996. J. Pharm. Sci., 85, pp. 670–679.
25. Kleinkort, J. A., and Wood, F., Phys. Ther., 55 (1975), pp. 1320–1324.
26. Kost, J., Levy, D., and Langer, R. 1989. In: Percutaneous Absorption: Mechanisms, Methodology, Drug Delivery (Bronaugh, R., and Maibach, H. I., eds.), Marcel Dekker, New York, pp. 595–601.
27. Kost, J. 1993. Clin. Mater., 13, pp. 155–161.
28. Kost, J., Pliquett, U., Mitragotri, S., Yamamoto, A., Weaver, J., and Langer, R., 1996. Pharm. Res., 13, pp. 633–638.
29. Liu, L.-S., Kost, J., D'Emanuele, A., and Langer, R. 1992. Macromolecules, 25, pp. 123–128.
30. Machluf, M., and Kost, J. 1993. J. Biomater. Sci., 5, pp. 147–156.
31. McElnay, J. C., Matthews, M. P., Harland, R., and McCafferty, D. F. 1985. Br. J. clin. Pharmacol., 20, pp. 421–424.
32. McElnay, J. C., Kennedy, T. A., and R., H. 1987. Int. J. Pharm., 40, pp. 105–110.
33. McEnlay, J. C., Benson, H. A. E., Harland, R., and Hadgraft, J. 1993. Pharm. Res., 4, pp. 1726–1731.
34. Menon, G., Bommanon, D., and Elias, P. 1994. Skin Pharmacol., 7, pp. 130–139.
35. Mitragotri, S., Edwards, D., Blankschtein, D., and Langer, R. 1995, J. Pharm. Sci., 84, pp. 697–706.
36. Mitragotri, S., Blankschtein, D., and Langer, R., 1995. In: Encyclopedia of Pharmaceutical Technology (Swarbrick, J., and Boylan, J., eds.), Vol. 14, Marcel Dekker, New York.
37. Mitragotri, S., Blankschtein, D., and Langer, R., 1996. Pharm. Res., 13, pp. 411–420.
38. Mitragotri, S., Blankschtein, D., and Langer, R. 1997. J. Pharm. Sci., 86, pp. 1190–1192.
39. Mitragotri, S., Farrell, J., Tang, H., Terahara, T., Kost, J., and Langer, R., J. Control. Rel. 63: 41–52, 2000.
40. Miyzaki, S., Mizuoka, O., and Takada, M. 1990. J. Pharm. Pharmacol., 43, pp. 115–116.
41. Mortimer, A. J. and Maclean, J. A. 1986. J. Ultrasound Med., 5(Suppl), p. 137.

42. Mortimer, A. J., Trollope, B. J., and Roy, O. Z. 1988. Ultrasonics, 26, pp. 348–351.
43. Novak, E. J. 1964. Arch. Phys. Med. Rehab., May, pp. 231–232.
44. Policoff, L. D. 1982. Orthop. Clin. North Am., 13, pp. 579–586.
45. Pottenger, J. F., and Karalfa, L. B. 1989. Milit. Med., 154, pp. 355–358.
46. Quillen, W. S. 1980. Athelet. Train., 15, pp. 109–110.
47. Simonin, J. P. 1995. J. Control. Rel., 33, pp. 125–141.
48. Skauen, D. M. and Zentner, G. M. 1984. Int. J. Pharm., 20, pp. 235–245.
49. Tachibana, K. and Tachibana, S. 1991. J. Pharm. Pharmacol., 43, pp. 270–271.
50. Tachibana, K. 1992. Pharm. Res., 9, pp. 952–954.
51. Tachibana, K. and Tachibana, S. 1993. Anesthesiology, 78, pp. 1091–1096.
52. Williams, A. R. 1990. Ultrasonics, 28, pp. 137–141.
53. Wing, M. 1981. Phys. Ther., 62, pp. 32–33.
54. Newman, J. T., Nellermo, M. D., and Crnett, J. L. 1992. J. Am. Pod. Med. Assoc., 82, pp. 432–435.
55. Coodley, G. L. 1960. Am. Pract., 11, pp. 181–187.
56. Moll, M. A. 1978. US Armed Forces Med. Serv. Dig., 30, pp. 8–11.
57. Hofman, D., and Moll, F. 1993. J. Control. Rel., 27, pp. 187–192.
58. Levy, D., Kost, J., Meshulam, Y., and Langer, R. 1989. J. Clin. Invest., 83, pp. 2974–2078.
59. Suslick, K. S. 1989. Ultrasound: Its Chemical, Physical and Biological Effects, VCH, New York.
60. Mitragotri, S., Ray, D., Farrell, J., Tang, H., Yu, B., Kost, J., Blankschtein, D., and Langer, R., 1999. J. Pharm. Sci. (in press).
61. Chen, T. 1988. Ph.D. thesis, (1998).

31
Electrotransport Systems for Transdermal Delivery: A Practical Implementation of Iontophoresis

Erik R. Scott, J. Bradley Phipps, J. Richard Gyory, and Rama V. Padmanabhan
ALZA Corporation, Minneapolis, Minnesota

I. INTRODUCTION

Electrotransport (ET) refers to the use of an electric potential to aid movement of molecules through biological tissues such as skin. Use of ET for drug delivery offers advantages over traditional parenteral drug delivery: ET is painless and noninvasive. Electrotransport devices are small enough to be worn unobtrusively with few restrictions on patient activity, and because drug delivery is controlled by the applied electrical current, preprogrammed and on-demand delivery profiles are possible.

Currently, the therapeutic use of ET has been limited to the local topical administration of drugs such as lidocaine and dexamethasone phosphate. In addition to these therapeutic uses, commercially available systems exemplifying the diagnostic application of ET also exist, such as the CF Indicator® (Scandipharm, Birmingham, AL) and the Webster Sweat Inducer (Wescor, Inc., Logan, UT) for the detection of cystic fibrosis. Although these examples demonstrate the successful commercial use of ET technology for *topical* delivery of compounds, transdermal ET systems for *systemic* administration of medicinal agents remain in the developmental stages. There is, however, heightened interest in this field because of potential medical and economical benefits offered by this technology, especially for meeting the delivery challenges posed by new biotechnology compounds.

A schematic of a typical transdermal electrotransport system (ETS) is shown in Fig. 1. A source of electrical energy, such as a battery, supplies electric current to the body through two electrodes. The first electrode, called the donor electrode, delivers the therapeutic agent into the body. The second electrode, called the counterelectrode, closes the electrical circuit. Each electrode is placed in ion-transmitting relation with its associated ionically conductive reservoir, normally present as a hydrogel. The reservoirs are placed in contact with the patient's skin and contain either the drug (for the donor electrode assembly) or a pharmacologically inactive electrolyte (for the counterelectrode assembly).

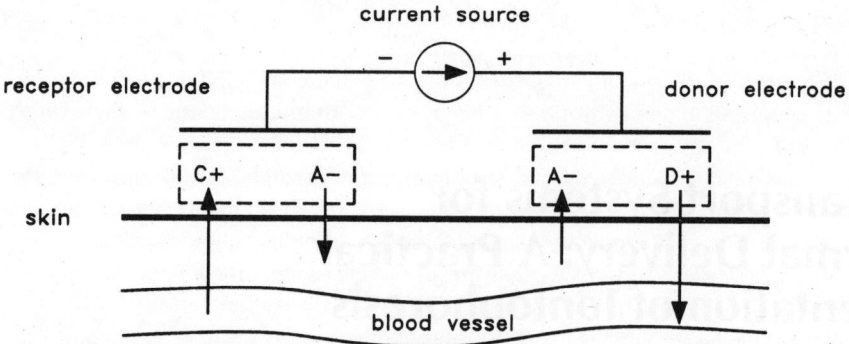

Figure 1 Schematic diagram of electrotransport device.

A. Overview of Electrotransport

This chapter focuses on the key aspects of transdermal ET system development, rather than presenting an overall review of ET technology. For a broad review of electrically controlled drug delivery, the reader is referred to a recent text by A. J. Banga (Banga, 1998) as well as the chapter by the same author contained in this volume. The greatest attention is paid to the most popular use of electrotransport, that of electromigration (also termed iontophoresis) for the delivery of drugs. The chapter begins with a discussion of two critical components of an electrotransport system: the electrodes and the formulation. These sections present a broad overview of existing technologies, as comprehensive reviews of these two subject areas are currently unavailable in the open literature. Then aspects of system integration and design are discussed, and finally clinical case studies that illustrate the successful implementation of these designs are presented.

The general term electrotransport encompasses several processes for moving molecules across the skin: electromigration, electro-osmosis, and electroporation. Electromigration is the movement of charged ionic species in response to an applied electrical field. This process is useful for delivering charged drug species. Electro-osmosis is the entrainment of bulk liquid, including species dissolved within it, by charged ions moving in an electric field. This process is useful for delivering both neutral and charged drug species. Electroporation is the temporary creation of aqueous pores through lipid bilayers by applying high-voltage pulses, e.g., approximately 50–1000 V, across the bilayers (Prausnitz et al., 1995; Zevert et al., 1995). This process is useful for delivering hydrophilic drug species. In any given ET system, one or more of these processes may occur simultaneously and to a different extent.

In addition to delivering substances *into* the body, ET may also be used to collect substances that are released *from* the body for subsequent diagnostic purposes. This is often referred to as reverse iontophoresis or reverse electro-osmosis. One example of reverse electro-osmosis is the collection and analysis of glucose from interstitial fluid of the skin for treatment of diabetes (Rao et al., 1995).

This chapter focuses on the design and formulation of ET systems that maximize drug delivery by electromigration. The movement of charges during electromigration is illustrated in Fig. 1. In this schematic, positively charged drug (D^+) and its counterion (A^-) are formulated for delivery from the anodic donor reservoir. The cathodic counterreservoir contains biologically acceptable cations (C^+) and anions (A^-). When current flows, drug ions migrate into the skin and endogenous chloride ions (Cl^-), migrate from the body into the donor reservoir. Simultaneously at the cathodic counterelectrode, anions migrate from the counterreservoir into the skin, while endogenous cations such as Na^+ migrate from the body into the counterreservoir. Note that local electroneutrality is preserved at all times throughout this process.

The therapeutic agent in ET systems must cross the skin, the body's natural barrier to foreign substances. The outermost layer of the skin, known as the stratum corneum, is the primary barrier to permeation of substances both into and out of the body. The stratum corneum's excellent barrier properties result from its unique structure: approximately 10–20 layers of flattened, keratin-rich cells bound together by lipid bilayers. In general, lipophilic species are capable of traversing the stratum corneum because of their ability to partition into the intercellular lipid region. However, most ionic substances that are likely candidates for ET are largely excluded from this region

With the relatively moderate voltages used in iontophoresis (e.g., 2–30 V), the nature and composition of the pathways in the skin remain matters of some debate. However, there is a growing body of evidence that the path of least resistance across stratum corneum is not spatially homogenous but rather consists of a distribution of localized regions (Cullander, 1992). These regions include endogenous shunt-like structures across the stratum corneum such as sweat ducts and hair follicles, but may also include pathways not associated with natural shunts. Direct physical measurements of the transport of model permeants through the skin of hairless and nude mice have shown that between 60% and 90% of the overall flux can be explained by such regions (Scott et al., 1995, 1993). Evidence also suggests that the opening of these shunt pathways may be reversible, provided the voltage threshold on the order of 1 to 10 V is not exceeded (Membrino et al., 1997).

For the delivery of charged drug substances by ET, the rate of transport is expressed by the Nernst–Planck equation. This equation contains terms for diffusion, electromigration, and bulk convection. However, under optimized ET conditions the electromigration contribution is often much greater than that of the other two, so the expression for delivery of a drug species is frequently simplified to include only the electromigration term. The mass flow of drug is thus related to the electric current, according to Faraday's principle:

$$N = (t_d IM)/(z_d F) \tag{1}$$

where

N = total rate of delivery (mol/s)
t_d = transport number (fraction of charge carried by drug)
I = current applied across skin
M = molecular weight
z_d = charge of drug molecule, and
F = Faraday's constant

It has been demonstrated experimentally that the rate of delivery is linearly proportional to the applied current over a wide range of currents (Phipps et al., 1989a). This indicates that, for a fixed drug formulation, t_d is a constant. However, the transport number is unique for each drug and is a function of the drug's mobility, charge, and concentration, as compared with those of other migrating species. This is expressed by the following formula:

$$t_d = \frac{\mu_d |Z_d| C_d}{\sum_i u_i |z_i| C_i} \tag{2}$$

where μ_d, z_d, and C_d are the mobility, charge, and molar concentration, respectively, of the drug species, and μ_i, z_i, and C_i are the mobility, charge, and concentration for each mobile ion that competes with the drug for transport across the skin barrier. Competing ions are those in the formulation that have the same sign of charge as the drug (i.e., competing co-ions), as well as those ions in the body that have the opposite sign as the drug (competing counterions).

The transport number determines delivery efficiency, i.e., the amount of drug delivered per unit charge passed across the skin. Because it is desirable to minimize current (for optimal biocompatibility and battery longevity), it is advantageous to develop a formulation that maximizes t_d. This can be accomplished by maximizing the mobility and concentration of drug species while minimizing—to the greatest extent possible—the mobility and concentration of the competing species. Simple measures to achieve this include incorporating the highest practical concentration of the drug in the formulation, as well as avoiding salts that produce mobile co-ions in the formulation. Even if both of these measures are taken, a t_d value of unity is still unattainable in practice because of endogenous counterions in tissue (e.g., Na^+ and Cl^-). However, the effect of competing counterions can be minimized by exploiting the skin's permselectivity. Permselectivity arises from the Donnan exclusion effect. The skin has an isoelectric point of about pH 4 (Rosendahl, 1942); a formulation pH below this value will result in increased transport of anions, and a formulation pH above this value will result in increased transport of cations. Thus, at physiological pH, skin is expected to be cation-selective.

II. ELECTRODES

A. Function and Overview of Requirements

The role of the electrodes in an ET system is to apply the driving force for ion migration across the skin. Electrodes are critical components of the overall system; serving as the bridge between the electric circuit and the drug formulation, they have both electrical and chemical functions. During ET therapy, electrodes undergo sustained chemical reactions; thus, the supply and removal of reactants need to be considered by the designer. ET electrodes are different from most other medical electrodes in this aspect. For example, medical potentiometric electrodes (such as those used for electrocardiograms or electroencephalograms) undergo no net reaction because no current is passed by the measurement equipment. In other applications such as cardiac pacing or transcutaneous electrical nerve stimulation (TENS), the applied voltage pulses are extremely brief (milliseconds or less), so the quantity of reaction products is not great, and therefore practical management of electrochemical reactions is achieved merely by constructing the electrodes from inert materials. With ET electrodes, however, inherently reactive materials are often deliberately chosen for reasons that will be described below. Because of their reactivity, and because electrodes contact the drug formulation directly and the patient's body indirectly, it can be a challenge to choose an electrode system that possesses adequate performance while avoiding adverse material and biological interactions during storage and use.

An ET system requires two electrodes: The donor (also known as the delivery or active) electrode contacts the drug reservoir. The counterelectrode (also known as the return or auxiliary electrode) contacts the counterreservoir and provides a return path for the current. The two reservoirs are separated from each other and contact skin over some known area. The electrodes apply an electric field across the skin by converting electric current (supplied by the battery) into ionic current (through the skin and body). In doing so, a faradaic reaction takes place at the electrode–electrolyte interface. As described previously in this chapter, there is a linear dependence of delivery on this current.

The polarity of the donor and counterelectrodes depends on the sign of the charge on the species to be delivered. To cause migration of positively charged species from the delivery reservoir, the donor electrode is the anode, and the counterelectrode is the cathode. For negatively charged species, the polarity is reversed, i.e., the delivery electrode is the cathode, and the counter is the anode.

A practical electrode system must meet a variety of performance, compatibility, and physical requirements (Cullander et al., 1993; Phipps, 1997b). It should not interfere with the delivery efficiency of the drug (amount of drug delivered per unit current), and it should operate at low voltage, have adequate longevity, and distribute the current evenly over the skin surface. The electrode will not interfere with the delivery efficiency of the drug if it does not contain or produce any competing ions (i.e., mobile ions of like sign as the drug species). For optimum compatibility, the electrode should be made of materials that are nontoxic and compatible with other formulation components (e.g., drug and other excipients), and should avoid generating reaction products that are toxic.

The two classes of electrode are nonconsumable and consumable. Nonconsumable electrodes are made from nonreactive materials, whereas consumable electrodes contain electroactive species that react during the passage of current.

B. Nonconsumable Electrodes

Early ET systems used materials that were not consumed during use. Commonly used materials included metals such as stainless steel or platinum (Tyle, 1986; Lindblad and Ekenvall, 1987). Although these nominally inert materials may have long lifetimes, they also have significant shortcomings.

The operation of an ET system necessitates redox reactions at the electrodes in proportion to the amount of charge passed. For nonconsumable electrodes, which contact an essentially aqueous electrolyte solution in an ET application, electrolysis of water is the likely redox reaction. The reaction at the anode is the following:

$$2H_2O \rightarrow 4H^+ + O_2\uparrow + 4e^- \qquad (E^0 = 1.229 \text{ V}) \qquad (3)$$

At the cathode, the prevalent steady-state reaction is the following:

$$2H_2O + 2e^- \rightarrow 2OH^- + H_2\uparrow \qquad (E^0 = -0.828 \text{ V}) \qquad (4)$$

Both of these reactions have a number of undesired consequences. The generation of H^+ and OH^-, according to Eq. 1 and 2, can shift the formulation pH, affecting both delivery efficiency (due to a shift in the skin permselectivity, formation of competitive ions, or alteration of the charge state of the drug) and skin tolerability. The gases that are produced can accumulate on the electrode or skin surface, interfering with the uniformity of current distribution. Furthermore, because these reactions take place at relatively high voltage, there is high power consumption and a risk of electrolytic decomposition of the drug or other excipients.

Nominally nonconsumable electrodes made from nonnoble metals, such as stainless steel, can release metal ions through direct oxidation at the anode, or indirectly by the creation of a caustic environment at the cathode. For example, nickel and chromium ions were found to be released from a medical-grade steel anode following a few minutes of iontophoresis at 400 $\mu A/cm^2$. These ions can be toxic to the body (Lindblad et al., 1986).

Chemical methods that mitigate the deleterious effects of unwanted reaction products can be divided into three categories: blocking their migration; neutralizing (e.g., buffering) them; and preventing their formation by inclusion of sacrificial redox species in the electrolyte. Blocking is achieved by isolating the electrolyte adjacent to the electrode from the drug formulation or from the body by using ion exchange or size-selective membranes or coatings (Sanderson and Deriel, 1988; Phipps, 1991; Haak, 1996). For example, an anion-selective coating at a nonconsumable electrode—methacrylamidopropyltrimethylammonium chloride copolymerized with methyl methacrylate—was found to prevent degradation of oxymorphone at electrode potentials up to 800 mV (Phipps, 1997b).

Buffering agents can partially compensate for the generation of acid and base, but their duration of efficacy (buffering capacity) is limited by the quantity of buffer species present, and the addition of excess buffer salts can result in ionic competition. Ion exchange polymers can effectively scavenge, neutralize, and immobilize generated reaction products (Sanderson and Deriel, 1988; Johnson and Lee, 1990); the advantage over simple buffer salts is that the polymer chains are immobile and therefore noncompeting.

Electrochemical methods can also be used to improve the function of nonconsumable electrodes. One method is to use electroactive counterions (Untereker et al., 1992). Alternatively, other soluble redox-active species can be incorporated into the electrolyte, such as metal salts of ferrocyanides (Phipps and Untereker, 1988) and hydroquinone (Lai et al., 1996). Another electrochemical way to manage acid and base generated at nonconsumable electrodes is using the weak acid or base form of the drug (Untereker et al., 1992). For example, the base form of the drug can be formulated in the electrolyte contacting the anode. Hydrogen ions generated by the anode will protonate the drug, creating drug cations that are subsequently delivered into the body by electromigration. Yet another means to manage acid or base production is to incorporate a set of secondary electrodes into the delivery or return reservoir that release H^+ or OH^- as needed to neutralize the acid or base generated by the primary electrodes (Phipps, 1997a).

C. Consumable Electrodes

As described above, design approaches have been devised for resolving the disadvantages of nonconsumable electrodes. While many of these schemes are simple in principle, their practical implementation becomes complex because of various physical, chemical, and biological requirements. An often simpler alternative is to use consumable electrodes. Also known as sacrificial electrodes, they contain redox species that undergo faradaic reaction during operation. Appropriate consumable electrodes will have redox reactions that take place at low potentials to avoid causing parasitic reactions (e.g., electrolysis of water, drug, or excipients) at the electrode surface. Also, the reactants and products of the redox reaction need to be managed in order to meet formulation and biological compatibility requirements.

A sacrificial electrode has a finite operational lifetime, or capacity, defined as the amount of charge that can be passed before the reactants are effectively depleted. The capacity of an electrode can be empirically determined, or it can be calculated from the following equation:

$$Q = \frac{umnF}{3.6M} \tag{5}$$

where

Q = capacity (mAh)
u = utilization (fraction of reacting species available for reaction)
m = mass of reactant (g)
n = number of equivalents of charge per mole of reactant (eq/mol)
F = Faraday's constant (96485 Coul/eq)

M = molecular weight of the reactant (g/mol), and the constant 3.6 is a conversion factor (Coul/mAh)

If depletion results in an open circuit, the electrode will cease to function. Otherwise, if an electrically conductive pathway remains, the electrode will continue to function under suboptimal conditions (i.e., at a higher voltage where other redox reactions, such as water electrolysis, take place).

It is advantageous to use materials and structures that achieve maximum utilization of the reactants, as this allows the electrodes to be thin while making the most economical use of the consumable reactant. Factors that limit utilization include a tendency for passivation of the active component (by formation of a uniform, insoluble, nonconductive product over the active surface), and formation of "islands" (electrical isolation of one or more active portions by nonuniform current distribution).

No single consumable electrode is ideal for all ET applications. Different materials meet different capacity needs, and because consumable electrodes consist of chemically reactive species, certain materials may be compatible with certain drugs or excipients but not all of them. The most popular electrodes are based on the silver/silver chloride redox couple. Silver and silver chloride have several advantageous characteristics: they are biocompatible, they perform well, and they have an established history of use in medical applications including sensing electrodes (e.g., electrocardiogram).

D. Silver as a Consumable Anode

The use of a silver anode in the presence of chloride or another halide ion in the electrolyte solution is an elegant solution to the electrode design problem for positively charged drugs.

Metallic silver anodically oxidizes according to the following reaction:

$$Ag(s) \leftrightarrow Ag^+ (aq) + e^- \qquad (E^0 = 0.800 \text{ V}) \qquad (6)$$

However, when chloride is present, it immediately coprecipitates with the silver ion according to the following:

$$Ag^+ (aq) + Cl^- (aq) \leftrightarrow AgCl(s) \qquad (K_{sp} = 1.78 \times 10^{-10} \text{ mol}^2/\text{kg}^2) \qquad (7)$$

The complete reaction is therefore:

$$Ag(s) + Cl^- (aq) \leftrightarrow AgCl(s) + e^- \qquad (E^0 = 0.222 \text{ V}) \qquad (8)$$

The final product, silver chloride, is electrically neutral and practically insoluble. Therefore, this system doesn't generate species that compete with cationic drugs for delivery. Because the equilibrium potential is low and the reaction is kinetically fast, the silver anode operates at low voltage, avoiding undesirable side reactions such as water splitting or electrochemical degradation of the drug or excipients. The rapid reaction kinetics and immobility of silver chloride make the system highly reversible. A reversible electrode system is especially attractive in an alternating-polarity ET system (i.e., one in which the drug is present in both electrode reservoirs and is delivered alternately from each as the current is reversed) (Lattin and Spevak, 1983). The electrode is effectively discharged on one phase of the cycle and recharged on the other phase, leading to extended capacity (Sage and Flower, 1995; Muller and Saunal, 1998).

Oxidation of silver to silver chloride does have some limitations. For example, the silver surface of the electrode gradually passivates as the silver chloride layer builds up, causing an increase in discharge voltage with use. This polarization process limits both the maximum allowable current density and the utilization of silver.

E. Chloride Ion Management with Silver Anodes

For the silver anode to work optimally, there must be sufficient chloride ion present to react with the silver ion. When the anode functions as a counterelectrode, there is little consequence to adding sodium chloride to the electrolyte for this purpose. However, when the anode is the donor electrode (i.e., delivers positively charged drugs), the addition of extraneous salts can lead to ion competition and reduced delivery efficiency. The preferred form of a cationic drug is therefore a chloride salt of the form DCl (where D is the drug species) (Phipps and Untereker, 1988; Untereker et al., 1996). Not all drug substances are normally obtained as chloride salts, but many can be converted to the chloride form by ion exchange or to the hydrochloride salt form by protonation of amine groups through addition of HCl.

Because chloride ion is consumed as it precipitates with silver ions, its concentration decreases over time as the electrode is used. Chloride must be present in the electrolyte in sufficient quantity to ensure proper operation of the electrode throughout the therapy. If the concentration of chloride drops to the point where chloride can no longer scavenge the free silver ions, there is the potential for silver to be delivered to the skin. Silver is considered to have minor toxicity, but significant delivery of silver to the skin can lead to permanent gray-blue local discoloration of tissue, a condition known as *argyria* (Hollinger, 1996). If a drug chloride salt is used, a simple method to ensure sufficient chloride content is to incorporate an excess amount of the drug salt. This method, while practical for inexpensive drugs, may be cost-prohibitive for expensive compounds such as peptides.

The amount of bulk chloride in the electrolyte required to avoid silver migration depends on many design factors, including the volume of the electrolyte, current density, duration of operation, the rate at which chloride is replenished from the body (i.e., the chloride transport number), and the conformation of the electrode and hydrogel. Because interaction among these factors is often complex, it is difficult to construct a generalized model purely from first principles. Rather, for a given electrode/matrix combination, it is often simpler to determine the threshold chloride concentration at which silver migration occurs and to then use a mass balance to compute the required starting composition. A helpful indicator of silver migration is the potential of the polarized silver electrode. As chloride becomes less abundant, the silver anode voltage increases in a nernstian fashion. Empirically, it has been found that operation of the anode above approximately 400 mV (vs. Ag/AgCl standard reference electrode) can lead to release of free silver ions (Phipps, 1997b).

If it is impossible to use the chloride salt of a drug or impractical to include it in the amount required to prevent silver migration, then two alternative methods can prevent the onset of silver migration without introducing mobile cations into the delivery reservoir. One is to block the silver by using anion-selective membranes or coatings, or chelating agents. Another is to precipitate the silver using chloride ion–containing resins (e.g., those with quaternary ammonium chloride functionality) in the gel matrix (Phipps et al., 1996).

F. Silver Chloride as a Consumable Cathode

The silver chloride cathode is depicted in Eq. 8 in reverse; silver chloride is reduced to form metallic silver and chloride ion. The silver chloride cathode shares many of the qualities of the silver anode, with some additional desirable traits: no electrolyte is depleted by its reaction; it is hydrophilic and therefore easily accessible by electrolyte; and the insoluble reaction product, metallic silver, is electrically conductive, eliminating problems of polarization or isolation of the redox species. Because of this combination of properties, the operating voltage of silver chloride decreases with use, and the utilization of a silver chloride cathode is frequently 100%.

Performance issues associated with the silver chloride cathode include the following: It is a poor electrical conductor and thus requires the addition of a current collector, and it releases chloride ions during use, which can compete with anionic drug species for delivery. Formulation compatibility issues can also arise with silver chloride cathodes, resulting from the formation of a small amount of silver ion. Silver ion is a moderate oxidizer (E^0 for the Ag/Ag^+ couple is 0.800 V), and it can bind to protein drugs (Merril, 1990). If an incompatibility exists between the drug or excipients and low concentrations of free silver, there are other options for using the two entities in the same product. One is to separate the silver chloride from the incompatible ingredient using a membrane. Another is to fabricate a "dry" matrix in which no water is introduced into the system until immediately before use. Various methods of hydrating dry matrices at the point of use have been proposed (Gyory and Peery, 1996).

Operation of the silver chloride cathode can lead to an accumulation of chloride ions in the electrolyte. When the electrode is a counterelectrode, chloride buildup is not problematic. However, for donor electrodes, the chloride ion is highly mobile compared with most drug species. Thus, the accumulation of chloride ion can lead to decreased drug flux because of ionic competition. For short-duration applications, this effect may be negligible. However, if the molar concentration of chloride approaches some appreciable fraction of that of the drug, competition will occur. A simple yet not always practical way to remain below this threshold fraction is to increase drug content. The amount of increase can be computed from a mass balance. The chloride accumulation rate is determined by the current, according to Faraday's law, and this can be compared with the drug content, which decreases linearly over time as drug is delivered to the body.

If there is no practical way to increase the drug content by a sufficient amount to avoid competition, then measures should be taken to immobilize the chloride ion. Such measures are analogous in principle to those described previously for preventing migration of other undesirable reaction products (membranes or coatings that physically block or chemically bind the chloride). For example, a cation-selective membrane located between the cathode electrolyte and the drug-containing reservoir will prevent chloride from mixing with the drug (Phipps, 1992). Just as the low solubility of silver chloride can be exploited to prevent silver migration from the anode by using polymers with quaternary ammonium chloride functionality, polymers having silver-exchanged carboxylic acid groups (i.e., R—COOAg) can be used to bind free chloride (Lai et al., 1996).

G. Beyond Silver and Silver Chloride

Other redox couples can have advantages over silver and silver chloride in some circumstances. The most obvious shortcoming of the silver/silver chloride couple is the competitive chloride ion formation effect when silver chloride is reduced. An alternative cathode could use a salt consisting of a reducible transition metal ion and a large polymeric anion. The immobile anion does not compete with the drug for delivery. An example of this system is Cu-AMPS (AMPS = acrylamidomethylpropanesulfonate). This electrode has been shown to deliver ketoprofen without the steady decrease in flux over time that is associated with silver chloride (Fig. 2) (Phipps, 1997b).

Electroactive polymers such as polyaniline and intercalation compounds such as sodium tungstate have also been proposed. With such systems, redox reaction of the host material is accompanied by incorporation of anions from the electrolyte. This is directly analogous to the capture of chloride during the oxidation of silver in that no competitive ions are formed. Convenient species to be available for capture would be biocompatible counterions of the drug such as sodium and chloride. Other noncompeting chloride ion sources were mentioned previously

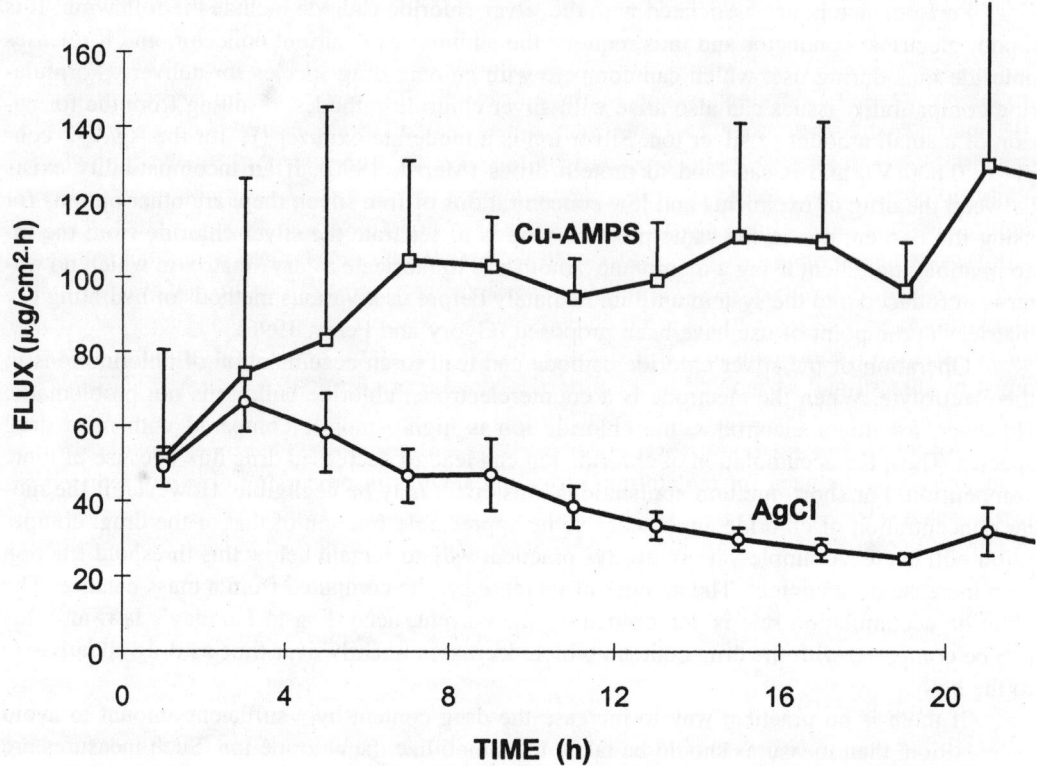

Figure 2 Comparison of in vitro flux of the anionic drug ketoprofen through human epidermis for Cu-AMPS and AgCl cathodes. Although the flux is identical for the two electrodes at early time points, it decreases within 5 h with the AgCl cathode, whereas no decrease is observed with Cu-AMPS. (Data from Phipps, 1997.)

in Section II. E. For a sodium ion source that presents no competing mobile anion species, sodium salts of ion exchange resins (e.g., Na-AMPS) can be used (Phipps and Untereker, 1988; Phipps et al., 1996).

H. Electrode Construction

In addition to the chemical aspects described above, the physical construction of electrodes can influence performance and biocompatibility. The exact design is driven by the application but some general principles can be applied. For example, in order to apply current evenly across the skin, the electrode should contact the entire area of the hydrogel, distal to the body. This naturally drives the design toward planar geometry. For electrodes that are more than a few square centimeters in area, the mechanical properties become important: a flexible electrode is less obtrusive when worn than one that is stiff.

Some electrode materials have desirable chemical and mechanical properties in their pure form. An example is silver, which can be formed into a thin foil. Silver's excellent electrical conduction lends uniform current distribution, and its high degree of flexibility allows it to be worn comfortably by the patient. If the delivery current density is higher than that which can be sustained by a planar foil, the surface area can be increased (and thus the current density at the electrode surface reduced) by using a silver screen or mesh (Phipps and Untereker, 1988).

Functional silver chloride–coated cathodes can be produced by anodic reaction of silver in the presence of chloride or by dip coating (Reddy, 1998). However, such layers are very brittle, inconvenient to produce, and subject to delamination from the silver unless the layers are very thin. An alternative to this approach is to make a composite film. Finely divided silver chloride powder can be cast in a film containing a polymeric binder and conductive filler, resulting in a flexible film with requisite electrical conductivity and electrochemical capacity. Films of adequate flexibility can be produced with silver chloride loading up to 40 vol %, yielding very thin materials with high capacity. For example, an electrode so constructed, with a thickness of only 0.015 cm, has been demonstrated to operate for 24 hours at a current density of 100 $\mu A/cm^2$ (equivalent to 2.4 mAh/cm^2) (Myers and Stahl, 1992). Foils or composite films must be die-cut and assembled into gel housings, with provisions for electrical connection to the current source.

An alternative method using a specialized type of composite electrode, i.e., the ink electrode, obviates the need for die cutting, providing savings in processing time and reduced material waste (Sibalis, 1989; Gyory, 1996; Jacobs and De Nuzzio, 1994). An ink consisting of the electroactive component (e.g., silver and/or silver chloride powder) is dispersed in a polymeric binder with a volatile solvent. The ink is then deposited in a pattern on a substrate using a variety of printing methods such as screen, gravure, or flexographic, followed by a thermal curing step. Ink electrodes are commonly used for other medical applications such as electrocardiography (Hoffman, 1987).

Additives can be used in composites. Hydrophilic agents can also be added to improve utilization by increasing the ability of electrolyte to gain access to electroactive components embedded in the polymer matrix (Myers and Stahl, 1992; Reddy, 1998). Also, ionic polymers, whose functions have been described earlier, can be formulated directly into the composite material rather than being used as coatings or gel components (Lai et al., 1996).

Other intriguing electrode structures have been disclosed in the patent literature. A plurality of closely spaced but electrically isolated electrodes can be activated in sequence, reportedly to improve biocompatibility of iontophoretic treatment (Sage, 1994). The anode and cathode materials can be chosen to form a galvanic couple (e.g., zinc/manganese dioxide) that provides a driving voltage for drug delivery without the need for an external battery (Horstmann, 1997). However, because of the potential stability window for water, the potential generated by such a system is limited to about 2 V. Because the skin has high electrical resistance, on the order of 10^4 ohm cm^2 (Scott et al., 1993), the voltage provided by such a couple may be too low to provide a therapeutic dosage. In an interesting variation on the intercalation electrodes, the drug itself may be formulated as a dopant ion in the redox polymer electrode and subsequently released during the redox reaction (Miller et al., 1986). While all of the above methods present interesting possibilities, the benefits of such constructions in practical delivery systems remain to be proved.

III. FORMULATION DEVELOPMENT

In an electrotransport system, the formulation refers to the ingredients in the drug gel and counter gel reservoir, which consist minimally of the solvent, the drug salt, and the hydrogel base polymer. A formulation may also include additives such as buffers, antimicrobial agents, antioxidants, and additional electrolyte salts or permeation enhancers. All of these can interact in a complex fashion to affect rate of delivery, biocompatibility, and product shelf life.

A. Solvent Selection

Drug solubility and stability, in addition to solvent biocompatibility, are obvious considerations when selecting a solvent for a pharmaceutical formulation. For an ET system, the effect of a solvent on the drug charge state is also an important consideration. Although a neutral drug molecule can be transported to the skin by electro-osmosis (Pikal, 1992), maximal drug delivery efficiency is usually achieved if the drug has a net electrical charge. For this reason, polar solvents with large dielectric constants are preferred. For example, the dielectric constants of water, glycerol, and ethanol are 80, 42, and 24, respectively. Use of solvents with large dielectric constants results in greater dissociation of the drug salt (i.e., less ion pairing), enhancing drug mobility during application of an electric field.

Because of its large dielectric constant and inherent biocompatibility, water is the most commonly used solvent in formulations for ET systems. Other cosolvents, such as ethanol, glycerol, polyethylene glycol, or polypropylene glycol, may be added to enhance drug solubility and drug stability, or to reduce the rate of water evaporation. Sanderson and colleagues (1989) used a 40:60 mixture of water and ethanol to enhance the solubility of dobutamine hydrochloride and demonstrated a twofold enhancement in dobutamine flux. However, addition of a cosolvent to enhance drug solubility may in some cases decrease the rate of delivery by electromigration if excessive ion pairing results.

Jadoul and co-workers (1997) studied the effect of adding ethanol and propylene glycol (PG) to aqueous solutions of fentanyl and metoprolol. They reported that drug flux was diminished by up to 80% for solutions containing 60% v/v ethanol or PG. A fourfold drop in formulation conductance was also measured, indicating that more ion association was occurring in the cosolvents. In addition, the solvent may have a direct effect on the skin, thus altering its permeability to drug ions (Gupta et al., 1994). In summary, the effect of a solvent or cosolvent on the drug solubility, ion interactions, and skin permeability are relevant when developing the formulation for an ETS.

B. Drug Salt Selection

In addition to the usual solubility, stability, and biocompatibility considerations, several unique aspects should be considered when selecting the drug salt for an ETS formulation. First, the counterion must be compatible with the electrochemical reactions occurring at the electrode. As noted in Section II, halide drug salts are preferred when using a silver anode. For example, fentanyl citrate is used in intravenous formulations, but citrate does not form an insoluble salt with electrochemically generated silver cation. For this reason, a formulation containing fentanyl hydrochloride was specifically developed for use in a patient-activated ETS for treatment of pain (Lattin et al., 1997). Clinical results using this formulation strategy are summarized in Section V.

As mentioned previously, it is important to consider the extent of drug salt dissociation when selecting a solvent. Therefore, for a particular solvent (e.g., water), selection of a drug salt that more fully dissociates will likely result in more efficient drug delivery. Using aqueous solutions of the acetate, sulfate, and hydrochloride salts of morphine, a correlation between drug salt dissociation and transdermal delivery has been observed (Corish et al., 1990). From conductance measurements it was determined that morphine hydrochloride was more fully dissociated in water than were the sulfate and acetate salts. The rate of morphine delivery, at currents ranging from 0.1 to 1 mA, was about 60% greater for the hydrochloride salt than for the sulfate and acetate salts.

Ion mobility (the velocity achieved by an ion per unit electric field) is largely determined by its ionic charge and by the extent of its physical interaction with the formulation or skin. The mobilities of a drug ion and its counterion in a formulation are likely to be different from their mobilities in the skin. In addition, the mobilities of ions that are endogenous in the skin (e.g., Na^+, K^+, Cl^-, HCO_3^-) are likely to be different in the two environments. Therefore, during electrotransport the ionic composition of the formulation in the vicinity of the skin can be substantially different than in the initial bulk composition (Burnette, 1989). As a result, it has been suggested that the drug counterion can alter the pH of the interface between the formulation and the skin, and thus alter transport efficiency (Sanderson et al., 1989). A twofold enhancement in transport efficiency for the succinate salts of verapamil, gallopamil, and nalbuphine relative to the hydrochloride salts was reported. This result was attributed to the ability of the weakly acidic succinate anion to buffer the boundary layer near the skin surface at about pH 4.8, thus avoiding significant hydronium ion competition.

The examples cited above illustrate that the drug salt can have a profound effect on drug transport from an ETS. Those developing an optimal formulation must therefore assess the effect of the drug counterion on system performance.

C. Matrix Selection

Use of drug dissolved in a liquid solvent is generally adequate for in vitro experimentation but is not optimal for use in a commercial product. Not only must the formulation be biocompatible, but it must also be readily incorporated into the ETS during commercial scale manufacturing, be easily applied by the user, and leave little or no residue on the skin. To achieve these goals, two fundamentally different matrix-based formulation strategies have been adopted for use in ETS.

In one approach, the drug solution is placed on an absorbent porous material. Candidate materials for these ET systems include hydrophilic fabrics composed of polyester or nylon, and hydrophilic porous films composed of polyurethane, polyvinyl alcohol (PVOH), or cellulose acetate (Okabe, 1997; Lloyd et al., 1994). To improve hydration kinetics and solvent retention, hydrophilic polymers and/or surfactants have been incorporated into the fabric or foam matrices (Beck et al., 1998). Examples of hydrophilic polymers are polyethylene oxide, PVOH, poly-N-vinylpyrrolidone, polyacrylamide, polyhydroxyethyl methacrylate, and polysaccharides such as hydroxyethylcellulose, modified starches, or natural gums. Nonionic surfactants such as Tween-20, Neodol 91-6, or Tergitol 15-S-7 can also be added to enhance the rate of hydration. The water-retentive properties of the polymers, combined with the structural integrity of a fabric or porous film, provide a composite matrix material that will readily absorb the drug solution during the manufacturing process or just prior to use by the patient. The addition of solvent just prior to use can enhance drug stability, particularly for polypeptides and proteins.

The second strategy, drug-containing hydrogels, provides an alternative to the absorption of drug solution by porous composite matrices (Webster, 1983). With the hydrogel approach, drug salt is mixed with a solvent and a network-forming polymer to form a viscous solution. The solution is then dispensed into a cavity containing an electrode of the appropriate polarity, and the polymer is crosslinked. To minimize degradation of the drug during the crosslinking process, physical crosslinking is preferred over chemical or radiation-induced crosslinking reactions. For example, PVOH can be dissolved in water, mixed with drug salt, and then frozen at about $-20°C$. When thawed, a soft, cohesive, water-rich hydrogel results (Hyon and Yoshito, 1988). Other hydrophilic polymers such as polyvinylpyrrolidone or polysaccharides (e.g., hydroxypropylmethylcellulose) can be added to modify the rheological, adhesive, or water-retentive properties of PVOH hydrogels (Jevne et al., 1986; Southam et al., 1996).

In general, polar nonionic polymers have been used as the matrix material in formulations for ET systems. Nonionic polymers are preferred because they typically do not have mobile ionic species and do not interact strongly with drug ions. However, some results of studies of drug ET from matrices composed of ionic polymers have been reported. For example, Gupta and co-workers reported a substantial reduction in cromolyn ET when a hydrogel composed of polyglyceryl methacrylate and water was employed, suggesting a strong interaction between the cromolyn anion and polymer (Gupta et al., 1994).

The transdermal ET of the 286 Dalton drug cation hydromorphone was enhanced by using a hydrogel formulation composed of water and poly-AMPS (Phipps et al., 1996). A hydrogel composed of water and the acid form of poly-AMPS was imbibed with a stoichiometric amount of hydromorphone base to form the hydromorphone salt of poly-AMPS. Hydromorphone hydrochloride was also added, and the hydrogel was placed in contact with a silver anode. Hydromorphone was delivered at a current density of 0.05 $mA \cdot cm^{-2}$ through dermatomed pig skin into a 0.1 M sodium chloride solution. The flux of hydromorphone from the poly-AMPS hydrogel was found to be about twice that of a nonionic PVOH hydrogel. This result suggests that migration of mobile chloride ions from the skin into the hydrogel was hindered by the presence of immobilized sulfonate anions (i.e., ionic repulsion or Donnan exclusion).

D. Excipient Selection

Excipients such as buffers, antimicrobials, antioxidants, and chelating agents may be required for optimal drug stability in ETS formulations. Several unique criteria ETSs must be considered in these systems.

As described in Section II, excipients can contact the electrodes of the system. Therefore excipients must be screened for their compatibility with the electrodes. Sacrificial electrodes (e.g., Ag and AgCl) often used in ETSs are particularly reactive. If inherently nonreactive electrodes are used (e.g., platinum or carbon), then the excipient can be exposed to a relatively large electric potential at the electrode–reservoir interface during system use. In such cases, excipients that are inherently stable or those that are electrostatically repelled from the electrode during use should be selected. Excipients are typically evaluated for their electrochemical stability using standard potentiometric techniques (e.g., cyclic voltammetry) before being selected for use in an ET formulation.

The effect of an excipient on drug transport must also be considered, especially if it is ionic. If the excipient has the same charge as the drug ion, then it will be delivered to the skin with the drug. In addition to the direct competitive effect on drug transport, the excipient may alter the permselectivity of the skin, causing a change in the drug transport efficiency. If an excipient of opposite charge to the drug ion is chosen, then the effect of the excipient counterion on drug transport must be determined.

Because ET formulations usually contain water, the use of lipophilic excipients may not be possible. Instead, salt forms of excipients are often employed in ET formulations. However, excipient salts often contain inorganic cations that are usually much more mobile than most drug cations. The detrimental effects of inorganic cations on the flux of drug cations have been well documented (Phipps et al., 1989b). In particular, since inorganic cations are depleted from the formulation more rapidly than the drug cations, the flux of the drug will not be constant but rather will increase with time during system use (Phipps et al., 1989b; Phipps, 1997b). The competitive effect of buffer anions on transport of anionic drugs has also been reported (Yoshida and Roberts, 1995).

Standard phosphate and citrate buffers have been successfully used in formulations for transdermal ET of drug ions (Hillman and Pawelchak, 1992). However, because small inorganic and organic ions frequently have a negative effect on drug flux due to competition, selection of a buffer can be challenging. Several unique buffering strategies have been developed specifically for use in ET systems. In one strategy, zwitterionic buffering agents are used at their isoelectric pH (Cormier et al., 1997). The net zero charge of the zwitterion largely avoids the ion competition effect. Two preferred zwitterionic buffers are N-2-hydroxyethylpiperazine-N-2-ethanesulfonic acid (HEPES) and 2-N-morpholinopropanesulfonic acid (MES).

Alternatively, the delivery of the buffer ion can be largely eliminated by using cationic buffers in the cathode reservoir and anionic buffers in the anode reservoir, so that the buffer ion moves away from the skin when an electric field is applied. In addition to common weak acids such as citric and phosphoric, the use of amino acids in the anode formulation has been suggested. Amino acids such as cysteine and histidine would be incorporated at neutral or basic pH, where they are predominantly anionic (Cormier et al., 1997).

In another buffering strategy, polymeric materials with pendant acid or base groups (e.g., carboxylic, phosphoric, amines) are dispersed in the formulation (Sanderson et al., 1989; Southam et al., 1996; Cormier et al., 1997). Examples of such polymeric buffers are polyacrylic acid and methacrylate/divinylbenzene copolymers (e.g., Amberlite IRP-64). The exceedingly high molecular weight of these polymers renders them essentially immobile in an electrical field. The counterion to the ionic resin must still be considered; preferably it should have the opposite charge of the drug to avoid ionic competition. Alternatively, the counterion to the drug ion can be specifically selected for its inherent buffering capability (Sanderson et al., 1989).

In all of these strategies, the goal is to minimize the mobility of the buffering agent, or its counterion, relative to that of the drug ion. This is accomplished by choosing buffers with no net ionic charge, by choosing buffers whose mobile species have a charge opposite that of the drug ion, or by increasing the molecular weight of the buffering agent.

Excipients may also be included in the formulation to enhance drug delivery efficiency. For example, Sanderson and colleagues (1989) reported a threefold enhancement in delivery of dobutamine after the skin site was pretreated with an anionic surfactant, sodium lauryl sulfate (SLS). They attributed the enhancement in flux to an increase in the negative charge on the skin because of neutralization of fixed positive charges in the skin and to hydrophobic binding of the surfactant to the skin. More specifically, Sanderson and co-workers proposed that an increase in negative charge within the transport pathway enhanced the migration of drug cations by hindering the migration of chloride ions from the body. They noted that, while SLS is not biocompatible, the charge–alteration strategy may be useful if other more biocompatible surfactants could be found.

Alternatively, Huntington and Cormier (1998) used nonionic surfactants, including dodecanol and 1,2-dodecanediol, to enhance the delivery of the anionic anti-inflammatory drug, ketoprofen. Since nonionic surfactants are not directly affected by the applied electric field, their use in ETS formulations may be preferred over ionic surfactants. Some drugs and excipients may cause excessive skin irritation (Ledger, 1992). Researchers have reduced skin irritation in humans by including an anti-inflammatory agent in the formulation (Cormier and Johnson, 1997; Ledger et al., 1997). Using the moderately irritating antiemetic drug metoclopramide, they demonstrated improved biocompatibility by adding hydrocortisone to the formulation. As little as 0.05% hydrocortisone in the formulation significantly reduced erythema at the skin site following treatment. They also reported that hydrocortisone had no effect on the transport of the metoclopramide cation.

E. Formulation pH Selection

Many drugs have a broad pH range in which drug solubility and stability are adequate for transdermal delivery by ET. However, optimal drug delivery and biocompatibility are usually restricted to a narrower range of formulation pH. As discussed previously, skin is a permselective membrane with an isoelectric point of about pH 4. For this reason, formulation pH can affect the selectivity of the skin to cations and anions. As formulation pH increases, skin becomes more negatively charged, thus favoring cation transport. Therefore, to maximize the transdermal flux of a cationic drug, the formulation pH should be as basic as is practical, limited by drug solubility, charge state, stability, and biocompatibility. By analogy, for anionic drugs, acidic formulations are generally preferred to take advantage of permselectivity.

The effect of formulation pH on skin permselectively has been clearly demonstrated (Nightingale et al., 1990): as the pH of a solution containing salicylate anion was increased from pH 4, to pH 6, and then to pH 8, the transdermal flux of salicylate anion at 200 $\mu A/cm^2$ decreased from 480, to 192, and then to 174 $\mu g\ h^{-1}\ cm^{-2}$, respectively. In contrast, with an identical increase in pH the flux of triethylamine cation increased from 117, to 170, and then to 303 $\mu g\ h^{-1}\ cm^{-2}$, respectively.

A formulation must provide adequate drug transport while ensuring good biocompatibility. Several investigators have found that formulation pH can have a substantial effect on skin irritation (Sanderson et al., 1989; Cormier et al., 1997; Cormier and Johnson, 1997; Ledger et al., 1997; Phipps et al., 1997). By measuring the redness at treated sites on hairless guinea pigs, Cormier and Johnson (1997) found that skin irritation was reduced by choosing different pH ranges for the anode and cathode formulations. For anode formulations, pH values between 4 and 10 produced the lowest skin responses. For cathode formulations, pH values of between 2 and 4 were least irritating.

Tables 1 and 2 illustrate the effect of anode and cathode formulation pH on skin resistance during treatment, and on skin redness at the anode and cathode sites measured 5 minutes after a 30-min application of 0.1 mA/cm^2. The anode formulations consisted of 3% w/w hydroxypropylcellulose, 0.1 M NaCl, 0.05 M citric acid, and sufficient sodium hydroxide to achieve the desired pH. The cathode formulation consisted of 3% w/w hydroxypropylcellulose, 0.1 M NaCl, 0.05 M L-histidine base, and sufficient hydrochloric acid to achieve the desired pH. Skin redness was measured using a chromameter (a-scale for red-green hue). Redness values were normalized by subtracting the redness measured at an untreated site from the redness measured at the treated site. For a normalized redness value of 1 or less, little or no erythema (i.e., redness) is evident to the human eye. Values of 1 to 3 are perceived as mild erythema, values of 3 to 7 appear as moderate erythema, and values of 7 or greater appear as severe or beet-red erythema.

As indicated by the data for both anode and cathode sites, skin resistance and skin redness are correlated. For anode sites, the citrate-buffered formulations resulted in lower resistance and redness when the pH was greater than about 4. In contrast, cathode sites contacting

Table 1 Average Skin Resistance and Normalized Skin Redness at the Anodic Site on Hairless Guinea Pigs (n = 4), Resulting from Use of Citric Acid Formulations

Formulation pH	Skin resistance (kohm·cm^2)	Skin redness (a-scale)
2.1	52	4.7
2.7	51	5.3
3.6	46	4.0
4.5	33	2.7
5.3	30	2.7
6.5	27	3.3

Source: Data from Cormier et al., 1997.

Table 2 Average Skin Resistance and Normalized Skin Redness at the Cathodic Site on Hairless Guinea Pigs (n = 4), Resulting from Use of L-Histidine Formulations

Formulation pH	Skin resistance (kohm·cm^2)	Skin redness (a-scale)
1.9	19	3.1
2.9	32	4.7
3.9	35	6.9
4.9	38	7.2
6.0	45	7.0
7.1	39	6.6

Data from Cormier et al., 1997.

the histidine formulations had lower resistance and redness values when the pH was less than about 4. These same trends have been observed in humans—greater skin irritation was found to be associated with larger efflux of potassium from the skin during current application (Phipps et al., 1997). Since the isoelectric point of skin is at about pH 4, the correlation between resistance, potassium efflux, and pH suggests that substantial concentration polarization within the viable epidermis may be occurring at particular pH values, resulting in high resistance, cellular release of cytoplasmic potassium, and skin irritation.

F. Selection of Electrolytes for Counterreservoir

An appropriate electrolyte for the formulation in contact with the counterelectrode must be selected that provides sufficient conductivity to minimize the voltage required during system use. The minimum conductivity, σ, needed to limit the voltage drop, ΔV, across a hydrogel formulation with a thickness of L and a cross-sectional area of A at a current of I is given by the expression:

$$\sigma = \frac{IL}{\Delta V A} \tag{9}$$

For example, a voltage drop of less than 1 V will occur across a hydrogel formulation with a thickness of 0.5 cm and a cross-sectional area of 5 cm^2 at a current of 0.5 mA, if the formulation has a conductivity of at least 50 μS/cm.

Since formulation conductivity is sensitive to solubility and ion pairing effects, it can be used to characterize alternative formulations during formulation development. Gangarosa and colleagues (1978) and Yoshida and Roberts (1995) provide examples of the effect of drug and electrolyte conductivity on formulation performance in ET systems.

In addition to rendering the formulation sufficiently conductive, the ion delivered from the nondrug formulation must be biocompatible. Irritation resulting from use of four inorganic electrolytes has been reported by Anigbogu and co-workers (1997). They reported that use of 0.9% NaCl or KCl in the anode reservoir at current densities of 0.5 mA/cm^2 and 1 mA/cm^2 for 1 h elicited no skin irritation in rabbits. In contrast, the use of 0.9% CaCl$_2$ or MgCl$_2$ caused moderate erythema.

Using weak acids and bases as electrolytes for the counterreservoir formulation at the proper pH (i.e., pH <4 for cathode formulations and pH >4 for anode formulations) provides adequate biocompatibility and low skin resistance (Cormier et al., 1997). Low skin resistance is advantageous since less voltage output is required from the control circuit, and therefore a smaller battery may be required, potentially reducing the size and cost of the ETS.

For current densities at or above 0.2 mA/cm^2, the sensation associated with transdermal ET is determined by the type of ion being delivered to the skin. When human subjects compared the sensation experienced during ET of different salt solutions applied to the right and left forearms, it was concluded that delivery of calcium caused less sensation than delivery of phosphate, magnesium, and zinc; which caused less sensation than delivery of chloride, acetate, citrate, and sulfate; which caused less sensation than delivery of lithium, potassium, and sodium. In general, multivalent ions were found to cause less sensation than monovalent ions (Phipps, 1993).

Sodium is commonly found in pharmaceutical formulations but may cause significant sensation if transdermally delivered by ET. Addition of small amounts of calcium to a sodium-rich solution was reported to dramatically reduce sensation at the anode site, suggesting that calcium may block nerve depolarization in the skin (Phipps, 1993). Less sensation during transdermal ET of calcium ion has also been reported. In addition, more erythema was observed when sodium was replaced by calcium in the anode formulation (Kalia and Guy, 1995). Others have obtained similar results (Anigbogu et al., 1997).

IV. SYSTEM DESIGN

A. Determining System Requirements

The design and manufacture of an ET system is more complicated than most other controlled drug delivery systems, such as extended release oral tablets or passive transdermal drug delivery systems. ET systems have many categories of components (e.g., circuitry, aqueous drug reservoir, outer housing, and means of attachment to skin), which all must be manufactured, stored, and, ultimately, made to function together.

The academic literature once broadly held that an iontophoretic drug delivery system could be designed so that many different drugs could be delivered using essentially the same controller and perhaps a few different-sized drug reservoirs/electrode assemblies. Several companies currently market products based on this approach, including Iomed (Phoresor) and EMPI (Dupel). These products have been useful for the delivery of lidocaine for the provision of local tissue anesthesia and for the delivery of sodium dexamethasone for the treatment of bursitis and other soft-tissue injuries typically treated with steroids. The widespread use of these products, especially outside supervised care settings, is limited for several reasons. They have a high initial cost that requires a sustained level of use to recoup the initial investment. The proper use of these systems is complicated and requires extensive training of doctors and staff. In general, these products are inconvenient to use because the appropriate current and duration of application must be determined for each application and the drug pad must be filled with the appropriate drug mixture prior to each treatment. Although these products are being marketed to clinics, their technically demanding user interface and overall complexity have limited their acceptance. A product is more likely to be widely accepted if it meets the following criteria: it is appropriately priced for the given therapy, requires little to no training to use, can be applied to home-based as well as clinic-based therapies, and is as simple to apply and use as a passive transdermal drug delivery system.

To achieve simplicity of use and wide acceptance, products ideally should be designed for specific therapeutic applications and be distributed as a system in which the drug and delivery mechanism are formulated together. Many needs and requirements must be considered in designing an iontophoretic delivery system for a specific drug. These needs can be categorized into three areas: therapeutic, functional, and user needs.

Therapeutic needs are requirements placed on system design due to the specific nature of the therapy. For example, if the therapy is site-specific, as in the case of delivery of an anti-inflammatory agent to a joint, then the system needs to be designed so that the drug reservoir both covers and conforms to the shape of that area. Table 3 lists a few of the therapeutic requirements that must be considered and their effects on system design.

The second requirement type, functional needs, is a requirement placed on system design that must be fulfilled if the system is to reliably deliver the requisite amount of drug in the desired profile. For example, the rate at which drug must be delivered to achieve the desired therapy along with the transport properties of that drug through skin will determine the overall skin contact area between the donor reservoir and the skin. Table 4 lists a few of the functional requirements that must be considered during system design and their effects on system design.

User needs are requirements placed on system design in order to create a system that meets the needs of all the users of the system. Users are not the only patients who rely on the system for their therapy; also involved are the physicians prescribing the therapy, the immediate caregivers responsible for overseeing the patient's therapy, and those responsible for paying for the therapy. For example, the design of a system must be appropriate for the level of dexterity that may be present in the intended population (e.g., children, the elderly). Table 5 lists a few of the user requirements that must be considered and their effects on system design.

A review of the design issues discussed above shows that many of the design attributes are affected by multiple needs. Therefore, making design decisions is often a complex process of balancing needs that may conflict with each other. Good solutions require a complete understanding of how the system will be used, who will be using it, what the expectations of the system will be, and what unique advantages ET will bring to this particular therapy.

Gathering this information is a multidisciplinary activity that should involve market researchers, clinical study personnel, industrial designers, and mechanical, electrical, material, and design engineers. Important sources of information include patients, physicians, and nurses, in one-on-one interviews and focus groups. Visits to the location where the system will be used should also be conducted to observe and understand the environment of use. Consultation with

Table 3 Effect of Therapeutic Needs on System Design

Therapeutic need	Design attribute
Site-specific application	Delivery area
	System shape
	Conformability
Amount of drug required and rate of delivery	Output current
	Duration of each dose
	Drug content
	Battery capacity
	Electrode capacity
	Compliance voltage
Prevention of drug overdose or underdose	Safety monitoring
	Audible/visual alarms
Total duration of therapy	Single-use vs. reusable design
	Multiple-day system design
	Waterproof vs. water-resistant design
Number of dosage levels	Optimized design (current, reservoir area, battery size, etc.) for each dosage level separately vs. a single design capable of all levels

Table 4 Effect of Functional Needs on System Design

Functional need	Design attribute
Shelf life	Selection of all materials, especially those in contact with the drug
	Storage conditions (dehydrated storage with reconstitution at the time of use vs. storage under refrigeration)
Drug delivery rate and therapy duration	Output current
	Battery capacity
	Drug content
	Electrode material and capacity
	Skin adhesive or other attachment mechanism
	Durability of system design
Biocompatibility	Selection of materials, especially those in contact with the body
	Maximum acceptable current density
	Maximum acceptable total current
	Flexibility
Manufacturability	Selection of materials
	Component design
	Process development
Packaging and distribution	Selection of materials
	Primary and secondary packaging
	Bundling in appropriately sized packages
	Labeling for distribution to single or multiple countries

opinion leaders within the therapeutic area can be used to identify shortcomings in the present common practice that may be solved through system design.

B. Electronic Components

The unique electrical nature of the delivery mechanism in ET allows a level of control and the possibility of providing information feedback that is not often available in other modes of drug delivery. As a result, special attention to the design of the electrical control scheme is warranted.

Two general approaches for the application of electric current are to control either the applied voltage or the current. A simple example of a controlled voltage circuit is a battery that applies a constant voltage to the system. However, as will be pointed out later, the skin resistance is neither constant between individuals nor static from the start to finish of a single application. Since the amount of drug delivered via ET is directly proportional to the current passed, a controlled-current approach is generally preferred.

The electrical control components of an ETS may be broken into three elements: power source, control circuitry (including added user interface features), and electrical attachment of the circuitry output to the anode and cathode electrodes.

C. Power for Portable Designs

The electrical power source for portable ET devices is a battery. Commercially available primary batteries have cell voltages that range from about 1.2 to 3.0 V. To overcome the resistance of the skin and achieve the desired current, it may be necessary to use higher voltages. Voltage

Table 5 Effect of User Needs on System Design

User need	Design attribute
Design appropriate for patient population	System complexity
	Maximum system size
	Aesthetic design
Current practice within the therapy	Expected features
	New features that may benefit current practice
	Meet or exceed expected safety profile
	Point of distribution (pharmacy or doctor's office) (affects packaging and labeling)
Cost-effective therapy	Single-use vs. reusable system design
	Selection of materials
	System complexity
	Number of added features
Circumstances of use	Flexibility
	Selection of materials
	Waterproof vs. water-resistant
User interface	Selection of materials
	Need for user-controlled buttons
	Information feedback (light-emitting diode vs. liquid crystal display)
	Management of system:
	Storage of system when not in use
	Storage of unused systems
	Disposal of used systems
	Replenishment of the power source (for reusable systems)

can be increased by combining cells in series or by using circuitry to transform the voltage at the cost of drawing a larger current from the battery. This additional current drain adds to the total battery capacity needed to provide the required therapy. Thus, the total battery capacity required is the sum of that needed to support the therapy plus any "overhead" associated with the electrical circuitry.

The additional current drain imposed on the battery by the supporting circuitry is difficult to predict until that circuitry is fully defined. The first objective of the circuitry is to control the amount of drug delivered. For example, for a zero-order (constant delivery) system, a specified current should be maintained regardless of the load or resistance provided by the application site. Computing the power requirement in this case is difficult because the resistive load of the skin depends on both the application site and the time elapsed since current has been initiated (Gyory and Phipps, 1997). Figure 3 shows the skin resistance at different application sites in response to the application of 1 mA to a 4-cm^2 area. Skin resistance remained constant at 545 $\pm$500 kΩ until current was applied. Even at 1 s following current application, the measured resistance had decreased significantly to 16 $\pm$4 kΩ. As time progressed, the resistance continued to fall and all sites appeared to approach a quasi-steady-state value, 10 $\pm$2 kΩ. Note the small relative standard deviation of the quasi-steady-state resistance (RSD 20%) compared with the initial resistance (RSD 92%). This indicates that all body sites tested tend toward a common resistance, despite the large differences that are present prior to application of current.

The high initial skin resistance significantly impacts system design. Because the start of current application is the time when skin resistance is highest, the initial resistance will determine the system voltage required to drive the desired current into the skin. For a typical initial

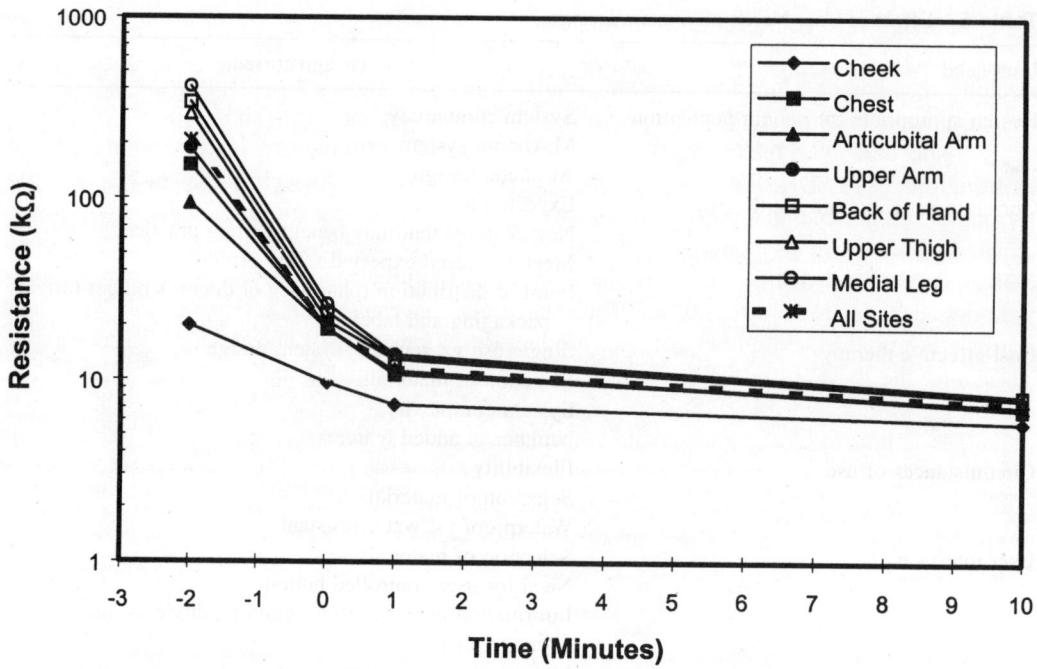

Figure 3 Skin resistance of various body sites as a function of time of current application. (Data from Gyory and Phipps, 1997.)

resistance, on the order of 500 kΩ, several hundred volts would be required to drive the full 1 mA. Therefore, systems having a lower voltage capability will operate below the desired current (i.e., they will be noncompliant) during the initial moments of current application. However, the resistance drops quickly, so that a voltage capability of about 10–20 V is sufficient to achieve compliance in an acceptably short time.

D. Control Circuitry Requirements

A controlled-current circuit does not require a high level of sophistication. A simple field effect transistor with a feedback resistor can control the current delivered from a battery at a constant value over a wide range of skin resistances. In some therapies, however, it is advantageous to vary the applied current in a controlled way to modulate the amount of drug delivered. For example, the constant delivery of leuteinizing hormone–releasing hormone (LHRH) or one of its analogs will diminish the body's production of estrogen or testosterone. In this mode, the continuous delivery of these compounds is used in the treatment of estrogen- and testosterone-dependent tumors such as breast and pancreatic cancer. However, LHRH pulsed into the body at 5–20 μg over 5 or 10 min once every 90 to 120 min enhances the production of estrogen in women; this treatment is used to treat some forms of infertility.

Other types of delivery requirements such as pulsed current, patient-controlled on-demand dosing, dose titration, ramp-up or ramp-down dosing, and other special waveforms can be addressed with control circuitry. However, these circuits can become very complicated, so that integrated circuits may be required to minimize system size. Size can be further reduced by using customized application-specific integrated circuits (ASIC), which incorporate both analog and digital circuitry (mixed-mode ASIC) into a single integrated circuit.

In addition to controlling the output current, it is often desirable to incorporate circuitry to increase the reliability and safety of the drug delivery system. Examples include redundant circuitry that guards against component failure, watch-dog timers that monitor the system and shut it down if failures are detected, current output monitors, and voltage monitors.

Visual and audio feedback information can be provided to the user by incorporating light-emitting diodes (LEDs), liquid crystal displays (LCDs), and piezoelectric transducers. This information can indicate that the system is working, show errors or warnings, signal system maintenance needs (such as battery replacement), or display the amount of drug that has been delivered. Although displays and other user interface features can enhance the therapy and provide new benefits over other dosage forms, they also have disadvantages, including increased power consumption, complexity of use, product development time and risk, and product cost. Therefore, the need and utility of each feature must be thoroughly analyzed prior to its inclusion in the product.

The ability of electrotransport to control drug delivery precisely gives rise to another advantage of its use—the opportunity to create closed-loop therapy. If an appropriate sensor is available to measure the biological response that the drug generates (e.g., to measure blood glucose levels in response to the delivery of insulin), then circuitry can be used to modulate the output current (hence drug delivery), based on the response of the sensor. In so doing, a complete closed-loop system is created which ensures that the proper amount of drug is delivered and avoids both over- and underdosing of the patient.

E. Circuitry Assembly

After the circuitry and power requirements have been defined, the appropriate components can be assembled using standard flexible circuit technology (flex circuits) or rigid polymeric circuit boards. Flex circuits permit systems that easily conform to the patient's body, but they can be prone to circuit trace breaks or solder bond breaks due to excessive flexing. Rigid polymeric circuit boards are more immune to trace and bond breaks but result in a more rigid final system. A combination of these technologies can be used in which the electrical components are isolated on several small rigid boards, which are interconnected by flexible circuits that contain only circuit traces (Gyory, 1996). An outer housing provides protection of internal components from the environment and creates an aesthetic and useful user interface.

F. Single-use vs. Reusable Designs

Depending on the therapeutic and user needs, the system can be of two general designs: (a) single-use or (b) reusable controller with disposable drug units. With a single-use system, the entire unit is disposed of or recycled at the completion of the application. An example of a single-use system and its major components is shown in Fig. 4. The greatest advantages of single-use system design are simplicity and ease of use for the patient. This is largely due to the integration of all components into a single package, eliminating any need for assembly at the point of use. However, even with the simplest electronic circuitry, single-use systems are relatively expensive compared with passive transdermal patches. Therefore, single-use systems are only appropriate in applications where simplicity and ease of use are critical to the therapy and the cost of therapy is justified by the advantages provided by ET drug delivery.

Reusable controllers with disposable drug units can be very economical, competing favorably on a cost basis with passive transdermal patches. However, the design of these systems and the user interface is typically more complex. Special design needs for reusable systems in-

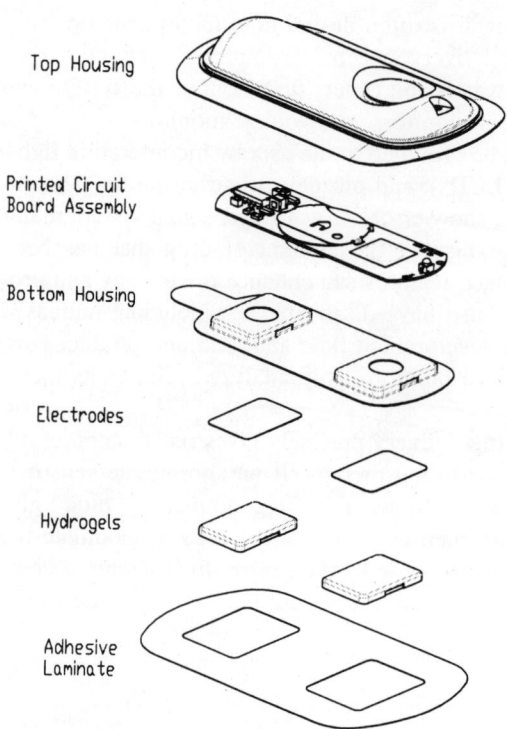

Figure 4 Exploded view of representative single-use electrotransport system showing major components. Top housing, printed circuit board assembly; bottom housing, containing reservoirs for placement of electrodes and hydrogels, and adhesive laminate.

clude ease of system assembly, secure mechanical and electrical connection between controller and drug unit, increased battery capacity for multiple days of therapy, design for replaceable batteries, memory retention during battery change, and capability to provide multiple dose levels with the same controller. An example of a reusable system and its major components is shown in Fig. 5.

G. Design Example: E-TRANS Lidocaine

A design example is provided to further demonstrate how therapeutic, functional, and user needs are translated into a product. The product concept was a small, self-contained system for the topical delivery of lidocaine that would be used to create a local anesthetic block for invasive procedures such as blood draws, intravenous (IV) catheter insertions, immunizations, wart removals, and skin biopsies. Although these procedures are performed on individuals of all ages, the pediatrics market was viewed as the predominant market for this product.

Market research and focus groups of doctors, nurses, and staff in pediatrics, dermatology, and oncology were conducted to determine which procedures could be enhanced by this product concept. Information was collected for required time to onset, duration, and depth of anesthesia for each procedure. In vitro formulation evaluation and phase I clinical testing were conducted to determine drug content, drug concentration, current requirements, and application time to achieve adequate anesthesia.

ET Systems for Transdermal Delivery

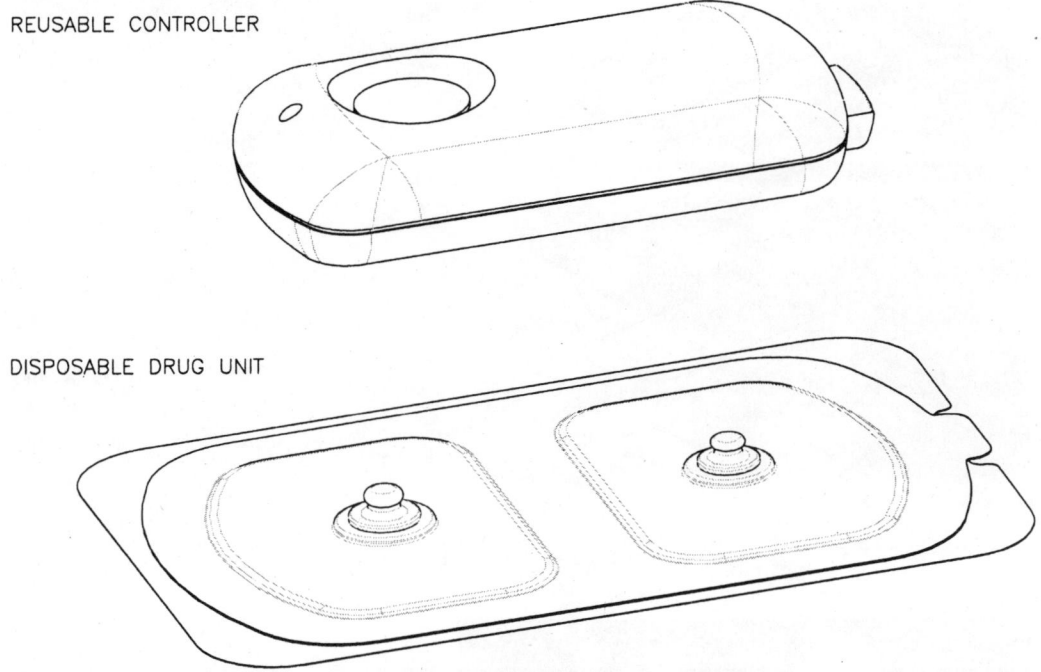

Figure 5 Illustration of electrotransport system with reuseable controller and disposable drug unit. The drug unit contains electrodes, drug and return reservoirs, and a skin adhesive. Conductive snaps make mechanical and electrical attachment between disposable unit and controller.

One therapeutic requirement identified in the clinical studies was that epinephrine must be added to the lidocaine hydrochloride drug reservoir to maintain anesthesia for at least 1 h. Epinephrine is a vasoconstrictor that decreases blood flow through capillaries in the skin. The reduced blood flow slows lidocaine removal from the local tissue area. Epinephrine is an organic base and is available as a bitartrate salt. Thus, at pH 5 both lidocaine and epinephrine are positively charged and will be codelivered from the positive anodic reservoir. Additional in vitro and in vivo experiments were required to determine the proper ratio of lidocaine and epinephrine to ensure the required extent and duration of anesthesia. Compatibility, stability, and microbial testing identified the additional excipients needed to ensure adequate stability and microbial purity of the product.

System design activities proceeded in parallel with the formulation work. A reusable controller with disposable drug unit approach was adopted to decrease the per-use cost. Based on the market research described previously, the predominant target procedures were identified and additional user-based research was conducted. Some relevant observations that were eventually translated into design specifications included: Onset of anesthesia must occur within 20 min; the anesthetized area should be about 4 cm^2 and have a length/width ratio of approximately 1:2; and the region for anesthesia is often curved and too small to accommodate both the delivery and the counterelectrode. In addition, because this product would replace an inexpensive injection or be used in place of no anesthesia, the ET delivery system must demonstrably make the procedure easier to perform, reduce the patient's or doctor's stress, or be demanded by the patient.

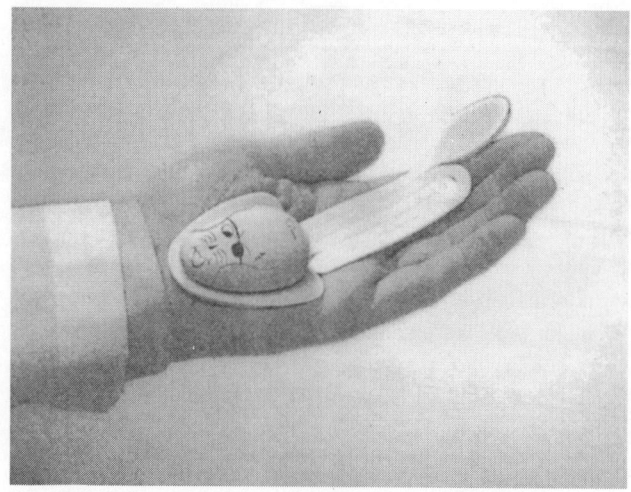

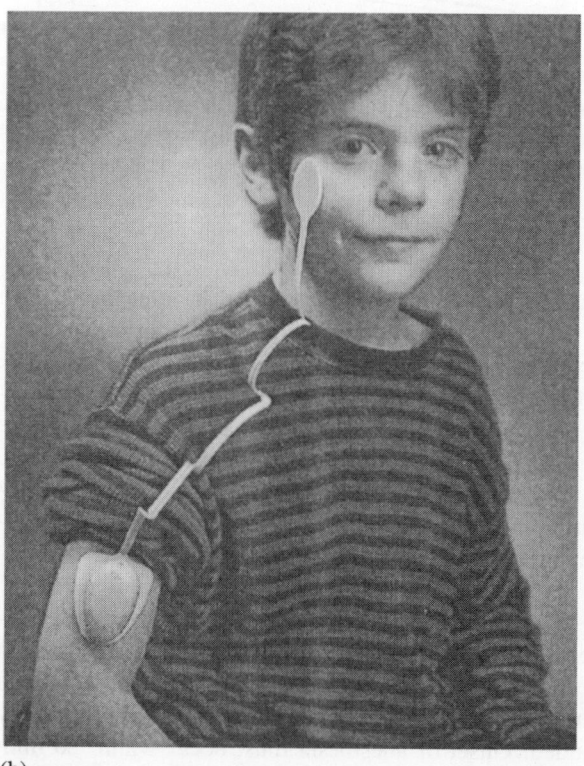

Figure 6 E-TRANS lidocaine delivery system. (a) Reusable controller connects to drug unit via serpentine connector. The oval drug reservoir is at the distal end of a serpentine connector, and the counter-electrode is located beneath the controller. (b) Illustration of system use on a patient.

This information led to the design shown in Fig. 6. The disposable drug unit features a small, flexible drug delivery reservoir that is connected to the return electrode via an extendable serpentine connector. This configuration allows the drug reservoir to be placed on a small, highly curved area (such as the back of the hand, crook of the elbow, or face), whereas the return reservoir is placed remotely on a larger and less contoured area of skin, such as the forearm, shoulder, or chest. The controller is placed over the return electrode, thus preventing its weight or rigidity from interfering with the placement of the drug delivery electrode.

The construction method for the disposable drug unit had to be appropriate for economic production of millions of units per year. As such, web-based handling with pick-and-place operations to apply snaps, foam reservoirs, and dispense the formulations, and a final die punch to remove the completed system from the carrier web were selected as the most appropriate manufacturing methods.

The electrodes consisted of a silver-containing ink that was preprinted onto the carrier web. Manufacture of the drug unit was further simplified by using the same electrode material at both anode and cathode. This meant that an appropriate buffer was required in the cathode formulation to prevent the formulation pH from increasing as a result of the hydrolysis reaction at the cathode.

Because lidocaine is being delivered at the drug delivery site, the sensation that would normally be associated with a high current density is blocked by the anesthetic. This allowed the system to operate at a greater current than would normally be acceptable in order to minimize the onset time for anesthesia. However, the counterreservoir did not benefit from this same effect. Therefore, the skin contact area of the return reservoir was increased to reduce the current density to an acceptable level. During the first minute of operation the controller applies a lower total current to further reduce sensation until the lidocaine begins to enter the skin. The current is then increased to its full level for the remainder of the application time.

The serpentine connector and the need to appeal to the pediatric market influenced the aesthetic design of the controller. Because the shape of the disposable drug unit with the serpentine connector extended suggested that of a mouse with a long tail, the shape, color, and graphics of the controller were chosen to evoke the shape of a mouse's body. Doctors and nurses can use this mouse imagery to create stories that help to put a pediatric patient completely at ease. The mouse motif helped to transform what was formerly the most stressful part of a procedure into the friendliest part.

Internal to the controller, two 3-V lithium coin cells placed in series were used to provide a 6-V power source. This voltage was boosted to a compliance voltage of 20 V to ensure that patients would receive the full intended current within a few seconds of initiating delivery. To preserve battery power, an internal switch was designed so that the batteries were connected to the rest of the circuitry only when the controller was attached to a disposable drug unit. These design choices allowed at least 100 uses for each set of batteries.

The cost of developing an ASIC was not warranted because the controllers will be manufactured at a much lower volume than the disposable drug units. Therefore, all off-the-shelf electrical components were used. Also because several very specific monitoring functions were required, a microcontroller allowed the most design flexibility during the development program. However, this added requirements for software development, verification, and validation to the development program.

A single LED was incorporated to provide a number of messages as feedback to the user. Through combinations of LED conditions of steady-on, steady-off, slow and rapid blinking, a reliable and intuitive means of indicating several messages was achieved. These messages are summarized in Table 6.

Table 6 LED Status Messages

Status message	LED response
Dose in progress	LED on solid
Dose complete	LED off
Application error/high skin resistance	LED rapidly flutters on and off
Low battery during dosing	LED on 3 sec, off 0.5 sec
Low battery after dosing complete	LED on 0.5 sec, off 3 sec
Dead battery	LED off
Other system error	LED flutters 3 sec, off 1 sec

The controller was designed to immediately start dosing when it is attached to a disposable drug unit (provided that the drug unit is attached to the skin); this eliminates the need for a "start" button on the controller. It is important to have the dose begin when the disposable unit is on a patient's body. An electrical circuit was therefore created that initiates dosing only after the controller detects that the system is applied to the patient. This is achieved by periodically applying a short voltage pulse to the electrodes, measuring the resultant current, and calculating the resistance across the electrodes using Ohm's law. As long as the calculated resistance is greater than a predetermined value, the controller does not initiate dosing. Once the system is properly applied to the body, the calculated resistance quickly drops, signaling the controller to initiate a treatment cycle.

The final system design results from thorough identification and careful consideration of the therapeutic, functional, and user needs. In the end, the design must meet as many needs as possible, but compromises are often required. Creativity and a multifunctional approach are important to achieving a successful solution.

V. CASE STUDIES IN CLINICAL ASSESSMENT OF SYSTEMIC DELIVERY

Electrotransport systems are evaluated for their ability to deliver drugs in an efficacious and safe manner. For drugs with proven histories of use by other delivery routes, the matter of efficacy, provided a target plasma level is reached, has generally been established. Also, systemic safety of these proven compounds is generally not at issue. However, skin tolerability at the site of delivery must be demonstrated for ET drug delivery.

Efficacy, the focus of this section, is assessed in terms of delivery rate, which in turn is determined by current and delivery efficiency. Using selected clinical case studies, a number of delivery attributes of ET technology discussed in earlier sections are exemplified. In vitro methodologies are discussed briefly to highlight useful correlations with observed in vivo findings. The examples comprise representative compounds with different physicochemical properties: fentanyl, a low molecular weight, cationic compound; ketorolac, an anionic compound; and two representative peptide drugs, LHRH and its analog.

A. Fentanyl

Fentanyl is a synthetic opioid widely used in anesthesia and analgesia. Passive transdermal delivery system are also marketed for the treatment of chronic pain (Duragesic, Janssen Pharmaceutica). For the transdermal product, each patch delivers fentanyl through the skin continuously over 72 h (Ahmedzai et al., 1994). For the management of acute pain, such as postoperative pain, the slow onset of action of fentanyl obtained under passive transdermal conditions, i.e., slow attainment of therapeutic blood levels, is not appropriate. Alternatively, ET delivery of fentanyl offers the advantages of quickly attaining therapeutic blood levels and thus offers a quick onset of action. In addition, the electrical nature of ET delivery offers patient actuation of drug delivery, which is not possible with passive delivery (Thysman et al., 1994). Fentanyl has a molecular weight of 336 D in the base form, aqueous solubility of about 24 mg/mL as the HCl salt, and a charge of +1 over a wide pH range.

E-TRANS™ (fentanyl) has been undergoing clinical evaluation (Gupta et al., 1998a, b) as a patient-controlled, transdermal delivery system for the treatment of acute postoperative pain. The prototype systems used in the clinical trials described here consisted of reusable, battery-operated devices capable of delivering on-demand user-activated current; they are different in design from the product that will be commercially marketed. The disposable fentanyl delivery platforms had silver anodes and silver chloride cathodes in intimate contact with hydrogel reservoirs. Two sizes of active anode hydrogel reservoir were used, containing either 5 or 10 mg (base equivalent) of the hydrochloride salt of fentanyl. In the two clinical studies summarized in this section, the hydrogel reservoir areas were either 2 or 5 cm^2 and the disposable drug units were applied to the upper outer arms of healthy volunteers. The opioid effects of fentanyl were blocked in the volunteers by oral administration of naltrexone every 12 h.

Clinical study 1 employed eight healthy volunteers in a three-treatment, sequential crossover, dose (current) escalation study design and evaluated continuous ET administration of fentanyl over 24 h at currents of 50, 100, and 200 μA. For the 5-cm^2 hydrogel area systems, these currents represent current densities of 10, 20, and 40 μA/cm^2, respectively. These current densities fall in the low end of the range of currents typically used in iontophoresis. Fentanyl serum concentrations were measured by gas chromatography/mass spectrometry over 24 h for the three currents and the results were plotted as shown in Fig. 7. Clinically relevant fentanyl serum concentrations were achieved fairly rapidly compared with passive systems, and the mean peak fentanyl serum concentration (C_{max}) increased approximately in proportion to the applied current. The AUC (area under the curve) values (representing the total amount of drug absorbed over the delivery period) also increased with increasing current, but the relationship was not linear, suggesting that delivery efficiency had some current dependence at the low current densities used in this study.

A second 24-h clinical study assessed intermittent delivery of fentanyl. In this study, the total applied currents (150, 200, and 250 μA) were similar to those employed in study 1. However, because the hydrogel area was smaller (2 cm^2), the current densities were greater than in study 1 (75–125 μA/cm^2 vs. 10–40 μA/cm^2). Study 2 was a four-treatment (three ET plus an IV treatment) crossover study, conducted in 12 subjects. All treatments involved drug delivery for the first 20 min of every hour for 24 h. The three ET treatments were 150, 200, and 250 μA each using 2-cm^2 drug hydrogel areas, whereas the IV treatment was 50 μg of drug infused over the first 20 min of every hour for 24 h (i.e., the identical pattern used for ET administration). Blood samples were collected, and serum fentanyl concentrations were measured using a specific radioimmunoassay. Results following the 0-, 12-, and 24-h treatments are shown in Fig. 8.

In Fig. 8, the gradual upward shifts in concentration over time indicate a baseline increase due to incomplete fentanyl clearance between the hourly doses. For all treatment types, serum fentanyl concentrations increased rapidly within a few minutes after beginning each dose. Despite the similarity in the rate of dose onset, close inspection reveals a difference in the rate of decrease in concentration between the IV and ET treatments. While the serum fentanyl con-

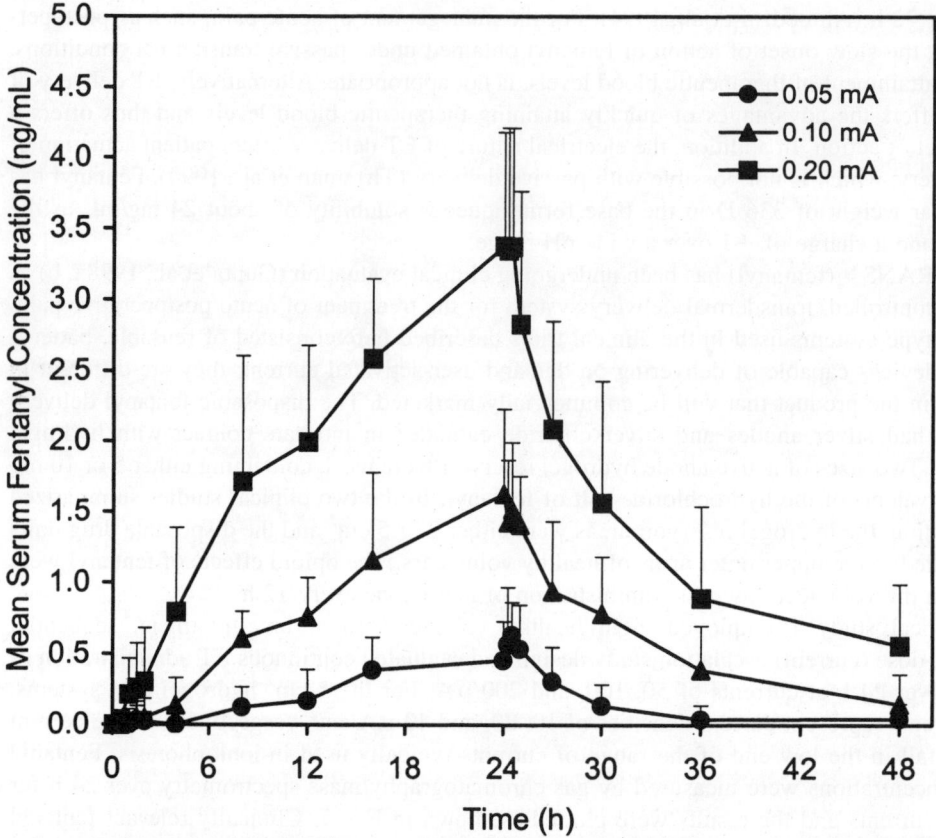

Figure 7 Mean (SD) serum fentanyl concentrations in eight healthy male volunteers receiving fentanyl continuously for 24 h at three different levels of current from an E-TRANS™ (fentanyl) system.

centration dropped immediately after cessation of the 20-min IV infusion, the concentration does not drop until approximately 10 min after cessation of current for the ET treatments. This apparent skin dampening effect following ET treatment has been observed with ET delivery of other drug substances as well.

The average drug input rate during the 20-min doses between hours 24 and 25 was 81, 108, and 138 µg/h/cm^2 for 150-, 200-, and 250-µA currents, respectively. These values, the mean C_{max} values, and the total AUC values (over the same time period) for the three ET treatments increased proportionally with current. These results agree with theoretical expectations (see Section I of this chapter) but contrast with study 1 results, where the AUC values did not increase proportionally with increases in applied current. The current densities used in study 1 may have fallen below some current density threshold, below which the transport number is not constant but rather decreases with decreasing current. If this hypothesis is true, then the threshold current density for fentanyl lies somewhere between the maximum current density of study 1 and the minimum current density of study 2, i.e., between 50 and 75 µA/cm^2.

In study 2, the coefficients of variation for the data from each of the three ET treatments were very similar to that obtained for the IV treatment. This suggests that ET delivery does not increase the observed intersubject variability in fentanyl pharmacokinetics over that of IV delivery.

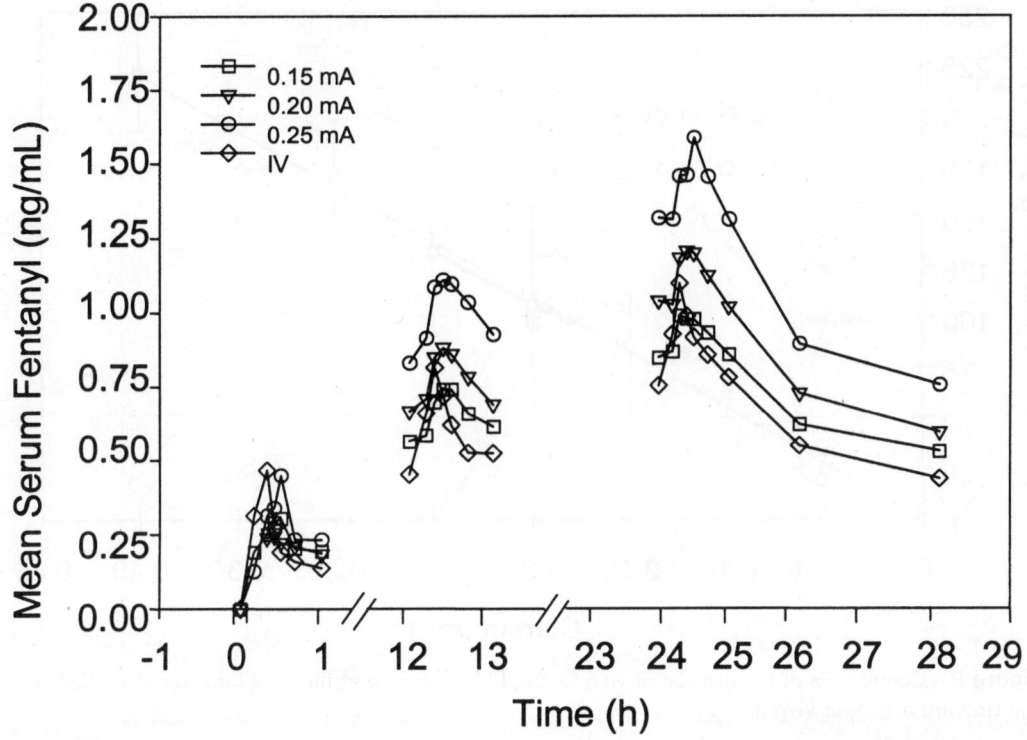

Figure 8 Mean serum fentanyl concentrations in 12 healthy volunteers (study 2) receiving fentanyl intermittently (20 min hourly over a 24-h administration period) from an E-TRANS™ (fentanyl) system (at three levels of current) and from IV fentanyl infusion (50 μg/20 min). Serum fentanyl concentrations were measured after the intermittent dose at 0, 12, and 24 h during E-TRANS™ treatments and the IV treatment.

The in vivo ET flux values for fentanyl calculated in this study agree closely with flux values obtained under in vitro conditions. In vitro transdermal experiments with fentanyl were conducted using custom, two-compartment permeation cells. Heat-stripped human epidermis was oriented so that the stratum corneum surface contacted the fentanyl hydrochloride solution in the donor compartment. The pH, concentration, and amount of fentanyl in the donor aqueous solution were essentially identical to that in the clinical ET system. The selection of appropriate in vitro conditions, particularly the composition and ionic strength of the receptor solution, are important to establish a good correlation with in vivo delivery data (Phipps and Gyory, 1992). The receptor compartment contained a 1:10 dilution of modified (without calcium or magnesium) Dulbecco's modified phosphate-buffered saline (DPBS, containing 0.15 M NaCl, prior to dilution), pH 7.4. This was selected to exhibit an in vitro fentanyl transdermal rate similar to the observed in vivo rate. The currents tested in vitro ranged from 0 to 400 μA and were applied to a silver anode and a silver chloride cathode using a galvanostat. The entire receptor compartment contents were collected every 15 min and analyzed for fentanyl by reversed-phase high-pressure liquid chromatography (HPLC). The data presented in Fig. 9 show that for fentanyl, proportionality exists for in vitro delivery data over a fairly broad range of current densities including very low values. Furthermore, a comparison of the in vitro and in vivo fentanyl ET flux data in Fig. 9 indicates an excellent correlation between the two.

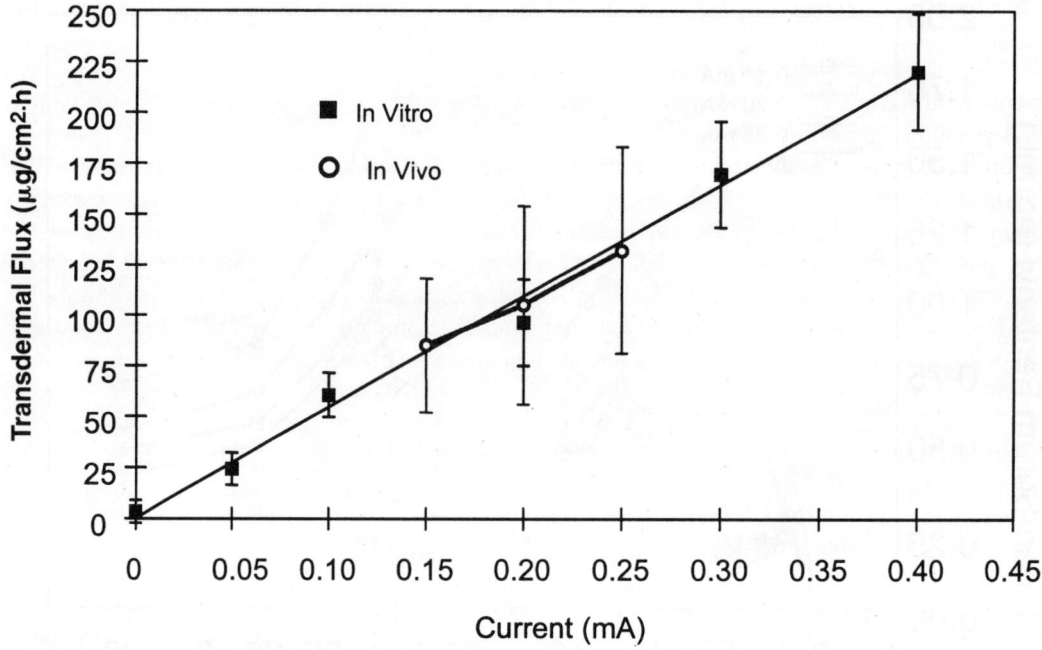

Figure 9 Comparison of in vitro and in vivo fentanyl electrotransport flux as a function of applied current (in vitro n = 5, in vivo n = 13).

B. Ketorolac

Ketorolac, a potent nonsteroidal anti-inflammatory analgesic, has a molecular weight of 255 D. It is available as a tromethamine salt and has excellent aqueous solubility (>500 mg/mL). In aqueous solution, ketorolac has a charge of -1 in the pH range of 5–7.5; hence, delivery studies were conducted using cathodic polarization. Ketorolac is available as a racemic mixture containing equal proportions of the (R) (inactive) and the (S) (active) enantiomers (Buckley and Brogden, 1990).

In vitro flux studies were initially conducted to select formulations that exhibited consistent 24-h delivery. Ketorolac as the tromethamine salt was formulated at relatively high drug concentration (100 mM) in PVOH hydrogels. In spite of this high drug concentration, in vitro drug flux was negatively impacted when the drug formulation was placed in contact with the silver chloride cathode because of the cathodic generation of chloride ions. However, acceptable and sustained in vitro flux of ketorolac was obtained over 24 h from systems in which the drug formulation was isolated from the cathode electrode. This was achieved by placing an electrolyte reservoir containing no drug directly against the cathode and separating the reservoir from the drug formulation with a cation-selective membrane.

With this system configuration, an in vitro transdermal ET ketorolac flux of about 40 $\mu g/cm^2/h$ was obtained using a receptor solution of phosphate buffered 0.015 M NaCl at a pH of 7 and a current density of 0.1 mA/cm^2. These results are for the racemic mixture of ketorolac. To investigate whether ET delivery was stereospecific, receptor solutions obtained from in vitro delivery experiments were also analyzed for the (R) and (S) enantiomers of ketorolac using a stereospecific HPLC assay. The samples consistently exhibited equal proportions of the two ketorolac enantiomers, suggesting an absence of preferential stereospecific electrotransport.

The absence of stereoselectivity agrees with a previously published report of non-stereospecific passive transport of an enantiomer (Roy et al., 1995a, b).

A pharmacokinetic study compared plasma ketorolac concentrations during 24-h treatments with ET, passive transdermal systems, and IV bolus injection. The study was conducted in a group of 12 healthy volunteers. The goal of this study was to deliver a dose of 24 mg of ketorolac from the passive and the ET systems. The ketorolac IV dose was a divided dose of 12 mg injected every 12 h over 24 h. The ketorolac clinical ET systems were identical in configuration to those used in the in vitro studies described above. For this study, a cathode area of 18 cm^2 and a current density of 0.1 mA/cm^2 were employed. The passive transdermal ketorolac system had a total area of 75 cm^2. Using a stereoselective HPLC assay, plasma concentrations of (R)- and (S)-ketorolac were measured over time. The amount of each enantiomer absorbed following ET and passive delivery was then calculated using the following equation:

$$N = AUC_{inf} \times C_{IV} \tag{10}$$

where N is the amount of drug absorbed; AUC_{inf} is the area under the curve, extrapolated to infinite time; and C_{IV} is the estimated IV clearance (calculated by dividing the IV dose by $AUC_{inf\text{-}IV}$).

Figures 10 and 11 show the mean plasma concentration–time profiles for the (R)- and (S)-ketorolac enantiomers for the three treatment groups. Following passive delivery, the mean amounts of (R)- and (S)- ketorolac absorbed (4.96 and 4.76 mg, respectively) were not

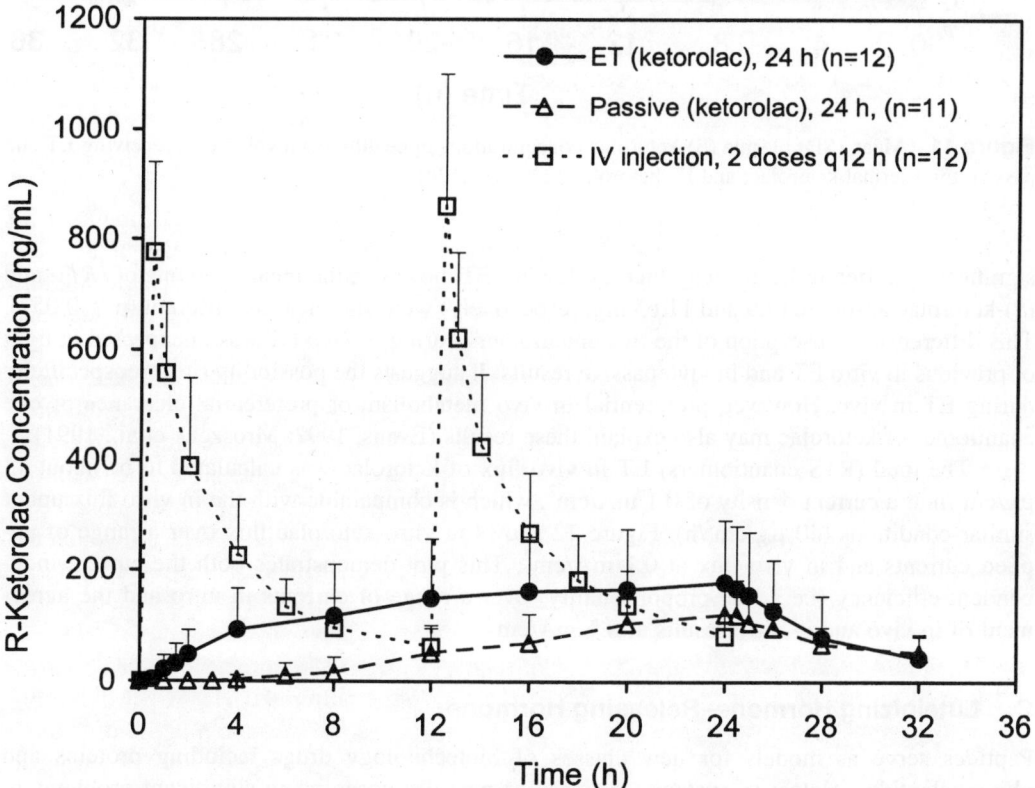

Figure 10 Mean (SD) plasma (R)-ketorolac concentrations in healthy male volunteers receiving ET and passive transdermal ketorolac, and IV ketorolac (2 doses q12h).

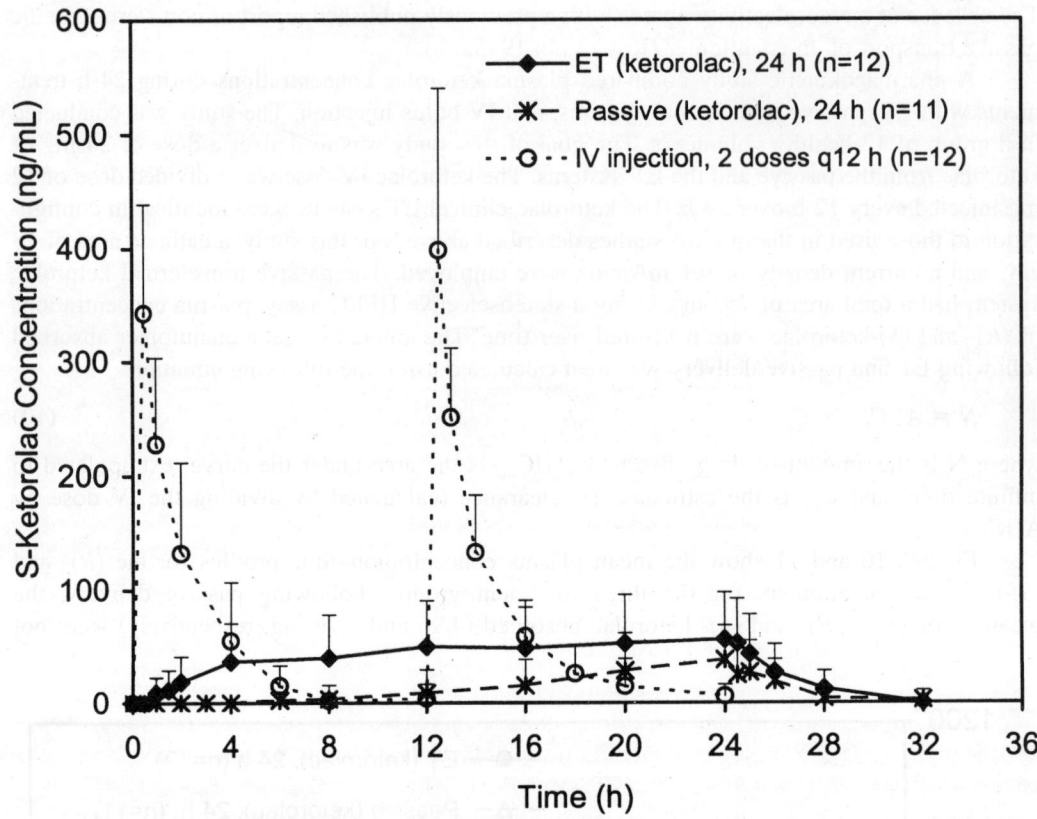

Figure 11 Mean (SD) plasma (S)-ketorolac concentrations in healthy male volunteers receiving ET and passive transdermal ketorolac, and IV ketorolac (2 doses q12h).

significantly different from each other. Following ET, however, the mean amounts of (*R1*)- and (*S*)-ketorolac absorbed (7.9 and 11.65 mg, respectively) were significantly different (p = 0.057). This difference in absorption of the two enantiomers during in vivo ET was unexpected in light of previous in vitro ET and in vivo passive results. It suggests the possibility of stereospecificity during ET in vivo. However, preferential in vivo metabolism or preferential clearance of one enantiomer of ketorolac may also explain these results (Evans, 1992; Mroszcak et al., 1991).

The total (R+S enantiomers) ET in vivo flux of ketorolac was calculated to be about 45 $\mu g/cm^2/h$ at a current density of 0.1 mA/cm^2, which is comparable with the in vitro flux under similar conditions (40 $\mu g/cm^2/h$). Figure 12 shows in vitro ketorolac flux over a range of applied currents and in vivo flux at 0.1 mA/cm^2. This plot demonstrates both the current-independent efficiency (i.e., dose proportionality) over a range of currents in vitro and the agreement of in vivo and in vitro results at 0.1 mA/cm^2.

C. Luteinizing Hormone–Releasing Hormone

Peptides serve as models for new classes of biotechnology drugs including proteins and oligonucleotides. However, systemic delivery of peptides poses many significant problems to pharmaceutical scientists. Because of their extensive metabolism in the gastrointestinal tract, peptides are not good candidates for oral administration. These compounds typically have large

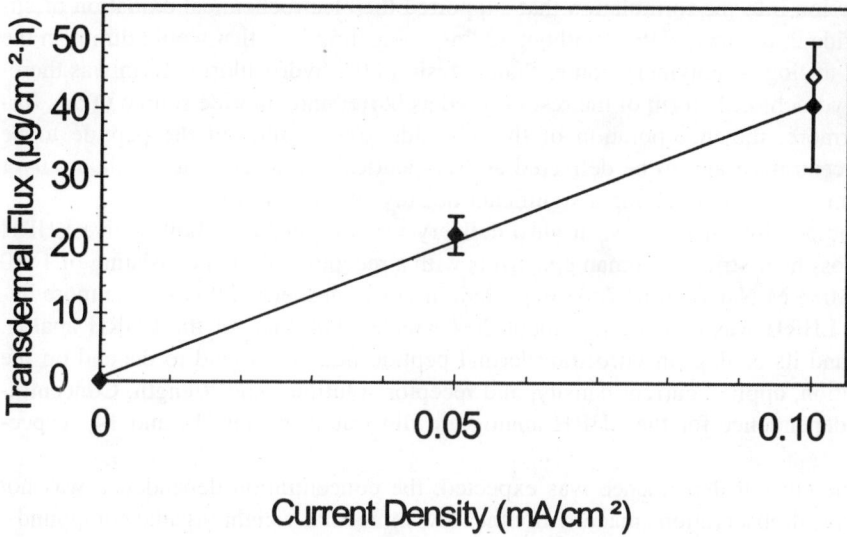

Figure 12 In vitro (solid diamonds) and in vivo (hollow diamond) ketorolac electrotransport flux. In vitro flux was measured at 0, 0.05, and 0.1 mA/cm^2, and in vivo flux was measured at 0.1 mA/cm^2.

molecular weights, are hydrophilic, and have net electrical charge. All of these qualities tend to negatively impact the passive transdermal flux, making LHRH a poor choice for passive transdermal delivery. However, the hydrophilic nature of these compounds and possession of net electrical charge makes them promising candidates for ET delivery (Delgado-Charro and Guy, 1995).

LHRH is a native reproductive hormone containing 10 amino acids with a molecular weight of approximately 1200 and a charge of +1 at near-neutral pH. Pulsatile delivery of LHRH by the hypothalamus stimulates the production of gonadotropins by the pituitary gland for the maintenance of normal female reproductive status. In contrast, continuous secretion of LHRH shuts down the reproductive axis.

In recent years, many highly potent and long-lived agonist and antagonist synthetic analogs of LHRH with different physicochemical properties have been synthesized; these are mainly used to eliminate the natural production of estrogen and testosterone in patients being treated for estrogen- and testosterone-dependent tumors. Pulsatile delivery of LHRH through infusion pumps (Lutrepulse, Ortho) has also been demonstrated to be an effective form of treatment for primary infertility of hypothalamic origin. Both of these therapies are invasive, requiring either multiple injections of slow-release depot formulations or an indwelling catheter. It is possible to achieve both the continuous and pulsed delivery profiles needed for these therapies using transdermal ET.

Published reports in the literature have demonstrated that continuous transdermal ET of LHRH is possible (Heit et al., 1993). Additionally, clinical success has also been obtained with continuous transdermal ET of leuprolide, a nine-amino-acid analog of LHRH (Meyer et al., 1990). The focus of the remainder of this section is the continuous ET delivery of a synthetic hydrophobic decapeptide LHRH analog and the pulsatile ET delivery of the hydrophilic native LHRH.

LHRH and its analog were incorporated into PVOH hydrogel formulations, and standard silver/silver chloride electrodes were employed. Because the native LHRH peptide was available as a chloride salt, creation of an ET-compatible hydrogel formulation was simple. However, since the LHRH analog was available only as the acetate salt, a method was required to introduce chloride ion into the formulation that supported the electrochemical oxidation of silver to silver chloride in the formulation without adding competing ions that would diminish the flux of the LHRH analog. A polymeric ion exchange resin in the hydrochloride form was therefore added. The hydrochloride form of the resin served as buffer and chloride source in this formulation. Furthermore, the incorporation of this chloride source allowed the peptide to be added at low concentration and to be delivered at therapeutically relevant rates without silver migration into skin and without having a significant negative effect on drug flux.

Using prototype clinical systems, in vitro delivery was evaluated for both native LHRH and its analog across heat-stripped human epidermis with a receptor solution consisting of 1:10 strength DPBS (0.015 M NaCl) at pH 7. As expected, in vitro transdermal flux for the more hydrophilic peptide LHRH was consistently about 20% greater than that for the LHRH analog. For both LHRH and its analog, in vitro transdermal peptide flux was found to depend on the peptide concentration, applied current density, and receptor solution ionic strength. Concentration and current dependence for the LHRH analog are illustrated in Figs. 13 and 14, respectively.

Although the current dependence was expected, the concentration dependence was not consistent with typical observations made with other low molecular weight organic compounds, in which delivery is constant over a large range of concentration. The observed concentration dependence of the flux may be due to the low concentrations used in this study (1–10 mM). At such low concentrations, the effect of ion competition may be strongly influenced by slight changes in drug concentration. Despite this phenomenon, there are compelling reasons to use such low concentrations with peptide drugs. These include the high cost of the drug, the well-known tendency of peptides to aggregate at higher concentrations, and the generally high potency of these drugs.

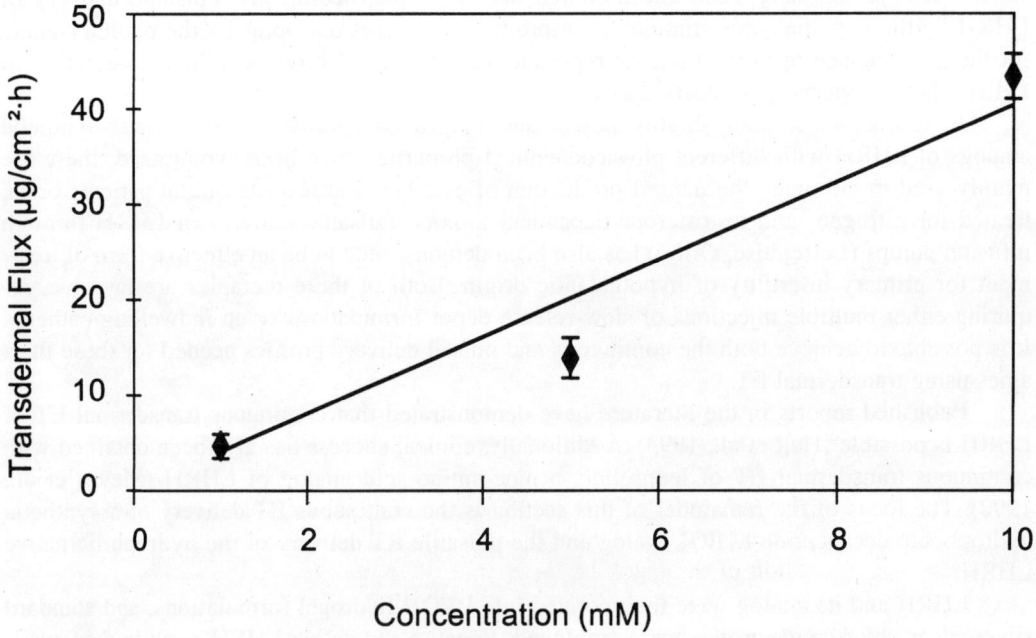

Figure 13 The effect of peptide concentration on in vitro steady-state electrotransport flux of a LHRH analog across human epidermis at 0.10 mA/cm^2 (n = 3).

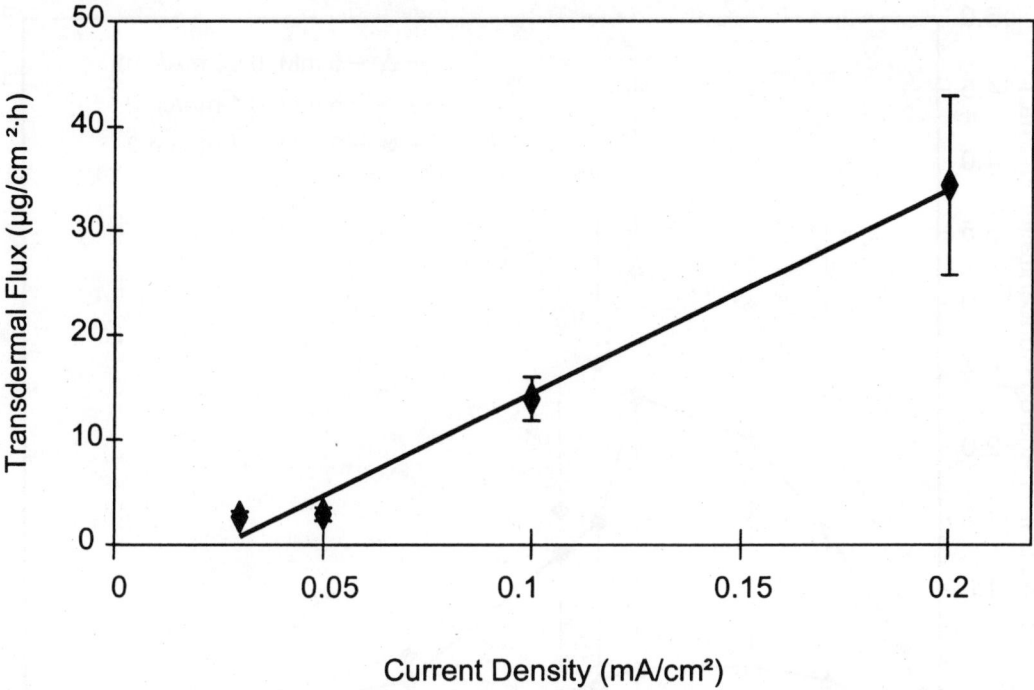

Figure 14 The effect of current density on in vitro steady-state electrotransport flux of an LHRH analog across human epidermis (n = 3, LHRH analog at 5 mM).

The effects of peptide concentration and current density were also evaluated in a clinical study with the LHRH analog. Formulation factors (i.e., current and drug concentration) had qualitatively similar results in vivo as they did in vitro. A reasonable in vitro/in vivo correlation was obtained. For example, a PVOH hydrogel formulation containing 5 mM LHRH analog resulted in an in vivo transdermal flux of 5 μg/cm^2/hr at 0.1 mA/cm^2 current density (Fig. 15). Under in vitro conditions, an identical formulation gave a transdermal flux of about 12 μg/cm^2/h across human epidermis into a 0.015 M NaCl DPBS receptor solution at pH 7.

The feasibility of delivering discrete pulses of LHRH using an ET system was also investigated in a clinical study in healthy male volunteers. The primary objective of the study was to determine the effects of various ET parameters, including pulse duration and current density, on plasma LHRH concentrations. The clinical prototype system employed was identical to systems that have been characterized for in vitro transport. The clinical system comprised an 8-cm^2 hydrogel formulation, which included 15 mM LHRH as the hydrochloride salt. Plasma samples were analyzed for both LHRH and the resultant luteinizing hormone (LH) using specific radioimmunoassays.

Plasma LHRH and LH concentrations obtained in eight subjects receiving one 15-min ET pulse every 2 h for 8 h at a current of 0.8 mA (0.1 mA/cm^2 current density) are shown in Fig. 16. The plasma LHRH concentration obtained following the administration of a single 5-μg IV bolus is also shown as a reference. These results demonstrate that pulsatile delivery of LHRH is possible using reasonable ET conditions. Significantly, the plasma LHRH profiles obtained with ETS are comparable to that obtained following IV bolus administration. The four consecutive 15-min pulses at 0.1 mA/cm^2 current density resulted in plasma LHRH pulses with

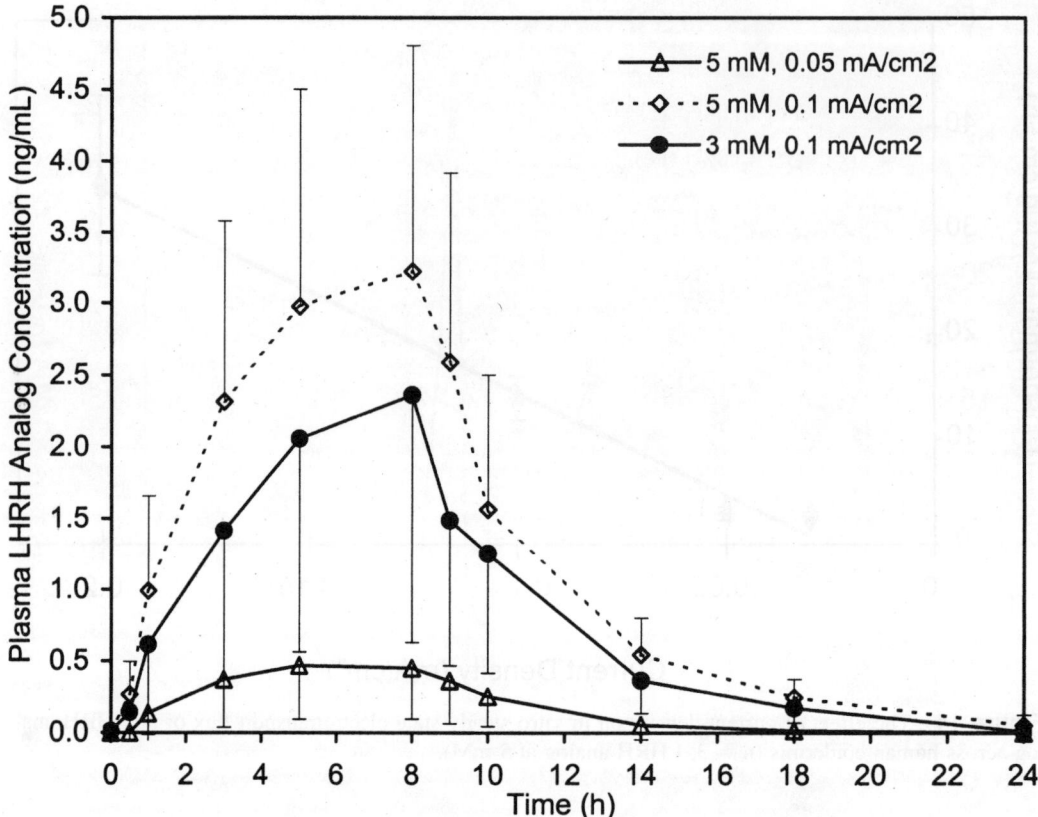

Figure 15 Mean (SD) plasma LHRH analog concentrations in healthy volunteers receiving ET LHRH analog; 4 cm^2, 8 h (n = 12).

sharp peaks (C_{max} up to 450 pg/mL). Plasma LHRH levels declined rapidly to negligible baseline values between ET pulses, consistent with IV administration but in contrast to subcutaneous injections (Handelsman et al., 1984). Following pulsatile ET delivery of LHRH, the pharmacodynamic plasma LH response also followed a pulsatile pattern with a mean C_{max} of about 26 mIU/mL. As was discussed earlier for fentanyl, the extent of variability in the LHRH ET delivery data was comparable with that obtained following IV administration.

In addition to the examples given above, other reports and reviews in the literature document drug delivery from ET systems using both in vitro and in vivo techniques (Banga and Chien, 1988; Singh and Maibach, 1994).

VI. CONCLUSION

Fundamental understanding of basic issues in electrotransport of drugs across skin has facilitated the process of designing practical commercial products. By defining these issues, a methodical approach to design is possible, resulting in products that are both therapeutically effective and likely to achieve acceptance in the marketplace. Delivery results demonstrate the ability of ET to deliver drugs in both a continuous and pulsatile fashion. Many of the special-

ET Systems for Transdermal Delivery

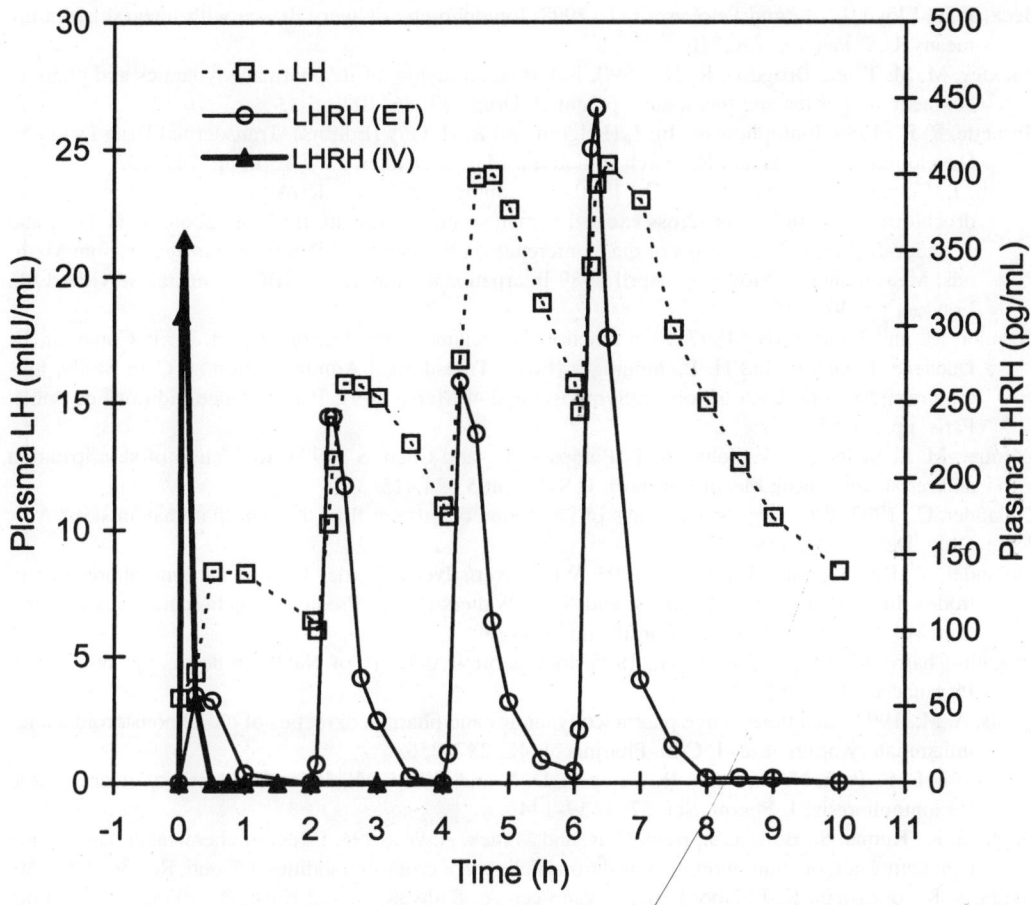

Figure 16 Mean plasma LHRH concentrations of healthy male volunteers receiving ET LHRH (0.1 mA/cm^2, 4 doses of 15 min every 2 h) and an IV LHRH bolus (5 μg). Mean plasma LH resulting from the ET LHRH treatment also plotted (n = 8).

ized formulation, component, and circuit-related solutions are described in the patent literature rather than in academic journals. This indicates a continued active commercial interest in the field of transdermal ET.

REFERENCES

Ahmedzai, S., Allan, E., Fallon, M., Finlay, I. G., Hanks, G. W., Hanna, M., Regnard, C. F. B. and Reilly, C., 1994. Transdermal fentanyl in cancer pain. J. Drug. Dev. 6: 93–97.

Anigbogu, A., Singh, P., Liu, P., Dinh, S. and Maibach, H., 1997. Effects of iontophoresis on rabbit skin in vivo. Pharm. Res. 14: S-308.

Banga, A. K., 1998. Electrically assisted transdermal and topical drug delivery. Taylor and Francis, London.

Banga, A. K. and Chien, Y. W., 1988. Iontophoretic delivery of drugs: fundamentals, developments and biomedical applications. J. Contr. Rel. 7: 1–24.

Beck, J. E., Lloyd, L. B., and Petelenz, T. J., 1998. Iontophoretic delivery device with integral hydrating means. U.S. Patent 5,730,716.

Buckley, M. M. T. and Brogden, R. N., 1990. Ketorolac: a review of its pharmacodynamics and pharmacokinetic properties and therapeutic potential. Drugs 39: 86–109.

Burnette, R. R., 1989. Iontophoresis. In: J. Hadgraft and R. H. Guy (Editors), Transdermal Drug Delivery: Developmental Issues and Research Initiatives, Marcel Dekker, New York, pp. 247–292.

Corish, J., Corrigan, O. I., and Foley, D., 1990. The iontophoretic transdermal delivery of morphine hydrochloride and other salts across excised human stratum corneum. In: R. C. Scott, R. H. Guy, and J. Hadgraft (Eds.), Proceedings of the Conference on Prediction of Percutaneous Penetration: Methods, Measurements, Modeling, April 1989 International Conference, IBC Technical Services Ltd., London, pp. 302–307.

Cormier, M. and Johnson, B., 1997. Skin reactions associated with electrotransport. In: P. Couvreur, D. Duchene, P. Green, and H. E. Junginger (Eds.), Transdermal Administration, A Case Study, Iontophoresis, a APGI/CRS European Symposium, 3–4 March 1997, Paris, France. Editions de Sante, Paris, pp. 50–57.

Cormier, M. J., Ledger, P. W., Johnson, J., Phipps, J. B., and Chao, S., 1997. Reduction of skin irritation and resistance during electrotransport. U.S. Patent 5,624,415.

Cullander, C., 1992. What are the pathways of iontophoretic current flow through mammalian skin? Adv. Drug. Del. Rev. 9: 119–135.

Cullander, C., Rao, G., and Guy, R. H., 1993. Why silver/silver chloride? Criteria for iontophoresis electrodes. In K. R. Brain, V. J. James, and K. A. Walters (Eds.), Prediction of Percutaneous Penetration; Vol. 3b. STS Publishing, Cardiff, pp. 381–390.

Delgado-Charro, M. B. and Guy, R. H., 1995. Iontophoretic delivery of Nafarelin across the skin. Int. J. Pharmaceut. 117: 165–172.

Evans, A. M., 1992. Enantioselective pharmacodynamics and pharmacokinetics of chiral nonsteroidal anti-inflammatory drugs. Eur. J. Clin. Pharmacol. 42: 237–256.

Gangarosa, L. P., Park, N. H., Fong, B. C., Scott, D. F. and Hill, J. M., 1978. Conductivity of drugs used for iontophoresis. J. Pharm. Sci. 67: 1439–1443.

Gupta, S. K., Kumar, S., Bolton, S., Behl, C. R. and Malick, A. W., 1994. Effect of chemical enhancers and conducting gels on iontophoretic transdermal delivery of cromolyn sodium. J. Contr. Rel. 31: 229–236.

Gupta, S. K., Bernstein, K. J., Noorduin, H., Van Peer, A., Sathyan, G. and Haak, R., 1998a. Fentanyl delivery from an electrotransport system: delivery is a function of total current, not duration of current. J. Clin. Pharmacol. 38: 951–958.

Gupta, S. K., Southam, M., Sathyan, G. and Klausner, M., 1998b. Effect of current density on pharmacokinetics following continuous or intermittent input from a fentanyl electrotransport system. J. Pharm. Sci. 87: 976–981.

Gyory, R. J., 1996. Electrotransport agent delivery device and method. U.S. Patent 5,380,271.

Gyory, R. J. and Peery, J. R., 1996. Iontophoretic delivery device and method of hydrating same. U.S. Patent 5,582,587.

Gyory, R. J. and Phipps, J. B., 1997. Effect of current density and current duration on the membrane resistance of skin. In: P. Couvreur, D. Duchene, P. Green, and H. E. Junginger (Eds.), Transdermal Administration, A Case Study, Iontophoresis, a APGI/CRS European Symposium, 3–4 March 1997, Paris, France. Editions de Sante, Paris, pp. 262–265.

Haak, R. P., 1996. Electrotransport device having improved cathodic electrode assembly. U.S. Patent 5,503,632.

Haak, R. P., Gyory, J. R., and Theeuwes, F., 1996. Device and method of iontophoretic drug delivery. U.S. Patent 5,496,266.

Handelsman, D. J., Jansen, R. P. S., Boylan, L. M., Spaliviero, J. A. and Turtle, J. R., 1984. Pharmacokinetics of gonadotropin-releasing hormone: comparison of subcutaneous and intravenous routes. J. Clin. Endocrinol. Metab. 59: 739–746.

Heit, M. C., Williams, P. L., Jayes, F. L., Chang, S. K. and Riviere, J. E., 1993. Transdermal iontophoretic peptide delivery: in vitro and in vivo studies with luteinizing hormone releasing hormone. J. Pharm. Sci. 82: 240–243.

Hillman, R. S. and Pawelchak, J. M., 1992. Apparatus and method for iontophoretic transfer. U.S. Patent 5,088,978.
Hoffman, K. C., 1987. Multi-element electrode. U.S. Patent 4,635,641.
Hollinger, M. A., 1996. Toxicological aspects of topical silver pharmaceuticals. Crit. Rev. Toxicol. 26(2): 255–260.
Horstmann, M., 1997. Galvanically active transdermal therapeutic system. U.S. Patent 5,685,837.
Huntington, J. A. and Cormier, M., 1998. Composition, device and method for electrotransport agent delivery. U.S. Patent 5,811,465.
Hyon, S. H. and Yoshito, I., 1988. Transdermal therapeutic composition. U.S. Patent 4,781,926.
Jacobs, N. A. and De Nuzzio, J. D., 1994. Iontophoretic drug delivery device electrode—has flexible backing member and active metal member covering part of inside surface. International Patent Publication WO 94/17853.
Jadoul, A., Regnier, V., and Preat, V., 1997. Influence of ethanol and propylene glycol addition on the transdermal delivery by iontophoresis and electroporation. Pharm. Res. 14: S308–S309.
Jevne, A. H., Vegoe, B. R., Holmblad, C. M. and Cahalan, P. T., 1986. Hydrophilic pressure sensitive biomedical adhesive composition. U.S. Patent 4,593,053.
Johnson, M. T. V. and Lee, N. H., 1990. pH buffered electrode for medical iontophoresis. U.S. Patent 4,973,303.
Kalia, Y. N. and Guy, R. H., 1995. The electrical characteristics of human skin in vivo. Pharm. Res. 12: 1605–1613.
Lai, Z., Kikunodai, C-S, Okabe, K., and Siego, S-K., 1996. High efficiency electrode system for iontophoresis. International Patent Publication WO 96/17649.
Lattin, G. A. and Spevak, R., 1983. Iontophoretic device with reversible polarity. U.S. Patent 4,406,658.
Lattin, G. L., Phipps, J. B., Southam, M. A. and Klausner, M., 1997. Evaluation of fentanyl delivery in humans using E-TRANS technology. In: P. Couvreur, D. Duchene, P. Green, and H. E. Junginger (Eds.), Transdermal Administration, A Case Study, Iontophoresis, a APGI/CRS European Symposium, 3–4 March 1997, Paris, France. Editions de Sante, Paris, pp. 365–368.
Ledger, P. W., 1992. Skin biological issues in electrically enhanced transdermal delivery. Adv. Drug Del. Rev., 9: 289–307.
Ledger, P. W., Cormier, M., and Campbell, P. S., 1997. Reduction of skin irritation during electrotransport delivery. U.S. Patent 5,693,010.
Lindblad, L. E. and Ekenvall, L., 1987. Electrode material in iontophoresis. Pharm. Res. 4: 438.
Lindblad, L. E., Ekenvall, L., Ancker, K., Rohman, H. and Oberg, P. A. 1986. Laser Doppler flow-meter assessment of iontophoretically applied norepinephrine on human finger skin circulation. J. Invest. Dermatol. 87: 634–636.
Lloyd, L. B., Beck, J. E., Petelenz, T. J. and Holt, C. H., 1994. Electrodes for iontophoresis. U.S. Patent 5,374,241.
Membrino, M. A., Orazem, M. E., Scott, E. and Phipps, J. B., 1997. Electrochemical impedance measurements for characterization of ion transport pathways in skin. In: P. Couvreur, D. Duchene, P. Green, and H. E. Junginger (Eds.), Transdermal Administration, A Case Study, Iontophoresis, a APGI/CRS European Symposium, 3–4 March 1997, Paris, France. Editions de Sante, Paris, pp. 313–317.
Merril, C. F., 1990. Silver staining proteins and DNA. Nature 343 (6260): 779–780.
Meyer, R. B., Kreis, W., Eschbach, J., O'Mara, V., Rosen, S. and Sibalis, D. 1990. Transdermal versus subcutaneous leuprolide: a comparison of acute pharmacodynamic effect. Clin. Pharmacol. Ther. 48: 340–345.
Miller, L. L., Blankespoor, R. L., and Zinger, B. 1986. Electrochemical controlled release drug delivery system. U.S. Patent 4,585,652.
Mroszcak, E., Combs, D., Tsina, I., Iam, Y., Massey, I., Chaplin, M. and Yee, J. 1991. Pharmacokinetics of (−)S and (+)R enantiomers of ketorolac in humans following administration of racemic ketorolac tromethamine. Clin. Pharmacol. Ther. 49: 126 (Abstract).
Muller, D. and Saunal, H., 1998. Iontophoresis device comprising at least one electrode assembly with a reversible composite electrode. U.S. Patent 5,807,305.
Myers, R. M. and Stahl, M. G., 1992. Iontophoretic delivery device. U.S. Patent 5,147,297.

Nightingale, J., Sclafani, J. and Kurihara-Bergstrom, T., 1990. Effect of pH on the iontophoretic delivery of ionic compounds, In: V. H. L. Lee (Ed.), Proceedings of the 17th International Symposium on Controlled Release of Bioactive Materials, 22–25 July 1990, Reno, Nevada. Controlled Release Society, Lincolnshire, IL, 17: 431–432.

Okabe, K., 1997. Interface for iontophoresis with hydrating mechanism,. U.S. Patent 5,628,729.

Phipps, J. B. and Untereker, D. F., 1988. Iontophoresis apparatus and methods of producing same. U.S. Patent 4,744,787.

Phipps, J. B., Padmanabhan, R. V. and Lattin, G. A., 1989a. Iontophoretic delivery of model inorganic and organic drug ions. J. Pharm. Sci. 78, 365–369.

Phipps, J. B., Sunram, J. M., and Padmanabhan, R. V., 1989b. The effect of extraneous ions on the transdermal iontophoretic delivery of hydromorphone. In: R. Pearlman and J. A. Miller (Eds.), Proceedings of the 16th International Symposium on Controlled Release of Bioactive Materials, 6–9 August 1989, Chicago, Illinois. Controlled Release Society, Lincolnshire, IL, 16: 50–51.

Phipps, J. B., 1991. Iontophoresis electrode. U.S. Patent 5,057,072.

Phipps, J. B., 1992. Iontophoresis apparatus and methods of producing same. U.S. Patent 5,084,008.

Phipps, J. B. and Gyory, J. R., 1992. Transdermal ion migration. Adv. Drug. Del. Rev., 9: 137–176.

Phipps, J. B., 1993. Method for reducing sensation in iontophoretic drug delivery. U.S. Patent 5,221,254.

Phipps, J. B., Howland, W. W., Jevne, A. H., and Holmblad, C., 1996. Device and method for iontophoretic drug delivery. U.S. Patent 5,558,633.

Phipps, J. B., 1997a. Method and apparatus for controlled environment electrotransport. U.S. Patent 5,591,124.

Phipps, J. B., 1997b. Electrode and Reservoir Design for Optimal Transdermal Delivery by Iontophoresis. In: P. Couvreur, D. Duchene, P. Green, and H. E. Junginger (Eds.), Transdermal Administration, A Case Study, Iontophoresis, a APGI/CRS European Symposium, March 1997, Paris, France. Editions de Sante, Paris, pp 30–39.

Phipps, J. B., Cormier, M. and Padmanabhan, R., 1997. In vivo ion efflux from humans and the relationship to skin irritation. In: P. Couvreur, D. Duchene, P. Green, and H. E. Junginger (Eds.), Transdermal Administration, A Case Study, Iontophoresis, a APGI/CRS European Symposium, 3–4 March 1997, Paris, France. Editions de Sante, Paris, pp. 289–291.

Pikal, M. J., 1992. The role of electroosmotic flow in transdermal iontophoresis. Adv. Drug Del. Rev. 9: 201–237.

Prausnitz, M. R., Corbett, J. D., Gimm, J. A., Golan, D. E., Langer, R. and Weaver, J. C., 1995. Millisecond measurement of transport during and after an electroporation pulse, Biophys. J. 68, 1864–1870.

Rao, G., Guy, R. H., Glikfeld, P., LaCourse, W.R., Leung, L., Tamada, J., Potts, R. O. and Azimi, N., 1995. Reverse iontophoresis: noninvasive glucose monitoring in vivo in humans. Pharm. Res., 12,1869–1873.

Reddy, V. N., 1998. Iontophoretic electrodes and surface active agents. U.S. Patent 5,792,097.

Rosendahl, T. 1942–43 Studies on the conducting properties of the human skin to direct current. Acta. Physiol. Scand. 5: 130–151.

Roy, S. D., Chatterjee, D. J., Manoukian, E. and Divor, A., 1995a. Permeability of pure enantiomers of ketorolac through human cadaver skin. J. Pharm. Sci. 84: 987–990.

Roy, S. D., Manoukian, E. and Combs. D. 1995b. Absorption of transdermally delivered ketorolac acid in humans. J. Pharm. Sci. 84: 49–52.

Sage, Jr., B. H., 1994. Electrode and method used for iontophoresis. U.S. Patent 5,284,471.

Sage, B. H. and Flower, R. J., 1995. International Patent Publication WO 95/09032.

Sanderson, J. E. and Deriel, S. R., 1988. Method and apparatus for iontophoretic drug delivery. U.S. Patent 4,722,726.

Sanderson, J. E., Reil, S. D. and Dixon, R., 1989. Iontophoretic delivery of nonpeptide drugs: formulation optimization form maximum skin permeability. J. Pharm. Sci. 78: 361–364.

Scott, E. R., Laplaza, A. I, White, H. S. and J. B. Phipps., 1993. Transport of ionic species in skin: contribution of pores to the overall skin conductance. Pharm. Res. 10: 1699–1709.

Scott, E. R., Phipps, J. B. and White, H. S., 1995. Direct imaging of molecular transport through skin. J. Invest. Dematol. 104: 142–145.

Sibalis, D., 1989. Disposable transdermal drug applicators. U.S. Patent 4,865,582.

Singh, P. and Maibach, H. I., 1994. Iontophoresis in drug delivery: basic principles and applications. Crit. Rev. Ther. Drug. Carr. Syst. 11: 161–213.

Southam, M., Bernstein, K. J. and Noorduin, H., 1996. Device for transdermal electrotransport delivery of fentanyl and sufentanil. International Patent Publication Number. WO 96/39222.

Thysman, S., Tasset, C. and Preat, V., 1994. Transdermal iontophoresis of fentanyl: delivery and mechanistic analysis. Int. J. Pharm. 101: 105–113.

Tyle, P., 1986. Iontophoretic devices for drug delivery. Pharm. Res. 3:318–326.

Untereker, D. F., Phipps, J. B. and Lattin, G. A., 1992. Iontophoretic drug delivery. U.S. Patent 5,135,477.

Untereker, D. F., Phipps, J. B. and Lattin, G. A., 1996. Iontophoretic drug delivery. U.S. Patent 5,573,503.

Webster, H. L. 1983. Iontophoresis electrode device with gel insert—has electrode plate in cup-like receptacle so that agar gel disc can protrude for pressing against patient's skin. US Patent 4,383,529.

Yoshida, N. H. and Roberts, M. S., 1995. Prediction of cathodal iontophoretic transport of anions across excised skin from different vehicles using conductivity measurements. J. Pharm. Pharmacol. 47: 883–890.

Zevert, T. E., Pliquette, U. F., Langer, R. and Weaver, J. C., 1995. Transdermal transport of DNA antisense oligonucleotides by electroporation. Biochem. and Biophys. Res. Commun. 212: 286–292.

32
Controlled Release Protein Therapeutics: Effects of Process and Formulation on Stability

Paul A. Burke
Amgen, Thousand Oaks, California

I. INTRODUCTION

A. Proteins as Therapeutics

Development of protein therapeutics is a long-standing focus of the biotechnology industry. Proteins currently marketed or undergoing clinical testing number in the hundreds (1) and include monoclonal antibodies, growth factors, cytokines, soluble receptors, and hormones. Proteins act specifically, and generally exert their effects at low concentrations. Despite these virtues, proteins exhibit low oral and transdermal bioavailabilities (2), necessitating delivery by injection (3). Because protein drugs are cleared rapidly from systemic circulation, injections must be given frequently (Table 1). This requirement is painful and inconvenient for the patient, and can result in noncompliance, compromising the efficacy of therapy.

One approach to reducing injection frequency has been to alter the pharmacokinetic properties of the molecule. Serum half-lives can be extended through covalent attachment of biocompatible polymers such as poly(ethylene glycol) (10–13), or through genetic engineering approaches such as increasing the levels of glycosylation (14) or creating fusion constructs (15). Covalently modified proteins may acquire unfavorable properties such as toxicity (16), immunogenicity, or lower bioactivity. In addition, they must be developed as completely new drugs. Furthermore, as with the parent molecule, clearance of a protein conjugate is first order. Peak exposure is many times the therapeutic level, resulting in waste and risking toxic overexposure in exchange for less frequent dosing.

The past decade has seen major advances in the systemic delivery of proteins and peptides by oral, transdermal, and pulmonary routes (2,17). To date, none of these systems has reached the market. Moreover, limits in net bioavailability may preclude their use with expensive drugs (18). The above technologies sometimes fail to address the fundamental issue that pulsatile delivery—regardless of route or frequency—is often not the best kinetic profile of drug exposure (19,20). Tailoring drug exposure to therapeutic need requires control of drug release into the systemic circulation. For many proteins, continuous maintenance of the drug concentration in a specific therapeutic window is optimal. This degree of control, achieved with zero-order systems, minimizes peak exposure and results in a lower cumulative dose. For proteins with very short half-lives or excessive systemic toxicity, sustained release may be required to

Table 1 Half-lives in Humans and Approved Dosing Frequencies of Several Recombinant Proteins

Protein	Serum half-life (h)	Weekly dosing frequency (4)
α-Interferon (5)	5.6	3
γ-Interferon (6)	0.6	3
Human growth hormone (7)	0.3	7
Erythropoietin (8)	6	3
Granulocyte colony-stimulating factor (8)	5	7
Granulocyte–macrophage colony-stimulating factor (9)	2	7

make commercial development attractive. In other cases, efficacy is enhanced. For example, in the treatment of acromegaly with octreotide, a sustained release formulation provided superior clinical efficacy (21). Likewise, sustained release of human growth hormone (hGH) was found more effective than conventional injections (22). For certain drugs maintenance of continuous drug levels is critical to avoid an adverse effect. Leuprolide acetate, a gonadotropin-releasing hormone superagonist, produces a potentially harmful spike in testosterone levels on initiation of therapy in prostate cancer patients (23). This can exacerbate symptoms and precludes use of the drug in certain patients. Giving the drug in a sustained release formulation prevents recurrence of the testosterone spike during the course of treatment (24).

B. Initial Reports of Protein Controlled Release

Given the limitations of protein drugs, interest in controlled release within the biotechnology industry unsurprisingly dates from its earliest days. However, the technical hurdles were thought insurmountable by many. Fickian diffusion of drugs through nonerodible hydrophobic polymers (such as ethyl vinyl acetate, EVA) was limited to compounds of much lower molecular weight and hydrophilicity. Poor biocompatibility was another problem. A further hurdle was the use of organic solvents, required by many encapsulation processes but long considered protein denaturants. The common knowledge that proteins are "very fragile and readily disrupted by heat and other seemingly mild treatments" (25) led many to conclude that they were incompatible with encapsulation using polymers of limited water solubility.

These challenges were first overcome by Langer and Folkman (26), who developed polymeric systems releasing model proteins for over 100 days. EVA matrices were rendered biocompatible by washing away polymer impurities prior to encapsulation. Protein release from the nonerodible matrix occurred by diffusion through aqueous-filled channels created by the protein particles (27). While organic solvents were used in processing, an encapsulated protein retained its activity as shown in an in vivo angiogenesis bioassay (26). Many subsequent reports of controlled protein release relate to bioassay development (28). This application of protein controlled release (where matrix erodibility is nonessential) continues to the present. The recent literature includes further examples of angiogenic bioassays (29–31), as well as pharmacological models of osseous repair (32) and inhibition of carcinogenesis (33).

C. From Proof of Concept to Clinical Candidates

The transition from nonerodible systems used in animal models to candidate formulations for clinical development has occurred over two decades. The Langer and Folkman report appeared in 1976 (26), while the first clinical testing of a controlled release protein formulation occurred only recently (34). The maturation of the field is attributable to several key developments. The availability of polymers that are both biocompatible and bioerodible made polymeric systems attractive for parenteral delivery. Copolymers of lactic and glycolic acid (PLGA) began to gain favor (35) in the late 1970s, and have since amassed a strong track record of biocompatibility (36). A further development has been in the area of protein stability. As the field has matured attention has turned to maintaining protein integrity at levels suitable for a pharmaceutical product. Proteins are large structures with complex architecture, possessing secondary, tertiary, and, in some cases, quaternary structure. They often have labile bonds and numerous chemically reactive groups on their side chains. While encapsulation processes designed for less complex molecules may retain some biological activity of a protein, this may be insufficient for a pharmaceutical. Disruption of native structure can lead to loss of activity or immunogenicity, presenting a safety concern. An understanding of the effects of organic solvent exposure on protein integrity, the result of 15 years of research, has illuminated the relationship between process, formulation, and stability. Better insight into factors affecting protein stability in the solid and aqueous states has also proved crucial.

Initial reports of macromolecule delivery using PLGA demonstrated feasibility using albumin and insulin (37). Advances in protein stabilization have come from studies with albumin (38–40) and lysozyme (40), as well as with vaccines. The past 3 years has seen a number of reports on vaccine stabilization in polymer delivery systems. In cases of passive immunity, an antibody is delivered either systemically or to a mucosal surface; integrity is necessary for efficacy, not for safety reasons (41). Similarly, with active immunization the presence of nonnative forms would not have an adverse effect, although sufficient integrity must be maintained to elicit an immunogenic response to the native antigenic structure (42). Stable microsphere formulations of subunit vaccines against HIV (43), hepatitis B (44), and tetanus (42,45–47) have been reported. Such advances in stabilization are critical to the development of single-administration vaccines (which exhibit biphasic release kinetics), an important public health objective (48).

In contrast to vaccines, therapeutics leave little room for compromise on integrity because antibody formation by a patient could potentially result in autoimmunity. The application of principles of protein stabilization can avert this risk. The recent literature includes multiple examples of formulations releasing human protein therapeutics for weeks with excellent integrity profiles (discussed below). Nearly all of these cases had as their goal systemic administration. Recent preclinical reports encompass similar examples, as well as an expanding list of new opportunities in areas such as tissue engineering and cancer therapy. Controlled release enables local administration of drugs to specific sites of action, an important capability for proteins. Intra- and perivascular delivery of angiogenic growth factors facilitates revascularization of heart tissue (49,50). A variety of growth factors are being used for regeneration of bone (51–53) and other tissues (54). Local delivery of cytokines is being pursued for tumor immunotherapy (55–57) and nerve growth factor has been administered intracranially (58). These applications will reach fruition only if protein stability challenges can be met. Of the many possible strategies for controlled delivery of proteins (59), to date only those based on PLGA have reached advanced stages of clinical development. These are the focus of the present review.

II. STABILIZATION TOWARD ENCAPSULATION

A. Overview of Encapsulation Processes

Encapsulation processes have been reviewed by Benoit et al. (60). The most common processes are those based on emulsions (solvent evaporation, solvent extraction or phase separation) or atomization [spray drying or spray freezing (61–63)]. These process options are considered in Fig. 1. Proteins may be encapsulated either as solids (Fig. 1A) or as aqueous solutions (Fig. 1B). In the former case, protein solids are usually obtained by lyophilization or spray drying of

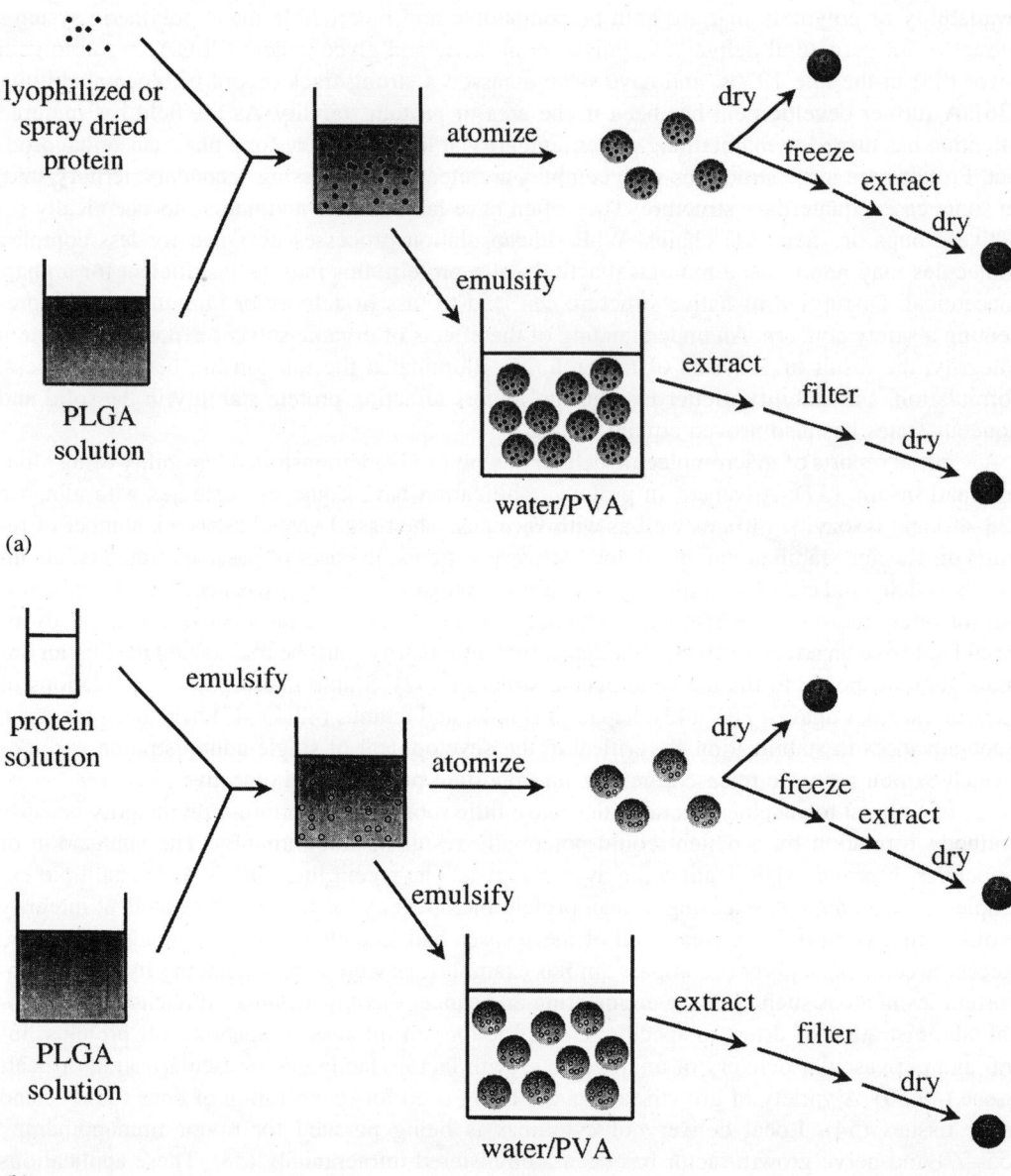

Figure 1 (A) Process options for encapsulation of water-soluble drugs in a solid form. Protein solids are created by lyophilization, precipitation, or spray drying. Solids are suspended in a solution of PLGA; methylene chloride and ethyl acetate are commonly used solvents. Microspheres are created by emulsification of the suspension, to form an s/o/w emulsion, or by atomization. (B) Encapsulation of protein solutions. Microspheres are created by forming a primary emulsion of protein solution in a polymer solution, followed by secondary emulsification in an aqueous continuous phase containing a stabilizer such as polyvinyl alcohol. Alternatively, the primary emulsion can be atomized. The remaining steps are the same as in A, except the final drying step removes both water and the polymer solvent.

Table 2 Stresses Imposed by Encapsulation Processes

Process	Stress		
	Solid–organic interfaces	Aqueous–organic interfaces and shear	High temperature
Double emulsion (w/o/w)		●	
Suspension emulsion (s/o/w)	●		
Spray dry	●	●	●
Spray freeze	●	●	

an aqueous protein solution, although precipitates have also been used (64). Solids are mixed with a solution of PLGA in an organic solvent. Nascent microspheres are formed by either atomization or emulsification. Atomized droplets can be dried directly (spray-drying process). Alternatively, droplets can be frozen, subjected to solid–liquid extraction to remove the polymer solvent, and subsequently dried [Alkermes ProLease spray-freeze process (62)]. In the case of suspension emulsification, the polymer solvent is removed by solvent evaporation or extraction. For all of these processes organic solvent exposure occurs at a solid–liquid interface between the protein particles and the polymer solvent. In the spray-freeze process, the protein is also exposed to a polymer nonsolvent (e.g., ethanol) during the extraction step. The encapsulation of aqueous protein solutions (Fig. 1B) differs in two major respects. First, the initial mixture of protein and polymer solutions requires emulsification, generating aqueous–organic interfaces as well as shear forces. Second, the final drying step imposes a phase change, from solution to solid, on the protein. Table 2 summarizes the stresses imposed by these processes.

B. How Organic Solvents Can Affect Protein Structure

The structural impact of encapsulation hinges on the physical forces stabilizing the native state and how process stresses, such as organic solvent exposure, affect them. Proteins are stabilized in their folded form by electrostatic interactions between oppositely charged residues, hydrogen bonding, van der Waals interactions, and the hydrophobic interaction (65). Interactions between charges are strongly influenced by the dielectric constant (D) of the medium according to Coulomb's law:

$$\Delta E = (Z_A Z_B \epsilon^2)/Dr_{AB}$$

where Z_A and Z_B represent the respective net charges of the interacting atoms, ϵ is one unit of electric charge, and r_{AB} is the distance between the charges. Dielectric constants vary widely among common PLGA solvents (Table 3).

The hydrophobic interaction is essentially the absence of a water interaction. In a folded protein, hydrophilic residues tend to partition to the outside surface of the protein, where they can hydrogen-bond with water molecules. In contrast, hydrophobic residues partition to the protein interior so as to avoid an unfavorable interaction with water. Hydrophobicity is frequently expressed as the logarithm of the partition coefficient (P) of a given entity between water and octanol, although alternative conventions can be used. Amino acid substituents have a wide range of hydrophobicities (Table 4), as do commonly used PLGA solvents (Table 5).

The addition of a *water-miscible* organic solvent to an aqueous protein solution will change the net dielectric constant, altering the energetics of coulombic interactions. In addition,

Table 3 Dielectric Constants of Some Commonly Used PLGA Solvents

Solvent	Dielectric constant
Water	80
Dimethylsulfoxide	45
Acetonitrile	39
Acetone	21
Methylene chloride	9.0
Ethyl acetate	6.0
Chloroform	4.8
Dioxane	2.2

Table 4 Hydrophobicities of Amino Acid Side Chains (65)

Amino acid	Substituent hydrophobicity constant, π^a
Ser	−1.03
His	−0.25
Ala	0.56
Met	−0.61
Val	1.53
Ile	2.04
Phe	2.01
Trp	2.14

^{a}Relative to Gly; $\pi = \log (P/Po)$.

Table 5 Hydrophobicities of Various Organic Solvents (66)

Solvent	log P
Dimethylsulfoxide	−1.3
Dioxane	−1.1
Acetonitrile	−0.33
Acetone	−0.23
Ethyl acetate	0.68
Chloroform	2.0

an increase of net solvent hydrophobicity will increase the tendency for hydrophobic residues to partition toward the surface as opposed to the hydrophobic core of a globular protein. As the organic solvent concentration increases, the protein conformation will change (67), although this can be preceded by precipitation. (Precipitation is most likely when the pH of the solution is near the protein isoelectric point.) Enzyme catalytic mechanisms have been characterized in aqueous–organic mixtures under cryogenic conditions (e.g., −100°C) (68). Cosolvent addition, required to effect freezing point depression, was not destabilizing due to the inverse relation between dielectric constant and temperature; the combined effects of cosolvent and decreased temperature offset one another.

The impact of organic solvents on protein structure is influenced by the order of component addition. Griebenow and Klibanov (69) added lysozyme powder to mixtures of acetonitrile in water. At acetonitrile contents of less than 60% the lyophilized powder dissolved, producing a solution. At higher acetonitrile contents a suspension resulted. As discussed above, one would expect increasing acetonitrile concentrations to destabilize coulombic interactions and alter solvent hydrophobicity, resulting in protein unfolding. The authors assessed protein unfolding by Fourier transform infrared (FTIR) spectroscopy, which measures secondary structure (Fig. 2). As expected, unfolding increased with acetonitrile content, but only if the mixture formed a solution. Under conditions where the protein remained as a suspension, a different result was observed. When lyophilized powder was added to *anhydrous* acetonitrile, the secondary structure was nearly identical to powder in the absence of solvent (Fig. 2). This seemingly counterintuitive finding is relevant to the design of protein-friendly encapsulation processes. The processes depicted in Fig. 1A start with addition of a protein powder to a water-free organic solvent. This step does not have the same structural consequences seen in monophasic cosolvent mixtures and is often benign.

C. Encapsulation of Protein Solids

1. Evidence for Structural Integrity in Organic Solvents

Evidence for protein structural integrity in anhydrous solvents has accumulated over the last 15 years, with the majority of studies coming from the field of nonaqueous enzymology (70). Enzymes suspended as powders exhibit catalytic activity in a wide variety of organic solvents,

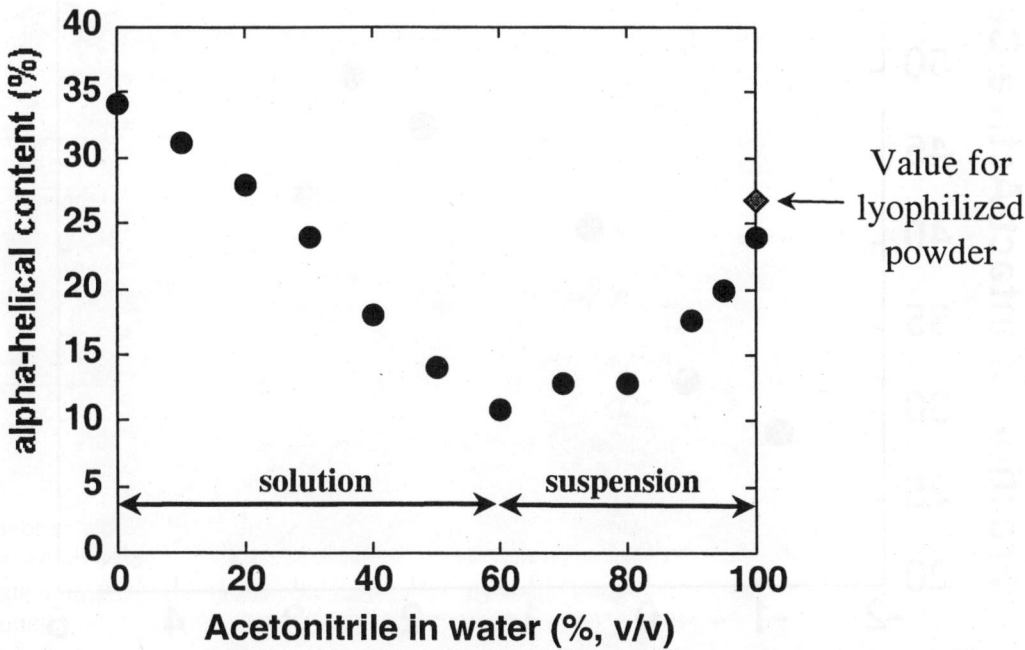

Figure 2 α-Helical content, measured by FTIR, of lysozyme in acetonitrile–water mixtures. Lyophilized lysozyme was added to cosolvents of various compositions. Loss of α-helical structure increased with acetonitrile concentration under conditions where the protein dissolved. At 100% acetonitrile, secondary structure was comparable to lyophilized powder in the absence of solvent. (Adapted from Ref. 69.)

suggesting retention of native structure. Solid-state nuclear magnetic resonance (NMR) spectroscopy provided the first direct evidence that an enzyme active site remained intact in organic solvents (71). Lyophilized α-lytic protease suspended in anhydrous acetone and octane retained its active center structure, while dimethylsulfoxide (which dissolves many proteins) disrupted it. These results were consistent with catalytic activity determinations in the same solvents. The active center structure of lyophilized α-chymotrypsin was also probed in a variety of organic solvents (72). Active center structure correlated with solvent hydrophobicity, with the most hydrophobic solvents being the most benign (Fig. 3). Active center disruption by hydrophilic solvents was likely due to removal of essential residual water molecules from the lyophilized protein (72). [Proteins retain some essential residual water following lyophilization (73).] Protein secondary structure in organic solvents has been characterized by FTIR (74), and 2D solution NMR has been used to deduce solvent effects on tertiary structure of lyophilized bovine pancreatic trypsin inhibitor (BPTI) (75). Tertiary structure in organic media has been directly observed by x-ray crystallography. Lyophilized protein powders are amorphous, and proteins cannot be crystallized from solvents in which they are insoluble. Hence, x-ray crystallographic evaluation starts with protein crystals in an aqueous mother liquor, followed by the gradual replacement of the medium with an organic solvent. Crystals of subtilisin required crosslinking

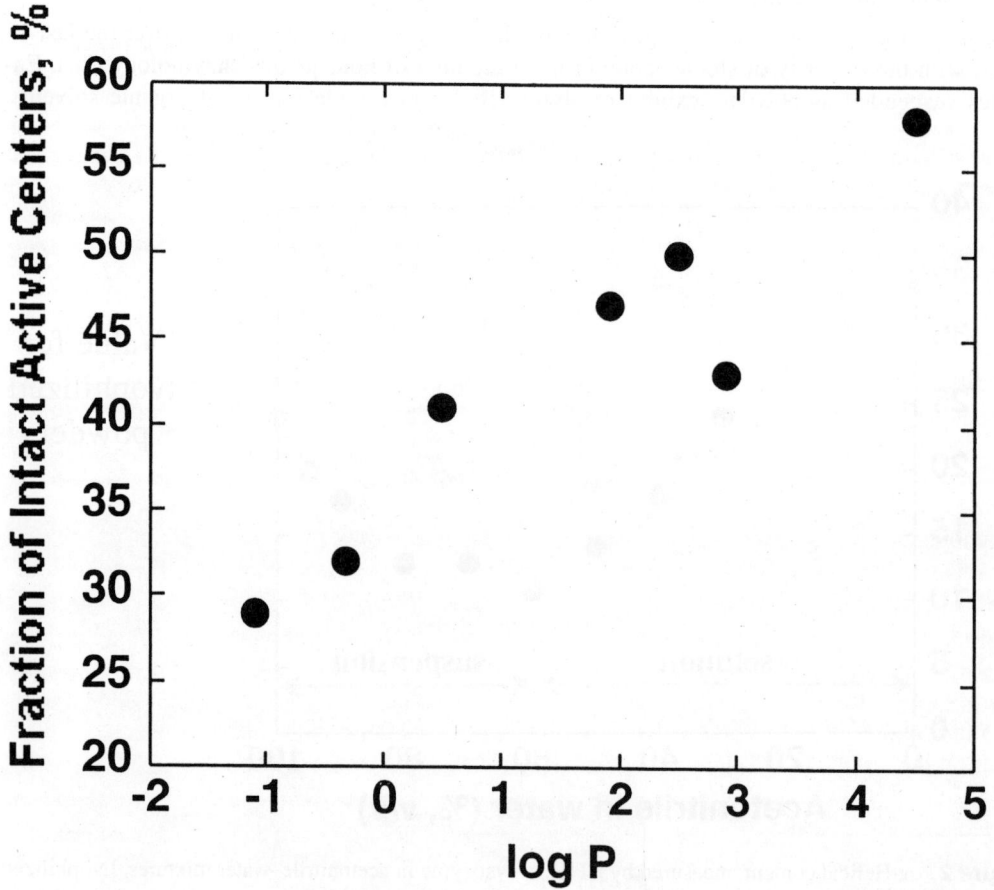

Figure 3 Integrity of chymotrypsin suspended in organic solvents of various hydrophobicities, expressed as log P. (Adapted from Ref. 72.)

prior to solvent exchange (76,77) to prevent disruption, while chymotrypsin crystals did not require crosslinking (78). These studies demonstrated remarkably little effect of the solvent on the structure, aside from some side chain rearrangements resulting in increased exposure of some hydrophobic groups in nonpolar solvents.

2. Why Don't Enzymes Unfold in Organic Solvents?

Given the known effects of organic solvents on electrostatic and hydrophobic interactions, one might wonder why proteins maintain their structure in nonaqueous milieu. The evidence shows that a lack of protein conformational mobility is responsible (79). While the native structure is not favored thermodynamically, protein rigidity prevents significant unfolding, resulting in a kinetic trap. Evidence from electron paramagnetic resonance (EPR) (80), solid-state NMR (81), and time-resolved fluorescence anisotropy (82) supports this hypothesis. The aforementioned crystallographic studies offer further support. A protein crystal's thermal factor is one measure of protein flexibility. Indeed, x-ray analysis of γ-chymotrypsin revealed lower thermal factors for protein atoms in hexane than in water (78). Increased order in the protein crystal lattice (evidenced by stronger diffraction) was observed in hexane, consistent with a more rigid structure. Interestingly, water molecules near the protein surface likewise showed reduced mobility in hexane, and the number of water molecules appearing in the structure was increased compared to aqueous conditions. Stronger interactions between the protein's polar groups in organic solvents apparently form the molecular basis for increased rigidity. In simulations of BPTI dynamics in chloroform, differences in flexibility were limited to specific regions of the protein (83). A substantial increase in intramolecular hydrogen-bonding interactions in chloroform was observed compared to water (83).

3. Stabilization of Protein Solids Toward Organic Solvents

The above discussion points to several principles for stabilizing protein solids toward organic solvent exposure. Since stability relies on a kinetic trap, the temperature and duration of solvent exposure should be minimized, although enzymes have been shown to exhibit remarkable thermostability in organic solvents (84). A kinetic trap relies on an energy barrier that prevents the structure from rearranging to a more thermodynamically favored one. Hence, the free energy of activation—rather than the free energy difference between the initial state and the denatured state—determines stability. Though counterintuitive, the least water-like solvents can be the most benign. To maximize protein rigidity, dielectric constant and water content should be *minimized*. Hydrophobic solvents minimize redistribution of residual water in protein solids while exogenous water acts as a plasticizer, resulting in protein unfolding (81). In light of these principles, some processes in Fig. 1A are more suitable than others, at least from a theoretical perspective. For example, in an s/o/w process water can partition to the solid protein particles. Iwata et al. (85) used an s/o/w process to encapsulate tumor necrosis factor-α (TNF-α) with methylene chloride as the solvent. Immediate hydration of the protein was observed, with a total loss of bioactivity.

In addition to the organic solvent, the properties of the protein solid influence stability. Based on the example above (Fig. 2), the protein particles obviously should be insoluble (69). As with the solvent, the residual water content in protein solids should be minimized (86). Lyoprotectants can be used to enhance protein stability toward organic solvent exposure. Ammonium sulfate and sucrose stabilized chymotrypsin toward lyophilization and protected against denaturation by hydrophilic organic solvents (72). Human growth hormone lyophilized with trehalose was stabilized toward an s/o/w encapsulation process (64) and toward encapsulation in a PLGA film (87). Inclusion of the lyoprotectant minimized loss of hGH secondary structure

Table 6 Postencapsulation Integrity of Human Therapeutic Proteins in Injectable, Biodegradable Sustained-Release Formulations: Proteins Encapsulated as Solids

Protein	Stabilization Strategy	Integrity (%)	Ref.
Erythropoietin	Protein colyophilized with ammonium sulfate	100	88
Nerve growth factor	None	94	89
Growth hormone	Protein colyophilized with trehalose or mannitol	96–100	64
Growth hormone	Encapsulated protein complexed and co-encapsulated with zinc	97	90
β-Interferon	None	100	91, 92
Vascular endothelial growth factor	None	100	31
Insulin	None	90	93
Tumor necrosis factor–α	Protein colyophilized with gelatin	99	85, 94

on organic solvent exposure (87). Similarly, TNF-α lyophilized with gelatin was stable toward acetonitrile exposure for up to 72 h (85). Table 6 summarizes several reports of postprocessing integrity of human proteins encapsulated as solids.

D. Encapsulation of Protein Solutions

1. Surface Denaturation

In contrast to the processes discussed above, organic solvent exposure occurs at an aqueous–organic interface when aqueous protein solutions are encapsulated (Fig. 1B). Proteins, being amphipathic, adsorb at interfacial surfaces in an unfolded state (95–97) and stabilize the primary emulsion in the absence of other surfactants (98,99). The fate of surface-denatured protein will impact the integrity of the final product. Protein adsorption is generally considered irreversible except at high interfacial pressure (95,97,100), although competitive displacement of proteins by surfactants can occur (101). The high local protein concentration at the interface accelerates intermolecular events such as aggregation, possibly resulting in precipitation, or disulfide exchange, resulting in covalent aggregates. Even in the absence of these events, structural changes can adversely affect storage stability, discussed below.

The polymer in the organic phase may also be surface-active. Boury et al. (102) characterized the interface of aqueous bovine serum albumin (BSA) and a solution of poly(D,L-lactide) (PLA) in methylene chloride. Analysis by a dynamic pendant-drop method indicated that a mixed interfacial layer resulted, with interpenetrating protein and polymer segments. Polymer (as opposed to protein) was preferentially displaced with increased interfacial pressure. Nihant et al. (99) observed interfacial coprecipitation of BSA and PLGA under similar conditions. The resultant surface protein concentration was 10- to 200-fold higher than in the absence of polymer.

A number of variables will influence the degree of surface denaturation. Droplet size will determine the available interfacial area. Surface tension will vary with the polymer solvent; Cleland and Jones (64) observed a higher recovery of monomeric hGH following emulsification with ethyl acetate than with methylene chloride, which may have been due to this effect. Surface denaturation of proteins can be exacerbated in the presence of shear (103), such as that generated by homogenization (104). Morlock et al. (105) found protein aggregation depended on the emulsification technique; a rotor/stator homogenizer gave the best results. Finally, surface denaturation of proteins is a time-dependent phenomenon (106); changes in secondary structure can occur over several hours after adsorption (107). This may impact large-scale manufacturing, where the duration of solvent exposure could increase on process scale-up.

2. Dehydration

The final drying step shown in Fig. 1B not only removes residual polymer solvent but also dehydrates the protein-containing droplets of the primary aqueous phase. Conventional protein formulations typically are dried by spray drying (108,109) or lyophilization (73). Both processes present potential threats to protein integrity. The freezing step of lyophilization can denature proteins. As ice crystals form, solutes are concentrated (73) resulting in crystallization and pH shifts in some cases. The ice–water interface generated on freezing can cause surface denaturation (110). In emulsion processes, the primary aqueous phase is saturated in the polymer solvent; methylene chloride and ethyl acetate, two common PLGA solvents, are soluble in water to 2% and 9%, respectively. These organic solutes will likely phase separate upon freezing, although this has not been studied. The drying step of lyophilization can result in conformational changes (111), although these are sometimes reversible on rehydration (112). To date microsphere drying has not been identified as a cause of protein denaturation, but few studies have examined this specific step. Cleland et al. (43) dried PLGA microspheres containing the HIV subunit vaccine gp120 by three different methods—under nitrogen, under vacuum, and by lyophilization. Though the integrity of gp120 released in a burst phase was unaffected, the burst magnitude was higher when the microspheres were lyophilized. (Lyophilization resulted in cracking of microspheres prepared from low molecular weight PLGA, a possible consequence of the expansion of entrapped water during freezing.) Fu et al. (113) examined the loss of α-helical (i.e., secondary) structure in BSA- and lysozyme-containing microspheres prepared by w/o/w and dried by lyophilization. Surface denaturation (such as might occur during emulsion formation) tends to alter tertiary as opposed to secondary structure (97). Hence the structural changes observed probably occurred on drying.

3. Minimizing Surface Denaturation and Dehydration Damage

Several approaches have been used to maximize protein integrity toward emulsion-based encapsulation processes. First, one can minimize the fraction of protein lost to the interface. For most proteins, interfaces will saturate at approximately 1 mg protein/m^2 (97). If adsorption is irreversible and the interface saturable, the amount of surface denatured protein will be fixed (provided droplet size is constant). In theory, by greatly increasing the protein concentration in the primary aqueous phase the percentage of protein lost to the surface will become insignificant (see Table 7). Cleland and Jones (64) found hGH and γ-interferon were stable toward a double emulsion process when encapsulated at concentrations of 100–400 mg/mL. (The primary aqueous phase included excipients, so the mechanism of stabilization likely involved multiple factors.) Use of highly concentrated protein solutions may not be appropriate for very potent

Table 7 Fraction of Surface-Denatured Drug Depends on the Fabrication Conditions[a]

Protein concentration (mg/mL)	Drug per unit interfacial area (mg/m^2)	Fraction of total drug at surface (%)
5	2	50
25	10	10
100	77	1.3

[a]Assumes 0.25-μm droplet size, 1 mg/m^2 at surface, 100% encapsulation efficiency.

or expensive drugs. Additionally, desorption of aggregates or precipitates from the surface would generate free interfacial area, invalidating the assumptions underlying this approach.

Inclusion of a surrogate protein with greater surface activity is an alternative strategy. Given a mixture of proteins, the most surface-active (e.g., albumin) will preferentially absorb (95,114). Relative rates of adsorption will also depend on component concentrations. Sah (114) recently showed inclusion of BSA improved recovery of lysozyme following emulsification with methylene chloride, although this was in the absence of polymer. This approach may have limited appeal for pharmaceuticals, where protein excipients derived from cartilage or blood, such as gelatin and albumin, are undesirable.

A number of authors have stabilized proteins toward emulsion processes by including nonprotein additives in the primary aqueous phase. In practice additives are often selected empirically. Stabilization derives from several potential mechanisms. Competitive adsorption between the protein and an added surfactant is the simplest (115,116); several investigators have included surfactants in the primary aqueous phase either to increase encapsulation efficiency (117) or to ameliorate surface denaturation (64,105). [The stabilization by surfactants of proteins toward air–liquid interfaces during spray drying occurs by the same mechanism (108,109).] Hydroxypropyl-β-cyclodextrin (HPCD) stabilized erythropoietin (EPO) against surface denaturation in a w/o/w process [105], and ovalbumin and lysozyme toward a methylene chloride–water interface in the absence of polymer (114). Competitive adsorption may have been responsible, and seems likely as the surface active excipient was present in vast excess. HPCD also binds to hydrophobic residues in proteins (118); competitive binding of the protein (with either HPCD or with the interface) may also play a role (105,114), but this has not been examined mechanistically. Polyethylene glycol (PEG) has also been observed to stabilize proteins toward the primary emulsification step (64). Though not established, stabilization likely resulted from a combination of PEG's slight surface activity and a strong steric component inhibiting monomer-to-monomer interactions at the surface, as demonstrated with granulocyte colony-stimulating factor (G-CSF) at an air–water interface (119). Small-molecule osmolytes, known stabilizers of proteins in solution (120, 121), have been used to stabilize a variety of proteins against double-emulsion processes. Trehalose and mannitol stabilized hGH against emulsification with methylene chloride and with ethyl acetate (64), and arginine stabilized EPO toward a w/o/w process (105). These excipients are known to result in preferential hydration of proteins, which could "shield" the protein from the aqueous–organic interface (64). An alternative mechanism is possible. Stabilizers shift the equilibrium between native and unfolded protein forms (N⇔U) toward the former (121,122).This equilibrium shift could be responsible for decreased surface denaturation protein unfolding is thought to precede adsorption (97), as depicted in Fig. 4. One consequence of preferential hydration is an increase in water surface tension (123). This could jeopardize the stability of the resultant emulsion, an issue not yet addressed in the literature.

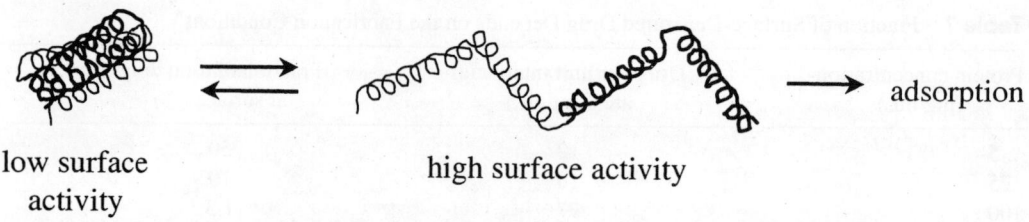

Figure 4 Schematic of protein surface adsorption.

Table 8 Postencapsulation Integrity of Human Therapeutic Proteins in Injectable, Biodegradable Sustained Release Formulations: Proteins Encapsulated as Solutions

Protein	Stabilization strategy	Integrity (%)	Ref.
Growth hormone	Maximized protein concentration; emulsion included trehalose or mannitol	95–98	64
Erythropoietin	Emulsion included hydroxypropyl-β-cyclodextrin and BSA	84	105
Nerve growth factor	Emulsion included carboxymethyldextran and BSA	<60	125
Nerve growth factor	Emulsion included HSA	~100	126, 127
γ-Interferon	Maximized protein concentration in emulsion; included trehalose	>90	64
Insulin	None	<40	93

BSA, bovine serum albumin; HSA, human serum albumin.

In addition to stabilizing proteins in solution, disaccharides such as trehalose, sucrose, maltose, and lactose protect against damage induced by dehydration (120), the required final step of the processes depicted in Fig. 1B. Trehalose stabilized hGH toward lyophilization (87), as evidenced by retention of secondary structure. Interestingly, this effect was not observed with hGH microspheres prepared by double emulsion with trehalose in the primary aqueous phase, where a substantial loss of α-helicity was observed in the dry product (124). One important caveat associated with carbohydrate stabilizers is the need to optimize sugar content; trehalose's protective effect is eliminated at very high concentrations (120). The stabilization approaches above have resulted in the encapsulation of multiple human proteins with good retention of integrity (Table 8).

E. Other Approaches

1. Alternative PLGA Encapsulation Processes

The principles discussed above pertain to alternative methods of encapsulation. The relevance to coacervation processes will be readily apparent (128). Super critical CO_2 has been used as an extraction solvent in atomization processes (60), applied by Young et al. (129) to the encapsulation of lysozyme. While lysozyme integrity following processing was not reported, independent work (130) showed that supercritical fluid precipitation of lysozyme had no negative consequences. Several groups have modified emulsion processes to reduce or eliminate water exposure during encapsulation. Sanchez et al. (131) encapsulated tetanus toxoid in a PLGA capsule with an oily core, using a s/o/o/w process developed with the twin objectives of avoiding water exposure of the antigen solids and providing pulsatile, rather than continuous, release kinetics. Iwata et al. (85,94) developed an anhydrous, multiphase s/o/o/o process for the encapsulation of solid particles of tumor TNF-α. High loading efficiencies and retention of bioactivity resulted when water was eliminated from the process.

Three recent reports introduce unusual protein–solvent exposure profiles with unknown structural consequences. Viswanathan et al. (132) developed a w/o/o process where the protein was precipitated by acetonitrile during encapsulation. The primary emulsion was prepared with PLGA dissolved in a cosolvent mixture of acetonitrile and methylene chloride. Secondary emulsification in a paraffin continuous phase effected the extraction of methylene chloride but not acetonitrile (which is immiscible with paraffin). The miscibility of acetonitrile and water resulted in phase inversion in the nascent microspheres, with formation of a polymer-rich phase and an acetonitrile/water phase in which the protein precipitates. The authors reported high loading efficiencies (>90%) for BSA and lysozyme encapsulated by this technique but did not report integrity following encapsulation. Park et al. (133) encapsulated lysozyme in PLGA using an o/w system, where protein and polymer were codissolved in dimethylsolfoxide. The generality of this approach remains to be seen; the denaturing effect of protein-dissolving organic solvents is well known (75,134). Moreover, the ability of proteins encapsulated in an unfolded form to regain their native conformation on release is unknown. Yewey et al. (135) developed a controlled release system (Atrigel) consisting of polymer, dissolved in either dimethylsulfoxide or N-methylpyrrolidone, and codissolved or suspended drug. Since the solvents used are biocompatible, the entire mixture can be injected directly. The system has been tested with a variety of proteins, but few integrity data have been reported.

2. Alternatives to PLGA

While to date the only bioerodible controlled release protein formulations to reach advanced clinical development have been based on PLGA, alternative systems remain an active area of research. Insulin-like growth factor I (IGF-I) was encapsulated in multivesicular liposomes (DepoFoam) (136). The encapsulation process is similar to the w/o/w process shown in Fig. 1B, with a lipid matrix substituting for PLGA. The integrity of IGF-I following encapsulation was examined by reversed-phase high-performance liquid chromatography (RP-HPLC) and sodium dodecyl sulfate polyacrylamide gel electrophoresis (SDS-PAGE), and found essentially unchanged. However, noncovalent aggregate formation was not characterized. Polyanhydrides, which exhibit surface, as opposed to bulk, erosion, are both biocompatible and erodible (137). Delivery of proteins using this promising class of polymers is the focus of recent work (138). A variety of hydrogels are under development for protein delivery, including alginates (139), as well as thermally reversible gels (140). Oil suspensions have been used to deliver bovine somatotropin, but to date this approach has been limited to veterinary applications (59). Possible stability advantages of these systems have yet to be fully assessed.

V. STABILIZATION TOWARD STORAGE

Bioerodible polyesters are generally water-labile, necessitating shelf storage under dehydrated conditions. Microsphere formulations require stability of both drug and polymer matrix. Storage stability, although frequently overlooked, will require increased attention as sustained release protein formulations move toward commercialization.

A. Polymer Stability Toward Storage

Stability of solids (whether protein or polymer) toward storage correlates with molecular mobility within the solid (73,141). For amorphous solids mobility is characterized by the glass transition temperature, T_g. In a matrix system, polymer and drug particles will exhibit separate T_g values if present in distinct phases; the lowest T_g will dictate the optimum storage temperature. The T_g of PLGA is a function of comonomer ratio and molecular weight, and is less than 50°C for the most frequently used compositions. T_g is strongly influenced by polymer purity. Blends of low and high molecular weight poly(DL-lactide) exhibited T_g values spanning more than 30°C (142). Bittner et al. (143) altered release kinetics in PLGA microspheres by either removing low molecular weight impurities from commercially available PLGA 50:50 or by adding unreacted lactide and glycolide. The T_g values of placebo microspheres made from pretreated polymers ranged from 22°C to 40°C. Polymer composition, and thus T_g, can be altered inadvertently during processing. A liquid extraction step can remove relatively soluble low molecular weight polymer impurities or residual monomer, resulting in a T_g higher than the polymer starting material. Partial hydrolysis during processing would have the opposite effect.

Residual solvent content (144) strongly influences polymer T_g in the final product. Residual solvent levels vary with process type and sometimes with scale (63). Encapsulation of protein solids by spray drying (Fig. 1A) involves only the polymer solvent, while other processes make use of mixtures of solvents (145) or a second extraction solvent (63). For emulsion processes involving an aqueous phase, residual moisture must also be considered (146). While organic solvent residuals in pharmaceuticals must not exceed safe levels (147), stability requirements may impose lower limits for solvents of low toxicity. The formulation can impact T_g if the polymer interacts with the encapsulated drug. Microspheres containing the synthetic peptide leuprorelin acetate (Lupron Depot) showed a substantial increase in T_g with increasing drug content (24). This effect, presumably due to an ionic interaction between the cationic drug and carboxylate end groups in PLGA, may be partially responsible for the 3-year shelf life of that product at room temperature (24).

Excessive polymer mobility in the stored microsphere product can have deleterious consequences. In the extreme case, particle agglomeration can occur, impacting injectability as well as product aesthetics. Lupron Depot microspheres are lyophilized from an aqueous mannitol solution to prevent interparticle contact during storage (24). On a smaller scale, morphological changes affecting internal pore structure are conceivable, although this has not been addressed in the literature. A change of internal morphology could impact water uptake upon hydration, influencing the rates of polymer erosion and drug release, and possibly protein integrity. Mobility impacts not only PLGA morphology but also its chemical stability. Polyesters can react chemically with amine-containing excipients or with the primary amino group side chains on proteins (150). These reactions can be avoided by optimization of storage temperature. γ-Irradiation, sometimes used for terminal sterilization of pharmaceuticals, causes degradation of PLGA and generates free radicals that can react with polymer or drug on storage (148,149). Microsphere formulations must be fabricated under aseptic conditions as a consequence (146).

B. Protein Stability Toward Storage

Protein stability in the dry state usually exceeds that in solution (73). The chemical reactions occurring in proteins under solid-state conditions have been reviewed recently (151), although storage stability of *encapsulated* proteins has received little attention. When proteins are encapsulated as solids (Fig. 1A), storage stability can be assessed prior to encapsulation, either before or after solvent exposure. This may aid identification of candidate formulations for encapsulation. Storage stability following processing will presumably mirror that of the starting material provided organic solvent exposure has no effect. Organic solvents can "strip" water from lyophilized proteins, possibly impacting storage stability (73,152).

Molecular mobility in protein solids is influenced by residual water (153) which acts as a plasticizer (151,154). As with polymers, mobility in amorphous protein solids is commonly characterized by the glass transition temperature. Yoshioka et al. (155) recently suggested T_g is too general a measurement of mobility in complex biomolecules, as it describes the matrix as a whole rather than its specific components. NMR relaxation was used to detect microscopically liquidized states in lyophilized protein formulations at least 20°C below T_g.

All of the reactions to which protein solids are susceptible are relevant to solid-state microsphere formulations (151). In an accelerated stability test of EPO microspheres prepared by double emulsion, Morlock et al. (105) noted a slight increase in covalent dimer content after 58 days at 37°C; the formulation included HPCD as a stabilizing excipient. The study did not include testing for other degradation products.

VI. STABILIZATION DURING RELEASE

Following storage of a depot formulation, the final hurdle is ensuring protein stability at body temperature after administration (*in situ* stability). The formulation must provide an environment maintaining bioactivity and integrity throughout the course of drug release.

A. Characterization of Released Protein

Stability during release is indicated by recovery of intact protein from the depot under relevant in vitro conditions. Test conditions (pH, temperature, ionic strength) should be physiological and must preserve the integrity of free (i.e., released) protein during the interval between sampling. Otherwise the source of degradants will be inconclusive. The generation of protons upon polyester hydrolysis requires a suitable combination of buffer strength and sampling frequency to maintain pH. The time required in vitro for complete recovery of encapsulated drug should mirror the formulation duration in vivo. This condition is elusive in practice since in vitro release rates vary substantially with the test conditions (24,156–158). Moreover, in vitro degradation of PLGA can be slower than in vivo (159), thereby affecting release rates in degradation-controlled systems. Once released, protein is characterized by a variety of chromatographic techniques and other assays, reviewed by Schwendeman et al. (160).

In vivo assessment of stability *in situ* requires calculation of drug bioavailability from the depot, i.e., the area under the serum drug concentration profile (3). Bioavailability of a parenteral depot formulation is expressed relative to an aqueous bolus injection of identical dose and route of administration (a "dose dump" control). If bioavailability is not linear with dose, comparison of depot and bolus formulations could give erroneous conclusions. A more precise control for a microsphere formulation is a subcutaneous infusion. In primates, the bioavailability of hGH from a microsphere formulation, ProLease hGH, was nearly 100% relative to a control consisting of an infusion plus a small bolus emulating the initial burst of drug from the microspheres (22). For protein drugs, serum concentration is usually determined by an immunoassay, which measures protein immunoreactivity but not necessarily structural integrity or bioactivity. Thus bioavailability should be supplemented with evidence of pharmacodynamic efficacy when possible.

B. Mechanisms of Protein Inactivation

In vitro release testing can result in recovery of degraded or aggregated protein, or, if insoluble aggregates form, no protein at all. Obviously, the ability to maintain protein integrity during microsphere fabrication and storage is no guarantee the protein will survive extended periods at physiological conditions. While protein solids are relatively thermostable, the drug will transition to a solution state *in situ*. Proteins inside microspheres will be susceptible to all of the chemical and physical degradation pathways occurring under normal storage conditions, whether in solution or solid form. These include aggregation (both covalent and noncovalent), oxidation, deamidation, peptide bond hydrolysis, β-elimination of disulfide bonds, and deglycosylation, as reviewed by several authors [122,160–162]. High local protein concentrations in microspheres (depending on the drug load) and a relatively high temperature can increase the likelihood of several of these events.

C. What Is the Internal Environment?

Further threats to protein integrity potentially stem from the microsphere itself, requiring an understanding of the internal microenvironment and how it changes over time. One potential threat is a gradual transition from solid to solution state. The vulnerability toward aggregation of solid proteins in environments of high water activity is well known (163,164). The rate of water uptake in the microsphere pore phase determines the time to transition from solid to solution state and, ultimately, the internal protein concentration. Pore structure following fabrication is visualized through freeze-fracture scanning electron microscopy (SEM); however, microsphere hydration produces a less tractable sample. Microstructure will vary with the extent of pore wetting, water uptake in the polymer phase, and, eventually, matrix erosion. Evidence from EPR studies suggests the transition from solid to solution state occurs within minutes of microsphere hydration (165). Recently, confocal laser scanning microscopy (CLSM) has been applied to microspheres after hydration. Optical sectioning of a sample results in planar images of submicometer thickness, enabling the construction of three-dimensional images. To date, CLSM has been used to characterize protein distribution in PLGA microspheres immediately following hydration (117,166,167). Schwendeman et al. (42) visualized rapid microsphere swelling using confocal microscopy; microspheres appeared to explode, presumably due to osmotic pressure differences. The dynamic evolution of pore morphology in hydrated PLGA disks in the absence of drug was recently reported (168). In porous PLGA systems, water will partition among pore and polymer phases, influencing the total aqueous volume accessible to the protein as well as the polymer hydrolysis rate (169). In addition to osmotic effects linked to the formulation salt content, process-related features, such as initial pore structure and connectivity with the surface, will likely impact these events. The relationship between the evolution of the microsphere internal environment and the resultant protein integrity is only beginning to emerge (126,156,165,170,171).

Acidification of the microsphere interior upon matrix degradation can jeopardize protein integrity. Carboxylic acids catalyze further polyester hydrolysis, presenting the risk that proton generation will exceed acid removal from the matrix by diffusion or neutralization by buffering components in the surrounding fluid. Removal of (acidic) polymer oligomers by diffusion from a PLGA mass depends on both oligomer size and the distance to the polymer mass surface. Oligomer removal also requires aqueous solubility in the medium, i.e., oligomers must be a few hundred daltons or less (172). The degradation of PLGA slabs has been shown to be heterogeneous, with a 200- to 300-μm-thick surface region comprising polymer less degraded than the core. Presumably any soluble oligomers generated in this layer are able diffuse away (173). The dimension of the surface region suggests acidification will not occur in microspheres less than 200 μm in diameter. The physical evidence resulting from studies of microspheres smaller than this diameter threshold is mixed, however. ^{31}P NMR has shown the PLGA microsphere interior is only marginally acidic (pH around 6.4) (174). Other studies suggest a more acidic microenvironment, which could denature some proteins (165,175,176). Differences in formulation and test conditions are likely responsible for the discrepancy.

Adsorption of the protein to the polymer surface is another putative event related to protein integrity within hydrated microspheres. Analogous to their adsorption at aqueous–organic interfaces, proteins can adsorb to hydrophobic polymer surfaces. The adsorption of albumin to PLGA films was recently characterized (177). The extent to which encapsulated proteins will adsorb to internal polymer surfaces is unknown, but the principles related to adsorption at liquid–liquid interfaces, discussed above, will apply. Whether or not the impermanence of PLGA surfaces, which ultimately degrade to lactic and glycolic acid, will render adsorption reversible has yet to be elucidated.

D. Stabilization Approaches

To date at least one dozen human protein therapeutics have been encapsulated and released from microspheres in a bioactive form (Table 9). The majority of cases employed specific strategies for protein stabilization, although the exact mechanism is often not fully understood. In some instances the recovery of bioactive protein from hydrated microspheres may be a residual benefit of stabilization toward processing as opposed to a deliberate effort to maximize stability *in situ*. The optimization of the integrity of protein released in vitro can be time consuming, requiring iterative formulation evaluation with real-time (i.e., not accelerated) testing accompanied by chromatographic characterization of released drug. Protein remaining inside

Table 9 Examples of Microsphere Formulations of Human Protein Therapeutics Releasing Bioactive Protein

Protein	Stabilization strategy	Integrity of released protein	Ref.
Erythropoietin	Various; see text	See text	88,105,178–180
Human growth hormone	Various; see text	See text	64,90,181–183
α-Interferon	Encapsulated protein complexed and coencapsulated with zinc	Immunoreactive protein released in vivo (rats) for 7 days	184
β-Interferon	None	50% bioactivity released at 5 weeks in vivo	91,92
γ-Interferon	Maximized protein concentration in emulsion; included trehalose	Bioactive protein released in vitro for one week	64, 158
Vascular endothelial growth factor	None	93% at day 21	31
Transforming growth factor–β	Protein colyophilized with demineralized bone and mannitol	~85% bioactivity released	185
Interleukin-2	Emulsion included HSA	100% bioactivity recovered at 35 days	186
Nerve growth factor	Emulsion included gelatin	Immunoreactive and bioactive protein released over 35 days	187
Granulocyte–macrophage colony-stimulating factor	Maximized protein concentrationin emulsion	Bioactive protein released in vitro for one week	188
Interleukin-1α	Emulsion included BSA	<50% bioactivity released over 20 days	55
Brain-derived neurotropic factor	Emulsifier included in polymer phase	Bioactive protein released over 30 days	189

Protein Therapeutics

the microspheres at the end of in vitro testing may also need to be extracted and analyzed if recovery is incomplete. Microsphere formulations of two proteins, hGH and EPO, have been the object of significant efforts by multiple groups. Sustained release formulations of these proteins, both developed by Alkermes, have reached advanced stages of clinical testing.

1. Erythropoietin

As discussed above, Morlock et al. (105) found that HPCD and BSA gave the best EPO integrity following a w/o/w encapsulation process (see Table 8). However, following the in vitro burst, no additional protein was released from the microspheres for 60 days. [Since in vitro often differs from in vivo behavior (182) this finding does not necessarily mean these formulations would not show sustained release in vivo.] To assess protein stability during the in vitro release test, the covalent aggregate content of EPO remaining inside the microspheres was characterized by SDS-PAGE analysis of microsphere extracts, prepared at various time intervals following microsphere hydration. For the formulation lacking stabilizers, the aggregate content inside the microspheres increased gradually with time; by day 32, over 50% of the total protein remaining was covalently aggregated. The results with stabilizer-containing formulations were not reported. EPO-containing microspheres fabricated by spray drying of a w/o emulsion similarly showed covalent aggregate formation during release (179). Recently, EPO was encapsulated in ABA triblock copolymers by w/o/w, consisting of hydrophobic A blocks (PLGA) and hydrophilic polyethylene oxide B blocks (178,180). The resultant microspheres showed enhanced water uptake, and presumably a more native-like internal microenvironment. The effect of this new material on the integrity of released protein has not yet been reported.

Zale et al. (88) encapsulated EPO using the ProLease spray-freeze process. A variety of EPO drug particle formulations were first prepared by lyophilization (Table 10). Microspheres were prepared with 10-kD PLGA 50:50, either blocked (terminal ester) or unblocked (terminal acid group), as shown in Table 11. In some cases, basic salts were coencapsulated with the drug

Table 10 Composition of EPO Drug Particle Formulations Used for Encapsulation (88)

Formulations (wt %)	Am1	Am4	Am7	Ma1	Ma3	Ma4	Zn1	Zn6
Erythropoietin	10.0	10.1	9.9	10.0	10.0	10.0	10.0	10.0
Ammonium sulfate	66.8	64.7	79.1	0.0	0.0	0.0	0.0	0.0
Zinc acetate	0.0	0.0	0.0	0.0	0.0	0.0	76.9	76.9
Mannitol	0.0	0.0	0.0	62.5	62.5	72.5	0.0	0.0
Sucrose	0.0	0.0	0.0	10.0	0.0	10.0	0.0	0.0
Maltose	0.0	0.0	0.0	0.0	10.0	0.0	0.0	0.0
5 mM citrate buffer (pH 7)	0.0	15.1	0.0	0.0	0.0	0.0	0.0	0.0
5 mM phosphate buffer (pH 7)	0.0	0.0	10.0	7.5	7.5	7.5	0.0	0.0
5 mM citrate / 5 mM phosphate buffer (pH 7)	22.1	0.0	0.0	0.0	0.0	0.0	0.0	0.0
10 mM bicarbonate buffer (pH 7)	0.0	0.0	0.0	0.0	0.0	0.0	13.1	12.1
Inulin	1.1	10.1	1.0	0.0	0.0	0.0	0.0	0.0
Glycine	0.0	0.0	0.0	10.0	10.0	0.0	0.0	0.0
Tween-20 surfactant	0.0	0.0	0.0	0.0	0.0	0.0	0.0	1.0

Table 11 Initial Burst Level and Duration of Erythropoietin (EPO) Release from Microspheres, as a Function of the Formulation (88)

Formula	EPO load (%)	Polymer/salt	Aggregate released (% init. load)[a]	Initial burst (%)[b]	Average release (%/day)[b]	Release duration (days)[b]
Zn1	10	Blocked / 10% MgCO$_3$	12	66	1.2	14
Zn1	10	Blocked / 10% ZnCO$_3$	22	46	1.7	28
Zn6	10	Blocked / 10% ZnCO$_3$	37	32	1.6	28
Am1	5	Unblocked / 10% MgCO$_3$	1	39	1.4	21
Am1	10	Blocked / 10% MgCO$_3$	2	71	0.3	3
Am4	5	Unblocked / 10% MgCO$_3$	1	29	1.1	21
Am4	5	Unblocked / none	1	35	0.9	28
Ma1	5	Unblocked / 10% MgCO$_3$	1	44	1.8	24
Ma3	10	Unblocked / 10% MgCO$_3$	1	71	1.3	21
Ma4	10	Blocked / 10% ZnCO$_3$	1	77	0.6	3

[a]In Hepes buffer; cumulative aggregate released as calculated by size exclusion chromatography.
[b]In Hepes buffer containing 2% sheep serum; data calculated by radioimmunoassay.

particles. These salts are thought to modulate the release rate and stabilize the protein by a buffering mechanism. All of the formulations exhibited acceptable protein integrity following encapsulation, with more than 98% monomer content by size exclusion chromatography (SEC) analysis. The microsphere formulations were evaluated in vitro for burst, protein release rate and duration, as well as integrity of protein released. In vitro testing was performed using Hepes buffer at 37°C, with periodic withdrawal and replacement of buffer. Samples were assayed by SEC and by radioimmunoassay.

The results, summarized in Table 11, reveal a striking formulation dependence of in vitro performance and, notably, the integrity of the protein released from the microspheres. To illustrate this point further consider two of the formulations examined, Zn1, containing zinc acetate as an excipient, and Am1, containing ammonium sulfate. Figure 5 shows in vitro test results for the former. Cumulative EPO monomer as well as total EPO (monomer plus soluble aggregates) were determined over the course of a 4-week study. The integrity of the protein released from the microspheres decreased steadily over the first 2 weeks, and between days 10 and 28 was only 50–60% monomeric. Consequently, while 60% of the total encapsulated EPO was recovered by day 28, only about 47% was released as monomer; the remainder was released as soluble aggregates (see Fig. 5). In contrast to the results obtained with the Zn1 formulation, EPO released from the Am1 formulation was nearly all monomeric, even in the fourth week of the study (Fig. 6). The cumulative aggregate released in optimized formulations was only 1% of the total initial encapsulated protein (Table 11). The mechanism of ammonium sulfate stabilization of EPO during in vitro release is not known definitively but is possibly related to salting out.

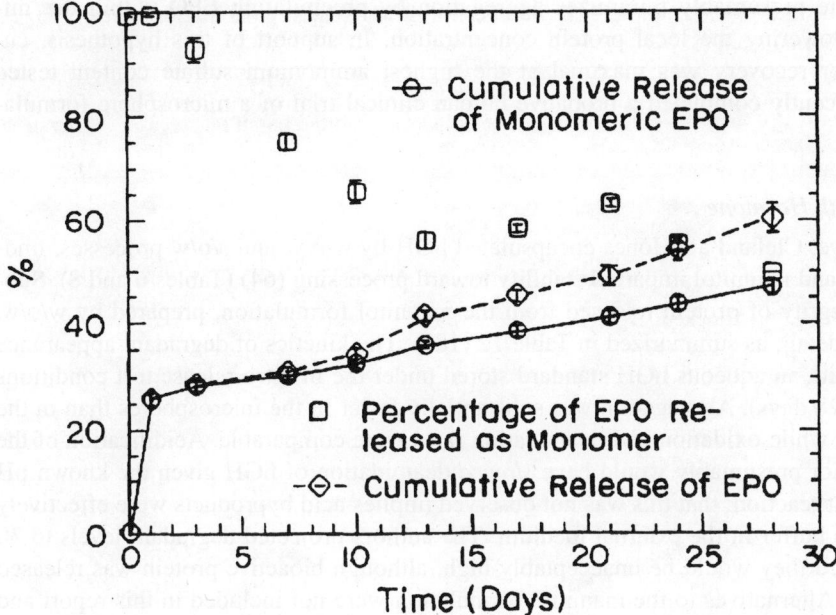

Figure 5 In vitro release of EPO from Zn1 formulation encapsulated in 10-kDa PLGA microspheres. Protein released between days 10 and 28 was 50–60% monomeric by SEC, resulting in a significant difference between the cumulative release profiles of total protein (dashed line) and monomer (solid line).

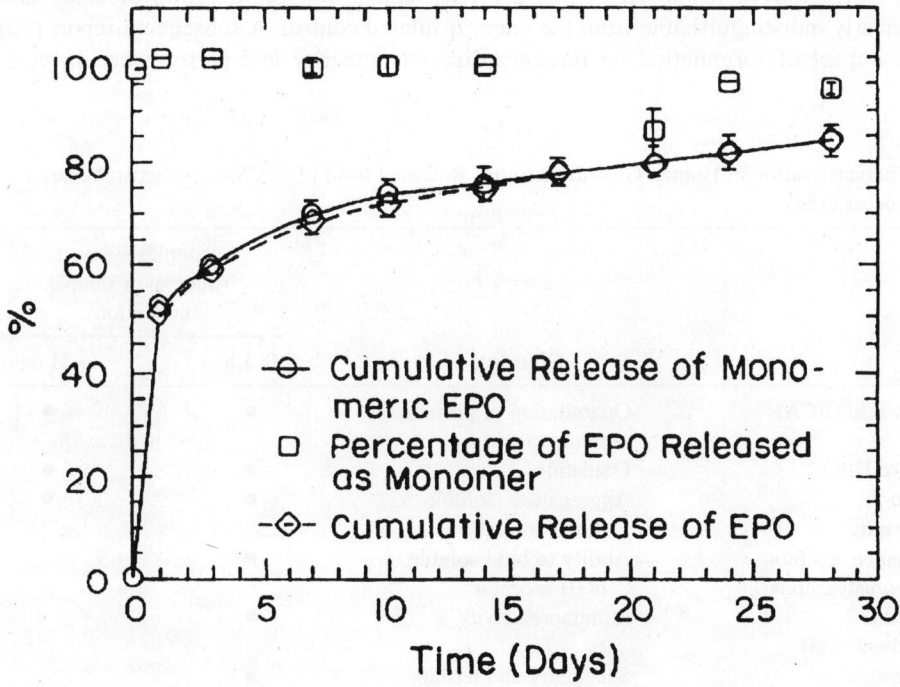

Figure 6 In vitro release of EPO from Am1 formulation encapsulated in 10-kDa PLGA microspheres. Protein released was more than 85% monomeric through day 28.

Ammonium sulfate presumably minimizes aggregation by precipitating EPO within the microspheres, thus lowering the local protein concentration. In support of this hypothesis, cumulative monomer recovery was maximal at the highest ammonium sulfate content tested (88). Alkermes recently completed a probative human clinical trial of a microsphere formulation of EPO.

2. Human Growth Hormone

As discussed above, Cleland and Jones encapsulated hGH by w/o/w and s/o/w processes, finding that trehalose and mannitol imparted stability toward processing (64) (Tables 6 and 8). Subsequently, the integrity of protein released from the mannitol formulation, prepared by w/o/w, was examined in detail, as summarized in Table 12 (183). The kinetics of degradant appearance were compared with an aqueous hGH standard stored under the in vitro release test conditions at pH 7.4 (37°C, 28 days). Aggregation was substantially faster in the microspheres than in the aqueous standard, while oxidation and deamidation rates were comparable. Acidification of the microsphere interior presumably would have *slowed* deamidation of hGH given the known pH dependence of that reaction; that this was not observed implies acid byproducts were effectively neutralized by the buffer in the external medium. The authors projected degradant levels to 30 days and concluded they would be unacceptably high, although bioactive protein was released as late as day 21. Alternatives to the mannitol formulation were not included in this report and thus the relevance of the protein phase composition to degradation rates is unclear.

Johnson et al. (181) used a spray-freeze process to encapsulate hGH, employing zinc as a stabilizing excipient. Zinc complexes with hGH to form a dimer with enhanced stability. Zinc is also present in the secretory granules of the pituitary, where hGH is normally stored at high concentrations (>50 mg/mL). Protein released through 28 days was collected and assayed by SEC, RP-HPLC, anion exchange HPLC, SDS-PAGE, and a cell proliferation bioassay and found to be nearly indistinguishable from the unencapsulated control. A subsequent report (90) assessed the impact of formulation on postencapsulation integrity and performance in vivo.

Table 12 Characterization of Human Growth Hormone Released from PLGA Microspheres Prepared by a w/o/w Process (183)

Assay	Objective	Samples assayed (interval of sample collection)	
		0–1 h	2–21 days
Bicinchoninic acid (BCA)	Quantitation of protein released	●	●
Reversed-phase HPLC	Oxidation	●	●
Size exclusion chromatography	Aggregation (soluble dimer formation)	●	●
High-performance receptor-binding chromatography	Ability to bind soluble hGH receptor	●	
Enzyme-linked immunosorbent assay	Immunoreactivity	●	
Circular dichroism	Secondary and tertiary structure	●	
Cell proliferation assay	Bioactivity	●	●

Polymer molecular weight and end-group chemistry were varied, as was the content of coencapsulated zinc carbonate, added to provide a source of zinc to maintain the protein in complexed form. One of the formulations was tested in monkeys; the relative bioavailability was nearly identical to a control group (22). The hGH ProLease formulation is currently awaiting regulatory approval and commercial launch.

The mechanism of zinc stabilization of hGH in microspheres was examined using FTIR spectroscopy (124). hGH secondary structure was examined after protein lyophilization, within the fabricated microspheres, and again following hydration. Zinc did not stabilize the protein against lyophilization, which caused some loss in α-helical content. A similar degree of disruption was observed in the fabricated microspheres. However, the protein refolded on microsphere hydration, resulting in an FTIR spectrum nearly identical to the protein in aqueous solution. This finding supports the hypothesis that zinc's stabilizing effect is specific to the period of drug release, after depot administration.

VII. CONCLUSIONS

Despite the synergy between the delivery needs of protein therapeutics and the capabilities of controlled release technology, the pairing of the two has been hindered by the stability challenges of these complex biomolecules. An understanding of the effects of organic solvents on protein structure has enabled the adaptation of encapsulation processes originally developed for less labile drugs. Recent reports (190,191) reveal a persistent belief in the incompatibility of proteins and organic solvents. Nevertheless the list of protein drugs encapsulated without consequence continues to grow. The final hurdle is maintenance of protein integrity and bioactivity at the depot site once in the body. Advances in protein stabilization have enabled the development of controlled release formulations of EPO and hGH meeting the integrity standards of pharmaceuticals. Other successes are sure to follow as the ability of controlled release to enhance the value of proteins as therapeutics becomes more widely appreciated.

ACKNOWLEDGMENTS

The author thanks Alex Klibanov and Bob Langer for inspiration, and Colin Pitt and Lisa Klumb for valuable comments on the manuscript.

REFERENCES

1. Struck, M. M., 1994. Biopharmaceutical R&D success rates and development times: a new analysis provides benchmarks for the future. Bio/Technology, 12: 674–677.
2. Wallace, B. M., and Lasker, J. S., 1993. Stand and deliver: getting peptide drugs into the body. Science, 260: 912–913.
3. Lee, H. J., 1995. Biopharmaceutical properties and pharmacokinetics of peptide and protein drugs. In: Taylor, M., and Amidon, G. (Editors), Peptide-Based Drug Design, American Chemical Society, Washington, D.C., pp. 69–97.
4. Arky, R., 1997. Physician's Desk Reference, 50th ed., Medical Economics Company, Montvale, NJ.
5. Zhi, J., Teller, S. B., Satoh, H., Koss-Twardy, S. G., and Luke, D. R., 1995. Influence of human serum albumin content in formulations on the bioequivalency of interferon alfa-2a given by subcutaneous injection in healthy male volunteers. J Clin Pharmacol, 35: 281–284.

6. Mordenti, J., Chen, S. A., and Ferraiolo, B. L., 1993. Pharmacokinetics of interferon-gamma. In: Kung, A. H. C., Baughman, R. A., and Larrick, J. W. (Eds.), Therapeutic Proteins. Pharmacokinetics and Pharmacodynamics, W H. Freeman, New York, pp. 187–199.
7. Harvey, S., 1995. Growth hormone metabolism. In: Harvey, S., Scanes, C. G., and Daughaday, W. H. (Eds.), Growth Hormone, CRC Press, Boca Raton, FL, pp. 285–301.
8. Cohen, A. M., 1993. Erythropoietin and G-CSF. In: Kung, A. H. C., Baughman, R. A., and Larrick, J. W. (Eds.), Therapeutic Proteins: Pharmacokinetics and Pharmacodynamics, W. H. Freeman, New York, pp. 165–186.
9. Stute, N., Furman, W. L., Schell, M., and Evans, W. E., 1995. Pharmacokinetics of recombinant human granulocyte–macrophage colony-stimulating factor in children after intravenous and subcutaneous administration. J Pharm Sci, 84: 824–828.
10. Knauf, M. J., Bell, D. P., Hirtzer, P., Luo, Z.-P., Young, J. D., and Katre, N. V., 1988. Relationship of effective molecular size to systemic clearance in rats of recombinant interleukin-2 chemically modified with water-soluble polymers. J Biol Chem, 263: 15064–15070.
11. Clark, R., Olson, K., Fuh, G., Marian, M., Mortensen, D., Teshima, G., Chang, S., and Chu, H., 1996. Long-acting growth hormones produced by conjugation with polyethylene glycol. J Biol Chem, 271: 21969–21977.
12. Tsutsumi, Y., Kihira, T., Tsunoda, S., Kamada, H., Nakagawa, S., Kaneda, Y., Kanamori, T., and Mayumi, T., 1996. Molecular design of hybrid tumor necrosis factor-alpha III: polyethylene glycol-modified tumor necrosis factor-alpha has markedly enhanced antitumor potency due to longer plasma half-life and higher tumor accumulation. J Pharmacol Exp Ther, 278: 1006–1011.
13. Sakane, T., and Pardridge, W. M., 1997. Carboxyl-directed pegylation of brain-derived neurotrophic factor markedly reduces systemic clearance with minimal loss of biologic activity. Pharm Res, 14: 1085–1091.
14. Macdougall, I. C., Gray, S. J., McEvoy, O., Breen, C., Jenkins, B., Browne, J., and Egrie, J., 1999. Pharmacokinetics of novel erythropoiesis stimulating protein (NESP) compared with epoetin alfa in dialysis patients. J Am Soc Nephrol, 10: 2392–2395.
15. Moreland, L. W., Baumgartner, S. W., Schiff, M. H., Tindall, E. A., Fleischmann, R. M., Weaver, A. L., Ettlinger, R. E., Cohen, S., Koopman, W. J., Mohler, K., Widmer, M. B., and Blosch, C. M., 1997. Treatment of rheumatoid arthritis with a recombinant human tumor necrosis factor receptor (p75)-Fc fusion protein. N Engl J Med, 337: 141–147.
16. Bendele, A., Seely, J., Richey, C., Sennello, G., and Shopp, G., 1998. Renal tubular vacuolation in animals treated with polyethylene-glycol-conjugated proteins. Toxicol Sci, 42: 152–157.
17. Patton, J., 1998. Breathing life into protein drugs. Nature Biotechnology, 16: 141–143.
18. Damms, B., and Bains, W., 1995. The cost of delivering drugs without needles. Biotechnology, 13: 1438–1440.
19. Dinbergs, I. D., Brown, L., and Edelman, E. R., 1996. Cellular response to transforming growth factor–beta 1 and basic fibroblast growth factor depends on release kinetics and extracellular matrix interactions. J Biol Chem, 271:29822–29829.
20. Hoffman, A., 1998. Pharmacodynamic aspects of sustained release preparations. Adv Drug Del Rev, 33: 185–199.
21. Lancranjan, I., Burns, C., Grass, P., Jaquet, P., Jervell, J., Kendall-Taylor, P., Lamberts, S. W. F., Marbach, P., Orskov, H., Pagani, G., Sheppard, M., and Simionescu, L., 1995. Sandostatin LAR: pharmacokinetics, pharmcodynamics, efficacy, and tolerability in acromegalic patients. Metabolism, 44: 18–26.
22. Sun, Y. N., Lee, H. J., Almon, R. R., and Jusko, W. J., 1999. A pharmacokinetic pharmacodynamic model for recombinant human growth hormone effects on induction of insulin-like growth factor I in monkeys. J Pharmacol Exp Ther, 289: 1523–1532.
23. Garnick, M. B., and Fair, W. R., 1998. Prostate cancer. Sci Am, Dec. 1998: 75–83.
24. Okada, H., 1997. One- and three-month release injectable microspheres of the LH-RH superagonist leuprorelin acetate. Adv Drug Deliv Rev, 28: 43–70.
25. Lehninger, A. L., 1982. Principles of Biochemistry, Worth Publishers, New York.
26. Langer, R., and Folkman, J., 1976. Polymers for the sustained release of proteins and other macromolecules. Nature, 263: 793–800.

27. Langer, R., 1980. Polymeric delivery systems for controlled drug release. Chem Eng Commun, 6: 1–48.
28. Langer, R. S., Rhine, W. D., Hsieh, D. S. T., and Bawa, R. S., 1980. Polymers for the sustained release of macromolecules: applications and control of release kinetics. In: Baker, R. W. (Ed.), Controlled Release of Bioactive Materials, Academic Press, New York.
29. Ko, C. Y., Dixit, V., Shaw, W. W., and Gitnick, G., 1997. Extensive in vivo angiogenesis from the controlled release of endothelial cell growth factor: implications for cell transplantation and wound healing. J Controlled Release, 44: 209–214.
30. Ozaki, H., Hayashi, H., Vinores, S. A., Moromizato, Y., Campochiaro, P. A., and Oshima, K., 1997. Intravitreal sustained-release of VEGF causes retinal neovascularization in rabbits and breakdown of the blood-retinal barrier in rabbits and primates. Exp Eye Res, 64: 505–517.
31. Cleland, J. L., Duenas, E. T., Kahn, J., Park, A., Daugherty, A., and Cuthbertson, A., 1997. Local controlled delivery of vascular endothelial growth factor provides neovascularization. Proc Int Sym Control Rel Bioactiv Mater, 24: 85–86.
32. Kim, H. D., and Valentini, R. F., 1997. Human osteoblast response in-vitro to platelet-derived growth-factor and transforming growth-factor-beta delivered from controlled-polymer rods. Biomaterials, 18: 1175–1184.
33. Mikhailowski, R., Shpitz, B., PolakCharcon, S., Kost, Y., Segal, C., Fich, A., and Lamprecht, S. A., 1998. Controlled release of TGF-beta(1) impedes rat colon carcinogenesis in vivo. Int J Cancer, 78: 618–623.
34. Vance, M. L., Woodburn, C. J., Putney, S., Grouse, J., Lee, H. J., and Johnson, O. L., 1997. Effects of sustained release growth hormone on serum GH, IGF-I and IGFBP-3 concentration in GH deficient adults. Endocrinol Metab, 4(Suppl A): 75.
35. Wise, D. L., Fellmann, T. D., Sanderson, J. E., and Wentworth, R. L., 1979. Lactic/glycolic acid polymers. In: Gregoriadis, G. (Ed.), Drug Carriers in Biology and Medicine, Academic Press, London, pp. 237–270.
36. Anderson, J. M., and Shive, M. S., 1997. Biodegradation and biocompatibility of PLA and PLGA microspheres. Adv Drug Deliv Rev, 28: 5–24.
37. Siegel, R. A., and Langer, R., 1984. Controlled release of polypeptides and other macromolecules. Pharm Res, 1: 2–10.
38. Hora, M. S., Rana, R. K., Nunberg, J. H., Tice, T. R., Gilley, R. M., and Hudson, M. E., 1990. Release of human serum albumin from poly(lactide-co-glycolide) microspheres. Pharm Res, 7: 1190–1194.
39. Igartua, M., Hernandez, R. M., Esquisabel, A., Gascon, A. R., Calvo, M. B., and Pedraz, J. L., 1998. Stability of BSA encapsulated into PLGA microspheres using PAGE and capillary electrophoresis. Int J Pharm, 169: 45–54.
40. Crotts, G., and Park, T. G., 1998. Protein delivery from poly(lactic-co-glycolic acid) biodegradable microspheres: release kinetics and stability issues. J Microencaps, 15: 699–713.
41. Kuntz, R. M., and Saltzman, W. M., 1997. Polymeric controlled delivery for immunization. Trends Biotechnol 15: 364–369.
42. Schwendeman, S. P., Tobio, M., Jaworowicz, M., Alonso, M. J., and Langer, R., 1998. New strategies for the microencapsulation of tetanus vaccine. J Microencaps, 15: 299–318.
43. Cleland, J. L., Lim, A., Barron, L., Duenas, E. T., and Powell, M. F., 1997. Development of a single-shot subunit vaccine for HIV-1._.4. Optimizing microencapsulation and pulsatile release of Mn rgp120 from biodegradable microspheres. J Controlled Release, 47: 135–150.
44. Uchida, T., Shiosaki, K., Nakada, Y., Fukada, K., Eda, Y., Tokiyoshi, S., Nagareya, N., and Matsuyama, K., 1998. Microencapsulation of hepatitis B core antigen for vaccine preparation. Pharm Res, 15: 1708–1713.
45. Tobio, M., Nolley, J., Guo, Y. Y., McIver, J., and Alonso, M. J., 1999. A novel system based on a poloxamer PLGA blend as a tetanus toxoid delivery vehicle. Pharm Res, 16: 682–688.
46. Johansen, P., Merkle, H. P., and Gander, B., 1998. Physico-chemical and antigenic properties of tetanus and diphtheria toxoids and steps towards improved stability. Biochim Biophys Acta Gen Subj, 1425: 425–436.
47. Audran, R., Men, Y., Johansen, P., Gander, B.,and Corradin, G., 1998. Enhanced immunogenicity of microencapsulated tetanus toxoid with stabilizing agents. Pharm Res, 15: 1111–1116.

48. Cleland, J. L., 1999. Single-administration vaccines: controlled-release technology to mimic repeated immunizations. Trends Biotechnol, 17: 25–29.
49. Lopez, J. J., Edelman, E. R., Stamler, A., Hibberd, M. G., Prasad, P., Caputo, R. P., Carrozza, J. P., Douglas, P. S., Sellke, F. W., and Simons, M., 1997. Basic fibroblast growth-factor in a porcine model of chronic myocardial-ischemia—a comparison of angiographic, echocardiographic and coronary flow parameters. J Pharmacol Exp Ther, 282: 385–390.
50. Arras, M., Mollnau, H., Strasser, R., Wenz, R., Ito, W. D., Schaper, J., and Schaper, W., 1998. The delivery of angiogenic factors to the heart by microsphere therapy. Nature Biotechnol, 16: 159–162.
51. Winn, S. R., Uludag, H., and Hollinger, J. O., 1998. Sustained release emphasizing recombinant human bone morphogenetic protein-2. Adv Drug Deliv Rev, 31: 303–318.
52. Puleo, D. A., Huh, W. W., Duggirala, S. S., and DeLuca, P. P., 1998. In vitro cellular responses to bioerodible particles loaded with recombinant human bone morphogenetic protein-2. J Biomed Mater Res, 41: 104–110.
53. Whang, K., Tsai, D. C., Nam, E. K., Aitken, M., Sprague, S. M., Patel, P. K., and Healy, K. E., 1998. Ectopic bone formation via rhBMP-2 delivery from porous bioabsorbable polymer scaffolds. J Biomed Mater Res, 42: 491–499.
54. Baldwin, S. P., and Saltzman, W. M., 1998. Materials for protein delivery in tissue engineering. Adv Drug Deliv Rev, 33: 71–86.
55. Chen, L., Apte, R. N., and Cohen, S., 1997. Characterization of PLGA microspheres for the controlled delivery of IL-1 alpha for tumor immunotherapy. J Controlled Release, 43: 261–272.
56. Egilmez, N. K., Jong, Y. S., Iwanuma, Y., Jacob, J. S., Santos, C. A., Chen, F. A., Mathiowitz, E., and Bankert, R. B., 1998. Cytokine immunotherapy of cancer with controlled release biodegradable microspheres in a human tumor xenograft SCID mouse model. Cancer Immunol Immunother, 46: 21–24.
57. Wiranowska, M., Ransohoff, J., Weingart, J. D., Phelps, C., Phuphanich, S., and Brem, H., 1998. Interferon-containing controlled-release polymers for localized cerebral immunotherapy. J Interferon Cytokine Res, 18: 377–385.
58. Saltzman, W. M., Mak, M. W., Mahoney, M. J., Duenas, E. T., and Cleland, J. L., 1999. Intracranial delivery of recombinant nerve growth factor: release kinetics and protein distribution for three delivery systems. Pharm Res, 16: 232–240.
59. Pitt, C. G., 1990. The controlled parenteral delivery of polypeptides and proteins. Int J Pharm, 59: 173–196.
60. Benoit, J.-P., Marchais, H., Rolland, H., and Velde, V. V., 1996. Biodegradable microspheres: advances in production technology. In: Benita, S. (Ed.), Microencapsulation: Methods and Industrial Applications, Marcel Dekker, New York, pp. 35–72.
61. Sefton, M., Brown, L., and Langer, R., 1984. Ethylene-vinyl acetate copolymer microspheres for controlled release of macromolecules. J Pharm Sci, 73: 1859–1861.
62. Gombotz, W., Healy, M., and Brown, L., 1991. Very low temperature casting of controlled release microspheres. US Patent 5,019,400.
63. Herbert, P., Murphy, K., Johnson, O., Dong, N., Jaworowicz, W., Tracy, M. A., Cleland, J. L., and Putney, S. D., 1998. A large-scale process to produce microencapsulated proteins. Pharm Res, 15: 357–361.
64. Cleland, J. L., and Jones, A. J. S., 1996. Stable formulations of recombinant human growth hormone and interferon-gamma for microencapsulation in biodegradable microspheres. Pharm Res, 13: 1464–1475.
65. Creighton, T. E., 1993. Proteins: Structures and Molecular Properties, W. H. Freeman and Co., New York.
66. Laane, C. 1987. Rules for optimization of biocatalysis in organic solvents. Biotechnol Bioeng, 30: 81–87.
67. Lapanje, S., 1978. Physicochemical Aspects of Protein Denaturation, John Wiley and Sons, New York.
68. Fink, A. L., and Geeves, M. A., 1979. Cryoenzymology: the study of enzyme catalysis at subzero temperatures. Meth Enzymol, 63: 336–352.

69. Griebenow, K., and Klibanov, A. M., 1996. On protein denaturation in aqueous-organic mixtures but not in pure organic solvents. J Am Chem Soc, 118: 11695–11700.
70. Klibanov, A. M., 1989. Enzymatic catalysis in anhydrous organic solvents. Trends Biochem Sci, 14: 141–144.
71. Burke, P. A., Smith, S. O., Bachovchin, W. W., and Klibanov, A. M., 1989. Demonstration of structural integrity of an enzyme in organic solvents by solid-state NMR. J Am Chem Soc, 111: 8290–8291.
72. Burke, P. A., Griffin, R. G., and Klibanov, A. M., 1992. Solid-state NMR assessment of enzyme active center structure under nonaqueous conditions. J Biol Chem, 267: 20057–20064.
73. Pikal, M. J., 1996. Freeze-drying of proteins: process, formulation and stability. In: Lee, V. H. L., (Ed), Peptide and Protein Delivery, 2nd ed., Marcel Dekker, New York.
74. Griebenow, K., and Klibanov, A. M., 1997. Can conformational changes be responsible for solvent and excipient effects on the catalytic behavior of subtilisin Carlsberg in organic solvents? Biotechnol Bioeng, 53: 351–362.
75. Desai, U. R., and Klibanov, A. M., 1995. Assesssing the structural integrity of a lyophilized protein in organic solvents. J Am Chem Soc, 117: 940–3945.
76. Fitzpatrick, P. A., Steinmetz, A. C. U., Ringe, D., and Klibanov, A. M., 1993. Enzyme crystal structure in a neat organic solvent. Proc Natl Acad Sci USA, 90: 8653–8657.
77. Schmitke, J. L., Stem, L. J., and Klibanov, A. M., 1997. The crystal structure of subtilisin Carlsberg in anhydrous dioxane and its comparison with those in water and acetonitrile. Proc Natl Acad Sci USA, 94: 4250–4255.
78. Yennawar, N. H., Yennawar, H. P., and Farber, G. K., 1994. X-ray crystal structure of gamma-chymotrypsin in hexane. Biochemistry, 33: 7326–7336.
79. Zaks, A., and Klibanov, A. M., 1988. Enzymatic catalysis in nonaqueous solvents. J Biol Chem, 263: 3194–3201.
80. Affleck, R., Xu, Z.-F., Suzawa, V., Focht, K., Clark, D. S., and Dordick, J. S., 1992. Enzymatic catalysis and dynamics in low-water environments. Proc Natl Acad Sci USA, 89: 1100–1104.
81. Burke, P. A., Griffin, R. G., and Klibanov, A. M., 1993. Solid-state nuclear magnetic resonance investigation of solvent dependence of tyrosyl ring motion in an enzyme. Biotechnol Bioeng, 42: 87–94.
82. Broos, J., Visser, A. J. W., Engbersen, J. F. J., Verboom, W., van Hoek, A., and Reinhoudt, D. N., 1995. Flexibility of enzymes suspended in organic solvents probed by time-resolved fluorescence anisotropy. Evidence that enzyme activity and enantioselectivity are directly related to enzyme flexibility. J Am Chem Soc, 117: 12657–12663.
83. Hartsough, D. S., and Merz, K. M., Jr., 1993. Protein dynamics and solvation in aqueous and non-aqueous environments. J Am Chem Soc, 115: 6529–6537.
84. Volkin, D. B., Staubli, A., Langer, R., and Klibanov, A. M., 1991. Enzyme thermoinactivation in anhydrous organic solvents. Biotechnol Bioeng, 37: 843–853.
85. Iwata, M., Tanaka, T., Nakamura, Y., and McGinity, J. W., 1998. Selection of the solvent system for the preparation of poly(D,L-lactic-co-glycolic acid) microspheres containing tumor necrosis factor-alpha (TNF-alpha). Int J Pharm, 160: 145–156.
86. Pikal, M. J., 1994. Freeze drying of proteins. In: Cleland, J., and Langer, R. (Ed.), Formulation and Delivery of Proteins and Peptides, American Chemical Society, Washington, pp. 120–133.
87. Carrasquillo, K. G., Costantino, H. R., Cordero, R. A., Hsu, C. C., and Griebenow, K., 1999. On the structural preservation of recombinant human growth hormone in a dried film of a synthetic biodegradable polymer. J Pharm Sci, 88: 166–173.
88. Zale, S. E., Burke, P. A., Bernstein, H., and Brickner, A., 1997. US Patent 5,716,644.
89. Cleland, J. L., and Duenas, E. T., 1997. Controlled delivery of nerve growth factor for local treatment of neuronal diseases. Proc Int Symp Control Rel Bioact Mater, 24: 823–824.
90. Johnson, O. L., Jaworowicz, W., Cleland, J. L., Bailey, L., Charnis, M., Duenas, E., Wu, C. C., Shepard, D., Magil, S., Last, T., Jones, A. J. S., and Putney, S. D., 1997. The stabilization and encapsulation of human growth-hormone into biodegradable microspheres. Pharm Res, 14: 730–1735.

91. Eppstein, D. A., 1986. Pathways to increasing efficacy of interferons: drug synergy and sustained release. In: Kurahara, C. G., Bruno, N. A., van Der Pass, M. A., Marsh, Y. V., and Schryver, B. B. (Eds.), Biology of the Interferon System 1985, Elsevier, New York, pp. 401–409.
92. Eppstein, D. A., and Schryver, B. B., 1990. US Patent 4,962,091.
93. Tabata, Y., Takebayashi, Y., Ueda, T., and Ikada, Y., 1993. A formulation method using D,L-lactic acid oligomer for protein release with reduced initial burst. J Controlled Release, 23: 55–64.
94. Iwata, M., Nakamura, Y., and McGinity, J. W., 1999. Particle size and loading efficiency of poly(D,L-lactic-co-glycolic acid) multiphase microspheres containing water soluble substances prepared by the hydrous and anhydrous solvent evaporation methods. J Microencaps, 16: 49–58.
95. Horbett, T., and Brash, J. L., 1986. Proteins at interfaces: current issues and future prospects. In: Brash, J. L., and Horbett, T. A. (Eds.), Proteins at Interfaces: Physicochemical and Biochemical Studies, American Chemical Society, Washington, D.C., pp. 1–33.
96. Phillips, M. C., 1977. The conformation and properties of proteins at liquid interfaces. Chem Ind, March 5: 170–176.
97. MacRitchie, F., 1978. Proteins at interfaces. Adv Prot Chem, 32: 283–311.
98. Nihant, N., Schugens, C., Grandfils, C., Jerome, R., and Teyssie, P. 1994. Polylactide microparticles prepared by double emulsion/evaporation technique. I. Effect of primary emulsion stability. Pharm Res, 11: 1479–1484.
99. Nihant, N., Schugens, C., Grandfils, C., Jerome, R., and Teyssie, P., 1995. Polylactide microparticles prepared by double emulsion-evaporation. 2. Effect of the poly(lactide-co-glycolide) composition on the stability of the primary and secondary emulsions. J Colloid Interface Sci, 173: 55–65.
100. Graham, D. E., and Phillips, M. C., 1979. Proteins at liquid interfaces. II. Adsorption isotherms. J Colloid Interface Sci, 70: 415–426.
101. Dickinson, E., 1998. Proteins at interfaces and in emulsions—stability, rheology and interactions. J Chem Soc Faraday Trans, 94: 1657–1669.
102. Boury, F., Ivanova, T., Panaiotov, I., Proust, J. E., Bois, A., and Richou, J., 1995. Dilational properties of adsorbed poly(D,L-lactide) and bovine serum albumin monolayers at the dichloromethane/water interface. Langmuir, 11: 1636–1644.
103. Maa, Y. F., and Hsu, C. C., 1997. Protein denaturation by combined effect of shear and air–liquid interface. Biotechnol Bioeng, 54: 503–512.
104. Maa, Y.-F., and Hsu, C., 1996. Liquid-liquid emulsification by rotor/stator homogenization. J Controlled Release, 38: 219–228.
105. Morlock, M., Koll, H., Winter, G., and Kissel, T., 1997. Microencapsulation of rh-erythropoietin, using biodegradable poly(d,l-lactide-co-glycolide): protein stability and the effects of stabilizing excipients. Eur J Pharm Biopharm, 43: 29–36.
106. Graham, D. E., and Phillips, M. C., 1979. Proteins at liquid interfaces. I. Kinetics of adsorption and surface denaturation. J Colloid Interface Sci, 70: 403–414.
107. Fang, Y., and Dalgleish, D. G., 1997. Conformation of beta-lactoglobulin studied by FTIR: effect of pH, temperature, and adsorption to the oil–water interface. J Colloid Interface Sci, 196: 292–298.
108. Mumenthaler, M., Hsu, C. C., and Pearlman, R., 1994. Feasibility study on spray-drying protein pharmaceuticals: recombinant human growth hormone and tissue-type plasminogen activator. Pharm Res, 11: 12–20.
109. Maa, Y. F., Nguyen, P. A. T., and Hsu, S. W., 1998. Spray-drying of air-liquid interface sensitive recombinant human growth hormone. J Pharm Sci, 87: 152–159.
110. Chang, B. S., Kendrick, B. S., and Carpenter, J. F., 1996. Surface-induced denaturation of proteins during freezing and its inhibition by surfactants. J Pharm Sci, 85: 1325.
111. Prestrelski, S. J., Tedeschi, N., Arakawa, T., and Carpenter, J. F., 1993. Dehydration-induced conformational transitions in proteins and their inhibition by stabilizers. Biophys J, 65: 661–671.
112. Griebenow, K., and Klibanov, A. M., 1995. Lyophilization-induced reversible changes in the secondary structure of proteins. Proc Natl Acad Sci USA, 92: 10969–10976.
113. Fu, K., Griebenow, K., Hsieh, L., Klibanov, A. M., and Langer, R., 1999. FTIR characterization of the secondary structure of proteins encapsulated within PLGA microspheres. J Controlled Release, 58: 357–366.

114. Sah, H., 1999. Stabilization of proteins against methylene chloride water interface-induced denaturation and aggregation. J Controlled Release, 58: 143–151.
115. Courthaudon, J. L., Dickinson, E., Matsumara, Y., and Clark, D. C., 1991. Competitive adsorption of beta-lactoglobulin + Tween 20 at the oil-water interface. Colloids Surf, 56: 293–300.
116. Chen, J., and Dickinson, E., 1995. Protein/surfactant interfacial interactions Part 3. Competitive adsorption of protein + surfactant in emulsions. Colloids Surf A: Physicochem Eng, 101: 77–85.
117. Rojas, J., Pinto, A.-H., Leo, E., Pecquet, S., Couvreur, P., Gulik, A., and Fattal, E., 1999. A polysorbate-based non-ionic surfactant can modulate loading and release of beta-lactoglobulin entrapped in multiphase poly(DL-lactide-co-glycolide) microspheres. Pharm Res, 16: 255–260.
118. Matsuyama, K., El-Gizway, S., and Perrin, J. H., 1987. Thermodynamics of binding of aromatic amino acids to alpha-, beta-, and gamma-cylodextrins. Drug Dev Ind Pharm, 13: 2687–2691.
119. Niven, R., 1996. Protein nebulization II. Stabilization of G-CSF to air-jet nebulization and the role of protectants. Int J Pharm, 127: 191–201.
120. Arakawa, T., Kita, Y., and Carpenter, J. F., 1991. Protein–solvent interactions in pharmaceutical formulations. Pharm Res, 8: 285–291.
121. Timasheff, S. N., 1992. Stabilization of protein structure by solvent additives. In: Ahern, T. J., and Manning, M. C. (Ed.), Stability of Protein Pharmaceuticals, Part B: In Vivo Pathways of Degradation and Strategies for Protein Stabilization, Plenum Press, New York, pp. 265–285.
122. Volkin, D. B., and Klibanov, A. M., 1989. Minimizing protein inactivation. In: Creighton, T. E. (Ed.), Protein Function: A Practical Approach, IRL Press, Oxford, pp. 1–24.
123. Timasheff, S. N., and Arakawa, T., 1989. Stabilization of protein structure by solvent additives. In: Creighton, T. E. (Ed.), Protein Structure: A Practical Approach, IRL Press, New York, pp. 331–345.
124. Yang, T. H., Dong, A. C., Meyer, J., Johnson, O. L., Cleland, J. L., and Carpenter, J. F., 1999. Use of infrared spectroscopy to assess secondary structure of human growth hormone within biodegradable microspheres. J Pharm Sci, 88: 161–165.
125. Krewson, C. E., Dause, R., Mak, M., and Saltzman, W. M., 1996. Stabilization of nerve growth factor in controlled release polymers and in tissue. J Biomater Sci Polym Edn, 8: 103–117.
126. Pean, J. M., Venier-Julienne, M.-C., Boury, F., Menei, P., Denizot, B., and Benoit, J. P., 1998. NGF release from poly(D,L-lactide-co-glycolide) microspheres. Effect of some formulation parameters on encapsulated NGF stability. J Controlled Release, 56: 175–187.
127. Pean, J. M., Venier-Julienne, M.-C., Filmon, R., Sergent, M., Phan-Tan-Luu, R., and Benoit, J. P., 1998. Optimization of HSA and NGF encapsulation yields in PLGA microparticles. Int J Pharm, 166: 105–115.
128. Thomasin, C., Merkle, H. P., and Gander, B. A., 1997. Physicochemical parameters governing protein microencapsulation into biodegradable polyesters by coacervation. Int J Pharm, 147: 173–186.
129. Young, T. J., Johnston, K. P., Mishima, K., and Tanaka, H., 1999. Encapsulation of lysozyme in a biodegradable polymer by precipitation with a vapor-over-liquid antisolvent. J Pharm Sci, 88: 640–650.
130. Winters, M. A., Knutson, B. L., Debenedetti, P. G., Sparks, H. G., Przybycien, T. M., Stevenson, C. L., and Prestrelski, S. J., 1996. Precipitation of proteins in supercritical carbon dioxide. J Pharm Sci, 85: 586–594.
131. Sanchez, A., Gupta, R. K., Alonso, M. J., Siber, G. R., and Langer, R., 1996. Pulsed controlled-release system for potential use in vaccine delivery. J Pharm Sci, 85: 547–552.
132. Viswanathan, N. B., Thomas, P. A., Pandit, J. K., Kulkarni, M. G., and Mashelkar, R. A., 1999. Preparation of non-porous microspheres with high entrapment efficiency of proteins by a (water-in-oil)-in-oil emulsion technique. J Controlled Release, 58: 9–20.
133. Park, T. G., Lee, H. Y., and Nam, Y. S., 1998. A new preparation method for protein loaded poly(D,L-lactic-co-glycolic acid) microspheres and protein release mechanism study. J Controlled Release, 55: 181–191.
134. Jackson, M., and Mantsch, H. H., 1991. Beware of proteins in DMSO. Biochim Biophys Acta, 1078: 231–235.

135. Yewey, G. L., Duysen, E. G., Cox, S. M., and Dunn, R. L., 1997. Delivery of proteins from a controlled release injectable implant. In: Sanders, L. M., and Hendren, W. (Eds.), Protein Delivery: Physical Systems, Plenum Press, New York, pp. 93–105.
136. Katre, N. V., Asherman, J., Schaefer, H., and Hora, M., 1998. Multivesicular liposome (DepoFoam) technology for the sustained delivery of insulin-like growth factor-I (IGF-I). J Pharm Sci, 87: 1341–1346.
137. Chasin, M., Domb, A., Ron, E., Mathiowitz, E., Langer, R., Leong, K., Laurencin, C., Brem, H., and Grossman, S., 1990. Polyanhydrides as drug delivery systems. In: Langer, R., and Chasin, M. (Ed.), Biodegradable Polymers for Drug Delivery, Marcel Dekker, New York, pp. 43–70.
138. Tabata, Y., Gutta, S., and Langer, R., 1993. Controlled delivery systems for proteins using polyanhydride microspheres. Pharm Res, 10: 487–496.
139. Gombotz, W. R., and Wee, S. F., 1998. Protein release from alginate matrices. Adv Drug Del Rev, 31: 267–285.
140. Bromberg, L. E., and Ron, E. S., 1998. Temperature-responsive gels and thermogelling polymer matrices for protein and peptide delivery. Adv Drug Deliv Rev, 31: 197–221.
141. Hancock, B. C., and Zografi, G., 1995. Molecular mobility of amorphous pharmaceutical solids below their glass transition temperatures. Pharm Res, 12: 799–806.
142. Bodmeier, R., Oh, K. H., and Chen, H., 1989. The effect of the addition of low molecular weight poly(dl-lactide) on drug release from biodegradable poly(dl-lactide) drug delivery systems. Int J Pharm, 51: 1–8.
143. Bittner, B., Ronneberger, B., Zange, R., Volland, C., Anderson, J. M., and Kissel, T., 1998. Bovine serum albumin loaded poly(lactide-co-glycolide) microspheres: the influence of polymer purity on particle characteristics. J Microencaps, 15: 495–514.
144. Bain, D. F., Munday, D. L., and Smith, A., 1999. Solvent influence on spray-dried biodegradable microspheres. J Microencaps, 16: 453–474.
145. Arshady, R., 1991. Preparation of biodegradable microparticles and microcapules. 2. Polylactide and related polyesters. J Controlled Release, 17: 1–22.
146. Niu, C. H., and Chiu, Y. Y., 1998. FDA perspective on peptide formulation and stability issues. J Pharm Sci, 87: 1331–1334.
147. Hubbard, W. K., 1997. International Conference on Harmonisation; Guidance on Impurities: Residual Solvents. Fed Reg, 62: 67377–67388.
148. Montanari, L., Costantini, M., Signoretti, E. C., Valvo, L., Santucci, M., Bartolomei, M., Fattibene, P., Onori, S., Faucitano, A., Conti, B., and Genta, I., 1998. Gamma irradiation effects on poly(DL-lactictide-co-glycolide) microspheres. J Controlled Release, 56: 219–229.
149. Bittner, B., Mader, K., Kroll, C., Borchert, H. H., and Kissel, T., 1999. Tetracycline-HCl-loaded poly(DL-lactide-co-glycolide) microspheres prepared by a spray drying technique: influence of gamma-irradiation on radical formation and polymer degradation. J Controlled Release, 59: 23–32.
150. Lin, W.-J., Flanagan, D. R., and Linhardt, R. J., 1994. Accelerated degradation of poly(epsilon-caprolactone) by organic amines. Pharm. Res, 11: 1030–1034.
151. Lai, M. C., and Topp, E. M., 1999. Solid-state chemical stability of proteins and peptides. J Pharm Sci, 88: 489–500.
152. Klibanov, A. M., 1997. Why are enzymes less active in organic solvents than in water? TIBTECH, 15: 97–101.
153. Hageman, M., 1992. Water sorption and solid-state stability of proteins. In: Ahern, T. J., and Manning, M. C. (Eds.), Stability of Protein Pharmaceuticals, Part A; Chemical and Physical Pathways of Protein Degradation, Plenum Press, New York, pp. 273–309.
154. Hancock, B. C., and Zografi, G., 1994. The relationship between the glass transition temperature and the water content of amorphous pharmaceutical solids. Pharm Res, 11: 471–477.
155. Yoshioka, S., Aso, Y., and Kojima, S., 1999. The effect of excipients on the molecular mobility of lyophilized formulations, as measured by glass transition temperature and NMR relaxation-based critical mobility temperature. Pharm Res, 16: 135–140.
156. Bodmer, D., Kissel, T., and Traechslin, E., 1992. Factors influencing the release of peptides and proteins from biodegradable parenteral depot systems. J Controlled Release, 21: 129–138.

157. Park, T. G., Lu, W., and Crotts, G., 1995. Importance of in vitro experimental conditions on protein release kinetics, stability and polymer degradation in protein encapsulated poly(D,L-lactic acid-co-glycolic acid) microspheres. J Controlled Release, 33: 211–222.
158. Yang, J., and Cleland, J. L., 1997. Factors affecting the in-vitro release of recombinant human interferon–gamma (rhIFN-gamma) from PLGA microspheres. J Pharm Sci, 86: 908–914.
159. Tracy, M. A., Ward, K. L., Firouzabadian, L., Wang, Y., Dong, N., Qian, R., and Zhang, Y., 1999. Factors affecting the degradation rate of poly(lactide-co-glycolide) microspheres in vivo and in vitro. Biomaterials, 20: 1057–1062.
160. Schwendeman, S. P., Cardomone, M., Brandon, M. R., Klibanov, A., and Langer, R., 1996. Stability of proteins and their delivery from biodegradable polymer microspheres. In: Cohen, S., and Bernstein, H. (Eds.), Microspheres/Microparticles: Characterization and Pharmaceutical Application, Marcel Dekker, New York, pp. 1–49.
161. Wang, Y.-C. J., and Hanson, M. A., 1988. Parenteral formulations of proteins and peptides: stability and stabilizers. J Parent Sci Technol, 42: S3–S26.
162. Manning, M. C., Patel, K., and Borchardt, R. T., 1989. Stability of protein pharmaceuticals. Pharm. Res, 6: 903–918.
163. Liu, W. R., Langer, R., and Klibanov, A. M., 1991. Moisture induced aggregation of lyophilized proteins in the solid state. Biotechnol Bioeng, 37: 177–184.
164. Costantino, H. R., Langer, R., and Klibanov, A., 1994. Moisture-induced aggregation of lyophilized insulin. Pharm Res, 11: 21–29.
165. Mader, K., Bittner, B., Li, Y. X., Wohlauf, W., and Kissel, T., 1998. Monitoring microviscosity and microacidity of the albumin microenvironment inside degrading microparticles from poly-(lactide-co-glycolide) (PLG) or ABA-triblock polymers containing hydrophobic poly(lactide-co-glycolide) A blocks and hydrophilic poly(ethyleneoxide) B blocks. Pharm Res, 15: 787–793.
166. Yan, C., Resau, J. H., Hewetson, J., West, M., Rill, W. L., and Kende, M., 1994. Characterization and morphological analysis of protein-loaded poly(lactide-co-glycolide) microparticles prepared by water-in-oil-in-water emulsion technique. J Controlled Release, 32: 231–241.
167. Lacasse, F. X., Hildgen, P., Perodin, J., Escher, E., Phillips, N. C., and McMullen, J. N., 1997. Improved activity of a new angiotensin receptor antagonist by an injectable spray dried polymer microsphere preparation. Pharm Res, 14: 887–891.
168. Tjia, J. S., and Moghe, P. V., 1998. Analysis of 3-D microstructure of porous poly(lactide-glycolide) matrices using confocal microscopy. J Biomed Mater Res, 43: 291–299.
169. Schmitt, E. A., Flanagan, D. R., and Linhardt, R. J., 1994. Importance of distinct water environments in the hydrolysis of poly(DL-lactide-co-glycolide). Macromolecules, 27: 743–748.
170. Zhang, Y., Zale, S., Sawyer, L., and Bernstein, H., 1997. Effects of metal-salts on poly(DL-lactide-co-glycolide) polymer hydrolysis. J Biomed Mater Res, 34: 531–538.
171. Burke, P. A., 1999. Characterization of delivery systems: magnetic resonance techniques. In: Mathiowitz, E. (Ed.), Encyclopedia of Controlled Drug Delivery, John Wiley and Sons, New York, pp. 228–234.
172. Vert, M., Li, S., Garreau, H., Mauduit, J., Boustta, M., Schwach, G., Engel, R., and Coudane, J., 1997. Complexity of the hydrolytic degradation of aliphatic polyesters. Angew Makromol Chemie, 247: 239–253.
173. Grizzi, I., Garreau, H., Li, S., and Vert, M., 1995. Hydrolytic degradation of devices based on poly(DL-lactic acid) size-dependence. Biomaterials, 16: 305–311.
174. Burke, P. A., 1996. Determination of internal pH in PLGA microspheres using ^{31}P NMR spectroscopy. Proc Int Symp Controlled Release Bioact Mater, 23: 133–134.
175. Shenderova, A., Burke, T. G., and Schwendeman, S. P., 1999. The acidic microclimate in poly-(lactide-co-glycolide) microspheres stabilizes camptothecins. Pharm Res, 16: 241–248.
176. Fu, K., Pack, D. W., Klibanov, A. M., and Langer, R., 2000. Visual evidence of acidic environment within degrading PLGA microspheres. Pharm Res, 17: 100–106.
177. Butler, S. M., Tracy, M. A., and Tilton, R. D., 1999. Adsorption of serum albumin to thin films of poly(lactide-co-glycolide). J Controlled Release, 58: 335–347.

178. Morlock, M., Kissel, T., Li, Y. X., Koll, H., and Winter, G., 1998. Erythropoietin loaded microspheres prepared from biodegradable LPLG-PEO-LPLG triblock copolymers: protein stabilization and in-vitro release properties. J Controlled Release, 56: 105–115.
179. Bittner, B., Morlock, M., Koll, H., Winter, G., and Kissel, T., 1998. Recombinant human erythropoietin (rhEPO) loaded poly(lactide-co-glycolide) microspheres: influence of the encapsulation technique and polymer purity on microsphere characteristics. Eur J Pharm Pharm Biopharm, 45: 295–305.
180. Pistel, K. F., Bittner, B., Koll, H., Winter, G., and Kissel, T., 1999. Biodegradable recombinant human erythropoietin loaded microspheres prepared from linear and star-branched block copolymers: influence of encapsulation technique and polymer composition on particle characteristics. J Controlled Release, 59: 309–325.
181. Johnson, O. L., Cleland, J. L., Lee, H. J., Charnis, M., Duenas, E., Jaworowicz, W., Shepard, D., Shahzamani, A., Jones, A. J. S., and Putney, S. D., 1996. A month-long effect from a single injection of microencapsulated human growth hormone. Nature Med, 2: 795–799.
182. Cleland, J. L., Duenas, E., Daugherty, A., Marian, M., Yang, J., Wilson, M., Celniker, A. C., Shahzamani, A., Quarmby, V., Chu, H., Mukku, V., Mac, A., Roussakis, M., Gillette, N., Boyd, B., Yeung, D., Brooks, D., Maa, Y. F., Hsu, C., and Jones, A. J. S., 1997. Recombinant human growth hormone poly(lactic-co-glycolic acid) (PLGA) microspheres provide a long lasting effect. J Controlled Release, 49: 193–205.
183. Cleland, J. L., Mac, A., Boyd, B., Yang, J., Duenas, E. T., Yeung, D., Brooks, D., Hsu, C., Chu, H., Mukku, V., and Jones, A. J. S., 1997. The stability of recombinant human growth-hormone in poly(lactic-co-glycolic acid) (PLGA) microspheres. Pharm Res, 14: 420–425.
184. Tracy, M. A., Bernstein, H., and Khan, M. A., 1998. US Patent 5,711,968.
185. Gombotz, W. R., Pankey, S. C., Bouchard, L. S., Ranchalis, J., and Puolakkainen, P., 1993. Controlled release of TGF-beta 1 from a biodegradable matrix for bone regeneration. J Biomater Sci Polym Ed, 5: 49–63.
186. Hora, M. S., Rana, R. K., Nunberg, J. H., Tice, T. R., Gilley, R. M., and Hudson, M. E., 1990. Controlled release of interleukin-2 from biodegradable microspheres. Bio/Technology, 8: 755–758.
187. Mendez, A., Camarata, P. J., Suryanarayanan, R., and Ebner, T. J., 1997. Sustained intracerebral delivery of nerve growth factor with biodegradable polymer microspheres. Meth Neurosci, 21: 150–167.
188. Pettit, D. K., Lawter, J. R., Huang, W. J., Pankey, S. C., Nightlinger, N. S., Lynch, D. H., Schuh, J. A. C. L., Morrissey, P. J., and Gombotz, W. R., 1997. Characterization of poly(glycolide-co-D,L-lactide)/poly(D,L-lactide) microspheres for controlled-release of GM-CSF. Pharm Res, 14: 1422–1430.
189. Mittal, S., Cohen, A., and Maysinger, D., 1994. In vitro effects of brain derived neurotrophic factor released from microspheres. NeuroReport, 5: 2577–2582.
190. Jameela, S. R., Suma, N., and Jayakrishnan, A., 1997. Protein release from poly(epsilon-caprolactone) microspheres prepared by melt encapsulation and solvent evaporation techniques—a comparative study. J Biomater Sci Polym Ed, 8: 457–466.
191. Franssen, O., and Hennink, W. E., 1998. A novel preparation method for polymeric microparticles without the use of organic solvents. Int J Pharm, 168: 1–7.

33
Solid-State Chemical Stability of Peptides and Proteins: Application to Controlled Release Formulations

Elizabeth M. Topp, Yuan Song, Ashley Wilson, Rong Li, and Richard L. Schowen
University of Kansas, Lawrence, Kansas
Michael J. Hageman
Pharmacia & Upjohn, Inc., Kalamazoo, Michigan

I. INTRODUCTION

Many of the newer drugs undergoing development and entering the marketplace are proteins or peptides. These drugs are both highly potent and susceptible to hydrolytic and enzymatic degradation in the gastrointestinal tract—characteristics that make them ideal candidates for parenteral controlled release formulation. For these formulations to be successful, however, they must not only deliver the therapeutic protein at the prescribed rate for the desired *in vivo* release period but also must preserve the activity of the protein during storage and release. Since proteins are subject to a variety of degradation reactions both in solution and in the solid state, the preservation of activity is a central challenge in their formulation.

This chapter reviews current issues related to the solid-state chemical stability of proteins and peptides. Proteins are subject to both chemical and physical instabilities; the former are the result of covalent modifications of specific amino acid residues, while the latter involve a loss of secondary and tertiary structure. The focus in this chapter is on chemical instability, since chemical changes can cause a loss of biological activity and can be the precipitating cause of physical instability. For a recent review of physical instability, the reader is referred to the article by Costantino et al. (1). In addition, the focus in this chapter is on the solid state, since most controlled release formulations are solids. While much of this literature involves freeze-dried (i.e., lyophilized) formulations and not controlled release devices, the mechanistic information it provides is applicable to the successful development of stable controlled release formulations as well.

The chapter begins with a general discussion of reaction kinetics in the solid state (Section II). This is followed by a review of common solid-state degradation reactions for peptides and proteins (Section III). These include oxidation, deamidation, chain scission, the Maillard reaction, and thiol–disulfide exchange. We then describe the physicochemical factors known to influence protein stability in the solid state: temperature, pressure, mobility in the matrix, water content, excipients, and effective pH (Section IV). Since many sustained and controlled release devices are based on polymer matrices, this is followed by a review of the effects of specific polymers on protein stability (Section V). Each of these sections concludes with a discussion of the implications of the information presented for the design of controlled release devices. An overall summary concludes the chapter (Section VI).

II. KINETICS OF SOLID-STATE REACTIONS

Reactions occurring within a solid or semisolid matrix are expected to be more similar to liquid state reactions than to those in crystalline solids. The relative rates of reaction in crystalline and amorphous solids are difficult to establish, however, since the factors determining reactivity are more complex in solids than in liquids. Transport processes such as diffusion are likely to be slower in all solid materials than in liquids, and are therefore more likely to compete with bond-making and bond-breaking steps in limiting the reaction rate. The reaction may be accelerated in amorphous materials by the presence of localized regions with high reactant concentrations and in crystals by packing forces compressing adjacent molecules. Internal molecular motions such as those required for cyclization reactions might be expected to be slowed relative to the reaction in solution due to friction in the more closely packed solid. However, if a molecule should be trapped in the solid state in a reactive conformation it may undergo more rapid reaction. Thus, while many individual cases can easily be interpreted, no broad generalizations are possible.

This section presents general information on reactivity in solid systems. First we discuss the kinetic laws that are used to treat data for solid-state reactions, and then we describe the calculation and interpretation of activation parameters. Applications to the design of controlled release system also are discussed.

A. Kinetic Laws

A kinetic law is a functional relationship between concentration and time. As a rule, such laws can be derived from mechanistic models for the chemical reaction that is responsible for the time-dependent variation in concentration. Consistency between experimental relationships and those predicted from specific mechanistic models is one test for the adequacy of the models in accounting for the data. Of course, consistency demonstrates only that the data do not falsify a particular model; it cannot guarantee that the model is positively correct.

Schmalzried identifies several basic kinetic situations that can apply to simple reactions in the solid state, such as a single homogeneous phase or two adjacent homogeneous phases that share an interface (2). These can be simplified for our purposes into the three cases listed below, with each leading to characteristic kinetic laws.

1. *Chemical reactions within a single solid phase.* Such reactions are not qualitatively distinct from those occurring in any other homogeneous phase, although their rate constants and mechanisms will reflect characteristics of the phase in which they occur. Their kinetic laws have familiar forms, however: unimolecular reactions display a simple exponential decay to an equilibrium or steady-state circumstance, for example.
2. *Interfacial reactions.* These occur at the juncture between two materials, so that transport of the materials to the interface is required for reaction. If this transport is not much faster than the reaction at the interface, the kinetic law must reflect the role of transport in the overall reaction.
3. *Multiphasic reactions.* These require diffusion of the reactants across an interface, with reaction occurring in one or more distinct solid phases. In this case, not only are the transport processes of possible significance, but the reaction itself may lead to changes in the medium in which the reaction occurs.

In some circumstances, then, the kinetics of a solid-state reaction may be quite simple. For example, one of the most thoroughly studied examples of peptide degradation is the cyclization of Asn or Asp residues to form a cyclic imide residue that then opens to two products (see Section III.B, Scheme 2). To date, this reaction has exhibited simple first-order kinetics in the reactant peptide in both solution (3,4) and solid states (5–7). Under conditions where the cyclic imide does not accumulate, the Asp product and isoAsp product also form in simple first-order fashion (3–7).

In the general case, however, solid-state reactions need not fall into any simple, single category because of local changes in concentrations and/or reaction conditions during the course of reaction. Shalaev and Zografi have reviewed cases in which phase transformations affect the kinetics of solid-state reactions (8). In such cases, the time–concentration profiles may contain as many as five stages depending on the solid-state miscibility or solubility of the species involved. Even the simple interconversion of cis- and trans-azobenzene at temperatures between the eutectic temperature of the cis/trans mixture and the melting point of the cis isomer exhibits a complex sigmoidal dependence of the fraction reacted on time. Shalaev and Zografi reanalyzed existing data for this temperature range to obtain first-order rate constants for the isomerization reaction in the solid and liquid states. Their treatment employed the Baum equation:

$$\text{Fraction reacted} = k_s M[\exp(Mt) - 1]$$
$$M = k_s/[\text{trans}] - k_a$$

where t is time, k_s and k_a are first-order rate constants for reaction in the solid and liquid phases, respectively, and [trans] is the concentration of trans-azobenzene.

More complex processes can require still more demanding analysis, as exemplified by the studies of Zografi et al. on the methyl transfer reaction of tetraglycine methyl ester (9,10). In these thorough studies, concentration–time profiles were obtained for the loss of reactant, formation of the final products tetraglycine, N-methyltetraglycine, and N,N-dimethyltetraglycine, and for the formation and disappearance of the intermediate compound N-methyltetraglycine methyl ester. The reaction was followed for crystalline material and material that had been lyophilized or milled. In the crystalline state, the reaction showed an autocatalytic acceleration in the rate until approximately 25% reaction. This phase of the reaction was analyzed assuming that the first-order rate constant for loss of reactant is a linear function of the total product concentration. Thereafter, this treatment failed to account for the observations. Data for the range 35–75% reaction were fit to a "contracting geometry" model, in which the rate of reaction was assumed to be equal to the rate of loss of the reactant crystalline phase. In this region, then, the phase transformation that accompanies reaction is directly coupled to the chemical conversion. The data are well described by the Avrami–Erofeev equation:

$$1 - [(1 - A)/3] = k(t - i)$$

where A is the fraction of reaction, i is an induction period, and k, although it has the dimensions of a rate constant, can be considered a fitting parameter.

B. Activation Parameters

There is a long history of measurement and interpretation of the temperature dependence of chemical reaction rates in both gas and condensed phases. The two most common formulations are the Arrhenius ("collision theory") equation,

$$k = A \exp(-E_a/RT)$$

and the Eyring ("transition state theory") equation,

$$k = (kT/h) \exp \{(S^{\ddagger}/R) \exp[-H^{\ddagger}/RT]\}$$

In these equations, k is the rate constant, T the absolute temperature, R the gas constant, **k** the Boltzmann constant, and h the Planck constant. The preexponential factor (A) and the activation energy (E_a) are usually considered to be temperature-independent in the Arrhenius equation, so that log (k) is predicted to be a linear function of 1/T. Similarly, in the Eyring equation, the entropy of activation ($S^{\ddagger}$) and the enthalpy of activation ($H^{\ddagger}$) are often assumed to be temperature-independent, so that log (k/T) should be a linear function of 1/T, although this assumption has not been employed universally. The two formulations are therefore formally inconsistent, but data for reactions in condensed phases are almost always so imprecise that both log (k) and log (k/T) often appear to be linear with respect to 1/T.

Most data for condensed phases are better interpreted with the use of the Eyring or transition state equation. The Arrhenius equation continues to be used in some gas phase studies, but it is rare for condensed phase results to be simply interpretable in Arrhenius terms. In contrast, physical interpretations of the entropy and enthalpy of activation are frequently possible and mechanistically informative. Thus the most reasonable procedure is to obtain these quantities from a fit of experimental rate constants to the Eyring equation. In principle, it is possible to first calculate A and E_a from a fit of rate constants to the Arrhenius equation and then convert these values to $S^{\ddagger}$ and $H^{\ddagger}$ for the mean experimental temperature, but this procedure is pointless and should not be used.

When the kinetic behavior is simple enough that a rate law derived from a mechanistic model can be fitted to the time–concentration profiles, meaningful activation parameters can be extracted from the temperature dependence of the rate constants present in the rate law. When empirical rate laws are used, the data may still be fitted to the Eyring equation. The resulting parameters then may be used to interpolate or extrapolate to the values of rate constants at temperatures where measurements were not carried out. Such extensions of the data usually assume a linear Eyring plot and may be quite reliable if there are good data at temperatures lower and higher than the interpolated point and at reasonably close temperatures. Extrapolations over a short range of temperatures may likewise be reliable. In contrast, extensions of temperature dependence data over wide ranges of temperature certainly cannot be relied on, whether or not the rate constants have an established molecular significance. In general, there is no warrant for an assumption of linearity in Eyring plots over wide ranges of temperature in any phase. Linearity of Eyring plots first requires that the values of the activation parameters ($S^{\ddagger}$ and $H^{\ddagger}$) be independent of temperature. This condition in turn requires that the heat capacity in the transition state be equal to that in the reactant state, an assumption that generally cannot be met. Even if this heat capacity requirement is met, nonlinear Eyring plots can arise from changes in rate-limiting step or changes in mechanism, as shown in Fig. 1.

Note from Fig. 1 that each of the two possible changes gives a unique diagnostic signal. If the nonlinearity arises from a change in rate-limiting step, then the actual rate at low temperature is slower than that predicted from high-temperature data. If the nonlinearity arises from a change in reaction pathway or mechanism, then the actual rate at low temperatures is faster than that predicted from high-temperature data. These are considerations that apply to reactions in all phases. They emphasize the many ways that error can afflict extrapolations of rate constants across broad temperature ranges.

There are particular problems that arise in polymeric and other solid-state phases that may undergo structural changes ("phase transitions") over the same range in which a constituent undergoes temperature-dependent reaction. In some cases, the phase transition may exert a medium effect on the constituent reaction, causing a change in the reaction mechanism and

Solid-State Stability of Peptides and Proteins

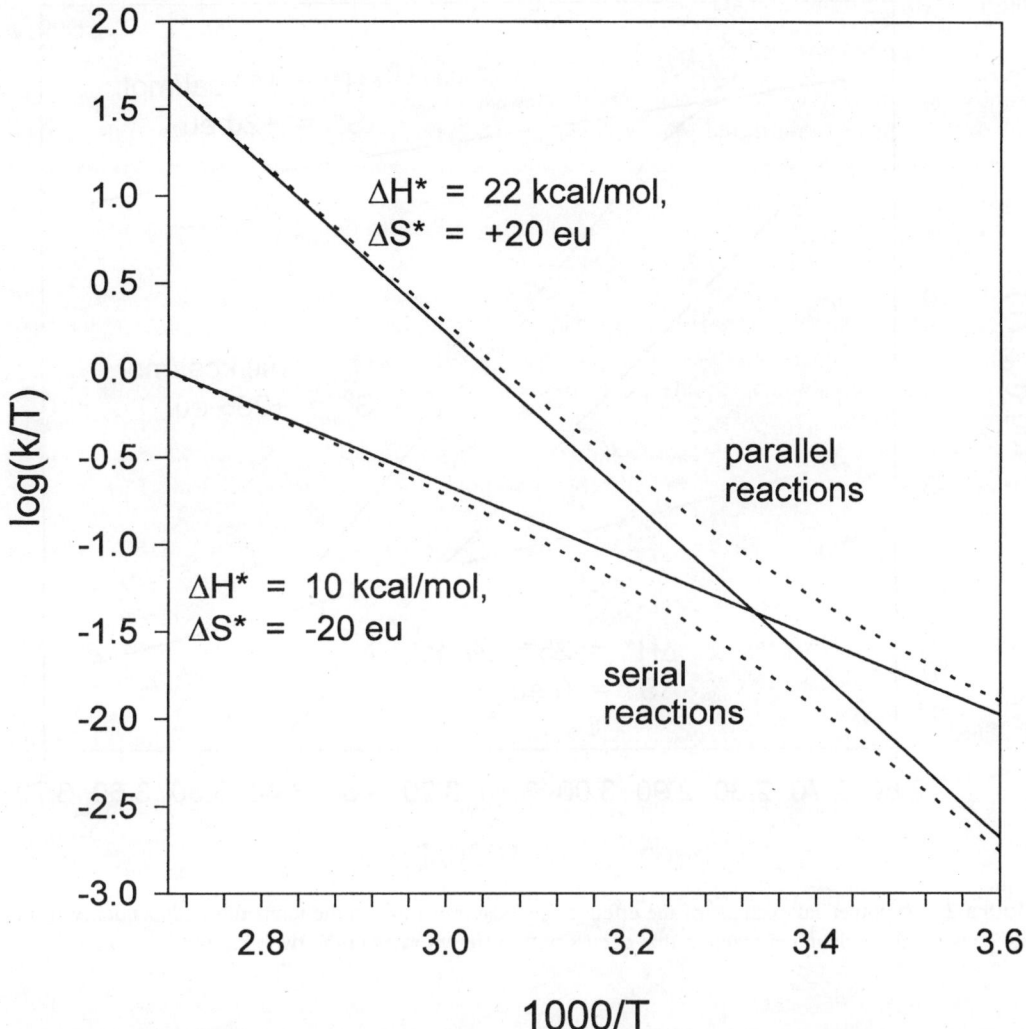

Figure 1 Hypothetical example of the nonlinear Eyring plots produced by a change in rate-limiting step along a pathway with two serial transition states and by a change in reaction mechanism between two pathways. The model consists of two processes in which a common reactant state is transformed to two different transition states: in one case, $\Delta H^{\ddagger} =$; 22 kcal/mol and $\Delta S^{\ddagger} = -20$ eu; in the other case, $\Delta H^{\ddagger} = 10$ kcal/mol and $\Delta S^{\ddagger} = +20$ eu. The two processes have equal rate constants when their $\Delta G^{\ddagger}$ values are equal, and thus at 300 K. The two solid lines give the Eyring plots for the two separate processes. When the two transition states are in series along a single reaction pathway, the overall reaction generates the lower dotted curve: the rate is always slower than the rate of either step and approaches the rate of the slower ("rate-limiting") step at temperatures far from the crossover point. When the two transition states are in parallel, each along its own reaction pathway, the overall reaction generates the upper dotted curve: the rate is always faster than the rate of either contributing pathway and approaches the rate of the faster ("dominant") pathway or mechanism at the extreme temperatures.

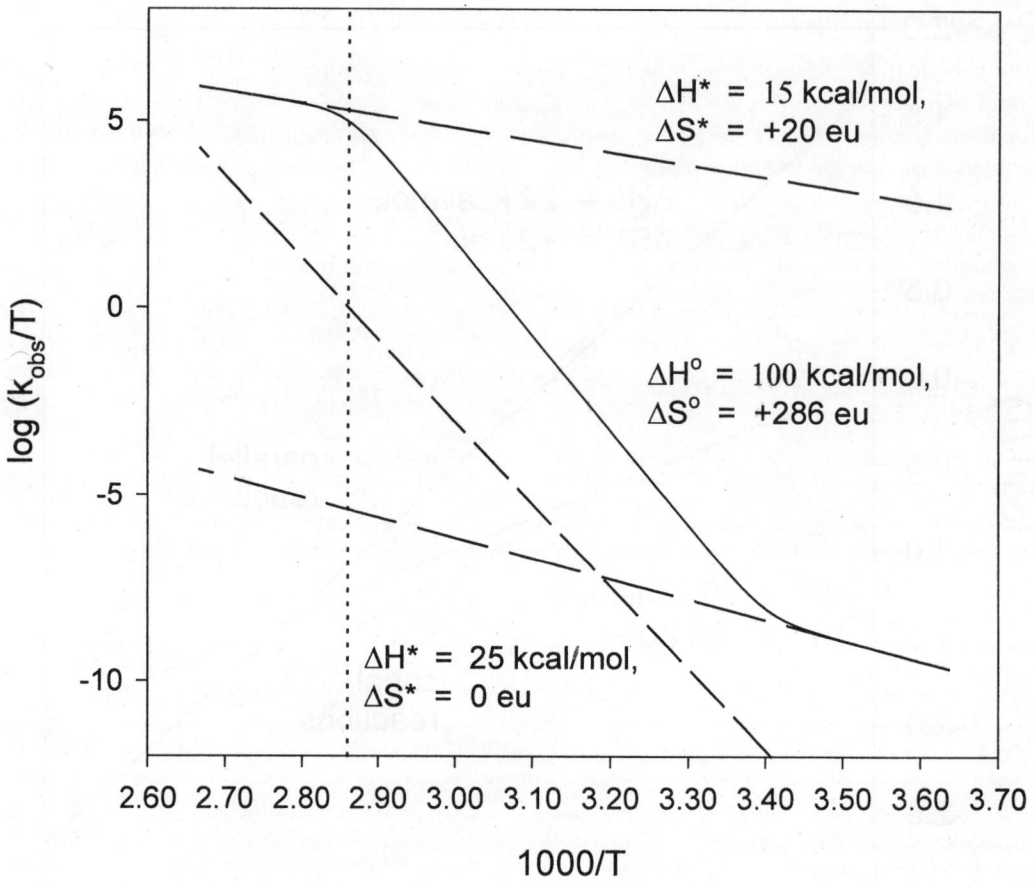

Figure 2 Hypothetical example of the effect of a phase transition on the temperature dependence of the rate constant for a chemical reaction that occurs with different rates in the two phases.

thus a change in the activation parameters. A case of this kind is shown in Fig. 2. The phase present at high temperature favors a much faster reaction than that found at low temperature. The result is that well below the transition temperature a major contribution to total reaction begins to arise from the small fraction of material in the high-temperature phase. The apparent activation parameters then correspond to the very large thermodynamic values associated with the phase transition. In such cases, mechanistic deductions from activation parameters are impossible without independent knowledge of the thermodynamics of the phase transition.

C. Product Formation and Distribution

There is little to add to the above discussion on these points. Product formation generally is subject to the same kinetic complexities as reactant loss. Product distribution is a result of the relative rates of the parallel reactions that generate the individual products. The kinetics and temperature dependencies of these reactions can be treated in the framework described above, but few general statements can be made.

D. Summary and Application to Controlled Release

The chemical degradation of peptides and proteins in typical controlled release devices is the result of specific reactions that occur in solid or semisolid media. In simple cases, kinetic data for these reactions can be interpreted using rate laws and expressions for the temperature dependence of the rate commonly employed for reactions in solution. Interpretation of the data can be complicated, however, by the existence of multiple solid phases or by temperature-dependent solid-state phase transitions. While mechanistic information can be derived from such kinetic data and can lead to rational strategies for protein stabilization, these complicating factors should be borne in mind to avoid misinterpretation.

III. CHEMICAL DEGRADATION REACTIONS OF PROTEINS AND PEPTIDES IN THE SOLID STATE

Several types of degradation reactions are known to affect peptides and proteins in the solid state. This section reviews the current literature on five of the more common solid-state degradation reactions: oxidation (Section III.A), deamidation (Section III.B), chain scission (Section III.C), the Maillard reaction (Section III.D), and thiol–disulfide exchange (Section III.E). References to more detailed reviews describing rates and mechanisms in the solution state are provided.

A. Oxidation

Potential oxidation sites in proteins and peptides are the side chains of Met, His, Cys, Tyr, and Trp residues (11). Of these, Met oxidation has probably been documented most extensively (Scheme 1). Met can be oxidized to Met sulfoxide in both the solution and solid states. Oxidation to Met sulfone can also occur, but this reaction usually requires more severe reagents and reaction conditions. Fransson et al. have documented Met oxidation in lyophilized formulations of human insulin-like growth factor I (hIGF-I), a small globular protein (MW = 7.65 kDa) (12).

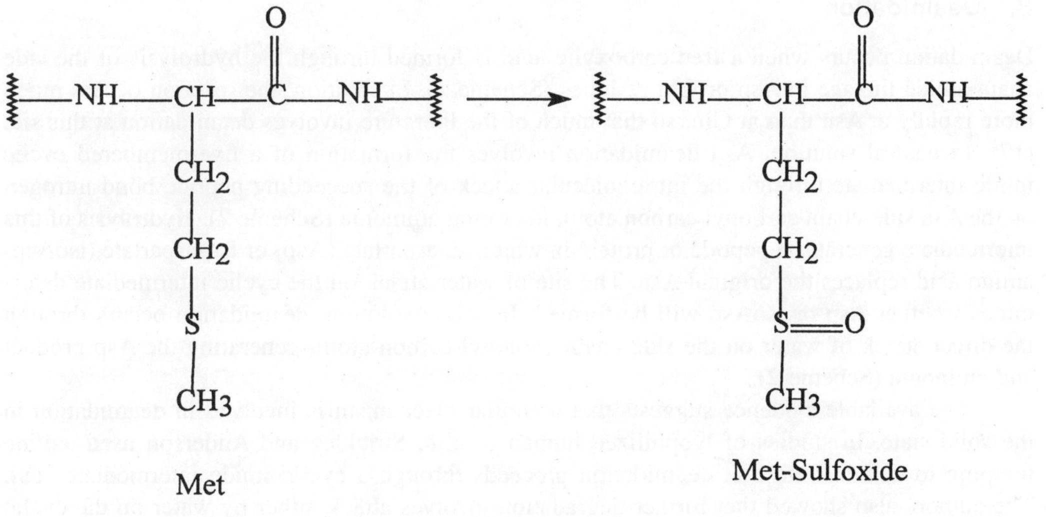

Scheme 1

The reaction was found to be second-order with respect to the amount of protein and dissolved oxygen. Interestingly, the reaction rate was similar in both solution and lyophilized formulations (12). The authors speculate that, although diffusion in the solid state is expected to be relatively slow, dissolved oxygen species present in the lyophilized matrix may have facilitated solid-state oxidation. The reaction rate was also found to be accelerated on exposure to light. Similarly, Pikal et al. studied the stability of lyophilized formulations of human growth hormone and observed significant oxidation at Met residues (13).

Townsend et al. have presented evidence for oxidative degradation of freeze-dried ribonuclease A (RNase), a 13.7-kDa protein (14). Stability studies were conducted with air or argon in the vial headspace, and in the presence of EDTA, antioxidants, or light. The primary instability observed was the formation of protein aggregates, as determined by size exclusion chromatography and by loss of soluble total protein in a Lowry assay. Aggregation was reduced in an argon atmosphere and by the inclusion of EDTA in the formulation, suggesting that oxygen and metal cations are involved in the degradation reactions. However, exposure to light and the inclusion of antioxidants in the formulation had little effect on the degradation rate. Given this evidence, the authors hypothesized that the mechanism of degradation involved oxidation, although the specific oxidative degradation products were not identified.

An unusual example of solid-state oxidation has been presented by Dubost et al., who studied oxidation in the lyophilized cyclic heptapeptide L-367,073, a potent fibrinogen receptor antagonist containing an aminomethylphenylalanine moiety (15). Degradation occurs by oxidative deamination of this derivatized amino acid, producing a benzaldehyde. Degradation increases at elevated temperature and in the presence of mannitol. The authors propose a mechanism in which reducing sugar impurities present in the mannitol act as oxidizing agents, forming Schiff base intermediates which then degrade. While the site of degradation in this study is a derivatized amino acid and not a naturally occurring one, the role of excipients in this oxidative degradation reaction is noteworthy.

Much of the literature on oxidation in peptides and proteins involves reactions in solution. For a summary of this literature, and for information on oxidation mechanisms and stabilization strategies, the reader is referred to the recent reviews by Li et al. (16) and by Schöneich et al. (17).

B. Deamidation

Deamidation occurs when a free carboxylic acid is formed through the hydrolysis of the side chain amide linkage in Asn or Gln residues (Scheme 2). In solution, the reaction occurs much more rapidly at Asn than at Gln, so that much of the literature involves deamidation at this site (17). In neutral solution, Asn deamidation involves the formation of a five-membered cyclic imide intermediate through the intramolecular attack of the succeeding peptide bond nitrogen on the Asn side-chain carbonyl carbon atom, liberating ammonia (Scheme 2). Hydrolysis of this intermediate generates a peptide or protein in which an aspartate (Asp) or iso-aspartate (isoAsp) amino acid replaces the original Asn. The site of water attack on the cyclic intermediate determines whether Asp or isoAsp will be formed. In acidic solution, deamidation occurs through the direct attack of water on the side chain carbonyl-carbon atom, generating the Asp product and ammonia (Scheme 2).

The available evidence suggests that a similar mechanism is involved in deamidation in the solid state. In studies of lyophilized human insulin, Strickley and Anderson used aniline trapping to demonstrate that deamidation proceeds through a cyclic imide intermediate (18). The authors also showed that further degradation involves attack either by water on the cyclic imide to generate the deamidated Asp_{A21} product, as in the solution state, or by an N-terminal

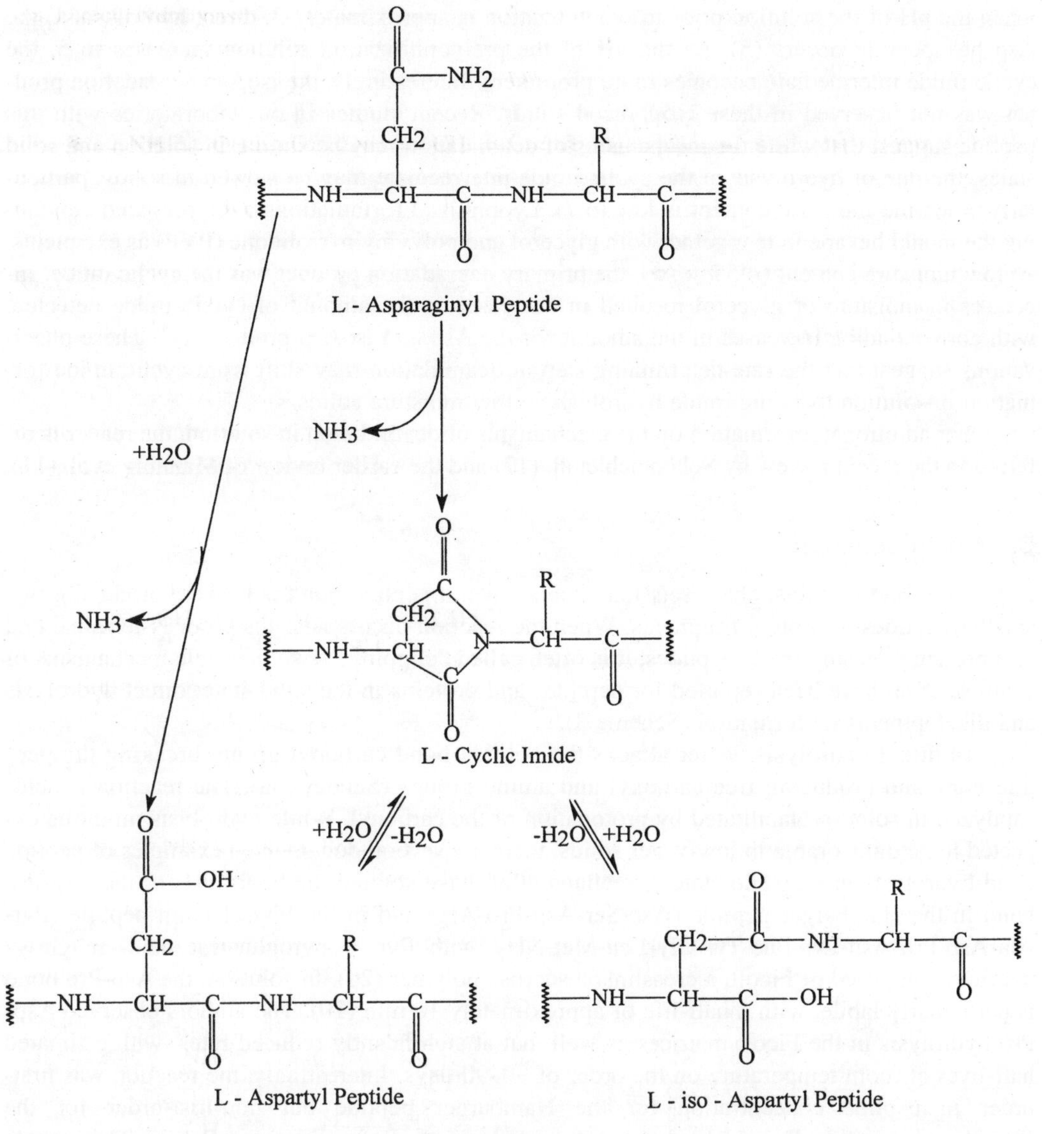

Scheme 2

[Scheme 2: Deamidation mechanism showing L-Asparaginyl Peptide converting via loss of NH₃ to L-Cyclic Imide, which hydrolyzes (+H₂O/−H₂O) to either L-Aspartyl Peptide or L-iso-Aspartyl Peptide; an alternative pathway shows direct hydrolysis of L-Asparaginyl Peptide with +H₂O and loss of NH₃ to give L-Aspartyl Peptide.]

primary amino group of a second insulin molecule to produce an insulin dimer. Studies of lyophiles prepared from solutions of pH 2–5 showed that the dependence of the reaction rate on this effective "pH" (i.e., the pH of the solution prior to lyophilization) paralleled that in solution. In similar studies, Pikal and Rigsbee also observed the Asp$_{A21}$ and dimerized degradation products, and further noted greater stability for insulin in the amorphous rather than the crystalline form (19). In earlier studies, Pikal et al. observed deamidation in lyophilized human growth hormone, but oxidized and deamidated products could not be resolved with the chromatographic methods used (13).

Studies with model peptides have provided additional evidence that the solution state deamidation mechanism shown in Scheme 2 applies in the solid state. In studies with a lyophilized model hexapeptide (Val-Tyr-Pro-Asn-Gly-Ala), Oliyai et al. demonstrated that when the pH of the solution prior to lyophilization is approximately 3, direct hydrolysis to the Asp hexapeptide occurs (5). As the pH of the prelyophilization solution increases to 5, the cyclic imide intermediate becomes more prominent. Interestingly, the isoAsp degradation product was not observed in these lyophilized solids. Recent studies in our laboratories with this peptide suggest that while the mechanisms of deamidation may be similar in solution and solid states, the rate of hydrolysis of the cyclic imide intermediate may be slowed in solids, particularly when the moisture content is low (6,7). Lyophilized formulations were prepared containing the model hexapeptide together with glycerol and polyvinylpyrrolidone (PVP) as excipients. At low moisture content (<5% w/w), the primary degradation product was the cyclic imide. Increases in moisture or glycerol resulted in decreases in the amount of cyclic imide detected, with corresponding increases in the amounts of the Asp and isoAsp products (7). These observations suggest that the rate-determining step in deamidation may shift from cyclic imide formation in solution to cyclic imide hydrolysis in low-moisture solids.

For additional information on the mechanisms of deamidation in solution, the reader is referred to the recent review by Schöneich et al. (17) and the earlier review of Manning et al. (11).

C. Chain Scission

In peptides and proteins, chain scission occurs when a peptide bond is broken, producing two smaller peptides or protein fragments. When the reaction occurs near the C- or N-terminal end of a protein releasing small peptides, it is often called "clipping." Two principle mechanisms of chain scission have been reported for peptides and proteins in the solid state: direct hydrolysis and diketopiperazine formation (Scheme 3).

In direct hydrolysis, water attacks the peptide bond carbonyl group, breaking the peptide bond and producing free carboxyl and amino groups (Scheme 3a). The reaction is acid-catalyzed in solution, facilitated by protonation of the carbonyl. While hydrolysis might be expected to be unfavorable in low-water solids, there are several documented examples of peptide bond hydrolysis in the solid state. Streefland et al. have studied the hydrolysis of the Asp-Pro bond in the Hamburger peptide (Asp-Ser-Asp-Pro-Arg) and in the Physalaemin peptide (Pyr-Ala-Asp-Pro-Asn-Lys-Phe-Tyr-Gly-Leu-Met-NH$_2$, with Pyr = pyroglutamic acid) in glassy matrices composed of Ficoll, a crosslinked sucrose polymer (20). In solution, the Asp-Pro bond is particularly labile, with a half-life of approximately 10 min (20). The authors observed Asp-Pro hydrolysis in the Ficoll matrices as well, but at significantly reduced rates, with estimated half-lives at room temperature on the order of 30–90 days. Interestingly, the reaction was first-order in peptide concentration for the Hamburger peptide but non-first-order for the Physalaemin peptide. Residual water content was low in both formulations (2–4%). The authors propose that carbohydrate polymer hydroxyl groups serve as proton donors in the reaction, effectively catalyzing hydrolysis in these low-water systems. However, this mechanism was not confirmed with studies of aprotic polymers.

A second example of peptide bond hydrolysis in the solid state is provided by the work of Li et al. on lyophilized formulations of human relaxin, a protein hormone consists of two polypeptide chains linked by disulfide bonds (21). The formulations contained various sugars (mannitol, glucose, or trehalose) as excipients. In solution, the primary degradation pathways involve oxidation of methionine residues and hydrolytic cleavage of the N-terminal Asp residue on the β chain. In contrast, in the lyophilized formulations the authors observed a significant amount of Trp-Ser cleavage at the C-terminal end of the β chain when glucose was used as the excipient. The authors proposed a mechanism involving initial reaction of the Ser hydroxyl with glucose producing a cyclic intermediate, followed by hydrolysis of the Trp-Ser bond. Thus, as in the studies by Streefland et al. (20), participation by an excipient in peptide bond hydrolysis in the solid state is proposed.

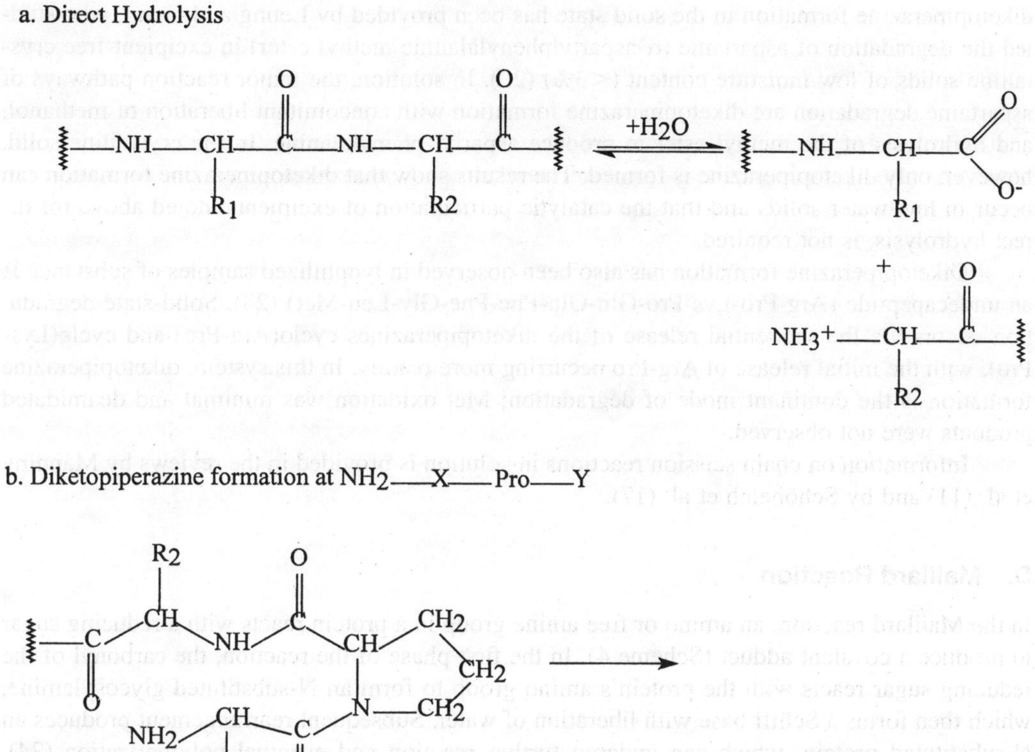

Solid-State Stability of Peptides and Proteins

a. Direct Hydrolysis

$$\sim NH-CH(R_1)-C(=O)-NH-CH(R_2)-C(=O)\sim \xrightleftharpoons{+H_2O} \sim NH-CH(R_1)-C(=O)O^- + NH_3^+-CH(R_2)-C(=O)\sim$$

b. Diketopiperazine formation at $NH_2-X-Pro-Y$

[Diketopiperazine formation reaction scheme showing cyclization of N-terminal X-Pro residues to form a diketopiperazine and a "Clipped" Protein]

Diketopiperazine   "Clipped" Protein

Scheme 3

A second important mechanism for peptide bond cleavage is diketopiperazine formation (Scheme 3b). The reaction occurs when a free N-terminal amino group attacks the carbonyl of the penultimate peptide bond. Cleavage of that bond results, producing a diketopiperazine from the two N-terminal amino acids, and a clipped peptide or protein that lacks these two residues. In solution, the reaction occurs readily for proteins with the N-terminal sequence H_2N-Gly-Pro, but it also may occur with other amino acids such as Val, Ile, and Ala. An example of diketopiperazine formation in the solid state has been provided by Leung and Grant, who studied the degradation of aspartame (α-aspartylphenylalanine methyl ester) in excipient-free crystalline solids of low moisture content (<3%) (22). In solution, the major reaction pathways of aspartame degradation are diketopiperazine formation with concomitant liberation of methanol, and hydrolysis of the methyl ester to produce aspartyl-phenylalanine. In the crystalline solid, however, only diketopiperazine is formed. The results show that diketopiperazine formation can occur in low-water solids and that the catalytic participation of excipients, noted above for direct hydrolysis, is not required.

Diketopiperazine formation has also been observed in lyophilized samples of substance P, an undecapeptide (Arg-Pro-Lys-Pro-Gln-Gln-Phe-Phe-Gly-Leu-Met) (23). Solid-state degradation occurs via the sequential release of the diketopiperazines cyclo(Arg-Pro) and cyclo(Lys-Pro), with the initial release of Arg-Pro occurring more readily. In this system, diketopiperazine formation is the dominant mode of degradation; Met oxidation was minimal and deamidated products were not observed.

Information on chain scission reactions in solution is provided in the reviews by Manning et al. (11) and by Schöneich et al. (17).

D. Maillard Reaction

In the Maillard reaction, an amino or free amine group in a protein reacts with a reducing sugar to produce a covalent adduct (Scheme 4). In the first phase of the reaction, the carbonyl of the reducing sugar reacts with the protein's amino group to form an N-substituted glycosylamine, which then forms a Schiff base with liberation of water. Subsequent rearrangement produces an N-substituted protein, which can undergo further reaction and eventual polymerization (24). The Maillard reaction is responsible for the nonenzymatic browning of foods (24) and is important in the solid state because the initial formation of the N-substituted glycosylamine occurs readily at low moisture content.

An example of the Maillard reaction in a pharmaceutical formulation has been provided by Li et al. in their studies of lyophilized formulations of human relaxin (21). In addition to the Trp-Ser chain scission reaction discussed above, the authors observed the formation of covalent adducts at Lys and Arg residues in formulations containing glucose. Tryptic digestion and liquid chromatography/mass spectrometry (LC/MS) confirmed that these adducts were Maillard reaction products. No degradation of relaxin was observed in studies using mannitol (a polyhydric alcohol) or trehalose (a nonreducing sugar) as excipients, a result that is consistent with the involvement of reducing sugars in the Maillard reaction (21).

Additional information on the Maillard reaction is provided in the review by Hageman (24).

E. Thiol–Disulfide Exchange

Biologically active proteins often contain disulfide bonds, which serve as crosslinks between or within polypeptide chains and are formed when the thiol groups of two Cys residues are oxidized. Disruption of these bonds can result in a loss of activity. One of the more common routes of disulfide bond disruption is thiol–disulfide exchange, which occurs when a free thiolate ion attacks the disulfide, producing a new disulfide bond and liberating the thiol group of a formerly bonded Cys residue (Scheme 5) (25). In solution, the rate of reaction is pH-dependent and is enhanced by the presence of nearby positive charges (25). In the solid state, thiol–disulfide exchange has been implicated in protein aggregation, which can result when the reaction occurs intermolecularly.

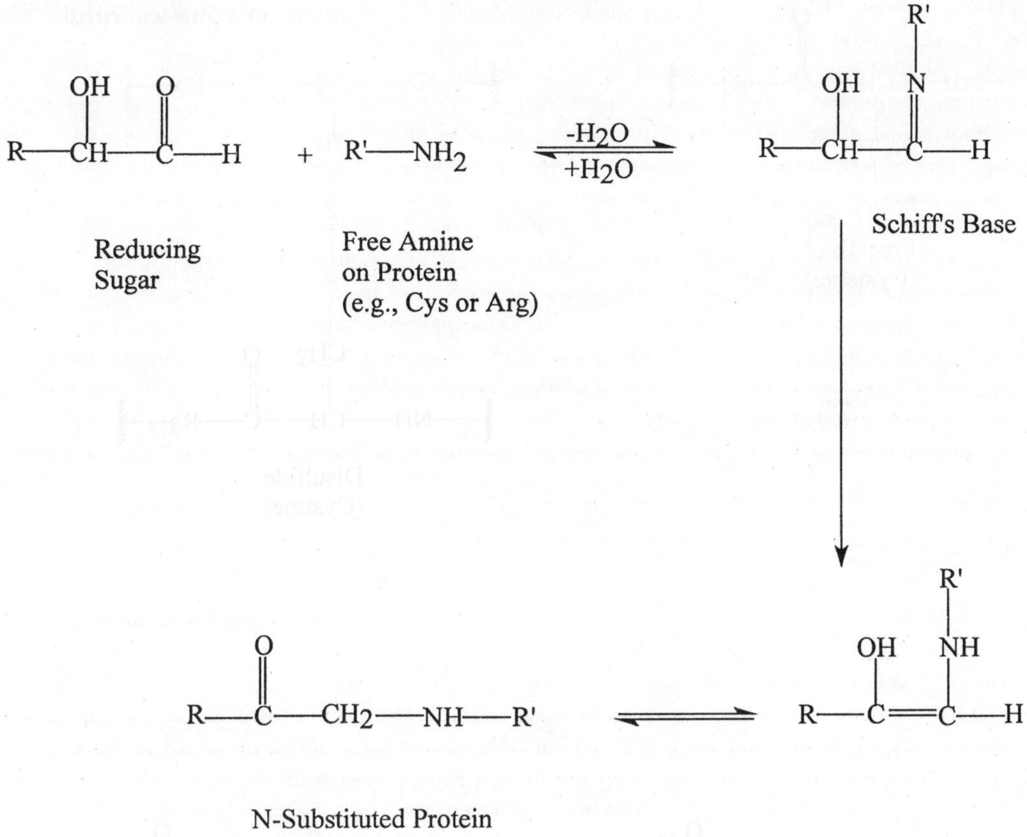
OH
O
R—CH—C—H
+
R'—NH2
-H2O
+H2O
OH
N
R'
R—CH—C—H
Reducing Sugar
Free Amine on Protein (e.g., Cys or Arg)
Schiff's Base
O
R—C—CH2—NH—R'
OH
NH
R'
R—C═C—H
N-Substituted Protein

Scheme 4

Thiol–disulfide exchange has been reported by Liu et al. for lyophilized formulations of bovine serum albumin, a 66-kDa protein with 17 disulfide bonds and one free thiol at a Cys residue (26). When the lyophilized protein was incubated in the presence of moisture, insoluble aggregates were formed. The aggregates were not affected by exposure to strong denaturants such as urea and guanidine hydrochloride but were solubilized by exposure to dithiothreitol, a preferred reducing agent for protein disulfides. Alkylation of the free thiol group with iodoacetamide prior to lyophilization completely prevented aggregate formation. The authors concluded that the presence of free thiols is both necessary and sufficient for aggregate formation, and proposed a mechanism involving intermolecular thiol–disulfide exchange (26). Formation of insoluble aggregates by thiol–disulfide exchange was also demonstrated for ovalbumin, glucose oxidase, and β-lactoglobulin (26).

In related work, this group investigated the aggregation of lyophilized insulin on exposure to moisture at elevated temperature (27). At 50°C and 95% relative humidity, insulin solubility decreased to approximately 25% of the initial value in 40 days. Partial solubilization of the aggregates was observed on exposure to guanidine hydrochloride and urea, and on exposure to dithiothreitol, indicating that both intermolecular disulfide bonds and non-covalent interactions are involved. Interestingly, the addition of cupric chloride to the formulation prior to lyophilization practically eliminated the formation of insoluble aggregates. The authors hypothesize that the stabilization is caused by the catalytic oxidation of free thiols by

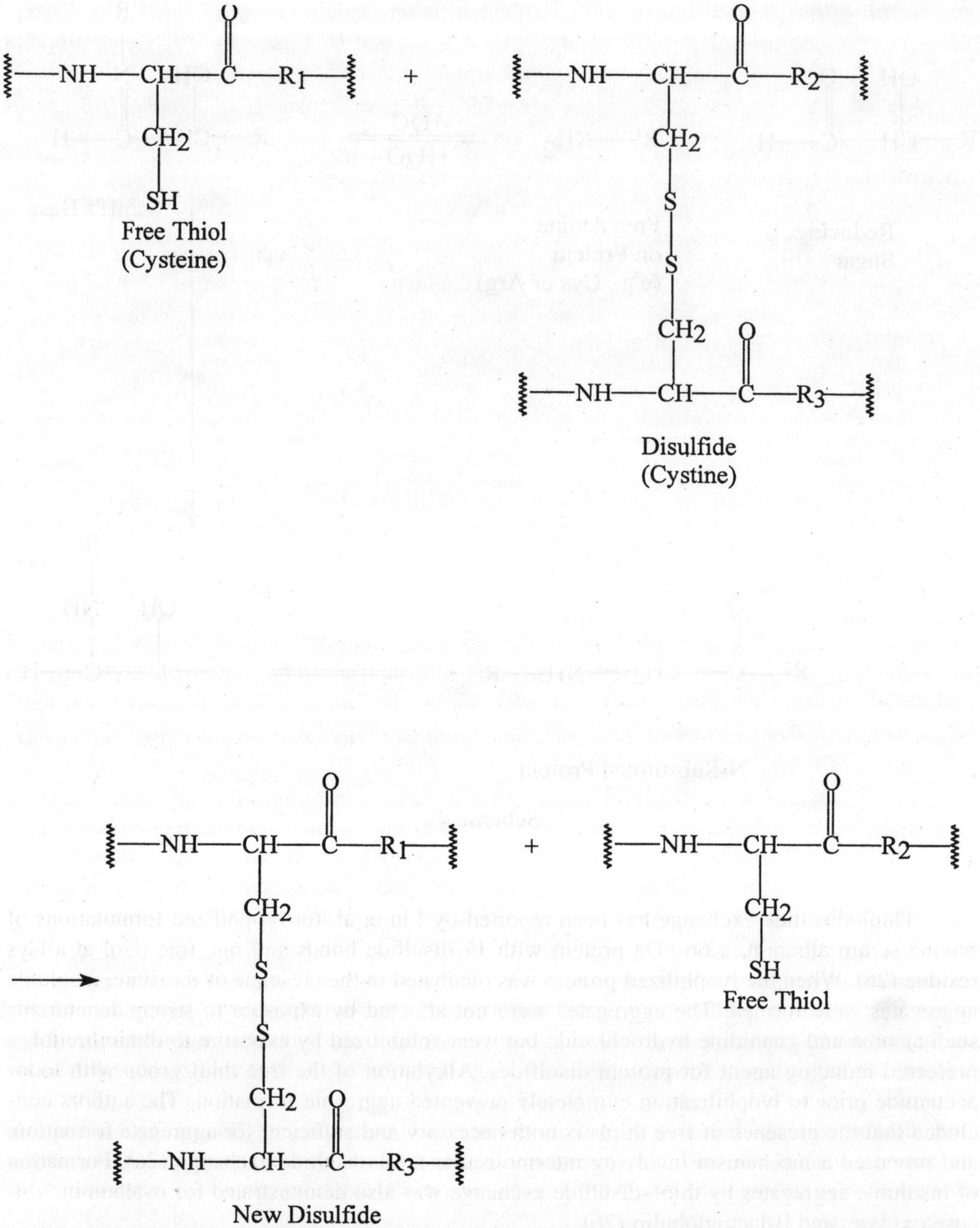

[Scheme 5: Thiol-disulfide exchange reaction showing free thiol (cysteine) reacting with a disulfide (cystine) to form a new disulfide and a new free thiol.]

Scheme 5

Cu^{2+}, preventing their involvement in thiol–disulfide exchange reactions. Although thiol oxidation can occur in the presence of other transition metal cations, Fe^{2+}, Fe^{3+}, Mn^{2+}, Ni^{2+}, and Co^{2+} were significantly less effective than Cu^{2+} in these studies.

For additional information on thiol–disulfide exchange reactions, the reader is referred to the review articles by Kosen (25) and Costantino (1).

F. Summary and Implications for Controlled Release

Several types of degradation reactions have been reported for peptides and proteins in the solid state. These include oxidation, deamidation, chain scission, the Maillard reaction, and thiol–disulfide exchange. Each has been observed in solid systems with relatively low moisture content and limited mobility. The successful development of a controlled release formulation of a particular protein may require information on the degradation reactions to which the protein is susceptible, so that the formulation can be stabilized effectively. For example, a protein that is prone to Met oxidation may require packaging under nitrogen, whereas susceptibility to aggregation caused by thiol–disulfide exchange may require reduced protein loading or inclusion of protecting excipients. Identifying and distinguishing the sites of degradation in a protein calls for adequate analytical methods; in some cases, several methods of analysis must be employed. These methods may include chromatographic and electrophoretic methods, circular dichroism, and tryptic digestion. For a comprehensive review of analytical methods for peptides and proteins, the reader is referred to the recent review by Hühmer et al. (28) or to an earlier version by Schöneich et al. (29).

IV. PHYSICOCHEMICAL FACTORS AFFECTING PROTEIN STABILITY IN THE SOLID STATE

The degradation reactions discussed in Section III can be influenced by the physical and chemical properties of the medium surrounding the protein. Properties that have been shown to affect protein degradation in the solid state are reviewed in this section. These include temperature (Section IV.A.), pressure (Section IV.B.), mobility in the matrix (Section IV.C.), water content (Section IV.D.), excipients (Section IV.E.), and effective pH (Section IV.F.).

A. Temperature

As discussed in Section II.B, the effect of temperature on the degradation of small organic molecules in solution often is described by the Arrhenius or Eyring rate laws, which although different in underlying theory often apply equally well to experimental data. While simple Arrhenius/Eyring behavior often is observed in the solid state as well, deviations from this behavior can occur due to secondary thermal effects that can accompany direct effects on chemical reactivity. Examples of these secondary effects include increased protein denaturation (unfolding) and increased mobility in the solid matrix (reduction in effective viscosity) with increased temperature. Because temperature changes can be experienced during the manufacture, storage, and administration of controlled release devices, thermal effects on protein stability are of considerable practical importance. For example, elevated temperatures can be encountered in processes such as spray drying, whereas temperatures below the freezing point of water are used in lyophilization. Either extreme may influence protein stability adversely.

Examples of Arrhenius/Eyring behavior in the solid state include isomerization at the Asp residue in the lyophilized hexapeptide Val-Tyr-Pro-Asp-Gly-Ala (30), chain scission at Asp-Pro bonds in Physalaemin and Hamburger peptides in Ficoll matrices (20), aminolysis in aspartame powders (22), and Asn deamidation in the hexapeptide Val-Tyr-Pro-Asn-Gly-Ala in PVP (31). In their studies of aspartame aminolysis, Leung and Grant contrasted the solid state activation energy of 265 ±6 kJ/mol with the solution state value of 70 kJ/mol and remarked that the significantly greater value in the solid state is evidence for a true solid-state reaction of the form (solid → solid + gas) (22). In our studies of Asn deamidation in PVP, Arrhenius behavior was observed in both glassy and rubbery polymer matrices, but the apparent activation energy in the glassy state (33 ± 4 kcal/mol) was significantly greater than in the rubbery state (24 ± 2 kcal/mol), perhaps reflecting restricted mobility in the more rigid glassy system (31).

An example of protein deactivation on freezing has been provided by Carpenter and Crowe, who studied cryoprotection of the enzyme lactate dehydrogenase by 28 different solutes (32). In the absence of added solute, 80% of the activity of the enzyme was lost during freeze–thawing. Solutes that were excluded from contact with the protein surface in solution, such as sucrose and poly(ethylene glycol), protected the enzyme from degradation during the freeze–thaw cycle, while increased degradation was observed for solutes that bound to the protein in solution. Based on these results, the authors concluded that the preferential exclusion hypothesis proposed by Timasheff for proteins in solution (33) applies to the frozen state as well (32).

For more general information on temperature effects on protein pharmaceuticals, the reader is referred to the review by Volkin and Middaugh (34).

B. Pressure

Tablets are prepared by compacting a drug-containing powder in a tablet press. High pressures during tabletting have been shown to cause a loss of activity in some enzymes and other biologically active proteins, a fact that has implications for the use of similar processing methods to prepare controlled release devices. A recent example of compaction-induced degradation of a protein has been provided by Wuster and Ternik, who studied activity losses in the enzyme catalase at applied pressures from 0 to 669 MPa (35). They observed a linear decrease in activity of the reconstituted enzyme as the compaction pressure increased from zero to 251 MPa, followed by a plateau region from 251 to 669 MPa in which additional increases in pressure caused no further losses in activity. The maximum loss in activity in the plateau region was approximately 30%. Though the mechanism of degradation was not determined, the authors suggested that the formation of local regions of increased pressure and/or temperature during compaction may be important. Additional examples of pressure-induced degradation are provided in the review by Groves and Teng, which describes compaction-induced activity losses for several proteins including urease, lipase, α-amylase, and β-glucuronidase (36).

C. Mobility in the Matrix

Molecular motion is required for most chemical reactions. For example, bimolecular reactions such as protein aggregation require the translational motion of the reactants toward each other (i.e., diffusion), whereas cyclic imide formation at an Asn residue, a unimolecular reaction, requires the flexional movement of the side chain carbonyl relative to the main chain (Scheme 2). Both translational and flexional motion can be hindered in the solid state, often with an attendant decrease in reaction rates. This fact has been employed in the development of solid formulations of peptides and proteins, which can serve to stabilize these labile molecules. In many solid systems, however, translational and/or flexional mobility is sufficient to allow undesirable degradation reactions to occur.

Several empirical methods have been used to measure molecular mobility in solids. In amorphous solids, the glass transition temperature (T_g) has been used as a semiquantitative indicator. At temperatures below T_g, the solid is said to be in the "glassy" state, and is rigid and brittle, with limited molecular mobility. Above T_g, the solid is in the "rubbery" state, with greater macroscopic flexibility and molecular mobility. Following the work of Williams et al. (37), many investigators have used the difference between the experimental temperature (T) and T_g as a measure of mobility. Thus, increasing values of the parameter $(T - T_g)$ indicate increasing mobility, with $(T - T_g) < 0$ corresponding to glassy solids and $(T - T_g) > 0$ corresponding to the rubbery state. Examples of studies in which $(T - T_g)$ has been related to solid-state protein degradation rates include the work of Bell and Hageman on diketopiperazine formation in aspartame (38), that of Streefland et al. on Asp-Pro bond cleavage in Ficoll (20), and our recent studies of Asn deamidation in polymer matrices (6,7). A correlation of reaction rate with $(T - T_g)$ and/or a significant increase in rate near T_g has been considered to be suggestive of a mobility-dependent reaction and has been observed in some cases (6,7), but not others (20,38). In addition, while it has been proposed that the production of a stable solid formulation of a protein requires only an amorphous excipient and a storage temperature below the formulation T_g (39), recent studies have contradicted this claim. For example, significant degradation in glassy formulations $(T < T_g)$ has been reported for a lyophilized formulation of the enzyme *Humicola lanuginosa* lipase (40), for Asn deamidation in a model hexapeptide in the presence of polymeric excipients (6), and for lyophilized formulations of IL-1 receptor antagonist (41).

The effect of polymer matrix mobility on the thermally induced unfolding of proteins has also been investigated (42). In these studies, the combined effects of moisture and matrix composition on the thermal stability of two lyophilized proteins, recombinant bovine somatotropin (rbSt) and lysozyme, were investigated in excipient systems containing sucrose, trehalose, sorbitol, glycerol, or PVP. Previous investigations of the impact of moisture alone on solid samples of rbSt (43) and other proteins (44) indicated that the temperature for denaturation (T_m) observed during differential scanning calorimetry was representative of a kinetically controlled unfolding transition of the protein. T_m values for unfolding of the pure protein decrease with the addition of most excipients or polymers at low moisture contents, indicating destabilization, whereas they increase with the same excipients or polymers at higher moisture contents, indicating stabilization. The stability toward unfolding in dehydrated or low-moisture systems correlated with the T_g of the excipient—an effect that the authors propose is due to the impact on the overall T_g of the matrix. This work suggests that the mode of conformational stabilization may depend on the moisture content and composition of the matrix.

Since T_g measures a bulk property of the system, the parameter $(T - T_g)$ provides no information on the mobility of individual species in a formulation and cannot discriminate between their translational and flexional movement. For this reason, several groups have employed nuclear magnetic resonance spectroscopy (NMR) to provide more detailed information on mobility at the molecular level and on its relationship to protein stability. Yoshioka et al. have related the spin-lattice relaxation times (T_1) for residual water to the inactivation of lyophilized formulations of β-galactosidase using ^{17}O NMR (45). More recently, this group has defined the critical mobility temperature (T_{mc}), a parameter based on the onset of liquid-like Lorentzian spin–spin relaxation (T_2) as measured by NMR, and has shown that the degradation of lyophilized γ-globulin is better correlated with T_{mc} than with T_g (46). Based on their studies on lyophilized DNase, insulin, and lysozyme, Separovic et al. have proposed that reduction in T_1 is related to the aggregation susceptibility of proteins during storage (47). These studies provide an alternative to T_g as a measure of mobility and in some cases begin to relate stability to the motion of specific components.

Information on the importance of mobility in solid protein formulations is provided in the review by Hageman (24). More general information on the amorphous state and the glass transition temperature is provided in the recent review by Craig et al. (48).

D. Water Content

Water may be present in solid-state formulations of peptides and proteins due to incomplete removal during processing (e.g., lyophilization), absorption of ambient moisture during storage, or exposure to bodily fluids following administration. In general, this residual or sorbed moisture can have a deleterious effect on protein stability. Examples of moisture-induced protein degradation in the solid state include aggregation and deamidation of lyophilized insulin (18,19,27); thiol–disulfide exchange and aggregation in bovine serum albumin (BSA), ovalbumin, glucose oxidase, and β-lactoglobulin (26); deamidation at Asn residues in model peptides (6,7); diketopiperazine formation in aspartame (38); and isomerization to isoAsp at Asp residues (30).

While the importance of water in solid-state protein stability has been established, the mechanism of its effect in a particular system is often unclear, in part because residual moisture can affect stability in more than one way. In degradation reactions in amorphous solids, residual water may (a) participate directly as a reactant or product, (b) serve as a solvent or medium in which the reaction occurs, or (c) act as a plasticizer, reducing the T_g and enhancing mobility in the solid matrix (49). In some cases, one of these mechanistic effects appears to be dominant. For example, the stabilization of lactate dehydrogenase by trehalose/borate mixtures has been attributed to the preferential sorption of residual water by borate preventing plasticization of the glassy matrix (50), suggesting that the primary role of water in this system is as a plasticizer. Similarly, our recent studies of cyclic imide ring opening in PVP matrices suggest that water serves primarily as a reactant in this system—a finding that is not surprising given that the reaction is hydrolytic (51).

More often, however, the data suggest that water has more than one mechanistic role in the solid-state degradation of a particular protein. For example, in their studies of the aggregation of lyophilized BSA, Liu et al. found a bell-shaped relationship between formulation water content and the degree of aggregation, with maximal aggregation at an intermediate value (26). They attributed the ascending portion of the curve to a water-induced enhancement in conformational mobility (i.e., plasticization), whereas the descending portion was attributed to dilution of the reactants (a solvent/medium effect). In contrast, in studies of insulin aggregation, Costantino et al. observed slow aggregation at low moisture content, which increased dramatically after a critical threshold value (6–23% w/w) (27). No decrease in aggregation rate was observed at high water content. The authors propose that water participates in this reaction both as a plasticizer and as a donor of hydroxide ions, which catalyze the thiol–disulfide exchange reaction (1,27). Finally, in our studies of Asn deamidation in PVP and poly(vinyl alcohol) (PVA) matrices, the reaction rate could not be correlated with either T_g or water activity alone but was well correlated with a dimensionless parameter that included both activity and T_g information, suggesting that water serves as both a plasticizer and a reactant or solvent in these systems (6).

Additional information on the role of water on protein stability in the solid state is provided in the reviews by Hageman (24) and by Groves and Teng (36). For a more general review of the role of water in solid-state drug stability, the reader is referred to the review by Shalaev and Zografi (49).

E. Excipients

Excipients are included in solid-state formulations of peptides and proteins to enhance stability during processing and storage, or to provide a matrix for controlled release. Compounds that are used as excipients include buffer salts, polymers, and sugars and other polyalcohols. Since polymeric excipients are important in controlled release, their effects on the stability of incorporated peptides and proteins are considered in detail in Section V. Similarly, buffer salts usually are added to control the effective pH in the solid, a topic that is discussed in Section IV.F. In this section, we provide a general introduction to excipient effects on solid-state stability.

The possible effects of excipients on solid state protein degradation reactions are similar to those of water (Section III.D.). An excipient may (a) act as a reactant or catalyst, (b) alter the physicochemical properties of the reaction medium, (c) alter mobility in the matrix by changing the glass transition temperature (T_g), or (d) interact with a protein to affect its structure. For example, Townsend et al. observed improved stability of lyophilized ribonuclease A when EDTA was included in the formulation and attributed this to the chelation of trace metal cations that catalyzed protein oxidation (14). In these studies, the excipient EDTA altered the physicochemical properties of the solid-state reaction medium (b above). Miller et al. observed that the stability of lactate dehydrogenase improved when trehalose/borate mixtures were used as excipients, rather than trehalose alone, and attributed this to the high T_g values of trehalose/borate (50), an effect related to the excipient's ability to alter mobility in the solid matrix (c). The stability of lyophilized *Humicola lanuginosa* lipase was enhanced by excipients such as trehalose and sucrose that had the capacity to hydrogen-bond to native protein, allowing retention of near-native conformation in the solid state (40)—an example of an excipient effect on protein structure (d).

As is the case with residual moisture, an excipient may have effects in more than one of the areas listed above, often with unintended results. For example, sugars that are added to lyophilized formulations as lyoprotectants may react with the protein during storage via the Maillard reaction, as observed by Li et al. for relaxin formulations containing glucose (21). Thus, an excipient added with the intent of altering the medium or its mobility (b or c) may inadvertently serve as a reactant (a). Similarly, protein degradation in controlled release devices fabricated with poly(lactide-co-glycolide) polymers has been attributed to an acidic microenvironment, formed during drug release by the biodegradation of the polymer (52–54). Here an excipient intended to alter mobility in the matrix (c) adversely affects the physiochemical properties of the reaction medium (b).

The use of excipients in solid-state formulations is further complicated by the fact that excipient crystallization or phase separation can occur and can reduce protein stability. In studies with β-galactosidase, Izutsu et al. observed crystallization of the cryoprotectants mannitol and inositol during freeze drying (55). While the amorphous forms of these excipients stabilized the protein against denaturation, aggregation, and loss of enzymatic activity, crystallization decreased their effectiveness (55). In later studies, this group observed that additives such as dextran and Ficoll, which prevented inositol crystallization, improved the retention of the enzyme's stability during freeze drying (94). Sarciaux and Hageman observed that formulations of bovine somatotropin were more resistant to sucrose crystallization at high protein concentrations, suggesting that the active protein itself can also serve to prevent excipient crystallization (57). Recently, Tzannis and Prestrelski studied the stabilization of trypsinogen by sucrose during spray drying and observed phase separation at high carbohydrate concentrations (58). The authors hypothesize that the formation of "sucrose-rich" and "protein-rich" phases reduced excipient/protein hydrogen bonding, promoting both protein degradation and sucrose crystallization.

F. Effective "pH"

Many of the degradation reactions discussed in Section III have been shown to be sensitive to pH in the solution state. For example, the rate of deamidation of a model peptide increases by four orders of magnitude as the pH increases from 4 to 10 (3), whereas oxidation of His is rapid at neutral solutions but quite slow at low pH (11). It is reasonable to expect that protein degradation reactions occurring in solid systems might display a similar sensitivity to hydrogen ion activity. Investigations of these effects are complicated by the fact that hydrogen ion activity is not easily measured in solids; in fact, pH technically is defined only in aqueous solution. However, several studies have demonstrated a correlation between the chemical stability of proteins and peptides in the solid state and the pH of the solution from which the solids were prepared, usually by lyophilization. These solids often are said to have an "apparent pH" equal to that of the initial solution. The apparent pH is sometimes designated by the symbol "pH," where the quotation marks are used to distinguish the apparent pH from true values measured in aqueous solution.

As noted above, there are several examples of "pH"-dependent degradation of proteins and peptides in the solid state. Oliyai et al. observed that the deamidation rate of an Asn-hexapeptide (Val-Tyr-Pro-Asn-Gly-Ala) increases as the "pH" increases from 5 to 8 (5). These studies also demonstrated that the effects of moisture level and temperature on deamidation rate are influenced by the "pH" value. The degradation of lyophilized human insulin is also quite sensitive to "pH" (18,19), with a 10-fold decrease in overall rate as the "pH" increases from 3 to 5 (18). For these studies of lyophilized insulin, total degradation included both deamidation and dimerization reactions (18). Increases in the oxidation of human growth hormone (13), and the formation of dimers of tumor necrosis factor (59) and in bovine somatotropin (24) in the solid state all increase with formulation "pH." In the case of bovine somatotropin, the increase in the rate of covalent dimerization of rbSt with increasing "pH" is attributed to the deprotonation of the lysine residues, which are more nucleophilic when deprotonated (24).

As with other excipients, buffer salts added to a solid formulation with the intent of controlling "pH" may have other, unintended effects. For example, buffer salts may have a catalytic effect on many protein degradation reactions, apart from their effect on pH. In a study on lyophilized RNase, Townsend and DeLuca showed that a buffer-free formulation had a 10% loss in activity over 120 days of storage at 45°C, whereas a formulation lyophilized from a 0.2 M buffer solution showed a nearly 40% loss during the same period (60). Similarly, Pikal et al. showed that sodium phosphate buffer concentration affected the chemical degradation and aggregation of lyophilized human growth hormone (13). The authors suggested that catalysis of oxidation by heavy metal contaminants in the buffer salts, or the preferential crystallization of phosphate buffer components during freeze drying with attendant "pH" shifts, may have been responsible (13). The latter hypothesis is a specific example of excipient crystallization in the solid state, here with undesired effects on "pH." In our recent studies of Asn-hexapeptide deamidation in PVP matrices, we have observed the formation of a formaldehyde adduct on the tyrosine residue of the Asp and isoAsp degradation products (61). Further investigation revealed that the formaldehyde was generated by the degradation of the Tris buffer [Tris(hydroxymethyl)aminomethane] at elevated temperatures used for the stability studies. In this case, degradation of a buffer component produced undesirable products, which further reacted with the incorporated peptide.

G. Summary and Implications for Controlled Release

The stability of solid formulations of peptides and proteins is affected by environmental factors such as temperature, pressure, moisture content, mobility in the solid matrix, excipients, and "pH." While the effects of these factors are often complex and few iron-clad rules can be applied in every situation, some general rules of thumb may be useful for the developer of controlled release systems. Stability generally decreases on exposure to elevated temperature, pressure, or moisture content (or relative humidity), although parabolic relationships between reactivity and moisture content have been observed (24). Glassy matrices often offer improved stability over rubbery matrices of similar composition. For controlled release, this suggests the selection of polymer/plasticizer systems with glass transition temperatures well above the storage and/or release temperatures, although this must be balanced against the desired release rate in diffusion-controlled devices. Based on the limited data available, the relationship between "pH" and degradation rate in the solid state often parallels the pH vs. rate relationship in solution, but shifted downward to slower rates. This suggests that, in the absence of solid-state data, buffer excipients should be chosen to achieve a "pH" near the pH of maximum stability observed in solution. Finally, the possibility of unintended chemical or physical effects of excipients should be borne in mind.

V. DEGRADATION REACTIONS IN SPECIFIC POLYMERS

This section reviews current information on the effects of polymers on the stability of incorporated peptides and proteins. Three specific categories of polymers are discussed: (a) the lactide/glycolide polymers (Section V.A), (b) dextrans and other polysaccharides (Section V.B), and (c) vinyl polymers (Section V.C). A final category summarizes the limited information on "other" polymers (Section V.D).

A. Lactide/Glycolide Polymers

Much of the recent literature on the chemical effects of polymers on peptide and protein stability involves the lactide/glycolide copolymers. These are of particular interest because they have been shown to be biocompatible and biodegradable, and are therefore desirable for use in implants and injectable microspheres. Degradation of these polymers occurs via chain scission to form lactic and/or glycolic acid, which may alter the local "microenvironmental" pH within the microspheres, with possible adverse affects on peptide and protein stability.

Several groups have reported increased rates of peptide and protein degradation in lactide/glycolide polymers (Scheme 6). For example, Johnson et al. studied the stability of atriopeptin III, a 24-amino-acid peptide, in poly(D,L-lactide-co-glycolide) (PLGA) microspheres at 40°C (52). When the peptide was dissolved in Tris buffer, no degradation was observed during 2 weeks of storage. However, PLGA microspheres stored at 95% relative humidity showed 20% degradation in 8 days, and microspheres stored in Tris buffer had no intact peptide remaining after 5 days (52). The investigators also noted the formation of different degradation products in microspheres than in solution, as evidenced by new peaks appearing on HPLC chromotograms (52), but the chemical composition of these products was not determined. They concluded that PLGA catalyzes the degradation of atriopeptin III and that the mechanism of degradation differs from that in solution (52).

Park et al. studied the degradation of carbonic anydrase (MW = 31 kDa) and BSA (MW = 66 kDa) in PLGA microspheres during protein release (53). During the release studies, the

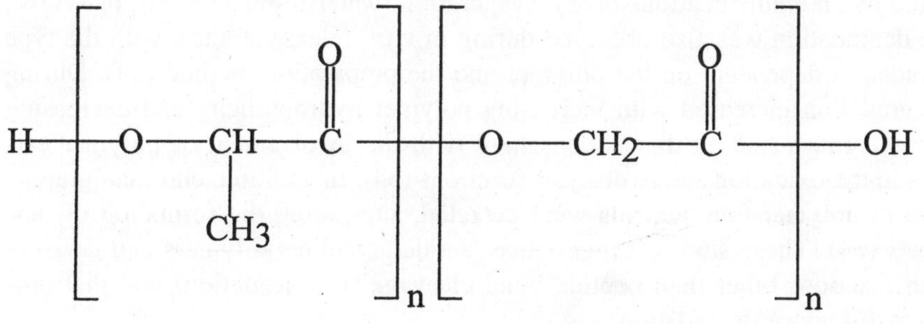

Scheme 6

microspheres were stored either (a) in a dialysis bag, which allowed for buffer exchange with the surrounding medium and maintained a constant pH of 7.4, or (b) in a closed tube, in which the pH decreased from 7.4 to 3 during the 1-month study due to the formation of lactic and glycolic acids by the degrading polymer. The authors observed that in the closed tube both proteins degraded to form products with reduced molecular weight. They postulated a polymer catalyzed degradation mechanism, in which "the protonated carboxylic acid end group of the polymer degradation products reacts with carbonyl group in the amide linkage, with subsequent cleavage of the peptide bond" (53). In related work (54), this group observed slow release of carbonic anhydrase from PLGA microspheres, which was attributed to protein aggregation and nonspecific adsorption within the microspheres. Aggregation was confirmed by SDS-PAGE; a loss of biological activity was also observed. The inclusion of excipients such as poly(ethylene oxide), gelatin, or pluronic led to more rapid and more complete protein release, suggesting that these afford some protection from degradation (54). The authors concluded that the low-pH microenvironment in PLGA may cause both peptide bond cleavage and aggregation of carbonic anhydrase, and that slow protein release was due to adsorption to PLGA (54).

Adsorption to PLGA has also been suspected for salmon calcitonin (SCT) (62) and for BSA (63). With SCT, in vitro binding studies suggested that 90% of the peptide was bound to PLGA in about 50 h and that the kinetics of adsorption varied with peptide concentration. Adsorption was assumed to occur through the interaction of the hydrophobic region of the peptide with the polymer and may have contributed to slow SCT release from PLGA microspheres (62). No degradation of SCT was observed in this system. In contrast, adsorption of BSA to PLGA may have contributed to its degradation (63). Crotts et al. observed the release of BSA from PLGA microparticles and found that approximately 35% of the released protein was aggregated after a day of incubation, with nearly 50% aggregated after 28 days of incubation. Studies using identical formulations of carboxymethylated BSA (CM-BSA), a modified BSA in which the free thiol groups are blocked, showed no significant aggregation. These results suggest that free sulfhydryl groups on the protein are necessary for aggregation, which was thought to occur by thiol–disulfide exchange reactions. Interestingly, the kinetics of aggregation appeared to differ in the microparticles and in polymer-free solutions. This difference was tentatively attributed to the presence of trace metal catalysts in the polymer.

Witschi and Doelker observed both oxidation and peptide bond cleavage when the peptide tetracosactide (24 amino acids, MW = 2933) was incorporated in poly(L-lactic acid) (PLA) or PLGA microparticles (64). The peptide is susceptible to oxidation at a methionine residue (Met4) and to peptide bond cleavage at several sites. The authors found severe peptide oxidation when the microparticles were prepared by spray drying using high molecular weight polymers such that no intact peptide was present in the finished microparticles. Microparticle preparation by a solvent extraction method also resulted in oxidation, but very low molecular weight PLGA seemed to afford some protection. Intact tetracosactide was recovered only from microparticles prepared by an emulsification/solvent evaporation (water-in-oil-in water, or WOW) technique. Peptide degradation was also observed during in vitro release studies, with the type and extent of degradation dependent on the polymer and the preparation method (64). During release, peptide degradation increased with increasing polymer hydrophilicity and decreasing polymer molecular weight, a finding that is consistent with the involvement of polymer carboxylic acid groups in the oxidation and hydrolysis reactions (64). In addition, chromatographic peaks not observed in polymer-free controls were detected, suggesting the formation of new degradation products (64). These studies suggest that lactide/glycolide polymers can catalyze protein degradation reactions other than peptide bond cleavage (i.e., oxidation) and that processing methods may influence degradation.

In contrast to these reports of protein degradation in PLGA, several recent studies suggest that it is possible to prepare stable protein formulations in lactide/glycolide polymers.

Cleland et al. used a double-emulsion process to prepare PLGA microspheres containing recombinant human growth hormone (rhGH) (65). During drug release into isotonic buffer (pH 7.4, 37°C), the rates of oxidation, diketopiperazine formation, and deamidation were equivalent to those in a solution control. The rates of rhGH aggregation were slightly higher in the PLGA microspheres than in solution; this finding was attributed to the higher rhGH concentrations in the microsphere interior. The authors inferred that the microenvironmental pH within the microspheres must be similar to that in solution in these studies, which they felt were representative of release conditions *in vivo* (65). In related studies, rhGH was stabilized in a PLGA microsphere formulation by forming an insoluble rhGH–zinc complex (66). *In vitro* release studies showed that rhGH activity was not affected by microsphere encapsulation with the zinc-containing formulation (66).

In summary, the use of lactide/glycolide polymers has been associated with peptide bond hydrolysis (53), thiol–disulfide interchange (63), methionine oxidation(64), and aggregation (54,62,63) of incorporated peptides and proteins. Some groups have attributed the degradation reactions to a changing microenvironmental pH caused by polymer (53,54,63), while others have found no evidence for such a pH change (65,66). Adsorption to lactide/glycolide polymers may contribute to degradation reactions for some proteins (63) but may serve only to prolong release for others (62). While instabilities have been reported, stable protein formulations have also been prepared using these polymers (65,66). Since the studies to date have used different proteins, processing techniques, and in vitro release methods, it is difficult to assess the specific role of the lactide/glycolide polymers with any accuracy. However, the variations in protein stability in PLGA systems suggest that factors other than polymer choice may affect drug stability. These may include the properties of the protein drug itself, other formulation variables, processing techniques, and the composition of the receptor fluid in release studies.

B. Dextrans and Other Polysaccharides

Polysaccharides such as methylcellulose, ethylcellulose, and dextran (Scheme 7) have been used as binders, suspending agents, and coating materials in pharmaceutical formulations. They are used less frequently in controlled release applications than the lactide/glycolide polymers, and considerably less information is available on their effects on peptide and protein stability. Recent results are summarized below.

Yoshioka et al. studied the effect of dextran molecular weight on the stability of bovine serum γ-globulin (BGG) in freeze-dried formulations (67) for a 50-fold range of dextran molecular weights (10 k, 40 k, 70 k, and 510 k). Aggregation of the incorporated BGG was used as a measure of protein instability, assessed by size exclusion chromatography (SEC) following storage of the formulations at 60°C (67). The authors observed a greater degree of protein

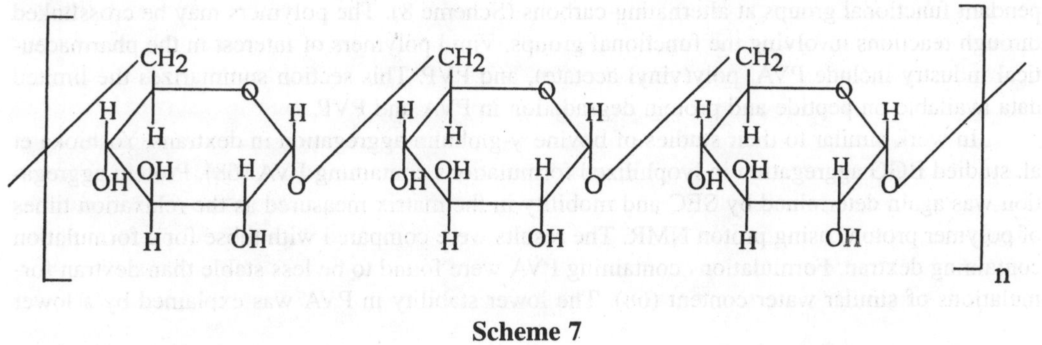

Scheme 7

aggregation in formulations containing low molecular weight dextrans. For example, the peak height ratio (i.e., the ratio of the aggregated SEC BGG peak height to that of the undenatured control) was nearly 0.4 for the 10-kDa dextran, but was greater than 0.8 for the 510-kDa dextran after 20 h of storage (67). This suggests that protein aggregates were twice as prevalent in the formulation with the lower molecular weight polymer. Within a formulation, higher water content further accelerated aggregation. To explain these results, the authors correlated protein stability with molecular mobility in the matrix (67), as indicated by the "molecular mobility changing temperature," T_{mc}, measured via proton NMR. Aggregation of BGG was found to correlate with the T_{mc} value, with higher rates of aggregation occurring in systems above the T_{mc}. Formulations containing higher molecular weight dextrans had a lower percentage of their polymer protons in the high-mobility state (P_{hm}) and had greater stability (67). The authors concluded that mobility in the dextran matrix, as indicated by T_{mc} and P_{hm}, is an important determinant of reactivity in this system (67). However, it should be noted that BGG aggregation is a multimolecular reaction involving at least two protein molecules of high molecular weight. Given this mechanism, it is perhaps not surprising that mobility in the polymer matrix is involved in reactivity. The importance of mobility in other types of protein degradation reactions, such as oxidation or deamidation, has not been fully established.

Interestingly, another recent study using carbohydrate polymers has demonstrated a mobility dependence. In their studies of Asp-Pro peptide bond cleavage in Physalaemin and Hamburger peptides in Ficoll matrices, Streefland et al. found that the Asp-Pro bond is more labile in Physalaemin than in Hamburger peptide. They also found that while the hydrolysis reaction is first order in peptide content for the smaller Hamburger peptide, it is not first order for the Physalaemin peptide (20). They concluded that peptide reactivity is related to mobility in the Ficoll glass and attributed the greater stability of the smaller peptide to a better fit of the peptide into the polymer matrix (20). However, this conclusion implies that factors other than mobility in the matrix may be important, since peptide fit into the matrix may involve specific interactions with the polymer. The difference in reaction order for the two peptides may also be indicative of more specific chemical effects. These issues were not addressed experimentally. Interestingly, the authors propose that the protons required for the acid-catalyzed peptide bond hydrolysis may be supplied by hydroxyl groups on the carbohydrate polymer, suggesting a catalytic role for the polymer in this reaction.

In summary, the limited data on peptide and protein stability in polysaccharides suggest that mobility in the polymer matrix is involved in aggregation (67) and peptide bond cleavage (20) reactions. In addition, a catalytic role for carbohydrate hydroxyl groups in the acid-catalyzed cleavage of peptide bonds has been suggested.

C. Vinyl Polymers

Vinyl polymers are essentially linear chains of carbon atoms linked by single bonds and having pendant functional groups at alternating carbons (Scheme 8). The polymers may be crosslinked through reactions involving the functional groups. Vinyl polymers of interest in the pharmaceutical industry include PVA, poly(vinyl acetate), and PVP. This section summarizes the limited data available on peptide and protein degradation in PVA and PVP.

In work similar to their studies of bovine γ-globulin aggregation in dextrans, Yoshioka et al. studied BGG aggregation in lyophilized formulations containing PVA (68). Protein aggregation was again determined by SEC and mobility in the matrix measured as the relaxation times of polymer protons using proton NMR. The results were compared with those for a formulation containing dextran. Formulations containing PVA were found to be less stable than dextran formulations of similar water content (68). The lower stability in PVA was explained by a lower

a. Poly (vinyl alcohol)

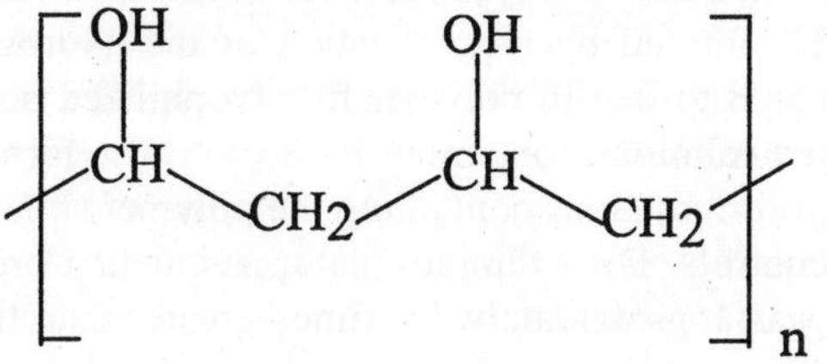

b. Poly (vinyl pyrrolidone)

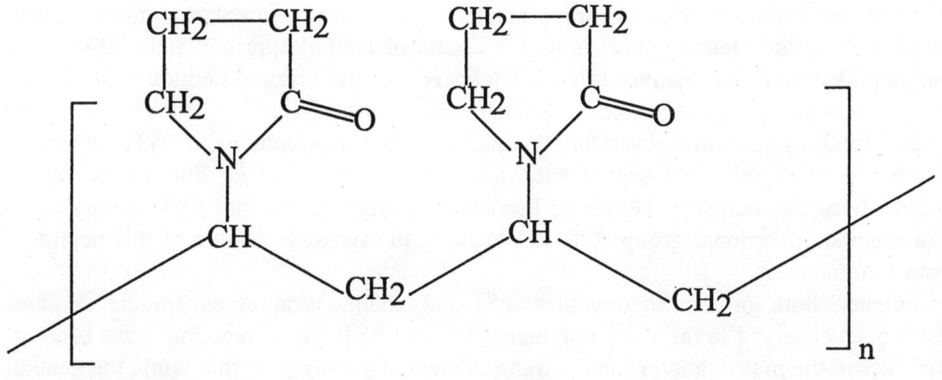

Scheme 8

"molecular mobility–changing temperature" (T_{mc}), with a value of less than 10°C for the PVA vs. 35°C for the dextran at comparable water content. The lower stability in PVA was thus attributed to higher molecular mobility in this polymer (68). Although this suggests that the T_{mc} is important for aggregation in this system, significant aggregation was observed in PVA formulations below T_{mc}. Differential scanning calorimetry studies demonstrated that PVA crystallized during storage at higher temperatures (about 60°C). The authors concluded that BGG aggregation is dependent on mobility in PVA matrices, as in the dextran matrices studied previously (68). The role of polymer crystallization and possible protein–polymer interactions were not addressed.

Recent studies in our laboratories have evaluated the stability of a model hexapeptide (Val-Tyr-Pro-Asn-Gly-Ala) in PVA matrices (69). In solution, the primary mode of degradation of this peptide is deamidation at the Asn residue, producing Asp and isoAsp containing hexapeptides (Scheme 2) (3). The peptide was incorporated into two types of PVA matrices: a semisolid hydrogel and a low-water content "xerogel" formed by lyophilization of the hydrogel. Peptide deamidation in these matrices was compared to that in polymer-free lyophilized powders and buffered solutions, and to that in buffered solutions containing PVA (69). The formulations were stored at 50°C for up to 122 days. All formulations containing the polymer showed more rapid deamidation than the polymer-free controls. For example, the apparent first-order deamidation rate constant in the PVA hydrogel was approximately 1.4 times greater than that in polymer-free solutions and 13 times greater than that in a lyophilized polymer-free powder (69). Interestingly, deamidation in the solid PVA xerogel and in the semisolid PVA hydrogel was more rapid than in polymer-free solutions (69).

To understand the mechanisms of the accelerated deamidation in PVA matrices, additional studies were conducted in which relative humidity (and therefore matrix water content) was carefully controlled and measured (6,7). The studies also used a second vinyl polymer, PVP, as a control to assess possible pendant group effects (6,7). The glass transition temperature, T_g, was also determined and was used as a measure of mobility in the polymer matrices. Deamidation rates were correlated with matrix water content and with a dimensionless T_g to determine the relative importance of mobility and water content in the reaction (6,7). Correlation of deamidation rates with dimensionless T_g, with water content, or with water activity yielded different curves for the two polymers (6). However, correlation of the deamidation rate with a dimensionless variable that incorporated both T_g and water content information gave a single curve applicable to both polymers (6). This finding suggests that both water content and mobility in the matrix are important in determining reactivity in these systems. Later studies at low water content and elevated temperature showed a kinetic plateau at approximately 20–40% of the original peptide remaining. Failure to completely recover the original peptide or its degradation products was also noted (i.e., a lack of closure of the mass balance) (31). Thesse results are consistent with formation of a reversible complex between the peptide and PVP, but the results of studies probing the existence of such a complex (e.g., dialysis, fluorescence spectroscopy) have been inconclusive. However, literature reports suggest that PVP readily complexes with aromatic functional groups (70–72), making the tyrosine residue of this peptide a possible site of interaction.

In summary, both protein aggregation (68) and deamidation at asparagine residues (6,7,31) have been observed in the vinyl polymers PVA and PVP. These reactions have been related to mobility in the matrix and/or matrix water content. This suggests that while the general physical environment provided by matrices of these polymers influences protein degradation, specific chemical or physical involvement has not been widely observed. However, the possibility of complexation of aromatic amino acids with the pyrrolidone residue of PVP has been raised, as noted above.

D. Other Polymers

The lactide/glycolide, polysaccharide, and vinyl classes of polymers discussed above enjoy widespread use in the pharmaceutical industry. There have been reports of peptide and protein stability in newer and less widely used polymer classes, such as the polyanhydrides; however, such reports have been sporadic and a coherent summary is not possible. Nevertheless, this section summarizes the available data on degradation reactions in these "other" polymers.

Ron et al. have reported the degradation of recombinant bovine somatotropin (rBST, 191 amino acids) and of zinc insulin in matrices of poly[1,3-bis(p-carboxyhydroxy) hexane anhydride], a very hydrophobic polymer, at 10% loading (73). They followed protein release into phosphate buffer (pH 7.4) under sink conditions and analyzed the resulting solution state protein concentrations by HPLC and radioimmunoassay. Prior to the experiments the authors suspected that rBST would be subject to decomposition and/or aggregation in the presence of moisture, and that amine groups on the proteins might interact with carboxylic acid groups produced as polyanhydrides degraded (73). Experimentally, they found no evidence for structural or chemical changes in rBST during 288 h of release. Furthermore, the cumulative release of rBST was affected by polymer hydrophobicity, with the least hydrophobic polymer showing less than 50% release and the most hydrophobic showing greater than 90% release (73). Similar results were obtained for insulin (73). The authors concluded that the polyanhydrides are inert with respect to degradation of these proteins and that modifying polymer hydrophobicity can control protein release rates (73).

Costantino et al. studied the stability of various bovine and human albumin preparations in the presence of fatty acids (74). As part of this larger study, they examined the release of bovine albumin and of S-alkylated bovine albumin from poly(fatty acid dimer: sebacic acid) matrices (74). Polymer disks were formed by compression molding at 9% albumin loading. Albumin release into phosphate buffer was monitored using a BCA assay. The authors' solution state experiments and prior published data suggest that albumin's stability toward aggregation is sensitive to fatty acid content and that binding to fatty acids may prevent aggregation (74). The S-alkylated albumin was used to test the involvement of thiol–disulfide exchange reactions in aggregation, since S-alkylation prevents thiol–disulfide exchange. Release profiles showed more rapid release of the S-alkylated albumin than the nonalkylated form, a result that is consistent with thiol–disulfide exchange–induced aggregation in the nonalkylated form (74). However, no confirmatory evidence for the suspected aggregation was presented.

E. Summary and Implications for Controlled Release

This section has reviewed the available data on peptide and protein degradation reactions in several classes of polymers. In lactide/glycolide polymers, several degradation reactions have been observed, including peptide bond hydrolysis, methionine oxidation, and aggregation. Some groups have attributed these reactions to a reduced microenvironmental pH within the degrading polymer matrix, caused by free lactic acid and/or glycolic acid monomers. Others who have produced stable protein formulations in these polymers have contested this. In the polysaccharides and vinyl polymers, the effects of the polymers on peptide and protein degradation reactions have been attributed in large part to physical effects on mobility with the matrix, although more specific interactions (e.g., complexation with PVP) have been suspected. The data on polyanhydrides and poly(fatty acids) are very limited, so that generalizations are not possible at this time. Based on this information, the developer of polymeric controlled release devices should be concerned with the effects of polymer selection on mobility within the device and with the resultant effects on protein stability. The possibility of more direct chemical or complexation effects should be borne in mind for certain polymers such as the lactide/glycolides and PVP.

VI. CONCLUSIONS

This chapter has reviewed the degradation of peptides and proteins in the solid state as it relates to the design of controlled release devices. In summary, the available literature has shown that a number of protein degradation reactions occur in the solid state, including oxidation, deamidation, chain scission, the Maillard reaction, and thiol–disulfide exchange (Section III). These reactions are affected by environmental and formulation variables, such as temperature, pressure, moisture content, mobility in the matrix, excipients, and effective pH in the solid (Section IV). Polymeric excipients, commonly used as platforms for controlled release, affect these degradation reactions by altering mobility in the solid state, although more specific interactions between proteins and polymers and/or their biodegradation products have been reported (Section V). As the discussion in this chapter has suggested, the design of controlled release devices can be informed by an understanding of these variables and their effects on protein stability in the solid state.

In concluding, we note that the available literature suggests several avenues for additional research. For example, while there have been many reports demonstrating an effect of mobility on solid-state protein degradation, little is known regarding the relative importance of mobility in different types of reactions. It seems reasonable to assume that reactions involving large reactant species (e.g., protein aggregation) should be more "mobility-dependent" than those with small reactants (e.g., oxidation), but this has not been demonstrated. Stabilization against these putative mobility-dependent reactions would rationally involve formulation changes such as a reduction in matrix T_g, while this would not be expected to be effective for a "mobility-independent" class. Other areas for research include the effect of protein secondary and tertiary structure on solid-state reactivity, the measurement of hydrogen ion activity in the solid state, and the development of stabilizing polymers and other excipients. Continued research to define the determinants of protein reactivity in solids, and to identify methods to prevent degradation, will improve our ability to design stable controlled release devices for this important class of drugs.

ACKNOWLEDGMENTS

Support for our work in this area has been provided by an NIGMS Biotechnology Training grant, by Pharmacia & Upjohn, Inc., and by NIH grant GM-54195.

REFERENCES

1. H. R. Costantino, R. Langer and A. M. Klibanov, Solid-phase aggregation of proteins under pharmaceutically relevant conditions. J. Pharm. Sci., 83/12: 1662–1669, 1994.
2. H. Schmalzried, Chemical Kinetics of Solids, VCH, New York, 1995, pp. 10–18.
3. K. Patel and R. Borchardt, Chemical pathways of peptide degradation. II. Kinetics of deamidation of an asparaginyl residue in a model peptide. Pharm. Res., 7: 703–711, 1990.
4. T. V. Brennan and S. Clarke, Spontaneous degradation of polypeptides at aspartyl and asparaginyl residues: effect of the solvent dielectric. Protein Sci. 2:331–338, 1993.
5. C. Oliyai, J. Patel, L. Carr and R. T. Borchardt, Solid state stability of lyophilized formulations of an asparaginyl residue in a model hexapeptide. J. Parent. Sci. Technol., 48: 167–173, 1994.
6. M. C. Lai, M. J. Hageman, R. L. Schowen, R. T. Borchardt and E. M. Topp, Chemical stability of peptides in polymers. I. Effect of water on peptide deamidation in poly(vinyl alcohol) and poly(vinyl pyrrolidone) matrices. J. Pharm. Sci., 88: 1073–1080, 1999.
7. M. C. Lai, M. J. Hageman, R. L. Schowen, R. T. Borchardt, B. B. Laird and E. M. Topp, Chemical stability of peptides in polymers. II. Discriminating between solvent and plasticizing effects of water on peptide deamidation in poly(vinyl pyrrolidone). J. Pharm. Sci., 88: 1081–1089, 1999.
8. E. Y. Shalaev and G. Zografi, Interrelationships between phase transformations and organic chemical reactivity in the solid state. J. Phys. Org. Chem., 9: 729–738, 1996.

9. E. Y. Shalaev, S. R. Byrn, and G. Zografi, Single-phase and heterophase solid-state chemical kinetics of thermally induced methyl transfer in tetraglycine methyl ester. Int. J. Chem. Kinet., 29: 339–348, 1997.
10. E. Y. Shalaev, M. Shalaeva, S. R. Byrn and G. Zografi, Effects of processing on the solid-state methyl transfer of tetraglycine methyl ester. Int. J. Pharm., 152: 75–88, 1997.
11. M. C. Manning, K. Patel and R. T. Borchardt, Stability of protein pharmaceuticals. Pharm. Res., 6(11): 903–918, 1989.
12. J. Fransson, E. Florin-Robertsson, K. Axelsson and C. Nyhlen, Oxidation of human insulin-like growth factor I in formulation studies: kinetics of methionine oxidation in aqueous solution and in solid state. Pharm. Res. 13(8): 1252–1257, 1996.
13. M. J. Pikal, K. M. Dellerman, M. L. Roy and R. M. Riggin, The effects of formulation variables on the stability of freeze-dried human growth hormone. Pharm. Res., 8(4): 427–436, 1991.
14. M. W. Townsend, P. R. Byron and P. P. DeLuca, The effects of formulation additives on the degradation of freeze-dried ribonuclease A. Pharm. Res., 7(10): 1086–1091, 1990.
15. D. C. Dubost, M. J. Kaufman, J. A. Zimmerman, M. J. Bogusky, A. B. Coddington and S. M. Pitzenberger, Characterization of a solid state reaction product from a lyophilized formulation of a cyclic heptapeptide. A novel example of an excipient-induced oxidation. Pharm. Res., 13(12): 1811–1814, 1996.
16. S. Li, C. Schöneich and R. T. Borchardt, Chemical instability of protein pharmaceuticals: mechanisms of oxidation and strategies for stabilization. Biotechnol. Bioeng., 48: 490–500, 1995.
17. C. Schöneich, M. J. Hageman and R. T. Borchardt, Stability of peptides and proteins. In: Controlled Drug Delivery: The Next Generation, K. Park (Ed.), ACS Books, Washington, DC, 1997, pp. 205–228.
18. R. G. Strickley and B. D. Anderson, Solid-state stability of human insulin. I. Mechanism and the effect of water on the kinetics of degradation in lyophiles from pH 2–5 solutions. Pharm. Res., 13(8): 1142–1153, 1996.
19. M. J. Pikal and D. R. Rigsbee, The stability of insulin in crystalline and amorphous solids: observation of greater stability for the amorphous form. Pharm. Res., 14(10): 1379–1387, 1997.
20. L. Streefland, A. D. Auffret and F. Franks, Bond cleavage reactions in solid aqueous carbohydrate solutions. Pharm. Res., 15(6): 843–849, 1998.
21. S. Li, T. W. Patapoff, D. Overcashier, C. Hsu, T. H. Nguyen and R. T. Borchardt, Effects of reducing sugars on the chemical stability of human relaxin in lyophilized state. J. Pharm. Sci., 85(8): 873–877, 1996.
22. S. S. Leung and D. J. W. Grant, Solid state stability studies of model dipeptides: aspartame and aspartylphenylalanine. J. Pharm. Sci., 86(1): 64–71, 1997.
23. U. Kertscher, M. Bienert, E. Krause, N. F. Sepetov and B. Mehlis, Spontaneous chemical degradation of substance P in the solid phase and in solution. Int. J. Peptide Protein Res., 41: 207–211, 1993.
24. M. J. Hageman, Water sorption and solid-state stability of proteins. In: Stability of Protein Pharmaceuticals: Part A—Chemical and Physical Pathways of Protein Degradation. T. J. Ahern and M. C. Manning (Eds.), Plenum Press, New York, 1992, pp. 273–310.
25. P. A. Kosen, Disulfide bonds in proteins, In: Stability of Protein Pharmaceuticals: Part A—Chemical and Physical Pathways of Protein Degradation. T. J. Ahern and M. C. Manning (Eds.), Plenum Press, New York, 1992, pp. 31–67.
26. W. R. Liu, R. Langer and A. M. Klibanov, Moisture-induced aggregation of lyophilized proteins in the solid state. Biotechnol. Bioeng., 37: 177–184, 1991.
27. H. R. Costantino, R. Langer and A. M. Klibanov, Moisture-induced aggregation of lyophilized insulin. Pharm. Res. 11(1): 21–29, 1994.
28. A. F. R. Hühmer, G. I. Aced, M. D. Perkins, R. N. Gursoy, S. D. S. Jois, C. K. Larive, T. J. Siahaan and C. Schöneich, Separation and analysis of peptides and proteins. Anal. Chem., 69: 29R–57R, 1997.
29. C. Schöneich, A. F. R. Hühmer, S. R. Rabel, J. F. Stobaugh, S. D. S. Jois, C. K. Larive, T. J. Siahaan, T. C. Squier, D. J. Bigelow and T. D. Williams, Separation and analysis of peptides and proteins. Anal. Chem., 67: 155R–181R, 1995.

30. C. Oliyai, J. P. Patel, L. Carr and R. T. Borchardt, Chemical pathways of peptide degradation. VII. Solid state chemical instability of an aspartyl residue in a model hexapeptide. Pharm. Res., 11/6: 901–908, 1994.
31. P. Berglund, The effect of temperature on peptide deamidation in polymer matrices, Master's thesis, Royal Danish School of Pharmacy, August 1998.
32. J. F. Carpenter and J. H. Crowe, The mechanism of cryoprotection of proteins by solutes, Cryobiology 225: 244–255, 1988.
33. S. N. Timasheff, The control of protein stability and association by weak interactions with water: how do solvents affect these processes? Annu. Rev. Biophys. Biomol. Struct., 22: 67–97, 1993.
34. D. B. Volkin and C. R. Middaugh, The effect of temperature on protein structure. In: Stability of Protein Pharmaceuticals: Part: A—Chemical and Physical Pathways of Protein Degradation. T. J. Ahern and M. C. Manning (Eds.), Plenum Press, New York, 1992, pp. 215–247.
35. D. E. Wurster and R. L. Ternik, Pressure-induced activity loss in solid state catalase. J. Pharm. Sci., 84(2): 190–194, 1995.
36. M. J. Groves and C. D. Teng, The effect of compaction and moisture on some physical and biological properties of proteins. In Stability of Protein Pharmaceuticals: Part A—Chemical and Physical Pathways of Protein Degradation. T. J. Ahern and M. C. Manning (Eds.), Plenum Press, New York, 1992, pp. 311–359.
37. M. L. Williams, R. F. Landel and D. J. Ferry, The temperature dependence of relaxation mechanisms in amorphous polymers and other glass-forming systems. J. Am. Chem. Soc., 77: 3701–3707, 1955.
38. L. N. Bell and M. J. Hageman, Differentiating between the effects of water activity and glass transition dependent mobility on a solid state chemical reaction: aspartame degradation. J. Agric. Food Chem., 42: 2398–2401, 1994.
39. F. Franks, R. H. M. Hatley and S. F. Mathias, Materials science and the production of shelf-stable biologicals. BioPharm. 4: 38–55, 1991.
40. L. Kreilgaard, S. Frokjaer, J. M. Flink, T. W. Randolph and J. F. Carpenter, Effects of additives on the stability of humicola lanuginosa lipase during freeze-drying and storage in the dried solid. J. Pharm. Sci., 88(3): 281–290, 1999.
41. B. S. Chang, R. M. Beauvais, A. Dong and J. F. Carpenter, Physical factors affecting the storage stability of freeze-dried interleukin-1 receptor antagonist: glass transition and protein conformation. Arch. Biochim. Biophys., 331: 249–258, 1996.
42. L. N. Bell, M. J. Hageman and C. M. Muraoka, Thermally induced denaturation of lyophilized bovine somatotropin and lysozyme as impacted by moisture and excipients. J. Pharm. Sci., 84/6: 707–712, 1995.
43. L. N. Bell, M. J. Hageman and J. M. Bauer, Impact of moisture on thermally induced denaturation and decomposition of lyophilized bovine somatotropin. Biopolymers, 35: 210–209, 1995.
44. Y. Fujita and Y. Noda, Effect of hydration on the thermal stability of protein as measured by differential scanning calorimetry: chymotrypsinogen A. Int. J. Peptide Protein Res., 18:12–17, 1981.
45. S. Yoshioka, U. Aso, K. Izutsu and T. Terao, Stability of β-galactosidase, a model protein drug, is related to water mobility as measured by ^{17}O nuclear magnetic resonance (NMR). Pharm. Res. 10(1): 103–108, 1993.
46. S. Yoshioka, Y. Aso and S. Kojima, The effect of excipients on the molecular mobility of lyophilized formulations, as measured by glass transition temperature and NMR relaxation-based critical mobility temperature. Pharm. Res. 16(1): 135–140, 1999.
47. F. Separaovic, Y. H. Lam, X. Ke and H. K. Chan, A solid state NMR study of protein hydration and stability. Pharm. Res., 15(12): 1816–1821, 1998.
48. D. Q. M. Craig, P. G. Royall, V. L. Kett and M. L. Hopton, The relevance of the amorphous state to pharmaceutical dosage forms: glassy drugs and freeze dried systems. Int. J. Pharm. 179: 179–207, 1999.
49. E. Y. Shalaev and G. Zografi, How does residual water affect the solid-state degradation of drugs in the amorphous state? J. Pharm. Sci., 85(11): 1137–1141, 1996.

50. D. P. Miller, R. E. Anderson and J. J. de Pablo, Stabilization of lactate dehydrogenase following freeze-thawing and vacuum drying in the presence of trehalose and borate. Pharm. Res., 15(8): 1215–1221, 1998.
51. A. Wilson, J. Dehadashti, E. M. Topp, R. T. Borchardt and R. L. Schowen, 1999 (unpublished data).
52. R. E. Johnson, L. A. Lanaski, V. Gupta, M. J. Griffin, H. T. Gaud, T. E. Needham and H. Zia, Stability of atriopeptin III in poly(D,L-lactide-co-glycolide microspheres), J. Contr. Rel., 17: 61–68, 1991.
53. T. G. Park, W. Lu and G. Crotts, Importance of in vitro experimental conditions on protein release kinetics, stability and polymer degradation in protein encapsulated poly(D,L-lactic acid-co-glycolic acid) microspheres, J. Contr. Rel., 33: 211–222, 1995.
54. W. Lu and T. G. Park, Protein release from poly(lactic-co-glycolic acid) microspheres: protein stability problems. PDA J. Pharm. Sci. Technol., 49(1): 13–19, 1995.
55. K. Izutsu, S. Yoshioka, T. Terao, Decreased protein-stabilizing effects of cryoprotectants due to crystallization. Pharm. Res. 10(8): 1232–1237, 1993.
56. K. Izutsu, S. Yoshioka, S. Kojima, Physical stability and protein stability of freeze-dried cakes during storage at elevated temperatures. Pharm. Res. 11(7): 995–999, 1994.
57. J. E. Sarciaux and M. J. Hageman, Effects of bovine somatotropin (rbSt) concentration at different moisture levels on the physical stability of sucrose in freeze-dried rbSt/sucrose mixtures. J. Pharm. Sci., 86(3): 365–371, 1997.
58. S. T. Tzannis and S. J. Prestrelski, Moisture effects on protein-excipient interactions in spray-dried powders. Nature of destabilizing effects of sucrose. J. Pharm. Sci., 88(3): 360–370, 1999.
59. M. S. Hora, R. K. Rana and F. W. Smith, Lyophilized formulations of recombinant tumor necrosis factor. Pharm. Res., 9:33–36, 1992.
60. M. W. Townsend and P. P. DeLuca, Stability of ribonuclease A in solution and the freeze-dried state. J. Pharm Sci, 79:1083–1086, 1990.
61. Y. Song, R. L. Schowen, R. T. Borchardt, and E. M. Topp, Formaldehyde production by Tris buffer in peptide formulations at elevated temperature. J. Pharm. Sci., submitted.
62. R. C. Mehta, R. Jeyanthi, S. Calis, B. C. Thanoo, K. W. Burton and P. P. DeLuca, Biodegradable microspheres as depot system for parenteral delivery of peptide drugs. J. Contr. Rel., 29: 375–384, 1994.
63. G. Crotts and T. G. Park, Stability and release of bovine serum albumin encapsulated within poly(D,L-lactido-glycolide) microparticles. J. Contr. Rel., 44: 123–134, 1997.
64. C. Witschi and E. Doelker, Peptide degradation during preparation and in vitro release testing of poly(L-lactic acid) and poly(DL-lactic-co-glycolic acid) microparticles. Int. J. Pharm., 171: 1–18, 1998.
65. J. L. Cleland, A. Mac, B. Boyd, J. Yang, E. T. Duenas, D. Yeung, D. Brooks, C. Hsu, H. Chu, V. Mukku and A. J. S. Jones, The stability of recombinant human growth hormone in poly(lactic-co-glycolic acid) (PLGA) microspheres, Pharm. Res., 14(4): 420–425, 1997.
66. O. L. Johnson, W. Jaworowicz, J. L. Cleland, L. Bailey, M. Charnis, E. Duenas, C. Wu, D. Shepard, S. Magil, T. Last, A. J. S. Jones and S. D. Putney, The stabilization and encapsulation of human growth hormone into biodegradable microspheres. Pharm. Res., 14: 730–735, 1997.
67. S. Yoshioka, Y. Aso and S. Kojima, Dependence of the molecular mobility and protein stability of freeze-dried gamma-globulin formulations on the molecular weight of dextran, Pharm. Res., 14(6): 736–741, 1997.
68. S. Yoshioka, Y. Aso, Y. Nakai and S. Kojima, Effect of high molecular mobility of poly(vinyl alcohol) on protein stability of lyophilized gamma globulin formulation. J. Pharm. Sci., 87(2): 147–151, 1998.
69. M. C. Lai, R. L. Schowen, R. T. Borchardt, and E. M. Topp, Deamidation of a model hexapeptide in poly(vinyl alcohol) hydrogels and xerogels. J. Peptide Res., 55: 93–101, 2000.
70. J. A. Plaizier-Vercammen and R. E. De Neve, Interaction of povidone with aromatic compounds I: Evaluation of complex formation by factorial analysis. J. Pharm. Sci., 69: 1403–1408, 1980.
71. J. A. Plaizier-Vercammen and R. E. De Neve, Interaction of povidone with aromatic compounds II: Evaluation of ionic strength, buffer concentration, temperature and pH by factorial analysis. J. Pharm. Sci., 70: 1252–1255, 1981.

72. J. A. Plaizier-Vercammen and R. E. De Neve, Interaction of povidone with aromatic compounds III: Thermodynamics of the binding equilibria and interaction forces in buffer solutions at varying pH values and varying dielectric constants. J. Pharm. Sci., 71(5): 552–555, 1982.
73. E. Ron, T. Turek, E. Mathiowitz, M. Chasin, M. Hageman and R. Langer, Controlled release of polypeptides from polyanhydrides, Proc. Natl. Acad. Sci. USA, 90: 4176–4180, 1993.
74. H. R. Costantino, L. Shieh, A. M. Klibanov and R. Langer, Heterogeneity of serum albumin samples with respect to solid-state aggregation via thiol–disulfide interchange. Implications for sustained release from polymers, J. Contr. Rel., 44: 255–261, 1997.

34
Growth Factor Release from Biodegradable Hydrogels to Induce Neovascularization

Yoshito Ikada
Faculty of Medical Engineering, Suzuka University of Medical Science, Suguka-city, Japan
Yasuhiko Tabata
Institute for Frontier Medical Sciences, Kyoto University, Kyoto, Japan

I. INTRODUCTION

Tissue engineering has increasingly attracted interest as a promising new technology to assist tissue regeneration at body defects as well as biological functions of damaged or injured organs. There are three factors necessary for tissue engineering: growth factors, cells, and materials for scaffolding. Since among them is growth factor of protein or glycoprotein, which is susceptible to proteolysis and denaturation, if the growth factor is administered in solution form into the body, one cannot always expect the biological function. Therefore, it is of prime necessity to develop dosage forms for in vivo prolongation of the biological activity. One possible way is to incorporate a growth factor into an appropriate matrix for achieving controlled release of the factor at the site of action over a long time period. Numerous studies have been performed on protein release by taking advantage of polymer matrices (1–5), but there is a problem before us in the protein release technology, i.e., loss in the biological activity of protein released. It has been demonstrated that this activity loss mainly results from protein denaturation and deactivation during a formulation process with a polymer matrix. When exposed to harsh environmental changes, such as heating and exposure to sonication and organic solvents, protein is generally denatured, losing its biological activity (6–8). Therefore, it is required to contrive a new formulation method for growth factor release under mild conditions to minimize protein deactivation. From this viewpoint, hydrogel is a preferable candidate for a release matrix because of its biosafety and inertness toward protein (9). However, it should be noted that the period of protein release from hydrogels is mostly as short as a day because of their diffusion-controlled characteristics (1,2,9,10).

It has been well recognized in the polymer science that a positively or negatively charged polyelectrolyte electrostatically interacts with an oppositely charged partner to form a polyion complex (11,12). It seems unlikely that all of the ionic interactions between the two polyelectrolytes with many charged groups are dissociated at the same time. As a result, in contrast to low molecular weight electrolytes, stable bonding will be formed between the oppositely charged polyelectrolytes without being easily dissociated. On the other hand, it is known that metal affinity chromatography is one protein separation method that is routinely used. This is based on the intrinsic nature of proteins to form a coordinate bond through metal chelation (13).

Various proteins can be separated and purified by this method with their biological activity remaining (14–16). Generally, the coordinate bond is not broken unless the environmental pH is changed rapidly. It is promising for long-term protein release to utilize these molecular interactions. A growth factor is immobilized to the biodegradable polymer chains constituting a hydrogel based on the interaction force to suppress the diffusional release. In this release system, the immobilized growth factor is released, accompanied by hydrogel degradation.

Figure 1 shows the conceptual scheme of growth factor release from a biodegradable hydrogel carrier on the basis of either polyion complexation or metal coordination. For example, a positively charged growth factor is electrostatically immobilized with negatively charged polymer chains constituting a hydrogel carrier. If an environmental change, such as increased ionic strength, occurs, the immobilized growth factor will be released from the drug–hydrogel formulation. Even if such an environmental change does not take place, degradation of the polymer hydrogel itself will result in growth factor release. It is possible that the growth factor immobilized through metal coordination is released from the hydrogel carrier as a result of the environmental pH change and hydrogel degradation. Because the latter is more likely to happen in vivo than the former in both cases, the hydrogel carrier should be prepared from biodegradable polymers. In this hydrogel system, growth factor release is thought to be based on hydrogel biodegradation, which can be regulated by changing the crosslinking extent of the hydrogels.

As the hydrogel material for controlled release of growth factor, it is absolutely necessary to employ a highly biosafe and water-soluble polymer. In addition, if biodegradability is required for the hydrogel, the material to be used will be restricted to natural polymers, such as proteins and polysaccharides. Therefore, as a hydrogel polymer, we selected gelatin that has been extensively used for industrial, pharmaceutical, and medical purposes. The biosafety of gelatin has been proved through its long clinical usage as a plasma expander, surgical biomaterials, and drug ingredients (17). Another unique advantage of gelatin as the hydrogel material is its electrical nature, which is modified by the treatment process of collagen (18). An alkaline process of collagen hydrolyzes the amide groups of the side chain, yielding gelatin having a high density of carboxyl groups, which render the gelatin negatively charged. This reduces the isoelectric point (IEP) of gelatin. To the contrary, such a hydrolysis does not occur by an acid process; consequently, the IEP of obtained gelatin remains similar to that of collagen, i.e., around 9.0.

Since the IEP of some growth factors is generally higher than 7.0, the acidic gelatin with an IEP of 5.0 is preferable as a biodegradable polymer for controlled release on the basis of polyion complexation. This acidic gelatin was chemically crosslinked to prepare a biodegradable hydrogel. As polysaccharide, we used biodegradable amylopectin which is one of the main components of starch, having been used for pharmaceutical, medical, and food applications as widely as gelatin (10). Since amylopectin is a nonpolar water-soluble polysaccharide, it is not expected to form a polyion complex with growth factor. Thus, for immobilization of growth factor through metal coordination, a metal-chelating residue was introduced to amylopectin, followed by chemical crosslinking to prepare a biodegradable hydrogel.

b-Fibroblast growth factor (bFGF) and vascular endothelial growth factor (VEGF) were selected as angiogenetic growth factors. They were immobilized to the acidic gelatin and derivatized amylopectin hydrogels based on polyion complexation and metal coordination, respectively. This chapter surveys our controlled release system of growth factor driven by hydrogel degradation and the superior vascularization effect to free growth factor. Few practical applications of growth factor release to tissue engineering are exemplified.

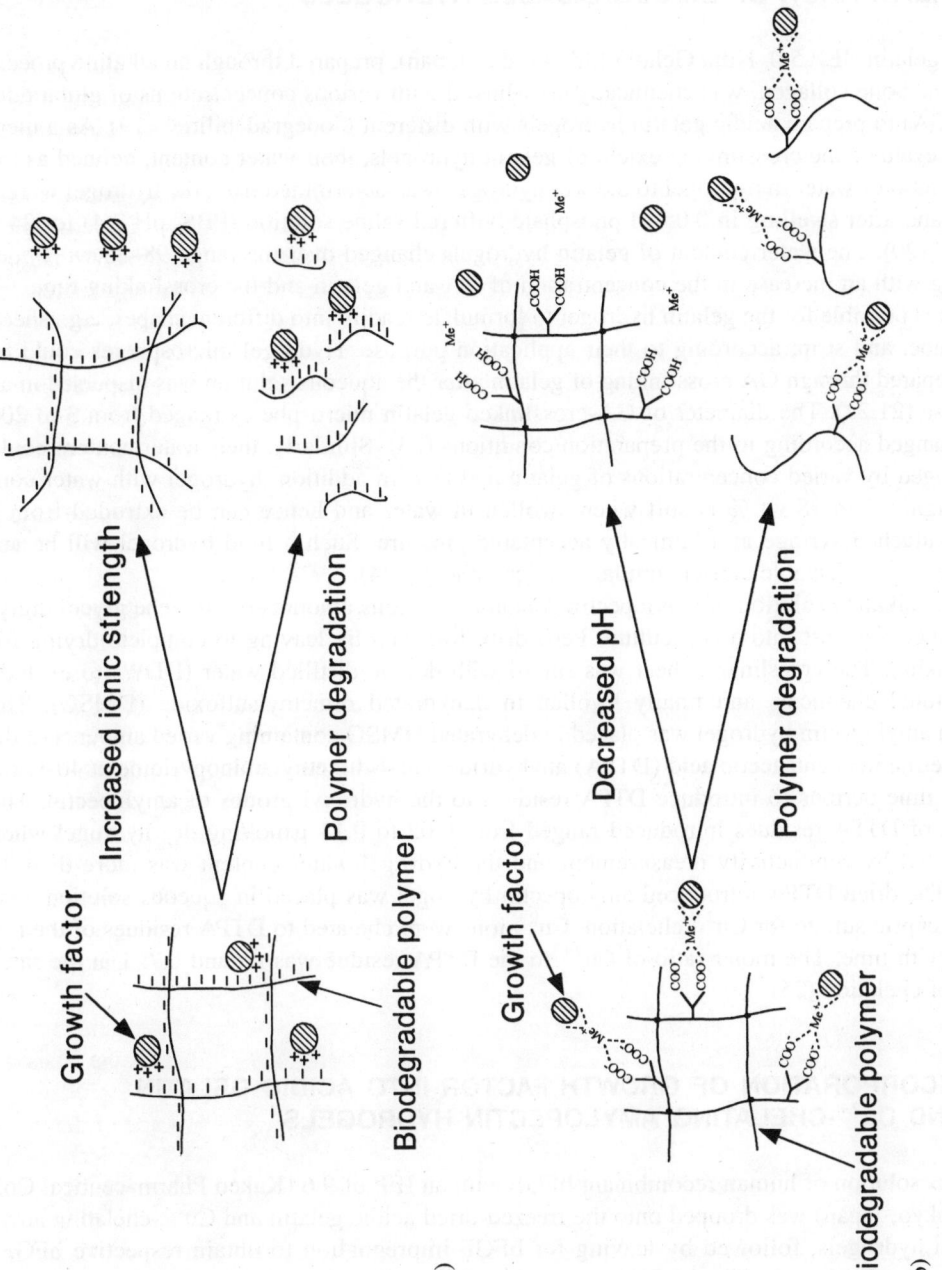

Figure 1 Release of growth factor from biodegradable polymer carrier on the basis of polyion complexation (a) and metal coordination (b).

II. PREPARATION OF BIODEGRADABLE HYDROGELS

Acidic gelatin (IEP 5.0, Nitta Gelatin Ltd., Osaka, Japan), prepared through an alkaline process of bovine bone collagen, was chemically crosslinked with various concentrations of glutaraldehyde (GA) to prepare acidic gelatin hydrogels with different biodegradabilities (19). As a measure to evaluate the crosslinking extent of gelatin hydrogels, their water content, defined as the weight ratio of water in hydrogel to the wet hydrogel, was determined from the hydrogel weight before and after swelling in 0.05 M phosphate-buffered saline solution (PBS, pH 7.4) for 24 h at 37°C (20). The water content of gelatin hydrogels changed over the range 98–85 wt %, decreasing with an increase in the concentration of GA and gelatin and the crosslinking time.

It is possible for the gelatin hydrogel to formulate readily into different shapes, e.g., sheet, disk, cube, and strip, according to their application purpose. Hydrogel microspheres could be also prepared through GA crosslinking of gelatin after the aqueous solution was dispersed in an oil phase (21,22). The diameter of GA-crosslinked gelatin microspheres ranged from 3 to 200 μm, changed according to the preparation conditions (23). Similarly, their water content could be changed by varied concentrations of gelatin and GA. In addition, hydrogel with water contents higher than 98 wt % is soft when swollen in water and hence can be extruded from a needle-attached syringe at a clinically acceptable pressure. Such a fluid hydrogel will be applicable as an injectable carrier, similar to microspheres (24).

An alkaline solution of amylopectin containing various amounts of ethylene glycol diglycidyl ether was cast into a cell culture Petri dish, followed by leaving to complete drying for crosslinking. The crosslinked sheet was rinsed with double-distilled water (DDW) to exclude the residual chemicals and finally swollen in dehydrated dimethylsulfoxide (DMSO). The swollen amylopectin hydrogel was placed in dehyrated DMSO containing varied amounts of diethylenetriaminepentaacetic acid (DTPA) anyhydride and 4-dimethylaminopyridine at 40°C for various time periods to introduce DTPA residues to the hydroxyl groups of amylopectin. The amount of DTPA residues introduced ranged from 0.02 to 0.14 μmol/mg dry hydrogel when quantitated by conductivity measurement and the hydrogel water content was more than 93 wt %. The dried DTPA-introduced amylopectin hydrogel was placed in aqueous solution containing cupric sulfate for Cu^{2+} chelation. Cu^{2+} ions were chelated to DTPA residues of the hydrogel with time. The molar ratio of Cu^{2+} to the DTPA residue was around 0.7:1 at the saturation of chelation (25).

III. INCORPORATION OF GROWTH FACTOR INTO ACIDIC GELATIN AND Cu^{2+}-CHELATING AMYLOPECTIN HYDROGELS

Aqueous solution of human recombinant bFGF with an IEP of 9.6 (Kaken Pharmaceutical Co., Ltd., Tokyo, Japan) was dropped onto the freezed-dried acidic gelatin and Cu^{2+}-chelating amylopectin hydrogels, followed by leaving for bFGF impregnation to obtain respective bFGF-incorporating hydrogels. The bFGF solution was fully sorbed into the dried hydrogels during the swelling process, irrespective of the hydrogel water content, because the solution volume was much less than that theoretically impregnated into each hydrogel.

Hydrogel preparation in the presence of growth factor leads to their activity loss, probably because of chemical crosslinking of gelatin (21). On the contrary, the present method, in which aqueous solution of growth factor was sorbed into pre-prepared hydrogels in a freeze-dried state, at least will prevent protein from chemical deactivation. This method is also effective in quantitatively incorporating growth factor into the hydrogel with high reproducibility, irrespective of the water content. The growth factor solution was found to be sorbed and homogeneously distributed in the interior of hydrogel (26).

IV. IN VITRO RELEASE OF BFGF FROM ACIDIC GELATIN AND Cu^{2+}-CHELATING AMYLOPECTIN HYDROGELS

When quantitated by heparin-affinity high-performance liquid chromatography (HPLC), intact bFGF was released in PBS at 37°C from the acidic gelatin hydrogel incorporating bFGF within 1 day up to about 30% of the initial loading, but thereafter no substantial release was observed. On the other hand, the hydrogel prepared from basic gelatin with an IEP of 9.0 exhibited almost complete release of the incorporated bFGF of intact form within a day. The similar trend on the bFGF release was observed for acidic gelatin hydrogels, irrespective of the shape and microsphere size (Fig. 2) (23). A sorption experiment revealed that basic bFGF was sorbed to the

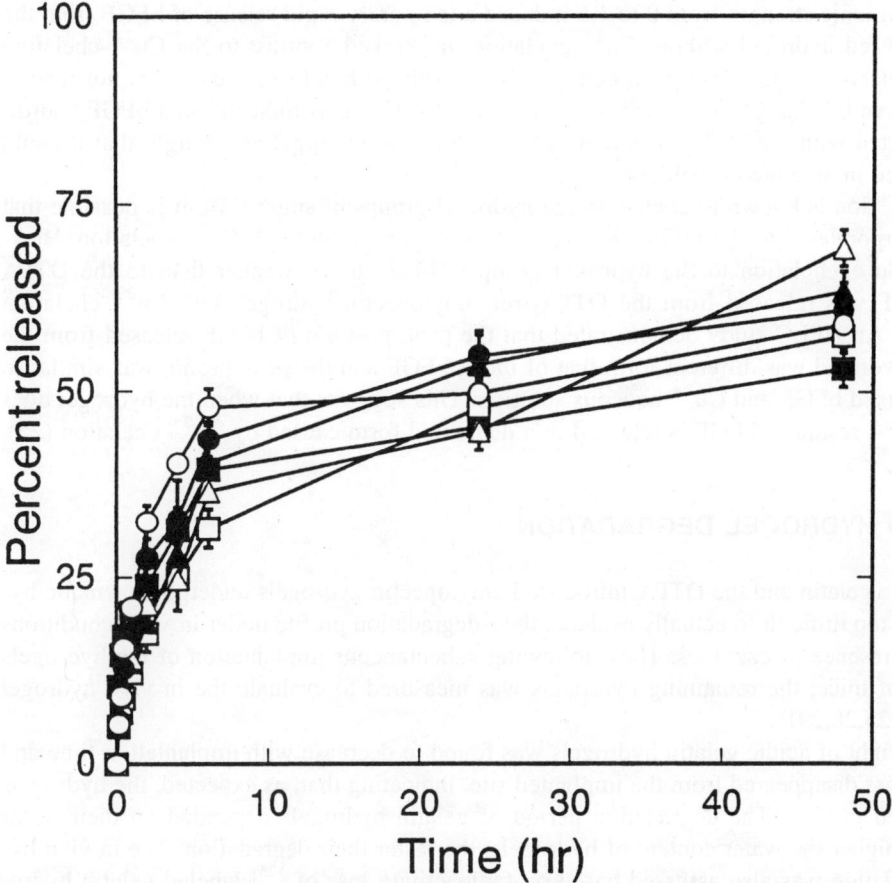

Figure 2 The in vitro profiles of bFGF release in PBS at 37°C from bFGF-incorporating acidic gelatin microspheres with diameters of (○) 3.2, (●) 10.2, (△) 22.5, and (▲) 71.2 and (□) 150.1 μm or a bFGF-incorporated acidic gelatin disc (8 mm in diameter, 2 mm thickness) (■). The water content of gelatin microspheres and disc is 95 vol% and 95 wt%, respectively.

hydrogel of acidic gelatin with time, irrespective of the hydrogel water content. The sorbed amount of bFGF decreased with the increased NaCl concentration of sorption solution, indicating that bFGF sorption to the acidic gelatin hydrogels is based mainly on the ionic interaction (26). These findings indicate that bFGF cannot be released from acidic gelatin hydrogels under in vitro nondegradation conditions because of polyion complexation of basic bFGF molecules with the acidic gelatin. It seems reasonable to suppose that this mechanism of bFGF release causes no dependence of hydrogel shape on the release profile. It is possible that all bFGF molecules are not always ionically complexed with the acidic gelatin constituting the hydrogel. Probably, the noncomplexed bFGF is released from the hydrogel during the initial period of release test, followed by no release of the ionically immobilized bFGF, whereas no formation between basic gelatin and basic bFGF leads to prompt release of all the bFGF molecules from the basic gelatin hydrogel.

In a bFGF release test, a DTPA-introduced amylopectin hydrogel incorporating bFGF with Cu^{2+} chelation exhibited approximately 10% of intact bFGF release in PBS or DDW at 37°C during the first hour, but thereafter no further release. A large initial release of the intact bFGF was observed from Cu^{2+}-free hydrogels, irrespective of DTPA introduction. An increase in the solution ionic strength from 0 to 1.5 induced a temporary rapid release of bFGF from the DTPA-introduced hydrogel without Cu^{2+} chelation, in marked contrast to the Cu^{2+}-chelating DTPA-introduced hydrogel. Since, in general, the coordinate bond once formed is not readily dissociated even by change in solution ionic strength (13–15). This indicates that bFGF coordinately interacted with the DTPA residue of the amylopectin hydrogel as strongly that it could not be released in an aqueous solution.

As Cu^{2+} ion is known to chelate to the hydroxyl groups of sugar (27), it is possible that bFGF is incorporated into the DTPA-free amylopectin hydrogel through Cu^{2+} chelation. However, since Cu^{2+} chelation to the hydroxyl group is likely to be weaker than to the DTPA residue, bFGF was released from the DTPA-free amylopectin hydrogel with Cu^{2+} chelation even in PBS. An HPLC study demonstrated that the peak position of bFGF released from the DTPA-free hydrogel was different form that of intact bFGF and the peak profile was similar to that of the mixed bFGF and Cu^{2+} aqueous solution. This suggests that when the hydrogel does not have DTPA residues, bFGF is released in a denatured form caused by Cu^{2+} chelation (25).

V. IN VIVO HYDROGEL DEGRADATION

Since both the gelatin and the DTPA-introduced amylopectin hydrogels undergo enzymatic hydrolysis, it is too difficult to actually evaluate their degradation profile under in vitro conditions even in the presence of enzymes. Thus, following subcutaneous implantation of the hydrogels in the back of mice, the remaining hydrogels was measured to evaluate the in vivo hydrogel degradation (25,28,29).

The weight of acidic gelatin hydrogels was found to decrease with implantation time and finally the mass disappeared from the implanted site, indicating that, as expected, the hydrogels were degraded in vivo. The degradation period of gelatin hydrogels depended on their water content: the higher the water content of hydrogels, the faster their degradation. The in vivo hydrogel degradation was also assessed based on radioactivity loss of ^{125}I-labeled gelatin hydrogels in the mouse subcutis. The time profile of the radioactivity loss was in good accordance with that of the weight loss. Change in the degradation period of hydrogels from 5 days to 5 weeks was possible when their water content was changed and their degradation profile was not influenced by bFGF incorporation. Gelatin microspheres were also degraded in vivo in the similar fashion (22). The radioactivity of ^{125}I-labeled DTPA-introduced amylopectin hydrogels with Cu^{2+} chelation decreased with implantation time, clearly indicating in vivo degradation of the hydrogels (25).

VI. IN VIVO GROWTH FACTOR RELEASE

To assess in vivo bFGF release, acid gelatin hydrogels incorporating ^{125}I-labeled bFGF were implanted subcutaneously into the back of mice and their residual radioactivity was measured at different time intervals (28,29). The residual radioactivity decreased with implantation time, without detection of radioactivity in the blood, indicating controlled release of bFGF from the bFGF-incorporating gelatin hydrogel around the implanted site. The decrement pattern of radioactivity depended on the hydrogel degradability in such a manner that the radioactivity was retained for a longer time as the hydrogel water content decreased. The time profile of bFGF radioactivity was in accordance with that of hydrogel radioactivity, irrespective of the hydrogel water content. The retention of bFGF in gelatin hydrogels with different water contents was found to be linearly related to that of the hydrogels (Fig. 3). It seems reasonable to suppose that bFGF was released from the gelatin hydrogel probably together with degraded gelatin fragments in the body as a result of hydrogel degradation.

DTPA-introduced amylopectin hydrogels incorporating ^{125}I-labeled bFGF with or without Cu^{2+} chelation were subcutaneously implanted to assess the in vivo bFGF release. The radioactivity of bFGF in the solution form decreased rapidly from the injected site within a day. More radioactivity was retained and for a longer time after implantation of DTPA-introduced amylopectin hydrogels incorporating ^{125}I-labeled bFGF with Cu^{2+} chelation than that of other

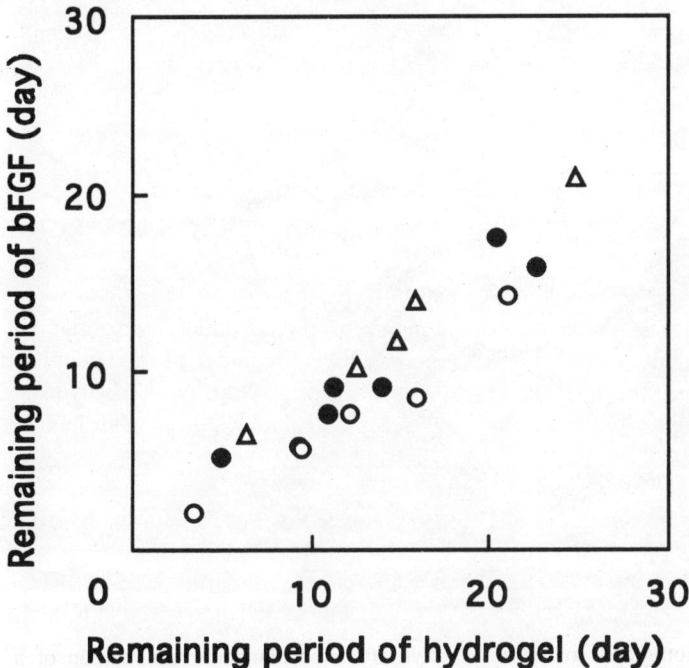

Figure 3 Relationship between periods of bFGF and gelatin hydrogel at which (○) 80, (●) 50, and (△) 20% of the initial radioactivity remain, after implantation of ^{125}I-labeled bFGF-incorporating acidic gelatin hydrogels with different water contents into the back subcutis of mice.

hydrogels, while any radioactivity of bFGF was not detectable in the blood. A correlation of the in vivo retention between bFGF and the hydrogel suggested bFGF release from the hydrogel based on hydrogel degradation (25).

VII. NEOVASCULARIZATION INDUCED BY BIODEGRADABLE HYDROGELS INCORPORATING GROWTH FACTOR

The most important concern on protein delivery is whether or not the protein released actually retains its biological activity. To evaluate this protein activity, in vitro culture techniques are normally employed because of their simplicity and convenience compared with in vivo animal experiments. However, no in vitro nondegradation experiment can be applied to our hydrogel release system. This is because the growth factor release is involved with the in vivo degradation of hydrogel matrices as described previously. Thus, the neovascularization effect following subcutaneous implantation of biodegradable hydrogels incorporating bFGF or VEGF was examined to assess their biological activity.

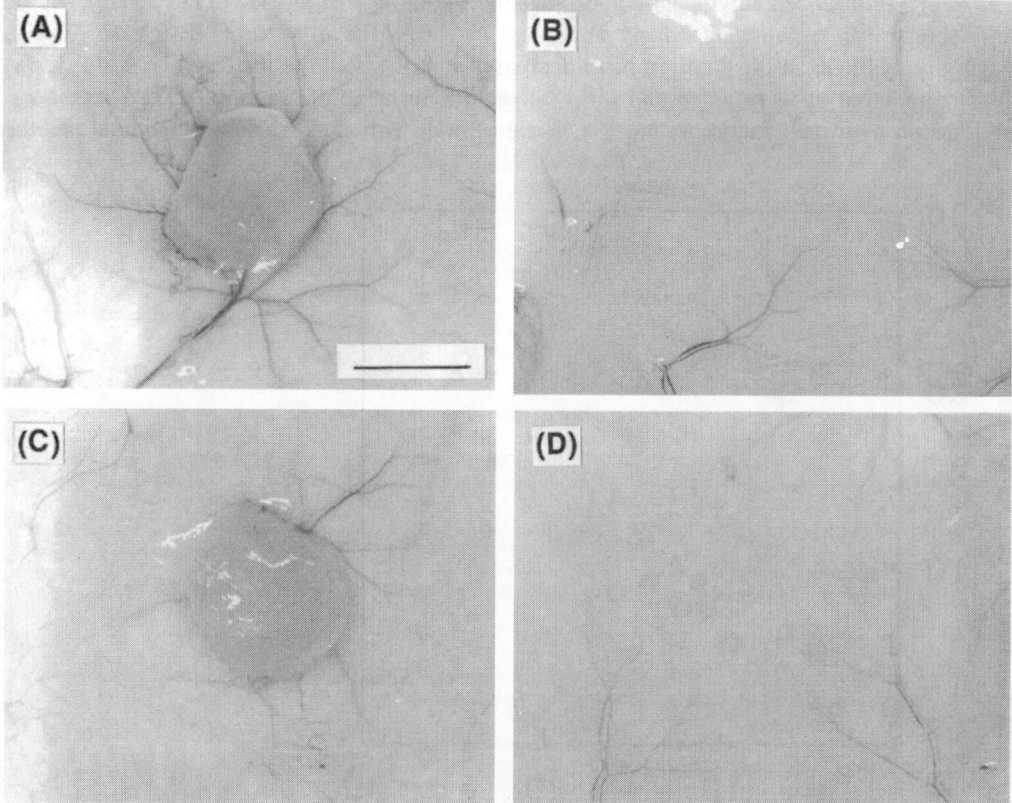

Figure 4 Optical microscopic photographs of tissues 7 days after subcutaneous implantation of a VEGF-incorporating acidic gelatin hydrogel and other agents. Mice were treated with (A) a gelatin hydrogel incorporating 2 μg of VEGF, (B) 2 μg of free VEGF, (C) a VEGF-free gelatin hydrogel, and (D) PBS. The back skin was torn off and photographs of the tissue around the treated site on the skin side were taken. The hydrogel water content was 95 wt%. A bar corresponds to 5 mm.

Remarkable vascularization was demonstrated around the implanted site of the acidic gelatin hydrogels incorporating bFGF by histological examination (20). bFGF-free gelatin hydrogels alone did not induce any vascularization. The bFGF-induced neovascularization effect notably increased within 1 day after hydrogel implantation and retained for 1 week at a significantly high level, followed by no detection at day 14. On the other hand, no vascularization was induced by injection of aqueous solution containing the same dose of bFGF as the bFGF hydrogel over the time range studied, which is similar to PBS-injected or untreated mice. No vascularization induction by bFGF solution, even at higher injection doses, is due to a rapid elimination of bFGF from the injected site. To the contrary, incorporation of bFGF into the acidic gelatin hydrogel enabled us to reduce the dose effective in inducing significant vascularization. Another angiogenetic growth factor, VEGF with an IEP of 9.5, was applied to the hydrogel release system on the basis of polyion complexation. Neovascularization was detected around the implanted site of a VEGF-incorporating gelatin hydrogel, in remarked contrast for free VEGF (Fig. 4).

Even after being implanted in the mouse subcutis for various time periods, bFGF-incorporating gelatin hydrogels still had the ability to induce significant neovascularization (Fig. 5). Their activity of neovascularization induction seemed to decrease as the preimplantation time was prolonged. Thus, this finding clearly indicates that the gelatin hydrogel system

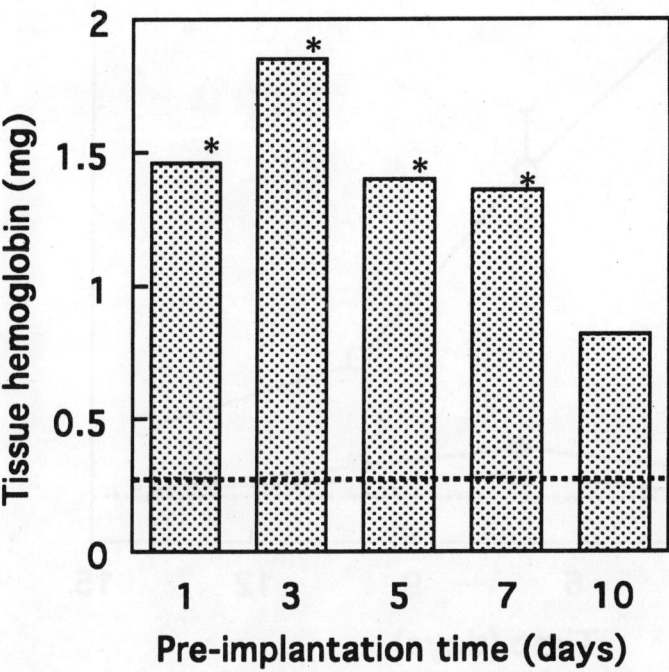

Figure 5 The time course of neovascularization induced by pre-implanted bFGF-incorporating gelatin hydrogels with a water content of 97.6%. The bFGF-incorporating gelatin hydrogels were pre-implanted into the back subcutis of mice, being placed in a diffusion chamber for various days described in the x axis. The bFGF-incorporating gelatin hydrogels explanted were again implanted without the diffusion chamber and their neovascularization was evaluated 3 days after implantation. The neovascularization effect was evaluated by measuring the amount of tissue hemoglobin around the implanted hydrogel. A dotted line indicates the tissue hemoglobin level in the corresponding area of untreated, normal mice. * indicates significant at $p < 0.05$ against the value of untreated, normal mice.

can release bFGF with the biological activity remaining even after placed in the body, although it is impossible to quantitatively assess the remaining percentage of the activity (28,29). Neovascularization was significantly induced by bFGF-incorporating gelatin hydrogels, irrespective of the water content, but the period of retained vascularization became longer with the decreased water content. This can be explained in terms of controlled release of bFGF. In our release system, the period of bFGF release is governed by the hydrogel degradability. The hydrogels with lower water content will be degraded in vivo more slowly and consequently release bFGF for a longer time than those with higher water content, resulting in the prolonged period of hydrogel-induced neovascularization.

The bFGF-incorporating acidic gelatin microspheres of injection type were effective in inducing remarkable vascularization (21,22). Neither bFGF in solution form nor bFGF-free gelatin microspheres alone induced vascularization at the injected site. In a time course study, the vascularization effect increased within a day of microsphere injection and was retained at a significantly high level to day 7, followed by gradual disappearance thereafter (Fig. 6). The

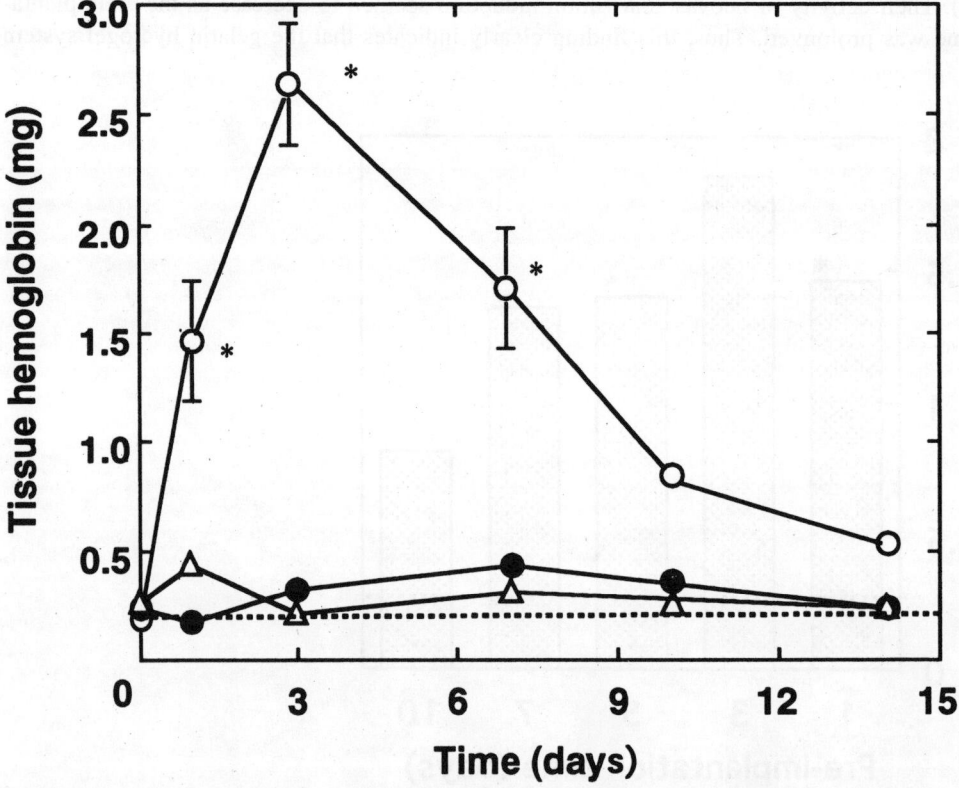

Figure 6 The time course of neovascularization effect induced by free bFGF and bFGF-incorporating acidic gelatin microspheres. Mice received subcutaneous injection of (○) gelatin microspheres incorporating 100 μg of bFGF, (●) 100 μg of free bFGF, and (△) bFGF-free gelatin microspheres. The neovascularization effect was evaluated by measuring the amount of tissue hemoglobin around the implanted hydrogel. A dotted line indicates the tissue hemoglobin level in the corresponding area of untreated, normal mice. The water content of microspheres was 95 vol%. *indicates significance at $p<0.05$ against the value of control mice at the corresponding day.

microspheres were completely resorbed around 14 days post injection. Thus, similar to the hydrogel system described above, this microsphere system exhibited a correlation in the time profile between the vascularization and hydrogel degradation, indicating controlled release of biologically active bFGF based on microsphere degradation.

DTPA-introduced amylopectin hydrogels incorporating bFGF with Cu^{2+} chelation induced significantly vascularization around the implanted site. This was in marked contrast to that without Cu^{2+} chelation. bFGF-free amylopectin hydrogels exhibited no vascularization, irrespective of Cu^{2+} chelation and DTPA introduction. The enhanced neovascularization effect was observed over 8 days from the third day of hydrogel implantation and thereafter disappearing with time, which correlated with the time profile of hydrogel degradation (25). It is likely that bFGF is released from this amylopectin hydrogel system according to the hydrogel degradation-driven mechanism as described in Fig. 1.

VIII. AN APPLICATION OF GELATIN MICROSPHERES INCORPORATING bFGF TO ISCHEMIC MYOCARDIUM

Yanagisawa-Miwa et al. (30) reported that during an acute myocardial infarction in a dog model, intracoronary administration of bFGF reduced the infarct size and increased the number of capillaries and arterioles in the treated territory. Periadventitial local delivery of bFGF by use of heparin-alginate beads improved a regional ventricular function in chronically ischemic myocardium of pigs with little systemic loss (31). Our hydrogel release system was applied to this therapeutic myocardial angiogenesis. When gelatin microspheres incorporating 100 μg of bFGF were subepicardially injected to several sites around the occlusion coronary artery of a dog model, the myocardial blood flow in the ischemic region was significantly increased, in remarked contrast to the same dose of free bFGF and bFGF-free, empty gelatin microspheres (Fig. 7). This clearly demonstrates feasibility of local bFGF delivery in improving collateral circulation at the myocardial infarct area.

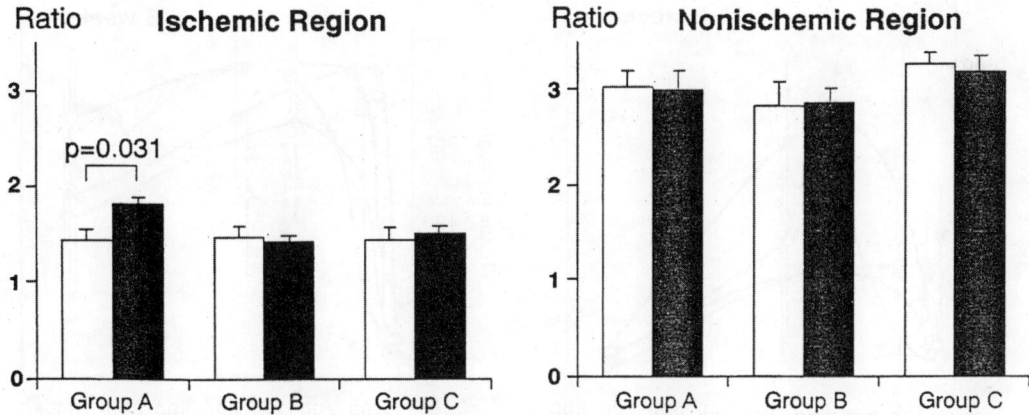

Figure 7 Change of regional myocardial blood flow in the ischemic and nonischemic regions of dog hearts before (□) and after bFGF treatments (■): bFGF-incorporating gelatin microspheres (Group A), bFGF in the solution form (Group B), and bFGF-free gelatin microspheres (Group C). The bFGF dose was 100 μg/dog.

IX. VASCULARIZATION INTO SCAFFOLD FOR TISSUE ENGINEERING

Porous biomaterials have been prepared from poly(lactic acid), its copolymers with glycolic acid, collagen, and hydroxyapatite to demonstrate the feasibility as scaffolds for cell seeding and tissue regeneration (32–38). The scaffolds have functioned expectedly as a temporary substrate for proliferation and differentiation of the cells seeded or have infiltrated from the surrounding host tissue, and have finally been integrated into or degraded in the regenerated tissue. However, the seeded cells do not always survive for a long time in a scaffold because oxygen and nutrients are not sufficiently supplied to the transplanted cells in the scaffold because of the poor diffusion. Such insufficient supplies will also prevent cell infiltration from the surrounding host tissue. It is promising for this end to induce neovascularization into the scaffold.

This vascularization was achieved by the gelatin hydrogel system for controlled release of bFGF. When homogeneously injected into poly(vinyl alcohol) (PVA) sponges with different pore sizes, followed by subcutaneous implantation, bFGF-incorporating gelatin microspheres appeared to have more markedly promoted the ingrowth of fibrous tissue accompanied by new capillary formation into sponges than free bFGF (Fig. 8). The sponge pore size had a great influence on the ingrowth of fibrous tissue into the sponges. The tissue ingrowth seemed to be highest around a pore size of 250 μm. The bFGF-incorporating gelatin microspheres enabled PVA sponges to form new capillaries therein at a higher rate and more deeply into the interior region than free bFGF. Enhanced capillary formation was noted for PVA sponges with medium pore sizes of 250 and 350 μm than with the smaller or larger sizes. These findings indicate that, even though incorporated in the PVA sponge, our release system of bFGF with gelatin microspheres incorporating bFGF induced neovascularization to a significantly higher extent than bFGF in the solution form. Empty gelatin microspheres induced neither tissue ingrowth nor neovascularization into sponges (39).

Such a vascularization procedure enabled transplanted hepatocytes to proliferate in a PVA sponge. A PVA sponge with a pore size of 250 μm was injected with bFGF-incorporating gelatin microspheres and then implanted at the rat mesentery, followed by 1-week implantation

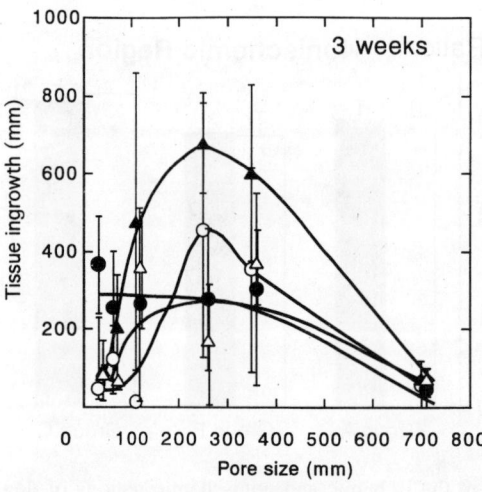 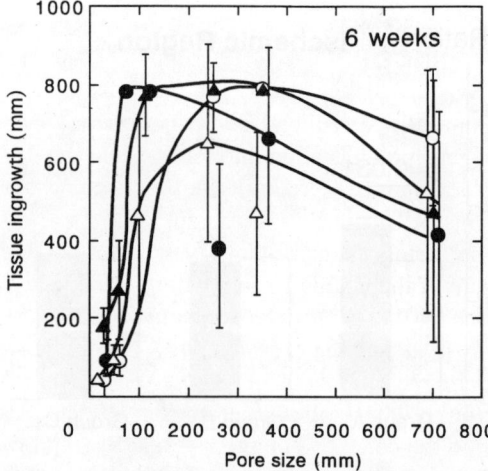

Figure 8 The effect of pore size on the ingrowth of fibrous tissue accompanied with new capillary formation into PVA sponges injected with PBS (○), free bFGF (●), empty gelatin microspheres (△), and bFGF-incorporating gelatin microspheres (▲). The sponge sections were viewed 3 and 6 weeks after implantation in the back subcutis of mice. The bFGF dose was 100 μg/mouse.

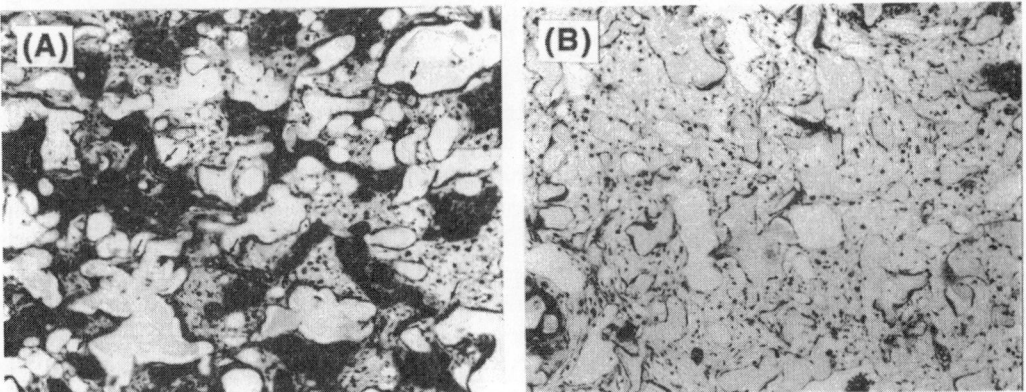

Figure 9 Histological observation of rat hepatocytes in the PVA sponge prevascularized by gelatin microspheres incorporating bFGF. Rat hepatocytes were injected into the PVA sponge which had been implanted at the rat mesentery for 7 days. The sponge was homogeneously injected with gelatin microspheres incorporating 100 μg of bFGF (A) and PBS (B). Arrows indicate capillaries newly formed in the PVA sponges. Histological sections were viewed at magnification of 100 following hematoxylin-eosin staining.

for vascularization into the sponge. Rat hepatocytes injected into the prevascularized sponge seemed to survive, whereas the cells died in the sponge without bFGF treatment (Fig. 9). This is because prevascularization induced by our release system was useful enough to provide the transplanted cells with oxygen and nutrients for their survival. It has been reported that hepatocytes seeded into porous biodegradable scaffolds survived in vivo when transplanted at the rat mesentery where blood vessels are abundant (33,34).

X. PROMOTED DERMIS REGENERATION BY GELATIN MICROSPHERES INCORPORATING bFGF

An acellular artificial skin called Pelnac, (Gunze Ltd., Kyoto, Japan) composed of an inner collagen sponge and an outer silicone layer, has been commercialized. The pores of the inner collagen sponge were infiltrated by fibroblasts and capillaries when it was placed on skin defects. This cell-infiltrated membrane was gradually converted to a connective tissue matrix similar to the dermis as the original network of collagen sponge was biodegraded. Postoperative contracture of the wound treated with the artificial skin was significantly less than that of the untreated one (40). The clinical investigation similarly revealed the advantageous results, but infection arose as another problem (41). A significant decrease in the infection rate may be due to expertise of clinicians in technology, taking into consideration that the material is prone to infection. It will be another promising strategy for reduced infection to accelerate neovascularization into the collagen sponge layer. Thus, the bFGF-incorporating gelatin microsphere was used for neovascularization in the collagen layer of Pelnac. When the Pelnac following homogeneous injection of the microspheres was grafted onto the full-thickness skin defect of guinea pigs, neovascularization as well as fibrous tissue ingrowth into the collagen layer was promoted to a significantly greater extent than that of the original Pelnac (Fig. 10). Neither granulation nor wound contraction by bFGF treatment was observed at the defect treated.

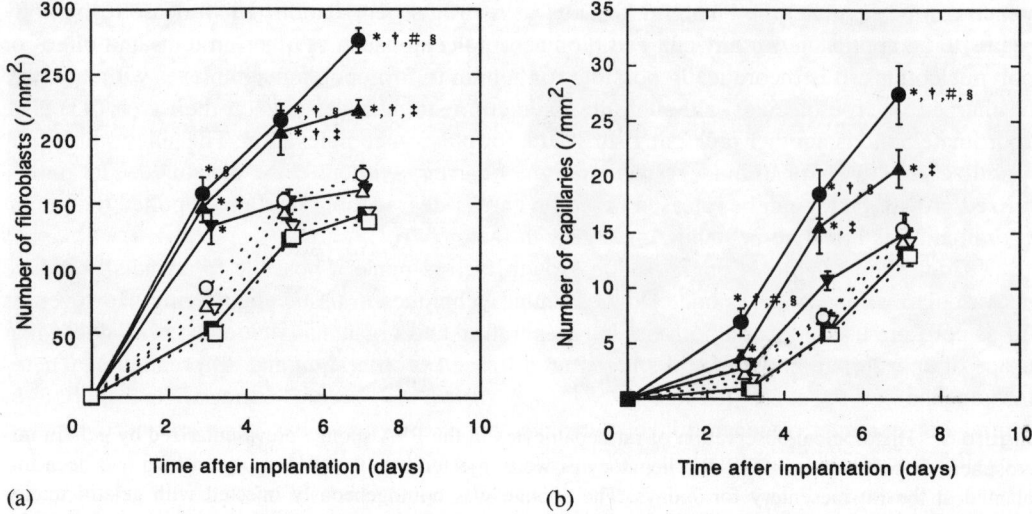

Figure 10 The time course of fibroblast infiltration (a) and new capillary formation (b) in the collagen sponge layer of acellular artificial skin, Pelnac® after grafting into the full-thickness skin defect of guinea pigs. The sponge was homogeneously injected with bFGF-free gelatin microspheres (■) and gelatin microspheres incorporating 10 (▼), 50 (▲), and 100 μg of bFGF (●) or PBS (□) and PBS containing 10 (▼), 50 (△), and 100 μg of bFGF (○).
*, $p < 0.05$ significant against the group of PVA sponges injected with bFGF-free gelatin microspheres
†, $p < 0.05$ significant against the group of PVA sponges injected with gelatin microspheres incorporating 10 μg of bFGF
#, $p < 0.05$ significant against the group of PVA sponges injected with gelatin microspheres incorporating 50 μg of bFGF
‡, $p < 0.05$ significant against the group of PVA sponges injected with 50 μg of free bFGF
§, $p < 0.05$ significant against the group of PVA sponges injected with 100 μg of free bFGF

XI. CONCLUSIONS

Regeneration and substitution of human tissues and organs by use of growth factors and cells are exciting and important scientific developments. This area is called *tissue engineering*, which requires controlled release of growth factors as one of the essential technologies. Necessity for controlled release of proteins will increasingly become larger in concert with their production on an industrial scale. However, little has been reported on technology that can achieve the controlled release of proteins under the maintenance of biological activity. The main reason may be that recombinant bioactive proteins, including growth factors, are at present expensive and still difficult to obtain even when available commercially. Our technology for the release of growth factor is based on the molecular interaction between the protein and the polymer constituting a hydrogel, as well as hydrogel degradation. Actually, such a release system is commonly observed in the body between growth factor and the extracellular matrix (ECM). It is known that the growth factor immobilized to the ECM through a certain intermolecular force is released based on enzymatic degradation of the matrix substance. Interaction with biological macromolecules existing in the ECM enables growth factor to regulate its biological functions (42). Therefore, it will be useful for controlled release of growth factor to learn such in vivo storage techniques. The gelatin hydrogel system described in this chapter is one that mimics natural release mechanisms. Biologically active growth factor is released over a certain period of time, which can be regulated by changing the rate of hydrogel degradation. This release technology seems to be applicable for any charged biomacromolecule, such as other proteins and oligo- or polynucleotides. It is theoretically possible for gelatin to form polyion complexes with any type of charged macromolecules, although the interaction strength depends on their type (43). The coordinate bond is another promising substitute for polyion complexation. This allows us to immobilize growth factor to biodegradable polymer carriers without being denatured. The immobilized growth factor can be released based on carrier degradation. It is also reported that metal coordination is effective in stabilizing a growth factor (44).

Controlled release of angiogenetic growth factors made it possible to artificially induce neovascularization, which is one of the essential techniques in tissue engineering. However, as far as cells are used to assist both tissue regeneration and organ substitution, it is no doubt that usage of appropriate growth factors is required for cell proliferation and differentiation. Therefore, technology for controlled release of growth factors will become increasingly important in future. For example, regeneration of cartilage, bone, and nerve has been enhanced through growth factor release, in remarked contrast to growth factor in the free form (19,45–49).

ACKNOWLEDGMENT

Research described in this chapter was supported by a grant from the Research for the Future Program of the Japan Society for the Promotion of Science (JSPS-RFTF96100203).

REFERENCES

1. Gombotz, W. R. and Pettit, D. K., 1995. Biodegradable polymers for protein and peptide delivery. Bioconj. Chem., 6: 332–351.
2. Banga, A. K., 1995. Therapeutic Peptides and Proteins, Formulation, Processing, and Delivery Systems, Technomic Publishing Co. Ltd., Basel, Switzerland.
3. Okada, H., 1997. Biodegradable microspheres for therapeutic peptide delivery, Adv. Drug Delivery Rev., 28: 1–170.
4. Cohen, S. and Bernstein, H., 1996. Microparticulate Systems for the Delivery of Proteins and Vaccines, Marcel Dekker, Inc., New York, USA.
5. Ikada, Y., 1998. Peptide release from polymer matrices. Adv. Drug. Deliv. Rev., 31(3): 183–318.
6. Hora, M. S., Rana, R. K., Nunberg, J. H., Tice, T. R., Gilley, R. M., and Hudson, M. E., 1990. Release of human serum albumin from poly(lactide-co-glycolide) microspheres. Pharm. Res., 7: 1190–1194.
7. Cohen, S., Yoshioka, T., Lucarelli, M., Hwang, L. H., and Langer, R., 1991. Controlled delivery systems for protein based on poly(lactic/glycolic acid) microspheres. Pharm. Res., 8: 713–720.
8. Tabata, Y., Takebayashi, Y., Ueda, T., and Ikada, Y., 1993. A formulation method using D,L-lactic acid oligomer for protein release with reduced initial burst. J. Controlled Release, 23: 55–64.
9. Park, K., Shalaby, W. S., and Park, H., 1993. Biodegradable Hydrogels for Drug Delivery. Technomic, Basel, Switzerland.
10. Dumitriu, S., 1996. Polysaccharides in Medical Applications, Marcel Dekker, New York.
11. Hara, M., 1993. Polyelectrolytes. Marcel Dekker, New York.
12. Dubin, P., Beck, J., Davies, R. M., Schulz, D. H., and Thies, C., 1994. Macromolecular Complexes in Chemistry and Biology. Springer-Verlag, Berlin.
13. Yip, T.-T. and Hutchens, T. W., 1994. Immobilized metal ion affinity chromatography. Mol. Biotechnol., 1: 151–164.
14. Porath, J., Carlsson, J., Olsson, J., and Belfrage, G., 1975. Metal chelate affinity chromatography: a new approach to protein fractionation. Nature, 258: 598–599.

15. Sulkowski, E., 1985. Purification of proteins by IMAC. Trend in Biotechnology, 3: 1–7.
16. Kroiher, M., Raffioni, S., and Steele, R. E., 1995. Single step purification of biologically active recombinant rat basic fibroblast growth factor by immobilized metal affinity chromatography. Biochim. Biophys. Acta, 1250: 29–34.
17. Zekorn, D., 1969. Modified gelatin as plasma substitutes. Bibl. Maematol., 33: 30–60.
18. Veis, A., 1964. The Macromolecular Chemistry of Gelatin. Academic Press, New York.
19. Tabata, Y., Yamada, K., Miyamoto, S., Nagata, I., Kikuchi, H., Aoyama, I., Tamura, M., and Ikada, Y., 1998. Bone regeneration by basic fibroblast growth factor complexed with biodegradable hydrogels. Biomaterials, 19: 807–815.
20. Tabata, Y., Hijikata, S., and Ikada, Y., 1994. Enhanced vascularization and tissue granulation by basic fibroblast growth factor impregnated in gelatin hydrogels. J. Controlled Release, 31: 189–199.
21. Tabata, Y. and Ikada. Y., 1995. Potentiated in vivo biological activity of basic fibroblast growth factor by incorporation into polymer hydrogel microsphere. Proc. 4th Jpn. Int. SAMPLE Symp., 4: 25–29.
22. Tabata, Y., Hijikata, S., Muniruzzaman, Md., and Ikada, Y., 1999. Neovascularization effect of biodegradable gelatin microspheres incorporating basic fibroblast growth factor. J. Biomater. Sci., Polym. Ed., 10: 79–94.
23. Tabata, Y., Morimoto, K., Katsumata, H., Yaguta, T., and Ikada, Y., 1999. Surfactant-free preparation of biodegradable hydrogel microspheres for protein release. J. Bioactive Biocompat. Polym., 14: 371–384.
24. Kang, H.-W., Tabata, Y., and Ikada, Y., 1999. Fabrication of porous gelatin scaffolds for tissue engineering. Biomaterials, 20: 1339–1344.
25. Tabata, Y., Matsui, Y., and Ikada, Y., 1998. Growth factor release from amylopectin hydrogel based on copper coordination. 56: 135–148.
26. Tabata, Y., Nagano, A., Muniruzzman, Md., and Ikada, Y., 1998. In vitro sorption and desorption of basic fibroblast growth factor from biodegradable hydrogels. 19: 1781–1789.
27. Dolezal, J., Klausen, K. S., and Langmyhr, F. J., 1973. Studies in the complex formation of metal ions with sugars. I. The complex formation of cobalt (II), cobalt (III), cupper (II) and nickel (II) with mannitol. Anal. Chim. Acta, 63: 71–77.
28. Tabata, Y., Nagano, A., and Ikada, Y., 1999. Biodegradation of hydrogel carrier incorporating fibroblast growth factor. Tissue Eng., 5: 127–138.
29. Tabata, Y. and Ikada, Y., 1998. Protein release from gelatin matrices. Adv. Drug Delivery Rev., 31: 287–301.
30. Yanagisawa-Miwa, A., Uchida, Y., Nakamura, F., Tomaru, T., Kido, H., Kamijo, T., Sugimoto, T., Kaji, K., Utsuyama, M., Kurashima, C., and Ito, H., 1992. Salvage of infarct myocardium by angiogenic action of basic fibroblast growth factor. Science, 257: 1401–1403.
31. Harada, K., Grossman, W., Friedmen, M., edelman, E. R., Prasad, P. V., Keighley, C. S., Manning, W. J., Sellke, F. W., and Simons, M., 1994. Basic fibroblast growth factor improves myocardial function in chronically ischemic procine hearts. J. Clin. Invest., 94: 623–630.
32. Freed, L. E., Marquis, J. C., Nohria, A., Emmanual, J., Mikos, A. G., and Langer, R., 1993. Neocartilage formation in vitro and in vivo using cells cultured on synthetic biodegradable polymers. J. Biomed. Mater. Res., 27: 11–23.
33. Mooney, D. J., Kaufmann, P. M., Sano, K., Mcnamara, K. M., Vacanti, J. P., and Langer R., 1994. Transplantation of hepatocytes using porous, biodegradable sponges. Transplant. Proc., 26: 3425–3426.
34. Robinson, B. P., Hollinger, J. O., Szachowicz, E. H., and Brekke, J., 1995. Calvarial bone repair with poroud D,L-polylactide. Otolaryngol. Head Neck Surg., 112: 707–713.
35. Wang J. W. and Aspenberg, P., 1996. Basic fibroblast growth factor promotes bone ingrowth in porous hydroxyapatite. Clin. Orthop. Rel. Res., 333: 252–260.
36. D. J. Mooney, D. J., K. Sano, K., P. M. Kaufmann, P. M., K. Majahod, K., B. Schloo, B., J. P. Vacanti, J. P., and R. Langer, R., 1997. Long-term engraftment of hepatocytes transplanted on biodegradable polymer sponges. J. Biomed. Mater. Res., 37: 413–420.
37. S. P. Andrade, S. P., R. D. P. Machado, R. D. P., A. S. Teixeira, A. S., A. V. Belo, A. V., A. M. Tarso, A. M., and W. T. Beraldo, W. T., 1997. Sponge-induced angiogenesis in mice and the pharmacolog-

ical reactivity of the neovasculature quantitated by a fluorimetric method. Microvasc. Res., 54: 253–261.
38. Chaignaud, B. E., Langer, R., and Vacanti, J. P., 1997. The history of tissue engineering using synthetic biodegradable polymer scaffolds and cells. In: A. Atala, D. J. Mooney, J. P. Vacanti, and R. Langer (Eds.), Synthetic Biodegradable Polymer Scaffolds, Birkhauser, Boston, pp. 1–14.
39. Yamamoto, M., Tabata, Y., Kawasaki, H., and Ikada, Y., 2000. Promotion of fibrovascular tissue ingrowth into porous sponges by basic fibroblast growth factor. J. Materilas Sci. Mater. Med. 11:1–6.
40. Suzuki, S., Matsuda, K. Isshiki, N., Tamada, Y., Yoshioka, K., and Ikada, Y., 1990. Experimental study of a newly developed bilayer artificial skin. Biomaterials, 11: 356–372.
41. Suzuki, S., Matsuda, K., Nishimura, Y., Maruguchi, Y., Maruguchi, T., Ikada, Y., Morita, S., and Morota, K., 1996. Review of acellular and cellular artificial skins. Tissue Eng., 2: 267–275.
42. Taipale, J. and Keski-Oja, J., 1997. Growth factors in the extracellular matrix. FASEB J., 11: 51–59.
43. Tabata, Y., Yamamoto, M., and Ikada, Y., 1997. Comparison of release profiles of various growth factors from biodegradable carriers. In: R. C. Thomson, D. J. Mooney, K. V. Healy, Y. Ikada, and A. G. Mikos (Eds.), Biomaterials Regulating Cell Function and Tissue Development, Materials Research Society Symposium Proceedings Vol. 530, Warrendale, PA, pp. 13–18.
44. Cunningham, B. C., Mulkerrin, M. G., and Wells, A. M., 1991. Dimerization of human growth hormone by zinc. Science, 253: 545–548.
45. Fujisato, T., Sajiki, N., Liu, Q., and Ikada, Y., 1996. Effect of fibroblast growth factor on cartilage regeneration in chondrocyte-seeded collagen sponge scaffold. Biomaterials, 17: 155–162.
46. Yamamoto, M., Tabata, Y., and Ikada, Y., 1998. Ectopic bone formation induced by biodegradable hydrogels incorporating bone morphogenetic protein. J. Biomater. Sci., Polym. Ed., 9: 439–458.
47. Hong, L., Tabata, Y., Yamamoto, M., Miyamoto, S., Yamada, K., Hashimoto, N., and Ikada, Y., 1998. Comparison of bone regeneration in a rabbit skull defect by recombinant human BMP-2 incorporated in biodegradable hydrogel and in solution. J. Biomater. Sci., Polym. Ed., 9: 1001–1014.
48. Tabata, Y., Yamamoto, M., and Ikada, Y., 1998. Biodegradable hydrogels for bone regeneration through growth factor release. Pure Appl. Chem., 70: 1277–1282.
49. Ide, C., Tohyama, K., Tajima, K., Endoh, K., Sano, K., Tamura, M., Mizoguchi, A., Kitada, M., Morihara, T., and Shirasu, M., 1998. Lone acellular nerve transplants for allogeneic grafting and the effects of basic fibroblast growth factor on the growth of regenerating axons in dogs: a preliminary study. Exp. Neurol., 154: 99–112.

35
Biopolymers for Release of Interleukin-2 for Treatment of Cancer

Debra J. Trantolo, Joseph D. Gresser, A. Ganiyu Jimoh, and Donald L. Wise
Cambridge Scientific, Inc., Cambridge, Massachusetts

James C. Yang
National Cancer Institute, National Institutes of Health, Bethesda, Maryland

I. INTRODUCTION

The objective of this study was to develop a means of locally delivering immunostimulatory proteins into tumors in order to enhance the immune response to these tumors. The delivery vehicle is based on the family of biodegradable, biocompatible polymers known as poly(lactic-co-glycolic acids) (PLGAs); the immunostimulatory protein is based on the immunomodulating cytokine known as interleukin-2 (IL-2). In pilot studies, a proprietary PLGA formulation of IL-2 was prepared and shown to maintain biological activity *in vitro*. The goal of these studies is to develop a controlled release approach for the 2- to 3-week treatment of cancer using only one long-acting dose of IL-2 incorporated into a biodegradable injectable polymer preparation. The active agent in this proposed system is IL-2; the biodegradable polymer carrier is PLGA. These initial studies deal with *in vitro* characterization and standardization of the biodegradable polymer preparations containing the selected cytokine and, importantly, the *in vivo* evaluation of prepared IL-2/polymer implants. Having shown that IL-2 can maintain biological activity, as demonstrated in *in vitro* pilot studies, the continued work will correlate that activity with total available protein and then establish the feasibility of tumor treatment by slow release IL-2 (SR-IL2) preparations. Feasibility will then be evaluated *in vivo* by measurement of the effects of SR-IL2 on augmentation of tumor-infiltrating lymphocyte (TIL) harvest, on modification of tumor growth patterns, and on stimulation of the immune response against a tumor antigen.

This work builds on pilot studies reported herein, carried out in collaboration with James C. Yang, M.D. and Christopher J. Bartels, M.D., under the direction of Stephen S. Rosenberg, M.D., Surgery Branch, National Cancer Institute, National Institutes of Health (NCI/NIH). Having established in related work that the controlled release of a number of traditional drugs and new biologicals are amenable to our proprietary formulation methods, we next will address the manipulation of processing parameters as a means of establishing uniform 2-to 3-week release of IL-2. Our pilot studies have shown that our injectable controlled release IL-2 system provides for substantial time periods of bioactive IL-2 release ranging from days to weeks. This 2-to 3-week system for cancer treatment clearly will alleviate significant problems in the logistics of using TILs and thereby "manually" enhancing the immune response to cancerous tumors.

II. BACKGROUND AND SIGNIFICANCE

Our overall goal is to develop means of locally delivering immunostimulatory proteins into tumors in order to enhance the immune response to those tumors. This immunologically favorable milieu is intended to foster the generation of T lymphocytes, which recognize and destroy tumors by the classical cellular arm of the immune response. Although this may lead to shrinkage of the treated tumor, it is unlikely to cause the destruction of other, distant tumors elsewhere in the body. Therefore, the strategy continues with the removal of the treated tumor and the immune cells propagated within it and the in vitro culture and expansion of those immune cells to large numbers. These TILs are then given into the bloodstream as a transfusion to treat tumors elsewhere in the animal (or patient). The latter part of this scenario has already been done in many patients within the Surgery Branch of the NCI and has shown dramatic effects in patients with incurable, metastatic melanoma (1–3). These results were obtained from tumors which had no cytokine enhancement or augmentation. Cambridge Scientific, Inc. and the NCI wish to pursue continued collaboration with respect to cytokine introduction (results of our pilot studies are given later). It is to be noted that earlier NIH/NCI staff utilized a simple collagen matrix, a diffusion-driven vehicle, to release IL at the site of an injected tumor and demonstrated that they could improve the therapeutic effects of TIL grown from those tumors in mice (4). However, the initial burst of protein release was high and the longer term release was minimal with this vehicle; it appeared far from optimal. Currently, release for a 2- to 3-week period is the objective. The immune response often requires this period for initiation, and the increasing number of immune cells puts increasing rather than decreasing demands on the cytokine substrates.

The cytokines of greatest interest are the following:

1. IL-2: Also known as T-cell growth factor, this 15,500 MW hydrophobic (native) glycoprotein is probably the most fundamental in augmenting a lymphocyte response to tumor. Although much of its effect can be obtained after the tumor is excised and placed with IL-2 in culture, it is possible that it has an important role early in the immune response such that local in vivo tumor instillation is still important. This cytokine is also the one available in the greatest quantity as a purified, nonglycosylated recombinant human protein that cross-reacts fully in the mouse. It is packaged as a lyophilized protein admixed with buffer constituents and sodium dodecyl sulfate (SDS) to solubilize the IL-2. It is this particular cytokine that we used in our pilot studies and will continue to use in our continued work, proposed herein. A review of other cytokines of potential future interest is given briefly in the following.

2. Interferon-γ (γ-IFN): This cytokine again has many functions, but those most important to our effort are the effects on the degree of expression of tumor antigens and major histocompatibility proteins on tumors. Both tumor-specific antigens and MHC molecules increase when tumors are exposed to γ-IFN, and this upregulation serves to make a tumor more immunologically "visible" to the immune system. Unfortunately γ-IFN is species-specific and thus the recombinant murine product must be used in preclinical studies and the recombinant human protein in clinical trials. Studies with murine tumors genetically altered to secrete murine γ-IFN have shown that the population of TIL obtained is therapeutically superior to control TIL, making this a particularly attractive candidate for study. Unfortunately, the murine γ-IFN supply is limited with, at most, milligram quantities available.

3. Granulocyte-macrophage colony-stimulating factor (GM-CSF): This cytokine again serves to stimulate the participants in early immune responses, with emphasis on the antigen-processing cell, typically a macrophage or dendritic cell. It is species-

specific, unlike IL-2, and murine material must be used for preclinical studies. It is also in short supply. Other experiments using immunization with tumors genetically altered to secrete GM-CSF show enhanced protection against tumor challenge by the wild-type unmodified parental tumor, suggesting that the augmented immune responses evoked will work against genetically unmodified tumors elsewhere. Experiments with systemic TIL therapy have not been done.

4. IL-6: Experience at NIH/NCI with IL-6 in a simple collagen matrix suggests that this lymphokine would also be an attractive one to study. It is not species-specific and human IL-6 will work in mouse models. Although the benefits of IL-6 were modest, the kinetics of the IL-6 release from matrix were far from satisfactory. Unfortunately, it is also in short supply.

By way of strategy, our team suggests initial development of an IL-2 sustained release formulation for in vivo murine testing. This product would use only human recombinant IL-2, which is available in the greatest supply. Murine models with tumors genetically modified to secrete IL-2 have shown impressive results in a mouse bladder tumor model. We make this recommendation because we believe the resulting product would require the least modification and revision when considering Food and Drug Administration (FDA) submissions and clinical testing.

Our overall plans, given in more detail later in this grant application, are briefly described in the following. We will first prepare and test IL-2/PLGA material for bioactivity testing in vitro and in vivo. Then we will inject this material in a microparticulate form into murine tumors in varying doses and schedules and compare the TIL growth from these tumors. Control tumors would be injected with IL-2 in a PLGA-free suspension. Then side-by-side titered efficacy studies would be done on these TIL populations in mice with metastatic tumors.

Based on our early pilot studies with IL-2, injectable PLGA/IL-2 microparticles will be used to test the cytokines. The total controlled release material needed would be relatively modest in the TIL augmentation experiments as only five animals need be maximally treated in each group, in each experiment, and on each dosage schedule. This would generate the TIL populations. Many more mice are needed to quantitatively test these TIL (but then these latter mice do not receive any controlled release material). To date our team has worked with vials of lyophilized IL-2. Each vial contains approximately 0.68 mg of protein which is 98.5% pure. Our overall objective is a controlled release formulation from this material that should have target characteristics of release for 2–3 weeks, with as sustained or steady release as possible, minimizing the initial release. The precise dose released is less important as long as the local concentration of the IL-2 is high enough to stimulate TIL; to determine one aspect of this a variety of doses were tested in animals. Because of these pilot studies, our project team is prepared to immediately continue the *in vitro* characterization and subsequent *in vivo* testing (in mice).

III. BACKGROUND ON CONTROLLED RELEASE

The research and development of biodegradable, biocompatible PLGA-based drug delivery systems is as follows. Early work focused on the delivery of "molecular drugs" where patient compliance or large-scale population treatment was a concern. In the last decade, while conventional molecular drugs still play a role in our delivery system development, work has focused on delivery of the newer "biologicals" where benign formulation methods and low-dose, parenteral delivery is required. This transition in the composition of the active agent coupled with increased regulatory scrutiny of delivery devices has led to development of low-temperature, nonsolvent formulation technologies for the delivery of active agents from PLGA-based dose forms (patent applicationsfor which have been submitted).

A. Molecular Drug Delivery

The first clinical application of a biodegradable drug delivery system in the United States was in the treatment of narcotic addictions (5–8). A removable spherical bead dose form was developed, which deterred patients from illicit removal but allowed for medical removal in emergencies requiring morphine administration. The final system, the first biodegradable delivery system approved by the FDA for clinical testing, was 70% naltrexone/30% PLGA-90:10. Another early project was done in collaboration with the Walter Reed Army Institute and investigated an injectable biodegradable controlled release system for malaria. This work, aimed mainly at overcoming compliance problems, dealt with a *dual-drug* system, which enabled synergistic drug effects resulting in much lower and thus more desirable drug doses. This work established the importance of polymer molecular weight and dispersity, as well as drug loading, in dosage forms of this type (9,10). Still another major project in the early years of delivery system development was one sponsored by the Population Council of Rockefeller University, and later by WHO, USAID, and NIH, which focused on fertility control (11,12). Investigated was a subcutaneous PLGA delivery system containing levonorgestrol for fertility regulation. Both implantable, removable rods and injectable powders were tested in small animals, dogs, and baboons for contraceptive activity and shown to be efficacious. These project examples underscore the long-standing interest and understanding of delivery system in terms of both the efficacy of the drug delivery system and the patient acceptance of the drug delivery system.

B. Biological Drug Delivery

The delivery of the new biologicals poses additional constraints on delivery system technology. While, indeed, it is true that lower doses of these drugs are usually required, it is also true that the biologicals are generally more sensitive to deactivation be it via denaturation, hydrolysis, etc. Thus, in any formulation, the first concern is the maintenance of biological activity. In work with these biologicals, nonsolvent incorporation methods have resulted in 100% recovery of activity with a number of biologicals, including follicle-stimulating hormone (FSH), IL-2, calcitonin, and luteinizing hormone–releasing hormone (LHRH), among others. Some examples of work on incorporation of sensitive peptide and protein drugs are summarized in Table 1.

Two types of formulation technologies have been practiced, one is referred to as "dry mix," the other as "polymeric foam," although the former has been under testing for a longer time. The reported IL-2 pilot work has exploited the use of both technologies for IL-2 incorpo-

Table 1 Peptide and Protein Drugs

Active agent	Application	Status
FSH	Superovulation in cattle	Rods tested in sheep for delivery, cows for efficacy (16-fold increase in ova vs. controls)
LHRH-agonist	Prostate cancer	Rods and powders tested in rats for delivery (6-month lifetime achieved)
IL-2	Tumor therapy	Powders tested in culture (1-week target delivery realized)
Calcitonin	Osteoporosis	Rods tested in sheep for delivery (2-week target delivery achieved)

ration. Comparison of data resulting from study of both methods allows selection of systems covering a wider range of loadings and durations than achievable by one technology.

C. Pilot Studies with IL-2/PLGA

Following is a summary of the status of the pilot studies being carried out in the collaboration between Cambridge Scientific, Inc. and the NCI.

1. IL-2 Used

The recombinant human IL-2 material was made by Dupont and carried no restriction on its use. Unfortunately, the exact composition of the vials was not available, except that they contained approximately 0.68 mg of IL-2 protein with buffer salts and a small amount of SDS. It is to be noted that NIH/NCI have used this material extensively, and its formulation and biological activity seem indistinguishable from other forms of commercially available IL-2.

2. Dry-Mix Preparation of SR-IL2

The contents of 12 vials of the Dupont IL-2 containing 0.68 mg of IL-2 per vial (as received by Cambridge Scientific from NCI) were combined with 3.25 g PLGA polymer in a glass jar that had been previously coated with a portion of the PLGA polymer. The mixture was rotated on a ball mill (without balls) for 24 h at 60 rpm to assure homogeneous distribution of IL-2 throughout the polymer. The IL-2/PLGA blend was loaded into a mold equipped with a 1.0-in.-diameter ram and a 1.0-mm-diameter extrusion die. The mixture was extruded under pressure using a Compac MPC 40-ID-3 hydraulic press. (These methods have been procedurally verified in previous Good Manufacturing Practice (GMP), work.) The IL-2/PLGA matrices were then ground and screened to less than 180 μm. The final formulation contained 0.25% IL-2 in PLGA.

3. Foam Preparation of SR-IL2

In formulating the foam-based IL-2 matrices, a polymer foam is first prepared. Then, following determination of the foam density, the foam is "loaded" with the drug. The IL-2-impregnated foam is extruded under pressure and the resulting matrix is ground and sieved as previously described. The foam matrices allow entrapment of the active agent within the pores of an open-celled polymer structure. A foam matrix distinguishes itself from a dry-mix matrix in its low initial burst of active agent and its lower rate of release.

A 452-mg polymer foam was impregnated under pressure with an aqueous solution containing 0.68 mg of the IL-2 in 20 mM phosphate buffer (pH 7.4). The solution impregnated foam was frozen and lyophilized at $-5°C$ to $7°C$ to constant weight. The IL-2/PLGA foam was extruded, ground, and sieved as previously described, yielding a final formulation 0.13% IL-2 in PLGA.

4. Results of Pilot Studies (Dry-Mixed Matrices)

It was first established by NIH/NCI (Dr. Yang) that the IL-2 from the above submitted samples of IL-2/PLGA was biologically active. However, there was still work to do on the kinetics of release from the initial dry-mixed IL-2 matrices. From the NIH/NCI assay of the Dupont IL-2, it was found that there was approximately 2366 U of IL-2 activity per microgram of protein. For the experimental results, discussed as follows, 40 mg of the IL-2/PLGA composite was suspended in 5 mL of complete medium (CM, which includes 10% fetal calf serum) at 37°C and

Table 2 Results of Pilot Studies on Dry-Mixed IL-2/PLGA Composites[a]

Time (hs)	Total IL-2 (U)
12	49,150
20	6,640
48	4,295
72	1,220
120	970
168	585
216	500
264 (11 days)	370

[a]IL-2 recovered in 11 days = 63,750 U or 26.9 μg.

the medium assayed at the time points listed in Table 2. Doctor Yang then centrifuged the tube and withdrew the medium and replaced it with 5 mL of fresh medium. The 5-mL aliquots were then assayed, and the total amount of IL-2 contained in the 5 mL was calculated; results are given in Table 2. (Note that Dr. Yang also did a similar experiment without changing the medium, (i.e., just sampling a tiny amount at successive times. However, that method showed very little change after the first 24 h.)

The results of the dry-mixed pilot studies may be explained as follows. As 40 mg of composite contains approximately 84 μg of IL-2 protein, then 32% of the total theoretical amount of IL-2 present eluted in 11 days. The data, presented in Fig. 1, show the rate of release of the 26.9 μg of activity that leached out over the 11 days, i.e., the release of IL-2 per hour at each of the time points tested (when the medium was changed). The graph is plotted in log form to better see the overall kinetics as well as the values at later time points when release was low. As is apparent, the initial burst was large; however, there was real and sustained release beyond a week. The assay has a reliable sensitivity down to 1 unit, but its interassay accuracy can be ±100% (due to the condition of the indicator cell line and the need for extensive serial dilutions). All values presented here were done in the same assay. Clearly, based on these pilot studies, the sustained release of IL-2 from IL-2/PLGA matrices was promising, but the initial burst is excessive. Note that with only fetal calf serum, saline, amino acids, and antibiotics present, we do not believe that degradation of the polymer was significant in the course of this study. The polymer does not undergo enzymatic lysis but rather only simple hydrolysis. We have now ways in which we can control this early large release of IL-2 by, for example, using a foam-

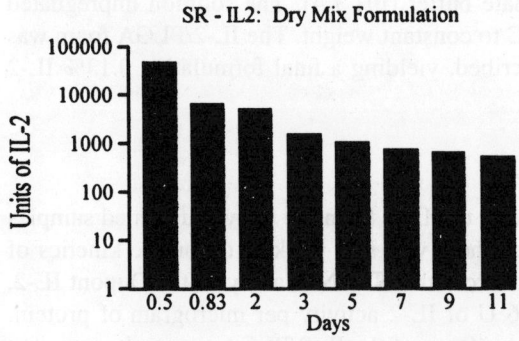

Figure 1 Results of pilot studies with dry-mixed IL-2/PLGA.

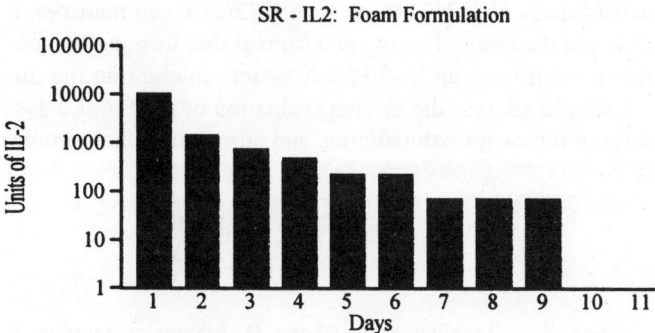

Figure 2 Results of pilot studies with foam-based IL-2/PLGA matrices.

based matrix. The IL-2/PLGA material for biological experiments, including histology in normal skin and multiple injections into tumors, should proceed immediately with work on a formulation with minimum early burst. This will almost certainly help in the animal experiments.

The results of pilot studies on foam matrices can be explained as follows: In order to slow the early burst of IL-2, foam-based IL-2/PLGA formulations were prepared. Fifty milligrams of the matrix (containing 0.065 mg IL-2) was weighed and placed in a 15 cm^3 conical tube with 5 mL CM. One milliliter aliquot samples were assayed daily and all medium was replaced daily. The results of the foam matrix IL-2 experiments are shown in Fig. 2. To compare, the total IL-2 released in the initial burst is substantially reduced in the foam-based samples. Correcting for the difference in total units available based on assayed mass (50 mg/assay with the dry-mixed samples and 40 mg/assay with the foam formulations), the total IL-2 released in the first 24 h is 55,790 U vs. 10,240 U for the dry-mix and the foam samples; thereafter, release is sustained for 9 days.

Release profiles for both systems yield release kinetics typical of diffusion-controlled matrix systems. A rapid initial release (early burst within 24 h) is followed by a slower release that is linear when plotted as cumulative percent release vs. the square root of time. Percent early burst and rate constants for the slow phases, calculated from the slopes of the kinetic plots, are given in Table 3.

These data indicate that the foam preparation releases more slowly in both the early burst phase and the slow controlled release phase. The early burst of IL-2 from the foam is only 20% as large as that for the dry-mixed preparation. Similary, the rate constant for release from the foam (following the 24-h early burst) is 37% as great as the rate constant for release from the dry mix. The fact that both systems display release kinetics in which cumulation percent release is proportional to the square root of time (following the early burst) is evidence that IL-2 release from PLGA is a diffusion-controlled process.

Although the initial target has been a 14-day release, it appears that further bioactivity testing is needed to confirm efficacy and determine whether any further modifications in the

Table 3 Percent Early Bursts and Rate Constants

	Foam	Dry Mix
Early burst (% release in first hours)	245.77	28.1
Sustained release phase rate constant, $h^{-1/2}$	0.058	0.156
(correlation coefficient)	(0.9917)	(0.9955)

formulation are necessary. On the basis of early NIH/NCI work with IL-2/collagen matrices, it is known that an early release of IL-2 is not desirable. Having determined that this can be controlled, the next steps are to investigate the utility of an IL-2/PLGA system in eliciting the immunoactivity that is desired. This work should address the in vivo evaluation of the SR-IL2 system in augmenting TIL harvest, modifying tumor growth patterns, and stimulating the immune response against a tumor antigen.

REFERENCES

1. S. A. Rosenberg, M. T. Lotze, J. C. Yang, S. L. Topalian, A. E. Chang, D. J. Schwartzentruber, P. Aebersold, S. Leitman, W. M. Linehan, C. A. Seipp, and D. E. White. Prospective randomized trial of high-dose interleukin-2 alone or in conjunction with lymphokine activated killer cells for the treatment of patients with advanced cancer, J. Natl. Cancer Inst., in press.
2. J. Weber, J. C. Yang, S. L. Topalian, D. R. Parkinson, D. J. Schwartzentruber, S. E. Ettinghausen, H. Gunn, A. Mixon, H. Kim, D. Cole, R. Levin, and S. A. Rosenberg. Phase I trial of subcutaneous interleukin-6 in patients with advanced malignancies, J. Clin. Oncol., 11, 449–506, 1993.
3. J. R. Lange, A. A. Raubitschek, B. A. Pockaj, W. F. Spencer, M. T. Lotze, S. L. Topalian, J. C. Yang, and S. A. Rosenberg. A pilot study of the cominbation of interleukin-2 based immunotherapy and radiation therapy, J. Immunol., 12, 265–271, 1992.
4. S. G. Marcus, L. D. Palmer, D. Perry-Lalley, J. J. Mule, S. A. Rosenberg, and J. C. Yang. The use of interleukin-6 to generate tumor-infiltrating lymphocytes with enhanced in vivo antitumor activity, J. Immunool., in press.
5. A. C. Sharon, and D. L. Wise. Development of drug delivery systems for use in treatment of narcotic addiction, in R. E. Willett, G. Barnett (Eds.), Narcotic Antagonists Naltrexone Pharmacochemistry and Sustained Release Preparation, NIDA Research Monograph, 28, DHHS publications (SM) No. 81-902, Washington, D.C., 1981.
6. R. H. Reuning, S. H. T. Liao, A. E. Staubus, S. B. Ashcraft, D. A. Downs, S. E. Harrigan, J. N. Wiley, and D. L. Wise. Pharmacokinetic quantitation of naltrexone controlled release from a copolymer delivery system, J Pharmaokinet. Biopharmaceut., 11, 369, 1983.
7. C. N. Chiang, L. E. Hollister, H. K. Gillespie, and R. L. Foltz. Clinical evaluation of a naltrexone sustained-release preparation, Drug Alcohol Dependence, 6, 1–8, 1985.
8. D. L. Wise, J. D. Gresser, and G. J. McCormick. Sustained release of a dual antimalarial system, J. Pharm. Pharmacol., 31, 201, 1979.
9. D. L. Wise, G. V. McCormick, and G. P. Willet. Sustained release of an anti-malarial drug using a copolymer of glycolic/lactic acid, Life Sci., 19, 867, 1976.
10. J. D. Gresser, D. L. Wise, L. R. Beck, and J. F. Hoses. Larger animal testing of an injectable sustained release fertility control system, Contraception, 17(3), 253, 1978.
11. J. D. Gresser, D. L. Wise, L. R. Beck, and J. F. Howes. Biodegradable cylindrical implants for fertility regulation in biodegradable delivery systems in contraception, 1, ESE Hafez (Ed.), Program for Applied Research in Fertility Regulation, Chicago, 1980.
12. P. R. J. Gangadharam, D. R. Ashtekar, D. C. Farhi, and D. L. Wise. Sustained release of isoniazid in vivo from a single implant of a biodegradable polymer, Tubercle, 72, 115–122, 1991.

36
Osmotic Drug Delivery from Asymmetric Membrane Film-Coated Dosage Forms

Mary Tanya am Ende, Scott M. Herbig, and Richard W. Korsmeyer
Pfizer Central Research, Groton, Connecticut

Mark B. Chidlaw
Bend Research, Inc., Bend, Oregon

I. INTRODUCTION

In this chapter we review the theory, design, and performance of asymmetric membrane film–coated systems that function by an osmotic drug release mechanism.

A. Oral Osmotic Systems

Osmotic drug delivery devices are composed of an osmotically active, drug-containing core dosage form surrounded by a rate-controlling, semipermeable membrane. The literature contains over 240 patented osmotic drug delivery systems, including variations in hydrogel driving layers (1). Osmotic drug delivery differs from diffusional-based systems in that the delivery of the active agent is driven by an osmotic gradient rather than by the concentration of drug in the device per se. Through the use of a semipermeable membrane and osmotic excipients, the rate of release of the drug can be made independent of such variables as pH and agitation rate. In addition, when properly designed, osmotic systems exhibit zero-order release of the drug because the drug content in the system (which is continuously depleting) does not affect the osmotic gradient. More sophisticated designs use a separate osmotic driving element ("push–pull" designs) or additional features, and can deliver the drug at increasing rates, introduce a delay before release begins, or achieve other release profiles (2). The design–performance characteristics of osmotic systems (pH and agitation–independence, reliable delivery profile) contribute to the robust clinical performance that is often observed with osmotic systems, including achievement of highly constant drug plasma concentrations, lack of a food effect, and, frequently, an *in vitro/in vivo* correlation (3–6).

The basic design of an elementary osmotic tablet is shown in Fig. 1. The drug is formulated in an osmotically active core and coated with a semipermeable membrane. The membrane is permeable only to water and not to the drug. The semipermeable membrane is pierced by a hole as shown. When this dosage form is placed in an aqueous environment, water is imbibed by osmosis and dissolves a portion of the drug. The imbibition of the water causes a slight

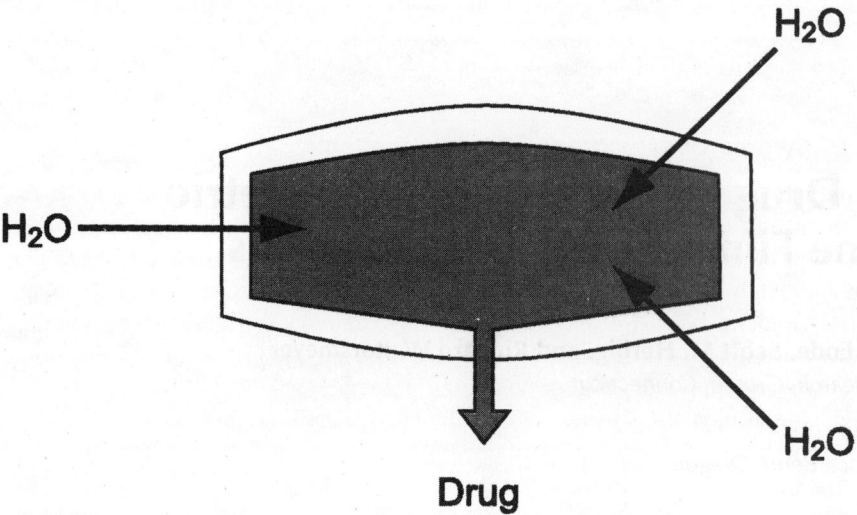

Figure 1 Schematic representation of an elementary osmotic tablet.

pressure rise inside the coated tablet, resulting in a convective flow of drug solution or suspension out through the delivery port. It is possible to design dosage forms so that drug release depends only on (a) the osmotic pressure of the drug core, (b) the thickness and permeability of the semipermeable membrane, and (c) the total area of the coating (6). All of these variables are under the control of the designer and do not vary under physiological conditions, leading to the robust performance alluded to above.

B. Marketed Products

While the concept of using osmotic pressure as a driving force for controlled release dates back at least to Rose and Nelson (1), the first successful pharmaceutical dosage forms were the Alza products based on the elementary osmotic pump concept. Later products were introduced based on the push–pull design in order to deliver higher doses of lower solubility drugs. Table 1 lists

Table 1 Marketed Osmotic Dosage Forms

Product name	Active	Design	Dose
Acutrim	Phenylpropanolamine	Elementary pump	75 mg
Alpress LP	Prazosin	Push–pull	2.5, 5 mg
Cardura XL	Doxazosin	Push–pull	4, 8 mg
Covera HS	Verapamil	Push–pull with time delay	180, 240 mg
Ditropan XL	Oxybutinin chloride	Push–pull	5, 10 mg
Dynacirc CR	Isradipine	Push–pull	5, 10 mg
Efidac 24	Pseudoephedrine	Elementary pump	60 mg IR, 180 mg CR
Efidac 24	Chlorpheniramine maleate	Elementary pump	4 mg IR, 12 mg CR
Glucotrol XL	Glipizide	Push–pull	5, 10 mg
Ivomec SR Bolus	Ivermectin	Push–pull	1.72 g total dose
Procardia XL	Nifedipine	Push–pull	30, 60, 90 mg
Sudafed 24-hour	Pseudoephedrine	Elementary pump	240 mg
Volmax	Albuterol	Elementary pump	4, 8 mg

IR, immediate release; CR, controlled release.

some osmotic dosage forms either that have been marketed or for which marketing approval is expected at the time of writing. The success of the osmotic approach to drug delivery is apparent from the number and diversity of products.

C. Features of Asymmetric Membrane Osmotic Systems

Asymmetric membrane (AM) film–coated delivery systems are a unique embodiment of osmotic devices in the use of phase inversion technology to create the semipermeable asymmetric membrane. As with other osmotic pumps, the AM drug delivery system releases the active ingredient by an osmotically controlled mechanism which, when properly constructed, delivers the active agent independently of pH or external agitation. The critical differentiating features that distinguish AM dosage forms from other osmotic devices are the high water permeability and controlled porosity resulting from the spray-coating process.

An elegantly simple appearing osmotic drug delivery technology developed jointly by Pfizer and Bend Research features an asymmetric membrane to control release (7). As the name indicates, the membrane structure is asymmetrical in nature and comprises a thin dense skin layer supported by a porous substructure as depicted in Fig. 2 (8). The membrane is formed by a phase inversion process controlled by the evaporation of a mixed solvent system.

There are several important advantages of the AM dosage form over previous osmotic technologies. The first benefit is that higher water flux and permeability of asymmetric membranes allows greater flexibility in designing faster release rates or incorporating lower solubility drug substances into the dosage form (8). Second, the skin layer porosity is easily controlled with selection of pore former type and concentration. Another advantage is the ability to fabricate AM dosage forms in conventional pharmaceutical process equipment without additional manufacturing complexities. Finally, the physical design of an AM dosage form is flexible—it is possible to adapt the technology to fabricate coatings on tablets or on small particles, or to fabricate osmotic capsules directly from the asymmetric polymer membrane.

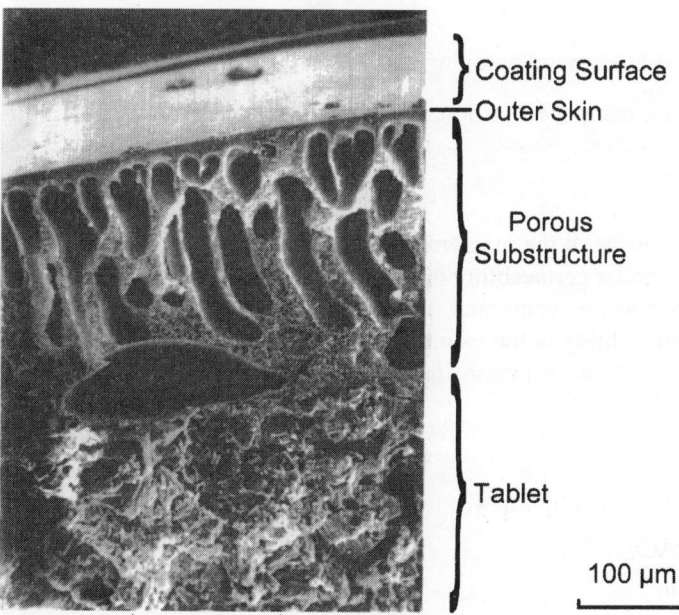

Figure 2 Scanning electron micrograph of asymmetric membrane tablet wall cross-section.

II. THEORY OF OSMOTIC DELIVERY FROM ASYMMETRIC MEMBRANE DOSAGE FORMS

Drug delivery from asymmetric membrane dosage forms is primarily controlled by the difference in osmotic pressure between the external fluid and drug-containing core of the dosage form. The mechanism of drug release from an AM tablet is illustrated in Fig. 3 and consists of imbibition of water through the membrane into the tablet core, dissolution of soluble components (including drug) in the core, and pumping of the solution out of pores in the membrane. The imbibition of water through the membrane is driven by its thermodynamic activity gradient between the external medium, e.g., receptor solution or gastric/intestinal fluids, and the osmotic agent(s) in the core. Dissolution of the soluble components within the core produces the activity gradient and establishes the osmotic pressure difference between the core and external environment. The approximately constant dosage form volume means that the volume of drug solution delivered will be roughly equal to the volume of water imbibed within a given time interval. As water diffuses into the core, the volume of the imbibed water creates a hydrostatic pressure difference across the membrane, which forces the solution out through the pores in the coating. Therefore, the rate of drug delivery will be constant as long as a constant osmotic pressure gradient is maintained across the membrane, the membrane permeability remains constant, and the concentration of drug in the expelled solution is constant. Sustained zero-order drug release can be achieved using AM devices while the concentration of dissolved drug within the fluid portion of the core remains constant. When the drug concentration in the core fluid falls below saturation, the release rate declines.

A comprehensive model describing drug release from an AM dosage form consists of osmotic and diffusional contributions. The diffusional contribution is derived from the fact that the asymmetric membrane is not perfectly semipermeable, and therefore a portion of drug is released by diffusion, primarily through pores in the coating. The total mass of drug delivered per unit time, $(dm/dt)_t$, is modeled by:

$$\left(\frac{dm}{dt}\right)_t = \left(\frac{dm}{dt}\right)_o + \left(\frac{dm}{dt}\right)_d \tag{1}$$

where $\left(\frac{dm}{dt}\right)_o$ is the mass released by osmotic pumping and $\left(\frac{dm}{dt}\right)_d$ is the mass released due to diffusion. The osmotic drug release component is described by Eq. 2.

$$\left(\frac{dm}{dt}\right)_d = \frac{AC}{h} P_w \Delta\Pi \tag{2}$$

Here A is the surface area of the device, h the membrane thickness, C the dissolved drug concentration in the core fluid, P_w the water permeability of the semipermeable membrane, and $\Delta\Pi$ the osmotic pressure difference across the membrane. The diffusional release component is dependent on the dissolved drug permeability in the membrane, P_d, the device surface area, A, the drug concentration in the core, C, and the membrane thickness, h, as described in Eq. 3.

$$\left(\frac{dm}{dt}\right)_d = \frac{P_d AC}{h} \tag{3}$$

The total drug release profile is described by Eq. 4.

$$\left(\frac{dm}{dt}\right)_t = \frac{AC}{h} P_w \Delta\Pi + \frac{P_d AC}{h} \tag{4}$$

Asymmetrical Membrane Film–Coated Dosage Forms

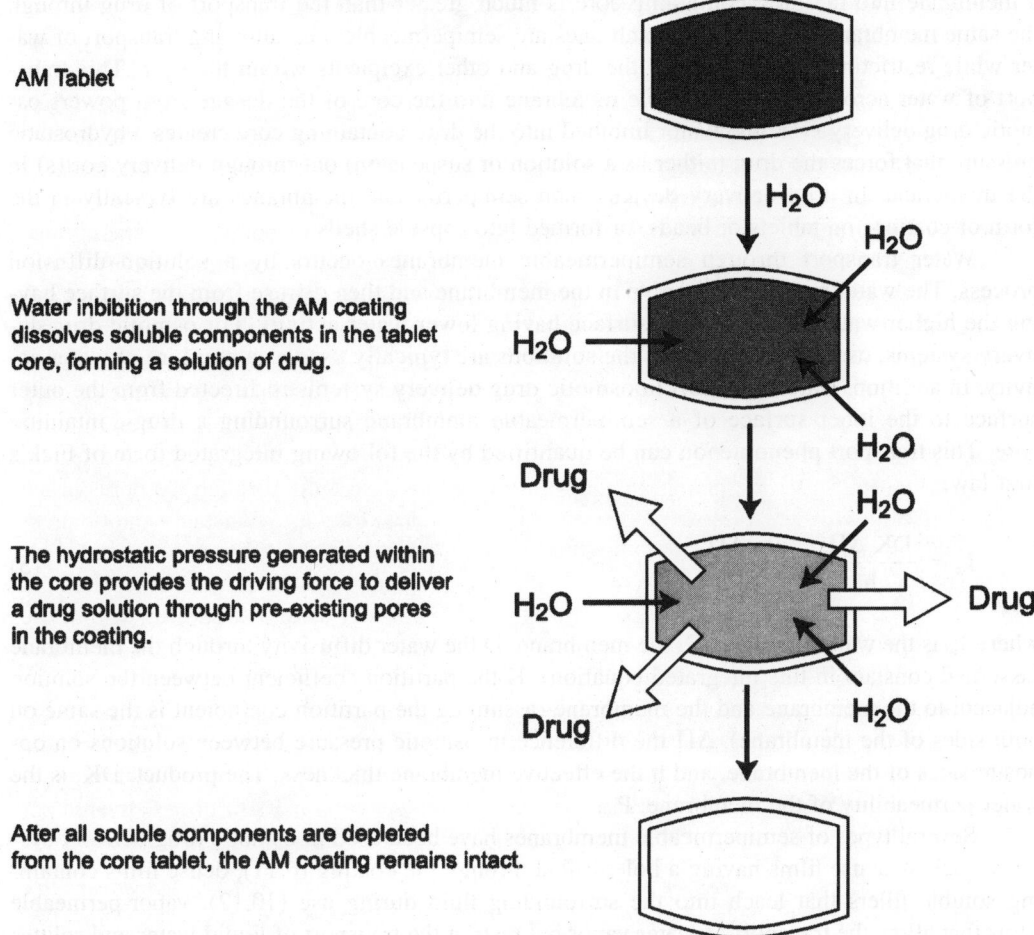

AM Tablet

Water inhibition through the AM coating dissolves soluble components in the tablet core, forming a solution of drug.

The hydrostatic pressure generated within the core provides the driving force to deliver a drug solution through pre-existing pores in the coating.

After all soluble components are depleted from the core tablet, the AM coating remains intact.

Figure 3 Mechanism of drug release from AM tablets.

The combination of both osmotic and diffusional release mechanisms has been addressed previously by Theeuwes for the simple osmotic pump (6) and by Zentner et al. for the controlled porosity osmotic pump (9,10). The dependence of AM dosage form drug release kinetics on the osmotic driving force is further discussed in the Section V. Depending on the AM properties, typical diffusional contributions to the overall quantity of drug released from AM devices ranges from less than 1% to 60%.

III. ASYMMETRIC MEMBRANE PROPERTIES

Membranes are primarily used for separation processes in many industries and function by controlling the rate of transport of various chemical species, allowing some to cross the membrane film much more rapidly than others. This fundamental function of membranes is also used in osmotic drug delivery systems. In osmotic drug delivery systems, the transport of water through a membrane into the drug-containing core is much greater than the transport of drug through the same membrane. Thus, these membranes are semipermeable, i.e., allowing transport of water while restricting the transport of the drug and other excipients within the core. This transport of water across a semipermeable membrane into the core of the dosage from powers osmotic drug delivery systems. Water imbibed into the drug-containing core creates a hydrostatic pressure that forces the drug (either as a solution or suspension) out through delivery port(s) in the membrane. In drug delivery devices such semipermeable membranes are typically in the form of coatings on tablets or beads, or formed into capsule shells.

Water transport through semipermeable membranes occurs by a solution–diffusion process. The water must first dissolve in the membrane and then diffuse from the surface having the higher water activity to the surface having lower water activity. For osmotic drug delivery systems, osmotic pressures of the solutions are typically used as a measure of water activity. In addition, water transport in osmotic drug delivery systems is directed from the outer surface to the inner surface of a semipermeable membrane surrounding a drug-containing core. This transport phenomenon can be quantified by the following integrated form of Fick's first law:

$$J_w = \frac{DK \, \Delta\Pi}{h} = \frac{P_w \, \Delta\Pi}{h} \tag{5}$$

where J_w is the water flux through the membrane, D the water diffusivity through the membrane (assumed constant in this integrated equation), K the partition coefficient between the solution adjacent to the membrane and the membrane (assuming the partition coefficient is the same on both sides of the membrane), $\Delta\Pi$ the difference in osmotic pressure between solutions on opposite sides of the membrane, and h the effective membrane thickness. The product, DK, is the water permeability of the membrane, P_w.

Several types of semipermeable membranes have been used in osmotic drug delivery systems, such as dense films having a hole drilled through the coating (6,11), dense films containing soluble fillers that leach into the surrounding fluid during use (10,12), vapor-permeable films that allow the transport of water vapor but restrict the transport of liquid water and solutes (13), and asymmetric membranes (7).

The first asymmetric membranes were invented for use in reverse osmosis (and later ultrafiltration) where the objective was to fabricate a highly permeable membrane, while maintaining permselectivity and sufficient mechanical strength to withstand the high pressures used in that separation process (14,15). The original concept was to form a single-membrane film consisting of a thick porous region to provide mechanical support and a thin dense region to provide permselectivity. While membranes for reverse osmosis need to be essentially defect-free (i.e., the dense region is completely nonporous to maintain permselectivity), osmotic drug delivery systems require at least one drug delivery port (one or more holes or pores) to allow the sustained release of either a drug solution or a suspension. Thus, it is possible to exploit process parameters and phase behavior of membrane-forming solutions to introduce a controlled porosity during the membrane formation step such that pores are formed in the dense region that function as drug delivery ports. An asymmetric membrane with controlled porosity eliminates the need for an additional process step to mechanically form holes (e.g., laser drilling) in the semipermeable membrane that function as drug delivery ports.

Asymmetric membrane coatings on tablets and beads and for use in capsules have been developed that, like asymmetric membranes used in separation technologies, consist of thick porous region supporting a thin dense region (8,16). Asymmetric membrane coatings for osmotic drug delivery systems can be made that are either imperforate or perforate. Perforations in the coating can be used as drug delivery ports. If imperforate, drug delivery ports can either be formed via mechanical means, e.g., drilling holes in the coating, or by rupturing the membrane via hydrostatic pressure generated in situ within the core. Typically, perforate asymmetric membrane coatings contain hundreds to thousands of pores that function as drug delivery ports. These pores typically range in size from tenths of a micrometer to several micrometers in diameter.

Asymmetric membranes used for osmotic drug delivery systems are unique in that the water permeability through these membranes is dependent on the structure of the membranes. Asymmetric membranes are made up of porous regions that comprise the bulk of the membrane and relatively thin dense regions. Thus, significant factors in determining the permeability of a given membrane is the porous nature of the membrane, and the thickness and extent of the dense regions, in addition to the composition of the membrane. Membrane structure is controlled by a combination of components in the solution used to form the membrane (e.g., coating solution) and processing conditions. Membrane structure can be consistently reproduced as has been demonstrated in making asymmetric membranes for separation processes and now as demonstrated in osmotic drug delivery systems.

IV. PROCESSING

An asymmetric membrane is composed of a thin, dense skin layer supported by a thicker, porous substructure layer. The first reported asymmetric membrane was developed for the reverse osmosis demineralization of saline water by Loeb and Sourirajan (17). The asymmetrical design of the membrane combined the advantages of high selectivity of a dense membrane with the high permeation rate of both the porous membrane and thin, dense membrane (18). The Loeb–Sourirajan type of asymmetric membrane processing was not amenable to pharmaceutical coating application onto core dosage forms. In the design of an osmotic drug delivery system that employed an asymmetric membrane to control drug release, new processing methods were developed by Cardinal et al. (7).

A. Development of Dosage Form Cores

1. Composition of Cores

During development of an asymmetric membrane dosage form, the first consideration is focused on the design of the core substrate. The core dosage form plays a pivotal role in the manufacturing process scale-up, quality, stability, and performance of the final product. The composition of the core dosage form dictates the osmotic driving force.

The ingredients formulated into the core generally include the drug substance, osmotic agent, binder/spheronizer, solubilizer, and lubricant. The selection of the excipients is dependent on the drug substance properties, such as solubility, and osmotic pressure. The critical core excipient affecting the drug release rate is the osmotic agent, as it affects the water flux through the semipermeable, asymmetric membrane into the core dosage form. A listing of potential osmotic agents compiled from previous publications (19,20) and our own laboratory measurements is located in Table 2. The osmotic agent is listed in descending order of osmotic pressure. Table 2 also lists one possible source for the osmotic agent and the designated grades of material (i.e., NF, USP, FCC). The osmotic agents must be carefully evaluated for each individual application considering the driving force/release rate target, stability, manufacturing capabilities, as well as in vivo concerns of chronic dosing and exposure.

Table 2 Summary of Osmotic Components, Osmotic Pressure, Sourcing Information, and Grades

Osmotic agents	Π (atm)	Source company	Grade
Sodium chloride	356	J. T. Baker (Phillipsburg, NJ)	USP
Fructose	355	Spectrum Quality Products, Inc. (New Brunswick, NJ)	USP
Potassium chloride	245	J. T. Baker (Phillipsburg, NJ)	USP, NF
Sucrose	150	Domino Sugar Corp. (Brooklyn, NY)	NF
Maleic acid	117	Spectrum Quality Products, Inc. (New Brunswick, NJ)	USP, NF, FCC
Potassium phosphate, monobasic	105	Spectrum Quality Products, Inc. (New Brunswick, NJ)	NF
Xylitol	104	Cultor Food Science (Thomson, IL)	FCC
D,L-Malic acid	95	Spectrum Quality Products, Inc. (New Brunswick, NJ)	NF
Sorbitol	84	Spectrum Quality Products, Inc. (New Brunswick, NJ)	NF
Dextrose	82	Spectrum Quality Products, Inc. (New Brunswick, NJ)	USP, NF
Citric acid	69	Archer Daniels Midland Company (Southport, NC)	USP
Tartaric acid	67	Spectrum Quality Products, Inc. (New Brunswick, NJ)	USP, NF, FCC
Ascorbic acid	54	J. T. Baker (Phillipsburg, NJ)	USP, FCC
Lactose-succinic acid	47	Quest International–Spectrum Quality Products	NF, USP-FCC
Mannitol	38	SPI Polyols (New Castle, DE)	Granular: USP
Mannitol	38	E. Merck–Germany (E. M. Industries, Hawthorne, NY)	Micronized: USP
Sodium phosphate, tribasic	36	FMC Chemical Products Group (Philadelphia, PA)	Anhydrous: FCC
Sodium phosphate, dibasic	31	Spectrum Quality Products, Inc. (New Brunswick, NJ)	Anhydrous: USP, NF
Sodium phosphate, dibasic	31	Spectrum Quality Products, Inc. (New Brunswick, NJ)	Monohydrate: FCC
Succinic acid	29	Spectrum Quality Products, Inc. (New Brunswick, NJ)	FCC
Sodium phosphate, monobasic	28	Ruger Chemical (Irvington, NJ)	Anhydrous: FCC, USP
Sodium phosphate, monobasic	28	J. T. Baker (Phillipsburg, NJ)	Monohydrate: FCC, USP
Lactose-adipic acid	26	Quest International–Monsanto	NF, USP-FCC
L-Arginine	26	Spectrum Quality Products, Inc. (New Brunswick, NJ)	NF, USP
Lactose	23	Quest International (Hoffman Estates, IL)	Anhydrous: NF, USP, PH, EUR, JP
Lactose	23	Foremost Ingredient Group (Baraboo, WI)	Monohydrate: NF
Fumaric acid	10	Haarman & Reimer Corp. (Elkhart, IN)	NF
Adipic acid	8	Monsanto (Pensacola, FL)	FCC

2. Processing of Dosage Form Cores

The physical forms of asymmetric membrane dosage form cores encompass encapsulation of blends or beads into AM capsule shells and application of the AM film coating onto core tablets or beads. The cores are processed using standard spheronizing, granulating, encapsulating, and tableting equipment used for conventional solid oral dosage forms (21,22).

3. Core Dosage Form Variables

Core dosage form variables that may impact the final drug product include the formulation components, physical and chemical properties of the components, as well as the processing methods (Table 3). The physicochemical and pharmacokinetic properties of the drug substance itself will determine the target release duration, dosage strength, core formulation requirements, and feasibility of AM delivery.

Excipient properties can influence the rate and extent of drug release. The excipient solubility and osmotic pressure determines its own rate of release from the AM dosage form. Insufficient quantities of a soluble component may result in early depletion that can lower the overall drug release amount. Such an effect can be detected by a lower plateau in the drug release profile compared to alternative formulations. An important aspect of the product quality is governed by the drug and excipient reactivity. Binary mixtures of the drug with candidate

Table 3 Core Dosage Form Variables and Potential Impact on Process or Product Performance

Core variable	Potential effect on final product performance
Drug physicochemical properties	Release rate
	Core formulation requirements
	Dosage strength per unit
Drug pharmacokinetic and absorption properties	Target release duration (extent of colonic absorption)
	Feasibility of dosage form
Excipient properties:	
Solubility and osmotic pressure	Release rate of drug and excipients
	Plateau in drug release due to early depletion of a critical excipient
	Dosage form size
	Stability
Hygroscopicity	Chemical stability due to increased mobility and/or reactivity
	Burst effect due to osmotic pumping during storage
Core design (type and shape)	Processing methods (core and coating)
	Surface area (for coating and releasing areas)
	Mixing in coating operation
	Coating permeability dependent on core size
Surface properties	Roughness (coating quality or appearance, and porosity of coating)
	Surface effects for coating adhesion
Core weight distribution	Coating level distribution
	Range in coating mechanical properties due to variable coating levels
	Range of release rates associated with variation in coating levels
Friability	Edge erosion during coating process
	Burst effect from eroded drug incorporated into coating

excipients are studied early in development using common accelerated stability procedures. The hygroscopicity of the core is another important variable as the absorption of water can increase mobility to facilitate certain types of chemical degradation mechanisms. The hygroscopicity of the core dosage form may also impact the initial rate of drug release, i.e., burst effect, if drug is convectively transported into the coating during a post coating drying operation or due to premature osmotic pumping. However, these situations are not commonly encountered in AM dosage forms.

In terms of physical dimensions, the core design and formulation define the dosage form size and shape. For example, a high-dose intermediate solubility drug may require an AM film–coated bead. The greater surface area-to-volume ratio for the bead can produce a faster drug release rate from the coated dosage forms. The core formulation and design can affect the desired coating permeability. Dosage form surface properties are critical in the wetting, spreading, and adhesion of the AM coating during application onto the core. The core surface roughness has been shown to affect the final coating quality and appearance of controlled release products (23).

Core formulation and manufacturing processes may affect the final product quality and performance in the following ways. Edge erosion (for tablets) or reduction in granule size (for beads) results in friable cores. The coated dosage form weight variability is a function of the ingoing core weight distribution. Poor blend flow during manufacturing translates to a variable core weight. Further processing of the cores to apply the AM coating results in an even broader final weight distribution. The extremes in coating levels associated with such a product can produce different release rates or coating mechanical properties. The impact of these process related issues on dosage form performance is a reflection of the need to develop and optimize the core with the final coated product in mind (23).

In order to compare the lead core formulations and identify the best formulation, prototype AM film-coated dosage forms are made by applying a highly permeable coating. The release characteristics of these coated prototypes are tested and stability studied using accelerated stability approaches (i.e., elevated temperature and/or humidity conditions). The stability and in vitro performance results are used to define the preferred core formulation.

B. Development of Asymmetric Membrane Coatings

The core dosage form is a major contributor in defining the rate of water flux into an AM dosage form. However, the rate of drug release is dictated by the composition of the asymmetric membrane. Once the core formulation is defined based on performance criteria set for the individual drug and target release profile, the coating formula can be altered to fine-tune the release profile. The main ingredients contained in an AM coating formulation include the film former, plasticizer or pore former, solvent(s), and nonsolvent(s).

1. Composition of AM Coatings

The polymer solution used to form the asymmetric membrane is prepared by dissolving the polymer of choice in a mixture of at least two solvents. The solvents are chosen to have differing boiling points and so that the more volatile solvent is a good solvent for the polymer and a less volatile solvent is a poor solvent or a nonsolvent for the polymer. When this solvent mixture evaporates, the progressive shift in composition (due to the differing boiling points of the solvents) from good solvent to poor solvent results in abrupt precipitation of the polymer (15). It is this abrupt precipitation that can be exploited to control porosity of the membrane.

Asymmetric membrane dosage forms have been fabricated from a wide range of polymers including cellulose derivatives, polysulfones, polyamides, polyurethanes, polypropylene, poly(vinyl chloride) polyvinyl alcohol, poly (vinylidene fluoride), ethylenevinyl acetate, ethylenevinyl alcohol, poly (methyl methacrylate) (7). The cellulose derivatives consist of cellulose esters or ethers containing mono-, di-, or triacyl esters in which the acyl group is two to four carbon atoms and lower alkyl ethers of cellulose where the alkyl group is one-to-four carbon atoms. Other cellulose derivatives employed in reverse osmosis membranes have been incorporated into asymmetric membrane dosage forms, such as cellulose nitrate, cellulose acetate phthalate, cellulose acetate methyl carbamate, cellulose acetate succinate, cellulose acetate trimellitate, cellulose acetate methylsulfonate, cellulose acetate p-toluenesulfonate, and cellulose methacrylates.

In order to improve the polymer elasticity and lower brittleness, plasticizers may be added to the coating formulation. The nature (hydrophobic/hydrophilic) of the plasticizer can affect polymer permeability and drug release rates. Generally, hydrophilic plasticizers (e.g., glycerol) increase the permeability and release rate while hydrophobic plasticizers, such as diethyl phthalate, reduce permeability and release rate. Partially soluble plasticizers can be employed to modulate these effects and include materials such as triacetin and triethyl citrate.

The pore former controls the porosity of the coating substructure as well as the dense film. The formation of the pore may result from evaporation of a volatile nonsolvent during the coating process or dissolution of the aqueous soluble pore former into imbibed water during dosage form operation. An example of a pore former evaporating during the coating process is water. Other aqueous soluble pore formers are formamide, acetic acid, glycerol, a (C_1–C_4) alkanol, sodium acetate, aqueous hydrogen peroxide, and polyvinylpyrrolidone (7). Nonsolvents, such as butanol and ethanol, may also act as volatile nonsolvent pore formers. As described in more detail by Kesting (15), the concentration of the nonsolvent pore former affects the coating permeability characteristics and morphology. Figure 4 depicts the effect of increased concentration of pore former on coating permeability and coating porosity (15).

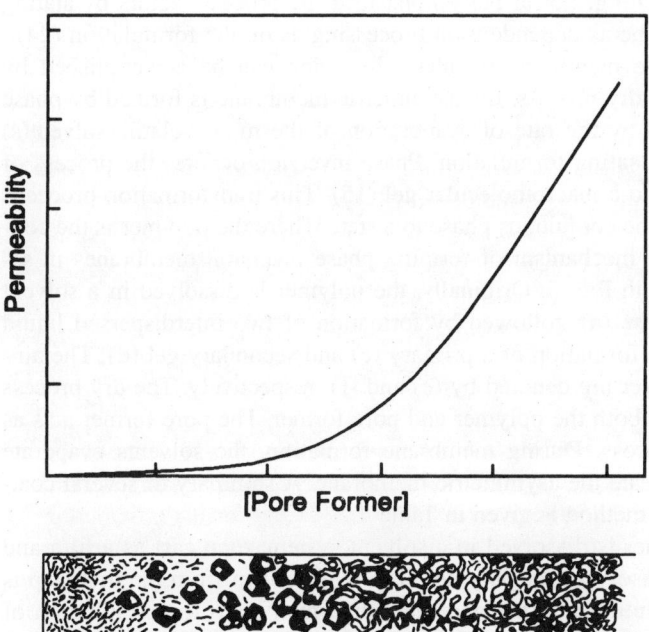

Figure 4 Relationship between cell type, skin thickness, concentration of pore former, and permeability in phase inversion membranes (15).

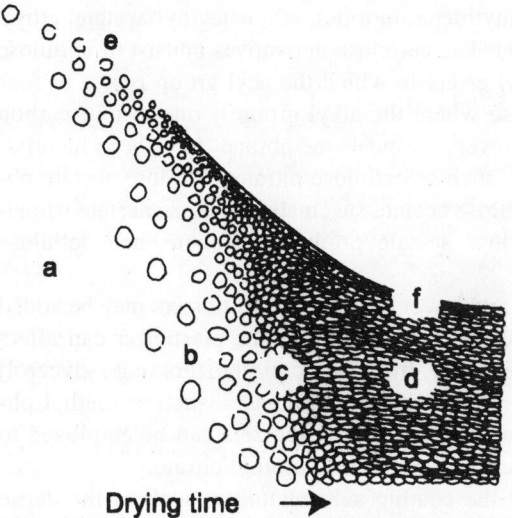

Figure 5 Schematic representation of the mechanism of phase inversion membrane formation: (a) a single phase solution; (b) two interdispersed liquid phases; (c) primary gel; (d) secondary gel; (e) air–solution interface; (f) skin (15).

2. Physical Forms and Coating Processes

The physical forms of the final drug product are typically capsules, tablets, and beads. The coating processes generally used in developing asymmetric membrane dosage forms include dip coating, spray drying, and spray coating. Porter has emphasized the process factors by stating that controlled release coatings can be as dependent on processing as on the formulation (24).

Preparation of the asymmetric membrane by phase inversion can be accomplished by either a wet or a dry process. In the dry process, the asymmetric membrane is formed by phase inversion of the polymer controlled by the rate of evaporation of the more volatile solvent(s) compared to the nonsolvent in the coating formulation. Phase inversion denotes the process of transforming a polymer in solution to a macromolecular gel (15). This transformation proceeds from a state in which the solvent is the continuous phase to a state where the polymer is the continuous phase. Kesting depicted the mechanism of forming phase inversion membranes in sequence with drying time, as shown in Fig. 5. Originally, the polymer is dissolved in a solvent system that constitutes a single phase (a), followed by formation of two interdispersed liquid phases (b). Further drying results in formation of a primary (c) and secondary gel (d). The air–solution interface and dense skin layer are denoted by (e) and (f), respectively. The dry process involves use of a solvent system for both the polymer and pore former. The pore former acts as nonsolvent for polymer in this process. During membrane formation, the solvents evaporate more rapidly than pore former to create the asymmetric membrane. A summary of several coating formulations applied by the dry method is given in Table 4.

In the wet process, the polymer is dissolved in a solvent system, then cast as a film and immersed into a quench bath of nonsolvent for polymer (15). The solvent from the first step is extracted from the cast polymer solution into the quench bath, which leads to precipitation of the polymer in a structured form (7). A listing of several coating formulations applied to capsules or tablets using the wet process is located in Table 5.

Table 4 Examples of Asymmetric Membrane Coating Formulations Applied Using the Dry Process (wt %) (7)

Coating Formulation ID	AA	BB	CC	DD
Coating Components				
Cellulose acetate	15			5
Ethylcellulose		11		
Cellulose acetate butyrate			31	
Acetone	47	75	52	55
Methyl ethyl ketone			14	
Methyl acetate				
Glycerol	1.9			
Ethanol	21.7			40
Butanol	11.8			
Water	2.6	14	3	

3. Dip Coating Capsules and Tablets

The manufacturing of AM capsule shells proceeds by a dip-coating process followed by immersion into a quench bath (wet process) or air drying (dry process) (7). The capsule consists of three parts including the shorter wider cap, longer thinner body, and sealing band. The capsule body and cap are formed by precipitation of the membrane onto a stainless-steel mold pin while dipping into the polymer coating solution, as shown in Fig. 6 (16).

As the mold pin is removed and immersed into the nonsolvent quench bath, the polymer undergoes phase inversion. The ratio of solvents to nonsolvents in the coating solution is designed so that phase inversion commences immediately after evaporation starts. The capsule shell is removed from the pin for subsequent processing into the final dosage form. Blends or uncoated beads are loaded into the AM capsule body, which is sealed to the cap with a band of polymer film. A semi-automated process for manufacturing the AM capsule shells was developed using the Zymate II robotic system with a throughput of 350 capsules/day. Further detail on the unit operations and setup can be obtained from Thombre et al. (16). Analysis of an AM capsule shell cross-section by scanning electron microscopy revealed that the dense skin region was 10–20 μm thick, compared to the porous substructure thickness of approximately 200 μm (Fig. 7).

Herbig et al. described dip-coated tablets with an AM coating solution composed of 15% cellulose acetate (CA-398-10, Eastman Chemicals, Kingsport, TN) dissolved in acetone and either formamide or glycerol (8). The dip-coated tablet was air-dried for 5 min and subsequently immersed in a water quench bath for 3 min. A final air drying step was performed for at least 12 h at ambient conditions. A cross-section of an AM coating applied to a tablet is shown by the scanning electron micrograph in Fig. 2. The outer skin layer extends 5–15 μm through the coating with approximately 200 μm porous substructure. The skin and porous regions in the asymmetric membrane compare well between the dip-coated AM capsules and the dip-coated AM tablets.

4. Spray Drying

Asymmetric membranes have been applied to beads, approximately 1 mm in diameter, using the following spray-drying technique: A slurry of the beads and polymer coating solution was sprayed through an external mixing air-atomizing nozzle (Spray Systems Co., Wheaton, IL,

Table 5 Examples of Asymmetric Membrane Coating Formulations Applied Using the Wet Process (wt %) (7)

Coating Formulation	A	B	C	D	E	F	G	H	I	J	K
Coating Components											
Cellulose acetate	15	15	15								
Ethylcellulose					15	2			2	3	
Cellulose acetate butyrate				12		10		15	13	12	
Cellulose acetate propionate							20				34
Cellulose acetate phthalate											
Cellulose acetate trimellitate											
Poly(vinyl alcohol)											
Ethylenevinyl alcohol											
Polyurethane											
Poly(vinylidene fluoride)											
Polysulfone											
Poly(methyl methacrylate)											
Polyamide											
Triethyl citrate		5									
Glycerol	8	3						5	5	5	10
Formamide				16	5	10	20	50			
Polyethylene glycol											
Acetic acid					25		9				
Acetone	49	49	52		55	48	51		50	50	56
Dimethylformamide											
Methyl acetate				48							
Ethanol	28	28	33			30		30	30	30	
Methanol				24							
Water											

Table 5 Continued

Coating Formulation ID	L	M	N	O	P	Q	R	S	T	U
Component										
Cellulose acetate									10	10
Ethylcellulose										
Cellulose acetate butyrate										
Cellulose acetate propionate	23.6								2	2
Cellulose acetate phthalate										
Cellulose acetate trimellitate										
Poly(vinyl alcohol)		15								
Ethylenevinyl alcohol			15							
Polyurethane				24.5						
Polyvinylidene fluoride					15	21.4				
Polysulfone										
Polymethyl methacrylate							25	25		
Polyamide										
Triethylcitrate										
Glycerol	7.3									
Formamide									10	10
Polyethylene glycol							10			
Acetic acid										
Acetone	43.6			75.5	85	78.6	65		48	48
Dimethylformamide										
Methyl acetate										
Ethanol	25.5	20	55					56	30	30
Methanol										
Water		65	30					19		

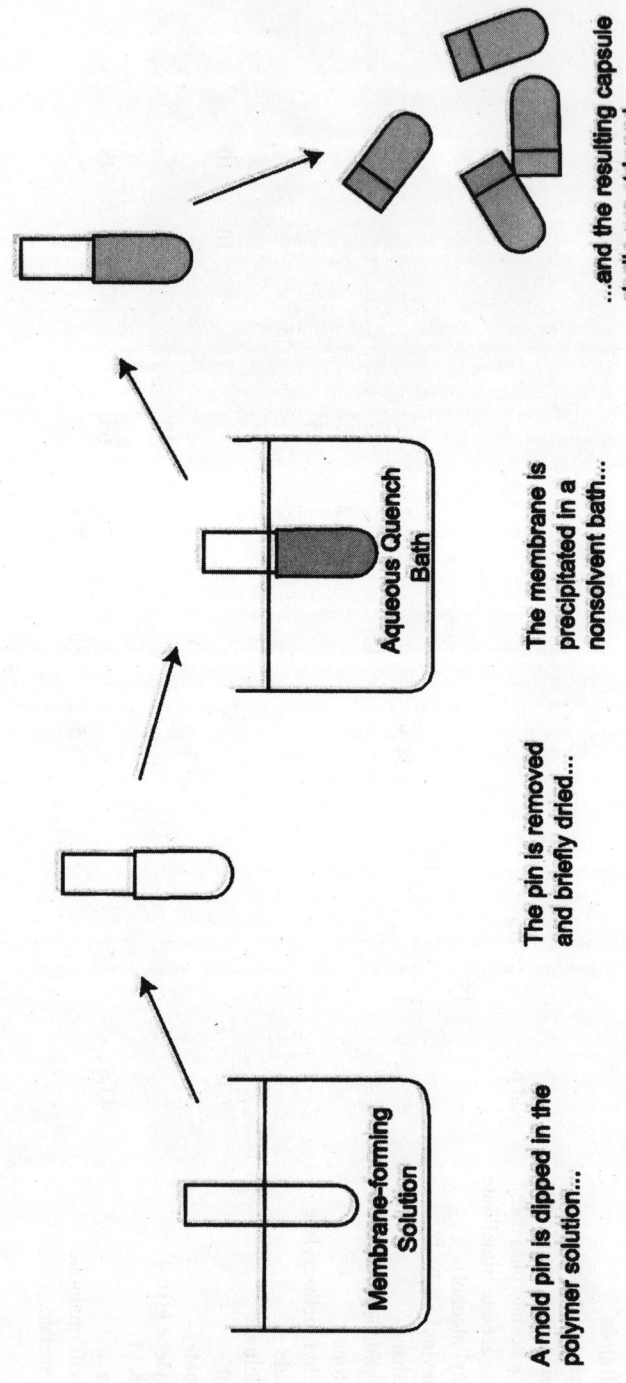

Figure 6 Dip-coating process manufacturing of asymmetric membrane capsules (16).

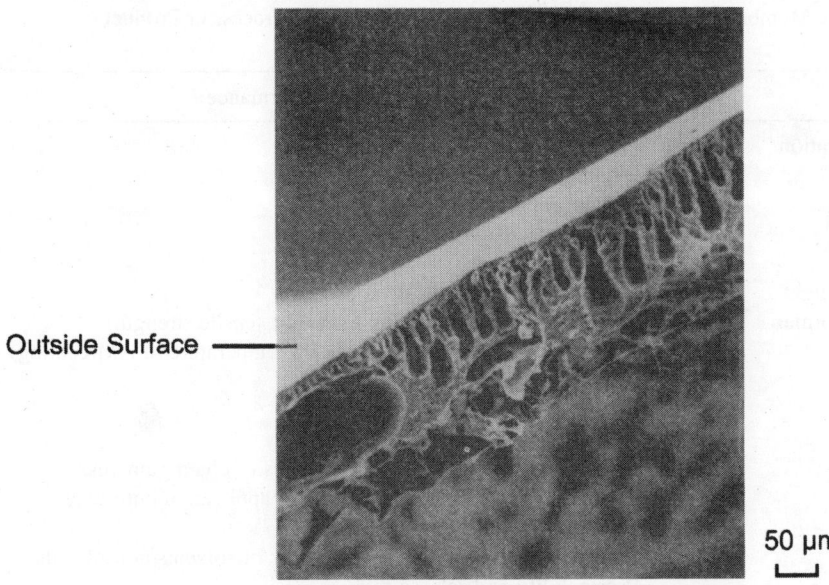

Figure 7 Scanning electron micrograph of asymmetric membrane capsule wall cross-section.

Model 100150) (7). The coating formulation contained 15 wt % cellulose acetate 398-10, 47% acetone, 21.7% ethanol, 11.8% butanol, 2.6% water, and 1.9% glycerol. The mixture of core beads and coating was heated to 40°C and sprayed at ambient temperature. The applied coating thickness ranged from 12 to 20 μm. Table 4 lists other coating formulations sprayed according to this method (7). The spray dry technique does not require a quench bath, and is categorized as a dry process method.

A method used to form macropores in the outer skin of the asymmetric membrane involves controlling the differential pressure across the nozzle assembly. The beads and polymer coating were prepared and transferred to a pressurized vessel at 40 psi. This pressurized slurry was sprayed from an airless nozzle, 3 mm diameter orifice, into room temperature air. The pressure difference resulted in bubble formation in the coating solution during coating precipitation (7). Elimination of the pressurization of the coating solution vessel resulted in a continuous dense outer skin layer.

5. Spray Coating

Conventional spray-coating techniques (25,26) have also been used to coat asymmetric membranes onto tablets or beads. An AM coating composed of 5% cellulose acetate, 55% acetone, and 40% ethanol was applied onto beads using a Wurster-type fluidized-bed coating system (7). The resultant coating appeared to be smooth and imperforate at a magnification of 4000. Spray-coating methods are classified as dry process techniques for AM coating formation.

6. AM Coating Formulation and Process Variables

AM coating variables that may affect the AM dosage form performance include formulation components, processing methods, and process parameters (Table 6). The coating formulation components and membrane properties will ultimately define the drug release rate. The polymer selection and its concentration in the coating dictates selection of the other coating components

Table 6 Asymmetric Membrane Coating Variables and Potential Impact on Process or Product Performance

Coating variable	Potential effect on final product performance
Polymer and concentration	Permeability
	Film coating mechanical properties
	Solvents/nonsolvents required
	Coating viscosity
	Drug release rate
Polymer molecular weight	Film-coating mechanical properties
Plasticizer and pore former	Mechanical properties (film elasticity, tensile strength)
	Physical properties (glass transition temperature of AM coating)
	Coating porosity
	Permeability and release rate
	Water sorption during storage/stability
Solvent	Spray conditions and thermodynamics of coating process
	Timing of phase inversion relative to application onto core
	Equipment requirements
Nonsolvent	Porosity dictated by relative volatility of solvents/nonsolvents
	Permeability and release rate
Dip coating (7,16):	
Quench bath composition	Rate of phase inversion
Pore former solubility in quench bath	Porosity
Air drying time	Permeability and drug release rate
Spray coating (22,24,25) and spray drying (7):	
Atomization pressure and flow rate	Porosity
Pattern air pressure	Coating weight variability
Drying air flow rate/volume	Coating adhesion and spreading
Distance between spray gun and cores	Surface appearance
Nozzle design	

(i.e., pore former, plasticizer, solvents, and nonsolvents). In addition to defining the coating formulation, the polymer affects the membrane and mechanical properties including permeability, solute selectivity, adhesion, tensile strength, and elasticity.

The plasticizer and pore former choice will be based on the polymer. These materials affect the mechanical properties of the membrane, such as the glass transition temperature and elasticity, as well as the coating porosity and water imbibition rate, which determines the drug release rate. In addition, these components may also affect water vapor transport rate, which can affect the stability and dosage form, shelf life, and storage requirements. The relative volatility of the solvent and nonsolvent affects the rate of polymer phase inversion during the coating application. Nonsolvents may also function as a pore former.

The coating process variables can affect the asymmetric membrane morphology and product performance. The coating process mass and energy balance should be optimized for proper formation of the membrane. Operating the process with excess humidity (overwet) produces a larger proportion of dense region that markedly reduces release rates. Low-humidity, or overdry, coating process conditions can result in a highly porous membrane with rapid release rates. Since the coating morphology and final release rate can be sensitive to process operating conditions, a thorough knowledge of the coating unit operation is necessary to successfully scale up AM dosage forms.

For dip-coating processes, important variables include the quench bath composition, pore former solubility in quench bath, and air drying time listed in Table 6. These variables control the rate of phase inversion and membrane porosity. The pore former is selected to be soluble in the quench bath to ensure leaching and pore formation occur. The critical variables in the formation of a porous asymmetric membrane using a spray-drying or coating approach are atomizing air pressure and flow rate, pattern air pressure, drying air flow rate and volume, and nozzle design.

Numerous spray-coating process variables have been studied for their impact on controlled release coated dosage forms (8,22,24–26). Asymmetric membrane film formation from a spray-coating process is critically dependent on the coating droplet size. The droplet size, density, and distribution vary with nozzle parameters, coating solution spray rate, and drying rate. Differences in nozzle design or dimensions, including liquid flow orifice diameter, atomizing fluid annulus area, and angle of pattern fluid source, affect the coating droplet size.

Altering the distance the coating droplet travels from the nozzle to the core substrate has been reported by Aulton and Twitchell to affect the droplet size (26). For aqueous-based coatings, increasing the nozzle gun–to–substrate distance results in increased droplet size due to coalescence. On the other hand, solvent-based coatings result in a decrease in droplet size with increased time in flight or distance due to solvent evaporation.

All parameters that affect the mass flow rate of coating solution or atomizing fluid through the nozzle can affect droplet size. The angle of pattern air side port relative to the atomized droplets determines the spray pattern used to control the spray zone (26). Narrow or overlapping spray zones from multiple nozzles produce an increased variability in final coating weight. These coating process variables are discussed in further detail by Porter and Bruno (25), Porter and Ghebre-Sellassie (22), and Aulton and Twitchell (26).

V. PERFORMANCE

A. In Vitro Performance

1. Effect of Media pH and Agitation on In Vitro Performance

To demonstrate the insensitivity of in vitro drug release to changes in dissolution media pH and agitation, pseudoephedrine tablets were coated with asymmetric membrane coating. These AM film–coated tablets contained 240 mg pseudoephedrine. The in vitro procedure for measuring drug release from AM tablets utilized the USP apparatus II, i.e., the paddle method. The dissolution vessels contained 900 mL of receptor solution maintained at 37 ± 0.5°C, with paddle agitation set at 50, 75, or 100 rpm. Samples periodically withdrawn from the vessels were analyzed by high-performance liquid chromatography (HPLC) to quantitate drug release with time.

The effect of media pH on drug release kinetics was investigated using five different dissolution media prepared according to USP 23. The five media included (a) distilled water, (b) 0.1 N HCI, (c) USP buffer with pH 4.5 (50 mM sodium acetate or 50 mM potassium biphthalate), (d) USP buffer with pH 6.8 (50 mM monobasic potassium phosphate), and

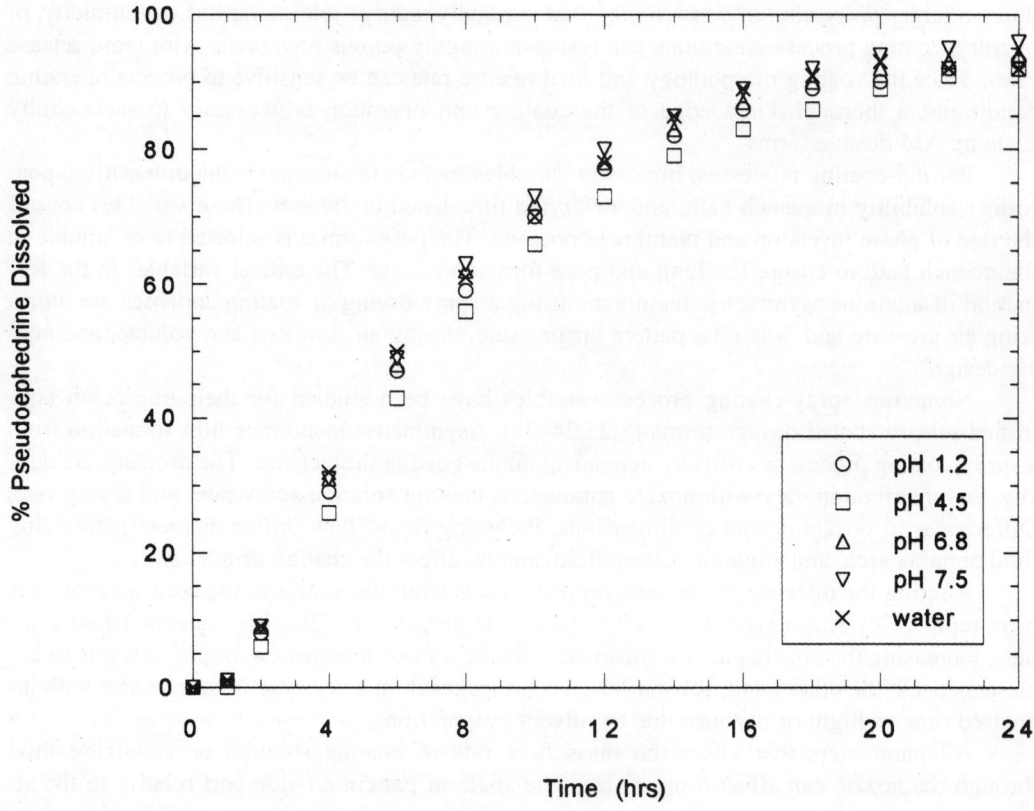

Figure 8 Effect of media pH on in vitro release of pseudoephedrine from 240-mg AM tablets into 900 mL medium with 50 rpm paddle agitation at 37°C (n = 12 tablets).

(e) simulated intestinal fluid without enzyme (pancreatin) with pH 7.5. The dissolution results are the average of 12 tablets. As the results show in Fig. 8, the pseudoephedrine release profile is unaffected by changes in the receptor media pH from 1.2 to 7.5 for constant agitation of 50 rpm. A similar media pH insensitivity for pseudoephedrine release from these tablets is seen at higher agitation rates of 75 and 100 rpm in Fig. 9 and 10, respectively. These results demonstrate the asymmetric membrane dosage form release kinetics is independent of dissolution media pH and agitation, characteristic of osmotic systems.

To further demonstrate the release independence of drug solubility in the dissolution media, doxazosin tablets were coated with asymmetric membrane coating. These tablets contained 2.5 mg doxazosin, 50 mg polyethylene glycol 1000, 50 mg adipic acid, 397.5 mg lactose (8). The AM coating formulation, composed of 15 wt % CA, 14 wt % formamide, and 71 wt % acetone, was applied by dip-coating the tablet into the polymer solution followed by quenching in a water bath. The dip-coated asymmetric membrane forms a porous substructure with an outer thin-skin layer as described in Section III.

Doxazosin release from AM tablets was performed in a manner similar to that described above. Two different receptor solutions were selected to study the effect of drug substance solubility on the in vitro release performance. Doxazosin solubility in simulated gastric buffer, pH 1.2, is 0.33 g/L compared to 0.006 g/L in simulated intestinal buffer, pH 7.5. The dissolution results are reported as the average of three replicate tablets. Doxazosin release rates into simu-

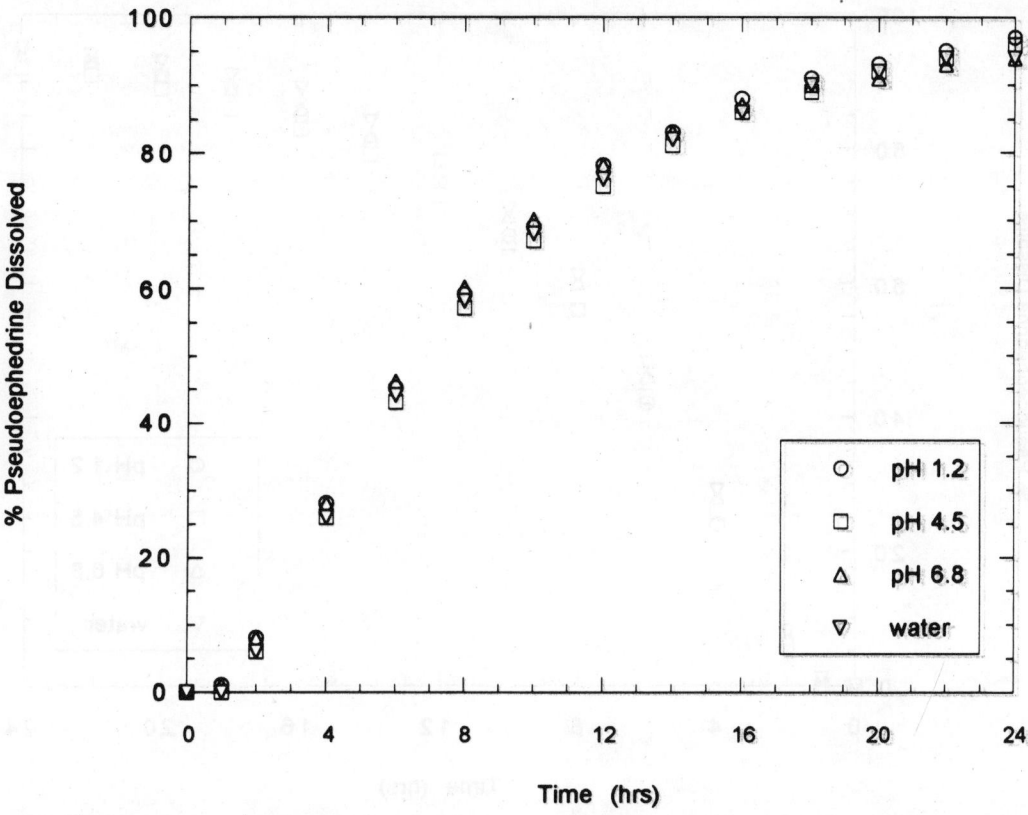

Figure 9 Effect of media pH on in vitro release of pseudoephedrine from 240-mg AM tablets into 900 mL medium with 75 rpm paddle agitation at 37°C (n = 12 tablets).

late gastric buffer and simulated intestinal buffer have the same values of 0.26 mg/h, as shown in Fig. 11. These results illustrate osmotic drug release from AM dosage forms is independent of drug solubility in the dissolution media.

2. *Effect of Intentional Defects in the Membrane on In Vitro Performance*

Studies were conducted to assess the effect of defects in the AM coating on the release kinetics. A highly soluble drug substance, pseudoephedrine HCl, was selected to facilitate the ease of detecting changes in the dissolution profile method. The solubility of pseudoephedrine in water is 2 g in 1 mL (27). The defects intentionally placed in the coating consisted of either a 2-mm hole or a 3-mm cut on the face of the AM film–coated tablet. The dissolution medium providing the greatest sink conditions, water, was selected for this study. As the results shown in Fig. 12 illustrate, pseudoephedrine release from AM tablets containing holes 2–3 mm in size is not different from the control dosage form. These results demonstrate that AM tablet release kinetics is independent of defects in the coating—a unique property of osmotic devices.

3. *Effect of Core Formulation Osmotic Pressure on In Vitro Performance*

To demonstrate the drug release rate dependence on the core osmotic pressure, doxazosin AM tablets were prepared. These tablets contained different core formulations to provide a range of

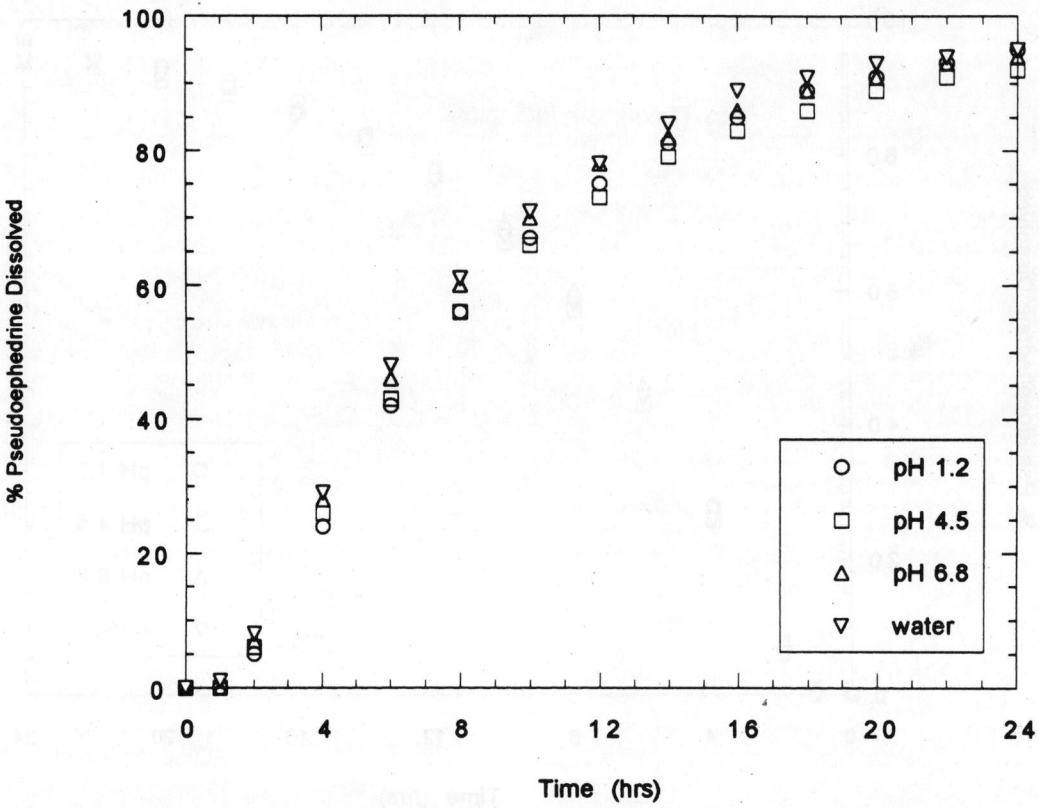

Figure 10 Effect of media pH on in vitro release of pseudoephedrine from 240-mg AM tablets into 900 mL media with 100 rpm paddle agitation at 37°C (n = 12 tablets).

osmotic pressures from 26 to 54 atm (Table 7) (8). The osmotic driving force, $\Delta\Pi$, was determined by subtracting the media osmotic pressure from the core tablet osmotic pressure. The dissolution medium used in these studies was simulated gastric fluid with osmotic pressure adjusted to 7 atm by addition of sodium chloride. The AM coating formulation and process used is the same as described previously for the doxazosin tablets. The steady-state release rates were determined at 10–60% release of total drug loading from 3 to 6 tablets per formulation. As shown in Fig. 13, doxazosin release rate (mg/h) increased from 0.2 to 0.6 mg/h with increased osmotic driving force from 19 to 47 atm. These results demonstrate that the mechanism of drug release from AM tablets is osmotically controlled.

4. Effect of Media Osmotic Pressure on In Vitro Performance

To demonstrate the release rate dependence on the dissolution media osmotic pressure, pseudoephedrine AM tablets were prepared with a single core formulation. The in vitro procedure for measuring drug release from these tablets utilized the USP II apparatus. The dissolution vessels contained 900 mL of water prepared with varying concentrations of sucrose to produce osmotic pressure of 0, 25, and 50 atm. The media osmotic pressure measurement was measured using a freezing point depression instrument. The dosage forms were withdrawn from the media at 2, 4, 8, 12, 16, and 24 h and assayed by HPLC for residual drug content. The amount of

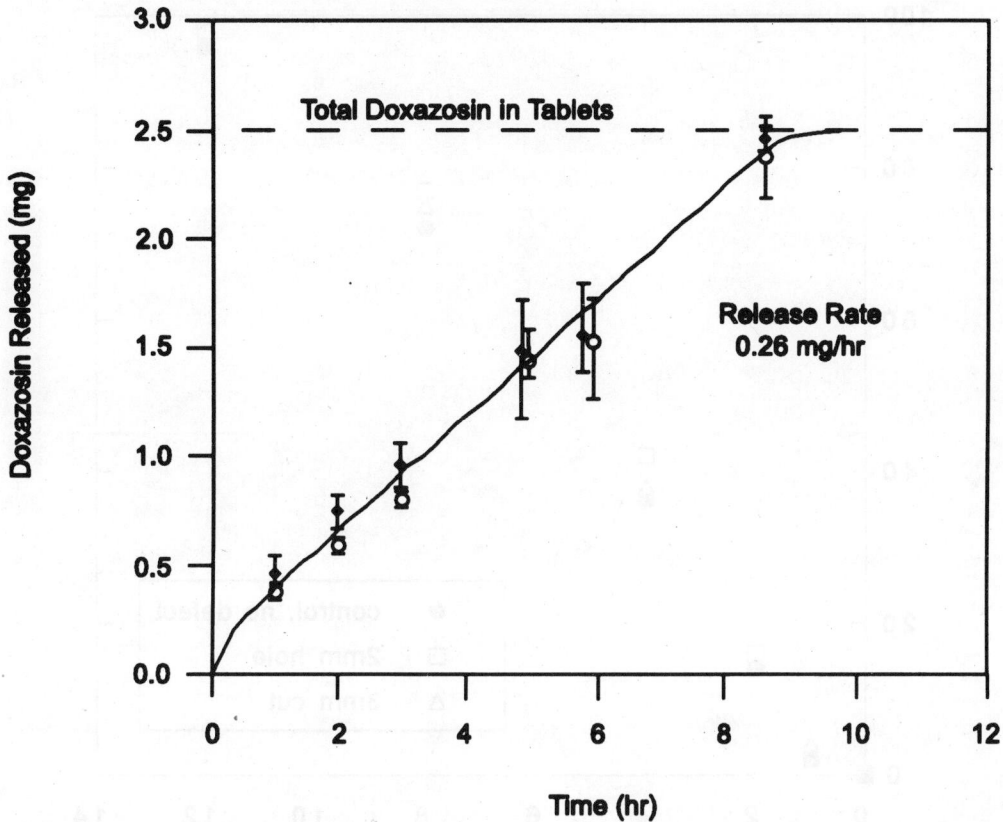

Figure 11 Release of doxazosin from AM tablets into 7.5-atm intestinal buffer (circle) or 7.5-atm gastric buffer (diamond) at 37°C. There are three replicates in each receptor solution (8).

drug release was calculated from the difference between the dose and amount remaining at each time point. The dissolution results are reported as the average of three tablets per assay time point.

As the results in Fig. 14 indicate, the drug release rate declined proportionally with increased media osmotic pressure. By extrapolation, osmotic release is completely shut off when the external media pressure exceeds 140 atm. The dependence of drug release rates on media osmotic pressure, and therefore changes in the overall osmotic driving force, is characteristic of osmotic delivery systems.

5. Effect of Bead Diameter on In Vitro Performance

The effect of bead diameter on release kinetics was assessed theoretically by varying three factors independently. The factors studied included the surface area–to–volume ratio, coating thickness, and size distribution. As illustrated by the data in Fig. 15, an increased average bead diameter resulted in a proportional decline in release rate from the AM beads, for beads coated to a constant thickness and distribution (standard deviation of 10% with normal distribution about the mean).

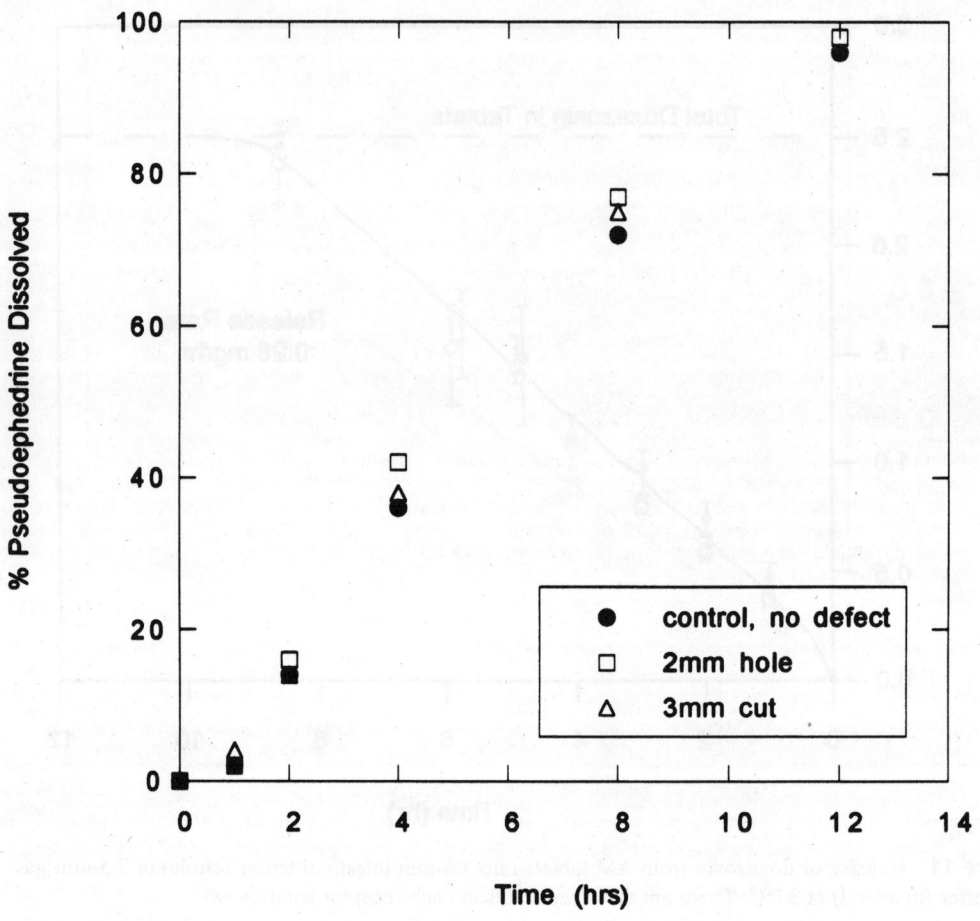

Figure 12 Effect of intentional defects in coating on pseudoephedrine release from AM tablets (2-mm hole or 3-mm cut).

Table 7 Four Different Core Formulations Prepared to Study Doxazosin Release Kinetics for a Range of Osmotic Driving Forces (8)

Formulation ID	Osmotic agent	Π_{core} (atm)	$\Delta\Pi$, driving force (atm)
1	Ascorbic acid	54	47
2	Lactose and succinic acid	47	40
3	Succinic acid	29	22
4	Lactose and adipic acid	26	19

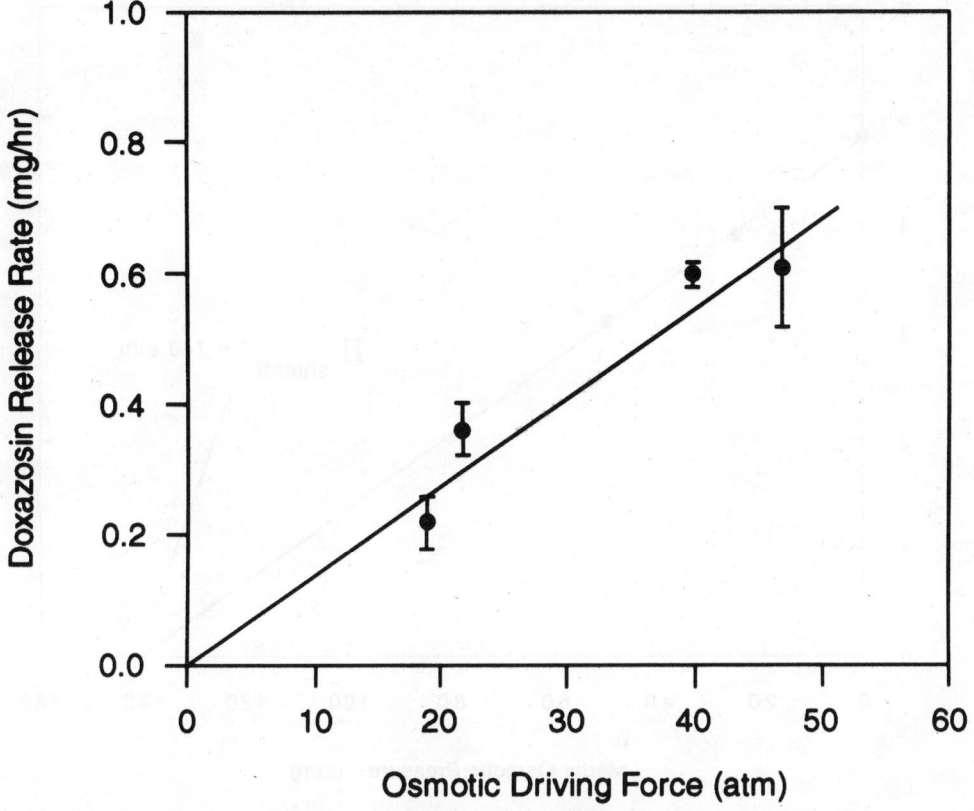

Figure 13 Release of doxazosin as a function of osmotic driving force (three replicates for each formulation and each tablet contained 2.5 mg doxazosin) (8).

As shown by the results in Fig. 16, the dependence of drug release rate on bead diameter was more significant for constant coating weight percent compared to constant coating thickness. This is attributed to the greater surface area per unit weight or volume of smaller beads. In addition, each small bead contains less total amount of drug, which reduces the release duration time when the release rate matches that of a larger bead. This translates to thinner coatings applied to the smaller beads and, consequently, increased release rates. An interesting example of the power of averaging can be seen by considering the average drug release profile resulting from a combination formulation of 50% 1-mm beads and 50% 3-mm beads. The resulting average in vitro profile aligns with the 2-mm beads in Fig. 16.

The effect of varying the standard deviation about one mean bead diameter (1-mm) on release was investigated. An increase in bead size distribution exhibited an overpowering influence from the larger, higher dose–containing beads (Fig. 17). The average release profile is shifted to longer release durations for the wider bead size distribution, as the smaller beads are exhausted. These results demonstrate the release kinetics from AM beads was dependent on bead diameter, coating weight percent, coating thickness, and size distribution.

Studies were conducted to experimentally assess the effect of bead diameter on drug release from AM-coated beads for an intermediate solubility drug substance (drug Y). The coating was applied using a Wurster fluidized-bed coater (Strea-1 Fluid Bed Coater, Aeromatic

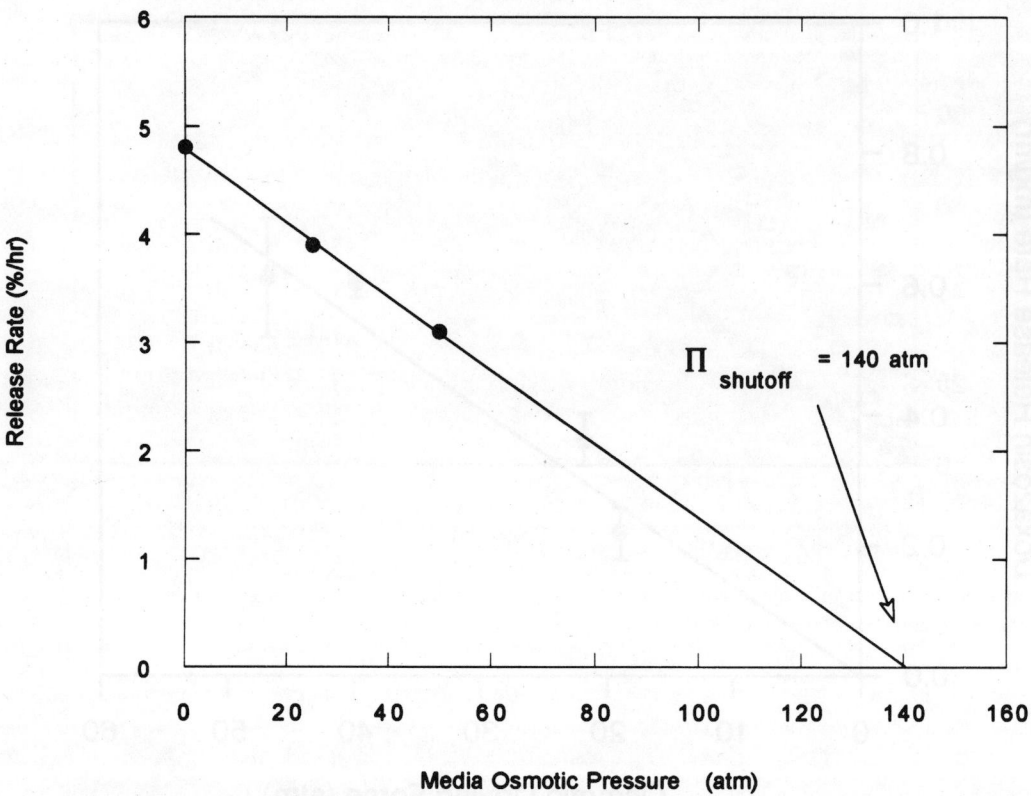

Figure 14 Effect of pseudoephedrine release rate from AM tablets as a function of external media osmotic pressure using sucrose in water at 37°C.

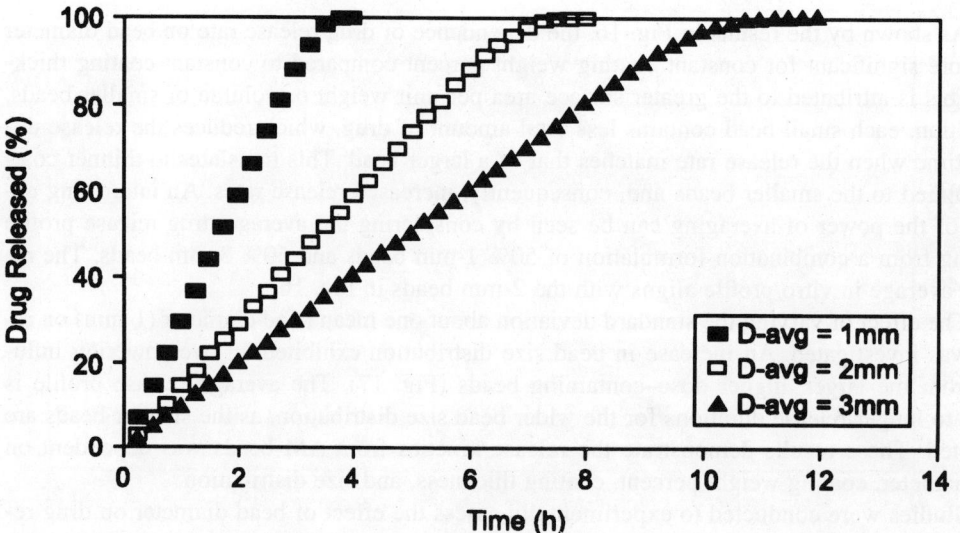

Figure 15 Effect of average bead diameter on drug release from AM beads while coating thickness (60 μm) and bead size standard deviation (10%) were held constant.

Asymmetrical Membrane Film–Coated Dosage Forms

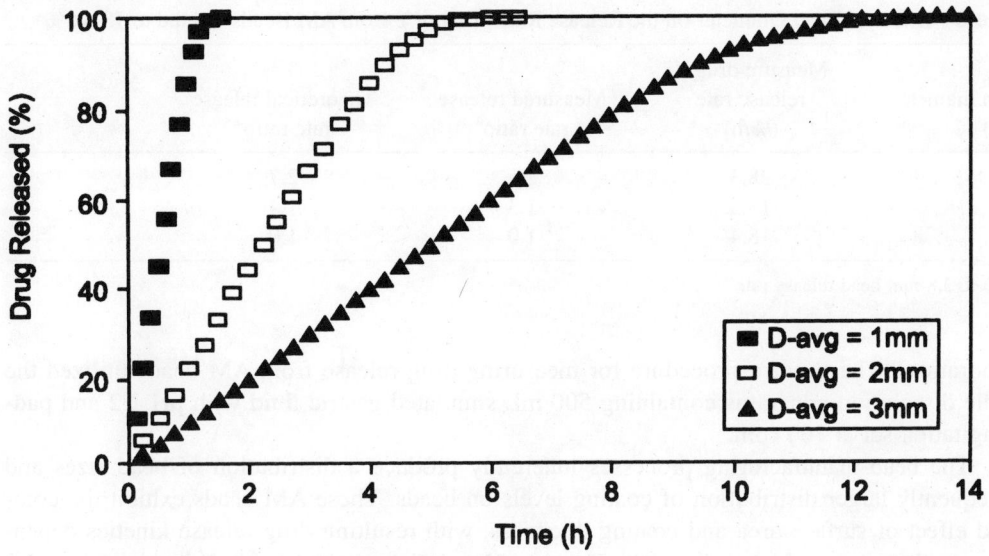

Figure 16 Effect of average bead diameter on drug release from AM beads while coating weight percent (13%) and bead size standard deviation (10%) were held constant.

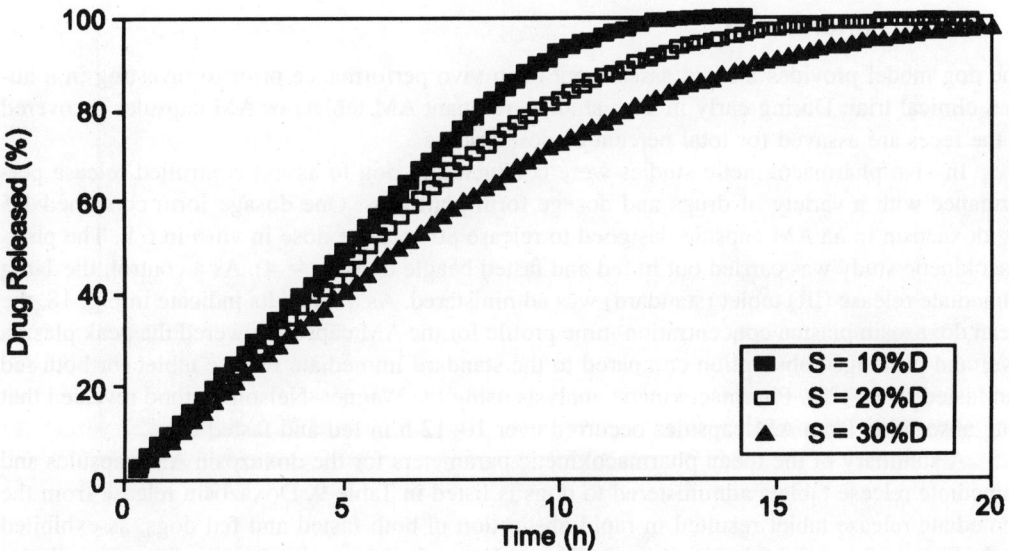

Figure 17 Effect of bead diameter size distribution on drug release from AM beads while coating weight percent (13%) and mean size diameter (1 mm) were held constant.

Table 8 Effect of Bead Diameter on the Release Rate of Drug Y from AM Beads Coated to 13 wt %

Mean diameter (mm)	Measure drug Y release rate (%/h)	Measured release rate ratio[a]	Theoretical release rate ratio[a]
2.3	38.3	2.5	2.7
3.2	19.5	1.3	1.4
3.8	15.4	1.0	1.0

[a]Ratio to 3.8-mm bead release rate.

Corporation). The in vitro procedure for measuring drug release from AM beads utilized the paddle dissolution apparatus containing 500 mL simulated gastric fluid with pH 1.2 and paddle agitation set at 100 rpm.

The bead-manufacturing processes inherently produce a distribution of bead sizes and subsequently larger distribution of coating levels on beads. These AM beads exhibit the combined effect of surface area and coating thickness, with resulting drug release kinetics dependence on the square of bead diameter. The mean bead diameters tested in this study were 2.3 mm, 3.2 mm, and 3.8 mm. Drug Y release rates were determined by linear fit to the initial 60% release and listed in units of %/h (Table 8). A comparison between the drug Y release rates from 2.3- to 3.8-mm beads and 3.2- to 3.8-mm beads is expected to be inversely proportional to the ratios of bead diameters squared, as described by Eq. 6.

$$\frac{\text{Rate}_1}{\text{Rate}_2} \propto \left(\frac{D_2}{D_1}\right)^2 \qquad (6)$$

The theoretical release rate ratios determined by the inverse square of the bead diameter ratio is closely matched by the ratio of measured release rates (Table 8). These results further demonstrate that release kinetics are dependent on the AM bead diameter.

B. In Vivo Performance

The dog model provides a rapid assessment of in vivo performance prior to investing in a human clinical trial. During early in vivo studies, remnant AM tablets or AM capsules recovered in the feces are assayed for total percent of dose release.

In vivo pharmacokinetic studies were conducted in dog to assess controlled release performance with a variety of drugs and dosage form platforms. One dosage form contained 1.5 mg doxazosin in an AM capsule designed to release 80% of the dose in vitro in 6 h. The pharmacokinetic study was carried out in fed and fasted beagle dogs (n = 4). As a control, the 1-mg immediate release (IR) tablet (standard) was administered. As the results indicate in Fig. 18, the mean doxazosin plasma concentration–time profile for the AM capsule lowered the peak plasma level and prolonged absorption compared to the standard immediate release tablet for both fed and fasted states (28). Pharmacokinetic analysis using the Wagner–Nelson method revealed that drug absorption from AM capsules occurred over 10–12 h in fed and fasted dogs.

A summary of the mean pharmacokinetic parameters for the doxazosin AM capsules and immediate release tablets administered to dogs is listed in Table 9. Doxazosin release from the immediate release tablet resulted in rapid absorption in both fasted and fed dogs, as exhibited by the T_{max} of 2.1 and 3.8 h, respectively. The AM capsule doxazosin pharmacokinetics reduced the maximum concentration from 9.1 to 6.9 ng/mL in fasted dogs and 6.6 to 5.3 ng/mL in fed dogs. The relative bioavailability of AM capsules compared to standard tablet was determined

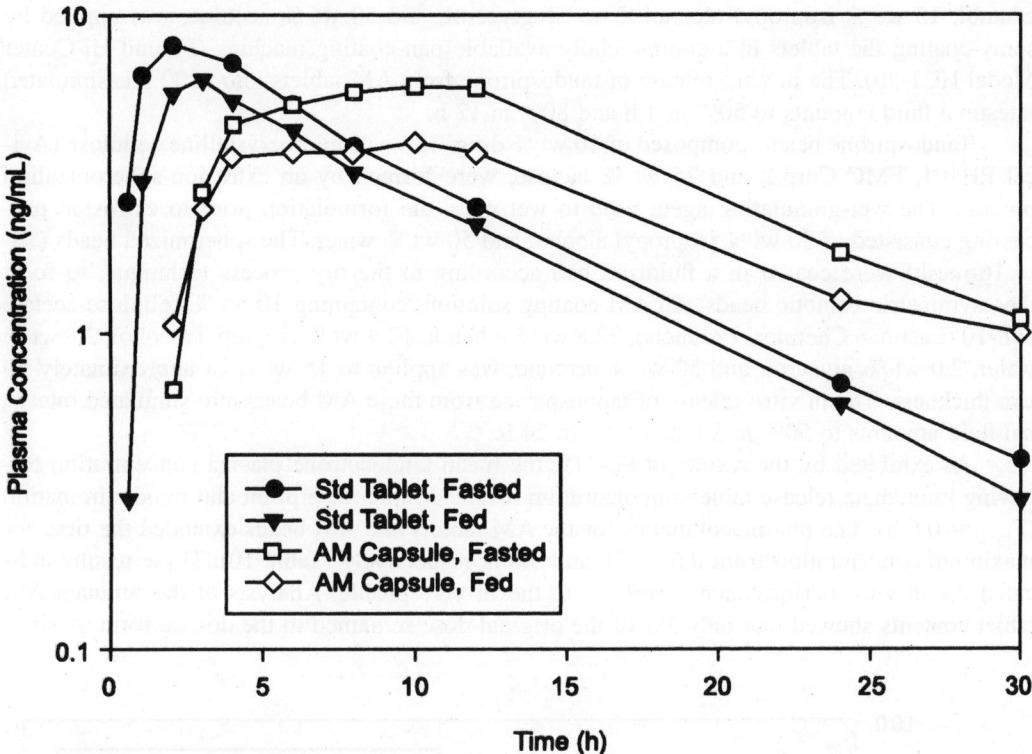

Figure 18 Mean plasma concentrations of doxazosin in dogs after oral administration of a standard 1-mg tablet or a 2-mg AM capsule in fed and fasted states (28).

to be 62% (fasted) and 56% (fed). These values are consistent with all drug being absorbed similarly to the IR tablet based on the analysis of remnant capsules recovered in the feces. The mean amount of drug remaining in the remnant AM capsules translated to in vivo release of 59% and 56% in fasted and fed dogs, respectively (28).

A pharmacokinetic study conducted in fasted dogs (n = 4) examined in vivo sustained release performance using two dosage form designs. In this investigation, 60 mg tandospirone was formulated into either a 12-h AM tablet or 24-h AM beads. The AM tablets contained 60 mg tandospirone, 300 mg citric acid, 200 mg lactose, 25 mg hydroxypropylcellulose (Klucel EXF), and 12 mg magnesium stearate. The AM coating, 10 wt % cellulose acetate, 22 wt %

Table 9 Mean Doxazosin Pharmacokinetic Parameters in Dogs (n = 4) After Oral Administration of a 1-mg Immediate Release (IR) Tablet or a 2-mg AM Capsule in Fed and Fasted States (28)

Formulation	Fed state	Dose (mg)	T_{max} (h)	C_{max} (ng/mL)	AUC(0-30) (ng h/mL)	RBA[a] (%)
IR tablet	Fasted	1	2.1	9.1	85	100
AM capsule	Fasted	2	9.0	6.9	106	62
IR tablet	Fed	1	3.8	6.6	65	100
AM capsule	Fed	2	7.0	5.3	73	56

[a]Relative to dose-adjusted IR tablet in same fed state.

ethanol, 13 wt % isopropyl alcohol, 5 wt % glycerol, and 50 wt % acetone, was applied by spray-coating the tablets in a commercially available pan-coating machine (Freund Hi-Coater Model HCT-30). The in vitro release of tandospirone from AM tablets into 1000 mL simulated intestinal fluid amounts to 50% in 4 h and 80% in 12 h.

Tandospirone beads, composed of 10 wt % drug, 15 wt % microcrystalline cellulose (Avicel PH101, FMC Corp.), and 75 wt % lactose, were formed by an extrusion-spheronization process. The wet-granulating agent used to wet mass the formulation prior to extrusion processing consisted of 50 wt % isopropyl alcohol and 50 wt % water. The spheronized beads (10- to 16-mesh) were coated in a fluidized bed according to the dry process technique, to form the asymmetric osmotic beads. An AM coating solution, containing 10 wt % cellulose acetate 398-10 (Eastman Chemical Products), 22.8 wt % ethanol, 12.4 wt % isopropyl alcohol, 2.8 wt % water, 2.0 wt % glycerol, and 50 wt % acetone, was applied to 15 wt % or approximately 50 μm thickness. The in vitro release of tandospirone from these AM beads into simulated intestinal fluid amounts to 50% in 8 h and 80% in 24 h.

As exhibited by the results in Fig. 19, the mean tandospirone plasma concentration following immediate release tablet administration revealed rapid absorption and rapid elimination (T_{max} = 0.6 h). The pharmacokinetics for the AM tablets and AM beads extended the time for maximum concentration from 0.6 to 2.8 and 5.8 h, respectively (Table 10). These results indicated the in vitro performance correlated to the in vivo profile. Analysis of the remnant AM tablet contents showed that only 3% of the original dose remained in the dosage form. A simi-

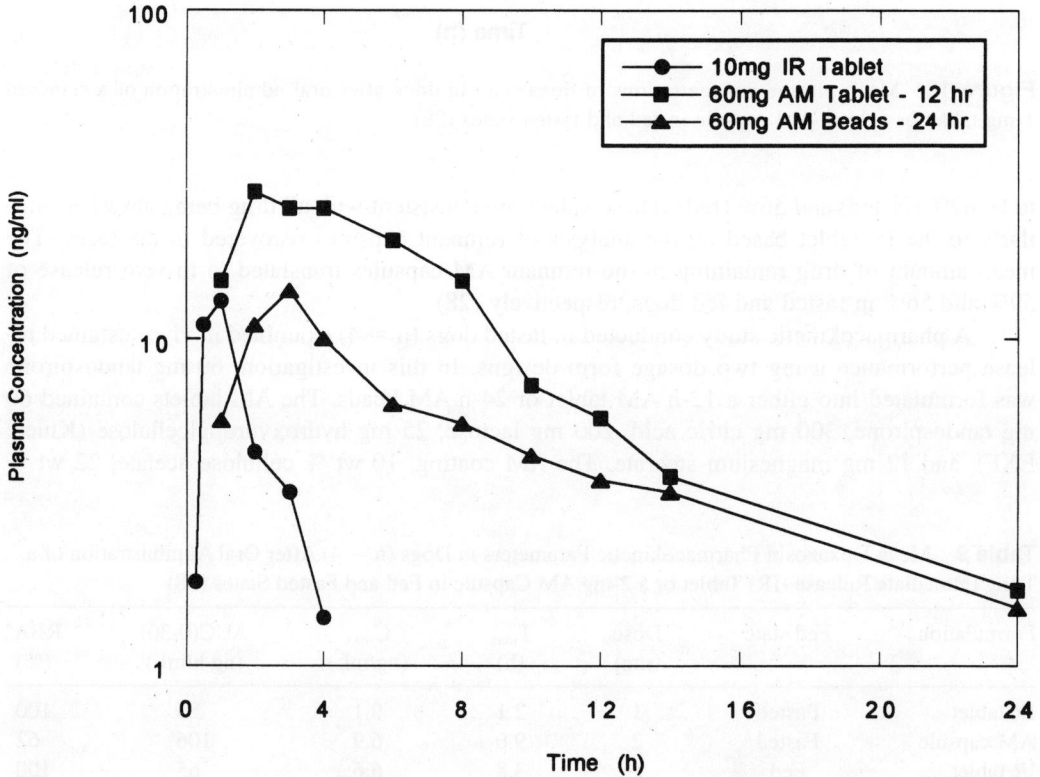

Figure 19 Mean plasma concentrations of tandospirone in dogs after oral administration of an immediate release (IR) tablet, an AM tablet with 12-h release, or AM beads with 24-h release (n = 4).

Table 10 Mean Tandospirone Pharmacokinetic Parameters in Dogs (n = 4) After Oral Administration of a 10-mg Immediate Release Tablet (IR), a 60-mg AM Tablet 12-h Release, or 60-mg AM Beads with 24-h Release

Formulation	Dose (mg)	T_{max} (h)	C_{max} (ng/mL)	$AUC_{(0-14)}$ (ng h/mL)	$AUC_{(0-inf)}$ (ng h/mL)(%)	RBA (%)
IR Tablet	10	0.6	18	20	22	100
AM Tablet–12 h	60	2.8	30	205	214	162
AM Beads–24 h	60	5.8	16	87	103	78

lar residual analysis was not performed for the AM beads, due to difficulty of total remnant bead recovery from the feces. These results demonstrated sustained delivery of tandospirone for the AM dosage forms compared to the immediate release tablet.

1. Comparison of Dog/Human Pharmacokinetics

To demonstrate the sustained absorption kinetics in dogs and humans, glipizide tablets were coated with an asymmetric membrane. These tablets contained 20 mg glipizide, 246 2 mg N-methyl glucamine, 69.2 mg microcrystalline cellulose, 69.2 mg spray-dried lactose, 8.5 mg hydroxypropylcellulose, and 10.9 mg magnesium stearate (7). The AM coating formulation, composed of 10 wt % cellulose acetate, 2% glycerol, 2.8% water, 12.4% n-butanol, 22.8% ethanol, and 50% acetone, was applied by spray-coating the tablets in a pan coater, HCT-30. The coating end point was achieved after 42.4 mg cellulose acetate, or 10 wt % CA, had been applied

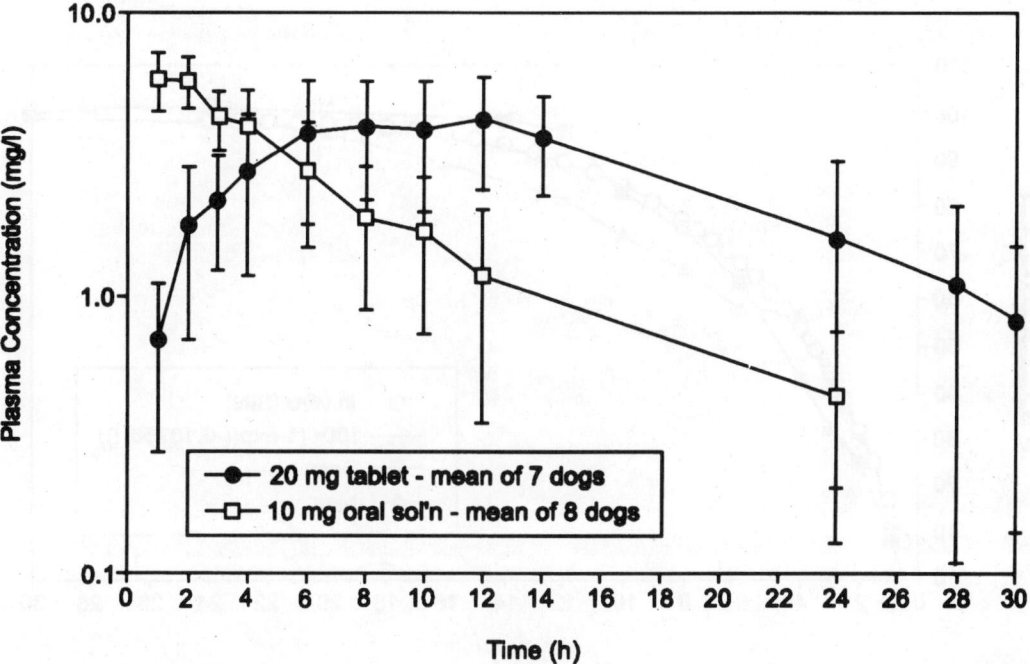

Figure 20 Mean plasma concentrations of glipizide in dogs after oral administration of a 10-mg oral solution (n = 8) versus a 20-mg AM tablet (n = 7) (29).

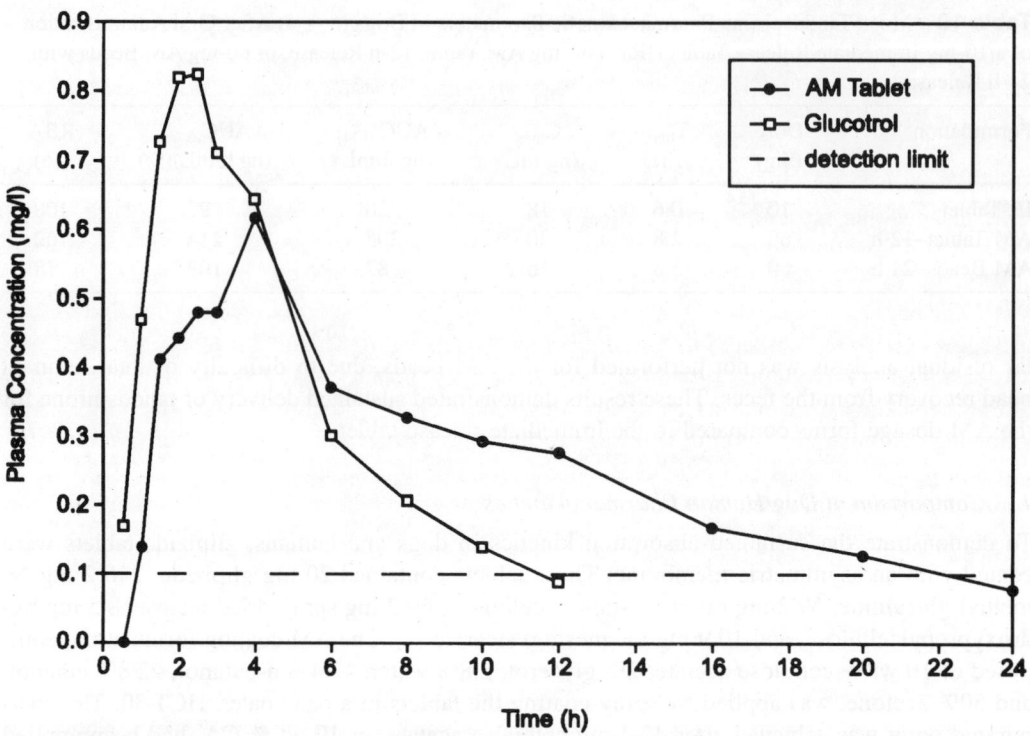

Figure 21 Mean plasma concentrations of glipizide in humans following oral administration of an AM tablet or a Glucotrol immediate release tablet (n = 6) (29).

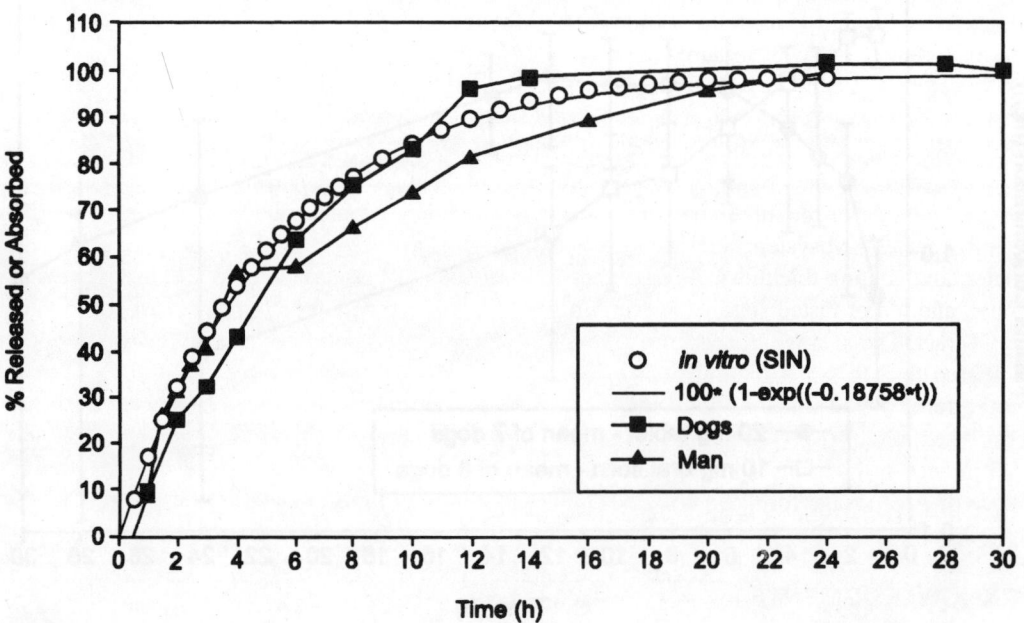

Figure 22 In vitro/in vivo comparison of glipizide AM tablets in dogs and humans. The elimination rate constant K_e was calculated from glipizide solution for dogs and from Glucotrol for humans (29).

per core tablet. The in vitro test procedure utilized the USP II apparatus with simulated intestinal fluid as media. In vitro release into simulated intestinal fluid indicated glipizide release from the AM tablets proceeded by a controlled fashion, with 50% dose release in 3.5 h and 90% delivered in 10–12 h.

The pharmacokinetic study of 20 mg glipizide AM tablets was carried out in fasted beagle dogs (n = 7) and compared to a 10-mg oral solution. As shown in Fig. 20, the mean glipizide plasma concentration–time profile for the AM tablet lowered the peak plasma level and prolonged absorption compared to the solution (29). Residual analysis of the recovered AM tablets indicated 90% of the dose was released in dogs.

The human clinical study was conducted to assess in vivo performance of the 20-mg glipizide AM tablet and compared to the commercial Glucotrol immediate release tablet. The study was designed as a randomized two-way crossover in six healthy male volunteers. These results further depict sustained plasma concentrations, extending T_{max} and lowering C_{max}, of glipizide following administration of an AM dosage form to humans (Fig. 21) (29). The in vivo drug absorption profiles in dogs and humans (scaled to total drug absorbed) correspond well to the in vitro release into simulated intestinal fluid (Fig. 22) (29). These results are consistent with the expected condition-independent release performance of osmotic dosage forms.

VI. CONCLUSIONS

In summary, the specific asymmetric membrane core and coating formulations and processing are tailored to the drug substance properties. This feature can require considerable development in the identification of a unique solubilizer or coating composition to achieve the desired performance. This required development can at times be a disadvantage, particularly for rapid assessment of dosage form feasibility for a new drug candidate. Although the development of the asymmetric membrane dosage form is complicated by the drug-specific nature, performance is robust, as expected for osmotic drug delivery systems.

Characteristic of osmotic drug delivery systems, the in vitro and in vivo performance of asymmetric membrane dosage forms is independent of many environmental conditions. In vitro drug release kinetics from AM devices is independent of media pH, agitation rate, drug saturation in dissolution media, and intentionally induced cuts in the membrane. Drug release is dependent on factors that affect the osmotic pressure gradient ($\Delta\Pi$), including the receptor solution osmotic pressure or the inner-core osmotic agent. Other key variables that influence drug release performance of AM systems include factors that alter surface area–to–volume ratio, e.g., bead diameter, and coating thickness. In vivo drug release from AM devices is independent of species, GI pH, and fed or fasted state. However, drug absorption can be a function of release location in the GI tract. The average transit time of a dosage form in the small intestines is 1 to 3 h in dogs, compared to 3 to 5.5 h for humans for fasted and fed conditions, respectively (30,31). Faster dosage form transit times in dogs may underestimate the overall exposure for the same dosage form when administered to humans. The dog model does provide a rapid assessment of in vivo performance prior to investing in a human clinical trial. In our experience, the in vivo performance of AM dosage forms corresponds well with the in vitro test results.

ACKNOWLEDGMENTS

The authors extend their gratitude to the following for their valuable contributions: Joel Bailie, Janet Bassett, Barbara Brockhurst, Mike Fergione, Christi Hostetler, Barbara Johnson, Marion

Johnson, Michael Likar, Gina Lorenz, Lee Miller, Kenroy Noicely, Cindy Oksanen, Mike Puz, and Avi Thombre for dosage form development and in vitro performance data, Mark Gardner, Steve Sutton, and Keith Wilner for human pharmacokinetic and in vitro/in vivo relationship results, and Bill Ballinger and Fred Falkner for dog pharmacokinetic results.

REFERENCES

1. Santus, G. and Baker, R. W., 1995. Osmotic drug delivery: a review of the patent literature. J. Controlled Release, 35: 1–21.
2. Wong, P. S., Felix, T., Ayer, A. D., and Kuczynski, A. L., 1992. Dosage form for time-varying patterns of drug delivery. US Patent 5,156,850.
3. Gupta, S. K., Atkinson, L., Theeuwes, F., Wong, P., and Longstreth, J., 1996. Pharmacokinetics of verapamil from an osmotic system with delayed onset. Eur. J. Pharm. Biopharm., 42: 74–81.
4. Grundy, J. S., and Foster, R. T., 1996. The nifedipine gastrointestinal therapeutic system (GITS). Evaluation of pharmaceutical, pharmacokinetic and pharmacological properties. Clin. Pharmacokine., 30: 28–51.
5. McClelland, G. A., Sutton, S. C., Engle, K., and Zentner, G. M., 1991. The solubility-modulated osmotic pump: in vitro/in vivo release of diltiazem hydrochloride. Pharm. Res., 8:88–92.
6. Theeuwes, F., 1975. Elementary osmotic pump. J. Pharm. Sci., 64: 1987–1991.
7. Cardinal, J. R., Herbig, S. M., Korsmeyer, R. W., Lo, J., Smith, K. L., and Thombre, A. G. March 18, 1997. Use of asymmetric membranes in delivery devices. US Patent 5,612,059.
8. Herbig, S. M., Cardinal, J. R., Korsmeyer, R. W., and Smith, K. L., 1995. Asymmetric-membrane tablet coatings for osmotic drug delivery. J. Controlled Release, 35: 127–136.
9. Zentner, G. M., Rork, G. S., and Himmelstein, K. J., 1985. The controlled porosity osmotic pump. J. Controlled Release, 1: 269–282.
10. Zentner, G. M., Rork, G. S. and Himmelstein, K. J., 1985. Osmotic flow through controlled porosity films: an approach to delivery of water soluble compounds. J. Controlled Release, 2: 217–229.
11. Swanson, D. R., Burday, B. L., Wong, P. S. L., and Theeuwes, F., 1987. Nifedipine gastrointestinal therapeutic system. Am. J. Med., 83: 3–10.
12. Baker, R. W., Smith, K. L. and Brooke, J. W., Delivery system. US Patent 4,769,027.
13. Cussler, E. L., Herbig, S. M., Smith, K. L. and van Eikeren, P. Osmotic devices having vapor-permeable coatings. US Patent 5,827,538.
14. Loeb, S. and Sourirajan, S., 1960. Report: UCLA 60–60.
15. Kesting, R. E. 1985. Phase-inversion membranes. In: Synthetic Polymeric Membranes: A Structural Perspective, 2nd ed. John Wiley and Sons, New York, pp. 237–286.
16. Thombre, A. G., Cardinal, J. R., DeNoto, A. R., Herbig, S. M., and Smith, K. L., 1999. Asymmetric membrane capsules-I. Development of a manufacturing process. J. Controlled Release, 57: 55–64.
17. Loeb, S. and Sourirajan, S., 1963. Sea water demineralization by means of an osmotic membrane. Adv. Chem. Ser., 38: 117–132.
18. Mulder, M., 1991. Basic Principles of Membrane Technology. Kluwer Academic, Dordrecht, The Netherlands.
19. Theeuwes, F. and Ayer, A. D., 1978. Osmotic device having composite walls. US Patent 4,077,407.
20. Baker, R. W., 1987. Osmotic and mechanical devices. In: Controlled Release of Biologically Active Agents. John Wiley and Sons, New York, pp. 132–155.
21. Lieberman, H. A., Lachman, L., and Schwartz, J. B., 1991. Pharmaceutical Dosage Forms: Tablets, Vols. 1–3, 2nd ed., Revised and Expanded, Marcel Dekker, New York.
22. Porter, S. C., and Ghebre-Sellassie, I., 1994. Key factors in the development of modified-release pellets. In: I. Ghebre-Sellassie (Ed.), Multiparticulate Oral Drug Delivery, Marcel Dekker, New York, pp. 217–284.
23. Aulton, M. E., 1995. Surface effects in film coating. In: G. Cole (Ed.), Pharmaceutical Coating Technology, Taylor and Francis Ltd., Bristol, PA, pp. 118–151.

24. Porter, S. C., 1989. Controlled-release film coatings based on ethylcellulose. Drug Dev. Ind. Pharm., 15: 1495–1521.
25. Porter, S. C. and Bruno, C. H., 1991. Coating of pharmaceutical solid-dosage forms. In: H. A. Lieberman and J. B. Schwartz (Eds.), Pharmaceutical Dosage Forms: Tablets, Vol. 3, Marcel Dekker, New York, pp. 77–160.
26. Aulton, M. E. and Twitchell, A. M., 1995. Solution properties and atomization in film coating. In: G. Cole (Ed.), Pharmaceutical Coating Technology, Taylor and Francis Ltd., Bristol, PA, pp. 64–117.
27. Benezra, S. A. and McRae, J. W., 1979. Pseudoephedrine hydrochloride. In: K. Forey (Ed.), Analytical Profiles of Drug Substances, Vol. 8, Academic Press, New York, pp. 489–507.
28. Thombre, A. G., Cardinal, J. R., DeNoto, A. R. and Gibbes, D. C., 1999. Asymmetric membrane capsules for osmotic drug delivery II. in vitro and in vivo drug release performance. J. Controlled Release, 57: 65–73.
29. Korsmeyer, R. W., Wilner, K. D., Ballinger, W. E. and Falkner, F. C., 1997. Asymmetric membrane tablets for delivery of glipizide. In: Proc. Int. Symp. Control. Rel. Bioactive Mater., 24, pp. 239–240.
30. Dressman, J., 1986. Comparison of canine and human gastrointestinal physiology. Pharm. Res., 3: 123–131.
31. Sako, K. and Mizumoto, T., 1996. Influence of physical factors in gastrointestinal tract on acetaminophen release from controlled-release tablets in fasted dogs. Int. J. Pharm., 137: 225–232.

37
Controlled Release Pain Management Systems

Vasif Hasirci
Middle East Technical University, Ankara, Turkey, and Northeastern University, Boston, Massachusetts

Dilek Sendil
Middle East Technical University, Ankara, Turkey

Leonidas C. Goudas and Daniel B. Carr
Tufts University School of Medicine and New England Medical Center Boston, Massachusetts

Donald L. Wise
Northeastern University, Boston, Massachusetts, and Cambridge Scientific, Inc., Cambridge, Massachusetts

I. INTRODUCTION

A. Pain

Pain, a nearly universal experience, is defined as "an unpleasant sensory and emotional experience associated with actual or potential tissue damage, or described in terms of such damage" by the International Association for the Study of Pain (Suri et al., 1997). The types and mechanisms of pain are given in Table 1. In addition to these, pain perception involves psychological components that may not be defined completely in physiological terms.

The awareness of pain is a highly important sensory function, since it alerts the organism to destructive or noxious stimuli. Pain receptors may be grouped as to whether they respond to mechanical, thermal, or chemical stimuli or to a wide variety of irritating chemicals such as bradykinin, histamine, and prostaglandins. There is a good deal of overlap, however, in receptor sensitivity to these different types of stimuli. Pain receptors, unlike most sensory receptors, do not adapt to a continuing stimulus. In fact, there is normally a decrease in pain threshold and increase in responsivity with time, so that the receptors become more sensitive to the pain (hyperalgesia). Nonadaptation to pain serves a protective function when the individual can remove the damaging stimulus or can get away from it. Nonadaptation might be highly detrimental to quality of life when the pain is caused by an incurable situation, such as certain forms of cancer.

At the spinal level, opioid analgesic function to impede pain impulses from entering the ascending pain tracts by inhibiting the release of the excitatory transmitter, substance P, from the sensory nerve endings in the dorsal horn. This modulation of transmission at the spinal level is a gating mechanism, the gate for pain being opened or closed depending on local enkephalin

Table 1 The Underlying Neural Mechanism of Pain. (WHO, 1996)

Type of pain	Mechanism	Example
Nociceptive	Stimulation of nerve endings	
Visceral		Hepatic capsule pain
Somatic		Bone pain
Muscle spasm		Cramp
Neuropathic	Damage to the control and peripheral nervous system	
Nerve compression	Ischemia via vasa nerovorum	
Nerve injury:		
Peripheral	Injury to peripheral nerve ("deafferentation pain")	Neuroma or nerve infiltration
Central	Injury to central nervous system	Spinal cord compression or poststroke pain
Mixed	Peripheral and central injury	Postherpetic neuralgia
Sympathetically maintained pain	Injury to sympathetic nerves	Some chronic postsurgical or posttraumatic pains

release as well as the action of other neurotransmitters in descending inhibitory circuit (Strand, 1983).

B. Opioid Receptors and Naturally Occurring Brain Opioids

A fascinating discovery is that the brain has *opioid* receptors, which have the ability to specifically bind opiates such as morphine and heroin. Snyder and Matthysse (1975) have shown that opioid receptors are concentrated in those areas of the spinal cord and brain concerned with the perception of pain, including the limbic system. These regions are also where opiates have their two main effects: *analgesia* (inhibition of pain sensation) and *euphoria* (elevation of mood).

Morphine does not occur naturally in the brain (at least in significant quantities), but a number of different peptides found in the brain have opioid activity. The smallest of these are the *enkephalins*, pentapeptides for which the entire amino acid sequence is known. The *endorphins* are larger peptides, such as β-*endorphin*, a 31-amino-acid peptide derived by cleavage from its precursor β-lipotropin, produced by the pituitary gland (Strand, 1983).

C. Causes of Pain

There are several causes of pain. When cancer is taken as the most important example of causes of chronic pain it is seen that pain may be caused by cancer itself (this is by far the most common). Pain could also be indirectly related to the cancer (e.g., muscle spasm, lymphedema) or be due to anticancer treatment (e.g., chronic postsurgical scar pain, chemotherapy-induced mucositis), or it may be caused by a concurrent disorder (e.g., osteoarthritis). Many patients with advanced cancer suffer from pain due to several of these causes. Cancer itself causes pain through:

Extension into soft tissues
Visceral involvement, often with obstruction
Bone involvement
Nerve injury
Rise in intracranial pressure

D. Pain Relief

Most pain can be controlled by pharmacological treatment with orally administered analgesics, either alone or supplemented with coanalgesic (adjuvant) drugs. With this conventional procedure only a small proportion of patients (10–20%) cannot be relieved properly and among these the most difficult are those with neuropathic pain. The World Health Organization (WHO), through its palliative care unit, has played a pivotal role in defining and disseminating the principles of cancer pain treatment. A simple stepwise approach embodied in the concept of the three-step analgesic ladder is the central idea of the so-called *WHO method of cancer pain relief* (Hanks, 1995; WHO, 1996):

The WHO Analgesic Ladder

A) Nonopioid Analgesics
Nonopioid analgesics represent the first step on the WHO analgesic ladder, where paracetamol (acetaminophen) or aspirin (*o*-acetylsalicylic acid) are used for the treatment of mild pain.

B) Weak Opioid Analgesics
Pain that is not controlled adequately with a nonopioid analgesic requires the addition of, or substitution by, a weak opioid such as codeine or dextropropoxyphene. The combination of a weak opioid with a nonopioid produces enhanced analgesia without the side effects associated with increasing the dose of the opioid.

C) Strong Opioid Analgesics
The last step in the ladder is the use of strong opioid analgesics such as morphine when pain is severe, especially in case of terminally ill patients.

E. Narcotic Analgesics

The term *opioid* refers to any natural or synthetic drug that has morphine-like pharmacological actions. The opioids are employed primarily for the relief of pain, but their use entails the risk of producing physical and sometimes psychological dependence. However, risk-free drugs that are effective against severe pain are not available. Opium is obtained from the milky exudate of the incised unripe seed capsules of the poppy plant, *Papaver somniferum*. The milky juice is dried in the air and forms a brownish, gummy mass. This is further dried and powdered to make the official powdered opium. Only a few poppy-derived alkaloids—morphine, codeine, papaverine, and noscapine—have clinical usefulness (Fig. 1). Of these, morphine, the alkaloid that gives opium its analgesic property, is used as a standard against which new analgesics are measured.

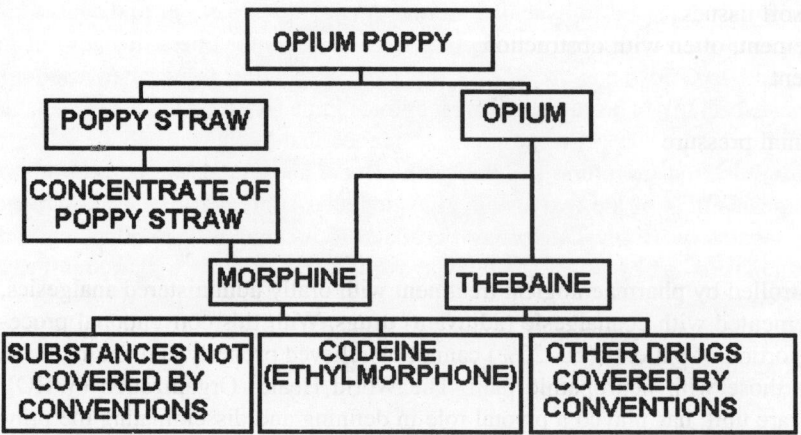

Figure 1 Production of opioid analgesics from the opium poppy (Angarola, 1990).

F. Mechanism of Action

Morphine and other opioids bind presynaptically on primary afferent terminals of the spinal cord dorsal horn, inhibiting the release of substance P and other neurotransmitters, thereby inhibiting pain transmission. Most opioids in clinical use, such as morphine, hydromorphone, and fentanyl, bind preferentially to μ opioid receptors, although others not yet in clinical use bind to δ receptors. Still other agents in clinical use, such as butorphanol or nalbuphine, bind to κ receptors although not with ideal selectivity. The potential advantage of opioids specific to non-μ receptors might be the lack of side effects seen with μ-receptor action, such as respiratory depression or constipation. Opioids are also recognized to act up on supraspinal sites to activate descending analgesic pathways and recently have been observed to decrease inflammation directly at the site of injury.

Local anesthetic drugs are categorized as membrane-stabilizing agents. These drugs reversibly block conduction of nerve impulses at the level of the axonal membrane. Impulses travel along the neuron by way of action potentials that are propagated by opening and closing sodium channels. Local anesthetics block impulses by interfering with the function of sodium channels along the membrane. When local anesthetic concentrations reach a threshold, membranes are stabilized as a result of blockage of all channels and prevent impulse generation and conduction. The size of the nerve fiber influences its sensitivity to local anesthetics. Small fibers tend to be blocked faster and at lower drug concentrations. Nerve fibers are categorized into three major classes: A fibers are myelinated somatic nerves, B fibers are myelinated autonomic nerves, and C fibers contain nonmyelinated axons. Both B and C fibers are small, generally less than 2 μm, but A varies in diameter between 4 and 20 μm. The A fibers are further divided into four groups: α, β, γ, and δ. The smallest A fibers, δ, are the carriers that initially signal tissue damage, sharp pain, and temperature. The B fibers innervate vascular smooth muscle (which has implications for cardiovascular effects associated with local anesthetic therapy). The C fibers are the more slowly conducting pain fibers, carrying the duller, throbbing pain. Fortunately, the C and A δ fibers are among the smaller fibers that are blocked more quickly and at lower local anesthetic drug concentrations than the larger motor fibers. This becomes critical when the goal is analgesia without anesthesia or motor impairment. Although all local anesthetics will block pain impulses to some degree before affecting motor function, some agents in this group have a greater ability to differentiate between sensory blockade and motor blockade.

Bupivacaine and the recently released ropivacaine are the agents most likely at low concentrations to differentially block pain fibers before affecting sensory or motor fibers. Because of its pain fiber selectivity and low cost bupivacaine is the local anesthetic most often used for chronic intraspinal use, especially in combination with opioids in the management of intractable cancer pain (Carr and Cousins, 1998). There is some evidence that analgesia may be potentiated when spinally administered morphine is given with a local anesthetic. This term *synergy* connotes that the analgesic effect of the two agents given together is greater than the combined effect of either drug separately. Bupivacaine may be added to an opioid-containing regimen when progressively increasing doses of opioid fail to relieve pain. Patients with a significant component of neuropathic or deafferentation pain may be more apt to require this combined approach (McGuire et al., 1995).

Some important analgesics are given below.

1. Morphine

Morphine is the prototype and standard of comparison for opioid analgesics (Fig. 2). The WHO has requested that oral morphine be part of the essential drug list and be made available throughout the world for cancer pain relief. Morphine and its surrogates produce their main effect on the central nervous system (CNS) and the bowel. It has been shown that morphine diminishes the rate of spontaneous release of acetylcholine (ACh) from nerve endings, in both the CNS and peripheral structures, without reducing its rate of synthesis. It also interferes with the release of ACh induced by electrical stimulation of the intestine, perhaps by an effect on postganglionic elements (Kosterlitz and Wallis, 1964). Similarly, opioids reduce the amount of ACh released by stimulation of cardiac postganglionic cholinergic fibers and of preganglionic fibers to the superior cervical ganglion. Morphine also appears to prevent the release of norepinephrine from postganglionic sympathetic fibers in the nictitating membrane. Although morphine does not prevent the release of catecholamines from postganglionic adrenergic fibers in the heart, it does decrease the myocardial chronotropic and inotropic response to stimulation by catecholamines. Morphine exerts in humans a narcotic action mainly seen as analgesia, drowsiness, changes in mood, and mental clouding. When morphine in the same dose is given to a normal, pain-free individual, the experience is not always pleasant. Sometimes dysphoria rather than euphoria results, consisting of mild anxiety or fear; frequently there is nausea and vomiting. Morphine also produces mental clouding characterized by drowsiness and inability to concentrate, difficulty in mentation, apathy, lessened physical activity, reduced visual acuity, and lethargy. As the dose is increased, these effects become more pronounced; increased drowsiness leads to deep sleep. Respiratory depression, the major toxic effect of morphine-like drugs, may also become more pronounced. But even large doses, particularly when given chronically, may not cause slurred speech or significant motor in coordination (Goodman, 1970).

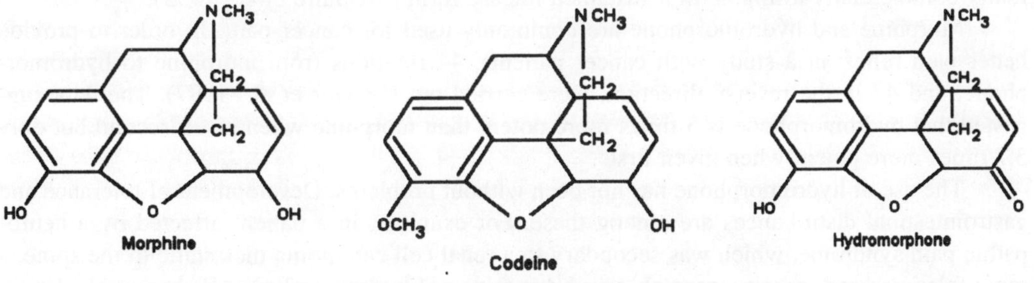

Figure 2 Structures of morphine, codeine, and hydromorphone (Sacerdote et al., 1997).

The clinical use of morphine may be influenced by new information about its active metabolites. Studies have demonstrated that morphine-6-glucuronide (M-6-G), a relatively minor metabolite by concentrations after single morphine doses, binds to opioid receptors and produces opioid effects with a higher potency than morphine itself. M-6-G appears in the plasma and cerebrospinal fluid of patients receiving morphine and accumulates in patients with renal insufficiency. In some patients with impaired renal function (e.g., creatinine level >2 mg/dL), high concentrations of M-6-G have been associated with opioid toxicity. A recent study suggests that M-6-G contributes to morphine analgesia even in patients with normal renal function (McGuire et al., 1995).

2. Codeine

The methyl ether of morphine, codeine, has only about 10% of the analgesic potency of morphine. Codeine itself has a plasma $t_{1/2}$ of 2.4 h, but free morphine also exists in the plasma after codeine administration. Thus it has been suggested that codeine acts as a slow-release prodrug producing low but sustained levels of morphine. The resulting morphine levels in the brain may be adequate for analgesia but less likely to induce abuse (Rogers et al., 1985). Although it is converted to morphine in the body before acting, it produces little euphoria and is of low addiction potential. In a study by Quiding et al. (1993), it was seen that four patients were unable to demethylate codeine to a detectable plasma concentration of morphine after 90 mg codeine. With those patients the analgesic effect during the first hours was better after 90 mg codeine than after 45 mg. Therefore, the investigators attribute some analgesic effect to codeine itself. In fact, codeine has been used for years as an alternative to aspirin for treating less severe pain and as a cough suppressant. It is given orally or by intramuscular injection (Rogers et al., 1985).

3. Hydromorphone

Hydromorphone is the oxidation product of morphine (Fig. 2). In this drug the C_6 hydroxyl group of the native opiate has been substituted with a carbonyl group, and a single bond introduced at C_{7-8}, yielding an antinociceptive potency that exceeds that of original compounds (Sacerdote et al., 1997). The usual starting dose is 1–2 mg by mouth (in contrast to 10–15 mg with morphine) or 1 mg by subcutaneous injection. The duration of action is 4–6 h (WHO, 1996).

Hydromorphone is, like morphine, a short half-life opioid and is used as an alternative to morphine by the oral and parenteral route in patients who require high doses or who have adverse reactions, such as histamine release, to morphine alone. It is more soluble than morphine and is available in a concentrated dosage form of 10 mg/mL. This preparation is intended for parenteral administration to the opioid-tolerant patient and, because of its high potential concentration, can be very useful when a subcutaneous infusion is the route of choice. It is not currently commercially available in a sustained release form (McGuire et al., 1995).

Morphine and hydromorphone are commonly used for cancer pain. In order to provide better pain relief, in a study with cancer patients, 44 rotations from morphine to hydromorphone, and 47 in the reverse direction, were carried out (Lawlor et al., 1997). The data suggested that hydromorphone is 5 times more potent than morphine when given second but only 3.7 times more potent when given first.

The use of hydromorphone has not been without problems. Development of tolerance and gastrointestinal disturbances are among these. For example, in a patient affected by a neuropathic pain syndrome, which was secondary to a renal cell carcinoma metastatic to the spine, a rapid tolerance and toxicity were observed due to use of hydromorphone (Vigano et al., 1996). A rotation to methadone led to a decrease of the morphine equivalent daily dose from 1050 to

36 mg, but after 4 months of good pain relief a switch back to hydromorphone was necessary due to worsening pain. The use of hydromorphone was, however, complicated by the onset of intractable nausea and sedation. In another study involving hydromorphone and morphine, in 119 bone marrow transplant patients the daily opioid consumption pattern showed a continual escalation during the first week of therapy for all groups, coincident with worsening mucositis (Coda et al., 1997). While morphine consumption reached a plateau by day 5, hydromorphone and sulfetanil consumption continued to rise until days 7 and 9, respectively. Sulfentanil requirement increased by 10-fold, compared with morphine and hydromorphone, whose requirements increased only 5-fold, suggesting the possibility of development of acute pharmacological tolerance.

4. Local Anesthetics

Local anesthetics are drugs that reversibly block the generation and transmission of action potentials in nerves. In the periphery, painful stimuli activate free nerve endings, which then transmit this information to the dorsal horn of the spinal cord via $A\delta/C$ fibers. These fibers are activated by harmful thermal, mechanical, and chemical stimuli from skin, subcutaneous tissues, joints, and muscles.

Clinically useful local anesthetics have an aromatic ring joined by an ester or aromatic link to a tertiary amine grouping and belong, respectively, to the chemically distinct amino ester and amino amide groups. A typical compound is bupivacaine (BPV), which is an amide-type local anesthetic used in primary clinical practice due to its blocking action for peripheral nerve conduction. However, various types of systemic toxic reactions often interfere with the full anesthetic potential of the drug. The present threshold of BPV toxicity is reported as 1.6 mg/mL of plasma.

The acute and most serious adverse effects of local anesthetics involve the cardiovascular and central nervous systems. They are usually caused by accidental intravascular or intrathecal injections, or a pronounced overdose. CNS symptoms of local anesthetic toxicity occur before cardiovascular symptoms and signs, and include numbness of the tongue, light-headedness, visual disturbances, and muscular twitching; more serious signs include convulsions, coma, respiratory arrest, and cardiovascular depression. CNS symptoms with the use of local anesthetics reveal that the threshold decreases with increase in the infusion rate because the maximum plasma concentration is directly proportional to the dose and inversely proportional to cardiac output and infusion time (Knudsen et al., 1997).

In a preclinical study, the effect on lipid dynamics and lipid–protein interactions in rat brain synaptosomal plasma membranes were investigated as possible mechanisms by which the local anesthetic BPV adversely affects nerve cell function (Kopeikina et al., 1997). Membrane-bound enzymes (Ca^{2+}/Mg^{2+}-stimulated ATPase, Na^+/K^+-stimulated ATPase, and acetylcholinesterase) were used as functional probes. The observations suggested that the drug can effect nerve cell function through asymmetrical perturbation of the membrane lipid structure and thus dysfunction of these enzymes.

However, bupivacaine when used as local anesthetic for spinal and epidural analgesia is reported to provide excellent anesthesia with minimal impairment of motor function even with very low concentrations. It blocks motor axons (preferentially ventral root in rats) (Dietz and Jaffe, 1997). However, the risk of hypotension, an adverse effect, must be considered after epidural application of this drug (McGuire et al., 1995).

There are few detailed studies about continuous administration of analgesics in humans for periods greater than 1–3 months. Local anesthetic blockade is generally regarded as a short-term analgesic technique for two reasons (a) secondary effects (sensory and motor blockade, symphatetic blockade, interference with urination and defecation) are deleterious in ambulatory patients, and (b) local anesthetic action may be associated with tolerance or tachyphylaxis. In a case study by Berde et al. (1990), continuous subarachnoid administration of bupivacaine for 7 months (with two brief interruptions) was carried out. This was done to provide relief of pain due to a spinal cord tumor that had already caused patient to be quadriparetic, without control of bowel or bladder function. Besides effective pain relief, this local anesthetic infusion provided a clear sensorium that the patient found invaluable and greatly improved her quality of life relative to systemic analgesia. These authors also suggested that the tolerance to local anesthetics may proceed more slowly when administered in the subarachnoid space than via other routes.

G. Methods of Drug Application in Pain Treatment

For the treatment of cancer pain there is no standard dose for opioid drugs. The right dose is that which brings relief to the patient because pain intensity and opioid responsivity vary from patient to patient. The range for oral morphine, for example, is from as little as 5 mg to more than 1000 mg every 4 h. Drugs used for mild to moderate pain have a practical dose limit because of their formulation or because of a disproportionate increase in adverse effects at higher doses (e.g., codeine) (WHO, 1996). More important parameters, however, are the way the pain reliever is administered and the form the drug is in, because through alterations in these, the plasma concentration of drugs and their distribution in the body can be modified to achieve different degrees of relief using the same dose. Commonly used and novel routes for drug administration are described below.

1. Oral Administration

The oral route is the simplest of all drug administration routes. Opioid analgesics are generally given by mouth and provide effective pain relief to most patients. Orally administered doses have a slower onset of action, relatively delayed peak time, and a longer duration of effect than those administered parenterally. For most oral formulations, the peak effect is typically achieved after 60 min. Although the oral route is generally preferable, it is not chosen in cases of impaired swallowing, gastrointestinal obstruction, or when there is a need for rapid onset of analgesia (McGuire et al., 1995).

The oral/parenteral analgesic potency ratio for morphine is stated as 1:3 to 1:6. Hydromorphone when given by mouth is 8 times more potent than morphine but only 6 times more potent by injection (WHO, 1996).

Morphine is the standard strong opioid analgesic for cancer pain relief. Given by mouth and by the clock, to prevent recurrence of pain, it may have to be maintained for long periods. In such instances, the dose (which may range widely from 2.5 mg to 2500 mg 4 hourly) is titrated against effect and there is no definite upper limit. An immediate release oral formulation of morphine is employed for short-term dose titration, where as controlled release morphine preparations are typically used for maintenance treatment (Hanks, 1995; WHO, 1996).

2. Rectal Administration

Morphine and other opioids may also be given per rectum. This is as effective as by mouth, but absorption is variable and can be affected by the condition of the mucosa, placement of the agent and use of lubricants. This route is not advised for use in patients with diarrhea or fecal incontinence (McGuire et al., 1995; WHO, 1996).

3. Subcutaneous Administration

When patients are unable to take an oral or a rectal drug, the subcutaneous route is an option. Repeated injections are unpleasant and should be avoided if possible. It is possible to place a fine-caliber needle under the skin after sterile preparation and to change needle sites every few days for an indefinite period. By injection, most patients need one-third to one-half of the previously satisfactory oral dose of many opioids. Morphine, hydromorphone, and levorphanol may all be given subcutaneously (WHO, 1996; Bruera, 1993).

4. Intramuscular Administration

The dose of opioids is the same as that for subcutaneous administration (WHO, 1996). Repetitive intramuscular (IM) injections are painful, are more erratically absorbed, and confer no pharmacokinetic advantage to the patient (McGuire et al., 1995).

5. Intravenous Administration

Opioids may also be given intravenously, either by bolus injection or by continuous infusion. The dosage is the same as the subcutaneous case (WHO, Geneva, 1996). This method of administration has the most rapid onset of action (usually less than 10 min for morphine). Repetitive parenteral bolus injections are usually effective but may be associated with prominent bolus effects such as toxicity at peak concentrations (McGuire et al., 1995).

6. Spinal Administration

The epidural and intrathecal routes provide pain relief with relatively few adverse effects. These routes are important with patients who experience severe adverse effects or who have pain that is poorly responsive to opioids. As spinal administration requires special expertise and equipment for catheter placement, these routes are practical for only a minority of patients cared for in specialized settings (WHO, 1996). The risk of infection and other complications also causes clinicians to employ intrathecal application of morphine in cancer pain only when all less invasive options have been exhausted. However, recent studies show that in long-term intrathecal morphine infusion more satisfactory pain relief is obtained with lower doses and fewer side effects, and a high degree of patient autonomy (Gestin et al., 1997).

Opioid selection for intraspinal delivery is influenced by several factors. Hydrophilic drugs, such as morphine and hydromorphone, have a relatively long half-life in cerebrospinal fluid (CSF), which results in substantial redistribution toward the brainstem. Rostral redistribution of hydrophilic opioids may increase the risk of supraspinally mediated adverse effects, such as sedation, confusion, nausea, and vomiting, but improve the likelihood of analgesia when pain is at sites rostral to the catheter tip or when pain is widespread (McGuire et al., 1995).

Pain may be defined as opioid-resistant in the face of intolerable adverse effects associated with inadequate analgesia. In this circumstance there are two possible solutions to improve analgesia and reduce adverse effects while still administering opioids alone. The first way is to change the route of administration of the opioid and second is the use of an alternative opioid agonist. As the route of application, spinal (epidural or intrathecal) has gained much attention due to evidence that analgesia may be obtained with much smaller drug doses, and an increased duration of action with lower adverse effects (particularly for intrathecal administration) than systemic use (Hanks et al., 1997).

High oral doses of morphine may cause disturbing adverse effects such as nausea, vomiting, sedation, hallucinations, and excessive sweating. Vainio and Tigerstedt (1988) have shown that for severe pain requiring high doses of morphine, equal pain relief with lower doses and less adverse effects can be achieved with epidural compared with oral morphine. But the epidural method requires expertise and close follow-up, besides having the possibility of technical problems. With time, the transdural transport of morphine can diminish and thus change its spinal availability. Subcutaneous infusion is another increasingly used method, and it is thought to reduce the incidence of adverse effects compared with oral morphine. Kalso et al. (1996) designed a study to evaluate the advantages and disadvantages of epidural morphine compared to the subcutaneous route. However, they observed no significant difference between the two routes in either effectiveness or adverse effects. Intracerebroventricular opioid therapy (ICV) is reported to be a rarely used option for the control of intractable pain due to cancer when systemic treatments have failed. It compares well with spinal opioid treatments in terms of efficacy, side effects, and complications (Ballantyne et al., 1996).

Intractable pain can be defined as uncontrollable pain despite aggressive use of conventional systemic opioids and adjuvant drugs. When all other appropriate analgesic therapies are tried with unrelieved pain, patients become candidates for intraspinal therapy. Lipid solubility of opioid is an important factor in spinal administrations. As lipid solubility increases, absorption of opioid from epidural space becomes faster. Conversely, when lipid-soluble drugs are delivered to the intrathecal space, they rapidly enter the systemic circulation by either capillary absorption in the spinal cord or back diffusion across the dura with absorption through venous structures in the epidural space. So it is suggested that more lipophilic agents offer less benefit when given spinally. Receptor affinity of a drug, along with the strength and duration of binding affects duration of analgesia. For example, morphine has a high affinity for its receptors and, therefore, has a long duration of action when used intraspinally. The molecular weight of these drugs also affects their distribution and thus effectiveness (McGuire et al., 1995).

7. Transdermal Administration

Certain drugs with a favorable oil/water partition coefficient, low relative molecular mass, and sufficient potency can be administered transdermally. Compliance of patients is generally very good as are the pharmacological results, but the cost of this method and its current limited availability restrict its use (WHO, 1996).

Transdermal application differs from the use of injectable microspheres in that in the former case the drug must penetrate the skin to be effective. Also the effect could be more localized depending on the site of application. A transdermal fentanyl patch for the treatment of chronic cancer-related pain is available to deliver dosages of 25, 50, 75, and 100 μg/h (Payne, 1998). Fentanyl was released from a 72-h reservoir by diffusion through a controlled release membrane to the skin, through which it is absorbed into the circulation. Unlike intravenous administration, where the plasma peak levels are reached in minutes with a plasma elimination half-life of 2–3 h, after the transdermal patch application peak levels are reached after 14 h and the half-life exceeds 24 h. When compared with oral morphine at doses effecting the same degree of pain relief, fewer gastrointestinal disturbances (nausea, vomiting, and constipation) and better alertness and sleep quality were observed. Thus the transdermal fentanyl patch was as effective as oral opioids in relieving cancer-related pain with a safety and side effect profile equal to or better than that of oral opioids. Patient acceptability was high, and the cost was lower than other methods required to deliver parenteral opioids.

8. Long-Term, Delayed, and Controlled Release Applications

Currently available local anesthetics and opioid analgesics have a relatively limited duration of activity (due to their short plasma half-lives), and some may cause severe toxicity due to their low LD_{50} values. In order to overcome this limited duration and provide pain management for longer periods, chronic drug delivery (mainly through infusions) has been put into practice. These generally involve infusion of medication at predetermined rates through a pump. Another approach is to modify the drug formulation and/or chemistry to provide delivery for prolonged periods such as 12 h instead of a typical 4-h application. The final and most promising one is the use of implantable or transdermal controlled release systems, which can provide drugs for periods extending to years. If prolonged, low doses of drugs could be used, then a variety of benefits might be observed. Prolongation of action, lowering of toxicity (as judged by LD_{50} values), and decreases in other side effects such as gastrointestinal disturbances, loss of alertness, and improved sleep quality would significantly benefit the patients. Development of tolerance might also be more gradual. Around-the-clock provision of medication would lead to stable and predictable plasma concentrations and would be convenient (and therefore increase compliance). The advantages of controlled release systems may be illustrated in the example of methadone maintenance of opiate addicts.

Methadone maintenance is an approach normally used as an antidote to opioid withdrawal. Here it achieves the following:

1. Reduces morbidity and mortality associated with intravenous drug use
2. Reduces or diminishes heroin use
3. Reduces HIV risk due to intravenous "street" drug injections
4. Is cost-effective (healthy people cost less to society)

Disadvantages of this treatment are:

1. Labor-intensive to administer under surveillance
2. Low initial treatment retention
3. Burdensome daily visits to clinics
4. High rate of relapse after termination
5. Inadequate treatment capacity
6. Illicit diversion of methadone

If an implantable controlled release system were to be introduced to deliver the methadone:

1. It would be easily implanted with a small incision.
2. The constant (or low) rate of drug release would minimize uncomfortable peaks and troughs.
3. It would eliminate hardware, personnel, and expense associated with subcutaneous or intravenous pumps.
4. Daily trips to clinics to receive daily methadone would be avoided.
5. The need for clinics would be minimized.
6. Illicit diversion would not be possible.
7. Since the antidote, naloxone, is available, in case of toxicity there would be no real danger.

Because methadone has analgesic properties, all of these advantages would also apply to cancer patients whose pain management programs cannot provide sufficient relief from pain due to fluctuations in dose, requirements for frequent administration, and the need for clinic care for administration of pain reliever.

Aside from the concept of methadone maintenance, continuous infusions are the presently accepted approach of provision of long-term medication. Thus, numerous studies along those lines are also being vigorously pursued. For example, in a case of severe cancer pain, 15 patients received two 48-h infusions of hydromorphone—one subcutaneous and one intravenous—using two infusion pumps, in randomly allocated order (Moulin et al., 1991). Pain intensity, pain relief, mood, and sedation showed no clinically or statistically significant differences. Side effects were slight and the morphine requirement for breakthrough pain was similar. Because of the simplicity, technical advantages, and cost effectiveness of continuous subcutaneous opioid infusion into the chest wall or trunk, authors suggested that intravenous opioid infusions for chronic therapy to be abandoned. Continuous subcutaneous infusion using portable infusion pumps appears to carry all the advantages of continuous intravenous infusion with the added benefits of greater mobility, management on an outpatient basis, and avoidance of the need for intravenous access. Some pumps are designed specifically for this purpose as low-tech, inexpensive, dedicated devices (Bruera, 1993).

Dahm et al. (1998) started testing the use of long-term continuous intrathecal opioid/BPV analgesia in a case not amendable to corrective surgery due to the absence of any reliable method for long-term treatment of severe pain following complications of hip arthroplasty. The uniqueness of their case is the length of the application, which exceeded 6 years. The patient was given 4.75 mg/mL bupivacaine and 0.015 mg/mL buprenorphine. The mean daily doses were 37 mg for BPV and 0.114 mg for buprenorphine. This intrathecal treatment with a local anesthetic and an opioid gave the patient 85–100% relief and mobility to carry out everyday activities (shopping, visits, etc.).

Various approaches to preparation of slow-release formulations of local anesthetics and opioids are available that allow patient mobility and avoid attachment of catheters of any type. Among the most promising of these are biodegradable polymer matrices and lipid-based systems (Renck et al., 1996). Although various formulations for morphine application are possible, modified release formulations are currently being intensively investigated. Some available sustained release forms are being prescribed with increasing frequency because of the convenience, continuous analgesia, and lower incidence of severity of morphine-related side effects. Oral controlled release morphine preparations provide analgesia with a duration of 8–12 h and allow the patients greater freedom from repetitive dosing, especially at night. Patients should be initially titrated on immediate release morphine and, once stabilized, administered the controlled release preparation. To manage breakthrough pain, immediate release morphine should also be made available to the patient. Recently, a sustained release morphine formulation called Kapanol (Glaxo Wellcome) has been developed. Both Kapanol and an earlier sustained release form called MS Contin (Purdue Frederick Co.) were designed as oral formulations with a 24-h and 12-h release duration, respectively. In a study comparing their performances, no significant difference was found between them in terms of any analgesic or pharmacodynamic parameters (Gourlay et al., 1997).

Similar to MS Contin, Codeine Contin was prepared as a sustained release form with a 12-h analgesic efficiency. Chary et al. (1994) showed that this formulation (150 mg/12 h) is equianalgesic to acetaminophen plus codeine (600 mg:60 mg every 6 h). They concluded that Codeine Contin sustained release form produces analgesia and side effects similar to that of a 60% lower cumulative dose of immediate release codeine every 12 h.

Since morphine is known to lead to adverse side effects, hydromorphone is prescribed as an alternative. It is 5 times as potent as morphine but it has a shorter elimination half-life, which causes 4-hourly administration of the drug. In order to prolong half-life and improve patient compliance, a controlled release form was prepared with 12-h activity as in the case of MS and Codeine Contin. This form was highly effective in the treatment of chronic severe cancer pain (Hays et al., 1994).

The use of oxycodone is also hampered by its short elimination half-life, which necessitates dosing every 4 h. In one study, 44 cancer patients were given controlled release oxycodone

(124 ± 22 mg/day) and controlled release hydromorphone (30 ± 6 mg/day) every 12 h for 7 days (Hagen and Babul, 1997). No differences were observed between Visual Analogue Scale pain intensities, categorical pain intensity, daily analgesic consumption, sedation scores, nausea scores, or patient preference. Two patients experienced hallucinations with hydromorphone, whereas none did with oxycodone. Controlled release oxycodone demonstrated excellent pharmacodynamic characteristics, analgesic efficacy, and safety as compared with controlled release hydromorphone.

In addition to these formulations, another category of drug carrier is available for delivery of local anesthetics and opioids. These are bilipid layered vesicles called *liposomes*. The action of even a "long-acting" local anesthetic, such as BPV, is limited to a few hours. Because an increase in drug dose could lead to systemic toxicity (especially CNS and cardiovascular effects), a liposomal drug delivery system resulting in a longer duration of action and reduced toxicity would be desirable. Lafont and Legros (1996) encapsulated BPV liposomes and showed that this resulted in lower and more sustained plasma levels than the free drug following a single epidural injection in rabbits. They also administered BPV liposomes epidurally to a patient and obtained complete analgesia for 11 h rather than the 4 h with plain BPV solution. No motor blockade or hemodynamic instability was observed with BPV liposomes.

In several other studies, local anesthetics were encapsulated to liposomes for topical application or administration around nerve structures to prolong their analgesic effects. Epidural and brachial plexus administration of BPV in liposomes led to a prolongation of human pain relief with minimal or no motor blockade. One potential source of concern is that the hydrolysis and oxidation products of lecithin, such as lysophosphatidylcholine and fatty acid free radicals and peroxides, have been demonstrated to be neurotoxic and cytotoxic. This possibility, however, has so far not occurred in any clinical trial. Malinovsky et al. (1997) assessed the histopathologic and blood–brain barrier changes occurring in the spinal cord after intracisternal administration of sterile, nonpyrogenic, and chemically well-defined lysophosphatidylcholine and peroxide-free liposomal BPV in rabbits. They found that injection of liposomal BPV increased the duration of motor block and produced no histopathologic medullary and blood–brain barrier lesions similar to that seen in control rabbits. Sustained release of BPV from liposomes is suggested as the most likely mechanism.

Liposomes were tested for their distribution in the body, too. After one extradural injection of 0.25% BPV 0.3 mL and ^{3}H-bupivacaine 0.005 mCi in multilamellar liposomes, no systemic radioactivity (plasma, liver, heart muscle) was obtained for 1 h, and the labeling was less than that of systemic distribution of plain BPV after 3 h (Boogaerts et al., 1995). In contrast, radioactivity in the lumbar spinal nerves peaked in the first hour and remained higher than that of plain bupivacaine for 4 h. No radioactivity was measured in CSF. Small unilamellar vesicles incorporating ^{3}H-cholesterol did not significantly label spinal nerves and central nervous structures, indicating that the mode of action of liposomal BPV did not involve uptake by nerve structures. Rapid uptake of radioactivity by spinal nerves suggested exchange of BPV between liposomes and nerve sheaths.

Liposomes containing local anesthetics have also been tested in mice. The duration of sensory block of the mouse tail was investigated using 1.1% BPV (Grant et al., 1994a). Sensory block was significantly prolonged with the liposomal formulation (130 ± 38 min) compared to plain bupivacaine (46 ± 11 min) or BPV with epinephrine (81 ± 28 min). The LD$_{50}$ for plain bupivacaine was significantly lower than that of the liposomal version (61 mg/kg vs. 291 mg/kg). The time for in vitro release of 50% of the drug through a dialysis membrane was markedly prolonged for the liposomal formulation (28 ± 9 min vs. 7 ± 1 min). Thus, the liposomal formulation of the local anesthetic was successful in prolonging the effect and had enhanced efficacy and safety. The same authors applied this approach to relieve postoperative pain in a mouse model via a liposomal morphine formulation (Grant et al., 1994b). The intraperitoneal lethal dose to cause death of 50% of the animals (LD_{50}) of free morphine was 400 mg/kg and the maximum safe dose (the dose that can be administered without causing any deaths) was 130 mg/kg. With the liposomal formulation even the highest dose administered (1650 mg/kg) did not cause death in any animal. Duration of analgesia was significantly prolonged with the highest dose (21.5 ± 5.3 h) compared with the maximum safe dose of free morphine (3.7 ± 0.75 h). *In vitro*, a slow release rate was observed from the liposomal preparation. Prolonged analgesia and decreased systemic toxicity for liposomal morphine were explained by sustained release of morphine from the liposomal depot.

In another study (Fletcher et al., 1997), BPV was encapsulated in poly(D,L,)-lactide microspheres. The encapsulation of BPV induced a dose-dependent increase in the duration of antinociception as compared with free BPV. Moreover, adverse effects of BPV, such as decreased blood pressure, were reduced in this system.

Even though durations of action are prolonged, the longest period with release systems or liposomes in general still does not exceed 24 h. In order to be truly able to free patients from frequent readministration, systems with longer release durations are needed.

Grossman and colleagues have developed a subcutaneous implant for controlled release of hydromorphone (Lesser et al., 1996; Grossman et al., 1997; Rhodes et al., 1997). This nonabusable, noninflammatory, biocompatible and nonbiodegradable implant delivered hydromorphone with near-zero-order kinetics; in other words, at a constant rate. The cylindrical implant consisted of a poly(ethylene–vinyl acetate) core and a poly(methyl methacrylate) coat with an opening along the axis. This was designed to provide an alternative to methadone maintenance for up to 90 days, especially for patients who were opiate addicts and who lived in remote areas or were unable to comply with periodic dosing regimens.

Biodegradability is important in that the release system does not need to be removed upon depletion.

A biodegradable, biocompatible, controlled release system for the delivery of local anesthetics to obtain prolonged, reversible nerve blockade when implanted or injected was developed by Sackler et al. (1998). The system consisted of microspheres of PLA and PLGA, among others, and was designed for the release of BPV as well as other local anesthetics.

In a similar study to develop a controlled release system, poly(D,L-lactide) and poly-(lactide-co-glycolide) microspheres were loaded with BPV and other local anesthetics (Le Corre et al., 1997). Encapsulation efficiency was found to be highly dependent on the lipophilicity of the drugs. The influence of molecular weight of PLGA on the release rate and on the release mechanism was found to depend on the drug and its physical state within the polymeric matrix. Diffusion-controlled release was evident in various formulations and was manifest as linearity of release as a function of square root of time.

Poly(lactic acid) microspheres prepared via solvent evaporation approach as a means to achieve sustained release of butamben, tetracaine, and dibucaine have been examined in vitro (Wakiyama et al., 1981, 1982a). The influence of preparation conditions on loading, and the rate of release from these microspheres were studied. Drug contents of about 25% and yields of ca. 75% were obtained. Diffusion-based release patterns were obtained. Release could be prolonged to about 600 h. The microspheres degraded significantly as shown by the scanning electron micrographs of specimens retrieved at the end of dosing.

Poly (D,L-lactic acid) microspheres containing lidocaine and dibucaine were prepared, and the drug release patterns as well as their anesthetic effects were examined (Wakiyama et al., 1982b). The release patterns of dibucaine from microspheres varied significantly among microspheres with different dibucaine contents, and the release mechanism of dibucaine from microspheres was greatly influenced by disintegration of the microsphere. *In vivo*, higher proportions of dibucaine were associated with a greater local anesthetic effect. The local anesthetic effect of dibucaine in microspheres lasted much longer (300 h) than that of the dibucaine hydrochloride solutions. As expected, the profile of the local anesthetic effect *in vivo* was different from the release profile *in vitro*.

PLGA is the most commonly used and most popular biodegradable polymer. Other groups have applied it to carry a combination of drugs. Microspheres prepared from PLGA 65:35 loaded with 75% w/w bupivacaine alone or with 0.05% w/w dexamethasone were prepared by solvent evaporation (Curley et al., 1996). The microspheres injected into rats produced sciatic nerve block ranging from 10 h to 5.5 days as shown with thermal sensory testing as well as motor testing. The presence of dexamethasone increased the block duration approximately 13-fold attesting to the possibility of increasing the duration of activity by the use of a combination of drugs, and the potential value of decreasing local inflammation.

Motor block was tested in rabbits that received the bupivacaine-loaded poly(D,L-lactic acid) microspheres via a chronically implanted epidural catheter (Malinovsky et al., 1995). Significant delay in reaching maximum effects and significant prolongation of motor block (244%) were observed when a dose of 5 mg of bupivacaine-loaded microspheres were injected.

Among other polymers tested are polycarbonate microspheres that were loaded with benzocaine, lidocaine, and dibucaine prepared by a solvent evaporation technique (Kojima et al., 1984). *In vitro* releases of up to 400 h with relatively constant rate was obtained. This is a sufficiently long duration for most acute pain management applications, such as after operations. As expected from the surface-to-volume ratio, decreasing the size increased the rate of release from these microspheres.

Another hydromorphone release system with hydrogel passages for drug delivery was designed for management of pain (Merrill et al., 1994). This time the polymers carboxymethylcellulose (CMC) and polyvinylpyrrolidone were used to make the core and the implant had a poly(ethylene oxide) coat with CMC gates to permit drug diffusion.

Polymer–local anesthetic matrices of other interesting types have also been constructed. 1,3-Bis(p-carboxyphenoxy)propane–sebacic acid anhydride (1:4) and bupivacaine were prepared by hot melt and compression molding (Masters et al., 1993). Local anesthetic release was achieved for 3–14 days depending on the choice of drug and processing condition. Twenty percent loaded devices achieved reversible neural blockade for 4 days in rats that received implants adjacent to their sciatic nerves.

H. Dual-Anesthetic Use

1. Logic of Dual Drug (Local Anesthetic and Opioid) Use [Partially Adapted from Carr and Cousins (1998)]

Opioid–local anesthetic interactions at the spinal level are now a cornerstone of daily clinical practice. Attempts to demonstrate postoperative benefits from systemic coinfusion of these agents have produced mixed results. Presently, as a result of compelling preclinical data, local anesthetics used to provide single-dose spinal anesthesia for surgery are supplemented with small doses of intrathecal opioid (e.g., meperidine, fentanyl, morphine) to secure postoperative analgesia. After major surgery or trauma, epidural infusion of a combination of local anesthetic plus opioid is now the worldwide standard by which other methods of acute pain management are judged. Many clinical reports attest to the safety and efficacy, particularly for movement-related pain, of such combinations in thousands of patients and indicate a reduction of side effects that would be expected if comparable degrees of analgesia were achieved by either drug alone. The value of such combinations for movement-related pain has led to their adoption outside the acute care setting for chronic management of cancer-related and nonmalignant pain. Keeping the concentration of bupivacaine below 0.1% minimizes the incidence of sensorimotor block during both acute and chronic infusion. Spinal application of nonopioid plus opioid analgesics may have not only a dose-sparing but also a tolerance-impeding effect.

2. *Advantages of Simultaneous Local Anesthetic–Opioid Use*
   1. Reduction of sensorimotor block caused by high local anesthetic concentration
   2. Economical, especially when they act synergistically
   3. Decreases the risk of tolerance development to opioids
   4. Provide a more effective pain management (local anesthetic during surgery and opioid for postoperative period) by using dual drug to manage different periods
   5. Capability to provide both rapid and prolonged pain management
   6. Reduction of side effects like toxicity, hypotension, sedation, nausea, vomiting, constipation

Although patients with intractable cancer pain had been studied previously during long-term infusion of morphine and bupivacaine, this method was undertaken as a last resort for severe pain despite the absence of toxicity of this mixture to the meninges, nerve roots, or spinal cord itself. Sjöberg et al. (1992) reinvestigated such problems with this mixture together with preservatives (sodium edetate and sodium metabisulfite). They carried out infusions of mixture via a subcutaneously tunneled Portex nylon catheter. In most patients catheter was coated with fibrin or by a whitish yellow fibrous cocoon. No cause of death other than cancer was found. Intrathecal administration of morphine in humans may cause adverse neurological symptoms (myoclonic jerking, hyperalgesia, and allodynia) if concentrations greater than 30 mg/mL or high bolus doses are used. Such neurotoxicity is attributed to a morphine metabolite, morphine-3-glucuronide, which might produce antiglycinergic effects at the spinal neurons. Bupivacaine potentiates spinal morphine antinociception. Long-term coinfusions of bupivacaine and morphine were therefore applied by both the epidural and subarachnoid routes for the treatment of refractory cancer pain. These achieved pain relief without clinically apparent signs of neurotoxicity (Sjöberg et al., 1992).

Besides chronic pains like that of cancer pain control of postoperative pain can also benefit from the use of extradural analgesia with bupivacaine and opioids alone or in combination. The addition of lipid-soluble opioids to bupivacaine results in improved analgesia and can reduce bupivacaine-related side effects. Cooper et al. (1993) demonstrated that combining extradural bupivacaine and fentanyl decreased analgesic requirements of each individual agent.

Comparative effects of using ketorolac or bupivacaine along with hydromorphone were investigated in relieving postoperative pain and on pulmonary function in patients after thoracotomy (Singh et al., 1997). They observed that both ketorolac and bupivacaine supplementation of hydromorphone patient-controlled epidural analgesia (PCEA) reduced the severities of pain on coughing and on movement compared with hydromorphone PCEA alone.

When epidural HM and epidural bupivacaine were followed by intramuscular hydromorphone the group that received only HM (epidural and intramuscular) had more side effects (nausea/vomiting and pruritis) than the patients that had epidural bupivacaine followed by intramuscular hydromorphone (Chestnut et al., 1986). This also is a proof of the utility of combination drugs.

Intrathecal opioids can provide labor analgesia but the onset of pain relief is slow. Bupivacaine causes less motor blockade than other local anaesthetics. Thus, they both have desirable properties that complement each other. Morphine and bupivacaine were, therefore, concomitantly used intrathecal on 55 patients (Wu et al., 1997). The results showed that a single injection of intrathecal morphine and bupivacaine provided rapid-onset and effective analgesia with manageable side effects and without major complications.

The usefulness of adding bupivacaine to an opioid administered by the epidural route is reported to have led to results inconsistent with others. In one study, patients undergoing open knee or ankle surgery with combined spinal–epidural anesthesia received postoperative analgesia via PCEA with sulfentanil alone or with 0.06% or 0.12% bupivacaine (Vercauteren et al., 1998). Patients receiving bupivacaine had better pain relief than those receiving only the opioid. The consumption of sulfentanil was significantly higher in the group receiving the opioid alone than in the group receiving both.

In progressive cancer syndromes that involve the spinal cord and vertebrae, severe back pain in combination with motor and sensory disturbances in the legs and problems with micturition can be observed (van Dongen et al., 1997). In these situations, increasing the dosage of systemic analgesics is considered first but this might be insufficient. Morphine and bupivacaine were intrathecally coadministered. Five patients showed symptoms of compression of the cauda equina or spinal cord shortly after the start of combined intrathecal administration of morphine and BPV in a dosage usually not associated with neurological symptoms. Epidural administration of hydromorphone was evaluated using a patient-controlled epidural analgesia delivery system in women undergoing cesarean delivery (Parker et al., 1992). In this case, however, concomitant use of a local anesthetic (BPV) or basal opioid infusion with hydromorphone via PCEA did not decrease the number of PCEA demands or delivered doses.

As a whole, it appears that the simultaneous use of local anesthetics and opioids is an effective pain management approach. The only problem is the modality (currently via pumps or injections) necessary to administer them. The future of pain management may involve the simultaneous delivery of local anesthetics and opioids, possibly along with other agents as well, through implantable controlled release systems.

ACKNOWLEDGMENT

This work was carried out while Professor Hasirci was on sabbatical leave from the Middle East Technical University, Ankara, Turkey, as a Fulbright Scholar at Northeastern University, Department of Chemical Engineering, Boston, MA. USA. Professor Hasirci wishes to acknowledge the assistance of his Ph.D. student Dilek Sendil, and colleagues Daniel B. Carr, M.D., Saltonstall Professor of Anesthesia and Medicine, Department of Medicine, Tufts University, School of Medicine, Boston, MA, USA and Donald L. Wise, Ph.D., Chairman, Cambridge Scientific, Inc. (and Cabot Chair Professor of Chemical Engineering, Emeritus, Department of Chemical Engineering, Northeastern University, Boston, MA, USA).

REFERENCES

S. Ahmedzai. Current strategies for pain control, Ann. Oncol., 8 (Suppl. 3), 21–24, 1997.
R. Angarola. Availability and regulation of opioid analgesics, Advances in Pain Research and Therapy, 16, Raven Press, New York, 1990.
J. C. Ballantyne, D. B. Carr, C. S. Berkey, T. C. Chalmers, and F. Mosteller. Comparative efficacy of epidural, subarachnoid and intracerebroventricular opioids in patients with pain due to cancer, Reg. Anesth., 21, 542–556, 1996.
C. B. Berde, N. Sethna, L. Conrad, M. B. Hershenson, and J. Shillito. Subarachnoid bupivacaine analgesia for seven months for a patient with a spinal cord tumor, Anesthesiology, 72, 1094–1096, 1990.

J. G. Boogaerts, N. D. Lafon, S. Carlino, E. Noel, P. Raynal, G. Goffinet, and F. J. Legros, Biodistribution of liposome-associated bupivacaine after extradural administration to rabbits, Br. J. Anaesth., 75(3), 319–325, 1995.

E. Bruera. Alternate routes for home opioid therapy, Pain: Clin. Updates, 1(2), 1–4, 1993.

D. B. Carr and M. J. Cousins. Spinal route of analgesia. Opioids and future options. In: Neural Blockade in Clinical Anesthesia and Management of Pain, 3rd Ed., eds. M. J. Cousins, P. O. Bridenbaugh, Lippincott-Raven Publ., 1998, pp. 915–983.

S. Chary, B. R. Goughnour, D. E. Moulin, W. R. Thorpe, Z. Harsanyi, and A. C. Darke. The dose response relationship of controlled-release codeine (codeine contin) in chronic cancer pain, J. Pain Sympt. Manage., 9(6), 363–371, 1994.

D. H. Chestnut, W. W. Choi, and T. Isbell. Epidural hydromorphone for post-cesarean analgesia, Obstet. Gynecol., 68(1), 65–69, 1986.

B. A. Coda, B. O'Sullivan, G. Donaldson, S. Bohl, C. R. Chapman, and D. D. Shen. Comparative efficacy of patient controlled administration of morphine, hydromorphone, or sulfentanil for the treatment of oral mucositis pain following bone marrow transplantation, Pain, 72(3), 333–346, 1997.

D. W. Cooper and G. Turner. Patient controlled extradural analgesia to compare bupivacaine, fentanyl and bupivacaine fentanyl in the treatment of postoperative pain, Br. J. Anaesth., 70, 503–507, 1993.

J. Curley, J. Castillo, J. Hotz, M. Uezono, S. Hernandez, J.-O. Lim, J. Tigner and M. Chasin. Prolonged regional nerve blockade. Injectable biodegradable bupivacaine/polyester microspheres, Anesthesiology, 84(6), 1401–1410, 1996.

P. O. Dahm, P. V. Nitescu, L. K. Appelgren and I. D. Curelaru. Six years of continuous infusion of opioid and bupivacaine in the treatment of refractory pain due to intrapelvic extrusion of bone cement after total hip arthroplasty, Reg. Anesth. Pain Med., 23(3), 315–319, 1998.

F. B. Dietz and R. A. Jaffe. Bupivacaine preferentially blocks ventral root axons in rats, Anesthesiology, 86, 172–180, 1997.

D. Fletcher, P. L. Corre, G. Guilbaud, and R. L. Verge. Antinociceptive effect of bupivacaine encapsulated in poly(D,L)-lactide-co-glycolide microspheres in the acute inflammatory pain model of carrageenin injected rats, Anesth. Analgesia, 84, 90–94, 1997.

Y. Gestin, A. Vainio, and M. A. Pegurier, Long-term intrathecal infusion of morphine in the home care of patients with advanced cancer, ACTA Anaesthesiol. Scand., 41, 12–17, 1997.

L. S. Goodman and A. Gilman. The Pharmacological Basis of Therapeutics, 4th ed., 1970.

G. K. Gourlay, D. A. Cherry, M. M. Onley, S. G. Tordoff, D. A. Conn, G. M. Hood and J. L. Plummer. Pharmacodynamics of twenty-four hourly Kapanol compared to twelve hourly MS Contin in the treatment of severe cancer pain, Pain, 69, 295–302, 1997.

G. J. Grant, K. Vermeulen, L. Langerman, M. Zakowski, and H. Turndorf. Prolonged analgesia with bupivacaine in a mouse model, Reg. Anesth., 19(4), 264–269, 1994a.

G. J. Grant, K. Vermeulen, M. I. Zakowski, M. Stenner, H. Turndorf, and L. Langerman. Prolonged analgesia and decreased toxicity with liposomal morphine in a mouse model, Anesth. Analg., 79(4), 706–709, 1994.

S. A. Grossman, K. W. Leong, G. J. Lesser, and H. Lo. Subcutaneous implant, US Patent 5,633,000 (1997).

N. A. Hagen and N. Babul. Comparative clinical efficacy and safety of a novel controlled release oxycodone formulation and controlled-release hydromorphone in treatment of cancer pain, Cancer, 79(7), 1428–1437, 1997.

N. Hagen, et al. Steady-state pharmacokinetics of hydromorphone and hydromorphone-3-glucuronide in cancer patients after immediate and controlled release hydromorphone, J. Clin. Pharm., 35(1), 35–37, 1995.

G. W. Hanks. Cancer pain and the importance of its control, Anti Cancer Drugs, 6(3), 14–17, 1995.

G. W. Hanks and K. Forbes. Opioid responsiveness, Acta Anaesthesiol. Scand., 41, 154–158, 1997.

H. Hays, N. Hagen, M. Thirlwell, H. Dhaliwal, N. Babul, Z. Harsanyi, and A. C. Darke. Comparative clinical efficacy and safety of immediate release and controlled release hydromorphone for chronic cancer pain, Cancer, 74(6), 1808–1815, 1994.

E. Kalso, T. Heiskanen, M. Rantio, P. H. Rosenberg, and A. Vainio. Epidural and subcutaneous morphine in the management of cancer pain: a double blind cross-over study, Pain, 67, 443–449, 1996.

K. Knudsen, M. B. Suurkula, S. Blomberg, J. Sjovall, and N. Edvardsson. Central nervous and cardiovascular effects of Y. V. infusion of ropivacaine, bupivacaine and placebo in volunteers, Brit. J. Anaesthesia, 78, 507–514, 1997.

T. Kojima, M. Nakano, K. Juni, S. Inoue, and Y. Yoshida. Preparation and evaluation in vitro of polycarbonate microspheres containing local anesthetics, Chem. Pharm. Bull., 32(7), 2795–2802, 1984.

L. T. Kopeikina, E. F. Kamper, I. Siafaka, and J. Stavridis. Modulation of synaptosomal plasma membrane-bound enzyme activity through the perturbation of plasma membrane lipid structure by bupivacaine, Anesthesia Analg., 85, 1337–1343, 1997.

H. W. Kosterlitz and D. L. Wallis. The action of morphine-like drugs on impulse transmission in mammalian nerve fibers, Br. J. Pharmacol., 22, 499, 1964.

N. D. Lafont and F. J. Legros. Use of liposome-associated bupivacaine in a cancer pain syndrome, Anaesthesia, 51, 578–579, 1996.

P. Lawlor, K. Turner, J. Hanson, and E. Bruera. Dose ratio between morphine and hydromorphone in patients with cancer pain: a retrospective study, Pain, 72(1–2), 79–85, 1997.

P. Le Corre, J. H. Rytting, V. Gajan, F. Chevanne, and R. Le Verge. In vitro controlled release kinetics of local anesthetics from poly(d,l-lactide) and poly(lactide-co-glycolide) microspheres, J. Microencapsul., 14(2), 243–255, 1997.

G. J. Lesser, S. A. Grossman, K. W. Leong, H. Lo, and S. Eller. In vitro and in vivo studies of subcutaneous hydromorphone implants designed for the treatment of cancer pain, Pain, 65(2–3), 265–272, 1996.

J. M. Malinovsky, D. Benhamou, M. Alafandy, J. M. Mussini, C. Coussaert, G. Courraze, M. Pinaud, and F. J. Legros. Neurotoxicological assessment after intracisternal injection of liposomal bupivacaine in rabbits, Anesthesia Analg., 85, 1331–1336, 1997.

J. M. Malinovsky, J.-M. Bernard, P. Le Corre, J.-B. Dumand, J.-Y. Lepage, R. Le Verge, and R. Souron. Motor and blood pressure effects from epidural sustained release bupivacaine from polymer microspheres: a dose–response study in rabbits, Anesthesia Analg., 81, 519–524, 1995.

D. B. Masters, C. B. Berde, S. Dutta, T. Turek, and R. Langer. Sustained local anesthetic release from bioerodible polymer matrices: a potential for prolonged regional analgesia, Pharm. Res., 10(10), 1527–1532, 1993.

D. B. McGuire, C. H. Yarbro, and B. R. Ferrell. Cancer Pain Management, 2nd ed., Jones and Bartlett, 1995.

S. Merrill, A. D. Ayer, N. Chadha, and A. L. Kuczynski. Hydromorphone therapy, US Patent 5,529,787 (1994).

D. E. Moulin, J. H. Kreeft, N. Murray-Parsons, and A. I. Bouquillin. Comparison of continuous subcutaneous and intravenous hydromorphone infusions for management of cancer pain, The Lancet, 137, 465–468, 1991.

R. K. Parker, Y. Sawaki, and P. F. White. Epidural patient-controlled analgesia: influence of bupivacaine hydromorphone basal infusion on pain control after cesarean delivery, Anesthesia. Analg. 75(5), 740–746, 1992.

R. Payne. Factors influencing quality of life in cancer patients: the role of transdermal fentanyl in the management of pain, Semin Oncol. 25(3, Suppl 7), 47–53, 1998.

H. Quiding, G. Lundqvist, L. O. Boreus, U. Bondesson, and J. Ohrvik. Analgesic effect and plasma concentration of codeine and morphine after two dose levels of codeine following oral surgery, Eur. J. Clin. Pharmacol. 44: 4, 319–323, 1993.

H. Renck and R. Wallin. Slow release formulations of local anesthetics and opioids, Curr. Opin. Anesthesiol., 9, 399–403, 1996.

D. J. Rhodes and S. A. Grossman. Hydromorphone polymer implant, J. Substance Abuse Treat., 14(6), 535–542, 1997.

H. J. Rogers, R. G. Spector, and J. R. Trounce. A Textbook of Clinical Pharmacology, Hodder and Stoughton Press, 1985.

P. Sacerdote, B. Manfredi, P. Mantegazza, and A. Paneria. Antinociceptive and immunosuppressive effects of opiate drugs: a structure related activity study, Br. J. Pharmacol., 121, 834–840, 1997.

R. Sackler, P. Goldenheim, and M. Chasin. Prolonged local anesthesia with colchicine, US Patent 5,747,060 (1998).

H. Singh, R. F. Bossard, P. F. White, and R. W. Yeatts. Effects of ketorolac versus bupivacaine co-administration during patient-controlled hydromorphone epidural analgesia after thorocotomy procedures, Anesthesia, Analg., 84(3), 564–569, 1997.

M. Sjöberg, P. Karlsson, C. Nordborg, A. Wallgren, P. Nitescu, L. Appelgren, L. E. Linder, and I. Curelaru. Neuropathological findings after long-term intrathecal infusion of morphine and bupivacaine for pain treatment in cancer patients, Anesthesiology, 76, 173–186, 1992.

S. Snyder and S. Matthysse. Neurosci Res. Program Bull. Opiate receptor mechanisms, 13(1), 1–166, 1975.

F. L. Strand. Physiology: A Regulatory Systems Approach, 2nd ed., Macmillan, N. Y. 1983.

A. Suri, K. S. Estes, G. Geisslinger, and H. Derendorf. Pharmacokinetic–pharmacodynamic relationships for analgesics, Int. J. Clin. Pharmacol. Ther., 35(8), 307–323, 1997.

A. Vainio and I. Tigerstedt. Opioid treatment for radiating cancer pain: oral administration vs. epidural techniques, Acta Anesthesiol. Scand., 32(3), 179–185, 1988.

R. T. M. van Donge, Ee R. van, and B. J. P. Crul. Neurological impairment during long-term intrathecal infusion of bupivacaine in cancer patients: a sign of spinal cord compression, Pain, 205–209, 1997.

M. P. Vercauteren, L. van der Bergh, S. L. Kartawiadi, K. van Boxem, and V. L. Hoffman. Addition of bupivacaine to sulfetanil in patient controlled epidural analgesia after lower limb surgery in young adults: effect on analgesia and micturition, Reg. Anesth. Pain Med., 23(2), 182–188, 1998.

A. Vigano, D. Fan, and E. Bruera. Individualized use of methadone and opioid rotation in the comprehensive management of cancer pain associated with poor prognostic indicators, Pain, 67(1), 115–119, 1996.

N. Wakiyama, K. June, and M. Nakano. Preparation and evaluation in vitro of polylactic acid microspheres containing local anesthetics. Chem. Pharm. Bull., 29, 3363–3368, 1981.

N. Wakiyama, K. Juni, and M. Nakano. Influence of physicochemical properties of polylactic acid on the characteristics and in vitro release patterns of polylactic acid microspheres containing local anesthetics, Chem. Pharm. Bull., 39(7), 2621–2628, 1982.

N. Wakiyama, J. Kazuhik, and M. Nakano. Preparation and evaluation in vitro and in vivo of polylactic acid microspheres containing dibucaine, Chem. Pharm. Bull., 39(10), 3719–3727, 1982.

WHO, Cancer Pain Relief with a Guide to Opioid Availability, 2nd ed., 1996.

J. L. Wu, M. S. Hsu, T. C. Hsu, L. H. Chen, W. J. Yang, and Y. C. Tsai. The efficacy of intrathecal coadministration of morphine and bupivacaine for labor analgesia, Acta Anaesthesiol. Sin. 35(4), 209–216, 1997.

38
Biodegradable Systems for Long-Acting Nestorone

Debra J. Trantolo, Yung-Yueh Hsu, and Joseph D. Gresser
Cambridge Scientific, Inc., Cambridge, Massachusetts

Donald L. Wise
Northeastern University, Boston, Massachusetts

A. J. Moo-Young
The Population Council, New York, New York

I. INTRODUCTION

The presence of a wide variety of fertility control methods provides different alternatives to cope with the diversity in human customs and preferences. Among fertile women, contraception can take many forms, but all have the same preferred outcome—the prevention of pregnancy. At this time, there is no method which can fit the definitions of "ideal" for fertility control (1). A major approach to improve the effectiveness, safety, and acceptability of steroid contraception is to develop long-acting preparations and delivery systems that can provide continuous medication at minimal daily doses sufficient to obtain a therapeutically adequate blood level to maintain their effectiveness. These systems have assumed a variety of forms, as injectable depot formulations, subdermal implants, and as intravaginal, intrauterine, and intracervical devices (2). Oral administration of steroids rapidly results in high blood levels that decrease with time, and repetitive doses must be given at frequent intervals to keep the blood levels in an efficacious zone. Steroid doses in excess of the optimum therapeutic range constitutes overmedication with the possibility of the appearance of dose-dependent side effects. Doses below the effective range result in contraceptive failure. Thus, a depot formulation would allow for controlled release from the injection site and result in the reduction of the total dose of the administered steroid for a prolonged period. In addition, a depot formulation reduces the chance of human errors by eliminating the need for repetitive self-administration (3).

The goal of this proposed study was to investigate a *biodegradable* depot formulation of an established progestin which can deliver steroid at a low efficacious dose for a sustained period. In the context of the proposed, the ultimate depot formulation is defined: a *biodegradable injectable* capable of controlling fertility for at least 6 months. The progestin used for investigation was Nestorone. Nestorone progestin is a potent 19-norprogesterone which is not biologically active when administered by the oral route. It has no estrogenic or androgenic activity (4). This steroid has been shown to be effective in inhibiting fertility at low doses when delivered through a single nonbiodegradable Silastic implant and appears to be an excellent candidate for contraception in lactating women because the infant would be free of the influence of the hormone excreted in the milk (5). The progestin excipient, i.e., delivery vehicle, is poly(lactic-co-glycolic) acid ("PLGA"), a polymer with an established history of biodegradability and biocompatibility for human use. The Nestorone/PLGA depot was formulated by a process shown to have performance characteristics superior to traditional PLGA technologies and now patented by Cambridge Scientific, Inc.

II. BACKGROUND ON LONG-ACTING CONTRACEPTIVE FORMULATIONS

Results from research on the use of steroidal formulations as long-acting injectable contraceptives, either progestogens alone for periods of more than 3 months or a progestogen–estrogen combination for a period of 1 month, started to appear in the literature in the mid-1960s. These developments have been reviewed in depth (6,7). The advantages of contraceptive depots are that they are highly effective, independent of coitus, long acting, easily administered, and assure regular contact with health services personnel. That latter may be a disadvantage for once-a-month preparations because visits to a clinic may be too frequent for many women. The major disadvantage of the existing progestogen-only formulations is the disruption of normal vaginal bleeding giving rise to unpredictable episodes of bleeding and spotting. With the once-a-month formulations, on the other hand, there are few discontinuations of use for these reasons. In the U.S. market, there are two depot formulations in current use: Depo-Provera and Norplant. Norplant, developed by the Population Council (personal communication with C. Wayne Bardin, M.D.), is a 5-year implant, but it is not degradable (it is a Silastic implant) and will not be included in this discussion. Depo-Provera is a degradable formulation designed to provide fertility control for 3 months. Depo-Provera has had a controversial history and was one of the first long-acting contraceptives to survive pharmacopolitical pressures (8). While Depo-Provera has been widely studied and there is no consistent trend in the contraindications with duration of use, certain subgroups of users show increased risks of side effects. Unfortunately, study differences have often been attributed to differences in efficacy between batches (8). Because Depo-Provera is formulated as an aqueous microcrystalline suspension, there can be major differences in the particle size distribution despite their being "micronized." The steroid can exist in several polymorphic forms which can influence the structure and hence the hardness of the crystals being micronized. Furthermore, the micronization process can be undertaken in several ways. Thus, very different particle size distributions can be obtained in which Depo-Provera preparations can be claimed to be micronized (8).

III. BACKGROUND ON NESTORONE CONTRACEPTIVE

Many breast-feeding women choose to use hormonal contraception rather than intrauterine devices or barrier methods. To satisfy their need, it is necessary to develop methods that do not interfere with breast-feeding and/or infant growth. Such methods should be devoid of estrogen (9–11) and the hormone, if excreted in the milk, should not be orally active. The synthetic progestin Nestorone (ST 1435) is very potent for inhibiting ovulation when it is administered parenterally (12,13), while it is ineffective when administered orally [unpublished observation from Noé (14)]. The low plasma concentration at which Nestorone suppresses ovulation and the lack of activity by the oral route made it a candidate for use as a contraceptive by lactating women, since the child would not be exposed to the action of the steroid present in the maternal milk (5,10).

Nestorone progestin (16-methylene-17 α-acetoxy-19-norpregn-4-ene-3,20-dione, hereafter referred to as Nestorone, a trademark of the Population Council), a potent contraceptive agent, devoid of certain properties exhibited by most other progestins. It does not affect serum lipoprotein patterns (15), sex hormone–binding globulin, or corticosteroid-binding globulin (16), and it is neither androgenic nor estrogenic. Unlike most other progestins, Nestorone while active when administered parenterally, is not active when given orally because of rapid first-pass hepatic metabolism (17). This steroid is, therefore, a suitable candidate to be developed as a contraceptive for lactating women, since Nestorone transferred through the mother's milk to the infant would be readily inactivated. Since Nestorone can be developed into various contraceptive dosage forms, such as subdermal implants, vaginal rings, and transdermals, it was important to establish how various conditions influence its stability. The stability of Nestorone in the solid state and in aqueous solutions was investigated (18) using reverse phase high-performance liquid chromatography. In the solid state, whether as a powder or when incorporated into Silastic implants, the steroid did not undergo detectable degradation even under severe experimental conditions. In solution, the drug underwent slow degradation that was dependent on temperature and pH of the medium.

The clinical performance and the in vivo release rate of a single 4-cm Nestorone subdermal implant have recently been investigated (4). Implants manufactured by two different procedures were compared. Volunteers were 70 healthy women of proven fertility. Forty women provided blood samples twice a week in the pretreatment cycle and for 5–6 weeks at 6-month intervals during treatment. Additional control cycles ($n = 31$) were studied in 19 Copper T users. No pregnancy occurred in 1570 woman-months. Nestorone plasma levels ($X \pm SE$) declined from 112 ± 8 to 86 ± 3 pmol/L (implant A) and from 145 ± 8 to 57 ± 5 pmol/L (implant B) from the first to the 24th month. Progesterone levels were <9.5 nmol/L in 166 (93%) of 178 blood samplings taken during treatment. Progesterone levels >16 nmol/L were found in only 7 sampling periods (3.9%) in treated women and in 70 (98.6%) of 71 control cycles. No ovulation occurred with Nestorone plasma levels above 105 pmol/L. No abnormal changes were observed in plasma lipoproteins or other clinical chemistry parameters during treatment. The implants were well tolerated. The most common complaint was the occurrence of irregular bleeding. Enlarged follicles found during pelvic examination in 8 subjects (11.4%) disappeared spontaneously in 10 days to 6 weeks. Implants were removed because of medial ($n = 10$, 14.3%) or personal reasons ($n = 6$, 8.6%) or at the 24th month of treatment ($n = 54$, 77.1%). The estimated average daily in vivo release rate of Nestorone was 45–50 μg/day. In summary, a single Nestorone subdermal implant was found to provide efficient contraceptive protection during 2 years.

IV. RATIONALE FOR THE PRESENT STUDY

Numerous investigators have published on the use of the polymers poly(lactic acid) and poly(glycolic acid) for drug delivery since the mid-1970s and, in particular, for the release of contraceptive steroids (19–21). Poly(lactic acid) and poly(glycolic acid) and their copolymers have been used in implants and as injectable microspheres or microcapsules. "Microspheres" (or "microparticles") represent a polymer–drug matrix which releases drug as the polymer erodes, and microcapsules represent a polymeric envelope through which the enclosed drug diffuses. The background to and the development of microspheres for releasing contraceptives has been discussed by Beck and Pope (22). Several approaches have been taken by different investigators, but a significant part of the work on contraceptive steroids was initially funded by the Program for Applied Research in Fertility Regulation (PARFR), and systems for the release of norethisterone, levonorgestrel, progesterone, ethinyl estradiol, and testosterone have been developed.

Matrix systems have the following advantages: they can be administered by either implantation (as rods) or injection (as particles); the rate and duration of drug release in vivo can be determined by the selection of microsphere size and the degree of loading of the steroid in the microspheres; they are completely biodegradable and do not cause irritation at the injection site. Preparations for which there have been the most extensive clinical trials are those releasing norethisterone (22). As yet, there have been only preliminary investigations undertaken with microsphere preparations of other steroids. Studies have been undertaken on several norethisterone preparations to optimize the formulations and dosages needed for long-acting cover, most focusing on 3-month systems.

Two approaches are being investigated to develop long-acting degradable fertility control preparations. The first is a simple aqueous microcrystalline suspension of contraceptive drugs; the second is to deliver the drug in a small biodegradable envelop (a "microcapsule") or support matrix (a "microparticle"). Development of microspheres was pursued initially by PARFR, then by Family Health International (FHI). While the crystalline suspensions may economical to prepare, they can potentially suffer from the batch-to-batch inconsistencies (8). Polymer depots may give better release characteristics, but they can be more complex to prepare and be even more difficult to reproduce batch to batch. On these bases, microencapsulation processes which yield these microcapsules will have higher costs than other contraceptive formulations (8), although the proven biocompatibility and degradability of the common polymer carrier, the PLGAs, bodes well for their continued investigation. A microparticle poly(lactic-co-glycolic acid) (PLGA) polymer system prepared using matrix technology is more cost-efficient because drug is conserved in the process; thus, if batch-to-batch reproducibility can be demonstrated, a rationale for the proposed depot technology is provided.

V. TRADITIONAL SOLVENT-BASED PLGA MATRIX DELIVERY

The first clinical application of a biodegradable drug delivery system in the United States was the application to treatment of narcotic addiction (23,24) in which Dr. Wise developed a removable "spherical bead" dosage form for this purpose with a 1-month designed lifetime. When the drug used in this implant, naltrexone, was formulated into the pamoate form, i.e., naltrexone palmoate, a 3-month lifetime resulted. The final system, as submitted to the National Institute on Drug Abuse, was the first biodegradable drug delivery system approved by the U.S. Food and Drug Administration (FDA) for clinical testing (25,26); and was a matrix of 70% by weight naltrexone/30% by weight PLGA copolymer of 90% L-lactic acid, 10% glycolic acid (molecular weight 35,000, synthesized using the nonmetallic catalyst para-toluenesulfonic acid (PTSA)). While demonstrating therapeutic efficacy for 4 weeks, in human trials the clinical utility of this system was limited by an "early burst" of drug which had a practical impact on implant size and lifetime (25).

Another early project done in collaboration with Walter Reed Army Institute investigated an injectable biodegradable controlled release system for the chemotherapeutic treatment of malaria (27,28). This work, aimed mainly to overcome the compliance problem dealt with a *dual*-drug system which enabled a synergistic effect resulting in much lower and thus more desirable drug doses. In this project, we established the importance of the effects on drug release rate of (a) polymer molecular weight, (b) ratio of drug to polymer in the final matrix dosage formulation, and (c) the importance of polymer molecular weight "dispersion," i.e., the distribution of molecular weights making up the polymer. In another early project on fertility control sponsored by the Population Council and later by the World Health Organization, the U.S. Agency for International Development, and the National Institutes of Health (NICHD), small cylindrical subdermal implants of PLGA polymers, containing levonorgestrol, were investigated which were evaluated in small animals, dogs, and baboons for contraceptive activity. Both removable rods and cryogenically ground powder forms suitable for application as long-acting injectables were produced and used with successful results (20,29). For example, in Fig. 1 is presented the results of the release of levonorgestrel from rats over an approximate 2-year period. Unfortunately, this promising work made use of organic solvents in implant formulation and these contribute to batch-to-batch release variations; additionally, while a long-acting system, this matrix technology was characterized by the typical early burst.

More recently, closely related worked on the controlled release of drugs for treatment of tuberculosis has been studied. Beginning with traditional solvent-based isoniazid/PLGA formulations, it was found that the equivalent of a single daily oral dose of isoniazid (INH), given as one biodegradable implant in vivo, achieves efficacious levels of free INH and the principal metabolite, acetyl isoniazid, for as long as 6–8 weeks both in serum and in urine (30). Furthermore, lung and liver extracts of animals obtained at 6 weeks after implantation showed high in vitro antimycobacterial activity against *M. tuberculosis* itself and *M. tuberculosis* contained within macrophages. All these data are comparable to those obtained from animals given a daily oral dose of 25 mg/kg of INH for the entire 6–8 weeks (30). Given the global impact of this work and the potential accounting for varied health and environmental regulations worldwide, focused work was continued on developing PLGA implants using a proprietary nonsolvent formulation process beginning with solvent-based design variables as a guide. This work has resulted in the development of a PLGA-based matrix technology which, although initially driven by client concerns over process and residual solvents, has also shown promise in improving on drug release patterns. These new techniques of sample preparation demonstrate much greater sample-to-sample reproducibility. Standard durations measured in replicate *in vitro* analysis are much smaller than those observed in standard solvent–cast matrix systems. In addition, extruded rods prepared without solvents give much smaller early bursts than those for typical matrix systems. The rapid early release of drug from controlled release delivery systems (frequently termed the "early burst") may account for a large fraction of the implanted dose within

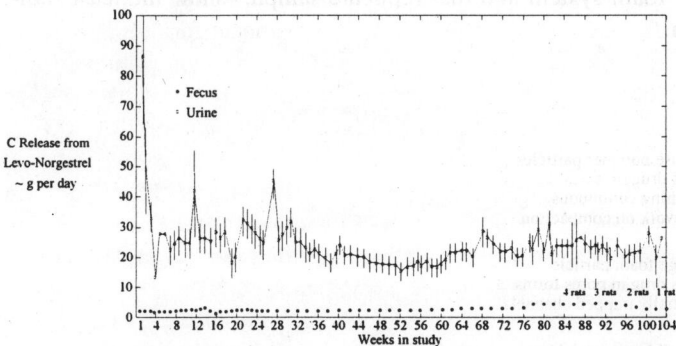

Figure 1 Rat urinary and fecal release of carbon-14 from levonorgestrel. Implant was 0.8 mm (1/33 in.) diameter cylinder, 50D,L-lactide/50L(+)-lactide copolymer of 180,000 mol wt, 50% levonorgestrel by weight. (From Ref. 20,29.)

the first several days or even within the first day post implantation. Although beneficial in some cases in that it rapidly builds up serum concentration of the drug, the early depletion can substantially reduce the expected lifetime. Studies have shown that the magnitude of the early burst is directly related to two factors: first, the density of the polymer excipient, and, second, the pressure at which the final dose form is extruded. The polymer, prepared as an open-celled foam by lyophilization, is cryogenically ground to retain a convenient particle size, e.g., 125–180 μm (microns). This size is substantially greater than the pore diameter (<40 μm) and permits the low-density particles to be impregnated with a solution of the *active* agent; the solvent is then removed by evaporation or by lyophilization, thus depositing the drug within the polymer pores. On compaction by extrusion the drug particles are effectively trapped within the polymer particles. Were the process of blending the drug with the polymer to be done without prior preparation of the low-density (0.1–0.3 g/cm^3) foam particles but rather with polymer ground from the usual, as received nonporous material with an absolute density of 1.2 g/cm^3 compaction would simply trap the drug between rather than within the polymer particle. Trapping active agent between particles rather than within them results in continuous polymer–grain boundaries through which the drug may diffuse. These drug loaded channels form conduits through which drug can be leached, thus accounting for the early burst. It is relevant to note that incorporation of the active agent in large blocks of foam prior to extrusion reduces the early burst, but not to the extent that prior grinding of the low-density polymer can achieve.

These observations are consistent with the model pictorialized in Fig. 2. Nonporous polymer particles allow formation of extensive drug networks between polymer particles (Fig. 2a). These channels are reduced by incorporating the drug into large foam structures, but as the pores are continuous within the foam, drug networks can still form it (Fig. 2b). It is only by grinding the foam that the pore lengths are shortened and blocked on compaction (Fig. 2c).

This model is consistent with data. The INH/PLGA system provides one example. INH/PLGA matrices were prepared by three methods: (a) solvent-casting; (b) dry mixing of micronized INH with high-density ground PLGA; and (c) incorporating INH into low-density PLGA. Results of these studies show that (a) the extruded low-density systems have the least early burst (5% within the first day); (b) the standard deviations are least for multiple replicates of the foam system at all time points; and (c) *in vitro* release of INH from the four systems follows Roseman–Higuchi kinetics, indicating that release behavior is that of typical diffusion-controlled matrix systems (31). Figure 3 compares release of isoniazid from matrices prepared with high-density ground polymer particle and low-density ground polymer foam particles (prepared from lyophilization of acetic *acid* polymer solutions). Note that the early burst is virtually eliminated in the low-density foam system and that replicate samples show the least standard deviation in the foam system.

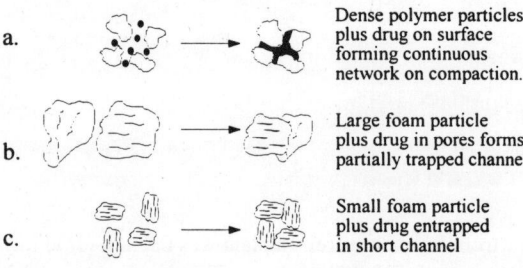

Figure 2 Model.

Biodegradable Systems for Long-Acting Nestorone

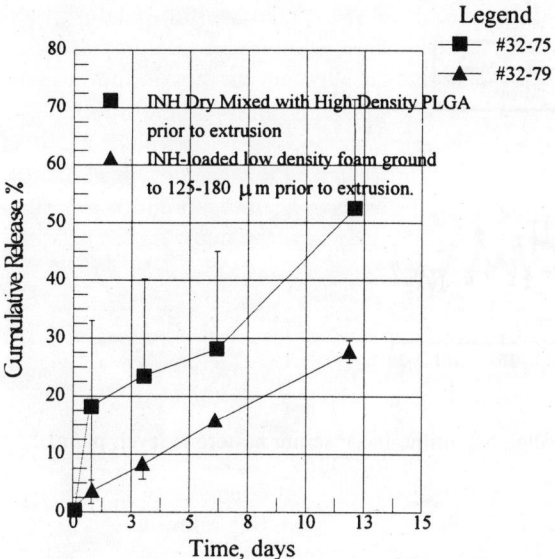

Figure 3 Comparison of cumulative release of isoniazid (INH) from dry mixed and foam formulations.

It is also noted that increasing the extrusion pressure reduces the early burst. This is consistent with reduction of porosity at higher pressures. Note that release rates increase with increasing porosity (32).

VI. PILOT STUDIES

The pilot studies were divided into two parts: (a) a small cylindrical implant and (b) an injectable system. Details on sample preparation for both implant and injectable systems follow.

A. Nestorone Bioerodible Implant Materials and Methods

The implant was made of PLA/PLGA copolymers and the active agent was Nestorone progestin (NES). The length and diameter (mean ± SD) of the implant was 10.14 ± 42 and 3.33 ± 0.08 mm, respectively. The NES drug load was 25.75 ± 0.50 mg (mean ± SD) and composed 25% of the total implant weight. The implant was manufactured by Cambridge Scientific (Belmont, MA). NES was supplied by a contract manufacturer.

1. Animals

Six female New Zealand white rabbits were used in this study. The animals were purchased from Hare Maryland Farms (Hewitt, NJ). Each animal was housed in an individual cage and was given food and water ad libitum, and exposed to 12 h of light and 12 h of darkness daily. The body weights of the animals at the beginning and conclusion of treatment were 4.36 ± 0.17 and 5.87 ± 0.05 kg (mean ± SD), respectively. One animal (104A) suffered a broken leg during the fourth month of treatment and was sacrificed.

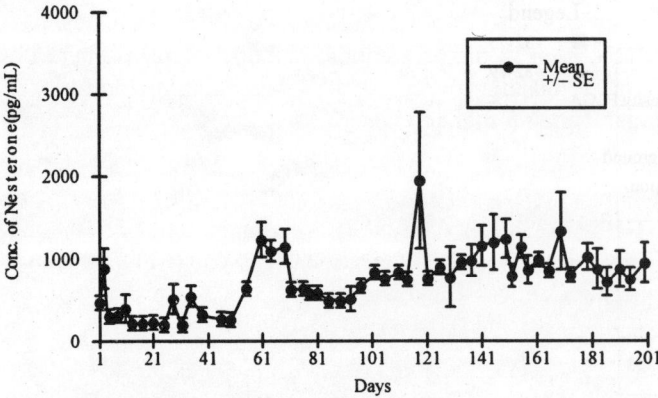

Figure 4 Nestorone implantable pellets (Cambridge Scientific, Inc.): serum nestorone level, pg/mL.

2. Implant Insertion

The animal was anesthetized. The abdominal area was shaved and prepared for surgery. A small stab wound, 4–5 mm, was made approximately 1–2 cm right of the midline and approximately 4 cm from the right axilla. The implant was loaded into a trocar fitted with a plunger. The trocar was introduced through the wound to about 3 cm, subdermally, and almost parallel to the surface of the skin. The implant was expelled by retracting the trocar along the axis of the plunger. The wound was doubly closed, first with a single stitch of 5-0 chronic gut suture, and second, externally with one or two stitches of 3-0 silk sutures. The animal was observed daily for adverse effects and to ascertain whether the implant was expelled from the animal. The duration of treatment was approximately 7 months.

3. Blood Collection

Blood was collected before treatment, daily for 5 consecutive days following implantation and thereafter twice weekly until the end of the study. Three millimeters of blood was drawn at each collection. Serum was prepared and stored at −20°C pending NES assay by radioimmunoassay (33).

4. Results

Steady-state serum levels of NES were achieved during the course of the study. Controlled sustained delivery of NES from PLA/PGA bioerodible implants was noted, based on the serum levels of NES (Fig. 4). The mean daily serum NES concentration during the first 50 days of treatment was 384.14 ± 47.14 pg/mL or 1036.79 ± 127.23 pmol/L (mean ± SE). The mean daily serum level of NES thereafter was 921.11 ± 49.18 pg/mL or 2486.08 ± 132.74 pmol/L (Mean ± SE). These blood levels are in excess of what is required to block ovulation in women. In women approximately 86–112 pmol/L of NES is needed to block ovulation (4). The 1-cm NES PLA/PGA bioerodible implant may have an effective life of 6 months. During the course of the study there were no adverse reaction at the implant site. At the end of the study, the implant did not maintain its integrity, but was found fragmented.

B. Nestorone Microspheres

NES microspheres, made from copolymers of PLA/PGA and containing 25% (w/w) of NES, were prepared by Cambridge Scientific. The NES was provided by the Population Council. The microspheres were less than 125 nm.

1. Suspension Vehicle

Each milliliter of the suspension vehicle used in the preparation of the NES microsphere injectable contained polyethylene glycol, 27.60 mg; Tween-80, 1.84 mg; sodium chloride, 8.3 mg; methylparaben, 1.50 mg; propylparaben, 0.5 mg; and water.

2. Nestorone Injectable

Six samples of NES microsphere (64-108-16 through 64-108-20) weighing a total of 530.8 mg with an equivalency of 132.7 mg NES were suspended in the suspension vehicle to give a final volume value of 5 mL. The NES concentration was 26.54 mg/mL.

3. Dose

The amount of NES administered to each rabbit was based on the body weight of the animal. The mean volume of the injectable preparation to be administered to the thigh muscle of the hind leg was 0.73 ± 0.02 mL (mean ± SE), and this was equivalent to 19.46 ± 0.56 mg NES (mean ± SE). Based on the body weight of each animal, the mean dose of NES administered was 4.25 ± 0.06 mg NES/kg body weight (mean ± SE). Before administration of the microspheres, the suspension is thoroughly shaken.

4. Animals

Six female New Zealand white rabbits were used in this segment of the study. There were purchased from Hare Maryland Farms following approval of the study protocol by the Institutional Animal Use Committee, of the Rockefeller University (New York, NY). Each animal was housed in its own individual cage and was fed standard Purina Rabbit Chow and given water ad libitum. The rabbits were exposed to 12 h of light and 12 h of darkness daily. The mean body weight (mean ± SE) of the animals at the beginning and conclusion of the study were 4.58 ± 0.11 and 6.27 ± 0.10 kg, respectively.

5. Blood Collection

Blood samples were drawn for NES assays, before treatment, daily for 5 consecutive days following intramuscular administration of the steroid, and thereafter twice weekly until the end of the study. Three milliliters of blood was collected at each sampling period from the central ear vein. Serum was prepared and stored at $-20°C$ pending NES assay by RIA (33).

6. Results

As shown in Fig. 5, within 1 h of the intramuscular administration of 4.25 ± 0.06 (mean ± SE) mg NES/kg, an extremely high concentration of the steroid was detected (13.04 ± 0.75 ng/mL, mean ± SE) in the serum. For 8 days serum NES concentrations were very high; then they declined rapidly to 91.17 ± 26.00 pg/mL within 28 days. Between days 28 and 196, the serum concentrations of the steroid displayed wide variations ranging from 6 to 241 pg/mL. For purposes of contraception, the serum levels of NES encountered in the first 28 days were more than adequate. The high variations in serum NES levels showed a spiking phenomenon, i.e., burst of NES release from the microsphere, which did not appear to be controlled, and this was judged unacceptable.

C. Polymer Selection and Characterization

Polymers and copolymers of lactic and glycolic acids are now commercially available in GMP form and were purchased. Extensive studies of these materials as matrices for controlled drug

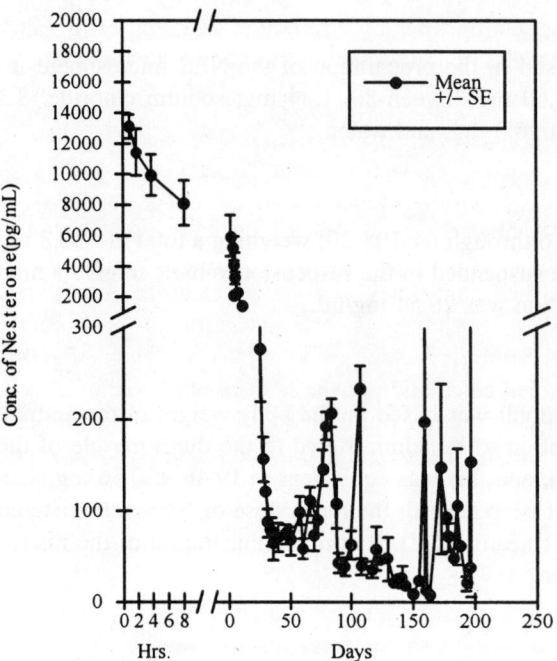

Figure 5 Nestorone injectable (Cambridge Scientific, Inc.): serum nestorone progestin levels, pg/mL.

release have shown that release rates for a particular drug may be controlled by proper selection of copolymer composition, i.e., the lactide-to-glycolide ratio, by the polymer molecular weight, and by the loading of the drug within the polymer matrix. Cutright (34) showed that the pure homopolymers, poly(lactic acid) and poly(glycolic acid), are the slowest to degrade in aqueous media, with increasing rates of degradation as the lactide glycolide ratio approached unity from either direction. Because hydrolytic degradation occurs by chain scission and creates progressively greater void volume as the hydrolysis products, lactic and glycolic acid monomers, diffuse from the matrix, the rate of drug diffusion is facilitated. Studies by Wise (2) have shown that increasing polymer molecular weight depresses the release rate for a given drug content. Again, the effect of diminishing the diffusional pathway by random chain scission is less pronounced for high molecular weight than for lower molecular weight polymers.

Based on earlier studies, 85:15 PLGA copolymer in GMP form (Boehringer-Ingelheim) was used. However, other copolymers, polymer molecular weights, polymer densities, and Nestorone loadings can be considered if modifications are needed. As shown in the citations of previously published work, these parameters can be changed to increase system lifetime as follows: (a) higher lactide-to-glycolide copolymer ratios, (b) higher molecular weight polymer, (c) lower polymer density, and (d) decreased loading of the active agent. Generally, changes in Nestorone loading and polymer density are first considerations because of the practical implications of using the initial characterized polymer lot. The polymers were characterized by verification of molecular weight by gel permeation chromatography (GPC) on a Waters Associates GPC equipped with a 600E system controller, a 410 differential refractometer, a 710 WISP autosampler, and an 825 Maxima software package for data handling. Separations were accomplished on two columns placed in series, an "Ultrastyragel Linear" (Waters) for low molecular weight polymer, using tetrahydrofuran as the mobile phase. Further characterization included determination of glass transition temperatures, melting points, and decomposition temperatures of both pure polymer and polymer/Nestorone composites by differential scanning calorimetry (DSC). Instrumentation includes a Mettler DSC 25 coupled with a Mettler TA 11 Processor.

D. Nestorone/PLGA Matrix Formulation and Quality Control

Delivery systems of Nestorone/PLGA were fabricated. PLGA "foams" are first prepared by lyophilization (freeze drying) of polymer solutions. Foam density (as low as 0.01 g/cm^3, whereas "melt" polymer is 1.3 g/cm^3), and void volume are a function of the concentration of the polymer in the solution. Foam structure was confirmed by scanning electron microscopy. Void volume and pore size distribution were determined by mercury intrusion porosimetry (MIP). Density was measured by standard gravimetric techniques as applied to solids. Together density and void volume measurements enabled calculation of the ratio of open to closed cell. Our examination of foams by these freeze-drying methods indicated a high percentage of open cell structure, but this was verified to determine the theoretical maximum loading of Nestorone within the open cells. The loading of Nestorone into the foams was accomplished by immersing blocks of foam in solutions of 50:50 (v/v) PBS: methanol adjusted to pH 7.4 Nestorone and forcing the Nestorone solution into the void volume by first degassing and then repressurizing to one atmosphere by admitting air. Target loading was 0.50% (w/w) in PLGA 85:15. Following loading, the foam is lyophilized. Loaded foams are homogeneous; however, this was verified by analysis of aliquot samples removed from both surfaces and interior portions of the foam. For this screening purpose, Nestorone was removed by dissolution in buffer and quantified by its ultraviolet absorption using HPLC. Final formulations were quantified to close the material balance on formulation parameters, as well as to quantify the retention Nestorone incorporated. Foams were extruded. PLGA extrusions were performed at a pressure of about 19,000 psi (7.5 tons on a 1-in.-diameter ram), and temperatures of approximately 45°C. In other work, results showed that the relationship between ln P and 1/T for extrusion is linear with a slope identified as the activation energy for viscous flow (32). Further, it was shown that release rate diminished with increasing extrusion pressure. Extrusions were conducted at 10,000, 20,000, 40,000, and 80,000 psi, and at minimum temperatures required (as low as 28°C). The result was an expanded implantable system. Extrudates were cryogenically ground to yield microparticulate powders as final dose forms for injectable system. The preparation and testing of each matrix was replicated to demonstrate batch-to-batch reproducibility. Quality control consists of verifying Nestorone loading and polymer molecular weight. Samples of extruded rod were dissolved in methylene chloride for polymer molecular weight determination by GPC, as described previously. After extraction of the methylene chloride solution with water, Nestorone content was verified as measured via HPLC (using a Waters Associate HPLC equipped with a 600/600E system controller, a 410 tunable absorbance detector, a 710 WISP autosampler, and a C-18 column).

1. Matrix Sterilization

Although sterilization can be achieved by exposure to steam, dry heat, or gas (ethylene oxide, propylene oxide, formaldehyde), these methods are not recommended for PLGA implants. Heat will bring the implants above their softening points (about 65°C) and at about 100°C will cause polymer flow. Elevated temperatures, especially in a moist environment, will cause extensive polymer degradation. Gaseous sterilization is preferable if effective degassing procedures can be developed. However, to avoid even traces of these gases in the implant, α irradiation is recommended. Wise has shown that a 2.5-Mrad dose from a cobalt-60 source is an effective sterilant (35) for a system composed of PLGA 90:10 beads containing 70% (w/w) naltrexone.

However, some polymer degradation was observed; molecular weight diminished by 20% as measured by GPC. Thus, *in vitro* release was measured on samples both before and after sterilization as was polymer molecular weight. The effect of irradiation on Nestorone will be determined by comparison of UV, infrared, and nuclear magnetic resonance spectra, and HPLC profiles with standards of known purity; polymer molecular weight will be determined via GPC. While this work did not specifically address the verification of sterilization protocols, the procedure approximated conditions specified in related Good Manufacturing Practices work.

VII. CONCLUSIONS AND RECOMMENDATIONS

Based on the present work, a biodegradable injectable controlled release Nestorone system appears to have merit. As noted, all work was done incorporating the nonsolvent, high-pressure extrusion technology. A major investigation requiring extensive *in vivo* testing, followed by marine samples made under GMPs and leading to clinical trials is needed. This work will therefore aim at system refinement with respect to loading and system duration. Release rates and duration can be adjusted by changing both loading and the lactide: glycolide monomer ratio of the PLGA.

REFERENCES

1. N. A. Haiba, M. A. El-Habashy, S. A. Said, E. A. Darwish, W. S. Abdel-Sayed, and S. E. Nayel. Clinical evaluation of two monthly injectable contraceptives and their effects on some metabolic parameters, Contraception, 39, 619, 1989.
2. G. I. Zatuchni. Contraceptive development for the future, in Symposium Proceedings on Long-Acting Contraception, Alexandria, Egypt, A. Goldsmith and M. Toppazada (Eds.), p. 8, 1983.
3. L. R. Beck. Pharmacological aspects of slow release in steroidal systems, in Symposium Proceedings on Long-Acting Contraception, Alexandria, Egypt, A. Goldsmith and M. Toppazada (Eds.), p. 24, 1983.
4. S. Díaz, V. Schiappacasse, M. Pavez, A. Zepeda, A. J. Moo-Young, A. Brandeis, P. Lähteenmäki, and H. B. Croxatto. Clinical trial with nestorone subdermal contraceptive implants, Contraception, 51, 33–38, 1995.
5. P. L. A. Lähteenmäki, S. Díaz, P. Miranda, H. B. Croxatto, and P. Lähteenmäki. Milk and plasma concentrations of the progestin ST 1435 in women treated parenterally with ST 1435, Contraception, 42, 555–562, 1990.
6. G. Benagiano, and F. M. Primiero. In: Long-Acting Steroid Contraception, 175, D. R. Mishell (Ed.), Raven Press, NY, 1983.
7. L. S. Liskin and W. F. Quillin. In Population Reports, Series K, No. 2, Population Information Program, George Washington University Medical Center, Washington, D.C., 1983.
8. P. E. Hall. Long-acting injectable formulations, in Fertility Regulation Today and Tomorrow, E. Diczfalusy and M. Bygdeman (Eds.), 119, Raven Press, NY, 1987.
9. H. B. Croxatto, S. Díaz, and O. Peralta, et al. "Fertility regulation in nursing women. IV. Long-term influence of a low-dose combined oral contraceptive initiated at day 30 postpartum upon lactation and infant growth, Contraception, 27, 13–25, 1983.
10. H. B. Croxatto and S. Díaz. The place of progesterone in human contraception, J. Steroid Biochem., 27, 991–994, 1987.
11. O. Peralta, S. Díaz, and G. Juez, et al. Fertility regulation in nursing women. V. Long-term influence of a low-dose combined oral contraceptive initiated at day 90 postpartum upon lactation and infant growth, Contraception, 27, 27–38, 1983.
12. E. M. Coutihno, A. R. DaSilva, and H.-G. Kraft. Fertility control with subdermal silastic capsules containing a new progestin (ST 4135), Int. J. Fertil., 21, 103–108, 1976.

13. M. Laurikka-Routti, M. Haukkamaa, and P. Lähteenmäki. Suppression of ovarian function with the transdermally given synthetic progestin ST 1435, Fertil. Steril., 58, 680–689, 1992.
14. G. Noé, A. Salvatierra, O. Heikinheimo, X. Maturana, and H. B. Croxatto. Pharmacokinetics and bioavailability of ST 1435 administered by different routes, Contraception, 48, 548, 1993.
15. H. Lithell, T. Ahren, V. Odlind, E. Weiner, B. Vessby, A. Victor, and E. D. B. Johansson. Effects of progestins on lipoprotein patterns, In: Bardin, E. Milgrom, and Mauvis-Jaris (Eds.), Progesterone and Progestins, Raven Press, New York, p. 421–432, 1983.
16. P. L. A. Lähteenmäki, G. L. Hammond, and T. Luukkainen. Serum non-protein bound percentage and distribution of the progestin ST-1435: no effect of ST-1435 treatment on plasma SHBG and CBG binding capacities, Acta Endocrinol. (Copenh), 102, 307–313, 1983.
17. P. L. A. Lähteenmäki. Intestinal absorpiton of ST-1435 in rat, Contraception, 30, 143–151, 1984.
18. S. M. Ahmed, F. Arcuri, F. Li, A. J. Moo-Young, and C. Monder. Accelerated stability studies on 16-methylene-17α-acetoxy-19-norpregn-4-ene-3,20-dione (Nestorone), Steroids, 60, 1995.
19. L. R. Beck, D. R. Cowsar, D. H. Lewis, J. W. Gibson, and C. E. Flowers. Am. J. Obstet. Gynecol., 135, 419, 1979.
20. J. D. Gresser, D. L. Wise, L. R. Beck, and J. F. Hoses. Larger animal testing of an injectable sustained release fertility control system, Contraception, 17(3), 253, 1978.
21. R. Gurney, N. A. Peppas, D. D. Harrington, and G. S. Banks. Drug Dev. Ind. Pharm., 7, 1, 1981.
22. L. R. Beck and V. Z. Pope. Res. Frontiers Fertil. Regul., 3(2), 1, 1984.
23. A. C. Sharon, and D. L. Wise. Development of drug delivery systems for use in treatment of narcotic addiction, R. E. Willett and G. Barnett (Eds.), Narcotic Antagonists Naltrexone Pharmacochemistry and Sustained Release Preparation, NIDA Research Monograph 28, DHHS publications (SM) No. 81-902, Washington, D.C., 1981.
24. D. L. Wise. Chapter 5 in Biopolymeric Controlled Release Systems: 1, D. L. Wise (Ed.), CRC Press, Boca Raton, 1984.
25. C. N. Chiang, L. E. Hollister, A. Kishimoto, and G. Barnett. Kinetics of a naltrexone sustained release preparation, Clin. Pharmacol. Ther., 36, 704, 1984.
26. R. H. Reuning, S. H. T. Liao, A. E. Staubus, S. B. Ashcraft, D. A. Downs, S. E. Harrigan, J. N. Wiley, and D. L. Wise. Pharmacokinetic quantitation of naltrexone controlled release from a copolymer delivery system, J. Pharmokinet. Biopharm., 11, p. 369, 1983.
27. D. L. Wise, G. V. McCormick, and G. P. Willet. Life Sci., 19, 867, 1976.
28. D. L. Wise, J. D. Gresser, and G. J. McCormick. J. Pharm. Pharmacol., 31, 201, 1979.
29. J. D. Gresser, D. L. Wise, L. R. Beck, and J. F. Howes. Biodegradable cylindrical implants for fertility regulation in biodegradable delivery systems in contraception, 1, ESE Hafez, Ed., Program for Applied Research in Fertility Regulation, Chicago, 1980.
30. P. R. J. Gangadharam, D. R. Ashtekar, D. C. Farhi, and D. L. Wise. Sustained release of isoniazid in vivo from a single implant of a biodegradable polymer, Tubercle, 72, 115–122, 1991.
31. Y.-Y. Hsu, J. D. Gresser, D. J. Trantolo, C. M. Lyons, and D. L. Wise. In vitro controlled release of isoniazid from poly(lactide-co-glycolide) matrices, J. Controlled Release, 131, 223–228, 1994.
32. J. G. DuChamp. Release of isoniazid from dry mixed extruded matrices, MS thesis (Chem. Eng.), Northeastern University, Boston, MA, 1992.
33. P. Lähteenmaki, E. Weiner, P. Lähteenmaki, E. Johansson, and T. Lukkainen. Contraception with subcutaneous capsules containing ST 1435. Pituitary and ovarian function and plasma levels of ST 1435, Contraception, 23, 65–75, 1981.
34. D. E. Cutright, B. Perez, J. D. Beasly III, W. J. Larson, and W. R. Posey. Degradation rates of polymers and copolymers of polylactic acids, Oral Surg., 37, 142–152, 1974.
35. D. L. Wise, et al. Advanced Drug Delivery, Reviews, 1, 19–39, 1987.

39
Preparation and Evaluation of Buprenorphine Microspheres for Parenteral Administration

William R. Ravis and Yuh-Jing Lin
Auburn University, Auburn, Alabama

Ram Murty
Murty Pharmaceuticals, Inc., Lexington, Kentucky

I. INTRODUCTION

Detoxification from opioid addiction is a long-standing medical and social problem. Treatments to date include methadone maintenance, maintenance on opioid antagonists, and clonidine for alleviation of withdrawal symptoms (1). The current project involves the formulation and evaluation of a narcotic partial agonist (buprenorphine) into a microsphere injectable delivery system that could be useful for withdrawal therapy in opioid-addicted individuals as well as prophylaxis (maintenance drug) against self-administration of opioids.

Buprenorphine is a semisynthetic opioid analgesic with partial agonist activity. Recently, buprenorphine has been used as an alternative to methadone in pharmacotherapy for opioid addiction. Like methadone, buprenorphine significantly suppresses opioid self-administration (2–4) and blocks the subjective effects of full opioid agonists such as hydromorphone (5). Unlike methadone, buprenorphine has minimal effects on respiration and is therefore a much safer drug than methadone (3). Buprenorphine also had better treatment retention rates when used as a maintenance drug in heroin addicts and resulted in fewer opioid-positive urine samples (6). Interestingly, depressive symptoms were also significantly decreased in opioid addicts maintained on buprenorphine (7). Another advantage of buprenorphine over methadone is that it produces minimal physical dependence and has a very mild withdrawal syndrome upon discontinuation (7,7–9). Buprenorphine is believed to have a lower abuse liability than methadone, despite the fact that it increases scores of "liking, good effects, euphoria" on scales designed to evaluate subjective drug effects (10,11). In countries where buprenorphine has been widely marketed, there have been cases of misuse, with addicts using either the parenteral form or preparing the sublingual tablets for injection (8,12,13).

Opioid antagonists have also been used to treat opioid addicts because they precipitate a short-lived but intense withdrawal. During maintenance therapy, they block the subjective effects of self-administered opioids. Buprenorphine has advantages over opioid antagonists because it does not precipitate withdrawal (14,15) and in fact may help alleviate withdrawal symptoms such as dysphoria and tension (16). Another advantage of buprenorphine over opioid antagonists is that retention during buprenorphine maintenance is excellent, whereas retention with opioid antagonists is quite low (17). Studies in both humans and nonhuman primates have shown that buprenorphine decreases self-administration of other opioids such as heroin and alfentanil. Interestingly, buprenorphine also decreases self-administration of benzodiazepines (2) and cocaine in humans (18). In preclinical studies, buprenorphine also significantly reduced the lethal effects of cocaine in mice (19).

One major disadvantage to the current use of buprenorphine in detoxification programs is its low and inconsistent oral absorption, making it impractical for daily oral dosing like methadone. As previously mentioned, the potential for abuse increases when buprenorphine is administered either parenterally or sublingually. A microsphere delivery system for this drug would (a) avoid oral absorption problems, (b) circumvent the abuse problems associated with sublingual and parenteral forms, and (c) address one of the major obstacles in agonist therapy, i.e., patient compliance.

The disposition and pharmacokinetics of buprenorphine has been examined in several species after various routes of administration. Following intravenous dosing, buprenorphine displays a distribution half-life of 2 min and a elimination phase half-life of 2–3 h (20,.21). This drug is nearly completely metabolized with a hepatic clearance approaching hepatic plasma flow. Buprenorphine is metabolized by N-dealkylation and subsequent conjugation of parent drug and metabolite with glucuronic acid (22). The product of dealkylation is the metabolite norbuprenorphine, which is believed to be active. Due to extensive hepatic and intestinal "first-pass" metabolism, buprenorphine displays very low systemic bioavailability following oral administration (23–26). After oral dosing, unchanged drug plasma concentration are very low. The bioavailability following intramuscular and sublingual administration is 40–90% and 31–58%, respectively (20,26). Intranasal bioavailability in humans is reported to be 48% (27). The bioavailability after the subcutaneous route is expected to be as good as that noted after intramuscular. Subcutaneous pellets of buprenorphine composed of cholesterol and glyceryl tristearate yielded peak drug concentrations in 4 weeks (28).

Due to the low dose and rapid metabolism of buprenorphine, the plasma concentrations are quite low and represent problems in the performance of in vivo disposition and pharmacokinetic studies. Sensitive assays based on radioimmunoassay (29) and high-performance liquid chromatography (HPLC) techniques with fluorescence (21) and electrochemical (30) detection have been employed in buprenorphine disposition studies in humans. Radiotracers have been frequently utilized in buprenorphine plasma, tissue, and urinary kinetics experiments in rats (28,31). The use of radiolabeled drug greatly improves the ability to perform disposition investigations in rats where sample volumes are small.

With the goal of buprenorphine release for 1–3 months, biodegradable microsphere delivery systems were prepared and investigated. Currently, the most promising and utilized polymers for developing controlled release parenterals are the biodegradable hydrophobic polymers, which include poly(D,L-lactide-co-glycolide) (PLGA), poly(ortho-esters), and polyanhydrides (32,33). PLGA polymers are hydrolyzed in the body to lactic and glycolic acids, which are easily metabolized by the body. Polymers of PLGA undergo bulk erosion, whereas the poly(ortho-ester) and polyanhydride polymers undergo surface erosion.

Dosage forms composed of PLGA polymers have been extensively studied and prepared as controlled drug release implants, pellets, and microsphere systems. While subcutaneous implant systems of PLGA polymers have been a popular approach for drug delivery, microsphere injectable forms would prevent implant removal by addicts being treated with the agonist. In addition, dosages of buprenorphine microsphere may be more easily adjusted than implant dosage forms. PLGA microspheres containing several agents have been investigated (34–41) and are perhaps the most promising from a regulatory point of view. Microspheres are spherical particles of less than 125 μm that can be easily suspended in a vehicle for parenteral administration through a conventional syringe and needle. The size, drug content, and drug release characteristics from microspheres of biodegradable polymers are dependent on the selection and amounts of components as well as the formulation methods. The microencapsulation processes commonly used are solvent evaporation and phase separation technique (33,37–40).

The primary objective of this study was to prepare and evaluate several microsphere systems of buprenorphine. The microspheres were formulated with different PLGA polymers. Numerous factors can influence drug release characteristics from microspheres including the polymer and its molecular weight, extraction/evaporation procedures, size and geometry of microspheres, and the drug form. Formulations, which varied in polymer, oil-in-water (o/w) preparation approach, and the methods used to remove the organic solvent, were prepared. Results of these studies would establish whether buprenorphine could be incorporated into a microsphere systems and whether these systems could provide drug release over several weeks.

II. METHODS

A. Preparation of Buprenorphine Microspheres

The microencapsulation process involved preparing an o/w emulsion in which drug and polymer are dissolved in the organic or methylene chloride phase. A drug/polymer ratio of 1:25 was selected based on the solubilities of the drug and polymer in the organic phase and the release range deserved.

Buprenorphine HCl was dissolved in methylene chloride with the selected PLGA polymer. This solution was added to purified water and vortexed for 10 s. Following mixing, the dispersion was added to a solution of poly(vinyl alcohol) (evaporation method) or isopropyl alcohol (extraction method) and mixed for 3 h. After centrifuging, the microspheres are washed three times with water. The microspheres were redispersed in water and then the mixture filtered. The precipitate was then either air-dried in a desiccator or lyophilized. In the case of microspheres containing ^{3}H-buprenorphine, labeled and unlabeled drug were added to methylene chloride prior to microsphere preparation. A table describing the components and preparation procedures for the 1:25 (drug/polymer) batches with both 50:50 PLGA and 85:15 PLGA polymers is provided in Table 1. The percentage yield was determined as the total weight of the formed microspheres divided by the weight of the initial starting components, polymer, and drug.

Table 1 Composition and Preparation Methods of Buprenorphine Microspheres

Formulation	PLGA polymer	Solvent removal	Drying method
A	50:50	Evaporation	Air
B	50:50	Evaporation	Lyo.
C	50:50	Extraction	Air
D	50:50	Extraction	Lyo.
E	85:15	Evaporation	Air
F	85:15	Evaporation	Lyo.
G	85:15	Extraction	Air
H	85:15	Extraction	Lyo.

B. Determination of Buprenorphine by HPLC Procedures

An HPLC method was developed that utilized a C-18 column and electrochemical detector. The mobile phase was 45% phosphate buffer pH 4.0 and 55% methanol, which was pumped at a rate of 1.0 mL/min. The electrochemical detector was set at 0.75V and 1 nA in oxidation mode. The detector was allowed to stabilize for 36 h prior to use. Standard curves were linear from 20 to 1000 ng/mL with a coefficient variation (CV) of 9%.

C. Determination of ^{3}H-Buprenorphine

The total radioactivity of samples obtained from dissolution and drug content experiments was determined by liquid scintillation counting. Aliquots (0.1 mL) of dissolution or content samples were added to scintillation cocktail and the total radioactivity determined in a scintillation counter. Concentrations and amounts of buprenorphine were estimated based on the specific activity of the mixture of labeled and unlabeled drug used to prepare the formulation.

D. Buprenorphine Content of Microspheres

Two-milligram quantities of microspheres were dispersed and extracted with ethyl alcohol for 24 h. Following centrifugation, aliquots were taken and analyzed by HPLC to determine buprenorphine content. For preparations containing ^{3}H-buprenorphine, the radioactivity of aliquots was determined to estimate drug content. The percentage of microsphere weight that was drug (% drug by weight) was calculated for each formulation. The % drug by weight was compared to the expected percentage of 4% (1:25) to obtain a value of percentage of drug incorporated.

E. Buprenorphine Release

Two-milligram quantities of buprenorphine microspheres were placed in a 25-mL phosphate pH 7.4 buffer maintained at 37°C in a water bath with constant shaking. Samples were drawn at 0, 0.167, 0.5, 1, 4, 9, 16, 32, 43, 49, and 60 days. Samples were filtered and the filter was rinsed to return undissolved microsphere to the dissolution media. Drawn samples were immediately analyzed by either HPLC or by total-radioactivity methods. Dissolution studies were conducted in triplicate.

F. Particle Size

The particle size and distribution of selected formulations were measured using a particle size analyzer (Model BI-90, Brookhaven Particle Sizer, Holtsville, NY). The average diameter was recorded as was the undersize distribution at 10%, 25%, 50%, 75%, and 90%.

G. Appearance and Morphology

Before and during microsphere dissolution experiments, the size and shape of microspheres were examined by scanning electron microscopy (SEM). Samples were dried and mounted on metal stubs with double-sided tape and then coated with gold. SEM (Model DSM 940, Zeiss, Germany) was performed at 2000x magnification and photographs were prepared.

III. RESULTS

Several approaches were used to prepare microspheres of buprenorphine and included varying the dispersion procedure, the polymer, extraction technique, and drying approach. Table 1 summarizes the methods and components of the eight microsphere products. Based on microscopic examinations (Fig. 1), vortexing of the emulsion yielded more uniform microspheres than sonification methods. Thus, vortexing was used for all preparation reported here.

Table 2 presents the percentage yield, the drug content as a percentage of total microsphere weight, and the percentage incorporation. The percentage yield was obtained based on the total amount of polymer and drug used and the final weight of dried microspheres. Yields were acceptable with mean values ranging from 58% to 68%. The choice of polymer or formulation procedure did not appear to alter the percentage yield results. With a 1:25 drug-to-polymer ratio and equal incorporation of drug and polymer into microspheres, the theoretical % of drug by weight would be 4%. The percentage of drug incorporated was less than theoretical, with a

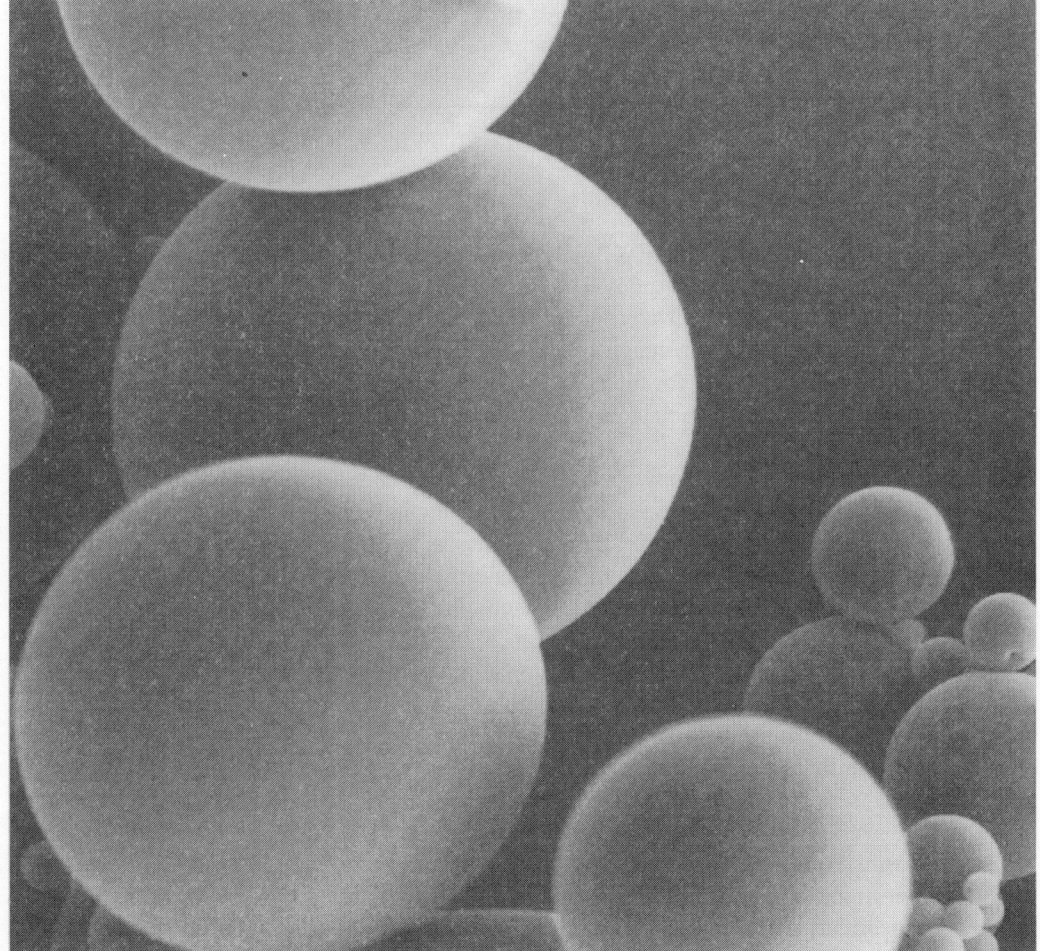

Figure 1 Scanning electron micrograph (2000x) of buprenorphine–PLGA microsphere formulation A prior to dissolution.

Table 2 Characteristics of Buprenorphine Microspheres

Formulation	% Yield by weight	% Drug by weight	% Drug incorporated	Average diameter (nm)	Cumulative range (nm) 25–75%
A	65 (5)[a]	1.23 (0.06)	27.3 (1.2)	4063	2396–5063
B	68 (4)	1.21 (0.11)	26.8 (2.5)	5237	1904–6407
C	63 (6)	0.93 (0.10)	21.1 (2.2)	2861	1889–3509
D	60 (3)	0.96 (0.13)	21.9 (3.0)	17101	3612–18552
E	58 (3)	0.85 (0.10)	18.7 (2.2)		
F	61 (4)	0.72 (0.12)	15.8 (2.8)		
G	64 (5)	0.83 (0.05)	18.6 (1.2)	2869	2394–3262
H	59 (6)	0.99 (0.04)	22.3 (0.9)	3550	1863–4454

[a]Mean (SD).

mean percentage for drug content of 0.72–1.23%. Formulation A and B, which contained 50:50 PLGA and utilized evaporation methods, had the highest percentage drug content. Use of these same procedures with 85:15 PLGA polymer produced microspheres with lower drug content. The drug incorporated as a percentage of the theoretical value (4%) ranged from 15.8% to 27.3%. Values of 15% or greater for the percentage incorporated relative to the theoretical value suggest reasonably good drug inclusion, as compared to studies with other drug microsphere systems.

Scanning electron microscopy photographs were obtained for freshly prepared microspheres and microspheres prior to dissolution, after 7 days of dissolution, and after 26 days of dissolution. The appearance of freshly prepared microspheres were similar showing spherical particles of varying size. Microspheres of formulation D (50:50 PLGA, extraction, lyophilization) appeared to be clustered and attached to each other. Photographs of formulation A before dissolution, after 7 days of dissolution, and after 26 days of dissolution are shown in Fig. 1–3, respectively. On day 7, some roughness was apparent on the microsphere surface, and by day 26 the surface appeared more porous and dented. The spherical shape of the microspheres was still clear on day 26 samples of most samples.

Particle size determination for six of the eight formulations demonstrated differences in particle size and size distribution between the products. Particle size distributions are illustrated in Fig. 4. The average diameter and the cumulative 25% to 75% range are provided in Table 2. Except for formulation D, the average particle diameter ranged from 2861 to 5237 nm. There was no demonstrable effect of polymer selection on particle size. In fact, with both polymers, the smallest particles were observed for microspheres prepared by extraction and air drying. Formulation D, which contained 50:50 PLGA polymer prepared by evaporation and lyophilization methods, displayed large particles and it was suspected that particle clumping was occurring.

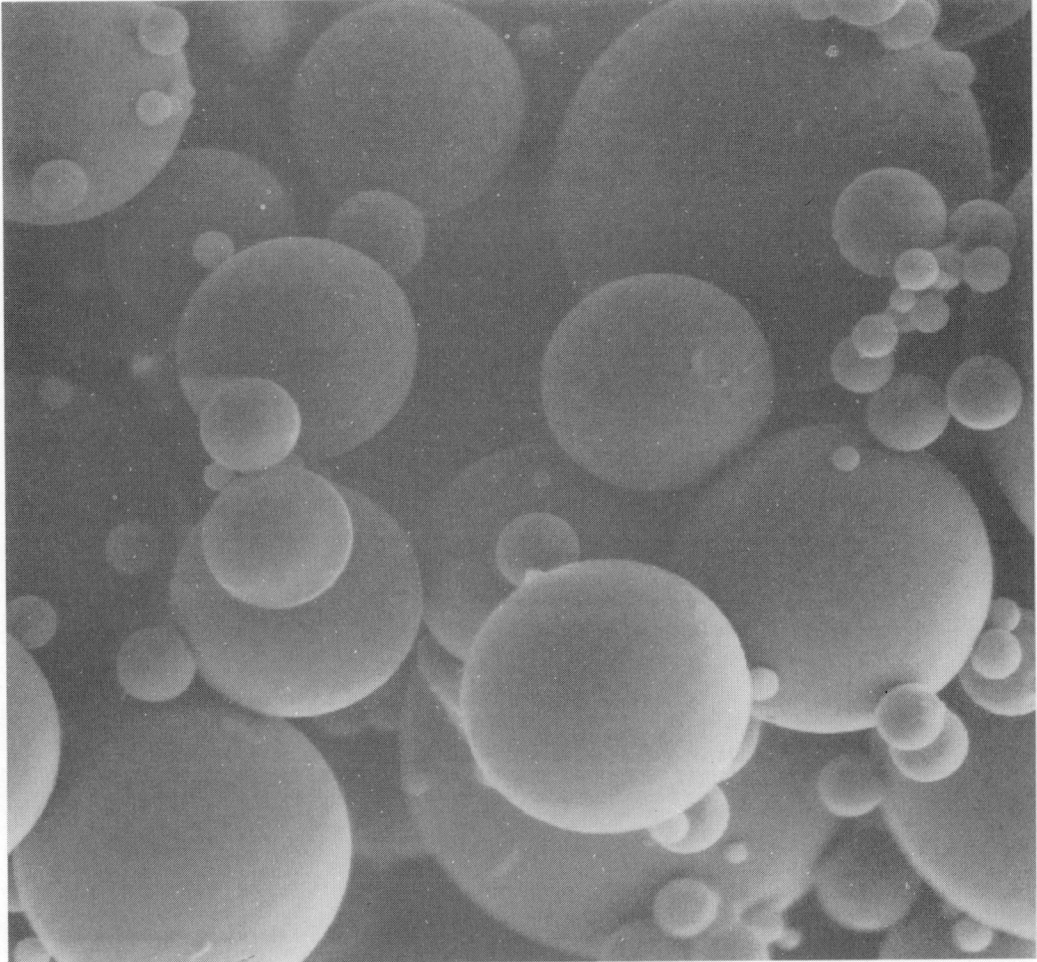

Figure 2 Scanning electron micrograph (2000x) of buprenorphine–PLGA microsphere formulation A after 7 days of dissolution at 37°C.

Dissolution studies were initially performed with microsphere containing only unlabeled buprenorphine. Cumulative amounts and percentage of dose released were estimated based on the concentration of buprenorphine in dissolution media as determined by HPLC methods using electrochemical detection. Electrochemical detection methods proved greatly superior to ultraviolet (UV) detection in terms of the least amount quantifiable and reproducibility. This improvement in sensitivity was needed for dissolution experiments since the concentration of buprenorphine was below UV detection limits due to this drug's low solubility in pH 7.4 buffer. Dissolution approaches were designed to maintain drug concentration less than 15% of the drug solubility in dissolution media. Thus, developing a sensitive HPLC method was critical.

Buprenorphine is reported to be quite stable at neutral pH values. However, our initial dissolution and stability experiments suggested that buprenorphine did degrade at a rate that would not be acceptable for long-term dissolution studies conduct at 37°C. Estimates of buprenorphine degradation half-life at 37°C in pH 7.4 phosphate buffer were 36 days. This rate of degradation did result in a considerable proportion of released drug degrading during the experiment and the

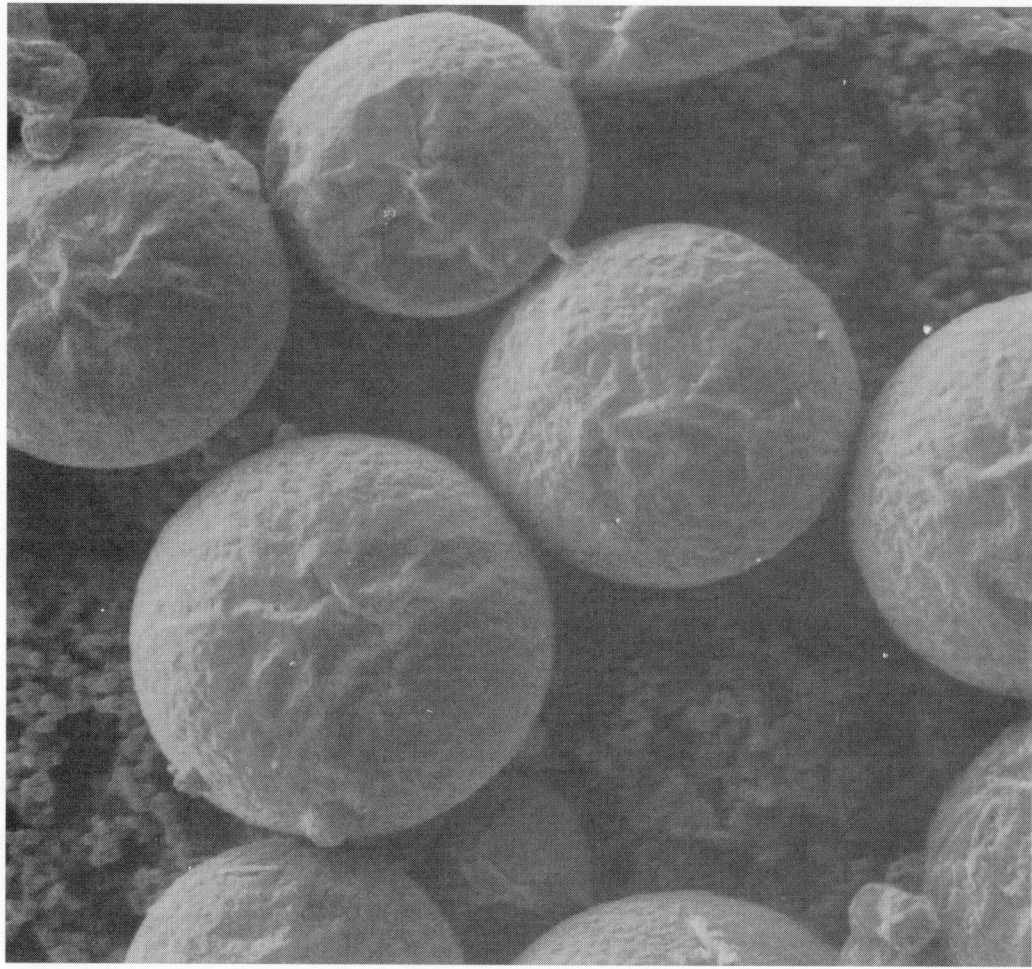

Figure 3 Scanning electron micrograph (2000x) of buprenorphine–PLGA microsphere formulation A after 28 days of dissolution at 37°C.

inability to correctly calculate cumulative amounts of drug released. For this reason, microsphere formulations of buprenorphine were again prepared with ^{3}H-buprenorphine. Content and microscopic studies suggested that these formulations were similar to the previously prepared microspheres. Dissolution studies were reinitiated with microspheres containing labeled drug. It was assumed that drug degradation occurred only with drug in solution and thus measures of total radioactivity in the dissolution media would permit the determination of drug release profiles.

Dissolutions of microsphere formulation prepared with labeled drug were performed under the same dissolution conditions and were conducted up for to 60 days. Burst effects were assessed from the percentage of the dose release in the first 4 days and constant release rates were determined over 4–60 days. The release rates for each dissolution run of the eight formulations were evaluated for order and the rate by linear regression of percentage of dose vs. time from 4 to 60 days. Figures 5 and 6 show the release profiles for formulations A–D (50:50 PLGA) and formulations E–H (85:15 PLGA), respectively. Table 3 presents the 4-day burst amounts expressed as the percentage of drug content, the zero-order release rate, and the

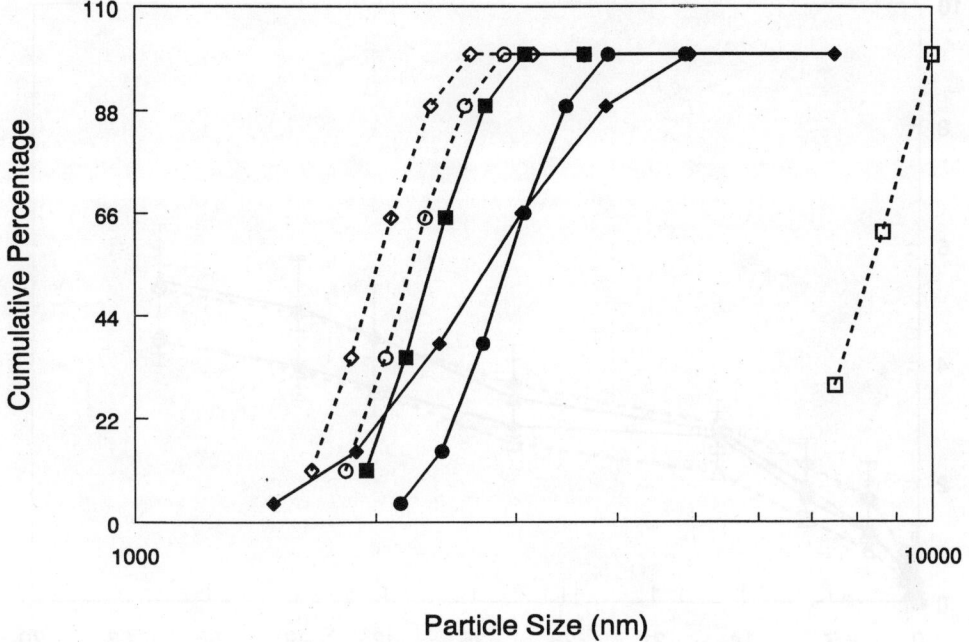

Figure 4 Particle size distributions of buprenorphine–PLGA microsphere formulations. ●(A), ○(B), ■(C), □(D), dc(G), ◇(H).

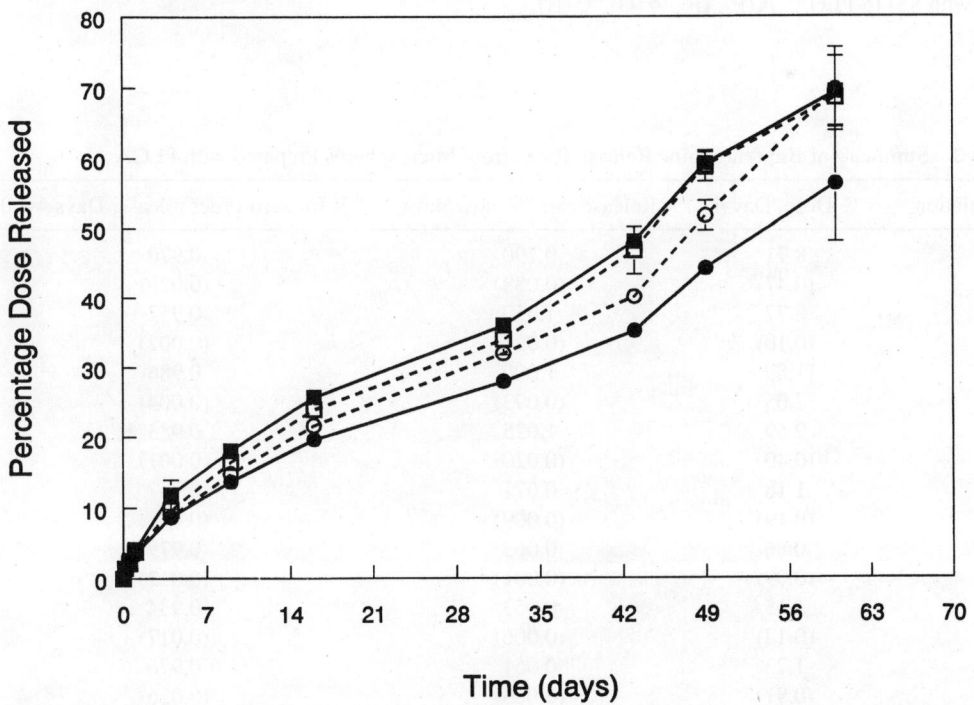

Figure 5 Cumulative percentage of dose released for buprenorphine microspheres formulations prepared with 50:50 PLGA. ●(A), ○(B), ■(C), □(D).

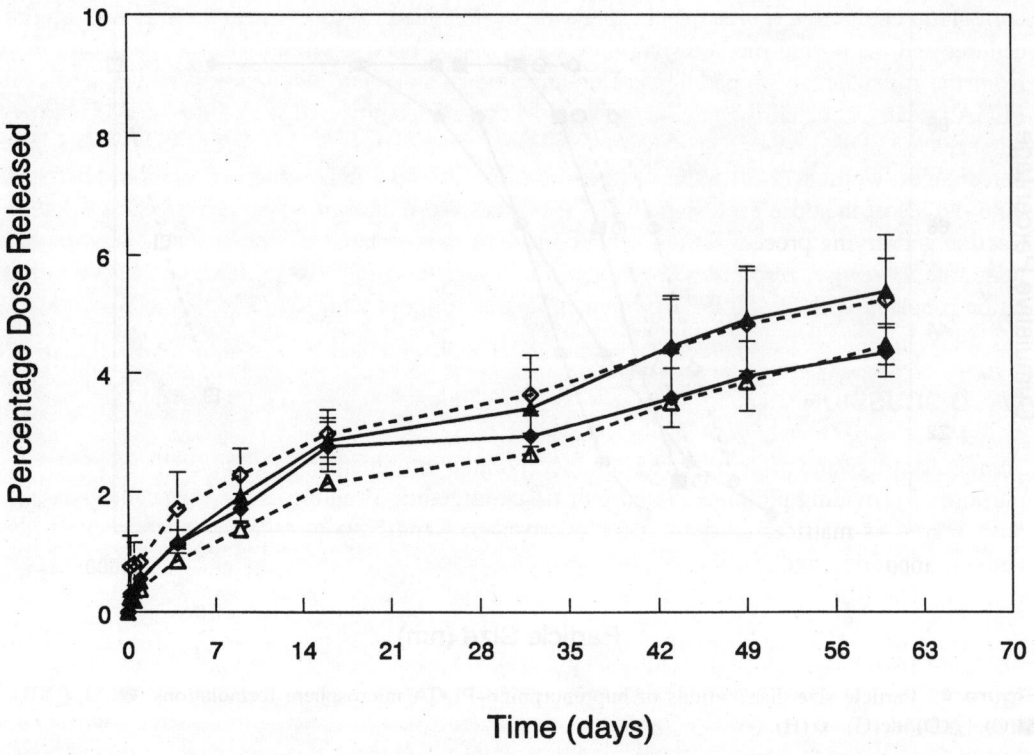

Figure 6 Cumulative percentage of dose released for buprenorphine microspheres formulations prepared with 85:15 PLGA. ▲(E), (F), ♦(G), ◇(H).

Table 3 Summary of Buprenorphine Release Rates from Microspheres Prepared with PLGA

Formulation	% Dose, Day 4	Release rate (% dose/day)	R for zero-order release, Days 4–60
A	8.71	0.790	0.970
	(0.47)[a]	(0.088)	(0.029)
B	8.77	1.050	0.952
	(0.10)	(0.021)	(0.002)
C	11.89	1.000	0.986
	(2.05)	(0.093)	(0.004)
D	9.69	1.025	0.983
	(0.40)	(0.020)	(0.001)
E	1.18	0.072	0.967
	(0.19)	(0.009)	(0.006)
F	0.86	0.063	0.979
	(0.09)	(0.001)	(0.012)
G	1.15	0.053	0.934
	(0.12)	(0.006)	(0.017)
H	1.73	0.061	0.976
	(0.81)	(0.006)	(0.026)

[a]Mean (SD).

correlation coefficient (r) for linear regression of this phase. As seen in Table 3, extraction procedures and the drying methods had little effect on the burst and release rate of buprenorphine from the microsphere preparations. The selection of polymer, either 50:50 PLGA or 85:15 PLGA, greatly affected the release profiles. Microspheres prepared with 50:50 PLGA showed burst release eight times greater than microsphere prepared with 85:15 PLGA. Four-day burst percentages were 8.71–11.89% of the dose for 50:50 PLGA microspheres compared to 0.86–1.17% of the dose for 85:15 PLGA formulations. Within each polymer group, solvent extraction and drying procedures did not produce changes on burst release or the 4- to 60-day release rate. Likewise, zero-order drug release was approximately 10–15 times greater for formulation prepared with 50:50 PLGA when compared to those with 85:15 PLGA.

IV. DISCUSSION

Numerous drugs and proteins have been incorporated into microsphere delivery systems for the purpose of providing prolonged release or tissue targeting. Erodible or biodegradable polymers have served as matrices or coating for microspheres and have included waxes, starches, fats, gelatin, albumin, and synthetic polymers composed of polylactic and polyglycolic acids (PLGA). The PLGA polymers have been popular because of their stability, physical characteristics, hydrophobic nature, and availability as varying molecular weights. The use or mixing of PLGA polymers of differing copolymer ratios (polylactic to polyglycolic acids) provides one approach to controlling the release of drug or protein from a microsphere delivery system. The most popular PLGA polymer for implants and microsphere dosage forms have copolymer ratios of 50:50, 75:25, and 85:15. In this study, PLGA polymers with copolymer ratios of 50:50 and 85:15 were used to prepare microspheres of buprenorphine that could potentially release drug over several weeks.

An injectable microsphere controlled release dosage form may not be a suitable or practical approach for all drugs or peptides due to the need to consider the drug's or peptide's chemical properties, pharmacokinetic profile, and therapeutic application. Buprenorphine has many physical and therapeutic characteristics that make it a good candidate for a parenteral microsphere delivery dosage form. Recognizing that buprenorphine has a short half-life of 2 h, maintaining constant therapeutic effects of buprenorphine as needed for addiction treatment would require this drug to be administered numerous times a day. Thus, a controlled release buprenorphine dosage form would have beneficial therapeutic outcomes when this drug is used during the treatment of drug addiction in patients. In addition, buprenorphine is not a good candidate for a sustained release oral dosage form due to its low systemic bioavailability following oral administration. This low oral bioavailability is a consequence of this drug's high hepatic clearance, leading to a substantial first-pass effect with extents of oral absorption of less than 15%. These pharmacokinetic features, along with the pharmacodynamic characteristics of buprenorphine, dictate the required dose necessary to treat addiction. Studies examining buprenorphine potential application in drug addiction therapy suggested sublingual daily doses of 8 mg. Considering that the sublingual bioavailability is approximately 0.5, a parenteral buprenorphine dose would be 4 mg/day. This low required dose for buprenorphine makes it feasible to incorporate a week or more dose into a microsphere release product intended for intramuscular or subcutaneous administration. With respect to other drugs used to treat addiction such as methadone (30 mg daily dose), buprenorphine dosage rates are substantially less. Many drugs whose therapeutic use could benefit from a parenteral controlled dosage form have daily dosing rates that are too large for possible consideration for a microsphere delivery formulations.

The physicochemical and drug release properties for a drug incorporated in microspheres are controlled by the particle size and distribution, the selected polymer and its molecular weight, the drug-to-polymer ratio, and the preparation procedures. The buprenorphine microsphere were prepared as drug in a polymer matrix with no drug encapsulation attempts. Solvent evaporation is one of the earliest and simplest approaches for incorporating drugs and peptides into microspheres of PLGA (33,37,40). In the simplest case where drug and polymer are soluble in a organic solvent, the drug and polymer are dissolved in the organic phase and then dispersed in an aqueous phase. This mixture is then mixed continuously whereas the organic solvent is evaporated and removed by heat or/and vacuum. After this step, the product would be drug incorporated in polymer matrix microspheres that are dispersed in an aqueous medium. As apparent from this solvent evaporation process, factors such as mixing method and speed, viscosity, and solvent removal technique contribute to the size, shape, degree of incorporation, and drug state characteristics of the formed microsphere. When a drug with significant hydrophilic properties is to be formulated in microspheres, low solubility of the drug in the organic phase, usually methylene chloride, could lead to very low or no drug inclusion in the polymeric microspheres. For such hydrophilic drugs and peptides, surface-active agents may be added to the mixture or double-emulsion procedures may be considered. Additional steps and components for incorporating hydrophilic agents require further optimization procedures and may possibly lead to greater product variability. It was decided that buprenorphine possessed enough lipophilic character to be prepared into microspheres by a single emulsion method without additional components.

Several procedural variables were considered and evaluated in preparing 1:25 buprenorphine microspheres with the two PLGA polymers. Electron microscopic scanning showed all formulations to contain spherical particles with no evidence of drug crystals. Mixing the polymer–drug emulsion by vortexing yielded microspheres in the size range of 2000 to 10,000 nm, whereas sonication methods proved unsuitable due to small particle size. Significant mixing is required to maintain a stable emulsion so that drug will be homogeneous in the polymer microsphere (39). Both mixing rate and emulsion viscosity will determine the size of emulsified droplets and thus the final microsphere size and distribution. The viscosity of the mixture is dependent on the concentration and ratios of the emulsion components, which included the selected polymer, drug, and emulsifier. Low polymer concentrations and low molecular weight polymers lead to lower viscosity mixtures and favor the formation of smaller microspheres. In this study, the polymer weight appeared not to affect the particle size since both 50:50 and 85:15 PLGA polymers produced microspheres of similar size. Although not studied, increasing drug concentration and decreasing the emulsifier have been noted to increase microsphere size (39). Comparison of solvent removal procedures (solvent extraction and solvent evaporation) did not appear to substantially alter the particle size. This is expected since these procedures are performed after the formation of the microspheres. With the exception of formulation D, the drying method did not affect the particle size. For formulation D, which was prepared with 50:50 PLGA followed by extraction, drying by lyophilization appeared to produced particle aggregation.

Based on a drug-to-polymer ratio of 1:25 and assuming that all drug and polymer was incorporated into microspheres, the theoretical drug content in the microspheres would be 4%. The content was determined by HPLC methods permitting the evaluation of any potential drug degradation during the microsphere preparation. The percentage by weight of drug in the final products ranged from 0.72% to 1.23%, which corresponds to percentages for theoretical incorporation rates of 15.8–27.3%. The percentage of drug incorporated was not affected by the choice of polymer, solvent removal methods, or drying technique. The total yields of the prepared microspheres were from 58% to 68% of the initial combined drug and polymer weight, and this suggests that buprenorphine is incorporated into the microspheres at a lower rate than the two PLGA polymers. Considering the aqueous and organic solubility of buprenorphine compared to PLGA polymers, the partitioning of the PLGA polymers into the organic phase of the emulsion mixture is probably greater than that of the drug. For these reasons, lower than theoretical drug content might be expected for buprenorphine microspheres prepared by these procedures. Some solvent evaporation approaches for preparing cisplatin microspheres have demonstrated percentages of incorporation efficiencies as high as 91% (39). The incorporation efficiency could potentially be improved by the addition of solubilizers to the emulsion or changing the ratio of drug to polymer.

The dissolution profile of the buprenorphine microspheres was determined for a period of 60 days. Buprenorphine is thought to be relatively stable at neutral pH values. Preliminary dissolution studies with unlabeled buprenorphine, however, demonstrated significant buprenorphine degradation in the dissolution medium by 10 days. To prevent the degradation of buprenorphine in the dissolution media, experiments in which all of the dissolution medium is removed after each sample time was considered. Unfortunately, by this approach, the low solubility of buprenorphine in the dissolution medium, its slow release from the microspheres, and the desire to maintain sink conditions resulted in drug concentrations below the HPLC sensitivity limits. The application of radiolabeled drug was considered as an alternative that would improve drug assay sensitivity and still maintain sink conditions. For these dissolution studies, it was assumed that while the drug was in the solid state within the microsphere, no drug degradation was occurring. Once the drug was release from the microsphere, drug degradation was no longer a consideration since total radioactivity in the dissolution media reflected the cumulative drug release. It was estimated based on a 36-day degradation half-life that by 60 days as much as 69% of the radioactivity was degraded buprenorphine products. The stability of the released drug in the dissolution media has been generally assumed in long-term dissolution studies of delivery dosage forms. As in this case, the analytical methods and dissolution approach may greatly affect the determined percentage released profile. When drug accumulation occurs in the dissolution medium and/or long sampling periods are used, the possibility of drug degradation effects on analytical procedures should be examined.

Delivery systems composed of PLA and PLGA polymers first undergo hydration and then erosion when placed in aqueous media. The degradation of the polymers is not enzymatic but results from the hydrolytic cleavage of esters group within the polymers. This hydrolysis process occurs with hydrated polymers and leads to a decrease in their molecular weight. Eventually, the polymer's molecular weight is low enough to allow the low molecular weight polymer to dissolve in the aqueous environment. After polymer hydration but before polymer dissolution, drug close to the microsphere's surface may be released to the aqueous media producing an initial burst period. With the erosion of the microsphere and the dissolution of drug, pores may develop in the intrastructure of the microsphere, further increasing the rate of polymer hydrolysis and drug dissolution. A burst followed by a slow-release phase is typical of controlled release dosage forms composed of high molecular weight polymers.

Dissolution profiles of the buprenorphine microspheres showed a rapid release or burst period during the first 4 days and then a slower release phase lasting more than 60 days. The burst and release rate after 4 days was related to the formulations, with the highest rapid release also showing the greatest prolonged release rate. Only the choice of polymer (50:50 PLGA or 85:15 PLGA) appeared to have an effect on the drug release profiles. Neither the solvent removal method nor the drying procedure appeared to influence the extent of the initial or the controlled release rate of buprenorphine. For microspheres prepared with 50:50 PLGA, the initial release up to day 4 was approximately 10% of content and the release after day 4 was approximately 1% per day. The microspheres prepared with 85:15 PLGA displayed a initial burst of 1% and a prolonged release rate of 0.06% of the dose per day. Electron microscopic examination of microspheres after 7 and 26 days of dissolution showed surface porosity appearing by day 7 and surface changes becoming greater by 26 days. The appearance of the microspheres is consistent with the drug release characteristics.

The studies demonstrate that buprenorphine can be incorporated into PLGA microspheres that will release drug in vitro over 60 days. Microsphere formulations with 50:50 PLGA released buprenorphine over 2 months, whereas 85:15 PLGA microsphere released drug at 6% the rate of the 50:50 PLGA microsphere and this was considered too slow. Varying the solvent removal and drying methods did not affect the incorporation efficiency or the drug release properties of the microspheres. Preparation of buprenorphine microspheres with 50:50 PLGA, solvent evaporation, and air drying thus far appears be the simplest and most consistent approach. The in vivo release of buprenorphine from these microsphere preparations needs to be evaluated to better understand the influence of polymers and preparation methods as well as in vivo to in vitro correlations for this microsphere dosage form.

ACKNOWLEDGMENT

This project was partially supported by Grant NIH 43DA-6-7055.

REFERENCES

1. Gold, M. S., 1993. Opiate addiction and the locus coeruleus. The clinical utility of clonidine, naltrexone, methadone, and buprenorphine. Psychiatr. Clin. North Am., 16(1): 61–73.
2. Seow, S. S., Quigley, A. J., Ilett, K. F., Dusci, L. J., Swensen, G., Harrison-Stewart, A., and Rappeport, L., 1986. Buprenorphine: a new maintenance opiate? Med. J. Aust. 144(8): 407–411.
3. Mello, N. K. and Mendelson, J. H., 1985. Behavioral pharmacology of buprenorphine. Drug Alc. Depend. 14(3–4): 283–303.
4. Kosten, T. R. and Kleber, H. D., 1988. Buprenorphine detoxification from opioid dependence: a pilot study. Life Sci., 42(6): 635–641.
5. Bickel, W. K., Stitzer, M. L., Bigelow, G. E., Liebson, I. A., Jasinski, D. R., and Johnson, R. E., 1988. A clinical trial of buprenorphine: comparison with methadone in the detoxification of heroin addicts. Clin. Pharmacol. Ther., 43(1): 72–78.
6. Johnson, R. E., Jaffe, J. H., and Fudala, P. J., 1992. A controlled trial of buprenorphine treatment for opioid dependence. JAMA, 267(20): 2750–2755.
7. Kosten, T. R., Krystal, J. H., Charney, D. S., Price, L. H., Morgan, C. H., and Kleber, H. D., 1990. Opioid antagonist challenges in buprenorphine maintained patients. Drug Alc. Depend., 25(1): 73–78.
8. Lewis, J. W., 1985. Buprenorphine. Drug Alc. Depend., 14(3–4): 363–372.
9. Woods, J. W., France, C. P., and Winger, G. D., 1992. Behavioral pharmacology of buprenorphine: issues relevant to its potential in treating drug abuse. NIDA Research Monograph. 121:12–27.
10. Bigelow, G. E. and Preston, K. L., 1992. Assessment of buprenorphine in a drug discrimination procedure in humans. NIDA Res. Monogr., 121: 28–37.
11. Pickworth, W. B.,11. Pickworth, W. B., Johnson, R. E., Holicky, B. A., and Cone, E. J., 1993. Subjective and physiologic effects of intravenous buprenorphine in humans. Clin. Pharmacol. Ther., 53(5): 570–576.
12. Arditti, J., Bourdon, J. H., Jean, P., Landi, H., Nasset, D., Jouglard, J., and Thirion, X., 1992. Buprenorphine abuse in a series of 50 drug addicts hospitalized at a Drug Dependence Evaluation hospital in Marseille. Therapie, 47(6): 561–562.
13. San, L., Tremoleda, J., Olle, J. M., Porta Serra, M., and de la Torre, R., 1989. Prevalence of buprenorphine use by heroin addicts undergoing treatment. Medicina Clinica, 93(17): 645–648.

14. Preston, K. L., Bigelow, G. E., and Liebson, I. A., 1988. Buprenorphine and naloxone alone and in combination in opioid-dependent humans. Psychopharmacology, 94(4): 484–490.
15. Johnson, R. E., Cone, E. J., Henningfield, J. E., and Fudala, P. J., 1989. Use of buprenorphine in the treatment of opiate addiction. I. Physiologic and behavioral effects during a rapid dose induction. Clin. Pharmacol. Ther., 46(3): 335–343.
16. Blom, Y., Bondesson, U., and Gunne, L. M., 1987. Effects of buprenorphine in heroin addicts. Drug Alc. Depend., 20(1): 1–7.
17. Cession, T. R., Morgan, C., and Kleber, H. D., 1991. Treatment of heroin addicts using buprenorphine. Am. J. Drug Alc. Abuse, 17(2): 119–128.
18. Cession, T. R., Rosen, M. I., Schottenfeld, R., and Ziedonis, D., 1992. Buprenorphine for cocaine and opiate dependence. Psychopharmacol. Bull., 28(1): 15–19.
19. Shulka, V. K., Goldfrank, L. R., Turndorf, H., and Bansinath, M., 1991. Antagonism of acute cocaine toxicity by buprenorphine. Life Sci., 49(25): 1887–1893.
20. Bullingham, R. E. S., McQuay, H. J., Moore, A., and Bennett, M. R. D., 1980. Buprenorphine kinetics. Clin. Pharmacol. Ther., 28(5): 667–672.
21. Ho, S. T., Wang J. J., Ho, W., and Hu, D. Y., 1991. Determination of buprenorphine by high-performance liquid chromatography with fluorescence detection: application to human and rabbit pharmacokinetic studies. J. Chromatogr., 570(2): 339–350.
22. Cone, E. J., Gorodetzky, C. W., Yousefnejad, D., Buchwald, W. F., and Johnson, R. E., 1984. The metabolism and excretion of buprenorphine in humans. Drug Metab. Dispos., 12(5): 577–581.
23. Brewster, D. M., Humphrey, M. J., and McLeavy, M. A., 1981. The systemic bioavailability of buprenorphine by various routes of administration. J. Pharm. Pharmacol., 33: 500–506.
24. Ravis, W. R. and Koster, A. Sj., 1989. Intestinal metabolism of narcotic analgesic, In: A. Sj. Koster, E. Richter, F. Lauterbach, F. Hartmann (Eds.), Progress in Pharmacology and Clinical Pharmacology, 7(2), Gustav Fischer Verlag, New York, pp. 273–287.
25. Mistry, M., and Houston, J. B., 1987. Comparison of intestinal and hepatic conjugation of morphine, naloxone, and buprenorphine. Drug Metab. Dispos., 15(5): 710–717.
26. Bullingham, R. E. S., McQuay, H. J., Dwyer, D., Allen, M. C., and Moore, R. A., 1981. Sublingual buprenorphine used postoperatively: clinical observations and preliminary pharmacokinetic analysis. Br. J. CLin. Pharmacol., 12: 117–122.
27. Eriksen, J., Jensen, N. H., Kamp-Jensen, M., Bjarno, H., Friis, P., and Brewster, D., 1989. The systemic availability of buprenorphine administered by nasal spray. J. Pharm. Pharmacol., 41(11): 803–805.
28. Pontani, R. B., Vadlamani, N. L., and Misra, A. L., 1985. Disposition in the rat of buprenorphine administered parenterally and as a subcutaneous implant. Xenobiotica, 15(4): 287–297.
29. Debrabandere, L., Van Boven, M., and Daenens, P., 1993. Development of a radioimmunoassay for the determination of buprenorphine in biological samples. Analyst, 118(2): 137–143.
30. Debrabandere, L., Van Boven, M., and Daenens, P., 1991. High-performance liquid chromatography with electrochemical detection of buprenorphine and its major metabolite in urine. J. Chromatogr., 564(2): 557–566.
31. Hand, C. W., Sear, J. W., Uppington, J., Ball, M. J., McQuay, H. J., and Moore, R. A., 1990. Buprenorphine disposition in patients with renal impairment: single and continuous dosing, with special reference to metabolites. Br. J. Anaesthesia, 64(3): 276–282.
32. Heller, J., 1993. Polymers for controlled parenteral delivery of peptides and proteins. Adv. Drug Deliv. Rev., 10: 163–204.
33. Burgess, D. J. and Hickey, A. J., 1994. Microsphere technology and applications. In: J. Swarbrick and J. C. Boylan (Eds.), Encyclopedia of Pharmaceutical Technology, Vol. 10. Marcel Dekker, New York, pp. 12–29.
34. Cohen, S., Yoshioka, T., Lucarelli, M., Hwang, L. H. and Langer, R., 1991. Controlled delivery systems for proteins based on poly(lactic/glycolic acid) microspheres. Pharm. Res., 8: 713–720.
35. Sanders, L. M., Kent, J. S., McRae, G. I., Vickery, B. H., Tice, T. R. and Lewis, D. H., 1984. Controlled release of a luteinizing hormone releasing hormone analogue from poly(d,l-lactide-co-Glycolide) microspheres. J. Pharm. Sci., 73: 1294–1297.

36. Sah, H. K. and Chien, Y. W., 1993. Evaluation of a microreservoir-type biodegradable microcapsule for controlled release of proteins. Drug Dev. Ind. Pharm., 19: 1243–1263.
37. Jeffery, H., Davis, S. S. and O'Hagan, D. T., 1993. The preparation and characterization of poly-(lactide-co-glycolide) microparticles. II. The entrapment of a model protein using a (water-in-oil)-in-water emulsion solvent evaporation technique. Pharm. Res., 10: 362–368.
38. Thies, C. and Bissery, M., 1984. Biodegradable microspheres for parenteral administration. In: F. Lim (Ed.), Biomedical Applications of Microencapsulation, CRC Press, Boca Raton, FL, pp. 53–74.
39. Spenlehauer, G., Valerate, M., and Band, J.-P., 1986. Formation and characterization of cisplatin loaded poly(d,l-lactide) microspheres for chemoembolization. J. Pharm. Sci., 75: 750–755.
40. Spenlehauer, G., Vert, M., Band, J.-P., and Boddaert, A., 1989. In vitro and in vivo degradation of poly(d,l-lactide/glycolide) type microspheres made by solvent evaporation method. Biomaterials, 10: 557–563.
41. Gopferich, A., Alonso, M. J., and Langer, R., 1994. Development and characterization of microencapsulated microspheres. Pharm. Res., 11: 1568–1574.
42. Alonso, M. J., Cohen, S., Park, T. G., Gupta, R. K., Siber, G. R., and Langer, R., 1993. Determinants of release rate of tetanus vaccine from polyester microspheres. Pharm. Res., 10: 945–953.

40
Prolonged Release of Hydromorphone from a Novel Poly(Lactic-co-Glycolic) Acid Depot System: Initial In Vitro and In Vivo Observations

Leonidas C. Goudas, Daniel B. Carr, and Richard M. Kream
New England Medical Center, Boston, Massachusetts and Tufts University School of Medicine, Boston, Massachusetts

Louis Shuster
Tufts University School of Medicine, Boston, Massachusetts

William M. Vaughan
Dental Research Detachment, U.S. Army, Great Lakes, Illinois

Joseph D. Gresser, Donald L. Wise, and Debra J. Trantolo
Cambridge Scientific, Inc., Belmont, Massachusetts

I. INTRODUCTION

The amelioration of pain with potent opioid analgesics may produce side effects, such as sedation, dizziness, or nausea, that impair functional activity for as long as pain relief is necessary. Nonetheless, opioid analgesics have an important clinical role that cannot always be filled by other agents such as nonsteroidal anti-inflammatory drugs or local anesthetics. When pain is severe and long-lasting, it may be desirable to administer a systemic opioid together with a regional local anesthetic. Side effects may be minimized and long-lasting relief achieved using controlled release implants for delivery of either type or both types of agent. Anesthetic formulations may be implanted at the wound or surgical site for local drug delivery. Analgesic formulations may be implanted at distant, nontraumatized sites for systemic drug delivery. By use of a biodegradable excipient, poly(lactic-co-glycolic) acid (PLGA), the implant need not be removed. Drug delivery can be adjusted to provide release for several days up to 2 weeks.

Controlled release pharmaceutical dosage forms offer several advantages over conventional dosage forms of the same drug. These include reduced dosing frequency, decreased incidence and/or intensity of adverse effects, greater selectivity of pharmacologic activity, and a more constant therapeutic effect. While it is not true that controlled release products have significant advantages in all cases, controlled release systems are attractive for certain subpopulations of patients where, for example, patient compliance or the logistics of drug administration is an issues.

Hydromorphone hydrochloride, a morphine derivative, has been used in the United States since the 1930s. Despite this long history, its dose–effect relationship is still being investigated.

Early reviews (1) indicated that hydromorphone was nine times more effective than morphine and faster acting. Recently, Coda, et al. determined that hydromorphone is five times more potent than morphine and has a shorter time to peak effect (2). In the last 10 years, new research has focused on alternate delivery routes. Bruera et al. in a double-blind study (3) compared the effectiveness of oral sustained release hydromorphone with immediate release hydromorphone in cancer patients who were experiencing pain. Their findings indicated that sustained release hydromorphone is as safe and as effective as the traditional immediate release dosage form. Similarly, Hayes et al. found controlled release hydromorphone in a 12-h formulation to be as effective as repeated doses of the standard 4-h formulation (4). In another study, subcutaneous infusion of high concentrations of hydromorphone was evaluated by Bruera, who found that hydromorphone can be safely administered in concentrations much higher than those that are commercially available (5). An ethylene vinyl acetate copolymer disk has been tested for delivery of hydromorphone, but it requires surgical insertion and is not biodegradable (6,7). Other implantable delivery systems for hydromorphone have been developed, but none to date combines ease of implantability, effectiveness of delivery, and the use of a bioresorbable polymer matrix.

II. MATERIALS AND METHODS

A. Drugs

Hydromorphone hydrochloride (HM) was obtained from Sigma Chemical Co. (St. Louis, MO). Upon receipt, the identity and purity of HM was confirmed by ultraviolet absorption spectra.

B. Poly-(Lactic-co-Glycolic) Acid (PLGA)

The polymers PLGA 50:50 (Resomer 506) and PLGA 85:15 (Resomer 858) were obtained from Boehringer-Ingelheim through its U.S. distributor, Henley Chemicals, Inc. (Montvale, NJ). PLGA 5O:50 is a copolymer of lactic and glycolic acids, with a mole ratio of 1:1, lactic to glycolic; PLGA 85:15 has a corresponding lactic-to-glycolic acid ratio of 85:15. On receipt of the polymers, molecular weight was confirmed by gel permeation chromatography (GPC) at Jordi Associates, Inc. (Bellingham, MA). The samples were analyzed in hexafluoroisopropanol (HFIP)/0.01 M sodium trifluoroacetate at a flow rate of 0.6 mL/min using a Jordi Gel DVB mixed-bed column, 25 cm $\times$ 10 mm (ID), at a column temperature of 40°C. The injection size was 100 μL of a 0.1% (w/v) solution. The samples were monitored at a sensitivity of 8X using a Waters Model 401 refractive index detector. Data acquisition and handling were accomplished with Viscotek TriSEC software. The following molecular weight data were reported: For PLGA 50:50, the initial molecular weight was 96,410. For PLGA 85:15, it was 177,840.

C. Depot Preparation

Matrices were prepared by a proprietary process described in U.S. Patent 5,456,917 (8). The polymer was prepared as a low-density foam by lyophilization of a polymer solution of specified concentration. The density of the resulting foam is a function of the concentration of the polymer in the solution. We have found glacial acetic acid to be a suitable solvent. Following production of the PLGA foam, the HM/PLGA depots were prepared via high-pressure extrusion of a blend of ground and sized polymer and HM.

1. Preparing the Foam

PLGA (3.00 g) was placed in glacial acetic acid (gl HAc, 75 mL) in a lyophilization flask (250 mL) used to contain the solution for freeze drying. The solution was stirred for 4 h until all of the polymer dissolved. The polymer solution then was frozen at $-78°C$ in a dry ice/isopropanol bath. Lyophilization was performed using a commercial freeze dryer at 0.1 mm Hg (Labconco, FD8). The foam density was determined to be 0.060 g/cm^3.

2. Grinding and Sieving the Foam

The polymer foam (1.0- to 1.5-g aliquots) was cryogenically ground in a Tekmar Model A-10 mill using dry ice in isopropanol as coolant. Sieving was done using standard Tyler mesh screens (180 and 125 μm) with pan and cover to collect the particles between 125 and 180 μm in diameter. A Syntron electric vibrator (sieve shaker) was used to remove the smaller particles, and the larger particles were returned to the mill for further grinding

3. Formulating PLGA and Hydromorphone Hydrochloride

To make the 25% (w/w) formulation of HM and polymer, 2.0706 g PLGA was mixed with HM (0.6902 g) in a covered glass jar (250 mL) and placed on a ball mill for 15 h (without grinding aids). The PLGA/25% HM powdered mixture was placed via a funnel into a steel mold capable of accepting a 25-mm-diameter cylindrical ram and fitted with a 1.2-mm-diameter die. The ram was inserted slowly and the die and mold were centered under a hydraulic cylinder (Compaq Model MPR 40-1). The mixture was heated to 60°C and compressed to compact the solid. A thermocouple was attached under the mold to monitor the temperature of the extrusion and a heating clamp placed around the outside of the mold. An extrusion force of 15 tons was applied to the 25-mm-diameter ram. The rod (1.3 mm diameter, approximately 40 cm long) was extruded at 64–66°C. Formulations containing 50% HM were similarly prepared.

D. *In Vitro* Release

In vitro drug (HM) release was measured in depots weighing approximately 10 mg. Each was immersed in 10 mL of pH 7.4 phosphate-buffered saline (PBS) at 37°C. Five replicates were analyzed. Release was measured spectrophotometrically at 280.1 nm using a Varian Cary 1 spectrophotometer. The extinction coefficient of HM at 280.1 nm was experimentally determined to be 4.207 absorbance units per unit concentration (mg/mL).

E. Studies in Mice

All studies were approved by the Animal Studies Committee of Tufts University School of Medicine. Groups of 10 mice (male, C57 Black/6J, Jackson Laboratories) weighing 20–25 g, housed five to a cage, were used to test the four different HM depots. Two control groups were included—one with a polymer-only implant, the other with no implant at all. Under methoxyflurane anesthesia, depots were implanted in the scapular region of the mice.

F. Studies in Rats

Sixteen male Sprague–Dawley rats were used for this study. The animals were delivered to the Animal Facilities of the Division of Laboratory Animal Medicine (DLAM) at Tufts University and housed two to three per cage under light/dark cycles of 12 h duration while water and rat chow was provided ad libitum. The average weight of the animals at the time of arrival was 200 g and at the time of *in vivo* testing was 250 g. Animal weight at the time of *in vivo* testing was used for the calculation of the desired delivery rate of hydromorphone and the preparation of rods.

Implantation of rods was performed under transient isoflurane anesthesia. Each animal was anesthetized and the lower dorsal area over the hind limbs was shaved and prepared with alcohol/betadine. A small incision was made and a 22-gauge trocar was placed through it into subcutaneous tissue. The rod was then placed inside the trocar and pushed to its tip using the corresponding stylet. The trocar then was advanced in the subcutaneous tissue plane to a distance that exceeded the length of the rod. While the the stylet was held steady, the trocar was withdrawn slowly, leaving the rod in the subcutaneous plane. The incision was closed with a 4-0 silk suture. Animals were allowed to recover from anesthesia and were returned to their cages.

G. Doses

The mice were dosed at a single level of 70 mg/kg HM, the total implant weight of 5 mg representing 1.25 mg HM. In the rat experiment, 15 animals were allocated to three groups (n = 5) to receive PLGA-HM implants. Two groups were implanted with rods containing 15 and 30 mg of HM (60 and 120 mg/kg), while the third group was implanted with rods containing no HM (placebo implants). An additional animal was implanted with a standard 2-mL volume capacity osmotic minipump filled with 20.8 mg/mL HM in sterile normal saline. This pump (Alzet, Palo Alto, CA) was designed to deliver volume at a rate of 5 µL/h when implanted subcutaneously. The dose selected to be delivered using the pump was 25 mg over a period of 10 days—an intermediate dose compared to the doses selected for the rods, which was intended to serve as a positive control.

1. Behavioral Analgesia Testing

The standard tail flick latency test was used to determine percentage of maximum possible analgesic response (% MPR). The % MPR was calculated as follows:

$$\% \text{ MPR} = [(\text{test latency} - \text{control latency})/(\text{cutoff} - \text{control latency})] \times 100$$

Test latency was defined as the time required for an implanted animal to respond to a heat (lamp) stimulus applied to its tail by removing the tail from the source of the stimulus. Control latency may refer either to unimplanted controls or to preimplant latency of the test animals. The cutoff is the maximum allowable duration of the heat stimulus as chosen by the investigator to avoid tissue damage. Animals were tested 30 min prior to implantation and daily thereafter for 10 days. Each daily assessment consisted of the average of three consecutive tail flick withdrawal latencies taken 3 min apart. All daily measurements were made at the same time of day.

2. Blood Sampling

After baseline testing and prior to implantation of rods, rats were held gently and a small (2-mm) superficial incision was made at the tip of the tail. Three to four drops of blood (0.3 mL approximately) were collected in labeled tubes and centrifuged for serum hydromorphone analysis. After collection of the sample the tip of the tail was gently compressed with a clean cotton swab for 5 min. At day 1 a second set of blood samples was collected 1 h after implantation. On alternate days until day 10, blood samples were collected following behavioral testing using the same technique. In that way residual surgical stress as well as technical difficulties relating to maintenance of patency of intravascular cannulas and sterility were eliminated. Blood was centrifuged for 5 min; then the supernatant serum was collected and frozen at $-80°C$ until analysis.

3. HM Determination in Rat Serum

Solid phase extraction of serum was performed by using Waters Oasis HLB extraction cartridges. The Oasis cartridges comprise a hydrophilic–lipophilic balanced copolymer that is a universal sorbent and allows high recoveries even if the cartridges are run dry. Exactly 100 µL (0.2 mg/mL) naloxone (used as an internal standard) was added to 100 µL of serum sample and the volume adjusted to 1.0 mL using PBS. The Oasis cartridges were primed using a vacuum filter with 1.0 mL methanol followed by 1.0 mL water. Finally, 1 mL of each sample was added to individual cartridges. The cartridges then were washed twice with 1 mL of water. The cartridges were eluted with 1 mL of methanol and samples collected. The methanol was evaporated to dryness under vacuum at 40°C. Until high-performance liquid chromatography (HPLC) analysis, dry samples were kept at $-20°C$. Samples were reconstituted in 100 µL of mobile phase and centrifuged for 5 min in order to remove any particulate contaminants.

4. HPLC and Electrochemical Detection Assays

Biochemical analysis of HM concentrations in serum samples was performed by HPLC combined with EC detection as optimized by our investigators. Other recent HPLC assays have been reported (2,9,10), but the sensitivity and/or the difficulty of implementation with each provided an impetus for us to develop a new method. The system consisted of a Waters 510 pump, a Waters U6K injector, an ESA Model 5100A coulometric detector, and a Hewlett Packard integrator. HM and naloxone standards were separated using a C-18 column (Rainin 4.5 × 150 mm, 5-µm particles) at a flow rate of 0.7 mL/min. A voltamogram was performed to determine the optimal settings for the detector. Maximum peak heights for the eluted substances were obtained with settings at $D1 = 3$ mV and $D2 = 4.5$ mV. The mobile phase consisted of 0.1 M KH_2PO_4 containing 10% acetonitrile. The pH was adjusted to approximately 3.2–3.3 using concentrated (70%) phosphoric acid. Retention times were approximately 6 and 12 min for hydromorphone and naloxone, respectively. The detector response was linear from 1 ng to 10 ng of standard compounds. Standard curves were constructed by plotting detector responses in units of peak height (or area under curve) vs. nanograms of standard. Recovery of extracted blood samples was tested in blood samples of naive rats spiked with varying amounts of 0.2 mg/mL HM and a known concentration of naloxone (internal standard).

5. Excision of Rods

At the end of the study period, mice and rats were sacrificed by cervical dislocation and the implants with surrounding tissue were excised. Implants were removed and examined for residual drug.

III. RESULTS AND DISCUSSION

In vitro release of hydromorphone from the PLGA 50:50 depots containing 25% (w/w) HM is shown in Fig. 1. Data are presented as cumulative percent release vs. time for separate experiments conducted on the same batch. Linear regressions of cumulative percent release vs. time

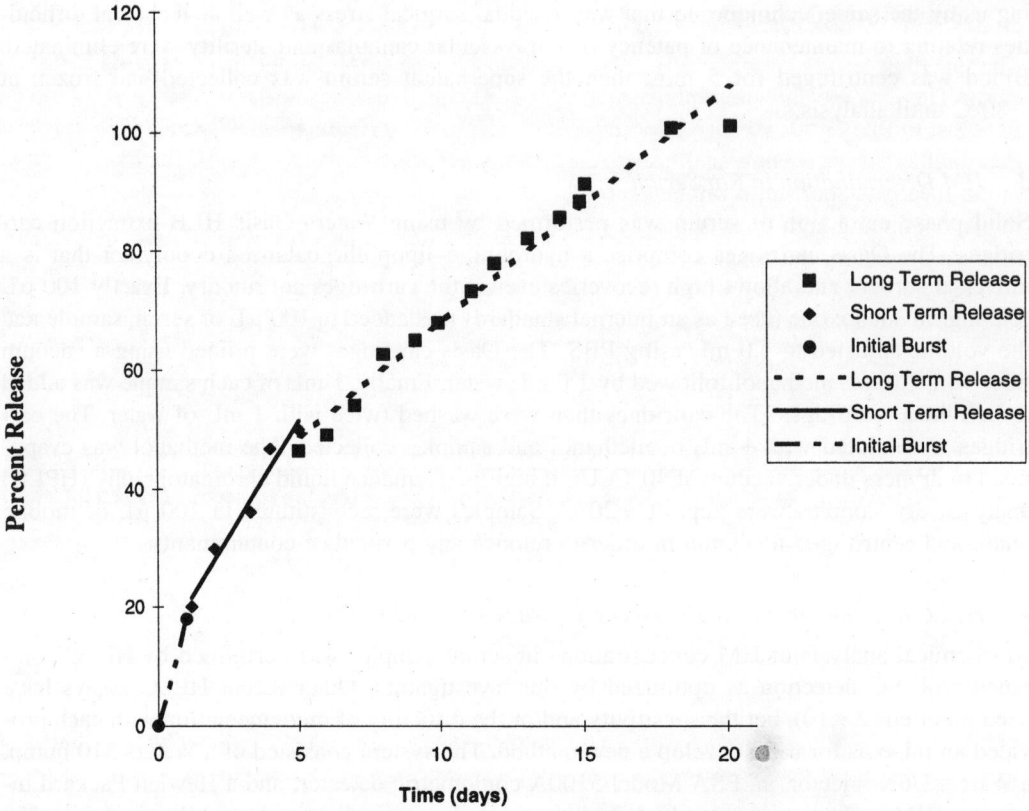

Figure 1 *In vitro* release of hydromorphone hydrochloride from PLGA 50:50/25% HM rods.

for days 1–5 and days 5–15 are shown in Fig. 1. The slopes within these time periods (mean daily percent release of five replicates) and correlation coefficients are shown in Table 1.

The high correlation coefficients indicate fairly constant release rates within each of these periods. From day 15, at which time 91.4% of the drug had been released, system depletion followed quickly with 100% release by day 18.

Within the first 29 h (short-term run), 20.2% of the HM rod had been released. Given the constancy of the release rates in the two time periods (days 1–5 and days 5–15), this "early burst" is acceptable—indeed, may be therapeutically desirable in that it delivers an initial loading dose. The overlay of the two curves, intersecting at day 5, is indicative of the reproducibility of the results.

Table 1 Slopes and Correlation Coefficients

Time interval (days)	Slope (% release/day)	Correlation coeff.
1–5	7.90	0.9824
5–15	4.38	0.9962

A. Behavioral Observations

The tail flick testing on mice was used to select the best formulation for proceeding to the rat study. The data are shown graphically in Fig. 2. The analgesic response as measured by the tail flick test to PLGA 50:50/25% HM and PLGA 85:15/50% HM are virtually identical and show measurable but decreasing analgesia to day 8 at which time analgesia was 16–18% of the maximum. Ideally, a short-term implant should show gradually decreasing analgesia with time rather than a continuing high level of analgesia followed by an abrupt drop. In clinical settings, such as after an operation, the usual intensity of pain declines with each postoperative day. Decreasing analgesia also allows the physician to judge the severity of residual pain over time. Both polymers have advantages and disadvantages as delivery vehicles. The PLGA 50:50 is more rapidly

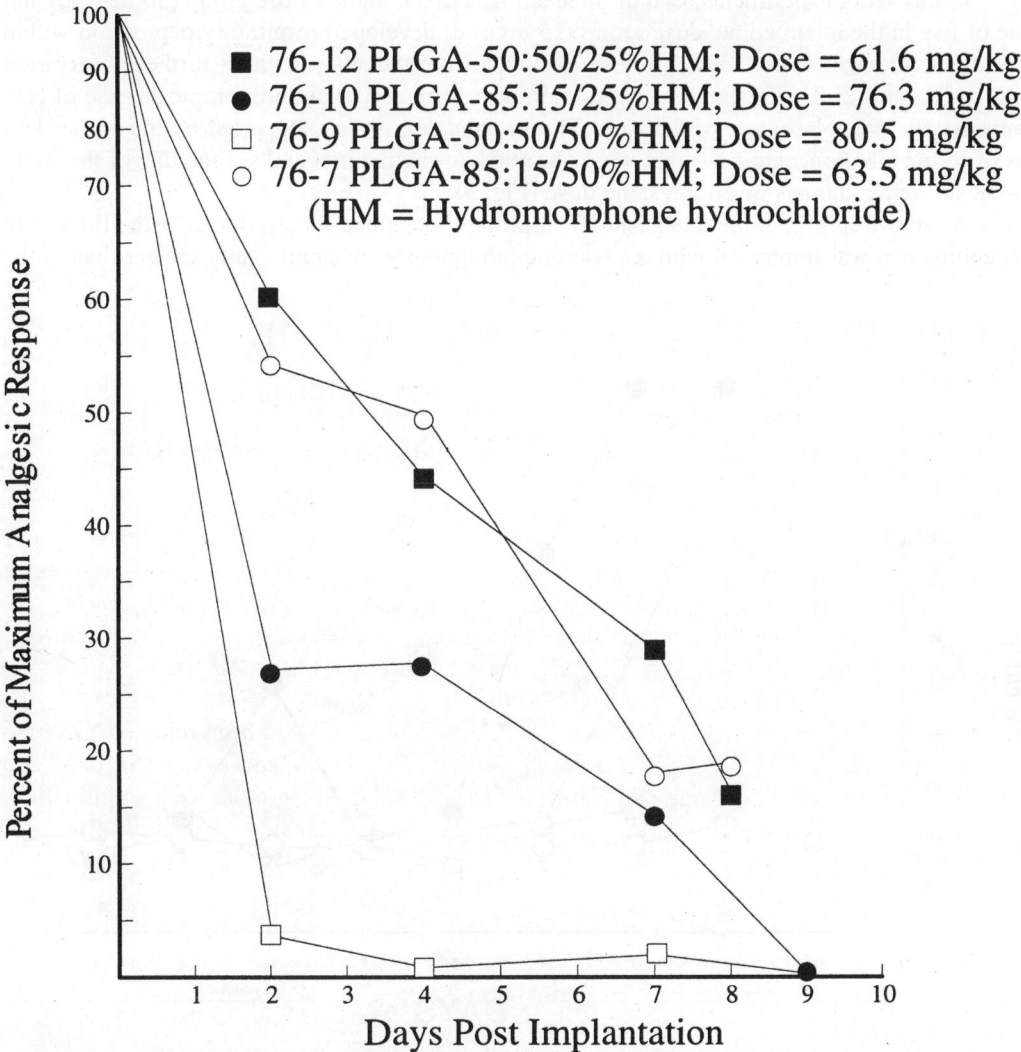

Figure 2 Analgesic responses in mice implanted with PLGA-HM rods vs. time. Analgesic responses were assessed using the tail flick withdrawal latency test.

resorbed. Although this is a desirable feature, the possibility of dumping (rapid release) at some point is increased. Release from the PLGA 85:15 is more gradual, except at high loadings. However, the slow *in vitro* release of HM from the 25% loaded PLGA 85:15 resulted in insufficient analgesia. On the other hand, insufficient late analgesia from the 50% loaded PLGA 50:50 may reflect early dumping and exhaustion of the HM. Therefore, these two systems were eliminated from further consideration. The PLGA 85:15 containing 50% HM, even though it gave a good analgesic effect, also released too rapidly. This system, therefore, was eliminated too. The remaining system, PLGA 50:50 containing 25% HM, gives both adequate analgesic response and acceptable *in vitro* release kinetics. It also has the virtue of being more rapidly resorbed.

The tail flick testing on rats is shown below. Percent MPRs for three different doses (n = 3 per dose) of HM-PLGA systems (0, 15, and 30 mg/rod corresponding to titrated doses of 0, 60, and 120 mg/kg based on an average rat weight of 250 g) are shown in Fig. 3 below.

In this set of experiments, two of three animals in the highest dose group (30 mg/rod) and one of five in the intermediate dose group (15 mg/rod) developed respiratory depression within 6 h after placement of the rods and were excluded from the study without further observation or blood sampling. This respiratory depression was attributed to an initial rapid release of HM immediately after placement of the rods. This explanation is also supported by the higher levels of serum HM concentrations that were observed during the first and second day of the study in the surviving animals given the same dose (Fig. 3).

As shown in Fig. 3, the analgesic effect in the groups that received rods with HM and in the animal that was implanted with the osmotic minipump were significantly greater than in the

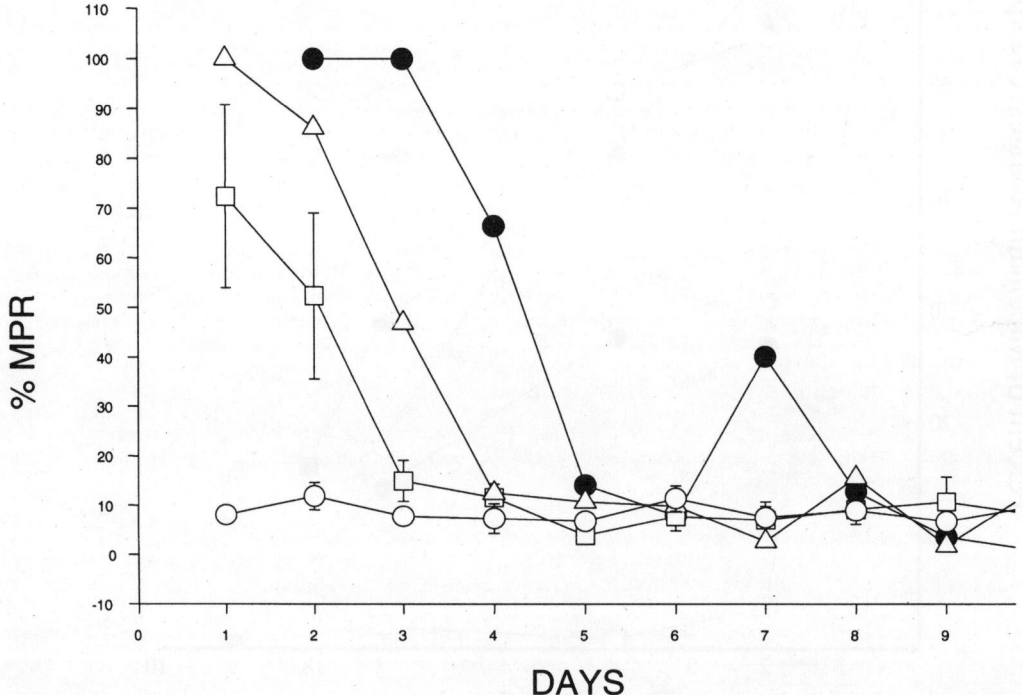

Figure 3 Analgesic responses in rats implanted with PLGA-HM rods vs. time. Analgesic responses over time were assessed using the tail flick withdrawal latency test. The doses of HM contained in the rods used were 0 mg, 15 mg, and 30 mg. An Alzet mini–osmotic pump was used as a control for sustained release.

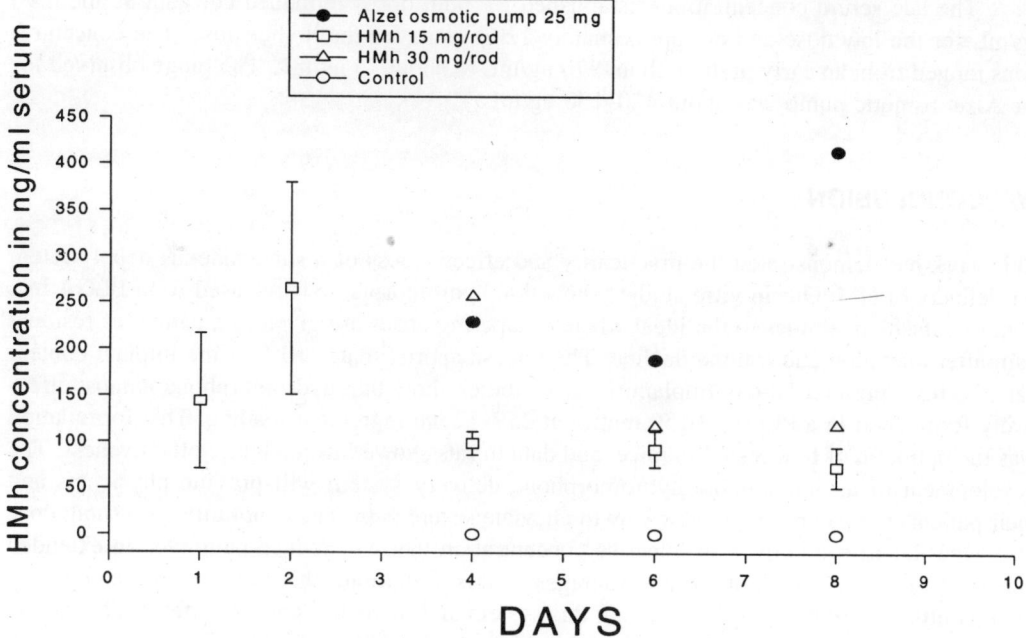

Figure 4 Serial concentrations of HM in rat serum vs. time.

control group (PLGA–no HM). This difference was observed until approximately day 4 of the study. No differences were observed between groups thereafter. The duration of analgesia in this set of experiments reflects the development of tolerance to the opioid actions. Such tolerance is predictable and is typically more pronounced when the experimental animals are subjected to minimal noxious stimulation, as opposed to patients with trauma or inflammation and ongoing severe pain.

The duration of analgesic effect was approximately 4 days. Corresponding concentrations of HM, determined using HPLC and EC assays as described above (see Section II), and are plotted versus time in Fig. 4. In the figure, error bars appear where the number of animals is more than one. Serum hydromophone concentrations in the control group (PLGA without HM) were less than detection.

As shown in Fig. 4, the higher initial serum concentrations are in accord with the higher initial release rates observed in vitro. Early and late serum concentrations and in vitro release rates are compared below in Table 2.

Table 2 Serum Concentrations and Release Rates During Prolonged (3-week) Depot Implantation

In vitro release		*In vivo* release	
Time interval (days)	% per day	Serum HM conc. (ng/mL)	
0–1	20		
1–5	7.9	Early	~150–200
5–20	4.4	Late	~90–120

The late serum concentrations established for both doses remained constant at about 90 ng/mL for the low dose and at approximately 120 ng/mL for the higher dose. The concentrations ranged from an early high of about 270 ng/mL to about 75 ng/mL. The range observed for the Alzet osmotic pump was about 420–180 ng/mL.

IV. CONCLUSION

This work has demonstrated the practicality and effectiveness of a subcutaneous depot system for delivery of HM. Our in vitro studies show that hydromorphone is released from PLGA in a nonlinear fashion, similar to the ideal whereby tapering doses are given to a patient as residual pain after operation and trauma decline. The release approximates 10% of the implant content per day, resulting in a 10-day implant. In vivo studies show that hydromorphone is most effectively formulated in a PLGA 50:50 matrix at 25% active ingredient loading. This formulation was the optimum of four tested in mice, and data in rats showed its analgesic effectiveness. The development of an implantable hydromorphone delivery system will provide physicians and their patients with a promising new way to alleviate severe pain. The depot utilizes a small dose of analgesic and can deliver an effective concentration that will reduce pain over an extended period of time after insertion. The advantages of this system are that, unlike other analgesics, there is little opportunity for abuse using this system and there are few side effects. This depot, by allowing extended release of potent analgesic, has great potential in the field of chronic pain management.

ACKNOWLEDGMENTS

Support for these studies was provided by the U.S. Department of Defense Contract No. DAMD17-96-C-6043 grant to Cambridge Scientific Inc., and the Department of Anesthesiology, New England Medical Center, Tufts University School of Medicine (L.C.G. and D.B.C.); the Richard Saltonstall Foundation (L.C.G., D.B.C., R.M.K., J.M.); the National Institutes of Health DA04128 (R.M.K.), training grant T32-MH-12294 (L.C.G. and R.M.K.). Finally, we thank Heinrich Wurm, M.D., Chairman, Department of Anesthesiology, Tufts University School of Medicine and New England Medical Center, for support and encouragement of these studies.

REFERENCES

1. H. Haas, E. Hohagen, G. Kollmannsperger. Vergleichende Untersuchungen mit Analgeticis. Arznein-Forsch., 3, 238–247, 1953.
2. B. Coda, A. Tanake, R. C. Jacobson, G. Donaldson, C. R. Chapman. Hydromorphone analgesia after intravenous bolus administration. Pain, 71, 41–48, 1997.
3. E. Bruera, P. Sloan, B. Mount, J. Scott, M. Suarez-Almazor. A randomized, double-blind, double-dummy, crossover trial comparing the safety and efficacy of oral sustained-release hydromorphone with immediate-release hydromorphone in patients with cancer pain. J. Clin. Oncol., 14, 1713–1717,1996.
4. H. Hayes, N. Hagen, M. Thirlwell, H. Dhaliwal, N. Babul, Z. Harsanyi, A. C. Darke. Comparative clinical efficacy and safety of immediate release and controlled release hydromorphone for chronic severe cancer pain, Cancer, 74, 1808–1816, 1994.

5. E. Bruera, T. MacEachern, K. Macmillan, M. Miller, J. Hanson. Local tolerance to subcutaneous infusions of high concentrations of hydromorphone: a prospective study, J. Pain Sympt. Manage., 8, 201–204, 1993.
6. G. J. Lesser, S. A. Grossman, K. W. Leong, H. Lo, S. Eller. In vitro and in vivo studies of subcutaneous hydromorphone implants designed for the treatment of cancer pain. Pain, 65, 265–272, 1996.
7. D. J. Rhodes, S. A. Grossman. Hydromorphone polymer implant. J. Substance Abuse Treat., 14, 535–542, 1977.
8. Wise et al. U.S. Patent 5,456,917 (1995).
9. M. Lou Stiles, L. V. Allen, S. J. Prince. Stability of deferoxamine mesylate, floxuridine, fluorouracil, hydromorphone, hydrochloride, lorazepam, and midazolam hydrochloride in polypropylene infusion-pump syringes, Am. J. Health Syst. Pharm., 53, 1583–1588, 1996.
10. T. G. Venkateshwaran, J. T. Stewart. "HPLC Determination of morphine–hydromorphone–bupivacaine and morphine–hydromorphone–tetracaine mixtures in 0.9% sodium chloride injection, J. Liq. Chromatog., 18, 565–578.

41

Incorporation of an Active Agent into a Biodegradable Cement: Encapsulation of the Agent as Protection from Chemical Degradation During Cure and Effect on Release Profile

Joseph D. Gresser, Debra J. Trantolo, and Hisanori X. Nagaoka
Cambridge Scientific, Inc., Cambridge, Massachusetts

Yung-Yueh Hsu and Donald L. Wise
Northeastern University, Boston, Massachusetts

Pattisapu R. J. Gangadharam
University of Illinois, Chicago, Illinois

I. INTRODUCTION

A. Background

The utility of bone cements has been recognized since 1951, when Charney first anchored an endoprosthesis with a self-curing poly(methyl methacrylate) (PMMA) cement (1). Acrylic bone cements currently available in the United States include Palacos R (Kulzer and Co. GmbH, FRG), Zimmer Bone Cement and Zimmer Low Viscosity Cement (Zimmer, Inc.), CMW Type I (CMW Laboratories, Blackpool, UK), and Surgical Simplex P (Howmedica Int. Ltd.). As an example of cement composition, the Surgical Simplex P is formulated to contain a mixture of PMMA and a copolymer of methyl methacrylate and styrene. Methyl methacrylate monomer (MMA) is used in the curing process, with benzoyl peroxide as initiator, N,N-dimethyl-p-toluidine (DMPT) as an accelerator to make possible low-temperature cure, and hydroquinone to inhibit premature polymerization.

Because the rate of infection following total joint replacement surgery may be as high as 11% (2), it has been of continuing interest to minimize this by incorporating various antibiotics into the cement for slow release at the surgical site. Marks et al. (2), while investigating the release of oxacillin, cefazolin, and gentamicin from both Simplex and Palacos cements, found that the three were released more rapidly and for longer periods from the Palacos than from the Simplex cement, and in microbiologically active form. In a comparison of several bone cements, Wahlig and Dingeldein (3) confirmed the use of Palacos R for release of gentamicin, observing continuous release for over 5 years in clinical trials.

Although other studies have also explored acrylic cements as carriers for antibiotics (4–7), the use of a resorbable cement has also been recognized in treatment of chronic bone infections such as bacterial osteomyelitis. However, Gerhart et al. (8) pointed out that PMMA is an inert material which if remaining at the implant site would require a second surgical procedure for removal. These investigators formulated a biodegradable cement using MMA to crosslink the unsaturated polyester poly(propylene fumarate) (PPF) and incorporated vancomycin or gentamicin into the cement before cure. Because PPF can be hydrolyzed at the ester linkage, the hydrolysis products (fumarate residues linked by MMA chains) would contribute to increased resorbability.

The development of a biodegradable cement was carried further by Wise et al. (9) who used PPF with vinylpyrrolidone (VP) as a crosslinking agent rather than MMA. The hydrolysis products of this cement should be more soluble by analogy with the solubility of polyvinylpyrrolidone (PVP) itself. Sanderson (10) reported use of a PPF/VP cement for controlled drug release and showed that drug release and polymer degradation occurred at equivalent rates with rates proportional to surface area, indicating that release from these crosslinked PPF matrices is controlled by surface erosion rather than by diffusion. Domb et al. (11) and Domb (12) investigated PPF/VP cements formulated with PPFs synthesized to specific molecular weights and with either carboxyl or hydroxyl end groups. The mechanical strength of the cement composites was found to be greater for those with carboxyl-terminated PPF chains than those with hydroxyl end groups, and also to increase with the degree of polymerization.

B. Objectives and Rationale

Incorporation of biologically active agents into materials which subsequently undergo in situ cure (hardening, polymerization) provides a means for ensuring continuous drug delivery at specific sites. Such materials have immediate orthopedic and periodontal applications.

These composite materials (the PPF/MMA and PPF/VP systems) undergo cure by a vinyl polymerization requiring the presence of monomer, accelerator, and initiator. The present system, a bone cement designed to be resorbable, uses the unsaturated polyester PPF and MMA as the monomer which via vinyl polymerization achieves cure by crosslinking to PPF. Benzoyl peroxide (BP) is the initiator and adjustment of the cure rate is provided by the accelerator DMPT. Other components (Tween-40 and water) are processing aids to improve viscosity and workability of the cement. Control of the release rate of the incorporated drug, in this case the antituberculosis drug isoniazid (isonicotinic acid hydrazide, or INH) is achieved by two methods: first, by incorporating the INH in a protecting envelope of poly(lactide-co-glycolide) 85:15 (PLGA 85:15 or, simply, PLGA), and second, by incorporating nonreactive fillers of varying solubility into the cement.

The versatility of such a cement depends on (a) the extent to which a variety of drugs may be incorporated without reaction of the drug with the free radicals generated in the cure reaction; (b) the ability to control release rates of the drug; and (c) the ability to control the rate of dissolution (resorption) of the cement.

We have approached these design problems as follows: The INH is absorbed into an open-celled PLGA foam previously prepared by lyophilization of solutions of PLGA. Aqueous solutions of INH are then forced into the void volume of the foam by cycles of evacuation and repressurization. The water is then removed by a second lyophilization, thus depositing INH microcrystals within the pores of the foam. The loading of INH depends only on the void volume (which in turn depends on the foam density) and on the concentration of drug in the impregnating solution. The fractional loading, F, is given by the equation

$$F = [1 + d_p d_f / C(d_p - d_f)]^{-1} \tag{1}$$

where d_p and d_f are the densities of the nonporous polymer and foamed polymer respectively, and C is the concentration of drug in the impregnating solution.

Following impregnation, the foam/drug composite is compacted under high pressure. The compressed disk or rod is then ground and sieved to isolate the 125- to 180-mm particle size range prior to incorporation into the cement.

By incorporating the drug into the PLGA, the drug has been protected from the reacting components of the cement and has been formulated as a controlled release system. Further modification of release rates is provided by the cement itself.

The highly compact INH/PLGA matrix particles are now ready for incorporation into the cement. In this form we speculated that the active agent, encapsulated in an envelope of PLGA, would be protected from the free radicals generated during the cure reaction. Reaction with the free radicals would be minimal because the cure time during which the cement changes from a viscous putty to a hard pellet is short (about 10 min). Reaction would occur only if the active agent diffused out of and/or radicals diffused into the INH/PLGA microparticle during cure. Evidence for this concept was derived from the kinetic plots of $F + (1 - F) \ln(1 - F)$ vs. t. For a well-behaved matrix system, these plots are linear with respect to time with a 0.0 intercept. If, on the other hand, active agent had to diffuse from the protecting PLGA envelope through the cement, then an induction period or lag time would be observed.

A second objective of this study was to evaluate the role of inert filler composition on both release of the INH and the rate of dissolution of the cured cement in water. Parameters of interest included both the filler solubility and the content of PLGA. PLGA served two functions: as a moderator of release by virtue of the INH and as a filler in the cement.

In summary, then, the major objectives of this study are to investigate the release profile of INH and the dissolution profile of the cement:

1. *Release Rate of INH:* The INH release rate is a function of INH loading and filler composition. Filler in this instance is defined as the combination of salts (calcium phosphate, calcium gluconate, calcium acetate) and PLGA in the cement. INH loading is defined in a dual sense: the weight percent INH in the PLGA and in the complete cement. INH release will be seen to depend on both loading and filler composition.
2. *Dissolution of the cement:* The dissolution of the cement depends on the rate of hydrolysis of the crosslinked PPF. This in turn depends on the entry of water into the cement. Entry of water is facilitated by dissolution of the soluble filler components.

II. EXPERIMENTAL

A. Materials

The following materials were purchased and used as received except as otherwise noted:

Material	Supplier	Catalog number	Lot number
Acetone, HPLC grad	Fisher Scientific	A949-4	943401
Methanol	Fisher Scientific	A452-4	945215
Tetrahydrofuran	Fisher Scientific		
Calcium phosphate, tribasic[a]	Aldrich Chem. Co.	23093-2	05304AF
Calcium acetate hydrate	Aldrich Chem. Co.	22763-3	01120KX
Calcium D-gluconate	Aldrich Chem. Co.	22764	05926EZ
Calcium propionate	Aldrich Chem. Co.	344451	04810KF
Benzoyl peroxide, 97%	Aldrich Chem. Co.	17998-1	06613KY
Methyl methracrylate, 99%	Aldrich Chem. Co.	M5590-9	03021BX

Material	Supplier	Catalog number	Lot number
Na dioctyl sulfosuccinate	Aldrich Chem. Co.	32358-6	03309PF
Tween-40[b]	Aldrich Chem. Co.	27435-6	05306JV
Isonicotinic acid hydrazide	Sigma Chem. Co.	I-3377	29F-0592
PLGA[c]	Boehringer-Ingelheim	640671	25054

[a]Hydroxyapatite.
[b]Polyoxyethylene (20) sorbitan monopalmitate.
[c]Poly(D,L-lactide-co-glycolide) 85:15 (lactide:glycolide wt. ratio = 85:15).

A sample of tribasic calcium phosphate was kindly sent by Dr. H. Ben-Bassat (Hadassah University Hospital, Jerusalem) for comparison with the purchased calcium phosphate. This sample, identified as HA-SAL1, was prepared by rapid precipitation from aqueous medium using microwave radiation. HA-SAL1 is a dense material having a Ca/P ratio of 1.55 (13). The nominal Ca/P ratio for the commercial hydroxy apatite is 1.67.

Isoniazid was used as received. Its melting range, 170.9–172.2°C, compared favorably with the reported melting point of 171.4°C (14).

B. PLGA Purification and Molecular Weight

PLGA was purified before use. PLGA solutions in acetone (50 mg/mL) were slowly added to at least a fivefold excess of methanol with continuous stirring. The fibrous precipitate was air-dried at room temperature for at least 2 days and then vacuum-dried at <1 mm Hg for at least 2 more days. The molecular weight distribution was determined by gel permeation chromatography (GPC) in a tetrahydrofuran mobile phase on a micro-Styragel 10^4-Å column by comparison with polystyrene standards. The weight average molecular weight (M_w) and polydispersity were respectively 107,790D and 1.02.

C. PPF Synthesis and Molecular Weight

PPF was synthesized by the direct esterification of fumaric acid with propylene glycol using p-toluenesulfonic acid as a catalyst by an adaptation of the procedure described by Sanderson (10) and reported by Gresser et al. (15). The molecular weight, determined by GPC, was 5364 with a dispersity of 1.013.

D. Preparation and Loading of PLGA Foam

PLGA foams were prepared by lyophilization (freeze drying) of polymer solution as previously described (22). The density of the resulting foam was 63.3 mg/cm^3.

The active agent, INH, was introduced into the foam via aqueous solutions of known concentration that were forced into the pores by a sequence of evacuation and pressurization cycles. The water was removed by a second lyophilization step, thus depositing microcrystals of INH in the pores. The final INH content depends only on the void volume (of which bulk density is a measure) and the concentration of the drug in the impregnating solution. The loading, f, as weight fraction of INH, is given by Eq. 1, where d_p and d_f are the densities of the nonporous and foamed polymer, respectively, and C is the concentration of INH in the impregnating solution.

Table 1 Nominal Composition of Standard Cement

Factor	wt. %
Part A:	
PPF	15[a]
Filler/PLGA-INH	42
Part B:	
Water	2
MMA/Tween 40/BP	32[b]
Part C:	
MMA/DMPT	9[c]

[a]PPF, poly(propylene fumarate), $M_w = 5364$ Da.
[b]A cosolution of methyl methacrylate (MMA), Tween-40, and benzoyl peroxide (BP) in a weight ratio of 82.7:10.8:6.5.
[c]A cosolution of N,N-dimethyl-p-toluidine in MMA in a weight ratio of 1.1:98.9.

E. Preparing the INH/PLGA Matrix for Incorporation into the Cement

Prior to incorporating the INH/PLGA composite into the cement, the porous matrix was compressed at 45°C and 10,000 psi (type MPC 40-ID-3 Compac hydraulic press) for approximately 16 h. The compressed matrix was then ground (Tekmar A10 mill) and sieved to retain the 125- to 180-μm size range. The highly compact INH/PLGA matrix particles were then ready for incorporation into the cement.

F. Blending Components of the Cement and Curing

The cement was prepared as a three-part formulation as shown in Table 1. Part A contained the PPF and fillers (the PLGA/INH matrix particles plus inert materials). Part B comprised the crosslinking agent (MMA), processing aids (water, Tween-40), and the initiator (BP). Part C contains the remaining MMA with accelerator (DMPT). As a three-part system, the components are stable when stored cold (−5°C). Although Part B contains both MMA and BP, no reaction was observed over a storage period of over a month.

    Parts A and B are mixed to a viscous putty-like consistency. Addition of Part C decreases the viscosity and allows rapid placement at the site of use. Cured pellets were prepared in Teflon-coated cylindrical molds (2.82 mm diameter by 9.7 mm length) at 37°C. Although pellets were removed after 24 h, cure is essentially complete in 10–20 min.

G. Cement Formulations

Eight variations of this formulation were prepared by varying the filler composition. Note that filler also includes the PLGA 85:15/INH matrix. Filler compositions are given in Table 2.

    Total filler content varied from 40.6% to 42.4% by weight. PLGA/INH filler was nominally either 10.5% or 21.0% with an INH content in the PLGA/INH of 8.9%, 18.9%, or 41.0%. The remainder of the filler consisted of combinations of insoluble calcium phosphate (either 0 or nominally 10%) and soluble filler (calcium acetate and/or calcium gluconate).

    Two hydroxyapatites were compared. Formulations 1, 2, and 3 incorporated a commercial tribasic calcium phosphate [hydroxyapatite $Ca_{10}(OH)_2(PO_4)_6$. The second HA, identified as HA-SAL1, was prepared by rapid precipitation from aqueous medium using microwave irradiation. This sample was received from Dr. H. Ben-Bassat of Hadassah University Hospital, Jerusalem (13).

Table 2 Filler composition, wt %.

Formulation	PLGA/INH[a]	INH in PLGA[b]	INH[c]	HA[d]	SAL. I[e]	CaGlu[f]	CaAc[g]	Total
1	10.5	8.9	0.9	11.0	—	10.4	10.5	42.4
2	10.4	18.9	2.0	10.4	—	10.4	10.5	41.7
3	10.5	41.0	4.3	10.4	—	10.5	10.5	41.9
4	10.1	18.9	1.9	—	10.2	10.2	10.1	40.6
5	20.8	18.9	3.9	—	—	10.5	10.5	41.8
6	20.8	18.9	3.9	—	—	20.7	—	41.5
7	21.0	18.9	3.9	—	10.5	10.5	—	42.0
8 (control)	21.0	0.0	0.0	—	—	21.0	—	42.0

[a]Total wt % PLGA 85:15/INH matrix in cement.
[b]wt % INH in the matrix.
[c]wt % INH in the cement = (a)(b).
[d]Hydroxyapatite.
[e]Experimental hydroxyapatite.
[f]Calcium gluconate.
[g]Calcium acetate.

H. In Vitro Release and INH Assay

In vitro release measurements were conducted in quintuplicate. Each pellet was immersed in 5 mL of distilled water held in 16 mm × 125 mm test tubes. Leaching was conducted at 37°C in a shaker bath (Precision Scientific) operated at 35 cycles/min. Distilled water was used as the leaching bath rather than phosphate-buffered saline (PBS) to prevent reaction of the calcium salts used as filler with the phosphate of the buffer.

INH was assayed by HPLC using a modification of conditions reported previously (16,17). Equipment consisted of Waters multisolvent dual pump 600/600E delivery system, 410 differential refractometer, 486 tunable UV-Vis absorbance detector, and 712 WISP autosampler. System operation was controlled by a Maxima 825 software program. Separations were performed on a C-18 column with a mobile phase consisting of 60% methanol/40% aqueous 0.01 M dioctyl sodium sulfosuccinate. The pH was adjusted to 3.0. A flow rate of 2.0 mL/min gave an INH retention time of 2.25 min.

I. Cement Dissolution Study

The role of filler in modifying the rate of release of INH is clearly demonstrated in Section III. With increasing filler solubility, increasing release rates were observed. The presence of soluble filler may also facilitate dissolution by allowing ingress of water to sites at which PPF hydrolysis occurs, i.e., at the ester linkages. The role of filler composition in promoting or retarding cement dissolution was examined by periodic measurement of weight loss.

The standard three-part formulation was again used in this study, but with the replacement of the PLGA-INH matrix with calcium salts of varying solubility. The standard formulation as used in this study is given in Table 3.

Fillers were either calcium phosphate (hydroxyapatite), calcium acetate, calcium propionate, or calcium gluconate. After mixing, the viscous cement was allowed to cure at 37°C in molds that produced cured pellets of nominally 12.3 × 5.7 mm, each weighing approximately 450 mg.

Dissolution studies were carried out at 37°C in distilled water rather than in PBS to avoid reaction of the soluble calcium salts with the phosphate of the buffer. Five pellets of each for-

Table 3 Standard Formulation for Grout Dissolution Studies

Factor	wt %
Part A:	
PPF	15.3 (M_w = 5364 Da)
Filler	42.3
Part B:	
Water	0.9
MMA/Tween40/BP	32.2 (wt. ratio = 82.7:10.8:6.5)
Part C:	
MMA/DMPT	9.3 (1.6% DMPT in MMA)

mulation were used. Pellets were withdrawn according to the schedule shown in Fig. 1. Bars indicate time in water after which they were dried to constant weight at 50°C and replaced in the bath. This schedule was maintained for 21 days and allowed us to make an increasing number of measurements at subsequent time points. Also by comparison of weight losses at a specific time, it was possible to assess the effect of drying on subsequent weight loss. Our data demonstrate that drying had no statistically significant effect on subsequent dissolution. Following this intensive 21-day study, all pellets were continued to day 118, during which interval they were periodically dried and weighed.

III. RESULTS AND DISCUSSION

A. *In Vitro* Release of INH from Cement Formulations

INH release has been treated by Roseman–Higuchi kinetics (18,19), which assumes a diffusion-controlled release mechanism. In a related investigation of INH release from PLGA matrices, we demonstrated the applicability of this analysis (20). Fractional release, F, as a function of time is given by

$$F + (1 - F)\ln(1 - F) = [4DC/ar^2]t = kt \quad (2)$$

where D = diffusivity of INH in the polymer
C = solubility of INH in the polymer
a = total initial content of INH in the matrix
r = rod diameter
k = combined rate constant, h^{-1}

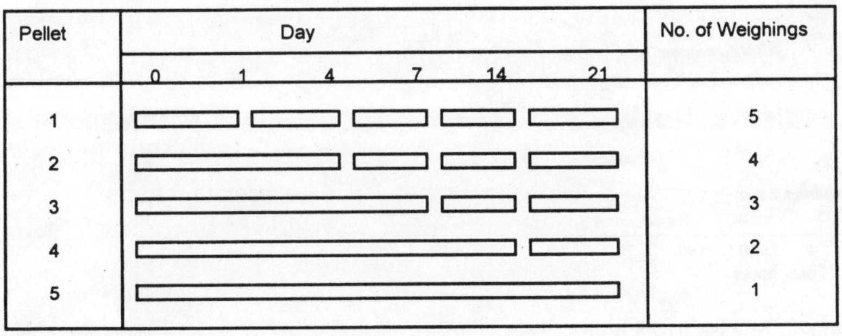

Figure 1 Schedule for drying and weighing.

Table 4 Rod Description, Early Time Combined Rate Constants, Intercepts, and Correlation Coefficients

Formulation	r, cm[a]	A, mg/cm^3[b]	[INH][c]	$k \times 10^{-3}$ h^{-1}[d,e]	Intercept $\times 10^{-3}$[d]	R[f]
1	0.264	8.9	0.94	0.86	−5.68	0.9456
2	0.263	18.9	1.97	0.99	−3.17	0.9893
3	0.261	41.0	4.31	2.74	−12.58	0.9879
4	0.268	18.9	1.91	0.63	−2.10	0.9915
5	0.264	18.9	3.93	9.04	−24.37	0.9943
6	0.267	18.9	3.93	5.76	−22.51	0.9608
7	0.263	18.9	3.97	3.82	−11.73	0.9966
8	—	—	—	—	—	—

[a]Rod diameter.
[b]Loading of INH in PLGA.
[c]Loading of INH in cement.
[d]Values to be multiplied by 10^{-3}.
[e]Early time rate constant.
[f]Correlation coefficient.

The effect of loading and filler composition on release was investigated by varying the filler/PLGA/INH composition in the standard formulation as given in Tables 1 and 2. Rod dimensions and loadings, as well as early time combined rate constants to 75 h as determined by linear regression of the Roseman–Higuchi plots, are given in Table 4. The kinetic plots are shown in Fig. 2. Release profiles, as percent cumulative release vs. time to 214 h, are shown in Fig. 3.

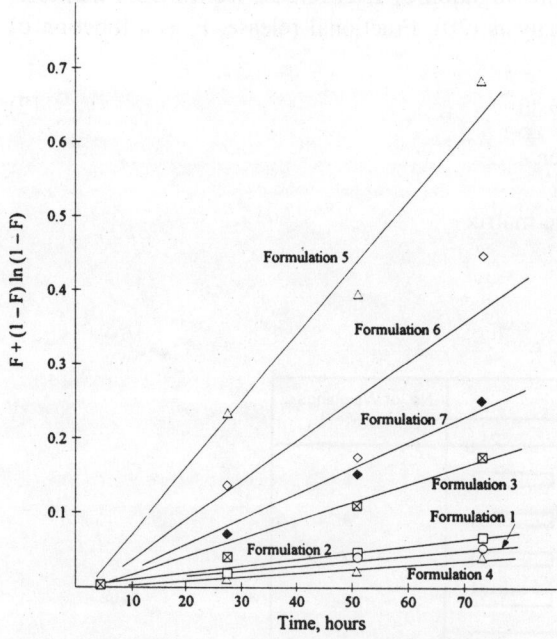

Figure 2 Kinetics of isoniazid release to 75 hours.

Incorporation of an Active Agent into a Biodegradable Cement

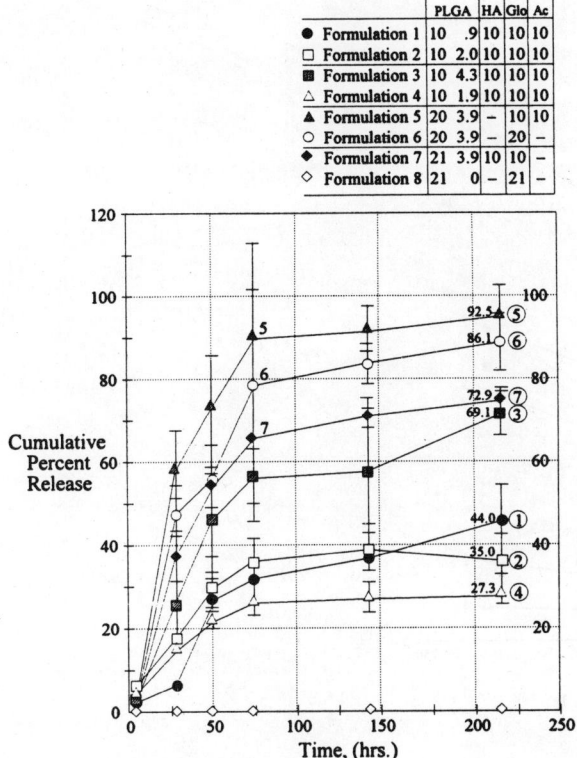

Figure 3 Cumulative percent release of isoniazid as a function of time.

Combined early time rate constants (k, h^{-1}) are given as the slopes of the plots of the release function [F + (1 − F)ln(1 − F)] vs time to 75 h as determined by linear regression analysis.

Diffusion coefficients were calculated from the slopes, which are defined in terms of parameters previously defined:

$$\text{slope} = k = 4CD/Ar^2 \tag{3}$$

Rod diameters and loadings are given in Table 3. We have taken loadings to be the initial quantity of INH in the PLGA. The solubility of INH was taken as to value in PLGA, 15 mg/cm^3. This is reasonable because initially there is no INH in the cement surrounding the PLGA particles.

Lag times, calculated from the linear regression of the release function vs. time as the ratio of intercept to slope, were used to calculate the mean diffusion path. Although the time lag equation was initially derived in 1920 and generalized by Barrer in 1939 (21), for treatment of membrane systems, we have assumed that the equation is applicable to a system in which drug-loaded particles are surrounded by a drug-free region. The time lag equation is given by

$$D = h^2/6\tau_\ell \tag{4}$$

where τ_l is the lag time and h may be interpreted as the equivalent membrane thickness or the mean length of the diffusion path.

The release profiles are given in Fig. 3 as percent cumulative release versus time. These data to 214 h are replotted in Fig. 4 as the release function F + (1 − F) ln(1 − F) vs. time. The

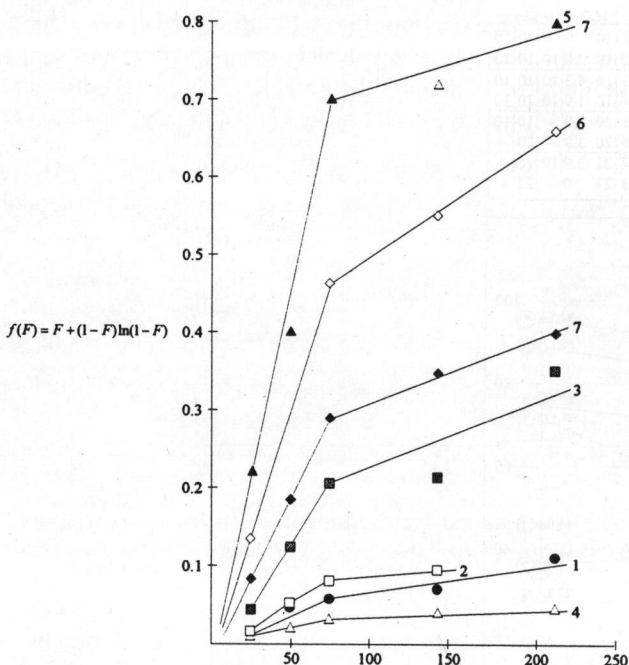

Figure 4 Kinetics of isoniazid release to 214 h.

release is seen to be biphasic with a sharp break in the slope at approximately 75 h. Early time (<75 h) rate constants and both early and late time (>75 h) diffusion coefficients are given in Table 5. Table 5 also includes calculated lag times and equivalent membrane thickness.

The first problem in interpreting these data is that the mean diffusion constant of INH from PLGA rods as reported by Hsu et al. (20) is 1.32×10^{-5} cm^2/h (3.67×10^{-9} cm^2/s), which is at the lower limit of the early time diffusion coefficients reported herein (0.90×10^{-5} cm^2/h). Hsu's work was done with intact extruded rods of 1.1–1.6 mm diameter. These rods were prepared by a dry-mixing technique in which micronized INH and ground PLGA (125–180 μm) powders were blended prior to extrusion. As expected, they observed no statistically significant dependence of the diffusion coefficient on rod diameter. However, the particulate INH/PLGA used in the present work for incorporation into the cement was prepared by low temperature grinding of INH/PLGA matrices.

Table 5 Release of INH from Matrix Particles Incorporated in Cement

Formulation	Diffusion constant, cm^2/h			lag time, h	Height, cm
	$k \times 10^{-3}$, h^{-1}	D (early)	D (late)		
1	0.86	0.899×10^{-5}	5.52×10^{-7}	6.605	1.89×10^{-2}
2	0.99	2.282×10^{-5}	2.03×10^{-9}	3.202	2.09×10^{-2}
3	2.74	13.377×10^{-5}	2.90×10^{-6}	4.591	6.07×10^{-2}
4	0.63	1.433×10^{-5}	1.26×10^{-8}	3.333	1.69×10^{-2}
5	9.04	40.953×10^{-5}	2.53×10^{-7}	2.696	8.15×10^{-2}
6	5.76	26.691×10^{-5}	1.28×10^{-6}	3.908	7.91×10^{-2}
7	3.82	17.175×10^{-5}	1.09×10^{-6}	3.071	5.62×10^{-2}

Recently, Hsu et al. investigated release of INH from injectable PLGA matrices. These matrices were prepared by incorporating the INH into a low-density open-celled PLGA foam prior to compaction, extrusion, and grinding. Approximating the irregularly shaped ground matrix particles as small cylinders allows a comparison of INH diffusion coefficients for PLGA matrices prepared by different techniques.

Method	D, cm^2/h	Ref.
Dry-mixed matrix, extruded rods	1.32×10^{-5}	Hsu et al. (20)
Injectable particles from extruded, ground foam	4.53×10^{-7}	Hsu et al. (22)
Present work	$1\text{--}40 \times 10^{-5}$	Nagaoka et al., this work
In water	21.0×10^{-3}	Baker and Lonsdale (23)

The approximate diffusion coefficient calculated for the injectable matrix prepared from compacted, foamed PLGA is about one-thirtieth that of the drug-mixed matrix rods. The particles incorporated into the cement (this work) were also prepared by incorporation into the PLGA foam. However, the calculated early time diffusion coefficients, ranging from approximately 1 40 $\times 10^{-5}$ cm^2/h, are 20–880 times larger than for the injectable particles. Why?

To answer this, it is instructive to compare the observed early time diffusion coefficients with that estimated for INH in water. Baker and Lonsdale (23) present diffusion coefficients in water for compounds ranging in molecular weight from 2.0 to almost 40,000 D. The relationship presented by them graphically is

$$\log D = -0.540 \log(\text{mol wt}) - 4.08 \tag{5}$$

This predicts a diffusion coefficient of

$$0.58 \times 10^{-5} \text{ cm}^2/\text{s} \ (21.0 \times 10^{-3} \text{ cm}^2/\text{h})$$

for a compound of molecular weight 137.2 (INH). Thus our early time values for diffusion through the cement are between those for diffusion of INH from PLGA particles (ground from rods prepared by extrusion of INH/PLGA foams) and for the estimated diffusion of INH in water.

These results are consistent with the following model.

- Incorporation of INH/PLGA matrix particles into a cement isolates the particles in a medium (the cement) devoid of INH.
- Upon entry of water into the cement and upon its further entry into the INH/PLGA particle, diffusion of INH begins, but it must traverse a drug-free zone prior to reaching the surface, which explains the observed lag times.
- However, diffusion is more rapid than from the PLGA alone. Apparently this is because on compounding the cement with MMA, the PLGA structure is partially dissolved by the MMA (PLGA is readily soluble in MMA). Thus, the observed early time diffusion coefficients are characteristic of INH passing through the porous cement, not through the PLGA.
- However, the Roseman–Higuchi plots show a biphasic pattern. Early time release is characterized by rapid diffusion through the cement but late time release is much slower with diffusion constants in the range $5.6\text{--}8.1 \times 10^{-10}$ cm^2/s. Note that in polystyrene the diffusion constant for INH is predicted to be $\approx 10^{-12}$ cm^2/s (23). This value may be compared with those of Hsu (manuscript in preparation) for INH in

PLGA injectable particles ($D = 1.26 \times 10^{-10}$ cm^2/s). Thus, Hsu's value is within the range observed by us for late time diffusion. We interpret this to mean that although the dissolution of INH/PLGA in the MMA allows some of the INH to be released into the cement during cure (and thus available for subsequent rapid release), a fraction is still protected by the PLGA. This fraction is probably given by the value of the abscissa at the breakpoint in the Roseman–Higuchi plots.

B. *In Vitro* Grout Dissolution

Table 6 presents weight loss and standard deviations for the 21-day study. These data are also displayed graphically in Fig. 5. The rate of weight loss increases in the order phosphate < gluconate < propionate < acetate. In this period the dissolution rates are given by the slopes of the linear regressions calculated from day 1 through day 21 (see Table 6). Choosing the phosphate cement as the arbitrary standard, the relative rates of dissolution in this interval are 1.0, 7.8, 13.3, and 19.3. Note that reported solubility data indicate that calcium acetate and propionate are water-soluble compounds; the gluconate has a limited solubility of 1 g/30 mL in cold water. The phosphate is quite insoluble.

Following day 21 measurements were continued periodically to day 118. Dissolution profiles to day 118 are displayed in Fig. 6. The slopes of the weight loss vs. time curve, giving the dissolution rates, are also given in Table 6.

Between days 21 and 118 the dissolution rate of the phosphate cement has decreased to a slow but constant 0.023% per day. The acetate cement in the interval day 35–118 is only slightly faster (0.049% per day), but by day 21 it has already lost about 45% of its initial weight, or virtually all of its filler. The slow dissolution probably reflects PPF hydrolysis and loss of hydrolysis products.

Between days 21 and 62 the propionate cement dissolution rate is about 0.33% per day. After day 62 the rate falls to 0.065% per day, i.e., only slightly faster than the late phase of the acetate cement. By day 62 the propionate cement has lost 50% of its weight, no doubt all of the filler plus some hydrolysis products.

The gluconate cement shows a constant dissolution rate of 0.11% per day following day 35. By day 118 it has lost only 33% of its original weight and thus is probably still in a rapid dissolution phase characterized by filler loss. Calcium gluconate is less soluble than the acetate and propionate, and thus it will be lost more slowly. The dissolution rate of the gluconate cement will probably reach a late slow phase also, when it has lost all of its filler.

Table 6 Summary of Percent Weight Loss as a Function of Time

Filler	Time, days					Linear regression	
	1	4	7	14	21	% day^{-1}	r
Phosphate	3.4	3.8 ± 0.4	3.9 ± 0.6	4.4 ± 0.6	5.1 ± 0.7	0.082	0.9893
Gluconate	6.5	10.0 ± 1.0	13.1 ± 1.8	16.2 ± 1.6	19.5 ± 2.3	0.62	0.9762
Propionate	11.0	19.4 ± 0.6	24.2 ± 4.2	30.3 ± 6.0	33.8 ± 8.8	1.06	0.9472
Acetate	16.2	21.5 ± 1.1	30.2 ± 2.5	40.6 ± 4.3	46.5 ± 7.3	1.54	0.9802

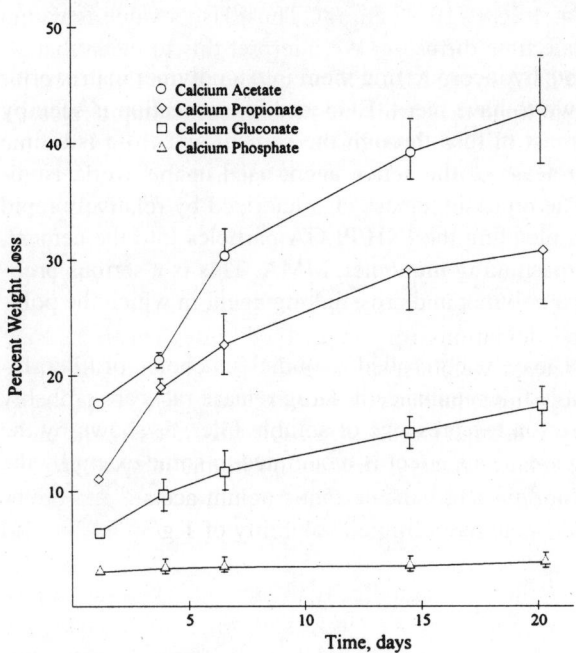

Figure 5 Cement dissolution to day 21.

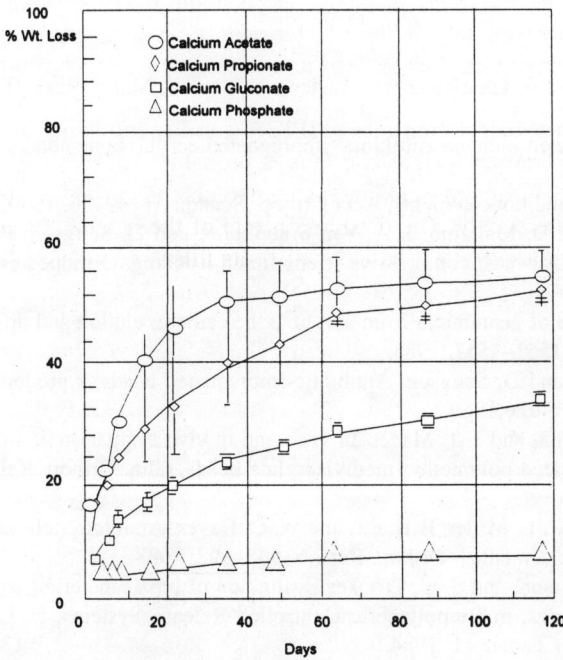

Figure 6 Cement dissolution to day 118.

IV. SUMMARY AND CONCLUSIONS

The concept of protecting labile active agents by incorporating them into a polymer matrix prior to blending the agent into a cement is shown to have merit. Evidence for protection is seen by (a) a lag time during which active agent must diffuse through the cement and (b) a late time diffusion constant more characteristic of release of the active agent used in this work, isoniazid, from PLGA than from the cement. The biphasic release characterized by relatively rapid release in the early phase suggests that on blending the INH/PLGA particles into the cement, some of the PLGA was dissolved in the crosslinking monomer, MMA. This is a serious problem which must be addressed by choosing a polymer and crosslinking agent in which the polymer is insoluble.

The rate of dissolution of the cement may be controlled by judicious choice of filler. Insoluble fillers retard dissolution; more soluble fillers enhance it. Drug release rates are probably more dependent on release from PLGA than on the presence of soluble filler, as shown by the late time portions of the release function curves. This effect is moderated to some extent by the presence of insoluble hydroxyapatite.

ACKNOWLEDGMENT

We thank the National Institutes of Health/National Institute of Allergy and Infectious Diseases (Grant No. 5 R01 AI27272-06 to D. L. Wise) and the National Institutes of Health/National Institute of Dental Research (Grant No. 5 R44 DE08880-03 to J.D. Gresser) for support of various aspects of this work.

REFERENCES

1. S. Saha and S. Pal. Mechanical properties of bone cement: a review, J. Biomed. Mater. Res., 18, 435–462, 1984.
2. K. E. Marks, C. L. Nelson, and E. P. Lautenschlager. Antibiotic-impregnated acrylic bone cement, J. Bone Joint Surg., 58-A, 358–364, 1976.
3. H. Walig and E. Dingeldein. Antibiotics and bone cements, Acta Orthop. Scand., 51, 49–56, 1980.
4. D. K. Kirkpatrick, L. S. Trachtenberg, P. D. Mangino, J. A. Von Fraunhofer, and D. Seligson. In vitro characteristics of tobramycin–PMMA beads: compressive strength and leaching, Orthopedics, 8, 1130–1133, 1985.
5. A. S. Baker and L. W. Greenham. Release of gentamicin from acrylic bone cement: elution and diffusion studies, J. Bone Joint Surg., 70-A 1551–1557, 1988.
6. S. L. Henry, G. J. Popham, P. Mangino, and D. Seligson. Antibiotic-impregnated beads, a production technique, Contemp. Orthop., 19, 221–226,1989.
7. K. Adams, L. Couch, G. Cierny, J. Calhoun, and J. T. Mader. In vitro and in vivo evaluation of antibiotic diffusion from antibiotic impregnated polymethyl-methylacrylate beads, Clin. Orthop. Rel. Res., 278, 244–252, 1992.
8. T. N. Gerhart, R. D. Roux, G. Horowitz, R. L. Miller, P. Hanff, and W. C. Hayes. Antibiotic release from an experimental biodegradable bone cement, J. Orthop. Res., 6, 585–592, 1988.
9. D. L. Wise, R. L. Wentworth, J. E. Sanderson, and S. C. Crooker Evaluation of repair materials for avulsive combat-type maxiollofacial injuries, in Biopolymeric Controlled Release Systems, D. L. Wise (Ed.), CRC Press, Boca Raton, FL, Chapter 11, 1984.
10. J. E. Sanderson. Bone replacement and repair putty material from unsaturated polyester resin and vinyl pyrrolidone, U.S. Patent 722,948 (1988).

11. A. J. Domb, C. T. Laurencin, O. Israeli, T. N. Gerhart, and R. Langer. The formation of propylene fumarate oligomers for use in bioerodible bone cement composites, J. Polym. Sci., A., 28, 973–985, 1990.
12. A. J. Domb. Poly(propylene glycol fumarate) compositions for biomedical applications, U.S. Patent 4,888,413, Dec. 19, 1989.
13. H. Ben-Bassat, B. Y. Klein, E. Lerner, R. Azoury, E. Rahamim, Z. Shlomai, and S. Sarig. An in vitro biocompatibility study of a new hydroxyapatite ceramic HA-SAL1: comparison to bioactive bone substitute ceramics, Cells Mater., 4, 37–50, 1994.
14. The Merck Index, 11th Ed., S. Budavari, (Ed.), Merck & Co., Inc., 1989.
15. J. D. Gresser, S.-H. Hsu, H. Nagaoka, C. M. Lyons, D. P. Nieratko, D. L. Wise, G. A. Barabino, and D. J. Trantolo. Analysis of a vinyl pyrrolidone/ poly(propylene fumarate) resorbable bone cement, J. Biomed. Mater. Res., 29, 1241–1249, 1995.
16. S. J. Saxena, J. T. Stewart, I. L. Honigberg, J. T. Washington, and G. R. Keene. Liquid chromatography in pharmaceutical analysis. 8. Determination of isoniazid and acetyl derivative in plasma and urine samples, J. Pharm. Sci., 66, 813–816, 1977.
17. J. T. Stewart, I. L. Honigberg, J. P. Brant, W. A. Murray, J. L. Webb, and J. B. Smith. Liquid chromatography in pharmaceutical analysis v: determination of an isoniazid-pyridoxine hydrochloride mixture, J. Pharm. Sci., 65, 1536–1539, 1976.
18. T. Higuchi. Mechanism of sustained release medication, J. Pharm. Sci., 52, 1145–1149, 1963.
19. T. J. Roseman. Release of steroids from a silicone polymer, J. Pharm. Sci., 61, 46–50, 1972.
20. Y.-Y. Hsu, J. D. Gresser, D. J. Trantolo, C. M. Lyons, P. R. J. Gangadharam, and D. L. Wise. In vitro controlled release of isoniazid from poly(lactide-co-glycolide) matrices, J. Contr. Rel., 31, 223–228, 1994.
21. R. M. Barrer. Permeation, diffusion and solution of gases in organic polymers, Trans. Farad. Soc., 35, 628–643, 1939.
22. Y.-Y. Hsu, J. D. Gresser, D. J. Trantolo, C. M. Lyons, P. R. J. Gangadharam, and D. L. Wise. Low density poly (dl-lactide-co-glycolide) foams for prolonged release of isoniazid, J. Contr. Rel., 40, 293–302, 1996.
23. R. W. Baker and H. K. Lonsdale. Controlled release: mechanism and rates, In: Controlled Release of Biologically Active Agents, A. C. Tanquary, R. E. Lacey (Eds.), p. 21, Plenum Press, New York, 1974.

42
The Pharmacoeconomic Value of Controlled Release Dosage Forms

L. B. Gardner
Paradigm Health Corporation, Concord, California

I. INTRODUCTION

Increasing awareness of the finite nature of health care resources and the competitiveness of the health care marketplace have resulted in closer scrutiny of costs and benefits of health care services by consumers and payers alike. Manufacturers and marketers of new pharmaceutical and medical technologies are now quite sensitive to the importance of assessing, documenting, and communicating the pharmacoeconomic "value" of their products or programs. Pharmacoeconomics is the study of the monetary and nonmonetary costs and benefits of pharmaceutical usage. Pharmacoeconomic value is inherent when a product produces actual cost savings as well as when a higher cost product is justified by its additional benefits.

Controlled release dosage forms have a significant potential to provide pharmacoeconomic value by producing greater clinical effectiveness and/or lower total treatment costs than existing alternatives. For example, zero-order delivery of a drug can produce greater clinical effectiveness by avoiding the subtherapeutic plasma concentrations that occur between doses of immediate release therapies. Zero-order delivery is often associated with a lower rate of side effects related to peak concentrations of drug in plasma. Recent innovations in drug delivery technology now also permit a variety of highly tailored controlled release drug delivery modalities, including site-specific delivery.

This chapter reviews basic pharmacoeconomic concepts and their application to the evaluation of controlled release dosage forms, discusses the mechanisms of the potential pharmacoeconomic benefits of controlled release dosage forms, summarizes selected recent publications reporting on pharmacoeconomic evaluations of controlled release products, and gives an overview of strategies for pharmacoeconomic assessment of new drug delivery modalities.

II. REVIEW OF BASIC PHARMACOECONOMIC CONCEPTS

An increasing emphasis on pharmacoeconomic value has challenged the health care industry to move beyond standard clinical trial studies that focus only on safety and efficacy. Although the Food and Drug Administration has not made pharmacoeconomic value a prerequisite for drug approval, acceptance of a new product by the marketplace now frequently depends on an evaluation of economic benefits and costs, and, often, quality-of-life effects as well.

Cost effectiveness depends on the relative effectiveness and relative cost of one alternative compared with others. A pharmaceutical product must demonstrate either a net cost savings or, if the product increases cost outlays, sufficient additional benefits (both economic and noneconomic) to justify the higher costs. Usually, a cost-effectiveness evaluation will compare a new product or health care program with an existing standard of care. Infrequently, a new product is developed that addresses a need not currently being met or a condition not currently being treated with any existing products. In this type of situation, the cost-effectiveness evaluation would compare the costs and benefits of the new technology with the costs and benefits of no treatment.

A pharmacoeconomic evaluation will focus either on direct costs alone, or on direct and indirect costs. With respect to evaluations of pharmaceutical products, direct medical costs include both the product acquisition charges (price paid by the payer) and any expenditures for medical care. Indirect costs include lost working days, decreased productivity, opportunity costs, and increased mortality. Even when the acquisition charges of one product are higher than those of another product, a reduction in the cost of associated medical care can result in lower total direct and/or indirect costs for the product with the higher price.

Examples of interventions that actually result in net cost savings are rare but do occur. (One example is screening programs for phenylketonuria.) More commonly, a novel intervention increases direct costs but also results in better outcomes. When improvements in indirect cost measures or quality of life occur, the results of effectiveness studies and quality-of-life assessments are included either by quantifying their dollar value or by being presented alongside the delineation of the cost savings or cost–effectiveness expected from use of the new product.

Economic assessments are meant to clarify the trade-offs between higher costs and greater benefits, or, occasionally, the degree to which costs are reduced when there are fewer benefits. Clearly, when a product costs more and produces fewer benefits, or costs less and produces more benefits, there is no need to perform a pharmacoeconomic evaluation (see Fig. 1).

The output of an analysis of costs and benefits is either a benefit–cost ratio or a cost–effectiveness ratio. When effectiveness is measured in terms of monetary savings, the analysis, although termed a "cost–benefit analysis," produces a ratio indicating the excess of incremental *savings* over incremental *costs*:

$$\frac{\Delta S}{\Delta C} = \frac{\text{TS new intervention} - \text{TS standard therapy}}{\text{C new intervention} - \text{C standard therapy}}$$

where TS is the total savings associated with either the new or the standard therapy, measured in monetary units, and C is the corresponding total costs.

When effectiveness is measured by nonmonetary benefits, such as in terms of increased life expectancy, the analysis is called a "cost–effectiveness analysis." Cost–effectiveness can be defined generically as:

$$\frac{\Delta C}{\Delta E} = \frac{\text{TC new intervention} - \text{TC standard therapy}}{\text{E new intervention} - \text{E standard therapy}}$$

where TC is the total health care costs associated with either the new or the standard therapy and E is the corresponding effectiveness measured in nonmonetary units. The result of a cost–effectiveness analysis is a delineation of the incremental *cost* per incremental unit of *effectiveness* associated with the new intervention, e.g., cost per year of life saved. If improvements in quality of life result without an increase in effectiveness, the cost–effectiveness analysis would simply report the amount and source(s) of the increases in cost along with a delineation of the associated improvements in quality of life.

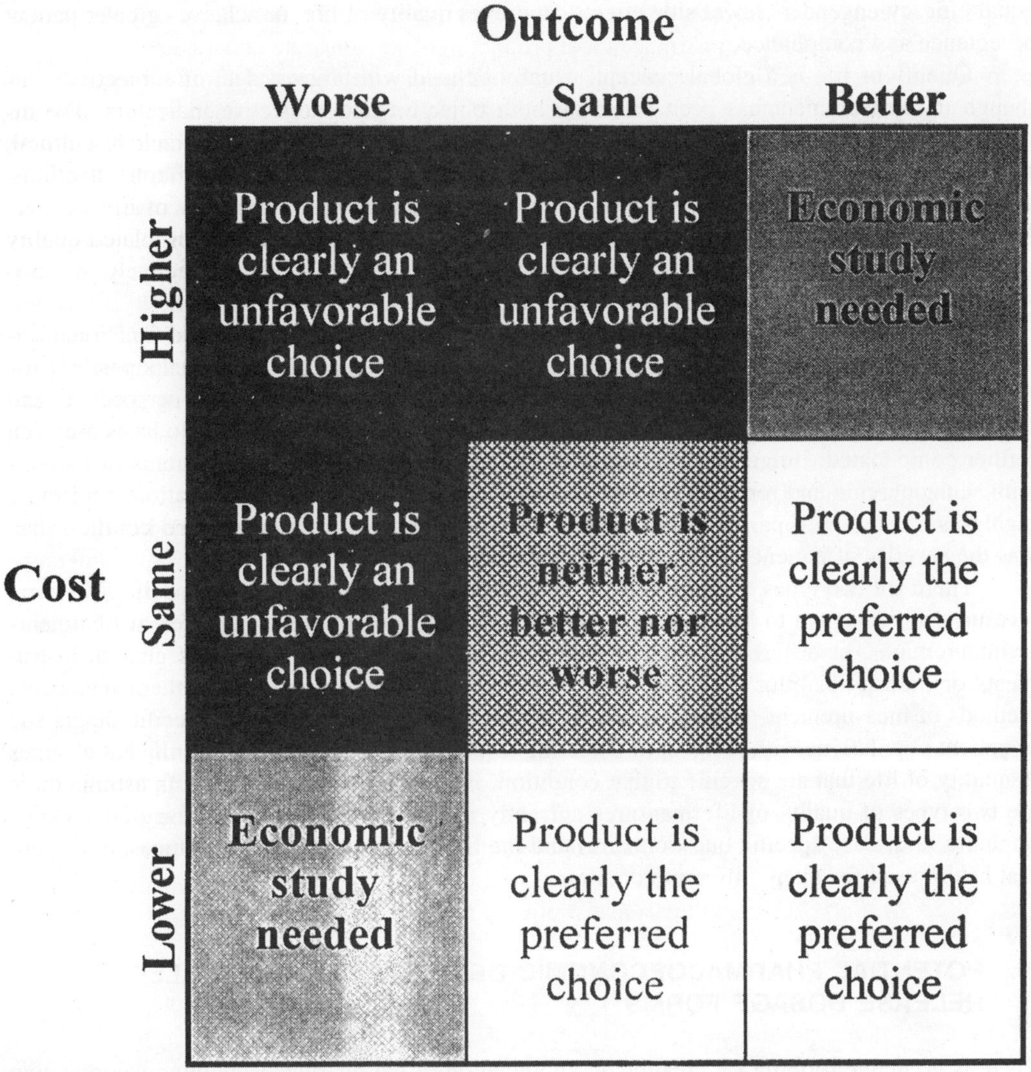

Pharmacoeconomics

	Outcome		
Cost	Worse	Same	Better
Higher	Product is clearly an unfavorable choice	Product is clearly an unfavorable choice	Economic study needed
Same	Product is clearly an unfavorable choice	Product is neither better nor worse	Product is clearly the preferred choice
Lower	Economic study needed	Product is clearly the preferred choice	Product is clearly the preferred choice

Figure 1 Cost/outcome map.

The following are factors that contribute to net cost–effectiveness:

Decreased product acquisition costs
Decreased costs of administering the product
Greater clinical effectiveness
Decreased frequency or costs of patient treatment or monitoring (including physician office visits)
Fewer adverse experiences requiring treatment

In drug development, a product that is efficacious (producing the desired results under controlled conditions among selected patient groups) is not always effective (producing the desired results in general usage under noncontrolled conditions). Greater clinical effectiveness *can* result from greater efficacy. Greater clinical effectiveness can also result when a product with equal efficacy engenders fewer side effects, improves quality of life, or achieves greater patient acceptance and compliance.

Quality of life is a global concept, usually defined with a great deal of subjectivity, although its measurement has been based on both objective and subjective indicators. The dimensions of quality of life span the full spectrum of human experience and include cultural, physical, psychological, spiritual, and social factors as well as fulfillment of role functions. These specific components of quality of life are known as "domains." Quality of life as it relates to specific medical conditions or treatments is often referred to as "health-related quality of life." It is important to note that quality of life can only be measured prospectively. A retrospective analysis will be unable to assess quality of life.

Quality of life is interrelated with and dependent on both health status and functional status. Subjective assessment of quality of life may be influenced by an individual's past experience, current health status, current pharmacoeconomic situation, expectations, perspective, and the context in which the assessment is conducted. Conditions with a psychiatric basis are even further complicated. Bulger (1993) evaluated the caregiving experiences of parents of patients with schizophrenia and reported that the parents' levels of burden and gratification were more highly associated with parent–child relationships, as measured by intimacy and conflict, than was the severity of patients' schizophrenic symptoms.

There are two types of quality-of-life measures: "general" and "disease-specific." General measures are designed to be used across a spectrum of different diseases, different treatments or interventions, or different groups of patients. The reliability and validity of general instruments or procedures, plus their extensive experience in empirical use, make them invaluable methods of measurement. Disease-specific measures are designed to assess specific diagnostic or patient populations with the goal of detecting responsiveness or clinically significant changes in quality of life that are specific to that condition. For example, for patients with asthma there are two types of quality-of-life measures currently in use: the St. George's Respiratory Questionnaire (a disease-specific questionnaire) and the Sickness Impact Profile (a measure of general health used for many different conditions).

III. POTENTIAL PHARMACOECONOMIC BENEFITS OF CONTROLLED RELEASE DOSAGE FORMS

There is no magic formula for creating an appreciation of net pharmacoeconomic value among clinicians, health care administrators, or payers. Claims for cost savings, cost–effectiveness, or a favorable benefit–cost ratio all need to be substantiated by credible scientific research and then clearly communicated to key audiences. Over the life of the product, initial claims for pharmacoeconomic value are reevaluated in the context of the accumulated experience of the product under actual conditions of use.

It has been known for many years that use of controlled release dosage forms can influence the costs and benefits of treatment compared with the same chemical entity in a non–controlled release dosage form (Arnold and Kaniecki, 1993). In most cases, both the price and the benefits of a controlled release product are higher than its non–controlled release counterpart. Many disease conditions respond better to zero-order delivery of a drug due to the absence of the subtherapeutic plasma concentrations that result from pulsed delivery of immediate release dosage forms. Hilleman et al. (1993) reported that only 78% of patients whose blood pressure was well controlled on long-acting nifedipine achieved control or tolerated therapy after being switched to an immediate release nifedipine dosage form.

Zero-order delivery can be associated with a lower rate of side effects in addition to potentially greater efficacy. Side effects often are related to peak concentrations of drug in plasma. To maintain adequate therapeutic levels when plasma concentrations decrease between dosing intervals, intermittently delivered products must often be consumed at very high doses (Zannad, 1995). In contrast, zero-order delivery avoids the "peak-and-trough" effect of intermittent delivery, often permitting less overall drug consumption.

However, the advantages of controlled release dosage forms are not limited to the ability to produce a zero-order delivery profile. Newer technologies can tailor drug delivery profiles to fit practically any therapeutic need, including delivery in circadian or pulsed patterns, delayed delivery, patient-controlled delivery, and site-specific delivery.

Another major potential benefit of controlled release dosage forms is improved patient compliance. Understanding of issues related to patient compliance has increased in recent years as drug dosing monitoring technology has improved the ability to detect noncompliance (Urquhart, 1996). Patient compliance is facilitated when there are fewer side effects or when dosing regimens can be simplified. The pharmacoeconomic benefit of greater compliance is clear in situations where inadequate compliance is the predominant cause of adverse effects. The adverse effects associated with reduced compliance might include lower cure rates or longer time to cure, increased medical care costs, decreased quality of life, or even the possibility that over time subtherapeutic plasma drug levels will promote the development of drug resistance.

IV. SUMMARY OF SELECTED PUBLICATIONS

A related article that was the predecessor of this chapter reviewed the existing literature on the pharmacoeconomic value of controlled release dosage forms (Saks and Gardner, 1997). That review summarized the results of a number of studies in selected therapeutic areas including cardiovascular therapy and pain management. Included were reports comparing sustained release and immediate release preparations (Skaer et al., 1993a, b), which showed that patients for whom a sustained release formulation of diltiazem was prescribed achieved a significant increase in compliance and a significant decrease in aggregate health care expenditures, compared with patients for whom an immediate release formulation was prescribed; and a report by Goughnour and associates (1991) comparing the acquisition, preparation, and administration costs of morphine sulfate extended release tablets (MS Contin) and morphine sulfate solution, which showed that although the acquisition cost of extended release tablets was considerably higher than that of morphine solution, the total daily cost of therapy with tablets was less than half that of therapy with solution. With respect to quality of life, review of a study of short-acting vs. controlled release products for cancer pain (Ferrell et al., 1989) revealed that controlled release analgesia achieved overall improved pain management.

A review of additional, more recent literature (Peters and Benfield, 1995; Glazer, 1996; Payne, 1998) supports the overall conclusion that controlled release products can result in greater effectiveness, equal or better safety and side effect profiles, greater patient acceptance, lower total direct treatment costs, and potentially decreased morbidity and mortality. Peters and Benfield (1995) reported that a controlled release antihypertensive was associated with a favorable effect on mortality and quality of life, and was more cost-effective than an alternative product with a lower price. Glazer (1996) reported that an extended release form of antipsychotic reduced total direct treatment costs among patients with a history of relapse and rehospitalization, using reasonable assumptions about prices, compliance, and rehospitalization rates. Payne

(1998) reported that use of controlled release analgesia resulted in lower costs, greater effectiveness, equal or better safety and side effect profiles, and greater patient acceptance.

V. OVERVIEW OF STRATEGIES FOR PHARMACOECONOMIC ASSESSMENT

Pharmacoeconomic research performed in conjunction with phase IIB or phase III clinical studies can facilitate timely and efficient assessment of the pharmacoeconomic value of a new drug product. If the pharmacoeconomic assessment is incorporated into the pivotal clinical studies, the investigators can capitalize on the rigor of the clinical study design, including the use of randomization and blinding. Pharmacoeconomic measures incorporated into the pivotal clinical studies entail much lower cost than a standalone pharmacoeconomic study.

However, incorporating the pharmacoeconomic assessment into the clinical study has a number of disadvantages. Clinical endpoints require much smaller sample sizes than do economic endpoints because clinical endpoints generally display much less inherent variability than do economic or social endpoints. Efficacy and safety trials often utilize a placebo comparator, but to establish pharmacoeconomic value the alternative used for comparison must be an existing standard of care rather than placebo. Finally, clinical study protocols usually require extensive diagnostic testing, a strict monitoring schedule, and other use of health care services that would not be performed in usual-care situations. Protocol-required expenses such as these are termed "protocol-induced demand" and clearly interfere with the assessment of pharmacoeconomic value. Frequently, invasive diagnostics or frequent recall visits will impinge on quality-of-life endpoints as well. For these reasons, evaluations of pharmacoeconomic value are best performed either as standalone studies during phase III or as part of more "naturalistic," postmarketing studies conducted after launch. Furthermore, when the pharmacoeconomic savings related to use of a product are expected to derive from better compliance leading to improved effectiveness, the data clearly are best collected as part of a standalone, naturalistic, postmarketing study that permits a degree of variation in compliance that ordinarily is not permitted during clinical trials.

It is important to understand the quality-of-life issues that arise in a usual-care setting. However, it is often still useful to pilot-test pharmacoeconomic data collection protocols during the clinical studies. The results, while not highly generalizable to usual-care conditions, can nevertheless inform the power calculations and help in developing the protocol for the standalone study. The results obtained from the phase III studies are very useful in planning the phase IV and postmarketing studies.

VI. CONCLUSION

Many, if not most, products come to market without a single well-controlled pharmacoeconomic study, let alone the two recommended by the March 1995 draft, "Principles for the Review of Pharmacoeconomic Promotion," circulated by the FDA. The initial perception of product value among key audiences is, therefore, typically driven solely by product price. The way to avoid obstacles to provider, payer, or formulary acceptance of a new product, especially one with a higher price than its counterparts, is to communicate, prior to and at the time of launch, the pharmacoeconomic value of the product along with its safety and efficacy.

Communicating the pharmacoeconomic value of a new medical technology before and during the initial product launch becomes a complex problem that must take into consideration many factors, including the following:

The lack of direct, "real-world" evidence of product costs and benefits
The natural skepticism of hospital, health care plan, and program administrators to manufacturers' cost–effectiveness claims
FDA guidelines on the promotion of pharmacoeconomic claims

In conclusion, Kranich et al. (1995) noted that an "a priori definition of the desired outcome of a medical intervention is of paramount importance for the evaluation of the actual treatment result." This statement can be translated into three guiding principles of pharmacoeconomics:

1. Cost–effectiveness depends on clinical effectiveness. If a product is not clinically effective, it can not be cost-effective, no matter how inexpensive or well tolerated by patients.
2. Cost–effectiveness is a relative phenomenon. It is assessed by comparing the incremental costs and benefits of one product or intervention with those of the next best alternative. Cost–effectiveness is not an absolute quality possessed by a product and cannot be assessed without reference to another alternative.
3. Economic evaluations can quantify cost savings or incremental benefits received for incremental costs, but not whether these benefits are worth the costs associated. Only the audience for whom the evaluation is being performed can make a determination as to value.

Preparing for and answering challenges about the pharmacoeconomic value of new medical technologies needs to be an ongoing process, one that starts by considering pharmacoeconomic factors during early evaluations of promising compounds and continues through pricing deliberations and the clinical trial program. Clinical studies of controlled release products should incorporate pilot testing of pharmacoeconomic data collection and the feasibility of assessing economic and quality-of-life endpoints. Ultimately, the process of establishing the pharmacoeconomic value of controlled release products will likely prove to be a good investment throughout the market life of these products.

REFERENCES

Arnold R. J. G. and Kaniecki, D. J. Selection of oral controlled-release drugs: a critical decision for the physician. South. Med. J. 1993, 86(2):208–214.
Bulger M. W., Wandersman A., Goldman C.R. Burdens and gratifications of caregiving: appraisal of parental care of adults with schizophrenia. Am. J. Orthopsychiatry 1993, 63(2):255–265.
Cole P. Pharmacologic and clinical comparison of cefaclor in immediate-release capsule and extended-release tablet forms. Clin. Ther. 1997, 19(4): 617–624.
Ferrell B., Wisdom C., Wenzl C., Brown J. Effects of controlled-released morphine on quality of life for cancer pain. Oncol. Nursing Forum 1989, 16(4):521–526.
Goughnour B. R., Arkinstall W. W. Potential cost-avoidance with oral extended-release morphine sulfate tablets versus morphine sulfate solution. Am. J. Hosp. Pharm. 1991, 48(1): 101–104.
Hilleman D. E., Mohiuddin S. M., Lucas B. D. Jr., Shinn B., Elsasser G. N. Conversion from sustained-release to immediate-release calcium entry blockers: outcome in patients with mild-to-moderate hypertension. Clin. Ther. 1993, 15(6):1002–1010.

Payne R. Factors influencing quality of life in cancer patients: the role of transdermal fentanyl in the management of pain. Semin. Oncol. 1998, 25(3 Suppl 7):47–53.

Peters D. H. and Benfield P. Metoprolol: a pharmacoeconomic and quality-of-life evaluation of its use in hypertension, post-myocardial infarction and dilated cardiomyopathy. Pharmacoeconomics 1995, 6(4):370–400.

Prisant L. M., Bottini B., DiPiro J. T., Carr A. A. Novel drug-delivery systems for hypertension. Am. J. Med. 1992, 93(Suppl 2A):45S–55S.

Saks S. R. and Gardner L. B. The pharmacoeconomic value of controlled-release dosage forms. J. Controlled Release 1997, 48:237–242.

Skaer T. L., Sclar D. A., Markowski D. J., Won J. K. Utility of a sustained-release formulation for antihypertensive therapy. J. Hum. Hypertens. 1993a, 7(5):519–522.

Skaer T. L., Sclar D. A., Robison L. M., Markowski D. J., Won J. K. Effect of pharmaceutical formulation for diltiazem on health care expenditures for hypertension. Clin. Ther. 1993b, 15(5):905–911.

Urquhart J. Patient compliance with crucial drug regimens: implications for prostate cancer. Eur. Urol. 1996, 29(Suppl 2):124–131.

Zannad F. Practical relevance of the 24-hour trough:peak ratio of antihypertensive drugs. J. Hypertens. 1995, 13(Suppl 2): S109–S112

Index

Absorption, extent of, 488–490, 515–516, 558–559
   improved enternal absorbtion of peptide drugs, 515–516
   locating absorption sites, 558–559
Acoustic streaming, of ultrasound transdermal drug delivery, 610
Accurate models (*see* Models, accurate, in controlled drug delivery systems)
Acrylate
   development of polymer networks, 47–64 (*see also* Photopolymerization technology)
Activation parameters, 695–698
Actual drug content, 400
Adhesives, 450–451, 559–560
   potential sites for adhesion or lodging, 559–560
Adsorbants, 278, 282
Agarose nanoparticles, 420–423 (*see also* Polysaccharide nanoparticles as novel drug carrier systems; Nanoparticulate controlled release systems for cancer therapy; Nanosuspensions; Solid lipid nanoparticles)
Air-suspension coating, 444–445 (*see also* Nanosuspensions)
Alginate nanoparticles, 414–417 (*see also* Polysaccharide nanoparticles as novel drug carrier systems; Nanoparticulate controlled release systems for cancer therapy; Nanosuspensions; Solid lipid nanoparticles)
α-interferon, 248–249
Alzet pumps, 230–239
   applications, 234–239
      antisense oligonucleotides, 235
      interleukins, 237–238
      nerve growth factor (NGF), 235
      octreotide, 238–239
   formulation parameters, 232–233
   implantation, 233–234
   system configurations, 230–232
   system design, 230

Analgesics, 789, 840
   narcotic, 789
Analysis of drug release, 193–194
Anesthetics, local, 793–794
Animal models, 477–478, 601–602, 778–783, 813, 815, 839–840, 844
Anionic gels, 70
ANN, optimization based on, 590–593
Anomalous transport, 184
Antibodies, 73, 278
   interactions, systems utilizing, 73
Antisense oligonucleotides, 235
Applications
   α-interferon, 248–249
   adsorbants, 282
   analgesics, 313
   antisense oligonucleotides, 235
   artificial cells, 281
   antibiotics, 310–311
   anticancerogens, 313
   antiepileptic drugs, 312–313
   antihypertensives, 313
   anti-inflammatory drugs, 311
   artificial cells, 281
   bronchodilators, 311–312
   converting liquids to free-flowing powders, 314
   dermis regeneration, 737–738
   diuretics, 312
   in drug delivery, 58–59, 92–95, 386–388, 541–544
   electrolyte replenishers, 314
   enzymes, 280
   factor IX, 249
   hormones and antibodies, 282
   to hydrogels, 136–137, 145–146
      infrared, 136–137
      Raman, 145–146
   ischemic myocardium, 735
   interleukins, 237–238, 743–750
   leuprolide implants, 243–246
   metal salts, 314
   nerve growth factor (NGF), 235
   octreotides, 238–239

[Applications]
  oily liquids, 281
  pain management, 787–803
  pharmaceuticals, 281
  pigments, 282
  polyelectrolytes, 281–282
  proteins, 280–281
  salmon calcitonin, 246–248
  sedative hypnotics, 314
  sulfa drugs, 312
  tissue engineering, 736–737
  tranquilizers, 313
  urinary antiseptics, 312
  vitamins, 314
Arginase, 280
Artificial cells, 281
Artificial neural networks for optimizing transdermal drug delivery systems, 583–593 (*see also* Transdermal drug delivery systems)
  multiobjective optimization, 586–587
  network structure, 584–586
  optimization based on ANN, 590–593
  promoting activity of MET, 587–589
  single-objective optimization, 586
Asparaginase, 280
Asymmetrical membrane properties, 755–757 (*see also* Osmotic systems)

Backing materials, 451
Balloon devices, 213
Barrier control, 562–563
Bead diameter, effect on performance, 773–778
β-fibroblast growth factor (bFGF), 729–736 (*see also* Growth factor release to induce neovascularization)
  in vitro release of, 729–730
Binding, 76–78, 853
  competitive, 76–78
  components, 853
Bioadhesive controlled release systems, 255–269, 458–459
  experimental techniques, 263–265
  interaction mechanisms, 258–259
  molecular modeling, 261–263
  mucin, structure and physiology of, 256–258
  mucoadhesive, 255–256
  recent developments, 265–266
  theories of, 259–261
Bioadhesive liposomal systems, 510–516
  improved enternal absorbtion of peptide drugs, 515–516
  mucoadhesive tests for partiuclate systems, 512–515

[Bioadhesive liposomal systems]
  polymer-coated liposomes, 511–512
Bioadhesive polymeric microparticulate systems, 516–523
  microsperes, 517–519
  mucoadhesive lactide/glycolide copolymer nanospheres, 519–523
Bioavailability, 347
Biocompatibility issues, 31–32
Biodegradable microparticles, characterization of, 113–119
Biodegradable polymers, 330–331, 728, 732–735 (*see also* Hydrogels; Nestorone)
  lactic/glycolic acid polymers, 330–331
  neovascularization induced by biodegradable hydrogels, 732–735
  preparation of biodegradable hydrogels, 728
Bioequivalence study, supporting waiver of, 542
Bioerodible implant materials and methods, 813–814
Biological drug delivery, 746–747
Biopolymers for release of interleukin-2 for treatment of cancer, 743–750 (*see also* Cancer therapy; Nanoparticulate controlled release systems for cancer therapy; Tumor models)
  background and significance, 744–745
  on controlled release, 745–750
    biological drug delivery, 746–747
    molecular drug delivery, 746
    pilot studies with IL-2/PLGA, 747–750
Biovectors, supramolecular, 423–425
Blood collection, 814, 815, 840–841
Bovine fibrinogen, 280
Bovine serum albumin (BSA), 67, 281, 402–407
  mechanisms of instability of bovine serum albumin, 402–407
    characterization of the denatured state, 402–404
    hypothesis for the mechanism of inactivation, 405–406
    kinetics of release and aggregation of, 402
    matching denatured states of, 404–405
    simulations of stresses, 404
    stabilization by neutralization of the acidic microclimate pH, 406–407
Buprenorphine microspheres for parenteral administration, 821–836
  discussion, 831–834
  methods, 823–824
    appearance and morphology, 824
    content of microspheres, 824
    determination of ^{3}H-buprenorphine, 824

Index

[Buprenorphine microspheres for parenteral administration]
    by HPLC procedures, 824
    particle size, 824
    preparation of, 823
    release, 824
  results, 825–831
Burkitt's lymphoma, 294

Calcium channel blocker (CCB), 433
Camptothecins, mechanisms of stabilization of, 394–402
  in PLGA microspheres, 394–395
  potential mechanisms, 395–402
Cancer therapy, 287–299, 743–750 (*see also* Biopolymers for release of interleukin-2 for treatment of cancer; Nanoparticulate controlled release systems for cancer therapy; Tumor models)
Canine model, in vivo study, 219–221
Carboxymethylcellulose (CMC), 140–141
Carcinoembryonic antigen (CEA), 297
Catalase, 280
Cavitational effects, of ultrasound transdermal drug delivery, 610–611
Cellulose derivatives as drug delivery carriers, 1–30 (*see also* Hydrophillic cellulose derivatives as drug delivery carriers)
Cement, 853, 854–855
  formulations, 853
  dissolution study, 854–855
Cetyltrimethylammonium bromide (CTAB), 294–295
Chain scission, 702–704
Charge couple devices (CCDs), 131, 144–145
Chelation, systems utilizing, 74
Chemical degradation reactions, 699–707
  chiral scission, 702–704
  deamidation, 700–702
  implications for controlled release, 707
  Maillard reaction, 704
  oxidation, 699–700
  thiol-disulfide exchange, 704–706
Chemical enhancement, and transdermal transport, 612–613
Chemically controlled systems, 173–174
Chemically crosslinked devices, 33–35
Chitosan nanoparticles, 417–420, 514, 520 (*see also* Polysaccharide nanoparticles as novel drug carrier systems; Nanoparticulate controlled release systems for cancer therapy; Nanosuspensions; Solid lipid nanoparticles)

[Chitosan nanoparticles]
  emulsification-based method, 419–420
  and polyanions, 418–420
Chloride ion management with silver anodes, 624
  (*see also* Electrodes)
Chymotripsin, 280
Circuit assembly, 638–639
  control circuitry requirements, 638–639
Coacervation separation methods, 301–328
  aqueous phase, 306–308
  organic phase, 308–309
Coatings, 444, 473, 760–769
  composition, 760–761
  dip, 763
  formulation and variables, 767–769
  pan, 444
  processes, 762
  spray, 767
  spray drying, 763–767
  technologies, 473
Codeine, 792
Colloidal drug delivery, 388, 555 (*see also* Drug delivery carriers)
  colloids and fine suspensions, 555
Colonic diversity, temporal control and, 561–562
Colonic transit, 483–484
Competitive binding, 76–78
Complexation
  between poly(methacrylic acid)/poly(ethylene glycol), 90–92
  in linear polymers, 90–91
  in polymer networks, 92
Complexing polymers in drug delivery, 89–98
  applications in drug delivery, 92–95
  complexation between poly(methacrylic acid)/poly(ethylene glycol), 90–92
  complexation in linear polymers, 90–91
  complexation in polymer networks, 92
  introduction, 89–90
Compression coating, 445
Concentration-dependent diffusion coefficients, 157–158
  effect of polymer morphology, 158
  thermodynamic considerations, 158
Controlled release devices and systems, 159–174, 431–463, 661–692 (*see also* Drug delivery carriers; Gamma scintigraphy and controlled release systems)
  chemically controlled systems, 173–174
  diffusion-controlled systems, 159–168
  drug delivery technologies, 1–46, 164–165, 175–177, 432–433, 541–542, 854–855, 860–861
  commercialized, 433

[Controlled release devices and systems]
    in development, 433–434
    intravenous, 432–433
    synthetic vs. natural polymers, 434
    tablets, 432
    toxicological considerations, 434–435
  implantable drug delivery systems, 452–457
    designs, 453–454
    fabrication, 456
    issues and opportunities, 456–457
    materials of use, 456
    polymer requirements, 455
    toxicological considerations, 454–455
  micro- and nanoparticle delivery, 287–299, 457–461
    injectable depot formulations, 459–460
    issues and opportunities, 460–461
    musocosal delivery, 458–459
  oral drug delivery systems, 435–445, 465–503, 505–525, 751–752, 794
    designs, 435–440
    fabrication techniques, 442–445
    functions of polymers, 441–442
    toxicological considerations, 440–441
  overview, 431–463
  protein therapeutics, 661–692
    stabilization during release, 676–683
    stabilization toward encapsulation, 663–674
    stabilization toward storage, 674–676
  swelling-controlled systems, 168–173
  transdermal drug delivery systems, 445–452, 567–581, 597–605, 617–659, 795
    delivery profiles and performance, 447–448
    designs, 445–447
    fabrication, 451–452
    issues and opportunities, 452
    polymer requirements, 449–451
    toxicological considerations, 447
Convolution and deconvolution, 529–532
Copolymers
  of PLA, PLAGA, and other materials, 119–120
  with ε-caprolactone, 120
  with poly(ethylene glycol) and poly(ethylene oxide), 119–120
Crosslinking
  by irradiation, 35
  using a freeze-thaw technique, 35–36
Crystal dissolution-controlled release systems, 38–39

Deamidation, 700–702
Degradation mechanisms, 102–105
  effect of ionic drugs, 104
  polymerization initiator, 105

Degradation reactions in specific polymers, 713–719
  dextrans and other polysaccharides, 715–716
  implications for controlled release, 719
  lactide/glycolide polymers, 713–715
  other polymers, 718–719
  vinyl polymers, 716–718
Dehydration, 671
Delivery technologies, 432–433 (*see also* Drug delivery carriers)
  commercialized, 433
  in development, 433–434
  intravenous, 432–433
  synthetic vs. natural polymers, 434
  tablets, 432
  toxicological considerations, 434–435
Denatured states, characterization of bovine serum ablumin, 402–404
Deposition and dispersion of formulations, 555–563
  barrier control, 562–563
  complex pharmacokinetics, 560
  locating absorption sites, 558–559
  potential sites for adhesion or lodging, 559–560
  resolving site of release and transit parameters, 557–558
  temporal control and colonic diversity, 561–562
Dermis regeneration, 737–738
Design
  of implantable drug delivery systems, 453–454
  of oral drug delivery systems, 435–440
  of transdermal drug delivery systems, 445–447, 634–644
    circuit assembly, 639
    control circuitry requirements, 638–639
    electronic components, 636
    E-TRANS lidocaine, 640–644
    power for portable designs, 636–638
    requirements, 634–636
    single-use vs. reusable designs, 639–640
Development of acrylate and methacrylate polymer networks, 47–64 (*see also* Photopolymerization technology)
Devices, heat-treated, 36–37
Dextrans and other polysaccharides, 715–716
Differential scanning calorimetry (DSC), 114–116
Diffusional effects during polymerization, 49–50, 441–442
Diffusion-controlled systems, 159–168, 436
Dimensionless parameters, 185–186
Dispersed drug, nonporous systems, 159–160

Index

Dispersed drug, porous systems, 164
Dissolution-controlled systems, 164–165, 175–177, 435–436, 541–542, 854–855, 860–861
   setting specifications, 541–542
Dissolved drug, nonporous systems, 160–161
Dissolved drug, porous systems, 164
Dog/human pharmacokinetics, 781–783
Dosage form cores, 757–760
   composition of, 757
   processing of, 759
   variables, 759–760
Doxorubicin, 293
Drug delivery carriers, 1–46, 168–173, 354–355, 431–461, 573–574 (*see also* Applications; Artificial neural networks for optimizing transdermal drug delivery systems; Controlled release systems; Complexing polymers in drug delivery; Hydrophillic cellulose derivatives as drug delivery carriers; Implantable drug delivery systems; Nanoparticles; Nanosuspensions; Osmotic systems; Polylactic and polyglycolic acids as drug deliver carriers; Poly(vinyl alcohol) as a drug delivery carrier; Smart polymers for controlled drug delivery; Transdermal drug delivery systems)
   definition, 431
   electrically assisted, 573–574
   formulations for drug delivery, 354–355
      oral, 355
      parenteral, 355
      peroral, 355
      topical, 354–355
   delivery technologies, 432–433
      commercialized, 433
      in development, 433–434
      intravenous, 432–433
      synthetic vs. natural polymers, 434
      tablets, 432
      toxicological considerations, 434–435
   implantable drug delivery systems, 452–457
      designs, 453–454
      fabrication, 456
      issues and opportunities, 456–457
      materials of use, 456
      polymer requirements, 455
      toxicological considerations, 454–455
   micro- and nanoparticle delivery, 108–119, 287–299, 457–461, 505–525
      injectable depot formulations, 459–460
      issues and opportunities, 460–461
      musocosal delivery, 458–459

[Drug delivery carriers]
   oral drug delivery systems, 435–445
      designs, 435–440
      fabrication techniques, 442–445
      functions of polymers, 441–442
      toxicological considerations, 440–441
   overview, 431–463
   swelling-controlled systems, 168–173
   transdermal drug delivery systems, 445–452, 567–581, 597–605, 617–659, 795
      delivery profiles and performance, 447–448
      designs, 445–447
      fabrication, 451–452
      issues and opportunities, 452
      polymer requirements, 449–451
      toxicological considerations, 447
Drug loading, effect on matrix characteristics, 16–18
Drug release, 4, 13–15, 193–194
   analysis of, 193–194
Drug solubility, effect on matrix characteristics, 19–24
Drug targeting to lymph nodes, 296–298
Dual drug system, 746, 801–803
   dual-anesthetic use, 801–803
      advantages of, 802–803
      logic of, 801–802
Duros implants, 240–249
   applications, 243–249
      α-interferon, 248–249
      factor IX, 249
      leuprolide implants, 243–246
      salmon calcitonin, 246–248
   formulation parameters, 242
   implantation, 242
   system configurations, 241–242
   system design, 240–241
Dynamic mechanical behavior, 53–54

Electrically stimulated pulsatile systems, 70–71 (*see also* Pulsatile systems)
Electrical exposure, adverse effects of, 572–573
Electrochemotherapy, 577
Electrodes, and iontophoresis, 620–627
   alternatives to silver and silver chloride, 625–626
   chloride ion management with silver anodes, 624
   construction, 626–627
   consumable, 622–623
   function and overview requirements, 620–621
   nonconsumable, 621–622
   silver, as a consumable anode, 623

[Electrodes, and iontophoresis]
    silver chloride, as a consumable cathode, 624–625
Electrolytes for counterreservoir, 633–634
Electro-osmosis, 568–569
Electrotransport mechanisms, 567–571, 613–614, 617–659 (*see also* Transdermal delivery of drugs)
    electro-osmosis, 568–569
    electroporation, 569–570, 613–614
    iontophoresis, 567–568
    pathways of delivery, 570
    pH control mechanisms, 571
    theoretical basis, 570–571
Encapsulation of the agent as protection from chemical degradation, 109–111, 667–673, 849–863
    experimental, 851–855
        binding components, 853
        cement formulations, 853
        cement dissolution study, 854–855
        incorporation into the cement, 853
        materials, 851–852
        PLGA purification, 852
        PPF synthesis and molecular weight, 852
        preparation and loading of PLGA foam, 852
        release and INH assay, 854
    of protein solids, 667–670
    of protein solutions, 670–673
    results and discussion, 855–861
        grout dissolution, 860–861
        release of INH, 855–860
    of water-soluble compounds, 109–111
Environmentally responsive systems, 71–73
Enzymes, 74, 278, 280
    systems utilizing, 74
Equilibrium swelling behavior of polymulti(meth)acrylates, 55–56 (*see also* Polymulti(meth)acrylates; Swelling)
Erosion, 457
Erythropoietin, 679–682
Ethylene-vinyl acetate copolymer, 67–68
E-TRANS lidocaine, 640–644
Excipients, 630–631, 710–711
    selection, 630–631
Extracellular matrix (ECM), 738–739 (*see also* Matrix characteristics; Matrix (monolithic) devices; Matrix tablets)
Extruded implants, 106

Factor IX, 249
Faraday's principle, 619
Fentanyl, 575, 644–647
Fibers, 105–106

Fickian, case II, and anomalous transport, 184
Fick's law of diffusion, 156–157
    solutions to, 157
Films, 107
Finite release volumes, 167–168
Floating devices, 212
Flow-through systems, 599
Fluorescent probe, pH-sensitive, 397, 406
Food excipient method, 212
Formation dynamics, 188–190
Formulations, 497–498, 554–563
    changes, 497–498
    deposition and dispersion of, 555–563
        barrier control, 562–563
        complex pharmacokinetics, 560
        locating absorption sites, 558–559
        potential sites for adhesion or lodging, 559–560
        resolving site of release and transit parameters, 557–558
        temporal control and colonic diversity, 561–562
    development, 627–634
        electrolytes for counterreservoir, 633–634
        excipient selection, 630–631
        matrix selection, 629–630
        pH selection, 631–633
        solvent selection, 628–629
    labeling, 554–555
        colloids and fine suspensions, 555
        particulate markers, 555
        solute phase markers, 554–555
Freeze-thaw technique, 35–36

Gamma scintigraphy and controlled release systems, 551–564 (*see also* Controlled release devices and systems; Drug delivery carriers)
    deposition and dispersion of formulations, 555–563
        barrier control, 562–563
        complex pharmacokinetics, 560
        locating absorption sites, 558–559
        potential sites for adhesion or lodging, 559–560
        resolving site of release and transit parameters, 557–558
        temporal control and colonic diversity, 561–562
    labelling formulations, 554–555
        colloids and fine suspensions, 555
        particulate markers, 555
        solute phase markers, 554–555
Gastric retention devices, 211–219, 440, 481–483

Index

[Gastric retention devices]
  emptying, 481–483
Gastrointestinal retentive microparticulate system, 505–525 (*see also* Drug delivery carriers; Oral drug delivery systems)
  bioadhesive liposomal systems, 510–516
    improved enteral absorption of peptide drugs, 515–516
    mucoadhesive tests for particulate systems, 512–515
    polymer-coated liposomes, 511–512
  bioadhesive polymeric microparticulate systems, 516–523
    microsperes, 517–519
    mucoadhesive lactide/glycolide copolymer nanospheres, 519–523
  intragastric floating microparticulate systems (microballoons), 506–510
Gel layer, boundaries of, 190
Glass transition temperatures, 54
Glucose, 280
Glucose-responsive insulin delivery, 76–81
GMP production, 365–372
  continuous large-scale production, 370–372
  of 50-kg batches, 369–370
  of 10-kg batches, 367–369
Grout dissolution, 860–861
Growth factor release to induce neovascularization, 725–741
  application to ischemic myocardium, 735
  dermis regeneration, 737–738
  incorporation of growth factor into acidic gelatin and hydrogels, 728–729
  in vitro release of bFGF, 729–730
  in vivo growth factor release, 731–732
  in vivo hydrogel degradation, 730–731
  neovascularization induced by biodegradable hydrogels, 732–735
  preparation of biodegradable hydrogels, 728
  vascularization into scaffold for tissue engineering, 736–737

H^+ determination of, 397–400
Heat-treated devices, 36–37
Hemoglobin, 280
Highly crosslinked polymers, control of the structure, 55
Histidase, 280
Hormones, 278, 282
Human growth hormone, 682–683
Human serum albumin, 280
Hydrogels, 136–137, 145–147, 211–223, 256–258, 730–731
  application of infrared to, 136–137

[Hydrogels]
  application of Raman to, 145–146
  in vivo hydrogel degradation, 730–731
  neovascularization induced by biodegradable hydrogels, 732–735
  preparation of biodegradable hydrogels, 728
  structural and compositional characterization, 146–147
  superporous, 211–221
    introduction, 211–213
    in vivo study in a canine model, 219–221
    principle and requirements, 213–214
    synthesis and characterization, 214–219
Hydromorphone, from a novel PLGA depot system, 792–793, 837–847
  materials and methods, 838–841
    depot preparation, 838–839
    doses, 840–841
    drugs, 838
    PLGA, 838
    studies in mice, 839
    studies in rats, 839–840
    in vitro release, 839
  results and discussion, 841–846
    behavioral observations, 843–846
Hydrophilic cellulose derivatives as drug delivery carriers, 1–30
  conclusion, 24–26
  effect of drug loading on matrix characteristics, 16–18
  effect of drug solubility on matrix characteristics, 19–24
  effect of substitution type on matrix characteristics, 5–15
    drug release, 13–15
    polymer erosion, 10–13
    swelling characteristics, 5–10
  experimental, 3–5
    compact preparation, 4
    drug release and polymer dissolution, 4
    materials, 3
    polymer disentanglement concentration, 4–5
    polymer hydrophilicity, 4
    polymer molecular weights, 3
    swelling and front movements, 4
  introduction, 1–3
  polymer hydrophilicity, 5
Hydrosols, 346
Hydroxyethylcellulose (HEC), 2–26
Hydroxyethyl methacrylate (HEMA), 138, 140
Hydroxypropylcellulose (HPC), 2–26
Hydroxypropylmethylcellulose (HPMC), 1–26

Iontophoresis, 567–568
Immobilized glucose oxidase in pH-sensitive polymers, 78–81
Implantable drug delivery systems, 452–457 (*see also* Drug delivery carriers)
  designs, 453–454
  fabrication, 456
  issues and opportunities, 456–457
  materials of use, 456
  polymer requirements, 455
  toxicological considerations, 454–455
Implants of PLAGA, 105–108, 813–814
  extruded, 106
  fibers, 105–106
  films, 107
  insertion, 814
  other implantable systems, 107–108
  tablets, 106
Inactivation, hypothesis for the mechanism of, 405–406
  kinetics of release and aggregation of, 402
  matching denatured states of, 404–405
  simulations of stresses, 404
Inflammation-responsive systems, 73
Infrared and Raman spectroscopy for characterization of controlled release systems, 131–153
  application of infrared to hydrogels, 136–137
  application of Raman to hydrogels, 145–146
  characterization of molecular interactions and diffusion, 139–142
  hydrogels, structural and compositional characterization, 146–147
  instrumentation for infrared, 133–135
  instrumentation for Raman, 144–145
  introduction, 131–132
  physical basis for infrared, 132–133
  physical basis for Raman, 142–144
  polymer chains, conformational and orientational characterization, 147–148
  polymerization process, characterization, 137–139, 148–149
  sampling techniques for infrared, 135–136
  sampling techniques for Raman, 145
INH, 854, 855–860
  assay, 854
  release of, 855–860
Initial release kinetics, effect of system history on, 168
Injectable depot formulations, 459–460
Instrumentation, 133–135, 144–145
  for infrared, 133–135
  for Raman, 144–145
Insulin, and glucose-responsive delivery, 76–81

Interaction mechanisms, 258–259
Interfacial polymerization reactions, 271–275, 694–695
  factors affecting, 274–275
  preparation by, 271–274
    solid core, 273
    water immiscible liquid core, 273
    water miscible liquid core, 273
Interferon-γ, 744 (*see also* Biopolymers for release of interleukin-2 for treatment of cancer; Interleukins)
Interleukins, 237–238, 743–750 (*see also* Biopolymers for release of interleukin-2 for treatment of cancer)
  pilot studies with IL-2/PLGA, 747–750
Interpulse skin impedance and resistance, 601
Intestinal transit, small, 483, 505–506
Intragastric floating microparticulate systems (microballoons), 506–510
Intramuscularly and intraperitoneally implants, 289–290
Intravenous delivery, 432, 795
Invertase, 280
Ionic drugs, 104
Ion exchange resins, 438–440
Iontophoresis, 617–659
  case studies, 644–654
  electrodes, 620–627
  formulation development, 627–634
  system design, 634–644
Irradiation, crosslinking by, 35
Ischemic myocardium, 735
Isoelectric point (IEP), 726–727

Kelvin equation and principle, 351
Ketorolac, 648–650
Kinetic gelation simulations, of network structure, 56–58
Kinetic laws, 694–695
Kinetics of release, 402, 488–490
  and aggregation of bovine serum ablumin, 402
Kinetics of solid-state reactions, 694–699 (*see also* Pharmacokinetics and pharmacodynamics)
  application to controlled release, 699
  activation parameters, 695–698
  kinetic laws, 694–695
  product formation and distribution, 698

Lactic/glycolic acid polymers, 330–331, 519–523, 713–715
Lactone fraction, 400
Leukemia, 294
Leuprolide implants, 243–246

Index

Lidocaine, 640–644
Linoleic acid, 612–613
Liposomes, 389, 510–516
  polymer-coated, 511–512
Liver, metastasis model, 290–291
Localized transport regions (LTRs), 599–602
Luteinizing hormone-releasing hormone, 650–654
Lymph nodes
  drug targeting to, 296–298
    efficacy in multidrug resistance, 291–294
    efficacy in tumor models, 288–291
    and oligonucleotide therapy, 294–296
Lymphoma, 294

Magnetic dosage forms, 67, 213
Maillard reaction, 704
Magnetically stimulated pulsatile systems, 67 (*see also* Pulsatile systems)
Markers, 554–555
  particulate, 555
  solute phase, 554–555
Mathematical modeling, 40–42, 156–157, 528–541 (*see also* Models)
  categories of correlations, 528
  development and evaluation of a correlation, 534–541
    case study, 538–541
    statistical assessment, 535–538
    study design, 534–535
  of diffusion processes, 156–157
    Fick's law of diffusion, 156
    solutions to Fick's law, 157
  dissolution specifications, setting, 541–542
  in vitro and in vivo correlations, 529–534
    convolution and deconvolution, 529–532
    mean time parameters, 532–534
    summary parameters, 534
Matrix characteristics
  effect of drug loading, 16–18
  effect of drug solubility, 19–24
  mobility, 708–709
  effect of substitution type, 5–15
    drug release, 13–15
    polymer erosion, 10–13
  sterilization, 817–818
  and swelling, 5–10, 194–198
Matrix (monolithic) devices, 159, 446–447, 451, 466–469, 470–471, 738–739, 817–818
  formulation and quality control, 817–818
  materials for, 470–471
Matrix tablets, swellable, 192–204, 470–472, 491–492, 495–496, 629–630

[Matrix tablets, swellable]
  free, 193–198
  reservoir systems, 203–204, 467, 471–472, 492–493, 633–634
    materials for, 471–472
  restricted, 198–203
  selection of, 629–630
Mechanical properties, 53–54
Membrane
  coatings, 760–769
    composition, 760–761
    dip, 763
    formulation and variables, 767–769
    processes, 762
    spray, 767
    spray drying, 763–767
  -controlled systems, 446, 449–451
  defects, intentional, 771
  osmotic pressure, 771–773
  permeability, 277
  properties, 276–278, 449–451, 771–773
  (reservoir) devices, 165
  stability, 277
  thickness, 276–277
MET, promoting activity of, 587–589
Methacrylate, development of polymer networks, 47–64 (*see also* Photopolymerization technology)
Methods of drug application, and pain management, 794–801
  intramuscular, 795
  intravenous, 795
  long-term, delayed, and controlled release, 796–801
  oral, 794
  rectal, 794
  spinal, 795–796
  subcutaneous, 795
  transdermal, 796
Methylcellulose (HMPC), 2–26
Micro- and nanoparticle delivery, 457–461 (*see also* Drug delivery carriers)
  injectable depot formulations, 459–460
  issues and opportunities, 460–461
  musocosal delivery, 458–459
Microballoons, 506–510
Microcapsules, 275–279 (*see also* Microencapsulation technology)
  properties of, 275–279
    flow properties, 279
    membrane properties, 276–278
    size and size distribution, 276
    surface morphology, 275–276
    ζ potential, 278–279

Microencapsulation technology, 271–285, 301–328 (*see also* Microcapsules)
  applications, 280–282, 310–318 (*see also* Applications)
    adsorbants, 282
    analgesics, 313
    antibiotics, 310–311
    anticancerogens, 313
    antiepileptic drugs, 312–313
    antihypertensives, 313
    anti-inflammatory drugs, 311
    artificial cells, 281
    bronchodilators, 311–312
    converting liquids to free-flowing powders, 314
    diuretics, 312
    electrolyte replenishers, 314
    enzymes, 280
    hormones and antibodies, 282
    metal salts, 314
    oily liquids, 281
    pharmaceuticals, 281
    pigments, 282
    polyeelectrolytes, 281–282
    proteins, 280–281
    sedative hypnotics, 314
    sulfa drugs, 312
    tranquilizers, 313
    urinary antiseptics, 312
    vitamins, 314
  coacervation separation methods, 301–302, 306–309
    aqueous phase, 306–308
    organic phase, 308–309
  core materials, 302–303
  factors affecting interfacial polymerization reactions, 274–275
  monomers and solvents used, 271
  phase boundary triangular diagrams, 304–305
    incompatible polymer addition, 304
    nonsolvent addition, 304
    polymer-polymer interaction, 304
    salt addition, 304
    temperature change, 304
  preparation by interfacial polymerization, 271–274
    solid core, 273
    water immiscible liquid core, 273
    water miscible liquid core, 273
  properties of microcapsules, 275–279
    flow properties, 279
    membrane properties, 276–278
    size and size distribution, 276
    surface morphology, 275–276

[Microencapsulation technology]
  ζ potential, 278–279
  storage conditions, 309–310
  using coacervation/phase separation, 301–328
Microgels and structural heterogeneity, 50
Microparticle drug delivery systems, 108–119, 457–461, 505–525 (*see also* Gastrointestinal retentive microparticulate system; Oral drug delivery systems; Particulate systems)
  behavior in vivo, 117–119
  characterization of biodegradable microparticles, 113–119
  preparation of particulate systems, 108–113
Microsphere preparation by solvent evaporation, 329–343, 517–519, 678–683, 737–738, 814–815, 821–836 (*see also* Buprenorphine microspheres for parenteral administration)
  biodegradable polymers, 330–331, 814–815
    lactic/glycolic acid polymers, 330–331
  dermis regeneration, 737–738
  solvent evaporation process, 332–338
    multiple emulsion, 336–338
    single emulsion, 332–336
Milling process, 346–347
Modeling (*see* Mathematical modeling)
Models, accurate, in controlled drug delivery systems, 155–181, 527–548 (*see also* Mathematical modeling; Solid oral controlled release dosage forms)
  conclusions and future directions, 178
  controlled release devices, 159–174
    chemically controlled systems, 173–174
    diffusion-controlled systems, 159–168
    swelling-controlled systems, 168–173
  convolution approach, 531–532
  deconvolution methods, 530–531
  introduction, 155–156
  mathematical modeling of diffusion processes, 156–157
    Fick's law of diffusion, 156
    solutions to Fick's law, 157
  other aspects of drug release modeling, 174–177
    dissolution-controlled systems, 175–177
    osmotic systems, 174–175
  polymer structure in modeling equations, 157–158
    concentration-dependent diffusion coefficients, 157–158
    effect of polymer morphology, 158
    thermodynamic considerations, 158

Index

Modulated drug release systems, 39–40
Molecular modeling, 261–263
Molecular drug delivery, 746
Molecular interactions and diffusion, characterization of, 139–142
Monomers, 271
Morphine, 75–76, 791–792
   -triggered naltrexone delivery system, 75–76
Mucin coating on the surface of superporous hydrogels, 217, 256–258 (*see also* Hydrogels)
   structure and physiology of, 256–258
Mucoadhesive dosage forms, 212–213, 255–256, 512–515, 519–523
   lactide/glycolide copolymer nanospheres, 519–523
   tests for particulate systems, 512–515
Multidrug resistance, efficacy of nanoparticulates, 291–294
Multiphase reactions, 694–695
Musocosal delivery, 458–459

Nanoparticulate controlled release systems for cancer therapy, 287–299 (*see also* Biopolymers for release of interleukin-2 for treatment of cancer; Cancer therapy; Controlled release devices and systems; Drug delivery carriers; Nanoparticles; Nanosuspensions; Polysaccharide nanoparticles as novel drug carrier systems; Solid lipid nanoparticles; Tumor models)
   drug targeting to lymph nodes, 296–298
   efficacy in multidrug resistance, 291–294
   efficacy in tumor models, 288–291
      in intramuscularly and intraperitoneally implants, 289–290
      in a liver metastasis model, 290–291
   introduction, 287–288
   nanoparticles made from poorly soluble drugs, 345–348
      hydrosols, 346
      NanoCrystals, 346–347
      nanosuspensions (DissoCubes), 348
   and oligonucleotide therapy, 294–296
Nanosuspensions, 345–357 (*see also* Controlled release devices and systems; Drug delivery carriers; Nanoparticulate controlled release systems for cancer therapy; Solid lipid nanoparticles)
   formulations for drug delivery, 354–355
      oral, 355
      parenteral, 355
      peroral, 355

[Nanosuspensions]
   topical, 354–355
   nanoparticles made from poorly soluble drugs, 345–348
      hydrosols, 346
      NanoCrystals, 346–347
      nanosuspensions (DissoCubes), 348
   poorly soluble drugs, 345
   production of, 348–350
   properties of, 351–354
      internal structure, 354
      physical long-term stability, 351
      saturation solubility, 351–353
Narcotic analgesics, 789
Neovascularization (*see* Growth factor release to induce neovascularization)
Nerve growth factor (NGF), 235
Nestorone, biodegradable systems for, 807–819
   background, 808–809
   pilot studies, 813–818
      bioerodible implant materials and methods, 813–814
      matrix formulation and quality control, 817–818
      microspheres, 814–815
      polymer selection and characterization, 815–817
   rationale for the present study, 809–810
   traditional solvent-based PLGA matrix delivery, 810–813
Network structure and mechanical properties, 53–55, 584–586
   control of the structure of highly crosslinked polymers, 55
   dynamic mechanical behavior, 53–54
   glass transition temperature, 54
   rubber elasticity analysis, 53
   volume shrinkage and aging, 54
Nonrelease controlling excipients, 497–498
Nonsolvent addition, 304
Nuclides, selected, 552

Octreotide, 238–239
Oil solvent diffusion (OSD), 519–520
Oily liquids, 278, 281
Oligonucleotides
   antisense, 235, 417
   delivery of, 576–571
   nanoparticulate therapy, 294–296
Opioid receptors and brain opioids, 788, 821
Optimization of drug delivery, 586, 590–593
   optimization based on ANN, 590–593
   single-objective optimization, 586

Oral drug delivery systems, 435–445, 465–503, 505–525, 751–752, 794 (*see also* Controlled release devices and systems; Drug delivery carriers; Gastrointestinal retentive microparticulate system; Osmotic systems; Solid oral controlled release dosage forms)
   common polymeric systems, 466–470
      matrix, 466–469
      osmotic pump, 469–470
      reservoir, 467
   designs, 435–440
   development technologies, 472–473
      coating technologies, 473
      spheronization and pelletization, 472–473
      tableting process, 472
   fabrication techniques, 442–445
   functions of polymers, 441–442
   materials used, 470–472
      for matrix systems, 470–471
      for osmotic pump systems, 472
      for reservoir systems, 471–472
   osmotic systems, 751–752
   postapproval changes, 496–499
      formulation changes, 497–498
      process changes, 498–499
   product and process development, 485–496
      formulation and process development, 491–496
      preformulation, 490–491
      system design consideration, 485–490
   research and development aspects, 465–503
   toxicological considerations, 440–441
   in vitro and in vivo considerations, 473–485
      animal models, 477–478
      feasibility assessment, 473–475
      pharmacokinetics and pharmacodynamics, 484–485
      studies in humans, 478–479
Organic solvents, 667–669
Osmotic systems, 174–175, 225–253, 436–438, 469–470, 472, 494–495, 751–785
   asymmetric membrane film-coated dosage forms, 751–785
      membrane properties, 755–757
      performance, 769–783
      processing, 757–769
      theory of, 754–755
   implantable, 225–253
      Alzet pumps, 230–239
      Duros implants, 240–249
      theory, 226–230
Ostwald-Freundlich equation, 352

Oxidase, 280
Oxidation, 699–700

Pain management systems, 787–803
   causes of pain, 788–789
   dual-anesthetic use, 801–803
      advantages of, 802–803
      logic of, 801–802
   methods of drug application, 794–801
      intramuscular, 795
      intravenous, 795
      long-term, delayed, and controlled release, 796–801
      oral, 794
      rectal, 794
      spinal, 795–796
      subcutaneous, 795
      transdermal, 796
   mechanism of action, 790–794
      codeine, 792
      hydromorphone, 792–793
      local anesthetics, 793–794
      morphine, 791–792
   narcotic analgesics, 789
   opioid receptors and brain opioids, 788, 821
   pain, 787–789
   relief, 789
Pan coating, 444
Paraaminohippuric acid (PAH), 68
Parameters, 532–534, 695–698 (*see also* Mathematical modeling; Models)
   activation, 695–698
   mean time, 532–534
   summary, 534
Parenteral administration (*see* Buprenorphine microspheres for parenteral administration)
Particle size analysis, 351, 824
Particulate systems, preparation of, 108–113, 555 (*see also* Microparticulate drug delivery systems)
   analysis of particulate degradation and drug delivery, 116–117
   analysis of particulate morphology, 114–116
   analysis of size and distribution, 113–114
   markers, 555
Partitioning, preferential, in the polymer, 401–402
Pendant chain systems, 174
Peptide delivery, 519–523, 575–576, 693–724 (*see also* Solid-state chemical stability of peptides and proteins)
Perfect sink conditions, 166–167

Index

pH, 72–73, 78–81, 396–400, 406, 571, 631–633, 711–712
  acidic, 396–400
  control mechanisms, 571
  -dependent degradation, 78–79
  -dependent solubility, 78
  -dependent swelling, 79–81
  effective, 711–712
  media, 769–771
  selection of, 631–633
  -sensitive systems, 72–73, 78–81, 397
Pharmaceuticals, 278, 281
Pharmacoeconomic value of controlled release dosage forms, 865–872
  basic concepts, 865–868
  potential benefits, 868–869
  summary of publications, 869–870
Pharmacokinetics and pharmacodynamics, 484–485, 508, 560, 781–783 (*see also* Kinetics of release; Kinetics of solid-state reactions)
  complex, 560
  dog/human, 781–783
Phase boundary triangular diagrams, 304–305
  incompatible polymer addition, 304
  nonsolvent addition, 304
  polymer-polymer interaction, 304
  salt addition, 304
  temperature change, 304
Phase markers, solute, 554–555
Phenylpropanolamine hydrochloride (PPA), 3, 13–14, 16–25
Photopolymerization technology, 47–64 (*see also* Polymerization)
  development of acrylate and methacrylate polymer networks, 47–64
    applications in drug delivery, 58–59
    equilibrium swelling behavior, 55–56
    kinetic gelation simulations, 56–58
    network structure and mechanical properties, 53–55
    preparation of, 49–53
    structure and applications, 47–48
Photostimulated pulsatile systems, 71 (*see also* Pulsatile systems)
Physicochemical factors, 707–713
  effective pH, 711–712
  excipients, 710–711
  implications for controlled release, 712–713
  pressure, 708
  mobility in the matrix, 708–709
  temperature, 707–708
  water content, 709–710
Pigments, 279, 282

Pig skin, 601 (*see also* Animal models)
Poly(acrylic acid) (PAA), 89–98, 520
Polyalkylcyanoacrylate (PACA), 292–294, 296
Polyamide microcapsules, 277
Polyamines, 272
Polybutylcyanoacrylate (PBCA), 289
Polyelectrolytes, 279
Polyelectrolytes, 281–282
Poly(ethylene glycol) (PEG), 89–98, 119–120, 141, 612–613
Poly(ethylene oxide) (PEO), 119–120, 418
Polyethylenimine (PEI), 415
Polylactic and polyglycolic acids as drug delivery carriers, 99–130, 378, 393–411, 456, 459–460, 519–523, 663, 673–677, 713–715, 743–750, 813–818, 822–823, 826–834, 838–846, 852 (*see also* Drug delivery carriers; Poly(lactide-co-glycolide) delivery systems)
  copolymers of PLA, PLAGA, and other materials, 119–120, 456
    with ε-caprolactone, 120
    with poly(ethylene glycol) and poly(ethylene oxide), 119–120
  degradation mechanisms, 102–105
    effect of ionic drugs, 104
    polymerization initiator, 105
    size, shape, and porosity, 104
  future opportunities utilizing poly(lactide-co-glycolide), 121–122
  microparticle drug delivery systems, 108–119
    characterization of biodegradable microparticles, 113–119
    preparation of particulate systems, 108–113
  preparation of PLAGA polymers, 100–102
  using implants of PLAGA, 105–108
    extruded implants, 106
    fibers, 105–106
    films, 107
    other implantable systems, 107–108
    tablets, 106
  utilizing PLAGA, 120–121
Poly(lactide-co-glycolide) delivery systems, 393–411, 456, 459–460, 663, 673–677, 713–715, 813–818, 822–823, 826–834, 838–846, 852 (*see also* Drug delivery carriers; Polylactic and polyglycolic acids as drug deliver carriers)
  mechanisms of instability of bovine serum ablumin, 402–407
    characterization of the denatured state, 402–404
    hypothesis for the mechanism of inactivation, 405–406

[Poly(lactide-co-glycolide) delivery systems]
  kinetics of release and aggregation of, 402
  matching denatured states of, 404–405
  simulations of stresses, 404
  stabilization by neutralization of the acidic microclimate pH, 406–407
 mechanisms of stabilization of camptothecins, 394–402
  in PLGA microspheres, 394–395
  potential mechanisms, 395–402
 purification of, 852
Polymerization, 50–51, 105, 137–139, 148–149 (*see also* Photopolymerization)
 kinetics, 50–51
 initiator, 105
 process, characterization, 137–139, 148–149
Polymers (*see also* Controlled release devices and systems; Drug delivery carriers; Photopolymerization; Polymerization; Smart polymers for controlled drug delivery)
 addition, incompatible, 304
 chains, characterization, 147–148, 815–817
 complex system, 76
 dissolution-controlled release systems, 37
 erosion, 10–13
 for controlled drug delivery, 443, 486–487
 morphology, 158
 networks, 47–64
 partitioning, preferential, 401–402
 -polymer interaction, 304
 properties and release, 441–442, 449–451
 selection and characterization, 815–817
 stability toward storage, 674–675
 structure in modeling equations, 157–158
  concentration-dependent diffusion coefficients, 157–158
  effect of polymer morphology, 158
  thermodynamic considerations, 158
 synthetic vs. natural, 434
Polymethyl methacrylate (PMMA), 89–98, 141, 145–148
Polymulti(meth)acrylates, 47–48
 preparation of, 49–53
  diffusional effects during polymerization, 49–50
  microgels and structural heterogeneity, 50
  polymerization kinetics, 50–51
  rate coefficients, 51–53
Polyphenols, 272

Polysaccharide nanoparticles as novel drug carrier systems, 413–429, 715–716 (*see also* Drug delivery carriers; Nanoparticulate controlled release systems for cancer therapy; Nanosuspensions; Solid lipid nanoparticles)
 agarose nanoparticles, 420–423
 alginate nanoparticles, 414–417
 chitosan nanoparticles, 417–420
  emulsification-based method, 419–420
  and polyanions, 418–420
 conclusion, 425–426
 dextrans and other polysaccharides, 715–716
 supramolecular biovectors, 423–425
Poly(vinyl alcohol) (PVA) as a drug delivery carrier, 31–46, 138–139, 736–737 (*see also* Drug delivery carriers)
 biocompatibility issues, 31–32
 mathematical modeling, 40–42
 PVA-based delivery devices, 32–40
  crystal dissolution-controlled release systems, 38–39
  modulated drug release systems, 39–40
  polymer dissolution-controlled release systems, 37
  swelling-controlled release systems, 33–37
Porous systems, 163–164
Porosity, 104
Postapproval changes, 496–499
 formulation changes, 497–498
 process changes, 498–499
Power for portable designs, 636–638
PPF, 850–852
 synthesis and molecular weight, 852
Prandtl equation, 351
Preformulation, 490–491 (*see also* Formulations)
Pressure, 708
Process changes, 498–499
Product formation and distribution, 698
Proteins, 279, 280–281, 661–692
 therapeutics, 661–692
  stabilization during release, 676–683
  stabilization toward encapsulation, 663–674
  stabilization toward storage, 674–676
Pseudoephedrine hydrochloride (PED), 3–26
Pulsatile systems, 67–71
 electrically stimulated systems, 70–71
 magnetically stimulated systems, 67
 photostimulated systems, 71
 ultrasonically stimulated systems, 68–70

Index

Quality, of product, 373–374
Qualification and validation of the manufacturing process, 372–373

Radiopaque marker and image analysis, 219
Raman spectroscopy (*see* Infrared and Raman spectroscopy for characterization of controlled release systems)
Rate coefficients, 51–53
Rate controlling membrane (RCM) systems, 446–451
Rectal drug delivery, 794 (*see also* Drug delivery systems)
Release kinetics, 488–490, 557–558 (*see also* Kinetics of release; Kinetics of solid-state reactions)
 resolving site of release and transit parameters, 557–558
Removal of solvents during particle preparation, 111–112
Reservoir systems, 203–204, 467, 471–472, 492–493, 633–634
 materials for, 471–472
Responsive hydrogels (*see* Hydrogels)
Rubber elasticity analysis, 53

Salmon calcitonin, 246–248
Sampling techniques, 135–136, 145
 for infrared, 135–136
 for Raman, 145
Salt addition, 304
Saturation solubility, 351–353
Self-regulated systems, 71–81
 environmentally responsive systems, 71–73
 glucose-responsive insulin delivery, 76–81
 systems utilizing specific binding interactions, 73–76
Silver, 623–626 (*see also* Electrodes)
 alternatives to silver and silver chloride, 625–626
 chloride ion management with silver anodes, 624
 consumable anode, 623
 consumable cathode, 624–625
Single-objective optimization, 586
Size of polymer samples, 104
Skin electroporation, 597–605 (*see also* Transdermal drug delivery systems)
 animal models, 601–602
 flow-through systems, 599
 interpulse skin impedance and resistance, 601
 theory, 598–599
 voltage measurements, 599–601

Skin impedance and resistance, 601
Skin source and study models, 571–572
Small intestinal transit, 483, 505–506
Smart polymers for controlled drug delivery, 65–87
 conclusion, 81–82
 introduction, 65–67
 pulsatile systems, 67–71
  electrically stimulated systems, 70–71
  magnetically stimulated systems, 67
  photostimulated systems, 71
  ultrasonically stimulated systems, 68–70
 self-regulated systems, 71–81
  environmentally responsive systems, 71–73
  glucose-responsive insulin delivery, 76–81
  systems utilizing specific binding interactions, 73–76
Sodium dodecyl sulfate (SDS), 380
Solid lipid nanoparticles, 359–391 (*see also* Nanoparticles; Nanosuspensions; Solid oral controlled release dosage forms)
 applications of, 386–388
 as a carrier system for controlled release of drugs, 377–391
 definition of, 379
 drug release and particle internal structure, 382–386
 excipients, status of, 380–381
 GMP production, 365–372, 381
  continuous large-scale production, 370–372
  of 50-kg batches, 369–370
  of 10-kg batches, 367–369
 historical background, 379–380
 introduction, 359–361
 laboratory-scale production, 361–365
 market situation, 388–389
 product quality, 373–374
 qualification and validation of the manufacturing process, 372–373
Solid oral controlled release dosage forms, 527–548 (*see also* Drug delivery carriers; Oral drug delivery systems)
 applications, 541–544
  limitations and considerations, 542–544
  setting dissolution specifications, 541–542
  supporting waiver of in vivo bioequivalence study, 542
 categories of correlations, 528
 development and evaluation of a correlation, 534–541
  case study, 538–541
  statistical assessment, 535–538
  study design, 534–535

[Solid oral controlled release dosage forms]
  mathematical methods, 529–534
    convolution and deconvolution, 529–532
    mean time parameters, 532–534
    summary parameters, 534
Solid-state chemical stability of peptides and proteins, 400–401, 693–724 (*see also* Peptides delivery)
  chemical degradation reactions, 699–707
    chiral scission, 702–704
    deamidation, 700–702
    implications for controlled release, 707
    Maillard reaction, 704
    oxidation, 699–700
    thiol-disulfide exchange, 704–706
  degradation reactions in specific polymers, 713–719
    dextrans and other polysaccharides, 715–716
    implications for controlled release, 719
    lactide/glycolide polymers, 713–715
    other polymers, 718–719
    vinyl polymers, 716–718
  kinetics of solid-state reactions, 694–699
    application to controlled release, 699
    activation parameters, 695–698
    kinetic laws, 694–695
    product formation and distribution, 698
  physicochemical factors, 707–713
    effective pH, 711–712
    excipients, 710–711
    implications for controlled release, 712–713
    pressure, 708
    mobility in the matrix, 708–709
    temperature, 707–708
    water content, 709–710
Solid-state reactions, kinetics of, 694–699
  application to controlled release, 699
  activation parameters, 695–698
  kinetic laws, 694–695
  product formation and distribution, 698
Solubility, 442
Soluble drugs, poorly, 345
Solvents, 108–109, 111–112, 183–188, 271, 273, 332–338, 519–520, 628–629, 665–670 (*see also* Microsphere preparation by solvent evaporation)
  evaporation, 108–109, 332–338
    multiple emulsion, 336–338
    single emulsion, 332–336
  organic, 667–670
  and protein structure, 665–667
  removal of during particle preparation, 111–112

[Solvents]
  selection of, 628–629
  transport in polymer matrices, 183–188
    dimensionless parameters, 185–186
    Fickian, case II, and anomalous transport, 184
    general characteristics, 186–188
    structural and compositional factors, 184–185
Sonophoresis, 608–611
  high-frequency, 609
  low-frequency, 608
  mechanism of, 609–611
  therapeutic frequency, 608–609
Spheronization and pelletization, 472–473
  tableting process, 472
Spinal drug delivery, 795–796 (*see also* Drug delivery carriers)
Spray drying, to prepare particles, 112–113, 444
Stabilization, and protein therapeutics, 661–692
  and encapsulation, 663–674
  during release, 676–683
  and storage, 674–676
Structural and compositional factors, 184–185, 442
  in swelling polymer systems, 184–185
Subcutaneous drug delivery, 795 (*see also* Drug delivery carriers)
Superporous hydrogels (*see* Hydrogels)
Supramoelcular biovectors (SMBVs), 423–425 (*see also* Polysaccharide nanoparticles as novel drug carrier systems)
Surface denaturation, 670–671
  minimization of, 671
Surface-enhanced Raman scattering (SERS), 145
Surface slipperiness of superporous hydrogels, 217–219
Swelling behavior, front movements, and drug release, 190–192
Swelling-controlled release systems, 33–37, 170, 183–209 (*see also* Drug delivery carriers)
  characteristics, 5–10
  drug release control and mechanisms, 188–192
    boundaries of gel layer and relevant fronts, 190
    formation dynamics, 188–190
    swelling behavior, front movements, and drug release, 190–192
  pH-dependent, 79–81
  solvent transport in polymer matrices, 183–188
    dimensionless parameters, 185–186
    Fickian, case II, and anomalous transport, 184